ACSM's
Resource Manual for Guidelines for Exercise Testing and Prescription

SIXTH EDITION

SENIOR EDITOR
Jonathan K. Ehrman, PhD, FACSM
ACSM Program Director^{SM}
ACSM Certified Clinical Exercise Specialist®
Henry Ford Hospital
Detroit, Michigan

SECTION EDITORS
Adam deJong, MA
ACSM Certified Clinical Exercise Specialist®
William Beaumont Hospital
Royal Oak, Michigan

Bonnie Sanderson, PhD, RN
ACSM Program Director^{SM}
ACSM Certified Clinical Exercise Specialist®
University of Alabama at Birmingham
Birmingham, Alabama

David Swain, PhD, FACSM
ACSM Program Director^{SM}
ACSM Certified Clinical Exercise Specialist®
Old Dominion University
Norfolk, Virginia

Ann Swank, PhD, FACSM
ACSM Program Director^{SM}
ACSM Certified Clinical Exercise Specialist®
University of Louisville
Louisville, Kentucky

Chris Womack, PhD, FACSM
ACSM Certified Clinical Exercise Specialist®
James Madison University
Harrisonburg, Virginia

ACSM's
Resource Manual for Guidelines for Exercise Testing and Prescription
SIXTH EDITION

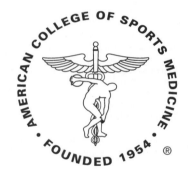

AMERICAN COLLEGE OF SPORTS MEDICINE

Wolters Kluwer | Lippincott Williams & Wilkins
Health

Philadelphia · Baltimore · New York · London
Buenos Aires · Hong Kong · Sydney · Tokyo

Acquisitions Editor: Emily Lupash
Managing Editor: Andrea M. Klingler
Marketing Manager: Christen D. Murphy
Production Project Manager: Cynthia Rudy
Creative Director: Doug Smock
Manufacturing Coordinator: Margie Orzech
Production Services: Aptara, Inc.

ACSM's Publications Committee Chair: Jeffrey L. Roitman, EdD, FACSM
ACSM Group Publisher: D. Mark Robertson

Sixth Edition
Copyright © 2010, 2006, 2001, 1998, 1993, 1988 American College of Sports Medicine

351 West Camden Street   530 Walnut Street
Baltimore, MD 21201   Philadelphia, PA 19106

Printed in China

Library of Congress Cataloging-in-Publication Data

ACSM's resource manual for guidelines for exercise testing and prescription / American College of Sports Medicine; [senior editor, Jonathan K. Ehrman]. — 6th ed.
    p. cm.
ISBN 978-0-7817-6906-8
1. Exercise therapy—Handbooks, manuals, etc. 2. Exercise tests—Handbooks, manuals, etc. I. Ehrman, Jonathan K., 1962-
RM725.R42 2010
615.8'2—dc22
                                                        2008047866

The publishers have made every effort to trace the copyright holders for borrowed material. If they have inadvertently overlooked any, they will be pleased to make the necessary arrangements at the first opportunity.

To purchase additional copies of this book, call our customer service department at (800) 638-3030 or fax orders to (301) 223-2320. International customers should call (301) 223-2300.

Visit Lippincott Williams & Wilkins on the Internet: http://www.lww.com. Lippincott Williams & Wilkins customer service representatives are available from 8:30 am to 6:00 pm, EST.

For more information concerning American College of Sports Medicine Certification and suggested preparatory materials, call (800) 486-5643 or visit the American College of Sports Medicine web site **www.acsm.org.**

9 8 7 6 5 4

I dedicate this book to my wife, Janel,
and children, Joshua, Jacob,
Jared, and Johanna.
I love you all very much.
May God bless you all.

JKE

Foreword

Advancing the profession of the exercise and fitness professional has been and remains a strategic priority for the American College of Sports Medicine (ACSM). During our sequential tenures as chair of the ACSM Committee on Certification and Registry Boards (CCRB), we appreciated that there are at least four key elements that need to be in place if one truly hopes to integrate the fitness or exercise professional into the general community of healthcare. These four elements include:

- a standardized curriculum to train and develop the knowledge, skills, and abilities that students interested in the field must acquire (i.e., academic accreditation)
- a standardized, national-level examination that evaluates and validates the proficiencies of relevant job-related knowledge, skills, and abilities (i.e., examination accreditation)
- an organized professional community (i.e., membership) to assist with continued education and advocate on behalf of the interests for the profession
- an industry-accepted, evidence-based body of knowledge that translates and supports the application of science (e.g., textbooks, papers, position stands, etc.)

Well, we are happy to report that much has transpired over the past 5 years—all of which gives the exercise professional great reason to celebrate.

First, ACSM, along with eight other professional organizations, helped create the Committee on the Accreditation for the Exercise Sciences (CoAES). In 2004, under the Commission on Accreditation of Allied Health Education Programs (CAAHEP), the CoAES developed the first-ever set of standards and guidelines for educational programs offering clinical and nonclinical curriculum in the fitness and exercise science-related fields (www.coaes.org). These standards and guidelines address the academic preparation requirements for personal trainers, health/fitness professionals and clinical exercise physiologists (CEPs).

Second, all four ACSM certification examinations have undergone third-party scrutiny and are now accredited through the National Commission for Certifying Agencies, under the National Organization for Competency Assurance (www.noca.org). The designation of NCCA accreditation demonstrates the integrity of the ACSM credentialing and certification process, in an industry that is forever interested in defining and ensuring the credibility and level of preparedness of its certified practitioners.

Third, and in addition to all of the organizational and advocacy efforts ACSM continues to undertake on behalf of all health/fitness professionals, in 2008 ACSM was instrumental in helping launch the *Clinical Exercise Physiology Association* (CEPA). CEPA (www.ACSM-cepa.org) now stands as an independent, national-level professional membership organization devoted exclusively to advancing the clinical exercise physiologist. CEPA does so by advocating on behalf of the profession, providing its members with continuing education and training, and working with other organizations and public policy makers to ensure that CEPs are fully integrated into the healthcare delivery team.

Finally, it is within the last of the above-mentioned four elements, the one that pertains to expanding the body of scientific knowledge, that this edition of *ACSM's Resource Manual* contributes. Drawing on the research, contributions, and teachings of many of the world's leading experts, we invite you to read and begin to apply the information found in this institutional classic—a resource that helped prepare and train both ourselves and so many of our colleagues over the years. Unlike other texts or journals, the *ACSM Resource Manual* provides, in one place, a comprehensive collection of information to prepare you in the field. Regardless of whether your career interests lie in the health/fitness or clinical settings, most all of the material in this book can contribute to your success as an exercise professional.

It is our expectation that the reader will find the information contained herein a most valuable resource. So dive in . . . and see first-hand why exercise is medicine.

Dino Costanzo, MA, FACSM
ACSM Program Director℠
ACSM Registered Clinical
Exercise Physiologist®
ACSM Exercise Test Technologist®
The Hospital of Central Connecticut
New Britain, Connecticut

Steven Keteyian, PhD, FACSM
ACSM Registered Clinical
Exercise Physiologist®
Henry Ford Hospital
Detroit, Michigan

Preface

The American College of Sports Medicine (ACSM) first published the *Guidelines for Exercise Testing and Prescription* (GETP) in 1975, shortly after beginning to offer professional certifications. The first edition of the *Resource Manual for Guidelines for Exercise Testing and Prescription* (RM) was published in 1988. Since then, four more editions of the RM have been published, with the expressed purpose of providing the evidence and advanced presentation of the GETP. It is the desire that this text will continue to serve as a preparatory guide for ACSM certification, continuing education, and teaching in the classroom. In this respect, it is an important aid for professionals at any level of ACSM certification.

Based on feedback from a user survey conducted in 2006 and from discussions at the kickoff meeting in Baltimore in June 2006, several new features were added to the RM6 that were not available in previous editions. Additionally, several items were also either updated or removed. The following paragraphs present these changes.

In 2006, as an initial step toward producing the next editions of the certification books, the ACSM Certification and Credentialing Review Board (CCRB) performed a job task analysis of health fitness and clinical exercise professionals and utilized this information to refine the knowledge, skills, and abilities (i.e., KSAs) list for both the Health Fitness Specialist and Clinical Exercise Specialist certifications. These new/updated KSAs were incorporated into this edition.

This sixth edition of RM is slightly modified in its organizational structure from previous editions. Sections I, II, and III are titled the same as sections I, II, and III in the GETP and include Health Appraisal, Risk Assessment, and Safety of Exercise; Exercise Testing; and Exercise Prescription, respectively. These sections are preceded in the RM by a Preliminary-Background Materials section, and followed by a section titled Supplemental-Programmatic and Professional Materials. The goal of this reorganization was to exactly follow the GETP sections while still providing the other pertinent information in the preliminary and supplemental sections. In addition, the GETP manuscript was completed well in advance of the RM, allowing for synching of the information contained in each text with a goal of reduced contrast on important issues.

An important new feature of this edition of the RM is the establishment of a KSA index. This index is located in the back of the RM immediately following the standard word index. This tool was designed with the preprofessional in mind who is preparing to take the Health Fitness Specialist, Clinical Exercise Specialist, or Registered Clinical Exercise Physiologist credentialing examination. The anticipated process is for the potential examinee to review the KSA list for their stated examination/certification level and to use the index to find specific topics in which the user requires additional understanding and/or study. The KSA index will lead them directly to the information, often presented in portions of several chapters, from which to review.

An additional feature of this edition of the RM is the development of several ancillary tools. The first is a PowerPoint slide package for each of the text's 51 chapters. These presentations are designed for those who plan to utilize the RM for classroom teaching. Each slide file has a presentation of the basic materials contained with the specific chapter. All of the tables, graphs, and figures in the RM are contained in these presentations.

The other ancillary is a test bank for each chapter. Again, this focuses on those who are using the RM in the classroom. Each chapter contains approximately 25 questions in multiple choice, true/false, and short answer format. Any or all of these questions can be easily copied by the user into an MS Word file for printing and use in classroom examinations.

Of note is the removal of the ACSM *Compendium of Physical Activities* from the appendix section. Although this was contained in the past several RM editions, the consensus of the senior editor and section editors was that this information can be easily obtained from its previous publication in the ACSM journal *Medicine and Science in Sports and Exercise*. For those wishing to obtain a copy of the *Compendium of Physical Activities,* the full reference is provided below (1).

As with previous editions, this edition of the RM attempts to provide the most up-to-date major references for each topic. These include position papers/statements, task force reports, consensus panel reports, guidelines, summaries of scientific conferences, and the like. In order to call out these references, they are highlighted in boldface within the reference list at the end of each chapter.

Finally, it was our goal, based on previous concerns, to improve the overall presentation of muscular fitness and resistance training information. The contributors of the three chapters devoted to this topic were given specific instructions to enhance this portion of the RM. We believe that you'll find this sufficiently enhanced.

We believe that the sixth edition of the *ACSM Resource Manual for Guidelines for Exercise Testing and Prescription* has addressed many of the suggestions provided by previous users. We hope that you'll find that it is appropriately updated and builds upon the wonderful work that has gone into the previous five editions of this extremely important text. We believe that you'll find this edition of the RM, along with the other simultaneously released ACSM certification texts, as one of the most important sources of information for preparing for professional certification and for providing important and vital continuing education.

COMMENT ON PROFESSIONAL PRACTICE

In the practice of any allied health profession, there is bound to be overlap across professions. For instance, both a health educator and a clinical exercise physiologist provide behavioral/lifestyle change information to patients with cardiovascular risk factors. With that in mind, the information provided in this text covers the gamut of required knowledge, skills, and abilities necessary for the practicing ACSM Health Fitness Specialist and Clinical Exercise Specialist, and a portion required by the Registered Clinical Exercise Physiologist. It is up to the individual practicing this information to apply it properly, which includes any direct interactions one has with patients or clients. It also is the responsibility of the individual practitioner to be familiar with any laws within his or her state jurisdiction that may limit the professional scope of practice.

Therefore, we urge all practicing exercise professionals (both clinical and nonclinical) to gain the knowledge provided in this text and others, while at the same time balancing the delivery or application of such information in a manner that is both prudent and consistent with both state and local regulations.

Jonathan K. Ehrman, PhD, FACSM

REFERENCE

1. Ainsworth BE, Haskell WL, Whitt MC, et al. Compendium of physical activities: an update of activity codes and MET intensities. *Med Sci Sport Exerc* 2000;32(9):S498–S516.

Acknowledgments

Certainly, an effort such as the *ACSM Resource Manual for Guidelines for Exercise Testing and Prescription* could not come to fruition without the dedicated assistance of many, many individuals.

The following section editors devoted significant time over the past 2.5 years, time taken from their work and personal lives, toward this effort. Their only compensation is the satisfaction that this effort was for the advancement of the college, and especially for those who will use this text as a resource to prepare for the ACSM certification examinations and to keep abreast of the current best evidence for exercise testing and prescription. So many, many thanks and adulations to:

Adam deJong, MA
ACSM Certified Clinical Exercise Specialist®

Bonnie Sanderson, PhD, RN
ACSM Program Director℠
ACSM Certified Clinical Exercise Specialist®

David Swain, PhD, FACSM
ACSM Program Director℠
ACSM Certified Clinical Exercise Specialist®

Ann Swank, PhD, FACSM
ACSM Program Director℠
ACSM Certified Clinical Exercise Specialist®

Chris Womack, PhD, FACSM
ACSM Certified Clinical Exercise Specialist®

Each of these individuals recruited and worked with an army of volunteer contributors who without their time, knowledge, and effort, this text would not be possible. Each of these contributors is listed on the contributors page in the front of this text. And all of us are grateful for the previous work of hundreds of other contributors in the previous five editions of this text. Although too numerous to list here, you can see their names in the previous five editions on the contributor pages. In many cases, it was they who laid the foundation for the current chapters that have been tweaked and updated from preceding editions.

In addition, a big thank you to all of the staff both at ACSM and the publisher (Lippincott Williams & Wilkins) for their consistent effort to get this book out on time. Especially thank you to Andrea Klingler at LWW and Beth Muhlenkamp at the ACSM for keeping me on track and beholden to the timeline. And thanks to Walt Thompson for the overall coordination of the certification texts and for completing the *ACSM Guidelines for Exercise Testing and Prescription*, 8th edition, text early enough to allow us to have ample time to complete our assignment of providing the supporting evidence for the Guidelines.

Additionally, thank you to the ACSM publications and CCRB (credentialing and publications subcommittee) committee members for their work on the KSAs and the job task analysis. And to all of the many reviewers who took time to carefully read the chapters and provide the many helpful suggestions to improve the overall text.

Finally, thank you to my colleagues Steven Keteyian and Clinton Brawner, who allowed me to bounce many ideas off of them over the past several years. Their insight, support, and advice were vital to me in the ups and downs of this entire process.

Jonathan K. Ehrman, PhD, FACSM
ACSM Certified Clinical Exercise Specialist®
ACSM Program Director℠

Contributors

Kent J. Adams
Department of Kinesiology
California State University
Chico, California
Chapter 3

Rafael Bahamonde, PhD, FACSM
School of Physical Education
Indiana University–Purdue University Indianapolis
Indianapolis, Indiana
Chapter 1

David Bassett, PhD, FACSM
ACSM Certified Clinical Exercise Specialist®
Department of Exercise, Sports and Leisure Studies
University of Tennessee
Knoxville, Tennessee
Chapter 12

Susan Beckham, PhD, FACSM
ACSM Program Director℠
ACSM Registered Clinical Exercise Physiologist®
ACSM Exercise Technologist®
Dallas Veteran Affairs Medical Center
Dallas, Texas
Chapter 50

Ghazelah Bigdeli, MD
Alleghany General Hospital
Pittsburgh, Pennsylvania
Chapter 23

Clinton A. Brawner, MS
ACSM Registered Clinical Exercise Physiologist®
ACSM Certified Clinical Exercise Specialist®
Preventive Cardiology
Henry Ford Hospital
Detroit, Missouri
Chapter 30

Cedric X. Bryant, PhD, FACSM
American Council on Exercise
San Diego, California
Chapter 48

Barbara Bushman, PhD
ACSM Program Director℠
ACSM Certified Clinical Exercise Specialist®
ACSM Certified Fitness Specialist
ACSM Certified Personal Trainer℠
Department of Health, Physical Education and
  Recreation
Missouri State University
Springfield, Missouri
Chapter 26

Brian W. Carlin, MD
Alleghany General Hospital
Pittsburgh, Pennsylvania
Chapter 23

Heather O. Chambliss, PhD, FACSM
Health, Exercise Science and
  Recreation Arrangement
University of Memphis
Memphis, Tennessee
Chapter 42

Dawn P. Coe, PhD
ACSM Certified Clinical Exercise Specialist®
Department of Health, Physical Education and
  Recreation
University of Tennessee
Knoxville, Tennessee
Chapter 41

Sheri R. Colberg, PhD
ACSM Exercise Test Technologist®
Exercise Science, Physical Education and Recreation
Old Dominion University
Norfolk, Virginia
Chapter 13

Christopher B. Cooper, MD
ACSM Health/Fitness Director®
David Geffen School of Medicine
University of California Los Angeles Medical Center
Los Angeles, California
Chapter 36

Laura Cupper, BSW, CCRC
Minto Prevention and Rehabilitation Centre
University of Ottawa Heart Institute
Ottawa, Ontario
Chapter 25

Adam deJong, MA
ACSM Certified Clinical Exercise Specialist®
Preventive Cardiology and Rehabilitation
William Beaumont Hospital
Royal Oak, Michigan
Chapter 20

Shawn Drake, PhD, PT
ACSM Program Director^{SM}
ACSM Certified Clinical Exercise Specialist®
Department of Physical Therapy
Arkansas State University
Jonesboro, Arizona
Chapter 18

Andrea L. Dunn, PhD, FACSM
Klein Buendel, Inc.
Golden, Colorado
Chapter 9

J. Larry Durstine, PhD
Department of Exercise Science
The University of South Carolina
Columbia, South Carolina
Chapter 38

Paul Estabrooks, PhD
Human Nutrition, Foods, and Exercise
Virginia Tech
Blacksburg, Virginia
Chapter 47

Maria A. Fiatarone-Singh, MD
School of Exercise and Sport Science
University of Sydney
Lidcombe, NSW, Australia
Chapter 41

Carl Foster, PhD
ACSM Program Director^{SM}
Department of Exercise and
    Sport Science
University of Wisconsin
LaCrosse, Wisconsin
Chapter 21

Barry Franklin, PhD
ACSM Program Director^{SM}
ACSM Certified Clinical Exercise Specialist®
Preventive Cardiology and Rehabilitation
William Beaumont Hospital
Royal Oak, Michigan
Chapter 20

Peter W. Grandjean, PhD, FACSM
ACSM Certified Clinical Exercise Specialist®
Department of Health and Human Performance
Auburn University
Auburn, Alabama
Chapter 46

B. Sue Graves, EdD, FACSM
ACSM Certified Health Fitness Specialist®
Department of Exercise Science & Health Promotion
Florida Atlantic University
Boca Raton, Florida
Chapter 5

Jennifer Guthrie, MS
StayWell Corporation
Auburn Hills, Michigan
Chapter 19

Patrick Hagerman, EdD
ACSM Certified Health Fitness Specialist®
Department of Exercise and Sport Science
University of Tulsa
Tulsa, Oklahoma
Chapter 19

Chad Harris
Department of Allied Health
Western New Mexico University
Silver City, New Mexico
Chapter 3

Jeffrey Hastings, MD
Institute for Exercise and Environmental Medicine
Presbyterian Hospital of Dallas and University of Texas
    Southwestern Medical Center
Dallas, Texas
Chapter 34

David L. Herbert, JD
David L. Herbert and Associates, LLC
Canton, Ohio
Chapter 51

William G. Herbert, PhD, FACSM
ACSM Program Director^{SM}
Human Nutrition, Foods, and Exercise
Virginia Polytechnic Institute and State University
Blacksburg, Virginia
Chapter 51

Julie M. Hughes
School of Kinesiology
University of Minnesota
Minneapolis, Minnesota
Chapter 39

Megan E. Jablonski, MS
Department of Psychological and Brain Sciences
University of Louisville
Louisville, Kentucky
Chapter 16

Patrick L. Jacobs, PhD, FACSM
Department of Exercise Science & Health Promotion
Florida Atlantic University
Boca Raton, Florida
Chapter 5

Rachel A. Jarvis, MS
ACSM Registered Clinical Exercise Physiologist®
ACSM Certified Clinical Exercise Specialist®
Edward Hospital
Naperville, Illinois
Chapter 35

Lyndon Joseph, PhD
University of Maryland School of Medicine
Division of Gerontology
Baltimore, Maryland
Chapter 8

Anthony S. Kaleth, PhD
ACSM Program Director^{SM}
ACSM Registered Clinical Exercise Physiologist®
ACSM Certified Clinical Exercise Specialist®
ACSM Certified Health Fitness Specialist
School of Physical Education
Indiana University–Purdue University Indianapolis
Indianapolis, Indiana
Chapter 1

Peter Kaplan, MD
Alleghany General Hospital
Pittsburgh, Pennsylvania
Chapter 23

Carol Kennedy-Armbruster, MS
ACSM Certified Health Fitness Specialist®
Department of Kinesiology
Indiana University
Bloomington, Indiana
Chapter 32

Steven J. Keteyian, PhD, FACSM
ACSM Registered Clinical Exercise Physiologist®
Preventive Cardiology
Henry Ford Hospital
Detroit, Michigan
Chapters 30,35

Abby C. King, PhD
Stanford Prevention Research Center
Stanford University School of Medicine
Stanford, California
Chapter 42

Duane Knudson, PhD, FACSM
Department of Physical Education and Exercise Science
California State University
Chico, California
Chapter 2

William J. Kraemer, PhD, FACSM
Department of Kinesiology
University of Connecticut
Storrs, Connecticut
Chapters 29,31

William E. Kraus, MD, FACSM, FACC
Duke University Medical Center
Durham, North Carolina
Chapter 11

Diana Lahue, RN, BSN
Research Medical Center
Kansas City, Missouri
Chapter 27

John Lee, MD, FACC
Research Medical Center
Kansas City, Missouri
Chapter 27

Benjamin Levine, MD
Institute for Exercise and Environmental Medicine
Presbyterian Hospital of Dallas and University of Texas
    Southwestern Medical Center
Dallas, Texas
Chapter 34

Shel Levine, MS, MSA
ACSM Certified Clinical Exercise Specialist®
School of Health Promotion and Human
    Performance
Eastern Michigan University
Ypsilanti, Missouri
Chapter 26

Beth A. Lewis, PhD
Health Partners Research Foundation
Minneapolis, Minnesota
Chapters 43,44

G. William Lyerly, MS
ACSM Certified Clinical Exercise Specialist®
ACSM Certified Health Fitness Specialist
Department of Exercise Science
The University of South Carolina
Columbia, South Carolina
Chapter 38

Bess H. Marcus, PhD
Department of Psychiatry and Human Behavior
Brown University
Providence, Rhode Island
Chapters 43,44

Bonita Marks, PhD, FACSM
ACSM Certified Clinical Exercise Specialist®
Department of Exercise and Sport Science
University of North Carolina
Chapel Hill, North Carolina
Chapter 10

Timothy Maynard, MS
ACSM Program Director℠
Providence Rehab and Wellness Center
Providence Hospital
Mobile, Alabama
Chapter 24

Peter A. McCullough, MD, MPH
Preventive and Nutritional Medicine
William Beaumont Hospital
Royal Oak, Michigan
Chapter 22

A. Lynn Millar, PT, PhD, FACSM
Department of Physical Therapy
Andrews University
Berrien Springs, Minnesota
Chapter 40

Nancy Houston Miller, RN, BSN
Stanford University School of Medicine
Palo Alto, California
Chapter 15

Geoffrey E. Moore, MD, FACSM
Cayuga Center for Healthy Living
Ithaca, New York
Chapter 38

Paul Nagelkirk, PhD
ACSM Certified Clinical Exercise Specialist®
School of Physical Education, Sport and Exercise
    Science
Ball State University
Muncie, Indiana
Chapter 6

Melissa A. Napolitano, PhD
Department of Kinesiology, Center for Obesity Research
    and Education
Temple University
Philadelphia, Pennsylvania
Chapters 43,44

Stefan M. Pasiakos, PhD
ACSM Certified Health Fitness Specialist
University of Connecticut
Department of Nutritional Science
Storrs, Connecticut
Chapter 4

James A. Peterson, PhD, FACSM
Healthy Learning/Coaches Choice
Monterey, California
Chapter 48

Moira A. Petit, PhD
School of Kinesiology
University of Minnesota
Minneapolis, Minnesota
Chapter 39

John P. Porcari, PhD
ACSM Program Director℠
ACSM Registered Clinical Exercise Physiologist®
Department of Exercise and Sport Science
University of Wisconsin
LaCrosse, Wisconsin
Chapter 21

Judith J. Prochaska, PhD, MPH
Department of Psychiatry
University of California
San Francisco, California
Chapter 45

Nicholas Ratamess, PhD
Department of Health and Exercise Science
College of New Jersey
Ewing, New Jersey
Chapter 17

Nancy R. Rodriguez, PhD, FACSM
Department of Nutritional Science
University of Connecticut
Storrs, Connecticut
Chapter 4

Jeffrey L. Roitman, EdD, FACSM
ACSM Program Director^SM
Research Medical Center
Kansas City, Missouri
Chapter 27

Lee M. Romer, PhD
Centre for Sports Medicine and
    Human Performance
School of Sport and Education
Brunel University
Uxbridge, Middlesex, England
Chapter 7

Alice Ryan, PhD
ACSM Certified Clinical Exercise Specialist®
University of Maryland School of Medicine
Division of Gerontology
Baltimore, Maryland
Chapter 8

James F. Sallis, PhD
Department of Psychology
San Diego State University
San Diego, California
Chapter 45

Paul Salmon, PhD
ACSM Certified Health Fitness Specialist
Department of Psychological and
    Brain Sciences
University of Louisville
Louisville, Kentucky
Chapter 16

Bonnie K. Sanderson PhD, RN, FAACVPR
ACSM Certified Exercise Specialist®
ACSM Program Director^SM
Department of Cardiovascular Services
University of Alabama at Birmingham
Birmingham, Alabama
Chapters 46,49

Patrick Savage, MS, FAACVPR
Cardiac Rehabilitation
Fletcher Allen Health Care
South Burlington, Vermont
Chapter 49

Matthew Saval, MS
ACSM Registered Clinical Exercise Physiologist®
ACSM Certified Clinical Exercise Specialist®
Preventive Cardiology
Henry Ford Hospital
Detroit, Michigan
Chapter 30

John R. Schairer, DO
Preventive Cardiology
Henry Ford Hospital
Detroit, Michigan
Chapter 35

Tom Spring, MS
ACSM Certified Clinical Exercise Specialist®
ACSM Certified Personal Trainer^SM
Preventive Cardiology and Rehabilitation
William Beaumont Hospital
Royal Oak, Michigan
Chapter 20

Thomas W. Storer, MD
David Geffen School of Medicine
University of California Los Angeles Medical Center
Los Angeles, California
Chapter 36

David P. Swain, PhD, FACSM
ACSM Program Director^SM
ACSM Certified Clinical Exercise Specialist®
Department of Exercise Science
Old Dominion University
Norfolk, Virginia
Chapter 28

Stephen J. Tharrett, MS
ACSM Program Director^SM
Club Industry Consulting
Highland Village, Texas
Chapter 48

Larry Verity, PhD
ACSM Certified Clinical Exercise Specialist®
Department of Exercise and Nutritional Sciences
San Diego State University
San Diego, California
Chapter 37

David E. Verrill, MS, FAACVPR
ACSM Program Director^SM
ACSM Registered Clinical Exercise Physiologist®
ACSM Exercise Test Technologist®
Presbyterian Hospital Pulmonary Rehabilitation
    Program
Charlotte, North Carolina
Chapter 49

Stella L. Volpe, PhD, RD, LDN, FACSM
ACSM Certified Clinical Exercise Specialist®
School of Nursing
University of Pennsylvania
Philadelphia, Pennsylvania
Chapter 33

Joseph M. Warpeha
ACSM Registered Clinical Exercise Physiologist®
ACSM Certified Clinical Exercise Specialist®
School of Kinesiology
University of Minnesota
Minneapolis, Minnesota
Chapter 39

Michael Whitehurst, EdD, FACSM
Department of Exercise Science &
    Health Promotion
Florida Atlantic University
Boca Raton, Florida
Chapter 5

Jessica A. Whiteley, PhD
Department of Exercise and Health Sciences
University of Massachusetts
Boston, Massachusetts
Chapters 43,44

Reviewers

Mark H. Bean, PhD
ACSM Program Director^SM
Mississippi University for Women
Columbus, Mississippi

Christopher Berger, PhD, CSCS
ACSM Certified Health Fitness Specialist
Instructor & Extension Coordinator
Kinesiology & Health Promotion
University of Kentucky
Lexington, Kentucky

Gordon Blackburn, PhD, FAACVPR
Program Director, Preventive Cardiology and
   Rehabilitation
Cardiovascular Institute
Cleveland Clinic
Cleveland, Ohio

Lee E. Brown, EdD, FACSM CSCS*D, FNSCA
ACSM Certified Health Fitness Specialist
Professor, California State University, Fullerton
Department of Kinesiology
Fullerton, California

Barbara N. Campaigne, PhD
Bloomington, Indiana

Susan Carter RN, BC, FAACVPR
Manager
HEARTEAM Cardiopulmonary Rehabilitation, CHF
   Center & Pacemaker Clinic
Bloomington Hospital
Bloomington, Indiana

James R. Churilla, PhD, MPH, CSCS
ACSM Program Director^SM
ACSM Registered Clinical Exercise Physiologist®
ACSM Certified Clinical Exercise Specialist®
ACSM Certified Health Fitness Specialist®
Assistant Professor of Exercise Physiology and Physical
   Activity Epidemiology
Athletic Training, Physical Therapy and Exercise Science
Brooks College of Health
University of North Florida
Jacksonville, Florida

Bernard A. Clark, III, MD, FACC
Chairman, Department of Medicine
Professor of Medicine, University of
   Connecticut School of Medicine
Associate Chief, Section of Cardiology
Saint Francis Hospital and
   Medical Center
Hartford, Connecticut

Kristine S. L. Clark, PhD, FACSM
Penn State University
University Park, Pennsylvania

Dino G. Costanzo, FACSM
ACSM Registered Clinical Exercise Physiologist®
ACSM Program Director^SM
ACSM Exercise Test Technologist®
Administrative Director
Health Promotion, Bariatrics, and
   Cardiology
The Hospital of Central Connecticut
New Britain, Connecticut

Michael H. Cox, PhD, FACSM
Chief Executive Officer
Central Maine Orthopedics
Auburn, Maine

Frederick S. Daniels, MS, MBA, HFD
President
CPTE Health Group, Inc.
Nashua, New Hampshire

Cathryn R. Dooly, FACSM
ACSM Certified Clinical
   Exercise Specialist®
Chair and Associate Professor
Department of Physical Education &
   Exercise Studies
Lander University
Greenwood, South Carolina

Julie J. Downing, PhD, FACSM
ACSM Health Fitness Director®
ACSM Certified Personal Trainer^SM
Central Oregon Community College
Bend, Oregon

Shawn Drake, PT, PhD, CSCS
ACSM Certified Clinical Program Director^{SM}
ACSM Exercise Specialist®
Associate Professor
Department of Physical Therapy
Arkansas State University
Jonesboro, Arkansas

Yuri Feito, MS, MPH
ACSM Registered Clinical Exercise Physiologist®
ACSM Certified Clinical Exercise Specialist®
Department of Exercise, Sport and
    Leisure Studies
University of Tennessee
Knoxville, Tennessee

Julianne Frey, MS
ACSM Registered Clinical Exercise Physiologist®
ACSM Certified Clinical Exercise Specialist®
Senior Clinical Exercise Physiologist
Cardiovascular Testing Department
Internal Medicine Associates
Bloomington, Indiana

V. F. Froelicher, MD
Professor of Medicine Stanford University
Palo Alto VA Medical Center
Palo Alto, California

Steve Glass, PhD, FACSM
ACSM Certified Clinical Exercise Specialist®
Associate Dean, Professor
Department Interdisciplinary Studies/
    Movement Science
Grand Valley State University
Allendale, Michigan

Fredric L. Goss, PhD, FACSM
ACSM Program Director^{SM}
University of Pittsburgh
Pittsburgh, Pennsylvania

Robert W. Gregory, PhD
Assistant Professor
Department of Physical Education
United States Military Academy
West Point, New York

Bryan Haddock, PhD
ACSM Health/Fitness Director®
ACSM Registered Clinical Exercise Physiologist®
ACSM Certified Health Fitness Specialist
California State University, San Bernardino
San Bernardino, California

David L. Herbert, JD
Attorney at Law
Member, David L. Herbert & Associates, LLC
Attorneys & Counselors at Law
Canton, Ohio

William G. Herbert, PhD, FACSM
ACSM Program Director^{SM}
Professor Emeritus
Department of Human Nutrition, Foods & Exercise
Virginia Tech
Blacksburg, Virginia

Martin D. Hoffman, MD, FACSM
Chief of Physical Medicine & Rehabilitation, VA
    Northern California Health Care System
Professor of Physical Medicine & Rehabilitation,
    University of California - Davis
Sacramento, California

Leonard A. Kaminsky, PhD, FACSM
ACSM Program Director^{SM}
ACSM Exercise Test Technologist®
Professor of Exercise Science, Director of the Clinical
    Exercise Physiology Program
Human Performance Laboratory
Ball State University
Muncie, Indiana

Steven J. Keteyian, PhD, FACSM
ACSM Registered Clinical Exercise Physiologist®
Program Director, Preventive Cardiology
Division of Cardiovascular Medicine
Henry Ford Hospital
Detroit, Michigan

Joanne B. Krasnoff, PhD
ACSM Certified Clinical Exercise Specialist®
Associate Director
Boston University Medical Center
Section Endocrinology, Diabetes & Nutrition
Boston, Massachusetts

Peter M. Magyari, PhD
ACSM Certified Health Fitness Specialist
Assistant Professor of Exercise Physiology
Brooks College of Health
University of North Florida
Jacksonville, Florida

Thomas P. Mahady MS, CSCS
Senior Exercise Physiologist
Cardiac Prevention & Rehabilitation Center
Hackensack University Medical Center
Hackensack, New Jersey

Jacalyn J. McComb, PhD, FACSM
ACSM Program Director^{SM}
ACSM Certified Clinical Exercise Specialist®
ACSM Exercise Test Technologist®
Professor in the Department of Health Exercise and
    Sport Sciences
Texas Tech University
Lubbock, Texas

Timothy R. McConnell, PhD, FACSM, FAACVPR
ACSM Program Director^{SM}
Chair
Department of Exercise Science
Bloomsburg University
Bloomsburg, Pennsylvania

Michelle Miller, MS, NSCA cPT
ACSM Certified Clinical Exercise Specialist®
Faculty
Department of Kinesiology
Coordinator, Fitness Specialist Undergraduate Degree
    School of HPER Indiana University Indiana
    University
Bloomington, Indiana

W. Allen Moore, Jr. PT, PhD
Assistant Professor
Department of Athletic Training and Physical Therapy
    University of North Florida
Jacksonville, Florida

Ann Cassidy Noonan, PT, EdD
Physical Therapy Program Director Department of
    Athletic Training and Physical Therapy University of
    North Florida Brooks College of Health
Jacksonville, Florida

Barbara Olinzock
Assistant Prof. of Nursing
University of North Florida
Jacksonville, Florida

Richard B. Parr, EdD, FACSM
ACSM Program Director^{SM}
Professor
Department of Exercise Science
Central Michigan University
Mount Pleasant, Michigan

Kenneth H. Pitetti, PhD, FACSM
Department of Physical Therapy
Wichita State University
Wichita, Kansas

Joel M. Press, MD
Reva and David Logan Distinguished Chair of
    Musculoskeletal Rehabilitation
Medical Director, Spine and Sports
    Rehabilitation Centers
Rehabilitation Institute of Chicago
Associate Professor, Physical Medicine and
    Rehabilitation
Feinberg/Northwestern School
    of Medicine
Chicago, Illinois

William S. Quillen, PhD, FACSM
University of South Florida
Odessa, Florida

Jeffrey L. Roitman, EdD, FACSM
ACSM Program Director^{SM}
Associate Professor, Director Exercise
    Science Program
Rockhurst University
Exercise Science
Kansas City, Missouri

Peter Ronai, M.S., NSCA CSCS-D, NSCA-CPT
ACSM Registered Clinical Exercise Physiologist®
ACSM Program Director^{SM}
ACSM Certified Clinical Exercise
    Specialist®
ACSM Exercise Test Technologist®
ACSM Certified Health Fitness
    Specialist®
Exercise Physiologist
Ahlbin Rehabilitation Centers
Bridgeport Hospital
Bridgeport, Connecticut

Dr. Robert D. Sawyer
Texas Tech University
Lubbock, Texas

Robert Shapiro, PhD, FACSM
Professor
Department of Kinesiology &
    Health Promotion
University of Kentucky
Lexington, Kentucky

Paul Sorace, MS
ACSM Registered Clinical Exercise Physiologist®
Clinical Exercise Physiologist
Hackensack University Medical Center
Hackensack, New Jersey

Ray W. Squires, PhD, FACSM, FAACVPR, FAHA
ACSM Program Director[SM]
ACSM Certified Clinical Exercise Specialist®
Professor of Medicine
Division of Cardiovascular Diseases and Internal
    Medicine
Mayo Clinic
Rochester, Minnesota

Jack E. Taunton, MD, FACSM
University of British Columbia
Allan McGavin Sports Medicine Centre
Vancouver, British Columbia

Donna J. Terbizan, PhD, FACSM
ACSM Certified Health Fitness Specialist®
ACSM Exercise Test Technologist®
Professor
Health, Nutrition and Exercise Sciences
North Dakota State University
Fargo, North Dakota

Paul D. Thompson, MD, FACSM
Hartford Hospital
Hartford, Connecticut

Vassilios G. Vardaxis, PhD
Department of Kinesiology
Indiana University
Bloomington, Indiana

David E. Verrill, M.S., FAACVPR
ACSM Registered Clinical Exercise Physiologist®
ACSM Certified Clinical Exercise Specialist®
ACSM Program Director[SM]
Clinical Exercise Physiologist
Presbyterian Hospital Pulmonary Rehabilitation Program,
Charlotte, North Carolina
CMC-NorthEast Medical Center Health and Fitness
    Institute,
Concord, North Carolina

Matthew Vukovich, PhD, FACSM
Associate Professor
EA Martin Program in Human Nutrition
South Dakota State University
Brookings, South Dakota

James S. Williams, PhD, FACSM
Texas Tech University
Lubbock, Texas

Contents

Preliminary Section: Background Materials

CHRISTOPHER WOMACK, PhD, FACSM, *Section Editor*

CHAPTER

1

Functional Anatomy

ANATOMICAL POSITION AND DEFINITIONS OF ANATOMICAL LOCATIONS AND PLANES

> **1.1.3-HFS: Knowledge of the following muscle action terms: inferior, superior, medial, lateral, supination, pronation, flexion, extension, adduction, abduction, hyperextension, rotation, circumduction, agonist, antagonist, and stabilizer.**

The **anatomical position** is the universally accepted reference position used to describe regions and spatial relationships of the human body and to make reference to body positions (e.g., joint motions). In the anatomical position, the body is erect with the feet together and the upper limbs hanging at the sides, palms of the hands facing forward, thumbs facing away from the body, and fingers extended (Fig. 1-1).

> > > **KEY TERMS**

Agonist: Muscle or muscle group that is the prime mover for a joint action.

Anatomical position: The universally accepted reference position used to describe regions and spatial relationships of the human body and to make reference to body positions.

Antagonist: Muscle or muscle group that opposes the action of the prime movers (agonist).

Appendicular skeleton: All of the bones that are found in the limbs of the body

Atrioventricular (AV) valves: Separate the atria from the ventricles. The right AV valve has three leaflets and is called the tricuspid valve. The left AV valve has two leaflets and is called the bicuspid (or mitral) valve

Auscultation: The act of listening to sounds of the body. A practitioner can use a stethoscope to assess blood pressure, heart rate, and heart and lung sounds by auscultation.

Axial skeleton: The bones of the skeleton that form the central or supportive core, including the bones of the skull, vertebral column, ribs, and sternum.

Contractile proteins: Specialized proteins found within muscle cells that interact with one another to cause muscle force production. The major contractile proteins are actin and myosin.

Joints: The articulations between bones, typically classified according to structure as being fibrous,

cartilaginous, or synovial. Synovial joints are the most common in the body.

Motor unit: A single somatic motor neuron and the group of muscle fibers innervated by it.

Muscle fiber architecture: The orientation of the muscle fibers to the longitudinal axis of the muscle. Terms commonly used to describe muscle fiber architecture include fusiform (longitudinal) and pennate (unipennate, bipennate, and multipennate).

Planes of motion: Orthogonally arranged planes that divide the human body and can be used to describe various body movements. The three planes of motion are commonly known as the sagittal, frontal, and transverse planes.

Regulatory proteins: Specialized proteins found within muscle cells that block the binding of the contractile proteins to one another and thus keep the muscle in a relaxed state. The regulatory proteins are troponin and tropomyosin.

Respiratory membrane: The membrane formed by the walls of alveoli and capillaries as they come in contact with one another in the lungs. The respiratory membrane is where diffusion of oxygen and carbon dioxide occurs within the lungs.

Synergist: Muscle or muscle group that assists the agonist in performing a joint action.

Ventilation: The act of breathing in (inspiration) and out (expiration) so that oxygen can be exchanged for carbon dioxide in the alveoli.

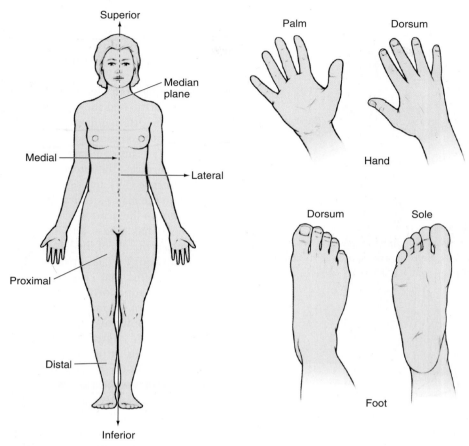

FIGURE 1-1. Anatomical position: the body is erect with the feet together, with the upper limbs hanging at the sides, palms of the hands facing forward, thumbs facing away from the body, and fingers extended. Typically, all anatomical references to the body relate to this position.

Another useful tool used to describe anatomical motions are the body planes, or **planes of motion**. There are three imaginary planes orthogonal to each other that pass through the body. The *sagittal plane* divides the body or structure into the right and left sides. The *frontal* or *coronal plane* divides the body or structure into anterior and posterior portions. The *transverse plane* (also called the *cross-sectional* or *horizontal plane*) divides the body or structure into superior and inferior portions (Fig. 1-2). Table 1-1 lists some terms commonly used to reference anatomical spatial relationships.

TABLE 1-1. DEFINITIONS OF ANATOMICAL LOCATIONS

TERM	DEFINITION
Anterior	The front of the body; ventral
Deep	Below the surface and not relatively close to the surface
Distal	Furthest point in distance from a given anatomic reference point
Inferior	Away from the head; lower
Lateral	Away from the midline of the body; to the side
Medial	Toward the midline of the body
Posterior	The back of the body; dorsal
Proximal	Closest point in distance to a given anatomic reference point
Superficial	Located close to or on the body surface
Superior	Toward the head; higher

CARDIOVASCULAR ANATOMY

> **1.1.1-CES: Describe and illustrate the normal cardiovascular anatomy.**

> **1.1.2-HFS: Knowledge of the anatomy and physiology of the cardiovascular system and pulmonary system.**

GENERAL COMPONENTS AND FUNCTIONS

The cardiovascular system is a continuous closed arrangement that includes a pump (the heart) and more than 60,000 miles of conduits (blood vessels) (28). The primary function of the cardiovascular system is to provide an environment for the transport of nutrients and

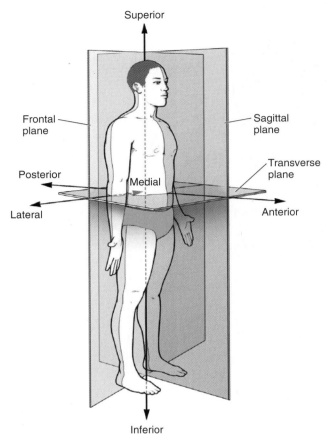

FIGURE 1-2. Anatomical planes of the body.

removal of waste products. The cardiovascular system assists with maintenance of homeostasis at rest and during exercise. The cardiovascular system performs the following specific functions (26,27,37):

1. transports oxygenated blood from the lungs to tissues and deoxygenated blood from the tissues to the lungs;
2. distributes nutrients (e.g., glucose, free fatty acids, amino acids) to cells;
3. removes metabolic wastes (e.g., carbon dioxide, urea, lactate) from the periphery for elimination or reuse;
4. regulates pH to control acidosis and alkalosis;
5. transports hormones and enzymes to regulate physiological function;
6. maintains fluid volume to prevent dehydration;
7. maintains body temperature by absorbing and redistributing heat.

The following sections provide an overview of the basic structures and functions of the heart and blood vessels.

Heart

Location and General Landmarks

The adult heart is approximately the size of a fist and weighs between 250 and 350 g (38). The heart is posi-

tioned obliquely within the thoracic cavity in a space known as the *mediastinum* (Fig. 1-3). It is anterior to the vertebral column and posterior to the sternum. The lungs flank the heart bilaterally and slightly overlap it.

The heart has four chambers; the two superior chambers are the *atria*, and the two inferior chambers are the *ventricles*. The external deep grooves of the heart (called *sulci*) define the boundaries of the four chambers of the heart (17,37). The coronary sulcus separates the atria from the ventricles; the interventricular sulcus separates the left ventricle (LV) and right ventricle (RV). The sulci also contain the major arteries and veins that provide circulation within the heart.

The heart has a base and an apex. The base of the heart consists mainly of the left atrium (LA) (11), part of the right atrium (RA), and parts of the proximal portion of the large veins that enter the heart posteriorly. The base is located superiorly and near the right sternal border at the level of second and third ribs. The apex of the heart is located inferiorly and to the left of the base at the level of the fifth intercostal space. Approximately two thirds of the mass of the heart is to the left of the midsagittal plane. As the heart is palpated at the apex (between the fifth and sixth ribs), the contraction can be easily felt. This is referred to as the *point of maximal intensity* (PMI) (26).

The superior border of the heart consists of both atria and the bases of the pulmonary trunk and the aorta. The right border is formed by the RA. The left border consists of the LV and a small part of the LA. The inferior border is formed primarily by the RV and a portion of the LV at the apex.

The heart is rotated to the left in the chest so that the anterior portion of the heart forms the sternocostal surface, which consists mainly of the RA and RV. The diaphragmatic surface consists mainly of the LV where it slopes and rests on the diaphragm.

Tissue Coverings and Layers of the Heart

The heart is covered by a double-walled, loose-fitting membranous sac called the *pericardium* (Fig. 1-4). The outer wall of the pericardium, the parietal pericardium, has both a fibrous (tough) layer and a serous (smooth) layer. The fibrous layer serves to strengthen the pericardium and anchor it within the mediastinum. The thin serous layer, called the visceral pericardium or *epicardium*, adheres to the fibrous layer of the parietal pericardium and forms a tight covering over the heart surface. Between the parietal and visceral layers is the *pericardial cavity*. The pericardial cavity contains *pericardial fluid*, which acts as a lubricant and reduces friction between the membranes during contraction. If the pericardium becomes inflamed, *pericarditis* (a condition characterized by painful adhesions) can result.

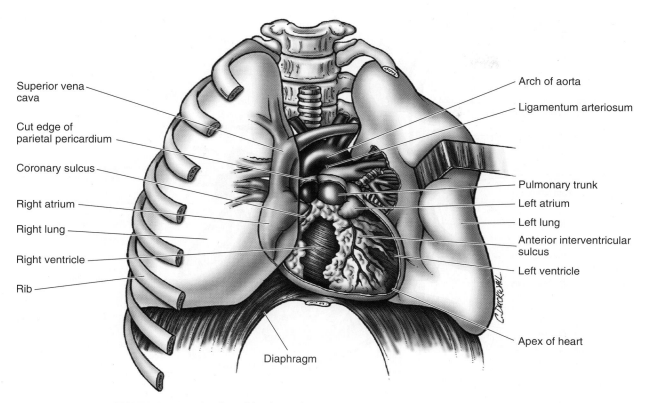

Superior vena cava

Cut edge of parietal pericardium

Coronary sulcus

Right atrium

Right lung

Right ventricle

Rib

Arch of aorta

Ligamentum arteriosum

Pulmonary trunk

Left atrium

Left lung

Anterior interventricular sulcus

Left ventricle

Apex of heart

Diaphragm

FIGURE 1-3. Anterior view of the thorax showing the position of the heart in the mediastinum.

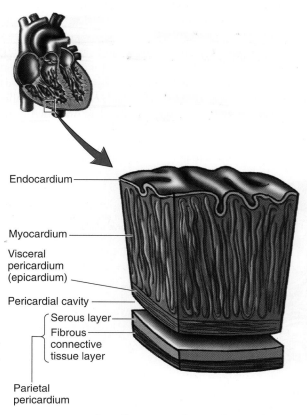

Endocardium

Myocardium

Visceral pericardium (epicardium)

Pericardial cavity

Serous layer

Fibrous connective tissue layer

Parietal pericardium

FIGURE 1-4. Endocardium, myocardium, and pericardium.

The thickest layer of tissue in the heart is the *myocardium*. The myocardium is composed of cardiac muscle. Within the myocardium is a network of crisscrossing dense connective tissue fibers called the *cardiac skeleton*. This cardiac skeleton provides insertion points for the fibers of the cardiac musculature, support for the valves of the heart, and some separation between the atria and the ventricles.

The inner layer of the myocardium is lined with a thin layer of endothelium called the *endocardium*. The endocardium forms the innermost lining of the walls of the various heart chambers as well as the heart valves. The endocardium joins with the endothelial linings of the blood vessels as they leave and enter the heart (35).

Heart Chambers, Valves, and Blood Flow

The heart is two pumps in a single unit with four chambers or cavities: the right atrium (RA), left atrium (LA), RV, and LV (Fig. 1-5). The right heart (RA and RV) and the left heart (LA and LV) make up the two pumps. The right side of the heart collects blood from the periphery and pumps it through the lungs (pulmonary circuit). The left side of the heart collects blood from the lungs and pumps it throughout the body (systemic circuit) (5,12,14,29,34).

The atria and ventricles of the heart are separated by the *interatrial septum* and the *interventricular septum*,

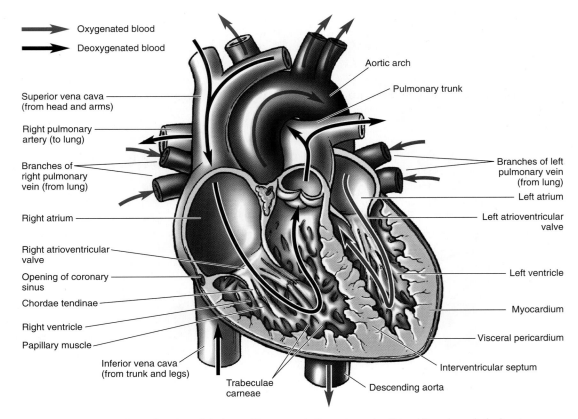

FIGURE 1-5. Frontal section of the heart. The arrows indicate the path of blood flow through the heart.

respectively. The atria are smaller and have thinner walls than the ventricles. The LV walls and interventricular septum are two to three times thicker than the RV walls. The thicker myocardium of the LV allows the left side of the heart to pump blood against the greater resistance offered by the large vascular tree that makes up the systemic circuit. Conversely, the RV only has to pump blood a relatively short distance through the pulmonary circuit.

The heart has four valves whose function is to maintain unidirectional blood flow. The **AV valves** separate the atria from the ventricles. The *semilunar valves* separate the ventricles from the aorta and pulmonary artery trunk. The AV valves are named for the number of leaflets, or *cusps*, formed by the endocardium (Fig. 1-6). Whereas the right AV valve has three cusps and is called the *tricuspid valve*, the left AV valve has only two cusps

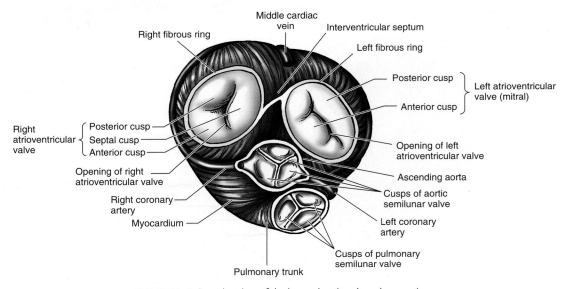

FIGURE 1-6. Superior view of the heart showing the valve openings.

and is called the *bicuspid* (or *mitral*) *valve*. The tricuspid valve controls the flow of blood from the RA to the RV, and the mitral valve controls blood flow from the LA to the LV. The cusps of the AV valves are attached to *chordae tendineae* (strong fibrous bands) that extend from the *papillary muscles*. The papillary muscles arise from folds and ridges of the myocardium that project into the ventricular chambers. During ventricular contraction, the papillary muscles shorten and pull the chordae tendineae taut; this prevents the AV valves from swinging back into the atria, thus preventing retrograde blood flow during ventricular contraction (18).

There are two semilunar valves in the heart, each with three cusps. The *pulmonary valve* lies between the RV and the pulmonary artery. The *aortic valve* is located between the LV and the aorta. The cusps of the semilunar valves prevent the backflow of blood from the arteries to the ventricles.

Blood flow through the heart is accomplished by the following sequence of events, beginning with the return of systemic blood to the RA:

1. venous blood flows into the RA via the superior and inferior vena cava, coronary sinus, and anterior cardiac veins;

2. the RA free wall (the contractile section of the RA heart wall) contracts and blood moves through the tricuspid valve into the RV;
3. the RV free wall contracts, the tricuspid valve closes, and blood flows through the pulmonary valve into the pulmonary artery and the branches of that system;
4. blood ultimately reaches the alveolar capillaries, where gas exchange occurs;
5. blood flows back to the LA via the pulmonary veins;
6. the LA free wall contracts and blood flows through the bicuspid valve and into the LV.
7. the LV free wall contracts, the bicuspid valve closes, and blood flows through the aortic valve into the aorta and its branches, where it is distributed to the coronary circulation and the systemic circulation (18,30,39,41).

Heart Blood Supply

Although the interiors of the heart chambers are continuously bathed with blood, only the endocardium is directly nourished. The myocardium is too thick to permit adequate diffusion of nutrients and oxygen to the cardiac muscle cells and epicardium. The functional supply of blood for the heart is delivered via the *left coronary artery* (LCA) and *right coronary artery* (RCA) (Figs. 1-7 and 1-8). The

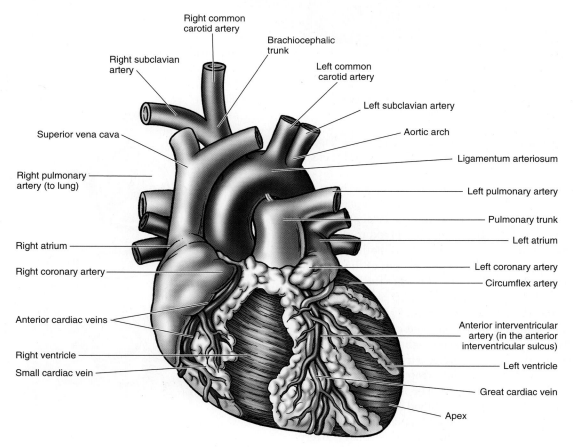

FIGURE 1-7. Anterior view of the heart.

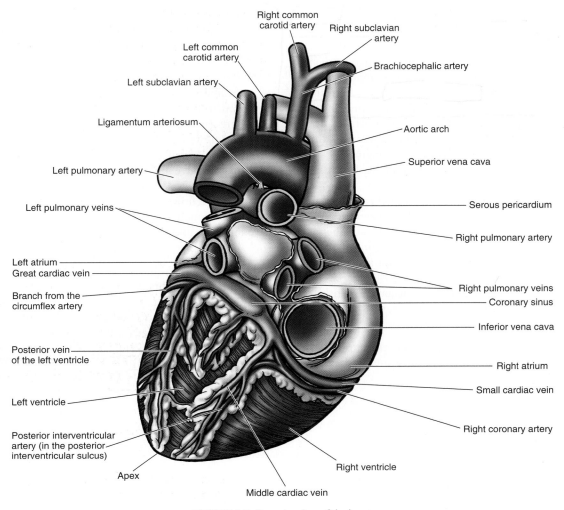

FIGURE 1-8. Posterior view of the heart.

coronary arteries arise from the *aortic sinus* at the base of the aorta just superior to the semilunar (aortic) valve cusps (Fig. 1-9).

The LCA angles toward the left side of the heart for about 1 to 2 cm before branching into the *left anterior descending* (LAD) coronary artery and the *circumflex artery* (CxA) (36). The LAD artery supplies blood to the interventricular septum and anterior walls of both ventricles. The CxA branches toward the left margin of the heart in the coronary sulcus and supplies blood to the laterodorsal walls of the LA and LV. Both the LAD artery and CxA curve around the left ventricular wall and supply small branches that interconnect (*anastomose*) with the RCA.

The RCA supplies blood to the right side of the heart as it follows the AV groove before curving to the back of the heart, giving off a *posterior interventricular artery* (*posterior descending artery*, or PDA). The RCA and PDA have numerous branches that supply blood to the anterior, posterior, and lateral surfaces of the RV and to the RA.

After blood circulates through the coronary artery system, which ends at the myocardial capillaries, it is

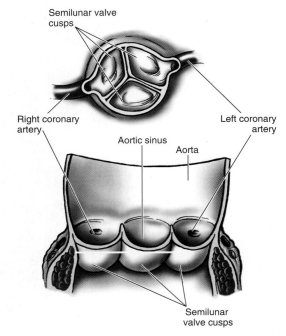

FIGURE 1-9. Origin of the coronary arteries.

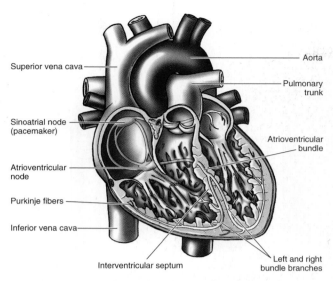

FIGURE 1-10. Electrical conduction system of the heart.

collected by the cardiac veins. The blood then travels a path similar to that of the coronary arteries but in the opposite direction. On the posterior aspect of the heart, the cardiac veins form an enlarged vessel, the *coronary sinus*, which empties the blood into the RA. Some smaller anterior cardiac veins also empty directly into the RA.

Conduction System of the Heart

> **1.4.3-HFS: Knowledge of the basic properties of cardiac muscle and the normal pathways of conduction in the heart.**

Cardiac muscle has intrinsic properties that allow it to depolarize and contract without direct neural stimulation. Cardiac cells interconnect end to end and form *intercalated discs* (27). These intercalated discs allow electrical impulses to spread from cell to cell and cause the myocardium to act as a single unit or functional *syncytium*. The components of the heart's conduction system include the *sinoatrial (SA) node*, the *AV node*, the *AV bundle (bundle of His)*, the *right* and *left bundle branches*, and the *Purkinje fibers* (Fig. 1-10).

The electrical impulse, which initiates cardiac contraction, begins at the SA node, or intrinsic pacemaker, of the heart. The cells of the SA node, which lie in the wall of the RA near the opening of the superior vena cava, depolarize spontaneously about 60–80 times per minute at rest (42). From the SA node, the electrical impulse spreads via internodal gaps through both atria until it reaches the AV node, which is located in the inferior part of the interatrial septum. The electrical impulse is delayed at the AV node for approximately 0.13 seconds to allow the atria to contract and fill the ventricles (42). The impulse then moves rapidly through the AV bundle (bundle of His), through the right and left bundle branches, and through the net-

work of Purkinje fibers in the myocardium of both ventricles. The Purkinje fibers are specialized fast-conducting cells that allow rapid conduction to the ventricles. This rapid conduction allows the ventricles to contract at approximately the same time.

The rate and forcefulness of heart contraction do not depend on intrinsic nerve stimulation; rather they are influenced by extrinsic factors such as autonomic nervous system control and hormone activity. Sympathetic nerves and hormones (e.g., norepinephrine and epinephrine) stimulate the atria and ventricles to beat faster (*chronotropic effect*) and more forcefully (*inotropic effect*). Parasympathetic nerves (vagi) control the atria and slow the heart rate.

Blood Vessels

After blood flows from the heart, it enters the vascular system, which is composed of numerous blood vessels. The blood vessels (a) form a closed system to deliver blood to the tissues; (b) help promote the exchange of nutrients, metabolic wastes, hormones, and other substances with the cells; and (c) ultimately return blood back to the heart.

Arteries carry blood away from the heart (Fig. 1-11). Large arteries branch into smaller arteries and eventually into smaller *arterioles*. Arterioles branch into capillaries, which allow the exchange of blood with various tissues (e.g., the digestive system, liver, kidneys). On the venous

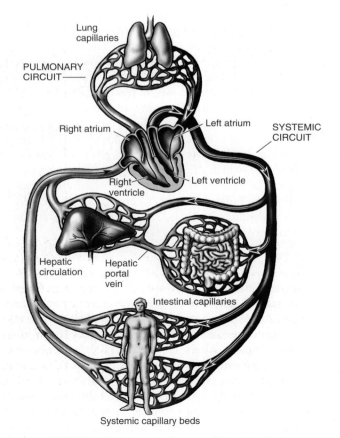

FIGURE 1-11. Schematic diagram of blood circulation.

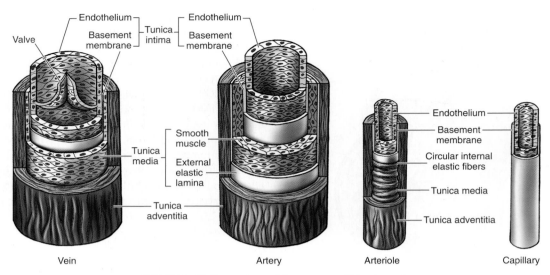

FIGURE 1-12. Comparison of the structure of blood vessels.

side of the circulation, capillaries converge into small *venules,* which converge to form larger vessels called *veins.* The large veins (e.g., superior and inferior vena cava, pulmonary veins) return blood to the heart.

The walls of the various blood vessels vary in thickness and size because of the presence or absence of one or more layers of tissues (Fig. 1-12). The *tunica intima* consists of the endothelium and a thin connective tissue basement membrane. The tunica intima is the only layer common to all of the blood vessels. The internal elastic lamina separates the tunica intima from the middle layer of smooth muscle fibers and elastic fibers known as the *tunica media.* The smooth muscle fibers of the tunica media can be influenced by neural control (parasympathetic and sympathetic nerves), hormones (e.g., acetylcholine, norepinephrine, epinephrine), or local factors (e.g., pH, oxygen levels, carbon dioxide levels), which can cause them to vasoconstrict or vasodilate. The external elastic lamina separates the tunica media from the outermost layer of connective tissue called the *tunica adventitia* (*externa*). The adventitia helps attach vessels to surrounding tissues (37).

Arteries

Arteries can be classified as *elastic* or *muscular* according to their size and function. Large arteries such as the aorta and those of the pulmonary trunk are called elastic arteries. The tunica media of these vessels is thick and contains many elastic fibers (see Fig. 1-12). The elastic nature of these arteries helps maintain pressure within the vessels. Other smaller arteries distribute blood throughout the body. These arteries are called muscular arteries and their tunica media contains primarily smooth muscle fibers. Muscular arteries are less distensible than elastic arteries.

Arterioles

Arterioles are arteries very small in diameter that deliver blood to the capillaries. They have lumens smaller than 0.5 mm, and their tunica media is largely composed of smooth muscle with scattered elastic fibers (37). Arterioles play a major role in regulating blood flow to the capillaries because of their ability to vasoconstrict or vasodilate. Also, changes in arteriole diameter can affect systemic blood pressure (BP).

Capillaries

Capillaries are microscopic vessels that connect the arterioles with the venules. Capillaries form dense networks that branch throughout all tissues. The average capillary is 1 mm in length and 0.01 mm in diameter, which is just large enough for a single red blood cell (RBC) to pass through (26) (Fig. 1-12). Capillaries have extremely thin walls made of a single layer of cells and a basement membrane. In contrast to the other blood vessels, capillaries do not have a tunica media or tunica adventitia. This unique characteristic allows for the exchange of materials between the blood and the tissue cells.

Venules and Veins

Venules, which form from capillaries, consist mainly of tunica intima and tunica adventitia. Venules collect blood from capillaries. *Veins* receive blood from the venules and have the same three tissue layers as arteries. However, the tunica media of the veins is thinner than that found in the arteries. In general, veins are thinner and more compliant than arteries and act as blood reservoirs. The walls of some veins, such as those in the legs, contain one-way valves that help maintain venous return to the heart by

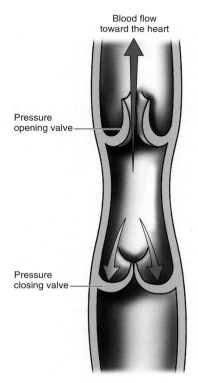

FIGURE 1-13. Valves of a vein.

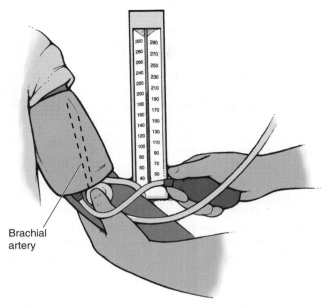

FIGURE 1-14. Positions of the stethoscope head and pressure cuff.

preventing retrograde blood flow even under relatively low pressures (Fig. 1-13). The valves in the veins are made up of folds of tunica intima (endothelium) and are similar in nature to the semilunar valves of the heart. A special type of vein formed by a thin layer of endothelial cells surrounded with dense connective tissue for support is called a venous sinus (e.g., the coronary sinus of the heart).

At rest, most (approximately 60%) of the blood volume is in veins and venules, which is why they are called blood reservoirs. Systemic capillaries hold only about 5% of the blood volume, and systemic arteries and arterioles hold about 15%. Blood stored in the veins and venules can be quickly redistributed to the arterial side via vasoconstriction, which is caused by smooth muscle located in the venous walls. The muscle pump provided by increased skeletal muscle activity, such as during exercise, can also assist in redistribution of the venous blood, thereby providing greater blood volume to the active muscles.

ANATOMICAL SITES FOR BLOOD PRESSURE AND HEART RATE DETERMINATION

> **1.1.43.-HFS: Ability to locate the anatomic landmarks for palpation of peripheral pulses and blood pressure.**

> **1.3.11-HFS: Ability to locate the brachial artery and correctly place the cuff and stethoscope in position for blood pressure measurement.**

The measurement of arterial BP before, during, and after an exercise test or training session is routine. The systolic BP (SBP) and diastolic BP (DBP) are taken to ensure patient safety and to obtain important diagnostic and prognostic information. The most common method used for the determination of BP is brachial artery **auscultation**. The brachial artery courses through a groove formed by the bifurcation of the triceps and biceps brachii muscles on the medial (inside) aspect of the upper arm (Fig. 1-14).

Health fitness professionals can assess peripheral pulses to obtain an index of resting heart rate, training bradycardia, or aerobic exercise intensity. Large, superficial arteries are preferable for pulse determination because they are easily palpable. Two conventional palpation sites are the common carotid and radial arteries. The right and left common carotid arteries are located on the anterior portion of the neck in the groove formed by the larynx (Adam's apple) and the sternocleidomastoid muscles (the large muscles on the lateral sides of the neck) just below the mandible (lower jaw) (28). The radial artery courses deep on the lateral (thumb side) aspect of the forearm and becomes superficial near the distal head of the radius (28). Radial pulses may be difficult to obtain in individuals with large amounts of subcutaneous fat over the palpation site. Pulses may be taken at any arterial site. Other palpation sites include the temporal (temple region of skull), popliteal (behind the knee), femoral (inguinal fold of groin), and dorsal pedis (top of foot) arteries. Lower extremity pulses may provide information regarding the adequacy of peripheral blood flow.

SUMMARY

The cardiovascular system is a closed system of pumps, valves, and conduits that coordinate both anatomical and physiological functions to maintain a constant internal environment. The heart is a hollow, four-chambered organ that works with the circulatory system to pump blood through elastic blood vessels to the lungs and systemic circulation. The compliance and elasticity of these blood vessels helps maintain BP at rest and during exercise. In times of increased cardiovascular work, the cardiovascular system functions in an even more sophisticated manner to meet those demands while it continues to maintain BP and meet tissue demand requirements.

RESPIRATORY ANATOMY

> **1.1.2-HFS: Knowledge of the anatomy and physiology of the cardiovascular system and pulmonary system.**

GENERAL COMPONENTS AND FUNCTIONS

This section describes the basic anatomy of the respiratory system as it relates to function. The lungs of an average-sized person weigh about 1 kg. However, if spread out, the tissue would occupy a surface area about the size of a singles tennis court (28). The anatomy of the respiratory system supports the basic function of exchanging carbon dioxide (CO_2), a by-product of cellular metabolism, and oxygen (O_2), which is necessary for cellular activity (32).

TABLE 1-2. STRUCTURAL COMPONENTS OF THE RESPIRATORY SYSTEM AND THEIR CORRESPONDING FUNCTION

STRUCTURAL COMPONENTS	FUNCTION
Respiratory center	Control of breathing
Peripheral chemoreceptors	Control of breathing
Afferent and efferent nerves	Control of breathing
Upper respiratory tract	Distribution of ventilation
Conducting airways	Distribution of ventilation
Respiratory bronchioles	Distribution of ventilation
Chest wall, respiratory muscles, and pleura	Ventilatory pump
Pulmonary arteries, capillaries, and veins	Distribution of blood flow
Functional respiratory unit	Gas exchange
Mucociliary escalator	Bronchial clearance
Alveolar macrophages	Lung clearance and defense
Lymphatic drainage	Lung clearance and defense

Other important functions include the production and metabolism of vasoactive substances and the filtration of systemic venous blood before entry into the LV. The structural components of the respiratory system (Fig. 1-15) are the framework for the corresponding functions of the system (Table 1-2) (2,7).

The respiratory system consists of two major divisions: the upper and lower respiratory tracts. Functionally, the

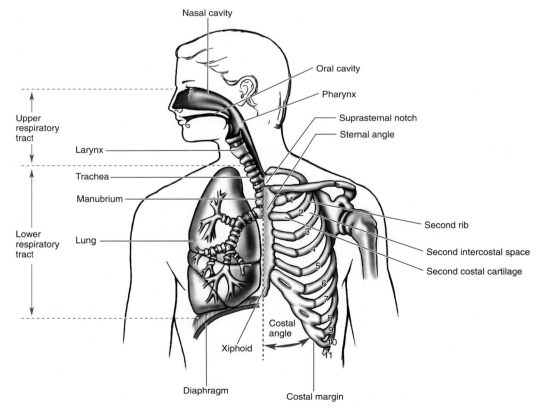

FIGURE 1-15. Respiratory system consists of an upper respiratory tract (nose, pharynx, and larynx) and a lower respiratory tract (tracheobronchial tree and lungs).

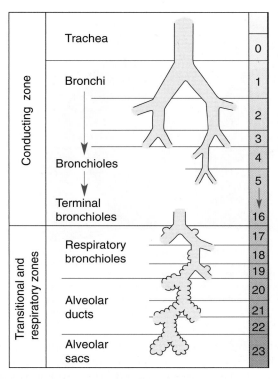

Trachea		0
Bronchi		1
		2
		3
Bronchioles		4
		5
Terminal bronchioles		16
Respiratory bronchioles		17
		18
		19
Alveolar ducts		20
		21
		22
Alveolar sacs		23

FIGURE 1-16. Branching of the airways starting from the trachea to the alveolar sacs. There are approximately 23 generations of branching in the tracheobronchial tree.

respiratory system can be separated in two portions: the *conducting portion*, which is a system of interconnecting cavities and tubes (i.e., the nose, mouth, pharynx, larynx, trachea, bronchi), and the *respiratory portion*, where the exchange of gases occurs (e.g., respiratory bronchioles, alveolar ducts, and alveoli) (Figs. 1-15 and 1-16).

Upper Respiratory Tract

The upper respiratory tract, which includes the nose, paranasal sinuses, pharynx, and larynx (see Fig. 1-15), acts as a conduction pathway for the movement of air into the lower respiratory tract. The function of these structures is to purify, warm, and humidify ambient air before it reaches the gas exchange units. During normal quiet breathing, inspired air is heated to body temperature and the relative humidity is increased to more than 90% during passage through the nose. Outside air goes into the nasal cavity via the nostrils. As air enters the nostrils, it passes through the vestibule, which is lined with skin that has coarse hairs that help filter out large dust particles. Air is then moved to the upper nasal cavity. The upper nasal cavity is lined with a membrane rich in capillaries, which are responsible for warming the air. *Mucus* secreted by cells moistens the air and traps dust particles. Mucus is removed by the cilia in the pharynx, where it is eliminated from the respiratory tract via swallowing or spitting. The pharynx (or throat) is a funnel-shaped tube about 13 cm

long that begins at the internal nares (internal nostrils), anterior to the cervical vertebrae and posterior to the nasal and oral cavities and larynx. The pharynx is made up of skeletal muscles and is lined with mucous membrane. It serves as a passage for air and food and as a resonating chamber for speech. The pharynx is divided by the soft palate into the *nasopharynx* and the *oropharynx*. The *epiglottis*, located at the base of the tongue, protects the laryngeal opening during swallowing. The *larynx* (or voice box) contains the vocal cords, which contribute to speech and participate in coughing. It also connects the pharynx with the next respiratory organ, the trachea, which is the first organ of the lower respiratory tract.

Lower Respiratory Tract

The lower respiratory tract begins in the *trachea* (windpipe) just below the larynx and includes the bronchi, bronchioles, and alveoli (see Figs. 1-15 and 1-16). There are approximately 23 generations of airways. The first 16 serve as conducting airways and the last 7 are respiratory airways ending in the approximately 300 million alveoli that form the gas exchange surface.

Trachea

The trachea, or windpipe, begins at the base of the neck and extends approximately 10–12 cm to an internal ridge called the *carina* (see Fig. 1-15), where it divides into the right and left main bronchi. It is anterior to the esophagus, extending from the larynx to about the fifth thoracic vertebra. The trachea consists of a series of anteriorly located horseshoe-shaped cartilaginous rings, which are closed posteriorly by a longitudinal muscle bundle. The mucous membrane of the carina is highly sensitive and is associated with the cough reflex.

Bronchi and Bronchioles

At the sternal angle, the trachea divides into *right* and *left primary bronchi*, which branch into the right and left lungs, respectively. The major bronchi contain cartilage that maintains the free passage of air as well as large numbers of mucous glands that produce secretions in response to irritation, infection, or inflammation. Once in each lung, the primary bronchi divide into smaller bronchi called *secondary (lobar) bronchi* because they go to each of the lobes of the lungs (three lobes in the right lung and two in the left lung) (Figs. 1-16 and 1-17). The secondary bronchi continue to branch into *tertiary (segmental) bronchi* (10 on the right and 10 on the left), then *bronchioles*, and end in *terminal bronchioles*. Beyond the terminal bronchioles are respiratory bronchioles, alveolar ducts, and alveoli (see Figs. 1-16 and 1-17). This branching is commonly referred as the *bronchial tree*. The structural makeup of the bronchial tree changes as it extends to its terminal branches. The C-shaped cartilage rings in the airway walls are gradually replaced by

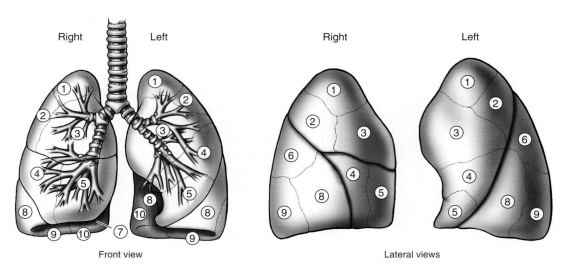

Right   Left   Right   Left

Front view

Lateral views

FIGURE 1-17. Structure of the tracheobronchial tree with corresponding lung segments, which originate from segmental bronchi. The right upper lobe contains segments 1 to 3, the right middle lobe contains segments 4 and 5, and the right lower lobe contains segments 6 to 10. The left upper lobe contains segments 1 to 5, and the left lower lobe contains segments 6 to 10.

smaller plates of cartilage and then totally disappear in the bronchioles. Smooth muscle makes up more of the airway wall as the cartilage decreases. In addition, the inside layer of epithelium experiences structural changes as there is a transition to squamous cells in the alveoli. This transition of the epithelium is important for facilitating gas exchange.

Alveoli

The respiratory bronchioles subdivide into *alveolar ducts,* which lead to *alveolar sacs* with alveoli. Alveolar sacs are air spaces or openings shared by two or more alveoli. *Alveoli* are cup-shaped pouches lined with type I and II epithelium surrounded by a thin elastic membrane for support. The *respiratory (alveolar-capillary) membrane* consists of the alveolar epithelium, the interstitium (containing the basement membrane), and the pulmonary capillary endothelial cells (Fig. 1-18). Type II epithelial cells, found primarily at the junctions of alveolar walls, produce *surfactant.* A thin layer of surfactant lines the alveolus and functions to lower the surface tension in the alveolus. This helps to prevent alveolar collapse.

Respiratory Gas Exchange

Gas exchange occurs by way of two anatomical structures, the functional respiratory unit and the alveolus. As illustrated in Figure 1-19, a terminal bronchiole enters the center of the functional respiratory unit accompanied by a pulmonary arteriole carrying deoxygenated blood from the body tissues and muscles. The arteriole divides into a rich network of pulmonary capillaries that lie adjacent to the alveolar walls and then drain into pulmonary venules and veins.

The exchange of respiratory gases takes place by passive diffusion across the respiratory membrane. The respiratory membrane wall is very thin, about 0.5 μm in thickness and 1/16th the diameter of a RBC. The combination of a large surface area and a thin respiratory membrane makes for rapid diffusion of the respiratory gases into and out of the blood.

Blood Supply to the Lungs

The pulmonary circulation is a low-pressure system with a normal mean pressure of approximately 15 mm Hg at rest. The lungs receive blood from the pulmonary arteries, which contain systemic venous blood from the RV, and

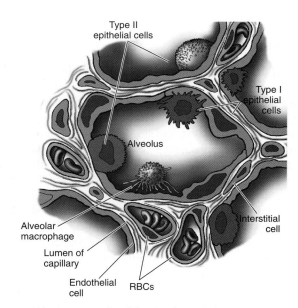

FIGURE 1-18. Major cells of the alveolus include epithelial cells (types I and II), endothelial cells of the pulmonary capillary, and alveolar macrophages. Also shown is a lumen of capillary with RBCs.

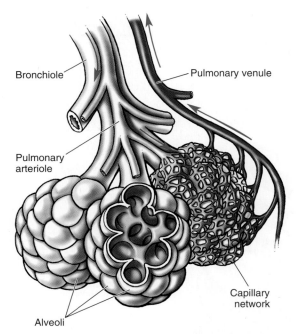

FIGURE 1-19. The functional respiratory unit consists of a bronchiole and corresponding blood supply; the pulmonary arteriole carries deoxygenated blood and the pulmonary venule carries oxygenated blood. The rich capillary network supplies the alveoli for the purpose of gas exchange.

bronchial arteries, which contain oxygenated blood from the LV (Fig. 1-20). The pulmonary arteries deliver blood to be oxygenated within the alveoli, and the blood within the bronchial arteries provides nourishment for the rest of the lung tissue.

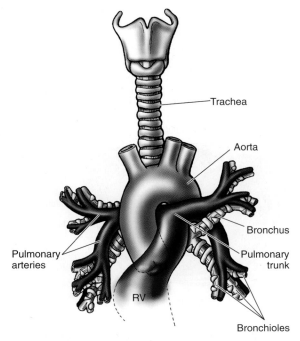

FIGURE 1-20. Major pulmonary arteries, which originate from the right ventricle (RV). Branches of the pulmonary arteries are adjacent to the bronchi and bronchioles.

Deoxygenated blood coming from the systemic circulation via the RA and RV of the heart passes through the pulmonary trunk and divides into the right and left pulmonary arteries. The pulmonary arteries divide into branches corresponding to the divisions of the bronchial tree and supply the pulmonary arterioles. In the lungs, blood releases CO_2 and gets replenished with O_2 (*respiratory gas exchange*). Oxygenated blood is then transported from the pulmonary capillaries to four pulmonary veins, which empty into the LA. The pulmonary veins also receive blood from the bronchial circulation, which accounts for a right-to-left shunt that normally occurs in the lungs and includes up to 5% of cardiac output. Oxygenated blood passes from the LA into the LV, where it is pumped into the coronary arteries of the heart and the systemic circulation via the aorta and its branches.

VENTILATORY PUMP AND MECHANICS OF BREATHING

The ventilatory pump consists of the chest wall, the respiratory muscles, and the pleural space (Figs. 1-21 and 1-22). These components of the ventilatory pump provide for the processes of *inspiration* (air moving into the lungs) and *expiration* (air moving out of the lungs). Breathing involves both inspiration and expiration so that **ventilation** (exchange of air) in the lungs is accomplished. Inspiration is initiated by activation of the respiratory muscles, particularly the diaphragm. The respiratory muscles increase the thoracic dimensions so that the pressure in the pleural space is lower than the outside atmospheric pressure. Air enters the lung until the *intrapulmonary* (inside the lung) gas pressure is equal to the atmospheric pressure. During expiration, the respiratory muscles relax and the thoracic dimensions decrease (i.e., the ribs fall back down and the diaphragm moves upward into the thorax), thus increasing intrapulmonary pressure relative to the outside atmospheric pressure. As a result, air flows from the lungs to outside the body, thus completing the process of breathing.

Chest Wall

The chest wall includes the intercostal muscles, which are considered respiratory muscles (see Fig. 1-21), and bones (the spine, ribs, and sternum). The ribs articulate with the spine so that the ribs can move upward and outward during inspiration and downward and inward during expiration. This movement contributes to the changes in thoracic volume that are critical for driving ventilation.

Respiratory Muscles

The muscles of respiration are the only skeletal muscles essential to life. The muscles of inspiration and expiration are illustrated in Figs. 1-21 and 1-22. The *diaphragm*, the major muscle of inspiration, is innervated by the *phrenic nerve*, which originates from the third to fifth cervical

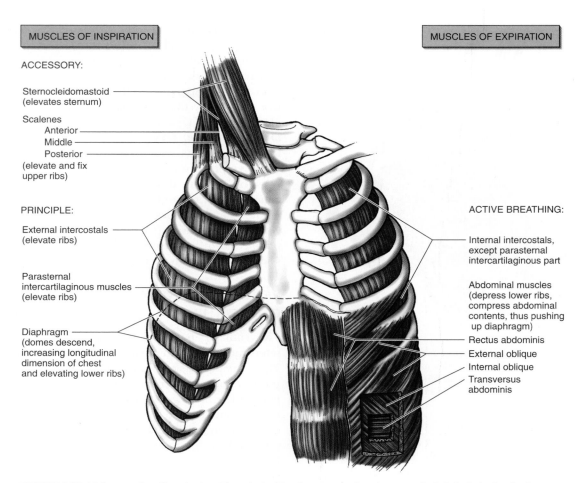

MUSCLES OF INSPIRATION

ACCESSORY:

Sternocleidomastoid
(elevates sternum)

Scalenes
    Anterior
    Middle
    Posterior
(elevate and fix
upper ribs)

PRINCIPLE:

External intercostals
(elevate ribs)

Parasternal
intercartilaginous muscles
(elevate ribs)

Diaphragm
(domes descend,
increasing longitudinal
dimension of chest
and elevating lower ribs)

MUSCLES OF EXPIRATION

ACTIVE BREATHING:

Internal intercostals,
except parasternal
intercartilaginous part

Abdominal muscles
(depress lower ribs,
compress abdominal
contents, thus pushing
up diaphragm)

Rectus abdominis
External oblique
Internal oblique
Transversus
abdominis

FIGURE 1-21. Major muscles of respiration. The principal inspiratory muscles, shown on the left, include the diaphragm, external intercostal muscles, and parasternal muscles. The principal expiratory muscles, shown on the right, include the internal intercostal muscles and the abdominal muscles (rectus, transversus, and internal and external oblique muscles).

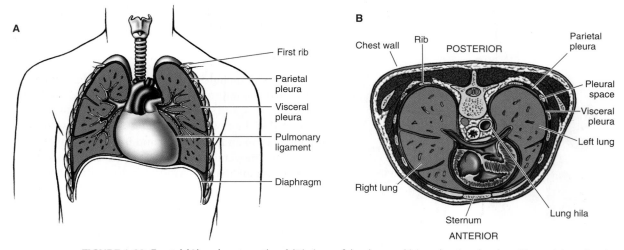

A

First rib

Parietal
pleura

Visceral
pleura

Pulmonary
ligament

Diaphragm

B

Chest wall   Rib   POSTERIOR   Parietal
                                   pleura

                                   Pleural
                                   space

                                   Visceral
                                   pleura

Right lung   Left lung

                                   Lung hila

Sternum

ANTERIOR

FIGURE 1-22. Frontal **(A)** and cross-sectional **(B)** views of the chest and lungs showing the pleural layers (visceral and parietal) and the pleural space. With inspiration, negative pressure develops in the pleural space. This allows air to move from the atmosphere into the tracheobronchial tree for gas exchange. The negative intrathoracic pressure also facilitates return of venous blood into the right atrium.

spine segments. Spinal cord transection caused by injury at or above this level compromises respiratory muscle function and, consequently, ventilation.

The diaphragm consists of a flat crural part (i.e., the domelike portion of the diaphragm) and vertical muscles called the *costal portion*. The diaphragm functions as a piston, with contraction and relaxation of the vertically oriented muscle fibers. With contraction, the crural portion moves downward and displaces the abdominal contents so that the abdomen moves outward. Expiration is normally passive (i.e., it requires no muscular work) under quiet breathing because of the elastic recoil of the lung tissue and gravity, which causes the ribs to fall back to their natural position. However, during active breathing, when ventilatory requirements are increased (e.g., during exercise), the muscles of expiration are recruited. The major muscles of expiration are the intercostal and the abdominal muscles (rectus abdominis, internal and external obliques, and transversus abdominis).

In patients with airflow obstruction (e.g., acute bronchoconstriction in asthma or emphysema), hyperinflation of the lungs stretches the lung tissue and leads to additional elastic recoil, forcing the crural portion of the diaphragm downward and shortening the vertical muscle fibers. This places the diaphragm at a mechanical disadvantage because of the altered length–tension relationship of these vertical muscle fibers.

Pleura

The visceral pleura (i.e., the inner layer that closely covers the lungs) and parietal pleura (i.e., the layer lining the inside of the chest wall and diaphragm) are thin membranes between the lungs and the chest wall; they converge at the lung hila (Fig. 1-22) (25). The pleural space, which lies between the visceral and parietal pleura, contains a small amount of fluid (Fig. 1-22). Because the pleural space is airtight and the chest wall and lung tissue pull against each other across the pleural space, negative pressure is produced at rest. During inspiration, both the visceral and parietal pleura expand outward, and increased negative pressure develops in the pleural space.

Air can enter the pleural space (i.e., the *pneumothorax*) by spontaneous rupture of a subpleural cyst or by trauma to the chest wall (e.g., a fractured rib with penetration of the parietal pleura). With a pneumothorax, the lungs collapse while the chest wall expands because of its intrinsic elastic properties. The parietal pleura contain abundant pain fibers, and irritation of this membrane by a pneumothorax or inflammation produces local chest pain exacerbated by motion of the pleura (e.g., deep inspiration).

SUMMARY

The major function of the respiratory system is the exchange of carbon dioxide and oxygen, which is necessary for metabolism. The respiratory system is divided functionally into conducting zones, which filter, warm, and moisten incoming air, and respiratory zones, where gas exchange occurs. Other important functions of the respiratory system include the production and metabolism of vasoactive substances and the filtering of particulate material before entry into the systemic circuit. The structural components of the respiratory system are the framework for these and other important functions at rest and with physical activity.

MUSCULOSKELETAL ANATOMY

GENERAL COMPONENTS AND FUNCTIONS

 1.1.1-HFS: Knowledge of the structures of bone, skeletal muscle, and connective tissues.

One of the primary objectives of regular exercise training is the improvement of musculoskeletal fitness. The physiological adaptations of muscle to exercise training may be manifested through increased muscle force production, muscular endurance, and resistance to injury. Inherent in designing effective training programs is a thorough understanding of muscle structure and function. This section provides a brief overview of the fundamentals of musculoskeletal anatomy. For in-depth study, the reader is referred to a variety of excellent sources (1,18,30,31,33).

Skeletal System (Axial Skeleton, Appendicular Skeleton, and Bone Tissue)

1.1.40-HFS: Ability to identify the major bones. Major bones include but are not limited to the clavicle, scapula, sternum, humerus, carpals, ulna, radius, femur, fibula, tibia, and tarsals.

Beyond supporting soft tissue, protecting internal organs, and acting as an important source of nutrients and blood constituents, the bones of the skeletal system serve as rigid levers for movement. The skull, vertebral column, sternum, and ribs are considered the **axial skeleton**; the remaining bones of the upper and lower limbs are considered the **appendicular skeleton**. The major bones of the body are illustrated in Fig. 1-23. The skeletal system consists of cartilage, periosteum, and bone (osseous) tissue. The structure of bone tissue can be explained using a typical long bone such as the humerus. The main portion of a long bone is the shaft, or *diaphysis* (Fig. 1-24). The ends of the bone are called the *epiphyses*. The epiphyses are covered by *articular cartilage*. Cartilage is a resilient, semirigid form of connective tissue that reduces friction in synovial joints and redistributes joint loads to a wider area, thus decreasing stresses sustained by the contacting joint surfaces. The region of mature bone where the diaphysis joins the epiphyses is called the *metaphysis*. In an immature bone, this region includes the *epiphyseal plate*, or *growth plate*. The *medullary cavity*, or marrow cavity, is the space inside the diaphysis. Lining the marrow cavity is the endosteum, which contains cells

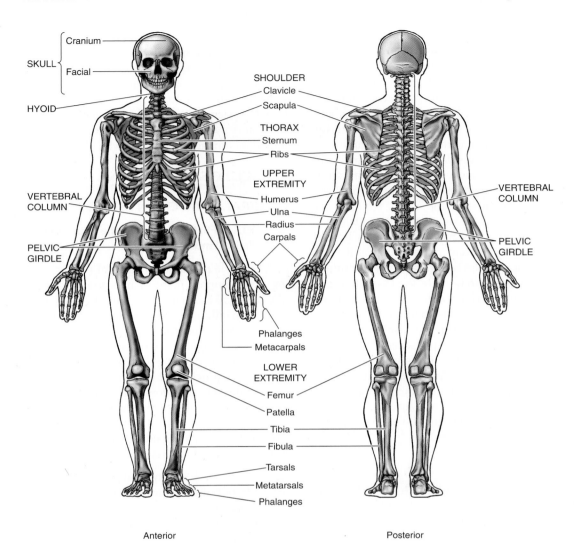

FIGURE 1-23. Divisions of the skeletal system.

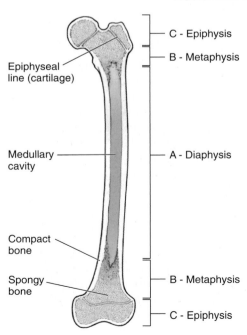

FIGURE 1-24. Bone anatomy.

necessary for bone development. The *periosteum* is a membrane around the surface of bones that are not covered with articular cartilage. The periosteum is composed of two layers, an outer fibrous layer and an inner highly vascular layer that contains cells for the creation of new bone. The periosteum serves as an attachment point for ligaments and tendons and is critical for bone growth, repair, and nutrition.

There are two types of bone: compact and spongy. The main difference is the amount of matter and space they contain. *Compact bone* contains few spaces and forms the external layer of all bones of the body and a large portion of the diaphysis of the long bones, where it provides support for bearing weight. In contrast, *spongy bone* is much less dense; it consists of a three-dimensional lattice composed of beams or struts of bone called *trabeculae*. The trabeculae are oriented to provide strength and counteract the stresses normally encountered by the bone. In some bones, the space within these trabeculae is filled with *red bone marrow*, which produces blood cells.

TABLE 1-3. CLASSIFICATIONS OF JOINTS IN THE HUMAN BODY

JOINT CLASSIFICATION	FEATURES AND EXAMPLES
Fibrous	
Suture	Tight union unique to the skull
Syndesmosis	Interosseous membrane between bone (e.g., the union along the shafts of the radius and ulna, tibia and fibula)
Gomphosis	Unique joint at the tooth socket
Cartilaginous	
Primary (synchondroses; hyaline cartilaginous)	Usually temporary to permit bone growth and typically fuse; some do not (e.g., at the sternum and rib [costal cartilage])
Secondary (symphyses; fibrocartilaginous)	Strong, slightly movable joints (e.g., intervertebral discs, pubic symphysis)
Synovial	
Plane (arthrodial)	Gliding and sliding movements (e.g., acromioclavicular joint)
Hinge (ginglymus)	Uniaxial movements (e.g., elbow, knee extension and flexion)
Ellipsoidal (condyloid)	Biaxial joint (e.g., wrist flexion and extension, radioulnar deviation)
Saddle (sellar)	Unique joint that permits movements in all planes, including opposition (e.g., the carpometacarpal joint of the thumb)
Ball and socket (enarthrodial)	Multiaxial joints that permit movements in all directions (e.g., hip and shoulder joints)
Pivot (trochoidal)	Uniaxial, biaxial and multiaxial joints that permit rotation (e.g., humeroradial joint)

Structure and Function of Joints in Movement

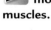 **1.1.4-HFS: Knowledge of the plane in which each movement action occurs and the responsible muscles.**

 1.1.41-HFS: Ability to identify the joints of the body.

Joints are the articulations between bones. Along with bones and ligaments, they constitute the articular system. *Ligaments* are tough, fibrous connective tissues that anchor bone to bone. Joints are typically classified as (a) *fibrous*, in which bones are united by dense fibrous connective tissue; (b) *cartilaginous*, in which the bones are united by cartilage; or (c) *synovial*, in which a fibrous articular capsule and an inner synovial membrane enclose a joint cavity filled with synovial fluid. Table 1-3 summarizes the joint classifications and provides examples in the human body.

Synovial (Diarthrodial) Joints

The most commonly occurring joint in the human body is the synovial joint. Figure 1-25 illustrates its unique capsular arrangement, which is of critical concern to exercise professionals. There are four distinct features of a synovial joint: (a) it has a joint cavity; (b) the articulating surfaces of the bones are covered with articular cartilage; (c) it is enclosed by a fibrous joint capsule; and (d) the capsule is lined with a *synovial membrane*. The synovial membrane produces *synovial fluid*, which provides constant lubrication during movement to minimize the wear and tear effects of friction on the cartilaginous covering of the articulating bones. Synovial joints are sometimes reinforced by ligaments. These ligaments are either separate or are a thickening of the outer layer of the joint capsule. Some synovial joints

have other structures such as articular discs (e.g., the meniscus of the knee). There are six major types of synovial joints that are classified by the shape of the articulating surface or type of movement allowed (see Table 1-3). Table 1-4 summarizes the major joints of the body, joint motions, and the plane in which these motions occur (Fig. 1-26).

Joints are typically well perfused by numerous arterial branches and are innervated by branches of the nerves supplying the adjacent muscle and overlying skin. Proprioceptive feedback and pain are important

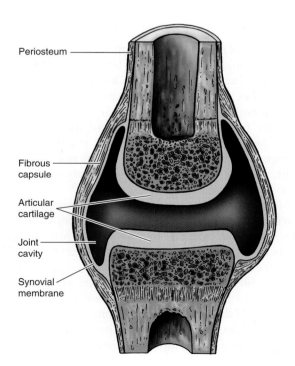

Periosteum

Fibrous capsule

Articular cartilage

Joint cavity

Synovial membrane

FIGURE 1-25. Synovial joint.

TABLE 1-4. MAJOR JOINT MOTIONS AND PLANES OF MOTION

MAJOR JOINT	TYPE OF JOINT	JOINT MOVEMENT(S)	PLANE
Scapulothoracic	Not a true joint	Elevation–depression	Frontal
		Upward–downward rotation	Frontal
		Protraction–retraction	Transverse
Glenohumeral	Synovial: ball and socket	Flexion–extension	Sagittal
		Abduction–adduction	Frontal
		Internal–external rotation	Transverse
		Horizontal abduction–adduction	Transverse
		Circumduction	
Elbow	Synovial: hinge	Flexion–extension	Sagittal
Proximal radioulnar	Synovial: pivot	Pronation–supination	Transverse
Wrist	Synovial: ellipsoidal	Flexion–extension	Sagittal
		Ulnar–radial deviation	Frontal
Metacarpophalangeal	Synovial: ellipsoidal	Flexion–extension	Sagittal
		Abduction–adduction	Frontal
Proximal interphalangeal	Synovial: hinge	Flexion–extension	Sagittal
Distal interphalangeal	Synovial: hinge	Flexion–extension	Sagittal
Interverterbral	Cartilaginous	Flexion–extension	Sagittal
		Lateral flexion	Frontal
		Rotation	Transverse
Hip	Synovial: ball and socket	Flexion–extension	Sagittal
		Abduction–adduction	Frontal
		Internal–external rotation	Transverse
		Horizontal abduction–adduction	Transverse
		Circumduction	
Knee	Synovial: hinge	Flexion–extension	Sagittal
Ankle: talocrural	Synovial: hinge	Dorsiflexion–plantarflexion	Sagittal
Ankle: subtalar	Synovial: gliding	Inversion–eversion	Frontal

joint sensations, which are a result of the high density of sensory fibers in the joint capsule. This feedback has obvious importance in regulating human movement and in preventing injury.

Joint Movements and Range of Motion

The degree of movement at a joint is typically called the *range of motion* (13). ROM can be *active* (AROM), the ROM that can be reached by voluntary movement, or *passive* (PROM), the ROM that can be achieved by external means (e.g., an examiner or device). Joint ROM is typically limited by the structure of the articulating bones (as in the limitation of elbow extension by the olecranon process of the ulna), ligamentous arrangement, and soft tissue limitations (as occurs in elbow and knee flexion).

Movement at one joint may influence the extent of movement at adjacent joints because a number of muscles and other soft-tissue structures cross multiple joints. For example, finger flexion decreases in the presence of wrist flexion because the muscles that flex and extend both the wrist and fingers are placed on slack and cannot generate enough tension to allow for full ROM. Tables 1-5 and 1-6 summarize major joint movements and the muscles that produce those movements, along with example resistance exercises for the muscles.

Muscular System

 1.1.19-HFS: Knowledge of the structure and function of the skeletal muscle fiber.

1.1.39-HFS: Ability to identify the major muscles. Major muscles include, but are not limited to, the following: trapezius, pectoralis major, latissimus dorsi, biceps, triceps, rectus abdominis, internal and external obliques, erector spinae, gluteus maximus, quadriceps, hamstrings, adductors, abductors, and gastrocnemius.

Bones provide support and lever systems for the body, but without muscles we would be unable to move. There are three types of muscle tissue: skeletal, cardiac (see "Heart—Location and General Landmarks": *myocardium*), and smooth muscle. Skeletal muscle is attached primarily to bones and is responsible for movement, stabilizing the body (maintaining posture), load distribution, shock absorption, and heat generation. Skeletal muscle tissue is under voluntary control and is referred to as *striated* because of the dark and light bands, which are visible under a microscope. In general, all muscle tissue has four important characteristics: (a) irritability, the ability to respond to stimuli, electrical or mechanical; (b) contractility, the ability to develop tension (does not imply length shortening); (c) extensibility, the ability to be stretched

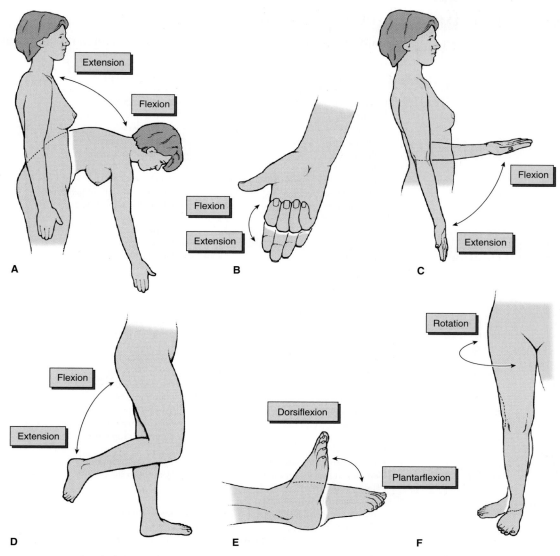

FIGURE 1-26. (A–E) Flexion and extension of various parts of the body. **(F)** Rotation of the lower limb at the hip joint.

or increase in length; and (d) elasticity, the ability to return to its original length after a stretch or compression.

Skeletal Muscle Macrostructure

The individual *muscle fibers* (muscle cells) that make up skeletal muscles are joined together by a hierarchical organization of several connective tissue membranes (Fig. 1-27). The outermost layer surrounding the whole muscle is the *epimysium*. Skeletal muscles are composed of multiple bundles of muscle fibers, varying in size from 15 to 150 muscle fibers. These bundles of muscle fibers are known as *fascicles* (an individual bundle is a *fasciculus*). A layer of connective tissue called the *perimysium* surrounds each fascicle. A third connective tissue layer known as the *endomysium* envelops

individual muscle fibers. Blood vessels, nerves, and lymphatic vessels pass into the muscle to reach the individual muscle fibers. An additional thin elastic membrane is found just beneath the endomysium and is called the *sarcolemma*. The sarcolemma is the true cell boundary and encloses the cellular contents of the muscle fiber, nuclei, local stores of fat, glucose (in the form of glycogen), enzymes, **contractile proteins**, and other specialized structures such as the mitochondria.

Skeletal muscles are anchored to the skeleton by extensions of the epimysium, perimysium, and endomysium. These connective tissues extend beyond the end of a muscle and converge to form *tendons*. In most cases, tendons are dense cords of connective tissue that attach a muscle to the periosteum of the bone. When the tendon

TABLE 1-5. MAJOR MOVEMENTS OF THE UPPER EXTREMITIES

JOINT	MOVEMENT	MAJOR AGONIST MUSCLES	EXAMPLES OF RESISTANCE EXERCISE
Scapulothoracic	Fixation	Serratus anterior	Push-up
		Pectoralis minor	Parallel bar dip
		Trapezius	Upright row
		Levator scapulae	Shoulder shrug
		Rhomboids	Seated row
Glenohumeral	Flexion	Anterior deltoid	Front raises
		Pectoralis major (clavicular head)	Incline bench press
	Extension	Latissimus dorsi	Dumbbell pull-over
		Teres major	Chin-up
		Pectoralis major (sternocostal head)	Bench press
	Abduction	Middle deltoid	Lateral raises, dumbbell press
		Supraspinatus	Low pulley lateral raise
	Adduction	Latissimus dorsi	Lat pull-down
		Teres major	Seated row
		Pectoralis major	Cable crossover fly
	Medial (internal) rotation	Latissimus dorsi	Back latissimus pull-down, bent row
		Teres major	
		Subscapularis	One-arm dumbbell row
		Pectoralis major	
		Anterior deltoid	Rotator cuff exercise, dumbbell press, parallel bar dip, front raise
	Lateral (external) rotation	Infraspinatus	External rotation
		Teres minor	
		Posterior deltoid	Back press, bent-over lateral raises
Elbow	Flexion	Biceps brachii	Curls
		Brachialis	Preacher curl
		Brachioradialis	Hammer curl
	Extension	Triceps brachii	Triceps dips, triceps extensions
		Anconeus	Triceps push-downs, tricep kickback
Radioulnar	Supination	Supinator	Dumbbell supination
		Biceps brachii	
	Pronation	Pronator teres, pronator quadratus	Dumbbell pronation
Wrist	Flexion	Flexor carpi radialis and ulnaris	Wrist curl
		Palmaris longus	
		Flexor digitorum superficialis	
	Extension	Extensor carpi radialis longus, Extensor digitorum	Reverse wrist curl brevis and ulnaris
	Adduction (ulnar deviation)	Flexor and extensor carpi ulnaris	Wrist curls, reverse wrist curl
	Abduction (radial deviation)	Extensor carpi radialis longus and brevis	Wrist curls, reverse wrist curl
		Flexor carpi radialis	

is flat and broad, it is called an *aponeurosis*. Tendons and aponeuroses provide the mechanical link between skeletal muscle and bone.

Skeletal muscles have different **muscle fiber architecture**, the arrangement of muscle fibers relative to the line of pull of the muscle. Muscles can have a *parallel* (or *fusiform*) *fiber arrangement* (i.e., the muscle fibers run in line with the pull of the muscle) or a *pennate arrangement* (i.e., the muscle fibers run obliquely or at an angle to the line of pull) (Fig. 1-28). Pennate muscles can be classified as *unipennate* (muscle fibers are located on only one side of the tendon, e.g., the vastus lateralis), *bipennate* (muscle fibers are located on both sides of a centrally positioned tendon, e.g., the rectus femoris), or *multipennate* (two or more fasciculi are attached obliquely and combine to form one muscle, e.g., the del-

toid). The muscle fiber architecture of a muscle can affect muscle force generation, velocity of shortening, and ROM. For example, muscles composed of long muscle fibers tend to have parallel arrangements and demonstrate greater ROM and velocity of shortening than pennate muscles. In contrast, pennate muscles are composed of large numbers of short fibers, providing a larger cross-sectional area capable of generating greater force production, but less ROM, than muscles with parallel fiber architecture.

Muscles also can be described by the number of joints they act upon. For example, a muscle that causes movement at one joint is *uniarticular* (e.g., the brachialis). Muscles that cross more than one joint are referred to as *biarticular* (having actions at two joints, e.g., the hamstring muscle group, biceps brachii) or *multiarticular*

TABLE 1-6. MAJOR MOVEMENTS OF THE LOWER EXTREMITIES

JOINT	MOVEMENT	MAJOR AGONIST MUSCLE(S)	EXAMPLES OF RESISTANCE EXERCISES
Intervertebral	Trunk flexion	Rectus abdominis	Sit-up, crunches, leg raise
		External obliques	Machine crunch
		Internal obliques	High pulley crunch
	Trunk extension	Erector spinae	Back extension, dead lift
	Lateral flexion	Rectus abdominis	Roman chair side bend
		External obliques	Dumbbell side bend
		Internal obliques	Hanging leg raises
	Rotation	External obliques	Broomstick twist
		Internal obliques	Machine trunk rotation
Hip	Flexion	Iliacus	Leg raise
		Psoas major	Incline leg raise
		Rectus femoris	Machine crunches
		Sartorius	Leg raise
		Pectineus	Cable adduction
	Extension	Gluteus maximus	Squat, leg press, lunge
		Hamstrings (semitendinosus, semimembranosus, long head of biceps femoris)	Leg curl (standing, seated, lying)
	Abduction	Tensor fasciae latae	Cable hip abduction
		Sartorius	Standing machine abduction
		Gluteus medius	Floor hip abduction
		Gluteus minimus	Seated machine abduction
	Adduction	Adductor longus, brevis, and magnus	Power squat
		Gracilis	Cable adduction
		Pectineus	Machine adduction
	Medial rotation	Semitendinosus	Leg curl (standing, seated, lying)
		Semimembranosus	Floor hip adduction
		Gluteus medius	Machine abduction
		Tensor fascia latae	
		Gracilis	
	Lateral rotation	Biceps femoris	
		Adductor longus, brevis, magnus	
		Gluteus maximus	
Knee	Flexion	Hamstrings	Leg curl (standing, seated, lying)
		Gracilis	
		Sartorius	
	Extension	Quadriceps femoris (rectus femoris, vastus lateralis, medialis, and intermedius)	Lunge, squat, leg extension
Ankle: talocrural	Dorsiflexion	Tibialis anterior	Ankle dorsiflexion against resistance
		Extensor digitorus longus	
		Extensor hallucis longus	
	Plantarflexion	Gastrocnemius, soleus, tibialis posterior	Standing calf raise, Donkey calf raise
		Flexor digitorum longus	Seated calf raise
		Flexor hallucis longus	
Ankle: subtalar	Eversion	Peroneus longus and brevis	Exercises against resistance
	Inversion	Tibialis anterior and posterior	Exercises against resistance

muscles. The main advantage of bi- and multiarticular muscles is that only one muscle is needed to generate tension in two or more joints. This is more efficient and conserves energy. In many instances, the length of the muscle stays within 100% to 130% of the resting length: as one side of the muscle shortens, the other side stretches, maintaining a near constant length. This property of bi- and multiarticular muscles enhances force production by optimizing the length–tension relationship. The major superficial skeletal muscles of the body are illustrated in Figures 1-29 and 1-30.

Skeletal Muscle Microstructure

Skeletal muscle fibers are approximately 10 to 100 μm in diameter and frequently many centimeters long. Each muscle fiber contains several hundred to several thousand regularly ordered, threadlike *myofibrils*. These myofibrils extend lengthwise throughout the cell and are connected to the plasma membrane by intermediate filaments. Myofibrils contain the apparatus that allows for contraction of the muscle cell, which consists primarily of two types of myofilaments: thick filaments (*myosin*) and thin filaments (*actin*). The myosin and actin filaments

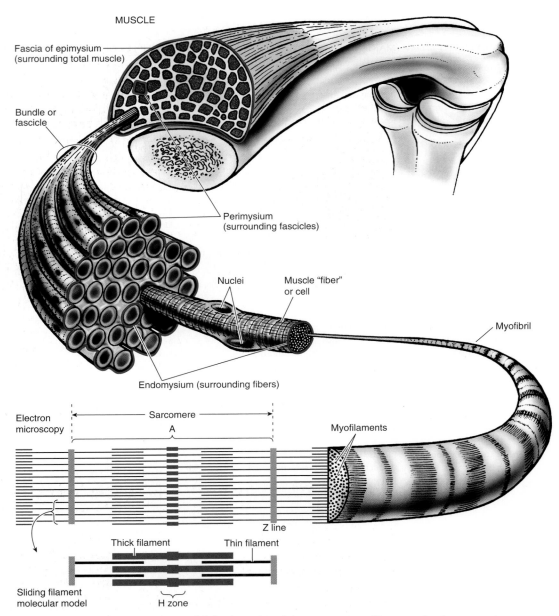

FIGURE 1-27. Cross-section of skeletal muscle and the arrangement of its connective tissue wrappings.

are arranged longitudinally in the smallest contractile unit of skeletal muscle, the *sarcomere*. Each myofibril is composed of numerous sarcomeres joined end to end at the *Z lines*. The dark *A band* represents the region that contains both thick myosin filaments and thin actin filaments. The *H zone* is the central portion of the A band that appears only when the sarcomere is in a resting state and it is occupied only by thick filaments (see Fig. 1-28). A thick filament contains approximately 200 myosin molecules with the heads of the molecules protruding outwards at regular intervals. They occur in the A band, where they overlap at either end with thin filaments. The thin filaments consist of the contractile protein *actin* and **regulatory proteins** *tropomyosin* and *troponin*. One end of

each actin filament is attached to a Z line, with the opposite end extending toward the center of the sarcomere, lying in the space between the myosin filaments. The actin protein has a binding site that, when exposed, serves as an attachment point for the myosin head. The site where the myosin head binds to the actin filament is known as a crossbridge. It is this arrangement of the myosin and actin filaments that give skeletal muscle its striated appearance.

Muscle Fiber Actions and Fiber Types

 1.1.20-HFS: Knowledge of the characteristics of fast and slow twitch muscle fibers.

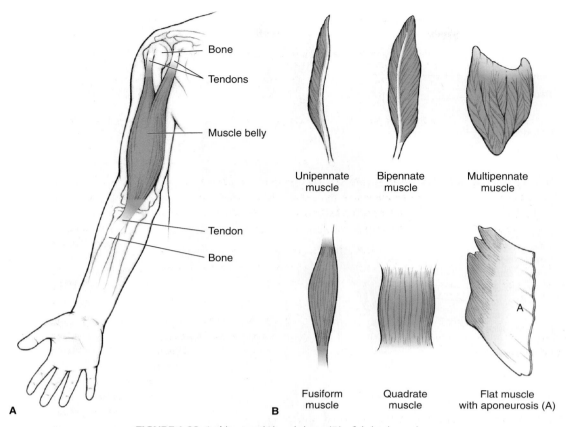

FIGURE 1-28. Architecture **(A)** and shape **(B)** of skeletal muscles.

 1.1.21-HFS: Knowledge of the sliding-filament theory of muscle contraction.

 1.1.22-HFS: Knowledge of twitch, summation, and tetanus with respect to muscle contraction.

Approximately 5% of skeletal muscle weight consists of the high-energy phosphates, key minerals, and energy sources needed for force production; an additional 20% of muscle is composed of protein, principally the contractile proteins *myosin*, *actin*, and *tropomyosin*. Water constitutes 75% of muscle composition (29). Physical training results in a significant alteration of these constituents, depending on the specific training stimulus.

Given the wide shift in blood supply shunted to active skeletal muscle during vigorous exercise, a highly efficient vascular bed must exist throughout muscles. Likewise, the body has the ability to enhance blood supply through formation of new capillary networks stimulated by physical training that involves endurance (or aerobic) training.

Skeletal muscles are controlled by the central nervous system (CNS), both through higher centers and individual spinal segments, and by proprioceptive structures (e.g., muscle spindles, Golgi tendon organs) inherent to the musculotendinous complex. The integration is complex yet remarkably efficient. Although it has never been conclusively proven, most evidence indicates that when stimulated to contract, muscle tissue shortens or lengthens because the myosin and actin myofilaments slide past each other without changing individual length (include reference(s) here). The contact between the actin any myosin filaments is known as *crossbridging*, and it controls shortening and lengthening of muscles during contraction. Box 1-1 summarizes the sliding-filament theory (19). This continual process of forming and releasing crossbridges permits the generation of tension. Force production continues as long as the muscle is stimulated, but the ability of the muscle to perform may be limited by intrinsic factors such as diminished production of adenosine triphosphate (ATP), decreased pH, and accumulation of metabolic by-products (see the discussion on fatigue in Chapter 3).

Three common terms describing muscle contraction are *twitch*, *summation*, and *tetanus*. *Twitch* refers to a single, brief muscle contraction caused by a single action potential traveling down a motor neuron. *Summation* is the addition of individual twitch contractions to increase the intensity of the overall muscle force. Progressive stimulation frequencies increase the amount of

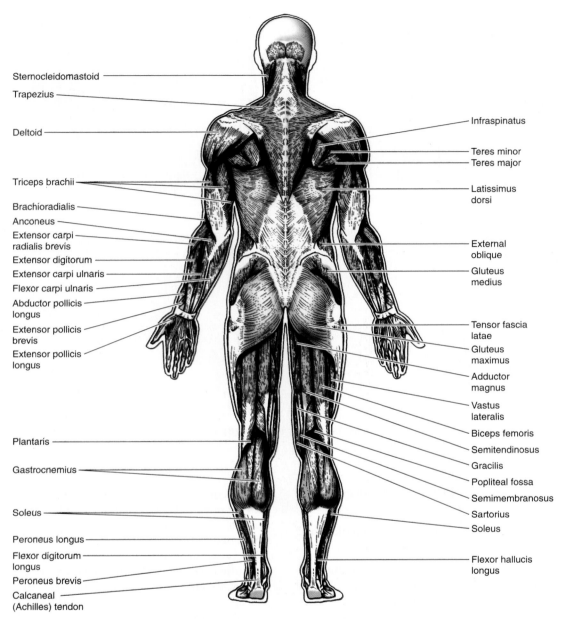

Sternocleidomastoid

Trapezius

Deltoid

Triceps brachii

Brachioradialis

Anconeus

Extensor carpi
radialis brevis

Extensor digitorum

Extensor carpi ulnaris

Flexor carpi ulnaris

Abductor pollicis
longus

Extensor pollicis
brevis

Extensor pollicis
longus

Plantaris

Gastrocnemius

Soleus

Peroneus longus

Flexor digitorum
longus

Peroneus brevis

Calcaneal
(Achilles) tendon

Infraspinatus

Teres minor
Teres major

Latissimus
dorsi

External
oblique

Gluteus
medius

Tensor fascia
latae

Gluteus
maximus

Adductor
magnus

Vastus
lateralis

Biceps femoris

Semitendinosus

Gracilis

Popliteal fossa

Semimembranosus

Sartorius

Soleus

Flexor hallucis
longus

FIGURE 1-29. Posterior view of superficial muscles.

force developed because the muscle cannot completely relax from the previous stimulus before the next stimulus arrives. As soon as the frequency of stimulation is high enough, full summation is achieved. This is referred to as *tetanus* and is the maximal amount of force the motor unit (i.e., all the muscle fibers innervated by a single motor neuron) can develop. At this point, muscle fiber stimulation is of such high frequency that it is unable to return to its resting length between contractions (29).

The human body has the ability to perform a wide range of physical tasks combining varying levels of speed, power, and endurance. No single type of muscle

fiber possesses the characteristics that allow optimal performance across this continuum of physical challenges. Rather, muscle fibers possess certain characteristics that result in relative specialization. For example, motor units of specific fiber types are selectively recruited by the body for speed and power tasks of short duration, whereas others are recruited for endurance tasks of long duration and relatively low intensity. When the task requires elements of speed or power but also has an endurance component, yet another type of muscle fiber is recruited.

These different fiber types, to be described more specifically later, should not be thought of as mutually

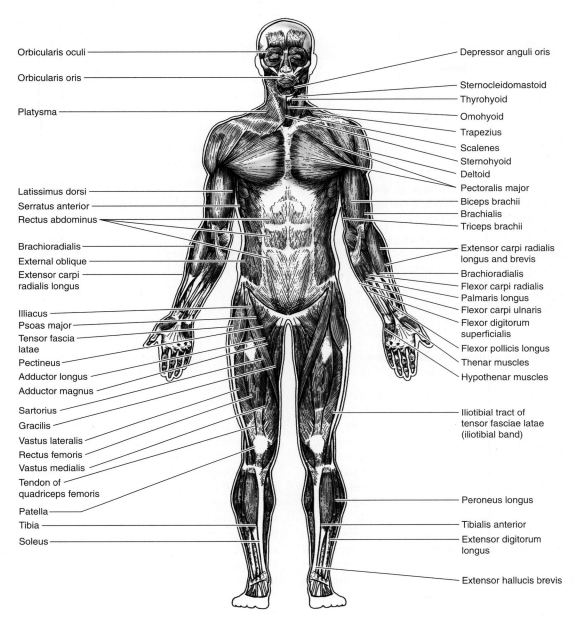

FIGURE 1-30. Anterior view of superficial muscles.

exclusive. In fact, intricate recruitment and switching occurs in muscle over the performance of many tasks, and fibers designed to be optimal for one type of task can contribute to the performance of another. The net result is a functioning muscle that can respond to a wide variety of tasks, and although the composition of a muscle may lend itself to performing best in endurance activities, it can still accomplish speed and power tasks to a lesser degree.

Fortunately, the human body can respond adequately to most physical tasks encountered in everyday living. In the presence of muscle impairment, specific training regimens may restore normal function. Likewise, normal

function can be enhanced through exercise training to accomplish physical tasks that are in excess of the demands of daily living, such as athletics (9,21).

Over the years, there has been a fair amount of controversy about the classification of muscle fiber types (3). In addition, questions remain about whether these fiber types can change in response to an intervention such as endurance training (8,16,20,22). In either case, there is general agreement that relative to exercise performance, two distinct fiber types—type I (slow twitch) and type II (fast twitch, in various forms)—have been identified and classified by contractile and metabolic characteristics (4,13). To illustrate the variation in fiber types within

BOX 1-1   SLIDING-FILAMENT THEORY OF MUSCLE CONTRACTION AND RELAXATION SUMMARY

RESTING MUSCLE

Calcium ions are bound to the SR

Tropomyosin–troponin complex blocks attachment sites for myosin; ATP is bound to myosin heads

MUSCLE CONTRACTION

Nerve impulse exceeding resting potential spreads across sarcolemma and down transverse tubules, causing release of calcium from the SR

Calcium binds with troponin, which permits actin and myosin to form crossbridges

Myosin ATPase is activated, splitting ATP; this transfer of energy causes movement of the myosin crossbridges and generates tension

Crossbridges uncouple when ATP binds to the myosin bridge

RELAXATION

Coupling and uncoupling continue until calcium concentration becomes insufficient

When the nerve impulse ceases, calcium is taken up the SR; actin and myosin return to a resting state

SR, sarcoplasmic reticulum; ATP, adenosine triphosphate.

---

humans, Table 1-7 lists fiber type distribution in elite athletes relative to the general population.

Type I Muscle Fibers   The characteristics of type I muscle fibers, listed in Table 1-8, are consistent with muscle fibers that are fatigue resistant. Thus, type I fibers are selected for activities of low intensity and long duration. Within whole muscle, type I motor units asynchronously contract; that is, in addition to their inherent fatigue resistance, endurance is prolonged by the constant switching that occurs to ensure unfatigued muscle as the exercise stimulus continues. Sedentary people have approximately 50% type I fibers, and this distribution is generally equal throughout the major muscle groups of the body (15). In endurance athletes, the percentage of type I fibers is greater, but this is thought to be largely a genetic predisposition, despite some evidence suggesting that prolonged exercise training can alter fiber type (Table 1-9) (6,10).

Essentially, those most successful at endurance activities generally have a high proportion of type I fibers, and this is most likely attributable to genetic factors enhanced through appropriate exercise training. From a metabolic perspective, type I fibers are those frequently called aerobic because the generation of energy for continued muscle contraction is met through the ongoing oxidation of available foodstuffs (carbohydrates and fats). Thus, with minimal accumulation of anaerobically produced metabolites, continued muscle contraction is favored in type I fibers.

Type II Muscle Fibers   At the opposite end of the continuum, individuals who achieve the greatest success in power and high-intensity speed tasks usually have a greater proportion of type II muscle fibers distributed through the major muscle groups. Because force generation is so important, type II fibers shorten and develop tension considerably faster than type I fibers (40). These fibers are typically thought of as type IIB fibers, the "classic" fast-twitch fiber. Metabolically, these fibers are the classic anaerobic fibers because they rely on energy sources intrinsic to the muscle, not the fuels used by type I fibers. When an endurance component is introduced, such as in events lasting upward of several minutes (800–1500 m running races, for example), a second type of fast-twitch fiber, type IIA, is recruited. As noted in Table 1-8, type IIA fibers represent an intermediate fiber type between the type I and type IIB fibers. Metabolically, although type IIA fibers have the ability to generate a moderately large amount of force, they also have some aerobic capacity, although not as much as type I fibers. This is a logical and

---

TABLE 1-7. MUSCLE FIBER COMPOSITION IN SELECTED POPULATIONS

SPORT	PERCENTAGE OF TYPE I (SLOW TWITCH)	PERCENTAGE OF TYPE II (FAST TWITCH)
Distance runners	60–90	10–40
Track sprinters	25–45	55–75
Weightlifters	45–55	45–55
Shot-putters	25–40	60–75
Nonathletes	47–53	47–53

Reprinted with permission from Powers SK, Howley ET. *Exercise Physiology*. Dubuque (IA): WC Brown; 1990. p. 160.

TABLE 1-8. STRUCTURAL AND FUNCTIONAL CHARACTERISTICS OF SLOW TWITCH (ST) AND FAST TWITCH (FT$_A$ AND FT$_B$) MUSCLE FIBERS

CHARACTERISTICS	FIBER TYPE		
	ST	FT$_A$	FT$_B$
Neural aspects			
Motor neuron size	Small	Large	Large
Motor neuron recruitment threshold	Low	High	High
Motor nerve conduction velocity	Slow	Fast	Fast
Structural aspects			
Muscle fiber diameter	Small	Large	Large
Sarcoplasmic reticulum development	Less	More	More
Mitochondrial density	High	High	Low
Capillary density	High	Medium	Low
Myoglobin content	High	Medium	Low
Energy substrates			
Phosphocreatine stores	Low	High	High
Glycogen stores	Low	High	High
Triglyceride stores	High	Medium	Low
Enzymatic aspects			
Myosin-ATPase activity	Low	High	High
Glycolytic enzyme activity	Low	High	High
Oxidative enzyme activity	High	High	Low
Functional aspects			
Twitch (contraction) time	Slow	Fast	Fast
Relaxation time	Slow	Fast	Fast
Force production	Low	High	High
Energy efficiency, "economy"	High	Low	Low
Fatigue resistance	High	Low	Low
Elasticity	Low	High	High

Courtesy of Fox EL, Bowers RW, Foss ML. *The Physiological Basis of Physical Education and Athletics*, 4th ed. Dubuque (IA): WC Brown; 1989. p. 110.

necessary bridge between the range of muscle fiber types and the ability to meet the variety of physical tasks imposed. Reference to the existence of the type IIC fiber is necessary in a complete description of human muscle fiber types. The IIC fiber has been described as a rare and undifferentiated muscle fiber type that is most likely involved in reinnervation of impaired skeletal muscle (24).

How Muscles Produce Movement

Skeletal muscle produces force that is transferred to the tendons, which in turn pull on the bones and other structures (skin). Most muscles cross a joint, so when a muscle contracts, it pulls one of the articulating bones toward the other. Usually, both articulating bones do not move

TABLE 1-9. ADAPTATIONS IN SKELETAL MUSCLE RELATIVE TO SPECIFIC TRAINING REGIMENS

MUSCLE FACTOR	TRAINING			
	SLOW TWITCH		FAST TWITCH	
	ST	ET	ST	ET
Percentage composition	0 or ?	0 or ?	0 or ?	0 or ?
Size	+	0 or +	++	0
Contractile property	0	0	0	0
Oxidative capacity	0	++	0	+
Anaerobic capacity	? or +	0	? or +	0
Glycogen content	0	++	0	++
Fat oxidation	0	++	0	+
Capillary density	?	+	?	? or +
Blood flow during work	?	? or +	?	?

ST, strength training; ET, endurance training.

0, no change; ?, unknown; +, moderate increase; ++, large increase.

Adapted with permission from Gollnick PD, Sembrowich WI. Adaptations in human skeletal muscle as a result of training. In Amsterdam E, editor. *Exercise and Cardiovascular Health and Disease*. New York: Yorke Medical Books; 1977. p. 90; and from McArdle W, Katch F, Katch V. *Exercise Physiology*, 4th ed. Baltimore: Williams & Wilkins; 1996. p. 334.

equally; one of the articulating bones stays more stationary. The attachment that is more stationary and usually more proximal (especially in the extremities) is called the *origin*. The muscle attachment that moves the most and is usually located more distally is called the *insertion*.

Levers   Mechanically, to produce movement, the muscles, joints, and bones work as a system of levers. The bone acts as the lever, the joint functions as the center of rotation (COR), and the muscles produce the force or effort (F) to move the lever. The resistance (R), or the force that opposes the movement of the lever, could be the weight of the body part or, as in the case of lifting weights, the external resistance provided by the weights. Levers are classified into three types according to the relative position of the center, axis of rotation, and the effort and resistance forces (Fig. 1-31). Third-class levers (Fig. 1-31C) are the most common type of levers in the human body and are designed for large ROM and speed of movement.

Muscle Actions   Muscle action is the result of neuromuscular activation that leads to the production of force and contributes to the movement or the stabilization of the musculoskeletal system (23). Muscle actions can be classified into three basic types: isometric, concentric, and eccentric. In an *isometric (or static) action,* the muscle generates force in the absence of joint movement, such as holding a dumbbell during a biceps curl without movement. An action in which the muscle length changes is often called *anisometric*. Concentric and eccentric actions are anisometric and in most cases dynamic muscle actions. A *concentric action* occurs when the muscle torque being generated exceeds the torque of the resistance force and the muscle shortens in length, such as the upward phase of a biceps curl. *Eccentric actions* occur when the torque generated by the muscle is less than the torque of the resistance force being encountered. This results in the active muscle lengthening rather than shortening. Eccentric actions are often used when muscles have to slow down body parts or oppose external resistance forces. Using the biceps curl example, the downward phase of this exercise requires eccentric action of the biceps brachii muscle.

Muscle Roles   Movements of the human body generally require several muscles to work together rather than a single muscle to perform all the work. Because muscles only pull and cannot push, most skeletal muscles are arranged in opposing pairs such as flexor–extensor, internal–external rotators, and so on. Muscles can be classified according to their roles during movement. When a muscle or group of muscles is responsible for the action or movement, it is called a *prime mover* or **agonist**. For example, during a biceps curl, the prime movers are the elbow flexors, which include the biceps brachii, brachialis, and brachioradialis muscles. The opposing group of muscles is called the **antagonist** (triceps brachii and anconeus). In addition, most movements also

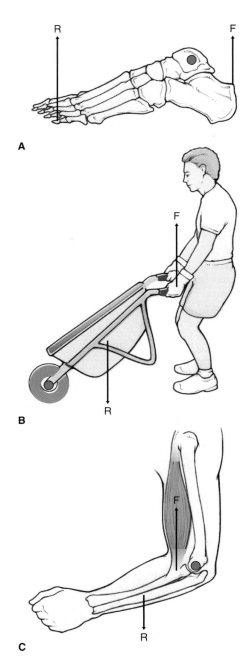

FIGURE 1-31. Examples of lever systems in the human body, where *F* is the exerted force, *R* is the reaction force, and the *red dot* (•) is the axis of rotation. Most musculoskeletal joints behave as third-class levers. **(A)** First-class lever, **(B)** second-class lever, and **(C)** third-class lever.

involve other muscles called **synergists**. The role of these muscles is to prevent unwanted movement, which helps the prime movers perform more efficiently. Synergist muscles can also act as fixators or stabilizers. In this role, the muscles stabilize a portion of the body against an external force. For example, the scapular muscles (e.g., rhomboids, serratus anterior, trapezius) must provide a stable base of support for the upper extremity muscles during a throwing motion.

Muscles and Exercise   Muscle actions produce force that causes joint movement during exercise. Exercise science and other healthcare professionals should have a good knowledge and understanding of which muscles are involved in the movements of the major joints. This knowledge is the basis for the development of exercise programs for use in training and rehabilitation (11). Tables 1-5 and 1-6 give a list of common resistance training exercises and the muscles involved (11).

SUMMARY

Besides contributing to body shape and form, bones perform several important functions, including support, protection, movement, and storage of essential nutrients and blood cell formation. Skeletal muscle is responsible for bodily movement, body stabilization, and heat production. It is composed of varying amounts of types I, IIA, and IIB muscle fibers whose quantity and distribution are largely genetic. Physical activity patterns and sports performance characteristics develop from the varying properties of muscle fibers, the organization and integration of fiber recruitment patterns, and the levers, bones, and joints through which the muscle fibers act. Although the conversion of muscle fiber types through either disuse or training and the splitting and generation of muscle fibers are somewhat controversial, what is known about exercise training and muscle fiber type is that specific training significantly enhances metabolic adaptations.

REFERENCES

1. Agur AMR, Grant JCB. *Grant's Atlas of Anatomy*. Philadelphia: Lippincott Williams & Wilkins; 2005.
2. Albertine KH, Williams MC, Hyde DM. Anatomy of the lungs. In: R.J. Mason et al., editors. *Murray and Nadel's Textbook of Respiratory Medicine*. Philadelphia: Saunders; 2005. p. 3–29.
3. Armstrong RB. Muscle fiber recruitment patterns and their metabolic correlates. In: E.S. Horton, and R.L. Terjung, editors. *Exercise, Nutrition, and Energy Metabolism*. New York: Macmillan; 1988.
4. Brooke MH, Kaiser KK. Muscle fiber types: how many and what kind? *Arch Neurol*. 1970;23:369–79.
5. Brooks G, Fahey T, Baldwin K. *Exercise Physiology: Human Bioenergetics and Its Applications*. New York: McGraw Hill; 2005.
6. Burke ER, Cerny F, Costill D, Fink W. Characteristics of skeletal muscle in competitive cyclists. *Med Sci Sports*. 1977;9:109–12.
7. Carrin B. Development and structure of the normal human lung. In: M. Turner-Warwick et al., editors. *Clinical Atlas: Respiratory Diseases*. Philadelphia: Lippincott-Gower; 1989. p. 1–14.
8. Chi MM, Hintz CS, Coyle EF, et al. Effects of detraining on enzymes of energy metabolism in individual human muscle fibers. *Am J Physiol*. 1983;244:C276–87.
9. Coggan AR, et al. Skeletal muscle adaptations to endurance training in 60- to 70-yr-old men and women. *J Appl Physiol*. 1992;72:1780–6.
10. Costill DL, et al. Skeletal muscle enzymes and fiber composition in male and female track athletes. *J Appl Physiol*. 1976;40:149–54.
11. Delavier F. *Strength Training Anatomy*. Champaign, IL: Human Kinetics; 2006. p. 144.
12. DeVries H, Housh T. *Physiology of Exercise for Physical Education, Athletics and Exercise Science*. Madison (WI): WCB Brown & Benchmark; 1994.
13. Edstrom L, Nystrom B. Histochemical types and sizes of fibres in normal human muscles: a biopsy study. *Acta Neurol Scand*. 1969;45:257–69.
14. Foss M, Keteyian S. *Physiological Basis for Exercise and Sport*. New York: McGraw Hill; 1998.
15. Fox EL, Bowers RW, Foss ML. *The Physiological Basis of Physical Education and Athletics*. Dubuque (IA): William C. Brown; 1989.
16. Gollnick PD, Armstrong RB, Sembrowich WL, et al. Glycogen depletion pattern in human skeletal muscle fibers after heavy exercise. *J Appl Physiol*. 1973;34:615–8.
17. Gray H. *Gray's Anatomy: The Anatomical Basis of Medicine and Surgery*. e-edition. New York (NY): Churchill Livingstone; 2005.
18. Hall-Craggs E. *Anatomy as a Basis for Clinical Medicine*. Baltimore: Williams & Wilkins; 1995.
19. Huxley HE. The structural basis of muscular contraction. *Proc R Soc Lond B Biol Sci*. 1971;178:131–49.
20. Jacobs I, Esbjörnsson M, Sylvén C, et al. Sprint training effects on muscle myoglobin, enzymes, fiber types, and blood lactate. *Med Sci Sports Exerc*. 1987;19:368–74.
21. Jansson E, Kaijser L. Muscle adaptation to extreme endurance training in man. *Acta Physiol Scand*. 1977;100:315–24.
22. Jansson E, Sjodin B, Tesch P. Changes in muscle fibre type distribution in man after physical training: a sign of fibre type transformation? *Acta Physiol Scand*. 1978;104:235–7.
23. Knudson DV, Morrison CS. *Qualitative Analysis of Human Movement*. Champaign (IL): Human Kinetics; 2002.
24. Komi PV, Karlsson J. Skeletal muscle fibre types, enzyme activities and physical performance in young males and females. *Acta Physiol Scand*. 1978;103:210–8.
25. Light RW. *Pleural Diseases*. Philadelphia: Lippincott Williams & Wilkins; 2007. p. xiii.
26. Marieb E, Hoehm K. *Human Anatomy and Physiology*. San Francisco: Benjamin & Cummings; 2007.
27. Martini F. *Fundamentals of Anatomy and Physiology*. San Francisco: Benjamin & Cummings; 2003.
28. McArdle W, Katch F, Katch V. *Essentials of Exercise Physiology*. Philadelphia: Lippincott Williams & Wilkins; 2005.
29. McArdle W, Katch F, Katch V. *Exercise Physiology: Energy, Nutrition, and Human Performance*. Philadelphia: Lippincott Williams & Wilkins; 2006.
30. Moore K, Agur A. *Essentials of Clinical Anatomy*. Philadelphia: Williams & Wilkins; 2007.
31. Moore KL, Dalley AF, Agur AMR. *Clinically Oriented Anatomy*. Philadelphia: Lippincott Williams & Wilkins; 2006.
32. Nilsestuen J. Pulmonary physiology. In: Berghuis P, Cohen N, Decker M, editors. *Respiration*. Redmond (WA): SpaceLabs; 1992. p. 1–11.
33. Olson TR, Pawlina W. *A.D.A.M. Student Atlas of Anatomy*. Baltimore: Williams & Wilkins; 1996.
34. Powers S; Howley E. *Exercise Physiology: Theory and Application to Fitness and Performance*. New York: McGraw Hill; 2006.
35. Schier D, Butler J, Lewis R. *Hole's Essentials of Human Anatomy and Physiology*. New York: McGraw Hill; 2006.
36. Sokolow M, McIlroy M, Cheitlin M. *Clinical Cardiology*. Norwalk (CT): Appleton & Lange; 1993.
37. Spence A, Mason E. *Human Anatomy and Physiology*. St. Paul (MN): West Publishing Co.; 1992.
38. Thibodeau G, Patton K. *Anthony's Textbook of Anatomy & Physiology*. St. Louis (MO): Mosby; 1999.
39. Thibodeau G, Patton K. *Anatomy and Physiology*. St. Louis (MO): Mosby; 2007.
40. Vrbova G. Influence of activity on some characteristic properties of slow and fast mammalian muscles. *Exerc Sport Sci Rev*. 1979;7:181–213.
41. Williams M. Cardiovascular and respiratory anatomy and physiology: responses to exercise. In: Baechle T, Earle R, editors. *Essentials of Strength Training and Conditioning*. Champaign (IL): Human Kinetics; 2000. p. 115–36.

42. Wilmore J, Costill D. *Physiology of Sport and Exercise*. Champaign (IL): Human Kinetics; 2004.

SELECTED REFERENCES FOR FURTHER READING

Aaberg E. *Muscle Mechanics*, 2nd ed. Champaign (IL): Human Kinetics; 2006.

Calais-Germain B. *Anatomy of Movement*. Seattle (WA): Eastland Press; 2003.

DeLavier F. *Strength Training Anatomy*, 2nd ed. Champaign (IL): Human Kinetics; 2006.

Floyd RT, Thompson CW. *Manual of Structural Kinesiology*, 16th ed. New York: McGraw-Hill; 2007.

Hamill J, Knutzen KM. *Biomechanical Basis of Human Movement*, 2nd ed. Philadelphia: Lippincott Williams & Wilkins; 2006.

Jenkins DB. *Hollinshead's Functional Anatomy of the Limbs and Back*, 8th ed. Philadelphia: WB Saunders; 2002.

Knudson DV, Morrison CS. *Qualitative Analysis of Human Movement*, 2nd ed. Champaign (IL): Human Kinetics; 2002.

Neuman, DA. *Kinesiology of the Musculoskeletal System*. St. Louis (MO): Mosby; 2002.

Oatis, CA. *Kinesiology: The Mechanics and Pathomechancis of Human Movement*. Philadelphia: Lippincott Williams & Wilkins; 2004.

INTERNET RESOURCES

- American Association of Anatomists: http://www.anatomy.org
- Anatomy on the Internet: http://www.meddean.luc.edu/lumen/Med Ed/ GrossAnatomy/anatomy.htm
- The Digital Anatomist Information System: http://sig.biostr. washington.edu/projects/da/
- Human Anatomy Online: http://www.innerbody.com/htm/body.html
- Muscles and Exercise Online: http://www.exrx.net/Lists/Directory. html
- NISMAT Exercise Physiology Corner: A Primer on Muscle Physiology: http://www.nismat.org/physcor/muscle.html
- Scottish Radiological Society: http://www.radiology.co.uk/srs-x/ index.htm
- University of California San Diego: Muscle Physiology: http://muscle.ucsd.edu/musintro/jump.shtml
- University of Michigan Muscles in Action: http://www.med.umich.edu/lrc/Hypermuscle/
- University of Washington Diagnostic Radiology Residency Programs Anatomy Modules: http://www.rad.washington.edu/ anatomy/index.html
- Vesalius: The Internet Resource for Surgical Education: http://www.vesalius.com/

Biomechanics

Exercise and sports medicine professionals often advise clients regarding modifying movement technique and using exercise or rehabilitation equipment. The discipline primarily involved in describing and understanding the mechanical causes of human movement is biomechanics. **Biomechanics** is the study and application of the motion of living organisms using the branch of physics known as mechanics. The study of forces and torques that cause movement is called **kinetics**, and the description of the resulting motion is called **kinematics**. This chapter summarizes how professionals can use their understanding of the causes of human motion (kinetics), the effects of forces on human tissues, and kinematic measurements of human motion to modify exercise prescriptions.

> > > KEY TERMS

Base of support: The area of the supporting surface of an object such as between and under the feet in standing or between the hands in a handstand.

Biomechanics: The study of the motion and causes of motion of living things and the application of mechanical principles.

Buoyancy: The floating force on an object immersed in a fluid.

Center of gravity: The location of a theoretical point that can be used to represent the total weight (mass) of an object.

Drag: The fluid force that acts parallel to the relative flow of fluid past an object.

Force: A push or pull that tends to modify motion or the shape of an object.

Friction: The force that acts parallel to and opposes motion between surfaces in contact.

Impulse: The effect of force acting over time.

Kinematics: The branch of mechanics that describes motion.

Kinetics: The branch of mechanics that explains the causes of motion.

Lift: The fluid force that acts at right angles to the relative flow of fluid past an object.

Mass: The quantity of matter in a body or substance.

Moment arm: The leverage of a force creating a torque or moment of force; the perpendicular distance between the line of action of the force and the axis of rotation.

Moment of force: The rotating effect of a force.

Moment of inertia: A measure of the resistance of a body to angular acceleration about a given axis.

Momentum: The quantity of motion of an object that is equal to the product of the mass and velocity of the object.

Normal reaction: The force acting at right angles between two surfaces in contact.

Stiffness: The measure of the elasticity of a material, defined as the slope of the stress–strain graph in the elastic region.

Strain: A measure of the deformation of a material when acted upon by a force.

Stress: The force per unit area in a material.

Torque: Another term used to refer to a rotating effect of a force. Mechanics of materials uses *torque* to refer to torsional (twisting about a longitudinal axis) moments.

Vector: A quantity that has both magnitude (size) and direction.

KINETICS

Understanding the causes of human movement requires an understanding of several kinetic variables. This section discusses the forces and torques that create and/or modify motion; introduces Newton's laws of motion, which describe the creation and/or modification of motion; and summarizes major forces that affect human movement.

FORCES AND TORQUES

 1.1.8-HFS: Knowledge of the biomechanical principles that underlie performance.

For a body segment to change its state of motion, a **force** must be applied. A **force** is a linear effect that can be defined as a push, pull, or tendency to distort. Forces can be represented by **vectors**. Forces have four important characteristics, two of which are the vector characteristics of magnitude (size) and direction. The other two characteristics are line of action and point of application.

Forces and the vectors used to represent them can be drawn as arrows with the length representing magnitude and the arrowhead indicating direction (Fig. 2-1). The International System of Units (SI) units of force magnitude are Newtons (N). The point of application of a force is the location at which the force acts on an object. The line of action is an imaginary line extending in both directions from the force vector (see Fig. 2-1). In most situations, multiple forces act on body segments, so vector addition techniques are needed to take into account the interacting magnitudes and directions. Adding vectors together determines a resultant vector. A vector can be also broken up into equivalent parts called *components*. For example, the forces between a runner's foot and the ground are usually resolved into right-angle components (Fig. 2-2).

Depending on how forces are applied to an object, they may cause three kinds of motion: (a) translation or linear motion; (b) rotation or angular motion; and (c) general motion, which is a combination of translation

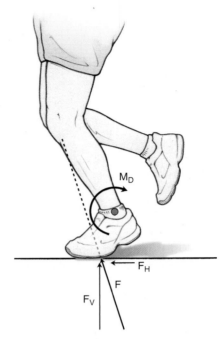

FIGURE 2-2. The ground reaction force (F) between a runner's foot in stance can be broken up into horizontal (F_H) and vertical (F_V) components. This ground reaction force acts off-center to the ankle joint axis and creates a dorsiflexing (M_D) moment of force or torque.

and rotation. A force acting through the center of mass of an object creates translation. Forces with a line of action not acting though the object's center of mass tend to create rotation and translation or general motion. The force F in Figure 2-2 does not act through the center of gravity of the runner, so it tends to create linear and angular motion of the body.

The measure of the rotary effect of a force is called a **moment of force** (M), which is commonly referred to as **torque**. A moment can be calculated as the product of the force and its **moment arm**, which is the perpendicular distance from the line of action of the force to the axis of rotation. The most common unit of a moment of force is Newton meters (Nm). Moments are also vector quantities that can be added to determine the net rotary effect of forces acting on an object. For instance, typical changes in the moment arm or leverage of the distal attachment of the biceps brachii at the elbow during flexion are illustrated in Figure 2-3.

NEWTON'S LAWS OF MOTION

Sir Isaac Newton developed three laws of motion that explain how forces create movement. The first law is the *law of inertia*, which states "a body continues in its state of rest, or uniform motion in a straight line, unless a force acts upon it." All objects have this innate property (inertia) that resists changes in state of motion. To move a motionless object, force must be applied to overcome its

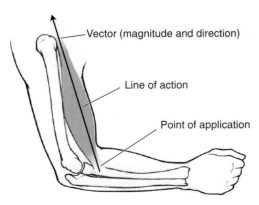

FIGURE 2-1. Vectors such as a force can be represented by an *arrow*. The four characteristics of a force are illustrated.

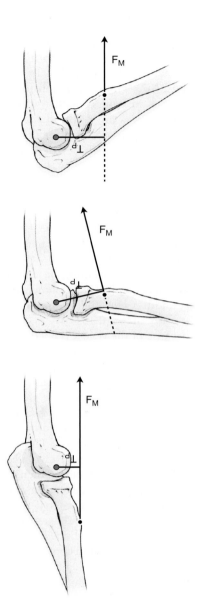

FIGURE 2-3. Schematic of the changes in the moment arm ($d_\perp$) at the elbow for the biceps brachii. The torque or moment of force the muscle can create is affected by both changes in force and moment arm ($T = F_M \cdot d_\perp$). The moment arm at the elbow for the long head of biceps would be affected by both shoulder and elbow joint rotation. (Note variation in the muscle angle of pull and the resulting moment arm.)

inertia and thus set it into motion. Likewise, the inertia of the moving object tends to keep it moving, so a force must be applied to either stop it or modify its motion.

The second law is usually called the *law of acceleration* and is represented by the mathematical formula $\Sigma F = ma$, where ΣF equals the sum of all forces in a given direction, m equals mass, and a equals acceleration in the same direction. This formula illustrates the relationship between kinetics and the resulting kinematics at any instant in time. The law says that "the acceleration an object experiences is proportional to the resultant force

acting on the object in that direction and is inversely proportional to the object's mass." This formula specifies the cause-and-effect relationship between forces and linear motion. Over intervals of time Newton's second law is expressed as the impulse–momentum relationship, where the change in momentum of any object in a direction is equal to the net impulse applied ($\Delta p = \Sigma J$) in that direction.

In angular motion, the law of acceleration is written as $\Sigma M = I\alpha$, where ΣM equals the sum of the moments acting on the object, I equals the moment of inertia of the object, and α equals the angular acceleration of the object. Newton's second law may be the most important because it defines the relationship between kinetics and kinematics, includes the inertia of objects (m and I), and provides for units of force. For example, a Newton of force is the linear effect that will accelerate 1 kg of mass (m) $1\ m \cdot s^{-2}$ (a). These two formulas are applied in biomechanical models to estimate the net forces and torques acting in linked segment models. This is called *inverse dynamics* because measures of kinematics (α) and body segment inertial properties (I) are used to calculate the net moments (ΣM) or forces creating the movement.

Newton's third law is called the *law of action–reaction*. This says that "for every force there is an equal and opposite force." In other words, forces do not act only on one body but are an interaction between two bodies. The law can be expressed mathematically as $F_{AB} = -F_{BA}$. When objects A and B interact, object A produces an equal and opposite effect on B. In turn, the second object, B, produces an equal and opposite effect on A. Positive and negative signs in mechanics refer to the direction of vector quantities. For example, during locomotion, the foot exerts a force every time it contacts the ground. However, the ground exerts an equal and opposite force on the foot (see Fig. 2-2). This is an important law of kinetics that shows that forces and torques are mutual interactions between objects.

IMPORTANT FORCES IN HUMAN MOVEMENT

> **1.1.4-HFS: Knowledge of the plane in which each movement action occurs and the responsible muscles.**

> **1.7.11-HFS: Knowledge of and the ability to describe exercises designed to enhance muscular strength and/or endurance of specific major muscle groups.**

Forces that create human motion can be external forces between parts of the body and the environment (i.e., the ground reaction forces in Fig. 2-2) or internal forces created by the musculoskeletal system. These forces can be classified many ways, but the forces that are most often considered in biomechanical analyses are described in this section.

Gravity is the vertical, attraction force between the earth and an object. The magnitude of this force is the body weight (BW) of the object. BW is proportional to mass from Newton's second law. Because gravitational acceleration is fairly constant on the earth (9.81 m/s/s), a barbell with a mass of 50 kg weighs 490.5 Newtons [$F_w = 50(9.81)$]. Skeletal muscles must skillfully balance the weight of body segments and external objects such as dumbbells to move in even the simplest exercise. Standing in the anatomical position, the weight force of the body interacts with the supporting force from the floor.

Contact between the human body and another object (e.g., catching a ball, jumping, wearing ankle weights) results in external forces that are often resolved into two important components: the **normal reaction** and **friction**. Friction (F_f) is the force acting parallel to the two surfaces in contact, and it acts in the opposite direction of the motion or impending motion (Fig. 2-4). The force acting perpendicular to the surfaces of contact is called the normal reaction (F_N) or normal force. In dry conditions, the sizes of these two forces are related by the simple formula $F_f = F_N \cdot \mu$, where μ is the coefficient of static friction. The coefficient of static friction is a dimensionless ratio that is experimentally determined and describes the frictional properties between the two interacting surfaces. For example, tennis shoes on sports surfaces typically have coefficients of static friction ranging from 0.4 to nearly 2.0 (46). When the two surfaces start to slide past each other, the friction force decreases, and a kinetic coefficient of friction must be used. Rotational friction can also be determined by how much moment of force must be applied to cause the surfaces to rotate against the other.

Some of the most important external forces in human movement are *ground reaction forces*. Ground reaction forces act between a person and the support surface on which that person moves, such as the foot of the runner shown in Figure 2-2. A force platform can be used to measure the changes in magnitude, direction, and point of application of the ground reaction forces during the period the foot is in contact with the platform. These ground reaction forces are resolved into three components relative to the person's direction of motion: the vertical (normal reaction) and two frictional components (anteroposterior and mediolateral). In running, the peak vertical ground reaction forces occur in midstance and are about 3 BW, and the peak anteroposterior forces are about 0.4 BW (42). If the coefficient of friction between this shoe and the platform surface was 0.8, then the maximum horizontal force that could be made before sliding would be 2.4 BW [$F_f = 0.8(3.0)$]. As such, there is little danger of slipping while running on dry surfaces. Frictional forces in wet conditions are much smaller than in similar dry conditions. A child running on a wet pool deck might only have 0.15 BW of friction [$F_f = 0.05(3.0)$] because of the very low coefficient of friction.

Examples of internal forces are *joint reaction forces*. In linked segment biomechanical models, these forces between adjacent segments are modeled using Newton's laws of motion. In a squat exercise, for example, the downward force on an intervertebral disc from the weight of the upper body has an equal and opposite (acting upward) force from the lower body. The most common methods of inverse dynamics use Newton's laws to determine net joint reaction forces and moments of force from measurements of segment acceleration and inertial parameters. Unfortunately, the joint reaction forces are a combination of joint, muscle, and ligament forces and do not represent the true bone-on-bone forces at joints (62). Actual bone-on-bone forces and contact pressures at joint surfaces are very difficult to calculate.

Important internal forces in human movement are elastic forces in muscles, tendons, and ligaments that contribute to joint reaction forces. Elastic forces often contribute to many movements and are created by the tendency of a deformed material to return to its original shape. The measure of the elasticity in a deformed material is called **stiffness** and is defined as the ratio of mechanical **stress** (σ) to **strain** (ε) in the linear (elastic) region of the curve. Figure 2-5 shows an idealized stress/strain curve. The slope of the linear portion of the graph (σ/ε) up to the yield point gives an indication of the stiffness of the material. Stress is defined as the force per unit area of the material, and strain is usually defined as the percentage change in length. For example, the maximal muscular strength of muscle is usually reported as a stress of 25 to 40 N/cm^2, and the typical elongation of the Achilles tendon in a maximal voluntary contraction is a strain of about 5% (23). Because the area of a deformed material changes, it is easier to ignore these small deformations and approximate stress–strain graphs with force–deformation graphs.

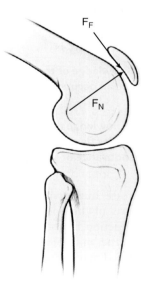

FIGURE 2-4. The contact force between two objects, such as at the patellofemoral joint, is often broken into friction (F_F) and normal reaction (F_N) components.

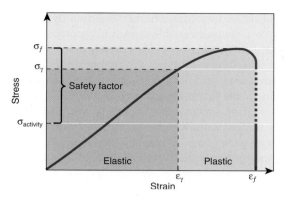

FIGURE 2-5. An idealized stress/strain curve. The elastic region is bounded by the yield point (designated by ε_y, σ_y). The plastic region is bounded by the yield point and the failure point (designated by ε_f, σ_f). The stress in musculoskeletal tissues in normal activity is much less than the yield point. The difference between the stress/strain of normal activities and the failure point is the safety factor. (Adapted with permission from Biewener AA, editor. *Biomechanics: Structures and Systems.* Oxford (UK): Oxford University Press; 1992.)

A stiff material is hard to deform (high force for small deformation) and therefore has high elasticity, tending to quickly return to its normal shape when an external force is removed. A material with low stiffness is called *compliant* because small forces can create larger deformations. Materials loaded in the elastic region of the curve return to their normal shape with minimal permanent change in shape. Stressing a material beyond the yield point and into the plastic region of the curve results in permanent change in the material's structure. Materials have an ultimate mechanical strength or failure point that represents the maximum force or stress a material can withstand before breaking. Stresses in the musculoskeletal system in normal activities are much lower than the yield point for these tissues, so there is a large safety factor (2) in most physical activities. Sometimes the mechanical strength of a material is documented as the total energy absorbed. Note that the mechanical strength of materials is different from muscular strength. This chapter refers to muscular strength as "strength" and uses "mechanical strength" to avoid confusion in terminology.

Most tissues have more complex stress/strain curves than the one shown in Figure 2-5. The curves are nonlinear, and the stiffness depends on the timing of force loading. This rate dependence of mechanical behavior is called *viscoelasticity*. Tissues of the musculoskeletal system have greater stiffness when they are loaded rapidly. This is a major reason why static stretching is preferred over ballistic stretching because a greater level of musculotendinous elongation can be reached using a smaller and safer amount of force. In normal and vigorous movements, however, muscles and tendons can be stretched like a spring, and a large percentage of this elastic energy can be recovered in subsequent shortening (1). This storage and recovery of elastic forces is just one mechanism of the important neuromuscular strategy called the *stretch–shortening cycle*. Many powerful movements are

naturally initiated with a countermovement that is stopped with an eccentric muscle action and immediately reversed to a concentric action in the intended direction of motion (34). For example, in the stance phase of sprinting, the plantar flexors are essentially eccentrically active in early stance, which serves to increase the force of the following concentric action in push-off.

Maybe the most important and complex internal forces affecting human movement are muscle forces. Muscles exert forces on the skeleton to create motion, stabilize posture, dampen vibration, or decrease the stress in bones created by other forces. Muscles create only tensile forces that pull on all attachments. Muscle forces also create torques about joints. The torques are always changing as the joint moves through the range of motion (ROM) because the moment arms change as joints rotate and because muscle force production is related to muscle length and velocity. Therefore, the torque a muscle group can make is a complex phenomenon that is a combination of tension variations attributable to contractile conditions and geometric–moment arm changes for muscles.

The amount of tension a muscle can create depends on excitation and mechanical factors related to muscle length and velocity. The *force–velocity relationship* dictates that the magnitude of muscle force depends on the rate of length change or muscle velocity (24). The faster a muscle shortens (concentric action), the less muscle force that can be created for the same level of excitation. On the other hand, the faster the active lengthening of muscle (eccentric action), the greater the muscle force. This relationship is illustrated in Figure 2-6. Note that the force potentials for all three muscle actions (eccentric, isometric, concentric) are defined by the graph. Training shifts the force–velocity graph upward but cannot change the pattern of decreased or increased force potential as muscle velocity changes. The actual force or tension in eccentric muscle actions is actually much higher (150%–180% of maximal isometric values) than illustrated in Figure 2-6.

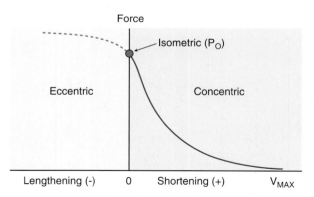

FIGURE 2-6. The force–velocity relationship of skeletal muscle illustrates skeletal muscle force potential for the rate of change of muscle length (velocity), so all three muscle actions can be visualized on the graph. (Adapted with permission from Knudson D. *Fundamentals of Biomechanics.* New York: Kluwer; 2003).

The *force–length relationship* indicates how the isometric force a muscle can create varies with its length (17,52). At intermediate lengths, muscles can produce the greatest force. Less force can be created in shortened conditions. Less active tension can also be created in lengthened conditions, but this is offset by increases in passive tension. In other words, the elastic force of stretched connective tissue and structural proteins within muscle generate tension that can be used to create subsequent motion. This passive tension is the discomfort that is felt in a vigorous stretch. Quite a bit of recent research has begun to document the complex interaction of active and passive sources of muscle tension (13,31) in muscle actions, and muscle force from passive tension can be used in some low intensity activities that do not have to be in the extremes of the range of joint motion (44).

Clinicians and researchers often assess muscle group strength using measurements from handheld or isokinetic dynamometers. A dynamometer is a machine that measures force or torque. Isokinetic dynamometers measure torque in conditions of nearly constant joint angular velocity. Isokinetic dynamometers allow muscle group strength to be defined for all points in the ROM isometrically or at various constant speeds of shortening or lengthening. The torque-angle or moment/angle curves created by these machines illustrate the strength curves of muscle groups integrating the many mechanical factors affecting muscle force (Fig. 2-7). Extensive normative data are available for most joints of the body (5), and these data are usually normalized to body mass and categorized for a variety of populations (e.g., age, gender, sport). Isometric (a special case of isokinetic: angular velocity = 0 deg/s) testing is a common method of muscular strength measurement because it controls for the velocity and length dependence of muscular tension.

Dynamic measurements such as the 1-RM (one repetition maximum) using various weights or resistance training machines are more commonly used field tests for estimating muscular strength because of the ease and low cost of these protocols. Another common dynamic muscular performance variable is muscular power. Peak musculoskeletal power output for a variety of movements can be measured by combining dynamometer and kinematic measurements and has been used to establish a range of training loads that maximize power output (7,10). These studies of muscular strength and power measurements are consistent with the fitness research showing three major expressions (static, dynamic, and explosive) of muscular performance (29).

Muscles rarely work in isolation because there are multiple muscles crossing most joints with similar and opposing anatomical actions. Determining the contribution of individual muscles to movements is very difficult, so often the hypothesized actions of muscles made in functional anatomy are incorrect. One reason for the difference is that muscles have actions at all joints, not just the joints they cross, because of the linked segments of the human body (61). The joint reaction forces acting at joints allow energy from a muscle to be transferred to segments quite distant from the segments to which the muscle attaches. Computer simulations of complex biomechanical models have begun to determine these complex actions of muscles in movements (60). Biomechanics uses a variety of research tools to validate these observations, including electromyography (EMG), movement kinematics, and direct measurements of forces in tendons. The use of EMG was one of the first technologies to show that muscular contributions to movement are more complex than hypothesized by anatomy (21). Recent EMG research has documented that many muscles have intramuscular segments (4), making them even more complicated than described in gross anatomy. The use of implanted force transducers in the tendons of animals and humans (14,33,35,54) and bright-mode ultrasound images of muscle and tendon length changes (30) are recent developments in that help confirm the complex actions of muscles in movement. In many normal movements, muscle fibers are able to act in high-force, nearly isometric conditions because the efficient

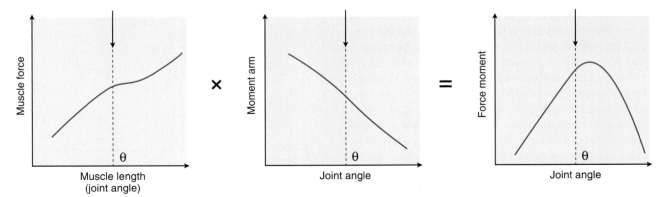

FIGURE 2-7. The joint moment/angle curve represents the strength curves of muscle groups. The shapes of these curves are a combination of muscular properties (similar to the force–length relationship) and muscle moment arms. (Adapted with permission from Zatsiorsky V. *Science and Practice of Strength Training.* Champaign (IL): Human Kinetics; 1995.)

stretch and recoil of passive connective tissues within the tendon and muscle minimize the shortening velocity of the muscle fibers (31). Muscle actions most often tend to occur in short bursts (25) timed to take advantage of external forces, gravity, and biomechanical geometry (12). This coordination of muscle activation or torques has been called passive dynamics, segmental interaction, or energy that can be transferred through joints (28,38,51,63). The integration of several kinds of biomechanical research is needed to develop a good understanding of how muscles create movement.

Other important forces affecting human movement are fluid forces. Fluid forces arise when people are submerged and move in water or air. There are three fluid forces: **buoyancy**, **lift**, and **drag**. Buoyancy is the supporting or flotation force of a fluid. Water exercise programs use the upward force of buoyancy to decrease the vertical loading in the joints of the lower extremities. This is an effective exercise modality for people with arthritis and people in rehabilitation programs.

When there is relative flow of a fluid past an object, the flow forces are resolved into two components: lift and drag. Lift acts at right angles to the relative flow, and drag acts in the same direction as the fluid flow and the opposite direction of the object moving through the fluid. Both of these forces increase with the square of the velocity of flow, so the resistance to body movements in water exercises increases dramatically with faster speeds of movement. There are a variety of assistive devices that increase buoyancy, lift, and drag to adjust resistance during water exercise. For example, a life vest increases a person's buoyancy so he or she can float in an upright position. Attaching fins to the feet would increase the lift provided by kicking movements, and specialized suits can decrease drag forces, thereby increasing swimming speed. Cyclists or swimmers follow directly behind other competitors (draft) to decrease the drag forces of the fluid rushing past them (9).

KINEMATICS

Biomechanics has a long history of studies documenting the kinematics of human movements. Although most of these studies have been two-dimensional analyses, more and more research has focused on documenting the three-dimensional movements of the body. Precise three-dimensional measurement of the motion of human segments and joints has been labor intensive and involves considerable technical complexity (62). However, kinematic studies have provided useful descriptive data in many areas of human movement. Kinematic data can be used to profile the technique of athletes (15,37), help workers avoid potentially injurious work movements (27), and document normal patterns of movement such as locomotion (47,57).

There are several limitations in modifying client movement to match normal, skilled, or elite kinematics. First, there are within- and between-person variabilities in movement technique. Despite the precision of kinematic measurements, there is subjectivity in determining what is considered normal or desirable given the variability of human movement. One example is the variation in running economy (mass normalized steady-state oxygen consumption for a given speed) that is fairly resistant to modifications in running technique (36,40,41). Runners naturally tend to select kinematics that maximize economy, so it is difficult to effectively modify running technique based on kinematics alone unless there is extreme deviation from normative technique. Second, kinematics measurements do not, in and of themselves, explain the causes of motion. In other words, nearly identical movements can have different muscular causes (58). For example, a physical therapist may help a patient with some muscular paralysis achieve a cosmetically normal walking pattern using other lower extremity muscles or orthotics. Therapists have been warned not to infer too much of the kinetic causes of walking from the kinematics of the patient's gait (22), and other exercise science professionals should also bear this in mind when qualitatively analyzing the kinematics of movements.

Despite the lack of explanatory power of kinematic measurements, useful information in kinematic studies can improve human movement. For example, the position and horizontal velocity of the whole-body center of mass relative to the base of support are important variables in theoretical models of stability and balance (49). The clinical value of static and dynamic measures of stance, however, is more controversial because these tests may not correlate with regaining postural control when body position is unexpectedly disturbed (48). More research on the kinematics of postural, locomotion, sport, and exercise movements may help improve the specificity of conditioning programs. This research may help inform the current emphasis on sensorimotor training in injured and athletic populations (19).

The decreasing cost and greater automation of kinematic calculations from video or position sensors may allow for the documentation of typical kinematics for more movements and with a wider variety of people (ages, skill levels, and disabilities). More examples of how kinematic data can be useful in improving human movement are summarized in the next section on the application of biomechanics in sports and exercise.

APPLICATION TO HUMAN MOVEMENT EXERCISE PRESCRIPTION

> **1.1.5-HFS: Knowledge of the interrelationships** among center of gravity, base of support, balance, stability, posture, and proper spinal alignment.

> **1.1.8-HFS: Knowledge of the biomechanical princi-** ples that underlie performance of the following activities: walking, jogging, running, swimming, cycling, weightlifting, and carrying or moving objects.

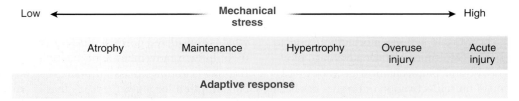

FIGURE 2-8. The continuum of mechanical stress imposed on tissue and the likely adaptive response.

> **1.7.29-HFS: Ability to identify proper and improper technique in the use of resistive equipment such as stability balls, weights, bands, resistance bars, and water exercise equipment.**

> **1.7.45-HFS: Ability to describe the advantages and disadvantages of various commercial exercise equipment in developing cardiorespiratory fitness, muscular strength, and muscular endurance.**

> **1.7.47-HFS: Ability to assess postural alignment and recommend appropriate exercise to meet individual needs and refer as necessary.**

KINETICS

In prescribing exercise, professionals select the resistance and intensity of movements to match the fitness level and goals of clients. It has been hypothesized that there is an optimal window of loading that healthy people should maintain, with loading greater than this window presenting a greater risk of injury (45). The idea can be viewed as a continuum (Fig. 2-8) between too little loading (resulting in musculoskeletal atrophy) and too much loading (resulting in injury). Unfortunately, this window is not easily defined for several reasons. It is difficult to measure or estimate the loads in body tissues in various activities, and once known, these loads will interact with other training variables (genetics, repetition, rest, nutrition, etc.) to determine a person's response.

Recently, some prospective studies have begun to address this issue. Fuchs et al. (16), for example, have shown that drop jump training can significantly increase bone mass in young children. More research on the forces involved in typical physical training activities could then help in the development of programs that not only build aerobic and muscular fitness but also promote long-term skeletal health. Research has also begun to link the exercise resistances used by older adults in weight training to increases in bone mass (8) and the kinds of training that create the largest increases in bone mechanical strength (56).

The mechanical variables related to external forces that have been measured to examine potential injury are the magnitude of the peak force, the rate of force development, and the repetition of loading. Figure 2-9 illustrates the difference in the vertical ground reaction force between heel–toe (rearfoot) and midfoot footstrike (42) patterns in running. The heel–toe running pattern has a passive peak or impact peak within the first 50 ms of contact from the heel striking the ground. The second peak force is the active peak force that corresponds to the reversal point of the down–up motion of the body near midstance. Note how the magnitude of the active peak force is about the same in both footstrike conditions, but there is usually a higher rate of force development in the heel–toe pattern compared with the midfoot pattern.

During normal physical activities, the magnitude of the peak ground reaction forces usually creates stresses in lower extremity tissues within the elastic range and, therefore, does not cause acute trauma or injury. The rate of force development is an important variable because of the viscoelastic nature of tissues. The greater the rate of loading, the more stiff the tissue and the greater the load reached before failure. The rate of force development is also clinically relevant because it determines the kind of

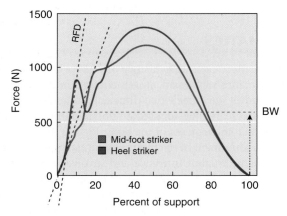

FIGURE 2-9. The vertical ground reaction force for heel and midfoot footstrike patterns. The heel–toe (rearfoot) footstrike pattern typically had a larger rate of force development (RFD) than the midfoot pattern. BW, body weight. (Adapted with permission from Hamill J, Knutzen KM. *Biomechanical Basis of Human Movement.* Philadelphia: Lippincott Williams & Wilkins; 2003.)

failure or fracture if loading goes beyond the elastic limit of the tissue. Studies of the kinetics of landing in Olympics gymnastics have been instrumental in changing rules and equipment that may help decrease the risk of injury to athletes (6).

Load repetition generally does not result in injury in normal physical activity in healthy individuals. It is possible, however, for long-term repeated impacts of high intensity to result in accumulation of microtrauma and the development of an overuse injury. *Overuse injuries* are usually the result of high-intensity activity over an extended period without adequate rest between training sessions. Because the long-term result of the mechanical stress of exercise can be either positive or negative, it is important for exercise professionals to be knowledgeable about symptoms of overtraining to reduce the risk of overuse injuries.

A promising area of biomechanics research involves the computer simulation of movements. In movements with simple performance criteria, computer simulations of biomechanical models can provide important information to optimize performance (20) and determine the effect of modifications in technique (26,59). One study found that increasing the strength of a muscle group did not automatically improve vertical jump performance unless the coordination of the model was adjusted to take advantage of the added strength (3). In the future, the integration of biomechanics and sports medicine research may enable professionals to define general guidelines for resistances and external force loading that result in desirable hypertrophy in tissues without elevated risk of injury.

KINEMATICS

Kinematic measurements of human movement may also have some use in defining desirable exercise and sports technique. Remember that earlier in the chapter it was noted that documenting what movement occurs (kinematics) cannot explain how the movement was created (kinetics). However, there are several ways that kinematic measurements can be used to help improve human movement.

There is some inherent value in documenting the kinematics of normal and skilled movement technique. This basic improvement in our understanding of what movements actually occur is important because many human movements are fast and difficult for professionals to see (32). Kinematic information on how movement changes with motor development (53) or learning (55) also helps the professional know what movements to look for with growth or practice. For example, kinematics measurements of walking gait have yielded data that is used (clinical gait analysis) to assist medical professionals in treating and monitoring progress for many

conditions (57). Knowing how much trunk lateral bending there is in normal walking helps therapists judge how much a patient has recovered. In sports, kinematic studies have improved the coaching of cricket bowling techniques and have significantly reduced intervertebral disc degeneration in athletes (11). Qualitative and quantitative kinematic analysis has also been used to remediate injuries and swing mechanics in golf (18,50). The kinematic prescription of maintaining approximately normal lordosis (lumbar curvature) minimizing transverse plane twisting is likely the safest spinal alignment in golf and most activities. Coaching this spinal position in lifting and sports movements evenly loads intervertebral discs and likely reduces the risk of injury.

Two more areas in which kinematic measurements have been applied in human movement are locomotion and lifting. Walking and running speed is a kinematic variable that is often used in modifying the intensity of exercise. Speed of locomotion is also strongly related to the biomechanical variables of gait, so coaches and therapists comparing walking or running technique over time need to evaluate clients at similar speeds. Locomotion is a highly skilled activity that requires considerable kinematic control to maintain balance. Weightlifting activities are often much slower and use more stable postures. A wide **base of support** and lower **center of gravity** increase stability but tend to decrease mobility. Whereas a squatting position favors stability over mobility, the upright, forwarding-leaning stance phase of running favors mobility. Both lifting and running require balance (the control over positioning the body), but the kinematics and geometry of the postures favor different objectives (stability vs. mobility).

An object's center of gravity is a theoretical point where the weight force of the object can be considered to act. The kinematics (variation in height and horizontal distance) of the center of gravity relative to the base of support is often studied to examine the balance exhibited by performer. Running requires a skilled bouncelike motion of the center of gravity over a very small base of support in stance. In a sit-to-stand movement, the body weight is slowly shifted over the base of support where there is a transition from primarily horizontal motion to a vertical or lifting motion (Fig. 2-10).

Kinematics provides useful information for defining safe lifting technique. When lifting boxes from the ground, the lifter should squat with a wide base of support. Spreading the feet apart helps maintain stability and allows the load to be carried close to the body, minimizing the moment arm and resistance torques for the lower back. The lifter should also keep the trunk straight (normal lordosis) and avoid exaggerated trunk lean. Performing the lift slowly with the legs and without

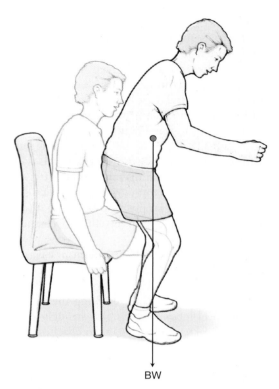

BW

FIGURE 2-10. The initial phase of the sit-to-stand movement involves trunk lean and horizontal weight shift to position the center of gravity over the new base of support (feet). The movement of the center of gravity in several directions is often used to study balance. BW, body weight.

axial trunk twisting are also important mechanical factors that minimize the risk of injury (39). Unfortunately, people unconsciously tend to stoop lift (lean over), probably because small weights can be lifted with passive back muscle and ligament forces and, therefore, less metabolic cost (Fig. 2-11B). Repetitive use of this lifting technique is dangerous because of the large moment arm for the resistances and uneven spinal loading. The 30 degrees of trunk lean in the squat lift illustrated in Figure 2-11A decrease the moment arms for weight forces of the box and upper body by one half (cos 60 deg = 0.5) from the stoop position, decreasing the gravitational torque loading on the lower back.

Statistical analysis of biomechanical data (including kinematics) has also been used to identify links between technique variables and performance (37). Therefore, kinematic measurements do hold promise in confirming the clinical observations of therapists and coaches, and these data may play a role in identifying key technique factors that can be used to improve human movement or reduce the risk of injury. However, kinematic data should be integrated with other studies (kinetics, EMG, training) to confirm that certain technique points are important and causative factors in performance or injury prevention.

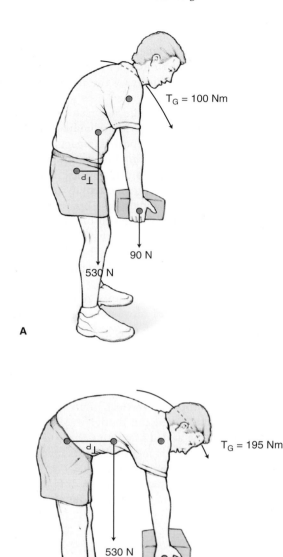

FIGURE 2-11. Squat lifting (A) is preferred over stoop lifting (B) because it decreases the gravitational torque (T_G) the lower back and hip extensors must balance. The kinematic variable of trunk lean is an important focus of observation because the angle of the trunk relative to gravity directly affects the moment arm ($d_\perp$) for the weight forces of the trunk and the box. A typical man decreases the gravitational torque about the hip from 195 Nm in the stoop lift to 100 Nm in the squat lift positions illustrated.

SUMMARY

The study of biomechanics is essential to sports medicine and exercise science professionals because it forms the basis for documenting human motion (kinematics) and understanding the causes of that motion (kinetics). The key mechanical variables that explain the creation of motion are force and moment of force (torque). Newton's three laws of motion are critical to understanding how human movement is created and how it can be improved. Key forces that affect human motion are gravity; friction; normal reaction; joint reactions; ground reactions; and elastic, muscular, and fluid forces. Biomechanics also provides information to help modify exercise through studies of the kinematics of human movement. These studies precisely document the motion of the body for a variety of movements and mover characteristics that professionals serve. The application of biomechanics in the prescription of exercise through the use of kinetic and kinematic data is being increasingly used to define desirable exercise intensities and movement amplitudes that create musculoskeletal adaptions with less risk of injury. Exercise science professionals typically use this biomechanical knowledge clinically in the qualitative analysis of exercise technique.

REFERENCES

1. Alexander RM. Tendon elasticity and muscle function. *Comp Biochem Physiol Part A*. 2002;133:1001–1.

2. Biewener AA, editor. *Biomechanics: Structures and Systems*. Oxford (UK): Oxford University Press: 1992.

3. Bobbert MF, van Soest AJ. Effects of muscle strengthening on vertical jump height: A simulation study. *Med Sci Sports Exerc*. 1994;26: 1012–20.

4. Brown JMM, Wickham JB, McAndrew DJ, Huang XF. Muscles within muscles: coordination of 19 muscle segments within three shoulder muscles during isometric motor tasks. *J. Electro Kines*. 2007;17: 57–73.

5. Brown LE, editor. *Isokinetics in Human Performance*. Champaign (IL): Human Kinetics; 2000.

6. Bruggemann GP. Improving performance and reducing injuries through biomechanics. *Olympic Rev*. 1998;22:9–10.

7. Cormie P, McCaulley GO, Triplett NT, McBride JM. Optimal loading for maximal power output during lower-body resistance exercises. *Med Sci Sports Exerc*. 2007;39:340–9.

8. Cussler EC, Lohman TG, Going SB, et al. Weight lifted in strength training predicts bone change in postmenopausal women. *Med Sci Sports Exerc*. 2003;35:10–7.

9. Delextrat A, Tricot V, Bernard T, et al. Drafting during swimming improves efficiency during subsequent cycling. *Med Sci Sports Exerc*. 2003;35:1612–9.

10. Dugan EL, Doyle TLA, Humphries B, et al. Determining the optimal load for jump squat: a review of methods and calculations. *J Strength Con. Res*. 2004;18:668–74.

11. Elliott BC, Kahangure M. Disk degeneration and fast bowling in cricket: an intervention study. *Med Sci Sports Exerc*. 2002;34: 1714–8.

12. Feldman AG, Levin MF, Mitnitski AM, Archambault P. Multimuscle control in human movements. *J Electromyo Kines*. 1998;8:383–90.

13. Finni T, Komi PV. Two methods for estimating tendinous tissue elongation during human movement. *J Appl Biomech*. 2002;18: 180–6.

14. Finni T, Komi PV, Lukkariniemi J. Achilles tendon loading during walking: application of a novel optic fiber technique. *Eur J Appl Physiol*. 1998;77:289–91.

15. Fleisig GS, Barrentine SW, Zheng N, et al. Kinematic and kinetic comparison of baseball pitching among various levels of development. *J Biomech*. 1999;32:1371–5.

16. Fuchs RK, Bauer JJ, Snow CM. Jumping improves hip and lumbar spine bone mass in prepubescent children: a randomized control trial. *J Bone Min Res*. 2001;16:148–56.

17. Gordon AM, Huxley AF, Julian JF. The variation in isometric tension with sarcomere length in vertebrate muscle fibers. *J Physiol*. 1966;184:170–92.

18. Grimshaw PN, Burden AM. Case report: reduction of low back pain in a professional golfer. *Med Sci Sports Exerc*. 2000;32:1667–73.

19. Gruber M, Gruber SBH, Taube W, et al. Differential effects of ballistic versus sensorimotor training on rate of force development and neural activation in humans. *J Strength Cond Res*. 2007;21:274–82.

20. Hatze H. Biomechanical aspects of a successful motion optimization. In: Komi PV, editor. *Biomechanics VB*. Baltimore: University Park Press; 1976. p. 5–12.

21. Hellebrandt FA. Living anatomy. *Quest*. 1963;1:43–58.

22. Herbert R, Moore S, Moseley A, et al. Making inferences about muscle forces from clinical observations. *Aust J Physiother*. 1993;39: 195–202.

23. Herzog W. Force-sharing among synergistic muscles: theoretical considerations and experimental approaches. *Exerc Sport Sci Rev*. 1996;24:173–200.

24. Hill AV. The heat of shortening and the dynamic constants of muscle. *Proc R Soc*. 1938;126:136–95.

25. Hof AL, Elzinga H, Grimmius W, Halbertsma JPK. Detection of non-standard EMG profiles in walking. *Gait Posture*. 2005;21: 171–7.

26. Holvoet P, Lacouture P, Duboy J. Practical use of airborne simulation in a release–regrasp skill on the high bar. *J Appl Biomech*. 2002;18: 332–44.

27. Hsiang SM, Brogmus GE, Courtney TK. Low back pain (LBP) and lifting technique—a review. *Int J Indust Ergonomics*. 1997;19:59–74.

28. Hunter JP, Marshall RN, McNair PJ. Segment-interaction analysis of the stance limb of sprint running. *J Biomech*. 2004;37:1439–46.

29. Jackson AS, Frankiewicz RJ. Factorial expression of muscular strength. *Res Quart*. 1975;46:206–17.

30. Kawakami Y, Abe T, Fukunaga T. Muscle-fiber pennation angles are greater in hypertrophied than in normal muscles. *J Appl Physiol*. 1993;74:2740–4.

31. Kawakami Y, Fukunaga T. New insights into in vivo human skeletal muscle function. *Exerc. Sport Sci Rev*. 2006;34:16–21.

32. Knudson D, Morrison C. *Qualitative Analysis of Human Movement*. 2nd ed. Champaign (IL): Human Kinetics; 2002.

33. Komi PV, Belli A, Huttunen V, et al. Optic fibre as a transducer of tendomuscular forces. *Eur J Appl Physiol*. 1996;72:278–80.

34. Komi PV, Nicol C. Stretch-shortening cycle of muscle function. In: Zatsiorsky V, editor. *Biomechanics in Sport*. Oxford (UK): Blackwell; 2000. p. 87–102.

35. Komi PV, Salonen M, Jarvinen M, Kokko O. In vivo registration of Achilles tendon forces in man, I: methodological development. *Int J Sports Med*. 1987;8:3–8.

36. Lake MJ, Cavanagh PR. Six weeks of training does not change running mechanics or improve running economy. *Med Sci Sports Exerc*. 1996;28:737–43.

37. Lees A. Biomechanical assessment of individual sports for improved performance. *Sports Med*. 1999;28:299–305.

38. Martin PE, Cavanagh PR. Segment interactions with the swing limb during unloaded and loaded running. *J Biomech*. 1990;23:529–36.

39. McGill S. *Low Back Disorders: Evidence-Based Prevention and Rehabilitation*. Champaign (IL): Human Kinetics; 2002.

40. Messier SP, Cirillo KJ. Effects of a verbal and visual feedback system on running technique, perceived exertion and running economy. *J Sports Sci*. 1989;7:113–26.

41. Morgan DW, Martin PE, Craig M, et al. Effect of stride length variation on oxygen uptake during distance running. *Med Sci Sports Exerc*. 1982;14:30–5.

42. Munro CF, Miller DI, Fuglevand AJ. Ground reaction forces in running: a reexamination. *J Biomech*. 1987;20:147–55.

43. Muramatsu T, Muraoka T, Takeshita D, et al. Mechanical properties of tendon and aponeurosis of human gastrocnemius muscle in vivo. *J Appl Physiol*. 2001;90:1671–8.

44. Muraoka T, Muramatsu T, Takeshita D, et al. Estimation of passive ankle joint moment during standing and walking. *J Appl Biomech*. 2005;21:72–84.

45. Nigg BM, Cole GK, Bruggeman GP. Impact forces during heel–toe running. *J Appl Biomech*. 1995;11:407–432.

46. Nigg BM, Luthi SM, Bahlsen HA. The tennis shoe—biomechanical design criteria. In: Segesser B, Pforringer W, editors. *The Shoe in Sport*, Chicago: Year Book Medical Publishers; 1989. p. 39–52.

47. Novacheck TF. The biomechanics of running. *Gait Posture*. 1998;7:77–95.

48. Owings TM, Pavol MJ, Foley KT, Grabiner MD. Measures of postural stability are not predictors of recovery from large postural disturbances in healthy older adults. *J Am Geriatr Soc*. 2000;48:42–50.

49. Pai YC. Movement termination and stability in standing. *Exerc Sports Sci Rev*. 2003;31:19–25.

50. Parziale JR. Healthy swing: a golf rehabilitation model. *Am J Phys Med Rehabil*. 2002;81:498–501.

51. Phillips SJ, Roberts EM, Huang TC. Quantification of intersegmental reactions during rapid swing motions. *J Biomech*. 1983;16: 411–417.

52. Rassier DE, MacIntosh BR, Herzog W. Length dependence of active force production in skeletal muscle. *J Appl Physiol*. 1999;86: 1445–1457.

53. Roberton MA, Konczak J. Predicting children's overarm throw ball velocities from their developmental levels in throw. *Res Quart Exerc Sport*. 2001;72:91–103.

54. Roberts TJ, Marsh RL, Weyand PG, Taylor DR. Muscular force in running turkeys: the economy of minimizing work. *Science* 1997;275:1113–1115.

55. Southard D. Change in throwing pattern: critical values for control parameter of velocity. *Res Quart Exerc Sport*. 2002;73:396–407.

56. Turner CH, Robling AG. Designing exercise regimens to increase bone strength. *Exerc Sport Sci Rev*. 2003;31:45–50.

57. Whittle M. *Gait Analysis: An Introduction*. 2nd ed. Oxford (UK): Butterworth-Heinemann; 1996.

58. Winter DA. Kinematic and kinetic patterns of human gait: variability and compensating effects. *Hum Mov Sci*. 1984;3:51–76.

59. Yeadon MR. The biomechanics of human flight. *Am J Sports Med*. 1997;25:575–580.

60. Zajac FE. Understanding muscle coordination of the human leg with dynamical simulations. *J Biomech*. 2002;35:1011–8.

61. Zajac FE., Gordon ME. Determining muscle's force and action in multi-articular movement. *Exerc Sport Sci Rev*. 1989;17:187–230.

62. Zatsiorsky VM. *Kinematics of Human Motion*. Champaign (IL): Human Kinetics; 1998.

63. Zatsiorsky VM. *Kinetics of Human Motion*. Champaign (IL): Human Kinetics; 2002.

SELECTED REFERENCES FOR FURTHER READING

Chaffin BD, Andersson GBJ, Martin BJ. *Occupational Biomechanics*. 4th ed. New York: Wiley; 2006.

Dvir Z, editor. *Clinical Biomechanics*. New York: Churchill Livingstone; 2000.

Hamill J, Knutzen K. *Biomechanical Basis of Human Movement*. 2nd ed. Baltimore: Lippincott Williams & Wilkins; 2003.

Hay JG. *The Biomechanics of Sports Techniques*. 4th ed. Englewood Cliffs (NJ): Prentice-Hall; 1993.

Knudson D. *Fundamentals of Biomechanics*. 2nd ed. New York: Springer Science; 2007.

Whiting WC, Zernicke RF. *Biomechanics of Musculoskeletal Injury*. Champaign, IL: Human Kinetics; 1998.

INTERNET RESOURCES

- American Society of Biomechanics: http://www.asbweb.org/
- Clinical Gait Analysis: http://www.univie.ac.at/cga
- Coaches' Infoservice: http://www.coachesinfo.com
- Exploratorium: Sport Science: http://www.exploratorium.edu/sport
- ExploreLearning: Motion and Force: http://www.explorelearning.com/index.cfm?method=cResource.dspResourcesFor Course& CourseID=330&CFID=461259&CFTOKEN=47919187
- Hosford Muscle Tables: Skeletal Muscles of the Human Body: http://ptcentral.com/muscles
- International Society of Biomechanics: http://isbweb.org
- International Society of Biomechanics in Sports: http://www.isbs.org

Exercise Physiology

This chapter presents a review of the acute responses of the body to the exercise stressor. Among the topics covered are the metabolic aspects of acute exercise, the acute cardiorespiratory responses to exercise, neuromuscular responses during exercise, the mechanisms of muscular fatigue, and the acute responses to exercise in varied environmental conditions.

> > > KEY TERMS

Acute mountain sickness (AMS): A sickness characterized by headaches, nausea, and lethargy that is related to acute exposure to altitude.

Cardiorespiratory: The collective systems of the heart, blood vessels, and lungs that function to circulate blood in the body and exchange gasses.

Central fatigue: The progressive reduction in voluntary drive to motor neurons during exercise.

Cold stress: The loss in heat either from the core or locally that is brought on by environment, metabolism, and clothing.

Concentric: When muscle length decreases during a muscle action.

Eccentric: When muscle length increases during a muscle action.

Electron transport chain: A series of chemical reactions in the mitochondria during which electrons from the hydrogen atoms of nicotinamide adenine dinucleotide (NADH) and flavin adenine dinucleotide (FADH) are transferred to oxygen. The electrochemical energy in this process is used in production of adenosine triphosphate (ATP) from adenosine diphosphate (ADP) and inorganic phosphate (Pi).

Energy metabolism: The net effect of chemical reaction in the body resulting in ATP production.

Glycolysis: A series of chemical reactions for the conversion of glucose to pyruvate and the anaerobic production of ATP.

Heat stress: An increase in core temperature collectively brought about by the environment, metabolism, and clothing.

Hemodynamics: The acute response of the blood flow and blood composition to changes in the activity state of the body.

Hypoxic ventilatory response: The increase in ventilation seen with acute altitude exposure as a result of reduced barometric pressure and lowered arterial oxygen pressure.

Krebs cycle: A series of chemical reactions in the mitochondria in which acetyl-coenzyme A (CoA) is oxidized, resulting in the production of 3 NADH, 1 FADH, 1 GTP, and 2 CO_2.

Maximal oxygen consumption ($\dot{V}O_{2max}$): The maximum rate of oxygen that can be used for production of ATP during exercise.

Motor unit: The motor neuron and the muscle fibers it innervates.

Muscle fatigue: The loss of force or power output in response to voluntary effort leading to reduced performance.

Peripheral fatigue: The loss of force and power that is independent of neural drive.

Primary pollutant: A direct source of pollution.

Secondary pollutant: A pollutant formed from the interaction of a primary pollutant with an environmental factor.

Size principle: The recruitment of motor units in order from smallest to largest according to recruitment thresholds and firing rates, resulting in a continuum of voluntary force.

TABLE 3-1. CHARACTERISTICS OF THE TWO MECHANISMS BY WHICH ATP IS FORMED

MECHANISM	FOOD OR CHEMICAL FUEL	OXYGEN REQUIRED?	RELATIVE ATP YIELD
Anaerobic phosphocreatine	Phosphocreatine	No	Extremely limited
Glycolysis	Glycogen (Glucose)	No	Extremely limited
Aerobic			
Krebs cycle and electron transport system	Glycogen, fats, proteins	Yes	Large

FUNDAMENTALS OF EXERCISE METABOLISM

At rest, a 70-kg human has an energy expenditure of about 1.2 kcal·min^{-1}; less than 20% of resting energy expenditure is attributed to skeletal muscle. However, almost all changes that occur in the body during exercise are related to the increase in energy metabolism, largely within the contracting skeletal muscle. For example, cardiac output increases as a direct linear function of whole-body metabolism. To meet the demands on the heart, a fourfold increase in myocardial blood flow and oxygen consumption takes place.

During intense exercise, total energy expenditure may increase 15 to 25 times more than resting values, resulting in a caloric expenditure of approximately 18 to 30 kcal·min^{-1}. Most of this increase is used to provide energy for exercising muscles, which may increase energy requirements significantly. Therefore, daily caloric expenditure can be changed dramatically by simply altering the amount of physical activity performed during a day. Muscle fibers contain the metabolic machinery to produce adenosine triphosphate (ATP) by three systems: creatine phosphate (CP), rapid glycolysis, and

aerobic oxidation of nutrients to carbon dioxide and water (oxidative phosphorylation).

The importance of the interaction of the aforementioned metabolic systems in the production of ATP during exercise should be emphasized. In reality, the energy to perform most types of exercise does not come from a single source but from a combination of anaerobic and aerobic sources (Fig. 3-1 and Table 3-1). The contribution of anaerobic sources (CP system and glycolysis) to exercise **energy metabolism** is inversely related to the duration and positively related to the intensity of the activity. The shorter and more intense the activity, the greater the contribution of anaerobic energy production. Conversely, the longer the activity and the lower the intensity, the greater the contribution of aerobic energy production. Although proteins are used as a fuel for aerobic exercise, carbohydrates and fats are the primary energy substrates during exercise in healthy, well-fed individuals. In general, carbohydrates are used as the primary fuel at the onset of exercise and during high-intensity work (39,40,56). However, during prolonged exercise of low to moderate intensity (longer than 30 minutes), a gradual shift from carbohydrate toward an increasing reliance on fat as a substrate occurs (Fig. 3-2) (56,62). The greatest amount of fat use occurs at about 60% of maximal aerobic capacity ($\dot{V}O_{2max}$) This section of the chapter focuses on muscle bioenergetics and exercise metabolism. A detailed review of bioenergetics and exercise metabolism is

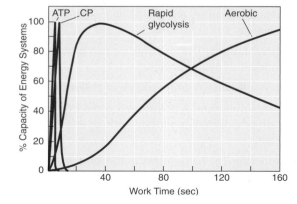

FIGURE 3-1. Interaction between anaerobic and aerobic energy sources during exercise, including adenosine triphosphate (ATP), creatine phosphate (CP), rapid glycolysis, and aerobic (oxidative phosphorylation). Note that whereas the energy to perform short-term high-intensity exercise comes primarily from anaerobic sources, the energy for muscular contraction during prolonged exercise comes from aerobic metabolism.

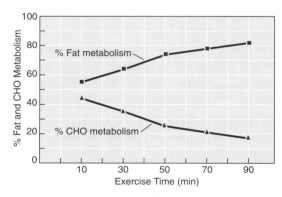

FIGURE 3-2. Alterations in substrate utilization during prolonged submaximal (<60% $\dot{V}O_{2max}$) exercise. CHO, carbohydrate. (Adapted with permission from Powers S, Byrd R, Tulley R, et al. Effects of caffeine ingestion on metabolism and performance during graded exercise. *Eur J Appl Physiol.* 1983;50:301.)

provided in the suggested reading section of this chapter. A brief discussion of the energy pathways and the metabolic response to various types of exercise follows.

ENERGY FOR SHORT-TERM EXERCISE

 1.1.9-HFS: Ability to define aerobic and anaerobic metabolism.

 1.1.10-HFS: Knowledge of the roles of aerobic and anaerobic energy systems in the performance of various activities.

ADENOSINE TRIPHOSPHATE (ATP)

The energy released through hydrolysis of the high-energy compound ATP to form adenosine diphosphate (ADP) and inorganic phosphate (Pi) powers skeletal muscle contractions. This reaction is catalyzed by the enzyme myosin ATPase:

$$\text{(Myosin ATPase)}$$
$$\text{ATP} \rightarrow \text{ADP} + \text{Pi} + \text{energy}$$

The amount of ATP directly available in muscle at any time is small, so it must be resynthesized continuously if exercise lasts for more than a few seconds.

CREATINE PHOSPHATE

The CP system transfers high-energy phosphate from CP to rephosphorylate ATP from ADP as follows:

$$\text{(Creatine kinase)}$$
$$\text{ADP} + \text{CP} \rightarrow \text{ATP} + \text{C}$$

This system is rapid because it involves only one enzymatic step (i.e., one chemical reaction); however, CP exists in finite quantities in cells, so the total amount of ATP that can be produced is limited. Oxygen is not involved in the rephosphorylation of ADP to ATP in this reaction, so the CP system is considered anaerobic (without oxygen).

RAPID GLYCOLYSIS

When **glycolysis** is rapid, it is capable of producing ATP without involvement of oxygen. Glycolysis, the degradation of carbohydrate (glycogen or glucose) to pyruvate or lactate, involves a series of enzymatically catalyzed steps (Fig. 3-3). The net energy yield of glycolysis, without further oxidation through aerobic metabolism, is two or three ATPs through substrate-level phosphorylation. The net production is two ATPs when glucose is the substrate and three ATPs when glycogen is the substrate. Although glycolysis does not use oxygen and is considered anaerobic, pyruvate can readily participate in aerobic production of ATP when oxygen is available in the cell. Therefore, in addition to being an anaerobic pathway ca-

Glucose
> Hexokinase

Glucose 6 – Phosphate
> Glucose 6 – Phosphate Isomerase

Fructose 6 – Phosphate
> Phosphofructokinase

Fructose 1,6 – Diphosphate
> Aldolase

Glyceraldehyde 3 – Phosphate + Dihydroxyacetone Phosphate
> Triophosphate Isomerase

Glyceraldehyde 3 – Phosphate
> Glyceraldehyde 3 – Phosphate Dehydrogenase

1,3 – Diphosphoglycerate
> Phosphoglycerate Kinase

3 – Phosphoglycerate
> Phosphoglucomutase

2 – Phosphoglycerate
> Enolase

Phosphoenolpyruvate
> Pyruvate Kinase

Pyruvate
> Lactate Dehydrogenase

Lactate

FIGURE 3-3. Enzymatic steps of glycolysis.

pable of producing ATP without oxygen, glycolysis can also be considered the first step in the aerobic degradation of carbohydrate.

ENERGY FOR LONGER DURATION EXERCISE

OXIDATIVE PHOSPHORYLATION

The final metabolic pathway for ATP production combines two complex metabolic processes, the **Krebs cycle** and **electron transport chain**; both occur inside the mitochondria. Oxidative phosphorylation uses oxygen as the final hydrogen acceptor to form water and ATP. Unlike glycolysis, aerobic metabolism can use fat, protein, and carbohydrate as substrates to produce ATP. The interaction of these nutrients is illustrated in Figure 3-4.

Conceptually, the Krebs cycle can be considered a primer for oxidative phosphorylation. Entry into the Krebs cycle begins with the combination of acetyl-coenzyme A (CoA) and oxaloacetic acid to form citric acid. The primary function of the Krebs cycle is to remove hydrogens from four of the reactants involved in the cycle.

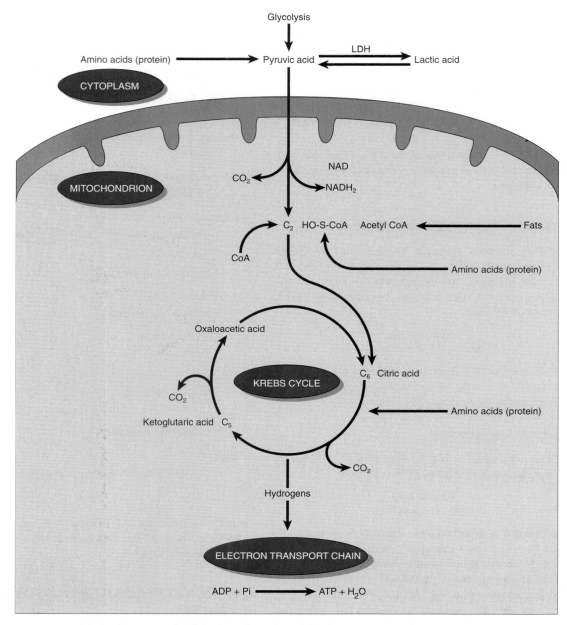

FIGURE 3-4. Relationship among glycolysis, the Krebs cycle, and the electron transport chain. CoA, coenzyme A; LDH, lactate dehydrogenase; NAD, nicotinamide adenine dinucleotide.

The electrons from these hydrogens follow a chain of cytochromes (electron transport chain) in the mitochondria, and the energy released from this process is used to rephosphorylate ADP to form ATP. Oxygen is the final acceptor of hydrogen to form water, and this reaction is catalyzed by cytochrome oxidase (see Fig. 3-4). Complete degradation of glucose by glycolysis and oxidative phosphorylation result in a net production of 38 ATP per glucose molecule, or 39 ATP when the glucose molecule is derived from glycogen. These ATP values for glucose degradation may vary slightly in some sources.

FAT METABOLISM

Oxidation of fat, which provides acetyl-CoA as substrate for the Krebs cycle, is possible through aerobic metabolism. Glycolysis can also interact with the Krebs cycle in the presence of oxygen by the conversion of pyruvate to form acetyl-CoA. Fats or triglycerides are lipids broken down to glycerol and fatty acids by hormone-sensitive lipase, which is inhibited by insulin and activated by catecholamines (epinephrine and norepinephrine) and growth hormone. Glycerol can be metabolized through glycolysis or used to make glucose. Free fatty acids enter the blood to be ultimately used as fuel in cells via a process known as β-oxidation. They may also be used as a precursor in the production of many substances such as cholesterol. Fatty acids must be activated using ATP and CoA and transported via the carnitine shuttle system to enter the mitochondria for oxidation. In the mitochondrial matrix, β-oxidation proceeds sequentially by cleaving off two carbon atoms at a time, forming acetyl-CoA, the substrate for the Krebs cycle. A 16-carbon fatty acid such as palmitate yields 129 ATP.

METABOLIC RESPONSE TO EXERCISE

TRANSITION FROM REST TO LIGHT EXERCISE

In the transition from rest to light exercise, oxygen uptake kinetics follow a mono-exponential pattern, reaching a steady state generally within 1 to 4 minutes (Fig. 3-5) (61). The time required to reach a steady state increases at higher work rates and is longer in untrained individuals than in aerobically trained individuals. Because oxygen uptake does not increase instantaneously to steady state at the onset of exercise, it is implied that anaerobic energy sources contribute to the meet the energy demand at the beginning of exercise. Indeed, evidence suggests that both the CP system and rapid glycolysis contribute to the overall production of ATP at the onset of muscular work (21). As soon as a steady state is obtained, however, the ATP requirements are met by aerobic metabolism. The term *oxygen deficit* has been used to describe inadequate oxygen consumption at the onset of exercise (see Fig. 3-5). Similar to short-term heavy exercise, the principal fuel used during the transition from rest to light exercise is muscle glycogen.

SHORT-TERM, HIGH-INTENSITY EXERCISE

The energy to perform short-term, high-intensity exercise (5 to 60 seconds in duration), such as weightlifting or sprinting 400 meters, comes primarily from anaerobic sys-

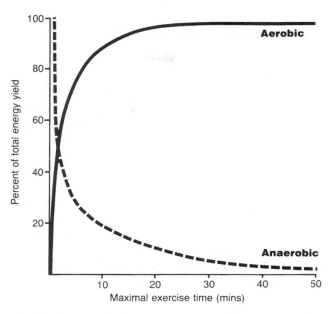

FIGURE 3-6. Relative contribution of aerobic and anaerobic metabolism during physical activity of increasing duration. In intense activities lasting 1.5 to 2.0 minutes, the ATP-CP and lactic acid energy systems generate approximately 50% of the energy, and aerobic metabolism supplies the remainder. A distance runner, on the other hand, derives essentially 98% of his or her energy from aerobic metabolism during a 50-minute training run.

tems (Fig. 3-6). Whether the ATP–CP system or glycolysis dominates the ATP production depends on the duration of the muscular effort. In general, energy for all activities lasting less than 5 seconds comes from the ATP–CP system. In contrast, energy to perform a 200-meter sprint (30 seconds) would come from a combination of the ATP–CP system and anaerobic glycolysis, with glycolysis predominating. The transition from the CP system to glycolysis is not abrupt but rather a gradual shift from one pathway to another as the duration of the exercise increases.

As illustrated in Figure 3-1, exercise bouts lasting longer than 45 seconds use a combination of the CP system, rapid glycolysis, and aerobic systems. For example, the energy required to sprint 400 meters (60 seconds) comes primarily (about 70%) from anaerobic sources (i.e., ATP, CP, rapid glycolysis), and the remaining ATP production is provided by aerobic metabolism. Carbohydrate (glycogen) stored in muscle is the principal fuel used during this type of exercise.

PROLONGED SUBMAXIMAL EXERCISE

Steady-state $\dot{V}O_2$ can usually be maintained during 10 to 60 minutes of submaximal continuous exercise. This rule has two exceptions. First, prolonged exercise in a hot and humid environment results in a steady drift upward of $\dot{V}O_2$ during the course of exercise (60). Second, continuous exercise at a high relative workload results in a slow rise in $\dot{V}O_2$ across time similar to that observed during exercise in

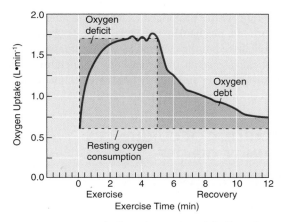

FIGURE 3-5. Oxygen uptake dynamics at onset and offset of exercise. See text for details.

a hot environment. In both cases, this drift probably occurs because of a variety of factors, such as rising body temperature and increasing blood catecholamines (34,59).

As depicted in Figure 3-2, both carbohydrate and fat are used as substrates during prolonged exercise. During prolonged low- and moderate-intensity exercise, there is a gradual shift from carbohydrate metabolism to the use of fat as a substrate. Explanations for this metabolic shift include the following: Fatty acids inhibit the Krebs cycle, leading to accumulation of citrate, which lowers phosphofructokinase (PFK) activity. This causes reduced uptake and oxidation of glucose. Carbohydrate metabolism regulates fat metabolism during exercise (17). The onset of exercise of low to moderate intensity produces a high glycolytic flux that slowly diminishes. The resulting glycolytic intermediates inhibit the carnitine transport system, thus preventing long-chain fatty acids from entering mitochondria for oxidation. Other factors that can affect the relative contribution of fat versus carbohydrate as energy substrate during prolonged exercise are nutritional status of the individual and the state of training.

PROGRESSIVE INCREMENTAL EXERCISE

> **1.1.9-CES: Plot the normal resting and exercise values associated with increasing exercise intensity (and how they may differ for cardiac, pulmonary, and metabolic diseased populations) for the following: heart rate, stroke volume, cardiac output, double product, arteriovenous O_2 difference, O_2 consumption, systolic and diastolic blood pressure, minute ventilation, tidal volume, breathing frequency, Vd/Vt, $\dot{V}_E/\dot{V}O_2$, and $\dot{V}_E/\dot{V}O_2$, FEV$_{1.0}$, SaO$_2$, blood glucose.**

Figure 3-7 illustrates the oxygen uptake during a progressive incremental exercise test. Note that oxygen uptake increases linearly with work rate until $\dot{V}O_{2max}$ is reached. After reaching a steady state, ATP used for muscular contraction during the early stages of an incremental exercise test comes primarily from aerobic metabolism. However, as the exercise intensity increases, blood levels of lactate increase (Fig. 3-8). Although much controversy surrounds

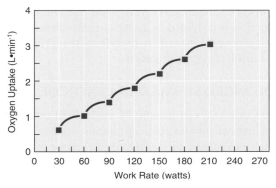

FIGURE 3-7. Changes in oxygen uptake as a function of work rate during incremental exercise.

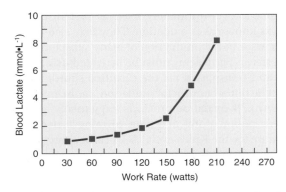

FIGURE 3-8. Changes in blood lactate concentrations as a function of work rate during incremental exercise.

this issue, many investigators believe that this lactate inflection point is a point of increasing reliance upon anaerobic metabolism brought about by the increased recruitment of type-II or nonoxidative fast-twitch muscle fibers.

Although the precise terminology is controversial, this sudden increase in blood lactate levels—termed the *anaerobic threshold* or *lactate threshold*—has important implications for the prediction of performance and perhaps exercise prescription. For example, it has been shown that the anaerobic threshold, used in combination with other physiological variables (i.e. $\dot{V}O_{2max}$), is a useful predictor of success in distance running (8). The lactate threshold may also prove to be a marker of the transition from moderate to heavy exercise for subjects and thus useful in exercise prescriptions.

RECOVERY FROM EXERCISE

Oxygen uptake remains elevated above resting levels for several minutes during recovery from exercise (see Fig. 3-5). This elevated postexercise oxygen consumption has traditionally been termed the *oxygen debt*, but more recently the term *elevated postexercise oxygen consumption* (EPOC) has been applied (34). In general, postexercise metabolism is higher after high-intensity exercise than after light or moderate work. Furthermore, postexercise remains $\dot{V}O_2$ elevated longer after prolonged exercise than after short-term exertion. The mechanisms to explain these observations are probably linked to the fact that both high-intensity and prolonged exercise result in higher body temperatures, greater ionic disturbance, and higher plasma catecholamines than in light or moderate short-term exercise (34).

METABOLIC OCCURRENCES DURING EXERCISE

LACTIC ACID THRESHOLD

Historically, increasing blood lactate levels during exercise have been considered an indication of increased anaerobic metabolism within the contracting muscle because of a lack of oxygen. If oxygen is not available in the mitochondria to accept hydrogen released during glycolysis, pyruvate must accept hydrogen to form lactate as an end product so that glycolysis can proceed. However, the hypoxia theory is controversial. Whether the end product of glycolysis is pyruvate or lactate also depends on other factors, including muscle fiber type and the speed of glycolytic flux. If glycolytic flux is extremely rapid, hydrogen production may exceed the transport capability of the shuttle mechanisms that move hydrogen from the cytoplasm (called *sarcoplasm* in muscle) into the mitochondria, where oxidative phosphorylation occurs without true hypoxia. When glycolytic hydrogen production exceeds the mitochondrial transport capability, pyruvate must again accept the hydrogens to form lactate so glycolysis can continue. During exercise, epinephrine (adrenaline) levels in the blood are elevated, which stimulates muscle *glycogenolysis* (breakdown of glycogen for fuel), increasing the rate of glycolysis. At rest and during low exercise intensities (<40% of maximal aerobic capacity), type I or slow-twitch muscle fibers are recruited predominantly. As the exercise intensity increases, more type II or fast-twitch fibers are recruited. This recruitment pattern has an important influence on lactic acid production. Conversion of pyruvate to lactate and vice versa is catalyzed by the enzyme lactate dehydrogenase (LDH), which exists in several forms (isozymes). Whereas type II muscle fibers contain an LDH isozyme that favors the formation of lactate, type I fibers contain an LDH form that promotes less conversion of pyruvate to lactate or even conversion of lactate to pyruvate. Therefore, more lactate formation occurs in type II fibers during exercise simply because of the type of LDH isozyme present, independent of oxygen availability in the muscle. Finally, type II fibers have higher activities of glycolytic enzymes than do type I fibers, indicating a greater potential of substrate flux through glycolysis.

In summary, debate over the mechanism or mechanisms responsible for muscle lactate production during exercise continues. It seems possible that any one or a combination of these possibilities (or lack of oxygen) may provide an explanation for muscle lactate production during exercise. The most important consequence of lactic acid production is that it immediately releases a proton (H^+), and unless this proton is buffered, a decrease in cellular pH results that may eventually disrupt enzyme function and muscle contraction and contribute to the characteristic muscle fatigue or pain that occurs with vigorous, intense exercise. However, blood lactate can also be used as a fuel by muscles and other tissues during and after exercise. Lactate concentrations can increase in the blood only when the rate of lactate production begins to exceed its removal. A detailed discussion of this topic is available from other sources (37,63,64, and see Brooks et al. in selected readings).

ANAEROBIC THRESHOLD

> **1.1.28-HFS: Knowledge of and ability to describe the implications of ventilatory threshold (anaerobic threshold) as it relates to exercise training and cardiorespiratory assessment.**

The onset of metabolic acidosis (i.e., anaerobic threshold, AT) during exercise, traditionally determined by serial measurements of blood lactate, can be determined noninvasively by assessment of expired gases during exercise testing, specifically pulmonary ventilation ($\dot{V}_E$), oxygen consumption ($\dot{V}O_2$), and carbon dioxide production ($\dot{V}CO_2$) (36). Oft-used methods are the modified V-slope and the ventilatory equivalents methods (36). This is often termed the ventilatory threshold (VT) and signifies the highest work rate or oxygen consumption at which the energy demands exceed circulatory ability to sustain aerobic metabolism. The physiology underlying the AT may be attributed, at least in part, to buffering of lactic acid by sodium bicarbonate in the blood, so that carbon dioxide is released in excess of that produced by muscle metabolism, providing an additional stimulus for ventilation. These biochemical alterations are summarized by the following reaction:

$$HLa + Na\ HCO_3 \rightarrow Na\ La + H_2CO_3 \rightleftarrows H_2O + CO_2$$

(lactic acid) (sodium bicarbonate) (sodium lactate) (carbonic acid)

Accordingly, values for $\dot{V}_E$ and carbon dioxide production increase out of proportion to the intensity of exercise performed (Fig. 3-9), suggesting an abrupt increase in serum lactate. This method correlates well with the lactate method and obviates measurement of lactate in repeated blood samples. An increase in the ventilatory equivalent for oxygen ($\dot{V}_E/\dot{V}O_2$) during exercise without a corresponding change in the ventilatory equivalent for carbon dioxide ($\dot{V}_E/\dot{V}CO_2$) has also been reported to be sensitive and reliable for determining the AT (36). There

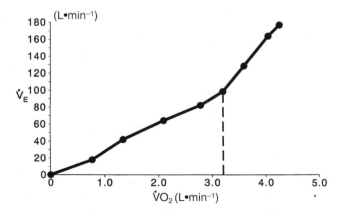

FIGURE 3-9. Relationship between intensity of exercise ($\dot{V}O_2$) and simultaneous, abrupt nonlinear increase in minute ventilation, signifying the anaerobic threshold. In this subject, the break point occurred at 3.20 L·min⁻¹, corresponding to 75% of measured $\dot{V}O_{2max}$ (4.25 L·min⁻¹).

is, however, controversy surrounding the mechanisms responsible for the AT (36,37,63,64). Increased lactate production may result from mechanisms not related to inadequate oxygen delivery. Another theory is that inflections in $\dot{V}_E$ and $\dot{V}CO_2$ are attributable to inadequate buffering at a fixed metabolic intensity, even when lactate production and oxygen uptake continue to increase linearly.

The AT from respiratory gas measurements is often expressed as a percentage of the $\dot{V}O_{2max}$. For example, a highly trained athlete with a $\dot{V}O_{2max}$ of 4.25 L·min^{-1} whose break point in $\dot{V}_E$ occurs at 3.20 L·min^{-1} has an AT corresponding to 75% of aerobic capacity (Fig. 3-10). This athlete should be able to maintain exercise intensities at less than 75% of $\dot{V}O_{2max}$ using a predominance of aerobic processes. Moreover, such exertion should be accomplished without inducing a significant increase in blood lactic acid and muscle fatigue. Although the AT typically corresponds to 55% ± 8% of the $\dot{V}O_{2max}$ in healthy untrained individuals, it normally occurs at a higher percentage of the $\dot{V}O_{2max}$ (i.e., 70%–90%) in physically trained subjects (8,36).

The $\dot{V}O_{2max}$ is recognized as an important predictor of performance in endurance events. However, several studies now suggest that the highest percentage of $\dot{V}O_{2max}$ that can be used over an extended duration without incurring significant increase in arterial lactate may be an even more important determinant of cardiorespiratory performance (8,36). This suggests that the AT may be critical in determining optimal race pace during endurance events.

HORMONAL RESPONSES TO EXERCISE

> **1.1.13-CES: Understand the hormonal (i.e., insulin, glucagon, epinephrine, norepinephrine, angiotensin, aldosterone, renin, and erythropoietin) responses to acute and chronic exercise.**

Several hormones are important to fuel usage during exercise. Subsequently, the response of the hormones important to metabolism change exercise intensity. Little change is seen during light exercise in catecholamines, glucagon, and growth hormone. Insulin exhibits a drop from resting levels. The percent change in insulin concentration from rest decreases at near maximum values but still remains below that of rest. As exercise intensity increases from moderate to maximum, an increase in the response of the catecholamines, glucagon, and growth hormone is seen.

MEASUREMENT OF METABOLISM AND OXYGEN CONSUMPTION

Traditionally, whole-body metabolism is measured via direct or indirect calorimetry. The principles behind these two strategies can be explained by the following relationship:

$$\text{Foodstuffs} + O_2 \rightarrow \text{Heat} + CO_2 + H_2O$$
(indirect calorimetry)   (direct calorimetry)

Heat is liberated as a consequence of cellular respiration and cell (e.g., muscular) work. Thus, heat production by the body allows a direct assessment of metabolism. Direct calorimetry requires that a subject be placed in an airtight chamber. As heat is released, the temperature inside the chamber increases. Typically, a circulating jacket of water used to transfer heat to the environment allows a means of determining the metabolic rate in joules or kilocalories.

Although direct calorimetry is a precise technique, construction of large chambers for measurement of metabolic rate in humans is prohibitively expensive. Also, heat produced by exercise equipment can complicate measurements using direct calorimetry. The principle of indirect calorimetry uses the measurement of oxygen

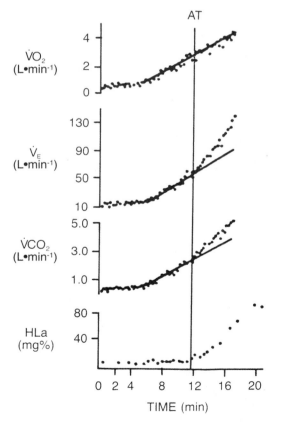

FIGURE 3-10. Relationship between intensity of exercise (oxygen consumption $\dot{V}O_2$) and simultaneous, abrupt nonlinear increases in serum lactate (HLa), carbon dioxide production ($\dot{V}CO_2$) and pulmonary ventilation ($\dot{V}_E$) occurring at the anaerobic threshold (AT). Exercise was initiated at minute 4. (Adapted with permission from Davis JA, Vodak P, Wilmore JH, et al. Anaerobic threshold and maximal aerobic power for three modes of exercise. *J Appl Physiol.* 1976;41:544–50.)

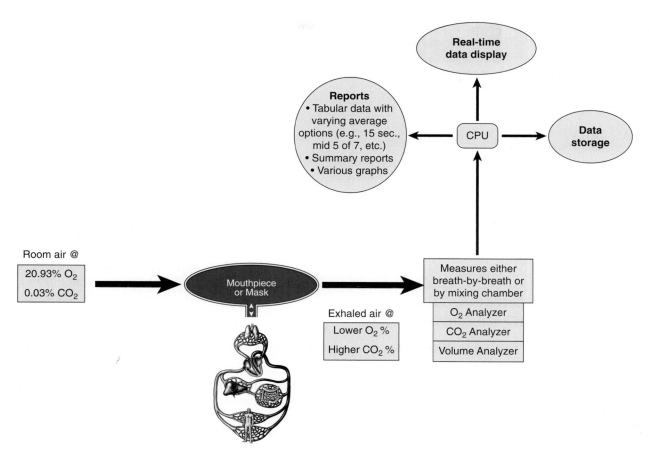

FIGURE 3-11. Open-circuit spirometry system interfaced with computer technology.

consumption ($\dot{V}O_2$) to determine metabolic rate. Using this method, metabolic rate in kilocalories can be estimated using the following formula:

Metabolic rate (kcal·min^{-1}) = $\dot{V}O_2$ (L·min^{-1}) × [4.0 + RQ]

Note: RQ = respiratory quotient

The most common method of measuring oxygen consumption uses open-circuit spirometry (Fig. 3-11). The volume of inspired oxygen is measured using a dry gas meter, turbine, or pneumotach. A one-way valve directs air through the mouth. Gas fractions are sampled and measured by oxygen and carbon dioxide analyzers on the expired side. Typically, analog voltages from the gas meter and analyzers are converted to digital information and fed into a microcomputer with $\dot{V}O_2$ calculated using the Haldane transformation of the Fick equation:

$$\dot{V}O_2 = \dot{V}_I \times F_IO_2 \; \dot{V}_I \times \left(\frac{[1 - F_EO_2 - F_ECO_2]}{[1 - F_IO_2 - F_ICO_2]} \right) \times F_EO_2$$

where

$\dot{V}_I$ = inspired ventilation

F_IO_2 = inspired oxygen fraction = 0.2093

F_ICO_2 = inspired carbon dioxide fraction = 0.0003

F_EO_2 = expired oxygen fraction

F_ECO_2 = expired carbon dioxide fraction

ENERGY COST OF ACTIVITIES

> **1.1.5-CES: Identify the metabolic equivalent (MET) requirements of various occupational, household, sport/exercise, and leisure time activities.**

The energy cost of many types of physical activity have been established. Activities that are vigorous and involve large muscle groups usually result in more energy expended than activities that use small muscle mass or require limited exertion. Estimates of energy expenditure have been previously obtained by measuring oxygen cost of these activities in an adult population (see Ainsworth in the Selected References for Further Reading).

Clinicians often use the term *metabolic equivalent* (MET) to describe exercise intensity. A single MET is equivalent to the amount of energy expended during 1 minute of seated rest. Therefore, exercise at a metabolic rate that is five times the resting $\dot{V}O_2$ rate is equivalent to 5 METs. In a strict sense, the absolute energy expenditure during exercise at a 5-MET intensity depends on the body size of the individual (i.e., a large person is likely to have a larger resting $\dot{V}O_2$ than a small person). For simplicity, individual differences in resting energy expenditures are often overlooked, and 1 MET is considered equivalent to a $\dot{V}O_2$ of 3.5 mL $O_2 \cdot kg^{-1} \cdot min^{-1}$; hence, 1 MET represents an energy expenditure of approximately 1.2 kcal $\cdot min^{-1}$ for a 70-kg person.

SUMMARY

Exercise metabolism is a reflection of each metabolic pathway as it contributes to the increased energy demands of activity and work. Substrates for energy production include carbohydrate, fat, and protein. The mix of these substrates during exercise metabolism depends on the intensity and duration of exercise and the conditioning of the individual.

NORMAL CARDIORESPIRATORY RESPONSES TO ACUTE AEROBIC EXERCISE

 1.1.13-HFS: Knowledge of the heart rate, stroke volume, cardiac output, blood pressure, and oxygen consumption responses to exercise.

1.1.15-HFS: Knowledge of the physiological principles related to warm-up and cool-down.

The energy requirements of exercising human muscle may increase substantially in the transition from rest to maximal physical exertion. Because the available stores of ATP muscle are limited and capable of providing energy to maintain vigorous activity for only several seconds, ATP must be constantly resynthesized to provide continuous energy production. Therefore, exercising muscle must possess a large capacity for increasing metabolic rate to produce sufficient ATP so that increased activity can continue. Energy production relies heavily on the respiratory and cardiovascular systems for the delivery of oxygen and nutrients and for the removal of waste products to maintain the internal equilibrium of cells. Warm-up activities prior to exercise help enhance blood flow to the active tissues and increase internal temperature, which is beneficial to energy production.

The purpose of this section is to review the normal **cardiorespiratory** responses to acute aerobic exercise with specific reference to energy systems, **hemodynamics**, posture, **maximal oxygen consumption ($\dot{V}O_{2max}$)**, the anaerobic threshold, dynamic versus isometric exertion, arm versus leg exercise, myocardial oxygen consumption, and the effects of physical conditioning. This information is vital to the understanding of the role of exercise physiology in the interpretation of diagnostic and functional exercise testing and the prescription of exercise in health and disease. The responses noted generally represent those of healthy individuals. Individuals with

cardiovascular, pulmonary, and metabolic disease may exhibit some similarities in the acute cardiorespiratory response with exercise. The magnitude of the responses may vary depending on the nature of the disease and disease severity. However, improvements in cardiorespiratory function in patients with a clinically manifest disease are possible with exercise training.

ACUTE CARDIORESPIRATORY RESPONSES TO EXERCISE

Many cardiorespiratory and hemodynamic mechanisms function collectively to support increased aerobic requirements of physical activity. The overall effect of changes in heart rate (HR), stroke volume (SV), cardiac output, blood flow, blood pressure (BP), arteriovenous oxygen difference, and pulmonary ventilation is to oxygenate the blood and ensure that it is delivered to the active tissues.

HEART RATE

Heart rate increases in a linear fashion with the work rate and oxygen uptake during dynamic exercise. The increase in HR during exercise occurs primarily at the expense of diastole (filling time), rather than systole (Fig. 3-12). Thus, at high exercise intensities, diastolic time may be so short as to preclude adequate ventricular filling. The magnitude of the HR response is related to age, body position, fitness, type of activity, the presence of cardiovascular disease, medications, blood volume, and environmental

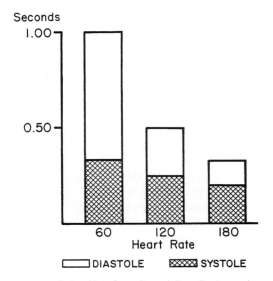

FIGURE 3-12. Relationship of systolic and diastolic time to heart rate (HR). Because coronary blood flow predominates during diastole, with increased HR, as during exercise, diastolic (perfusion) time is disproportionately shortened. (Adapted with permission from Dehn MM, Mullins CB. Physiologic effects and importance of exercise in patients with coronary artery disease. *J Cardiovasc Med.* 1977;2:365–87.)

factors such as temperature and humidity. In contrast to systolic BP (SBP), which usually increases with age, maximum attainable HR decreases with age. The equation of 220 – age provides an approximation of the maximum HR in healthy men and women, but the variance for any fixed age is considerable (standard deviation about ± 10 bpm).

STROKE VOLUME

The SV (volume of blood ejected per heart beat) is equal to the difference between end-diastolic volume (EDV) and end-systolic volume (ESV). Whereas the former is determined by HR, filling volume (preload), and ventricular compliance, the latter depends on two variables: contractility and afterload. Thus, a greater diastolic filling (preload) increases SV. In contrast, factors that resist ventricular outflow (afterload) result in a reduced SV.

Stroke volume at rest in the upright position generally varies between 60 and 100 mL·beat^{-1} among healthy adults, and maximum SV approximates 100 to 120 mL·beat^{-1}. During exercise, SV increases curvilinearly with work rate until it reaches near maximum at a level equivalent to approximately 50% of aerobic capacity, increasing only slightly thereafter. Within physiological limits, enhanced venous return increases EDV, stretching cardiac muscle fibers and increasing stroke volume (i.e., stroke work; Frank-Starling mechanism). Additionally, stroke volume can be increased by an increase in contractile state or ejection fraction (EF), which is the percentage of the EDV that actually leaves the ventricle during systole. EF is computed by the following:

$$EF = \left[\frac{SV}{EDV}\right] \times 100$$

Ejection fraction is normally 65% ± 8%. Increases in SV during exercise result from both the Frank-Starling mechanism and decreased ESV (Fig. 3-13). The latter is

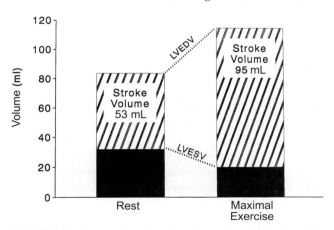

FIGURE 3-13. Changes in stroke volume from rest to maximal upright exercise is shown in young, healthy men. LVEDV, left ventricular end-diastolic volume; LVESV, left ventricular end-systolic volume. (Adapted with permission from Poliner LR, Dehmer GJ, Lewis SE, et al. Left ventricular performance in normal subjects: a comparison of the responses to exercise in the upright and supine position. *Circulation.* 1980;62:528–34.)

attributable to increased ventricular contractility, secondary to catecholamine-mediated sympathetic stimulation. The magnitude of these changes depends on several variables, including ventricular function, body position, and the intensity of exercise. Moreover, at a higher HR, SV may actually decrease because of the disproportionate shortening in diastolic filling time (Fig. 3-12).

CARDIAC OUTPUT

The product of SV and HR determines cardiac output. Cardiac output in healthy adults increases linearly with increased work rate, from a resting value of approximately 5 L·min^{-1} to a maximum of about 20 L·min^{-1} during upright exercise. However, maximum values of cardiac output depend on many factors, including age, posture, body size, presence of cardiovascular disease, and the level of physical conditioning. At exercise intensities up to 50% $\dot{V}O_{2max}$, the increase in cardiac output is facilitated by increases in HR and SV. Thereafter, the increase results almost solely from the continued increase in HR.

BLOOD FLOW

At rest, 15% to 20% of the cardiac output is distributed to the skeletal muscles; the remainder goes to the visceral organs, the heart, and the brain (44). With exercise, myocardial blood flow may increase four to five times; blood supply to the brain is maintained at resting levels. As much as 85% to 90% of the cardiac output is selectively delivered to working muscle and shunted away from the skin and the splanchnic, hepatic, and renal vascular beds. This redistribution of blood away from the visceral organs during exercise is caused by the sympathetic and hormonal (i.e., norepinephrine) influences on arterial smooth muscle and the resulting vasoconstriction. In active skeletal muscle, the exercise hyperemia is partly caused by local factors influenced by the increase in metabolism. Decreases in PO_2 and increases in norepinephrine and endothelial cell shear stress in the arterial intima cause the release of *nitric oxide*, which was formerly termed *endothelial-derived relaxing factor* (EDRF). Nitric oxide exerts a vasodilatory effect on arteries and arterioles that supply the working muscles. In addition, it appears that venules paired to arterioles may release EDRFs in response to ATP release from red blood cells (RBCs). These venular EDRFs diffuse to arterioles and influence vasodilation and, therefore, blood flow (44).

BLOOD PRESSURE

There is a linear increase in SBP with increasing levels of exercise, approximating 8 to 12 mm Hg per MET, where 1 MET = 3.5 mL O_2·kg^{-1}·min^{-1}. Maximal values typically reach 190 to 220 mm Hg (6). Nevertheless, maximal SBP should not be allowed to be greater than 250 mm Hg (6). Diastolic BP (DBP) may decrease slightly or remain unchanged; thus, pulse pressure (SBP minus DBP) generally increases in direct proportion to the intensity of exercise.

Because BP is directly related to cardiac output and peripheral vascular resistance, it provides a noninvasive way to monitor the contractile performance, or pumping capacity, of the heart (6). Until automated devices are adequately validated, the BP response to exercise should be taken manually with a cuff and a stethoscope (4). A SBP that fails to increase or decreases with increasing workloads may signal a plateau or decrease in cardiac output, respectively. Exercise testing should be terminated in persons demonstrating exertional hypotension (SBP toward the end of a test decreasing to less than baseline standing level or SBP decreasing 20 mm Hg or more during exercise after an initial increase). This response has been shown to correlate with myocardial ischemia, left ventricular dysfunction, and an increased risk of cardiac events during follow-up (29).

ARTERIOVENOUS OXYGEN DIFFERENCE (a-VO$_2$ DIFF)

Oxygen extraction by tissues reflects the difference between oxygen content of arterial blood (about 20 mL $O_2 \cdot 100^{-1}$ mL $\cdot$ dL^{-1} at rest) and the oxygen content of venous blood (about 15 mL $O_2 \cdot$ dL^{-1}), yielding a typical arteriovenous oxygen difference (CaO$_2$ − CvO$_2$) at rest of 5 mL $O_2 \cdot$ dL^{-1}. This approximates a use coefficient of 25%. During exercise to exhaustion, the mixed venous oxygen content typically decreases to 5 mL $\cdot$ dL^{-1} blood or lower, thus widening the arteriovenous oxygen difference from 5 to 15 mL $\cdot$ dL^{-1} blood, corresponding to a use coefficient of 75%.

PULMONARY VENTILATION

> **1.1.29-HFS: Knowledge of and ability to describe the physiological adaptations of the pulmonary system that occur at rest and during submaximal and maximal exercise following chronic aerobic and anaerobic training.**

Pulmonary ventilation ($\dot{V}_E$), the volume of air exchanged per minute, generally approximates 6 L$\cdot$min^{-1} at rest in the average sedentary adult man. At maximal exercise, however, $\dot{V}_E$ often increases 15- to 25-fold over resting values. During mild to moderate exercise intensities, $\dot{V}_E$ is increased primarily by increasing tidal volume, whereas increases in the respiratory rate are more important to augment $\dot{V}_E$ during vigorous exercise. For the most part, the increase in pulmonary ventilation is directly proportional to the increase in somatic oxygen consumed ($\dot{V}O_2$) and carbon dioxide produced ($\dot{V}CO_2$). However, at a critical exercise intensity (usually 47% to 64% of the $\dot{V}O_{2max}$ in healthy untrained individuals and 70% to 90% of the $\dot{V}O_{2max}$ in highly trained subjects), $\dot{V}_E$

increases disproportionately relative to $\dot{V}O_2$ paralleling the abrupt nonlinear increases in serum lactate and $\dot{V}CO_2$ (8,36). This suggests that pulmonary ventilation is perhaps regulated more by the requirement for carbon dioxide removal than by oxygen consumption and that ventilation is not normally a limiting factor to aerobic capacity. However, in highly trained male athletes exercising at high intensities (>80% $\dot{V}O_{2max}$), reductions in PaO$_2$ have been documented. Furthermore, female athletes have exhibited reduction in PaO$_2$, and the reductions began to occur at lower exercise intensities than with the male athletes. The exact mechanisms leading to the hypoxemic conditions are still being investigated. However, diffusion limitations, ventilation–perfusion inequalities, and limits to maximal flow rates may contribute to the occurrence of hypoxemia (42,58). With training, the ventilatory response to submaximal exercise may be reduced by approximately 25% for a given workload. With maximal exercise, maximal minute ventilation may increase up to 25% following training.

CARDIOVASCULAR DRIFT

Steady-state upright exercise is characterized by changes in cardiovascular response despite the constant work rate. SV and mean arterial pressure progressively decrease, and HR progressively increases. Traditionally, it was thought that the increase in HR may be attributed, at least in part, to alterations in sympathetic blood flow control mechanisms, increased shunting of blood to the periphery (skin) for cooling, and decreased central blood volume (particularly in warm environments). However, it now appears that there is not a strong association between cutaneous blood flow and SV. Rather, the decrease in SV results from increased HR whereby diastolic filling time and end-diastolic volume is reduced. Exercise during which dehydration occurs also contributes to cardiovascular drift, particularly if the dehydration leads to hypovolemia and hyperthermia. These conditions contribute to decreased SV and increased HR, respectively, thereby influencing the cardiovascular drift (18).

FACTORS INFLUENCING ACUTE CARDIORESPIRATORY RESPONSES TO EXERCISE

> **1.1.3-CES: Identify the cardiorespiratory responses associated with postural changes.**

> **1.1.6-CES: Knowledge of the unique hemodynamic responses of arm versus leg exercise, combined arm and leg exercise, and of static versus dynamic exercise.**

> **1.1.10-CES: Discuss the effects of isometric exercise in individuals with cardiovascular, pulmonary, and/or metabolic diseases.**

> **1.1.12-HFS: Ability to describe normal cardiorespiratory responses to static and dynamic exercise in terms of heart rate, stroke volume, cardiac output, blood pressure, and oxygen consumption.**

POSTURE

Posture has an effect on venous return and preload, particularly during brief bouts of physical exertion. At rest, EDV is highest when the body is recumbent. It decreases progressively as one shifts into sitting and standing postures. During exercise in the supine position, EDV remains largely unchanged. Thus, alterations in preload have little influence in increasing SV in this type of exercise. During exercise in the upright posture, EDV increases at intensities less than 50% $\dot{V}O_{2max}$. However, at higher exercise intensities, EDVs and SVs may decrease in some subjects (16).

DYNAMIC VERSUS STATIC EXERTION

> **1.1.26-HFS: Knowledge of the response of the following variables to acute static and dynamic exercise: heart rate, stroke volume, cardiac output, pulmonary ventilation, tidal volume, respiratory rate, and arteriovenous oxygen difference.**

Dynamic, or isotonic, activity (physical exertion characterized by rhythmic, repetitive movements of large muscle groups) results in increased oxygen consumption and HR that parallels the intensity of activity, as well as an increase in SV. There is a concomitant progressive increase in SBP with maintenance of or a slight decrease in DBP; thus, pulse pressure increases.

Blood is shunted from the viscera to working skeletal muscle, where increased oxygen extraction increases systemic a-vO_2 diff. Thus, dynamic exercise imposes a volume load on the myocardium, which is the basis for a cardiac training effect. In contrast, isometric or static exertion involves sustained muscle contraction against a fixed load or resistance with no change in length of the involved muscle group or joint motion. The cardiovascular response to isometric exertion is apparently mediated by a neurogenic mechanism (50). Activities that involve less than 20% of the maximum voluntary contraction (MVC) of the involved muscle group evoke a modest increase in SBP, DBP, and HR. During contractions greater than 20% of the MVC, HR increases in relation to the tension exerted, and there is an abrupt and precipitous increase in SBP. The SV remains essentially unchanged, except at high levels of tension (>50% MVC), where it may decrease. The result is a moderate increase in cardiac output, which is nevertheless high for the accompanying magnitude of increased metabolism. Despite the increased cardiac output, blood flow to the noncontracting muscle does not significantly increase, probably because of reflex vasoconstriction. The combination of vasocon-

TABLE 3-2. COMPARISON OF THE RELATIVE HEMODYNAMIC RESPONSES TO DYNAMIC AND STATIC EXERTION

	DYNAMIC (ISOTONIC)	STATIC (ISOMETRIC)
Cardiac output	+ + + +	+
Heart rate	+ +	+
Stroke volume	+ +	0
Peripheral resistance	−	+ + +
Systolic blood pressure	+ + +	+ + + +
Diastolic blood pressure	0−	+ + + +
Mean arterial pressure	0+	+ + + +
Left ventricular work	Volume load	Pressure load

+, increase; −, decrease; 0, unchanged.

striction and increased cardiac output causes a disproportionate increase in SBP, DBP, and mean BP. Thus, a significant pressure load is imposed on the heart, presumably to increase perfusion to the active (contracting) skeletal muscle. A comparison of the relative hemodynamic responses to dynamic and isometric exercise is shown in Table 3-2.

The magnitude of the pressor response to isometric exertion depends on tension exerted relative to the greatest possible tension in the muscle group, as well as muscle mass involved (50,54). Thus, a relatively mild isometric contraction by weakened upper extremities may evoke an excessive pressor response. The increased myocardial demands are camouflaged by the relatively low aerobic requirements, so the usual warning signs of overexertion (tachycardia, sweating, and dyspnea) may be absent. In persons who have impaired coronary blood flow, a marked pressure increase may lead to threatening ventricular arrhythmias, significant ST-segment depression, angina pectoris, ventricular decompensation, and in rare instances, sudden cardiac death (7).

ARM VERSUS LEG EXERCISE

At a fixed power output (kgm·min^{-1} or watts [W]), HR, SBP, DBP, rate–pressure product (HR times SBP), $\dot{V}_E$, $\dot{V}O_2$, respiratory exchange ratio, and blood lactate concentration are higher, and SV and AT (the latter expressed as a percentage of aerobic capacity) are lower during arm exercise than leg exercise (30). Because cardiac output is nearly the same in arm and leg exercise at a fixed oxygen uptake, elevated BP during arm exercise is believed to reflect increased peripheral vascular resistance. During maximal effort, physiological responses are usually greater during leg exercise than arm exercise, except when subjects are limited in their ability to perform leg work by neurological, vascular, or orthopedic impairment of the lower extremities (4,30).

The disparity in cardiorespiratory and hemodynamic response to arm exercise versus leg exercise at identical

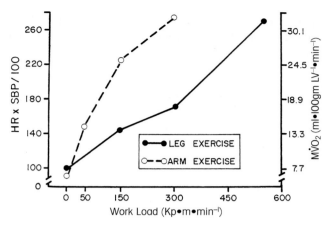

FIGURE 3-14. Mean rate–pressure product and estimated myocardial oxygen consumption (MV̇O₂) during arm (*broken line*) and leg (*solid line*) exercise. MV̇O₂ is estimated from its hemodynamic correlates, heart rate (HR) multiplied by systolic blood pressure (SBP). (Adapted with permission from Schwade J, Blomqvist CG, Shapiro W. A comparison of the response to arm and leg work in patients with ischemic heart disease. Am Heart J. 1977;94:203–8.)

work rates appears to be attributable to several factors. Mechanical efficiency (i.e., the ratio between the output of external work and caloric expenditure, or V̇O₂) is lower during arm exercise than leg exercise (30). This may reflect the involvement of smaller muscle groups and the static effort required with arm work, which increases V̇O₂ but does not affect the external work output. The higher rate–pressure product and estimated myocardial oxygen consumption at a fixed external work rate for arm work compared with leg work (Fig. 3-14) is believed to reflect increased sympathetic tone during arm exercise, perhaps mediated by reduced SV with compensatory tachycardia, concomitant isometric contraction, vasoconstriction in the nonexercising leg muscles, or all of these factors (66).

V̇O₂ₘₐₓ during arm exercise in men and women generally varies between 64% and 80% of leg V̇O₂ₘₐₓ (30). Similarly, maximal cardiac output is lower during arm exercise than leg exercise, and the maximal HR, SBP, and rate–pressure product are comparable or slightly lower during arm exercise. The latter, however, has relevance to arm exercise training recommendations, particularly training intensity. Accordingly, an arm exercise prescription that assumes a maximal HR equivalent to leg exercise testing may result in an overestimation of the training HR. As a general guideline, the prescribed HR for leg training should be reduced by approximately 10 bpm for arm training (4,30).

MAXIMAL OXYGEN CONSUMPTION

> **1.1.17-HFS: Knowledge of the physiological adaptations that occur at rest and during submaximal and maximal exercise following chronic aerobic and anaerobic exercise training.**

> **1.1.18-HFS: Knowledge of the differences in cardiorespiratory response to acute graded exercise between conditioned and unconditioned individuals.**

The most widely recognized measure of cardiopulmonary fitness is maximal oxygen consumption or V̇O₂ₘₐₓ. This variable is defined physiologically as the highest rate of oxygen transport and use that can be achieved at maximal physical exertion. Somatic oxygen consumption (V̇O₂) may be expressed mathematically by a rearrangement of the Fick equation:

$$\dot{V}O_2 = HR \times SV \times (\text{a-vO}_2 \text{ diff})$$

where

$\dot{V}O_2$ = oxygen consumption
(mL $O_2 \cdot kg^{-1} \cdot min^{-1}$)
HR = heart rate (bpm)
SV = stroke volume (mL·beat⁻¹)
(a-vO₂ diff) = arteriovenous oxygen difference

Thus, it is apparent that both central (i.e., cardiac output) and peripheral (i.e., arteriovenous oxygen difference) regulatory mechanisms affect the magnitude of body oxygen consumption.

Typical circulatory data at rest and during maximal exercise in a healthy, sedentary 30-year-old man and a similarly aged world-class endurance athlete are shown in Table 3-3. The absolute resting oxygen consumption (250

TABLE 3-3. HYPOTHETICAL CIRCULATORY DATA AT REST AND DURING MAXIMAL EXERCISE FOR A SEDENTARY MAN AND A WORLD-CLASS ENDURANCE ATHLETE: 30-YEAR-OLD SUBJECTS

CONDITION	OXYGEN CONSUMPTION (L·min⁻¹)	OXYGEN CONSUMPTION (mL·kg⁻¹·min⁻¹)	CARDIAC OUTPUT (L·min⁻¹)	HEART RATE (bpm)	STROKE VOLUME (mL·beat⁻¹)	ARTERIOVENOUS OXYGEN DIFFERENCE (mL·dL⁻¹ blood)
Sedentary man (70 kg)						
Rest	0.25	3.5	6.1	70	87	4.0
Maximal exercise	2.50	35.0	17.7	190	93	14.0
World-class endurance athlete (70 kg)						
Rest	0.25	3.5	6.1	45	136	4.0
Maximal exercise	5.60	80.0	35.0	190	184	16.0

mL·min^{-1}) divided by body weight (70 kg) gives the resting energy requirement, 1 MET (about 3.5 mL·kg^{-1}·min^{-1}). This expression of resting $\dot{V}O_2$ is extremely important in exercise physiology (14), independent of body weight and aerobic fitness. Furthermore, multiples of this value are often used to quantify respective levels of energy expenditure. For example, running at a 6-mph pace requires 10 times the resting energy expenditure; thus, the aerobic cost is 10 METs, or 35 mL O_2·kg^{-1}·min^{-1}.

The 10-fold increase in oxygen transport and use in the sedentary individual is contrasted by a 23-fold increase in the endurance athlete, corresponding to a $\dot{V}O_{2max}$ of 35 mL·kg^{-1}·min^{-1} and 80 mL·kg^{-1}·min^{-1}, respectively. Increased aerobic capacity in trained athletes appears primarily as the result of increased maximal cardiac output because of a greater increment in HR and SV rather than an increased peripheral extraction of oxygen. Because there is little variation in maximal HR and maximal systemic arteriovenous oxygen difference with training, $\dot{V}O_{2max}$ virtually defines the pumping capacity of the heart. Therefore, it is of major importance in the cardiovascular evaluation of the individual.

$\dot{V}O_{2max}$ may be expressed on an absolute or relative basis, that is, in liters per minute, reflecting total body energy output and caloric expenditure (i.e., 1 L = 5 kcal) or by dividing this value by body weight in kilograms. Because large persons usually have larger absolute oxygen consumptions by virtue of larger muscle mass, the latter allows a more equitable comparison between individuals of different body mass. This variable, when expressed as milliliters of oxygen per kilogram of body weight per minute or as METs, is widely considered the single best index of physical work capacity or cardiorespiratory fitness (4,8).

DETERMINATION OF THE MAXIMAL OXYGEN CONSUMPTION

 1.1.8-CES: Describe the methodology for measuring peak oxygen consumption (VO$_{2peak}$).

Maximal oxygen consumption is usually determined by measuring the volume and oxygen content of expired air, corrected to standard temperature and pressure dry (STPD), using the following equation:

$$\dot{V}O_2 = \dot{V}_E(F_IO_2 - F_EO_2)$$

where
  $\dot{V}_E$ = expired air (L·min^{-1})
  F_EO_2 = directly measured fraction oxygen in expired air
  F_IO_2 = directly measured fraction oxygen in inspired air (normally 0.2093)

Traditionally, $\dot{V}O_2$ has been measured using an open circuit or Douglas bag technique. However, automated systems are widely available to measure $\dot{V}O_2$ and related respiratory variables in real-time during exercise testing.

Because it is often inconvenient to measure the $\dot{V}O_{2max}$ directly, physiologists have sought to estimate aerobic capacity from the peak treadmill speed and grade, or cycle ergometer work rate, expressed as kilogram·meters per minute (also see Chapter 21 and GETP8 Chapter 5). The conventional Bruce protocol is perhaps the most familiar and widely used treadmill protocol with normative data on oxygen consumption so that aerobic capacity may be estimated from the workload attained (Fig. 3-15) (12). However, when a multistage protocol, such as the Bruce protocol, is used to predict the $\dot{V}O_{2max}$, aerobic capacity may be markedly overestimated (31). One recent advance in test methodology that can overcome many of the limitations of incremental exercise testing is ramping (57). Ramp protocols involve a nearly continuous and uniform increase in aerobic requirements that replaces the stage approach used in conventional exercise tests. With ramping, the gradual increase in demand allows for a steady increase in cardiopulmonary responses.

MYOCARDIAL OXYGEN CONSUMPTION

1.1.7-CES: Define the determinants of myocardial oxygen consumption (i.e., heart rate $\times$ systolic blood pressure = double product OR rate–pressure product) and the effects of acute exercise and exercise training on those determinants.

Determinants of myocardial oxygen consumption ($M\dot{V}O_2$) include HR, myocardial contractility, and the tension or stress developed in the ventricular wall. Wall tension reflects a combination of SBP and ventricular volume and is inversely related to myocardial wall thickness (Fig. 3-16). During exercise, increased HR is the major contributor to increased myocardial oxygen demand. In contrast, oxygen supply is primarily facilitated by increased coronary blood flow enabled by decreased coronary vascular resistance with only a modest increase in an already substantial myocardial oxygen difference.

Several investigators have reported excellent correlations between measured $M\dot{V}O_2$ (expressed as milliliters of oxygen per 100 g of left ventricle per minute) and HR and rate–pressure product, where $M\dot{V}O_2 = 0.28\,HR - 14$ (r = 0.88) or $M\dot{V}O_2 = ([0.14 \times HR \times SBP] / 100) - 6.3$ (r = 0.92) (48, 55). HR alone is limited in its ability to assess $M\dot{V}O_2$, especially when SBP is markedly elevated; this may occur during upper extremity work involving isometric or isodynamic efforts.

Exercise-induced angina and significant ST-segment depression ($\geq$1 mm) usually occur at the same rate–pressure product in an individual with ischemic heart

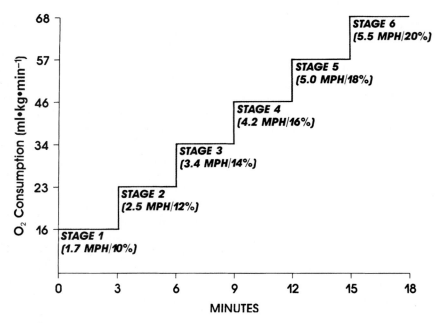

FIGURE 3-15. The standard Bruce treadmill protocol showing progressive stages (speed, percentage grade) and the corresponding aerobic requirement, expressed as mL·kg·min⁻¹.

disease. This suggests the existence of an ischemic threshold at which myocardial oxygen demand exceeds myocardial oxygen supply. The rate–pressure product also provides an estimate of maximal workload that the left ventricle can perform. It has been suggested that an adequate rate–pressure product during maximal exercise is greater than 25,000; however, this may be influenced by age, clinical status, and medications, especially β-blockers (4).

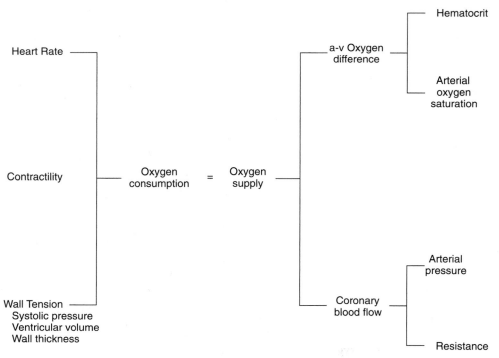

FIGURE 3-16. Determinants of myocardial oxygen demand and supply.

FACTORS AFFECTING THE ACUTE NEUROMUSCULAR RESPONSES TO RESISTANCE EXERCISE

Understanding the factors that affect acute resistance exercise stimuli is important in gaining insight into different resistance training protocols. Acute physiological changes are directly related to the configuration of external demands of resistance exercise, so resistance exercise protocols must be specific to the physiological systems targeted.

PHYSIOLOGY OF RESISTANCE EXERCISE

 1.1.23-HFS: Knowledge of the principles involved in promoting gains in muscular strength and endurance.

NEUROMUSCULAR ACTIVATION

The stimulus for muscle activation comes from a high-level central control command signal originating from the premotor cortex and the motor cortex. The signal is relayed through a lower-level controller (brainstem and spinal cord) and transformed into a specific motor unit activation pattern. To perform a specific task, the required motor units meet specific demands for force production by activating associated muscle fibers (22). Various feedback loops modify force production and provide communication to other physiological systems, such as the endocrine system. The high- and low-level commands can be modified by feedback from peripheral sensory or higher central command.

MOTOR UNIT ACTIVATION

 1.1.7-HFS: Knowledge of the stretch reflex and how it relates to flexibility.

The functional unit of the neuromuscular system is the **motor unit**. It consists of the motor neuron and the muscle fibers it innervates. Motor units range in size from a few to several hundred muscle fibers. Muscle fibers from different motor units can be anatomically adjacent to each other; therefore, a muscle fiber may be actively generating force while the adjacent fiber moves passively with no direct neural stimulation. When maximal force is required, all available motor units are activated. Another adaptive mechanism affected by heavy resistance training is the muscle force affected by different motor unit firing rates and frequencies.

Motor unit activation is also influenced by the **size principle**. This principle is based on the observed relationship between motor unit twitch force and recruitment threshold. Specifically, motor units are recruited in order according to recruitment thresholds and firing rates, resulting in a continuum of voluntary force. Whereas type I motor units are the smallest and possess the lowest recruitment thresholds, type IIa and IIb motor units are larger in size and have higher activation thresholds. Therefore, as force requirements of an activity increase, the recruitment order progresses from type I to IIa to IIb motor units. Thus, most muscles contain a range of motor units (type I and II fibers), and force production can span wide levels. Maximal force production requires not only the recruitment of all motor units, including high-threshold motor units, but also recruitment at a sufficiently high firing rate. It has been hypothesized that untrained individuals cannot voluntarily recruit the highest-threshold motor units or maximally activate muscles. Furthermore, electrical stimulation has been shown to be more effective in eliciting gains in untrained muscle or injury rehabilitation scenarios, suggesting further inability to activate all available motor units. Thus, training adaptation develops the ability to recruit a greater percentage of motor units when required.

Few exceptions to the size principle have been identified; however, some advanced weight lifters and other athletes may not require the order of recruitment stipulated by the size principle. It may be possible to inhibit low-threshold motor units yet activate high-threshold ones to enhance rate of force development and power production. This hypothesis emerged from observations during rapid, stereotyped movements and voluntary eccentric muscle action in humans. The central nervous system (CNS) can also limit force by engaging protective inhibitory mechanisms. For example, the Golgi tendon organs detect tension on the tendons from muscular contractions and elicit an inhibitory neuron response to limit muscular contraction. Training induced opposition of this inhibitory response may improve force production. Muscle spindles respond to stretch on the muscle. Rapid lengthening results in a contraction of the agonist muscle. This response is known as the stretch reflex and may be seen with dynamic or ballistic flexibility exercise. Thus, training may result in changes in fiber recruitment order or reduced inhibition, which assists in the performance of certain types of muscle actions.

MUSCLE FIBER TYPES

Several nomenclatures have been used to classify skeletal muscle fibers, including color (red or white), contraction speed (type II or type I), oxidative or glycolytic enzyme content (fast glycolytic, fast oxidative glycolytic, or oxidative), combination schemes (fast glycolytic), and myosin adenosine triphosphatase (ATPase) content (type I, IIa, IIb).

It is evident that exercise-induced changes in muscle have great plasticity (32,68). This is caused partly by a complex, yet readily adaptable group of contractile and regulatory proteins. Studies have focused on the myosin molecule and examination of fiber types. Fiber typing by myosin ATPase has been the most popular classification system (32,68). Figure 3-17 illustrates the continuum of

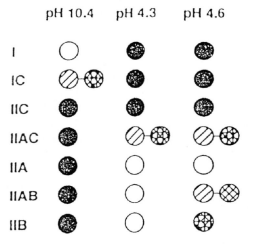

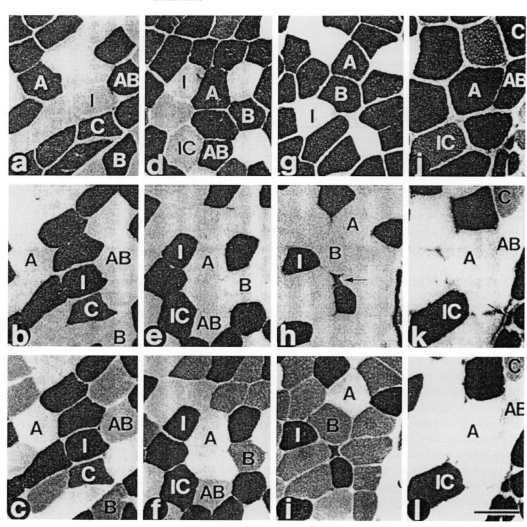

FIGURE 3-17. Myosin ATPase classification system. Staining profile and example fiber micrograph at 4.6 pH$^+$. (Courtesy of Robert Staron, Ohio University, Athens, OH.)

human muscle fiber types from the most oxidative (type I) to the least oxidative (type IIB) fibers.

Three major types of polypeptide chains, including a heavy chain and two types of light chains, constitute the myosin molecule. The complexity of the system allows for different expression of isomyosin forms with different heavy- and light-chain compositions. The differential myosin expression is of interest because it is related to muscle function and adaptation. A link between the myosin ATPase fiber type distribution and myosin heavy-chain content in skeletal muscle has been investigated by examining relationships for entire biopsy samples or single fibers. The relative percentage of myosin heavy chain (MHC I, MHC IIa, MHC IIb) is highly correlated with the corresponding percentage of muscle fiber types (I, IIA, IIB) in both men and women (32).

MUSCLE SORENESS

> **1.1.16-HFS: Knowledge of the common theories of muscle fatigue and delayed onset muscle soreness (DOMS).**

Muscle soreness may occur after an acute resistance training session. The exact mechanisms of muscle soreness remain speculative. Soreness is typically observed after excessively intense resistance training. It is most dramatic in relatively inexperienced or novice weightlifters. However, experienced weightlifters have soreness with novel exercise or excessive progression of intensity.

Several investigations demonstrate that eccentric exercise precipitates delayed-onset muscle soreness (DOMS). Eccentric contractions may damage the basic ultrastructure of the muscle cell. The focal point of the damage is the Z disk, a structural component that anchors the contractile protein actin.

The loss of structural integrity of the Z disks may be the stimulus leading to the associated symptoms. The appearance of DOMS ranges from 24 to 48 hours after exercise and may last up to 10 days. Symptoms of DOMS include local muscular stiffness, tenderness, local edema, limited range of motion caused by edema, and pain, which varies from low-grade ache to severe pain. Severity and location of discomfort specifically relate to the muscles used. The reason for increased soreness associated with eccentric training is unclear. However, one bout of eccentric exercise appears to result in protection from excessive soreness from another bout for up to 5 to 6 weeks in untrained or novice individuals. Thus, a slow progression in intensity is critical to limit soreness. It appears that excessive soreness develops from using resistance greater than the concentric one repetition maximum (1-RM).

HEMODYNAMIC RESPONSES TO ACUTE RESISTANCE EXERCISE

HEART RATE AND BLOOD PRESSURE

Heart rate and BP increase during dynamic resistance exercise using machines, free weights, or isokinetics. Peak BP response is higher during weight training in which a concentric and an eccentric phase occur than during isokinetic exercise (28). BP and heart rate may increase quite dramatically, with peak BPs of 320/250 mm Hg and heart rates of 170 bpm for a two-legged leg press at 95% of 1-RM to voluntary concentric failure with a Valsalva maneuver. HR and BP responses are also significant when the Valsalva maneuver is limited.

Peak BP and HR normally occur during the last several repetitions of a set to voluntary concentric failure. BPs are higher during sets at submaximal resistance to voluntary failure than at 1-RM. In dynamic resistance exercise, BP but not HR increases during the concentric rather than the eccentric portion of a repetition. In addition, BP increases with active muscle mass, but the increase is not linear (28).

STROKE VOLUME AND CARDIAC OUTPUT

Stroke volume (determined by electrical impedance) is not significantly elevated to more than resting during the **concentric** phase of resistance training exercise (with or without a Valsalva maneuver). However, during the **eccentric** phase, SV is significantly increased to more than resting (with or without a Valsalva maneuver) and is significantly greater than during the concentric phase of a repetition (28).

During both the concentric and eccentric phases of a repetition, cardiac output may be increased. For example, cardiac output during squatting exercise may increase to approximately 20 L during the eccentric phase but be only 15 L during the concentric phase. However, during exercise involving smaller muscle mass (e.g., knee extension), cardiac output may be elevated to more than resting only during the eccentric phase. The differing response between eccentric and concentric phases may result in no overall change from rest in mean cardiac output and SV during exercise involving a small muscle mass. Heart rate is not significantly different between the concentric and eccentric phases. Because SV is significantly greater during the eccentric than the concentric phase of a repetition, the higher cardiac output during the eccentric phase is caused by increased SV.

CALORIC COST OF RESISTANCE EXERCISE

The caloric cost of resistance exercise can be increased both during and after exercise. The caloric costs of an acute exercise session have been studied in a variety of protocols from single exercises to multiple exercise circuits. The caloric cost ranges from 14 to 75 kcal·kg^{-1}·day^{-1}. It appears that the caloric cost of resistance exercise is related to the amount of muscle mass activated (choice of exercises), the length of the rest period, the intensity of the exercise, and the ability to tolerate higher volumes of total work (28).

SUMMARY

The acute physiological stress of the neuromuscular system during resistance exercise is related to external demands. These demands are created by acute program variables that dictate the acute resistance exercise protocol. Careful consideration of these variables affecting the demands allows optimization of the exercise prescription for resistance exercise (see Chapter 29).

MECHANISMS OF MUSCULAR FATIGUE

> **1.1.24-HFS: Knowledge of muscle fatigue as it relates to mode, intensity, duration, and the accumulative effects of exercise.**

The causes of muscle fatigue has interested exercise scientists for more than a century, yet definitive fatigue agents have yet to be identified. **Muscle fatigue** is the loss of force or power output in response to voluntary effort leading to reduced performance. It is accepted that both central and peripheral fatigue factors contribute to fatigue. Whereas **central fatigue** is the progressive reduction in voluntary drive to motor neurons during exercise, **peripheral fatigue** is the loss of force and power that is independent of neural drive. The nature and extent of muscle fatigue clearly depend on the type, duration, and intensity of exercise, along with the fiber type composition of the muscle, individual fitness level, and environmental factors. For example, fatigue experienced in high-intensity, short-duration exercise depends on factors that differ from those precipitating fatigue in endurance activity. Similarly, fatigue during tasks involving heavily loaded contractions (e.g., weightlifting) probably differs from that produced during relatively unloaded movement (running and swimming). This section focuses primarily on muscle fatigue resulting from two general types of activity: short-duration, high-intensity exercise and longer duration, endurance exercise.

SHORT-DURATION, HIGH-INTENSITY EXERCISE

Fatigue during short-duration, high-intensity exercise may result from impairment anywhere along the chain of command from upper brain areas to contractile proteins (Fig. 3-18). Although the preponderance of evidence

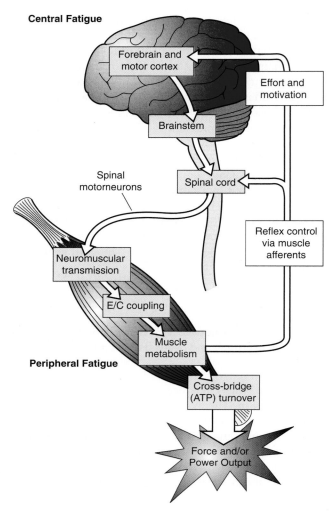

FIGURE 3-18. Chain of command for muscular contraction. Impairment along this pathway may be associated with fatigue. ATP, adenosine triphosphate; E/C, excitation–contraction.

suggests that a dysfunction within the muscle itself (peripheral mechanisms) is the most likely cause of fatigue under these circumstances, central deficits in motor drive (central mechanisms) may also occur.

PERIPHERAL MECHANISMS

During heavy exercise, the high level of anaerobic metabolism occurring results in decreases of ATP and CP and increases in the levels of hydrogen ion (H^{+}), Pi, ADP, and lactate. Theoretically, decreases in ATP level could contribute to fatigue because ATP supplies immediate energy for force generation in the muscles as well as provides for normal sodium–potassium pump and sarcoplasmic reticulum (SR) functioning. However, cell ATP concentration rarely decreases to less than 60% to 70% of the pre-exercise level, even in cases of extensive fatigue (11), and it is likely that fatigue produced by other factors reduces the ATP use rate before ATP becomes limiting (20,23).

Furthermore, the declines in CP concentration and tension during contractile activity follow different time courses, making a causal relationship between CP and fatigue unlikely (20).

Although the increase in ADP, Pi, and H^+ ions during intense contractile activity may cause fatigue by direct inhibition of ATP hydrolysis (26,27), the majority of evidence points to the effects of elevated H^+ (52). More specifically, H^+ appears to produce fatigue via the following mechanisms:

1. Inhibition of crossbridge actomyosin ATPase and ATP hydrolysis
2. Inhibition of phosphofructokinase and thus the glycolytic rate
3. Competitive inhibition of Ca^{2+} binding to troponin C, reducing crossbridge activation
4. Inhibition of the SR ATPase, reducing Ca^{2+} reuptake and subsequently Ca^{2+} release (67)
5. Increase of the threshold of free Ca^{2+} required for contraction, particularly in fast-twitch fibers (26,27)

As evidenced by the preceding discussion, the primary sites of fatigue are within the muscle and do not generally involve peripheral nerves or the neuromuscular junction (NMJ). The observation that fatigued muscles generate the same tension whether stimulated directly or by the motor nerve argues against NMJ fatigue. However, there are several possible sites within the excitation–contraction (E-C) coupling sequence of a muscle cell where disruptions during heavy exercise may induce fatigue. Specifically, the resting membrane potential is frequently altered, resulting in a reduced action potential (AP) amplitude and an increased AP duration that may ultimately effect Ca^{2+} release and contractile strength (11,27).

CENTRAL MECHANISMS

The possibility that specific brain mechanisms can reduce the magnitude of descending motor drive has received the least attention as a possible mediator of muscular fatigue even though willingness to maintain central motor drive (e.g., willingness to maintain a maximal effort) probably contributes to fatigue in most people during activities of daily life. It has been postulated that because failure to produce the necessary force during fatigue is usually preceded by increased perceived effort, the CNS processes are at least as likely to contribute to fatigue as are those that lie within the muscle (23,27).

During fatiguing contractions, there is inhibition of central motor drive (9,27,70). Using a technique called transcranial magnetic stimulation (TMS) (38), it has been shown that the electrical stimulus reaching the muscle after magnetic stimulation of the motor cortex (motor-evoked potential) is suppressed after fatiguing exercise. Furthermore, a prolonged silent period after TMS has been demonstrated (9). These changes are not influenced by muscle afferent feedback and can result from altered voluntary drive to the motor cortex as well as intrinsic cortical processes (9,70). The genesis of central fatigue may involve inadequate neural drive by the motor cortex at the highest levels of the brain.

ENDURANCE EXERCISE

Numerous factors have been linked to fatigue resulting from prolonged endurance activity, including depletion of muscle and liver glycogen, decreases in blood glucose, dehydration, and increases in body temperature. Undoubtedly, each of these factors contributes to fatigue to a varying degree, the relative importance depending on environmental conditions and the nature of the activity. Mechanisms that involve various neurotransmitters and neuromodulators have also recently been proposed to explain possible CNS involvement in fatigue during prolonged exercise. This section reviews some of these factors. In particular, carbohydrate depletion, alterations in SR function, and increased brain serotonin are discussed.

GLYCOGEN DEPLETION

It has long been suggested that the rate of carbohydrate use depends on the intensity of work. This belief was based on the observation that the respiratory exchange ratio (RER) increases from rest to exercise. The early theories have been confirmed by direct measurements of glycogen use at different work intensities. The rate of body carbohydrate usage depends not only on intensity but also on the state of fitness. At a fixed workload, trained individuals have lower RERs, deplete glycogen more slowly, and can work longer than untrained individuals (8,36). High-carbohydrate diets and ingestion of carbohydrate drinks during exercise can delay fatigue by increasing the availability and oxidation of carbohydrates. These observations support the hypothesis that depletion of carbohydrate stores causes muscular fatigue during endurance activity. However, the exact mechanism is not known. Low muscle glycogen concentration may reduce NADH production and electron transport, drain intermediates of the Krebs cycle, or reduce fat oxidation, the effects of which would be to inhibit ATP production and cause fatigue (8).

It is also possible that central fatigue occurs in conjunction with carbohydrate depletion during prolonged exercise. Carbohydrate ingestion throughout exercise may attenuate the onset of negative CNS changes involving serotonin (discussed in more detail later in this section). However, the effects of carbohydrate feedings on central fatigue mechanisms and the well-established beneficial effects on the contracting muscle are difficult to distinguish. It seems apparent that future efforts should focus on the mechanisms by which glycogen depletion causes fatigue.

OTHER FACTORS

Glycogen depletion is probably not an exclusive fatigue factor during endurance exercise. Other potential candidates include disruption of important intracellular organelles, such as the mitochondria, the SR, or the myofilaments (27). The role of mitochondrial damage in fatigue is controversial (53).

The contractile proteins and, particularly, myofibril ATPase activity appear relatively resistant to change with endurance exercise (53). Ca^{2+} uptake by the SR vesicles, however, is depressed in the slow- and fast-twitch red region of the vastus lateralis, which suggests uncoupling of the transport or a leaky membrane, allowing Ca^{2+} flux back into the intracellular fluid. In addition to these functional changes, it has been demonstrated that exhaustive endurance exercise structurally damages the SR (69). The exact nature of this change and its effect on muscle function has not been elucidated.

In one study, a prolonged swim produced a significant decrease in glycogen concentration in slow type I, fast type IIA, and fast type IIB fibers of muscles, but the type IIB fibers exhibited no fatigue and no change in any of the contractile or biochemical properties measured (53). The apparent explanation is that the type IIB (fast white glycolytic) fiber is recruited less frequently during endurance activity, but glycogen use is similar to other fiber types despite fewer total contractions. It is apparent that muscle fatigue during endurance activity is somehow related to the degree of muscle use and is not entirely dependent on glycogen depletion.

In some cases, fatigue is characterized by a period of prolonged recovery during which force may be depressed for days. This low-frequency fatigue (LFF) (13) is caused by disruption of the E-C coupling process, perhaps because of excessive production of reactive oxygen species or prolonged exposure to high levels of intracellular Ca^{2+} (1,72).

The long recovery period after LFF may be related to the time required for refolding of damaged proteins or the replacement of degraded proteins (72). Protein degradation could produce swelling and thus lead to muscle soreness. The time course of recovery from muscle soreness (i.e., days) exceeds that observed for most forms of fatigue but correlates well with recovery from LFF and reflects the time required to synthesize new muscle proteins.

Of the many proposed causes of central fatigue during prolonged exercise, the role of brain serotonin has generated the most interest. A review of the mechanisms involved in the control of brain serotonin synthesis and turnover at rest and during exercise (Fig. 3-19), along with its well-known influence on depression, sleepiness, mood, and pain, make it a particularly attractive candidate (10).

Concentrations of serotonin and 5-hydroxyindole acetic acid (5-HIAA) (a major metabolite) increase in several brain regions during prolonged exercise and peak at fatigue (35,71). The administration of serotonin agonist and antagonist drugs decreases and increases, respectively, run times to fatigue in the absence of any apparent peripheral markers of muscle fatigue (35).

SUMMARY

Both CNS and muscle mechanisms are likely to contribute to fatigue. After short-duration, high-intensity exercise, recovery in force production usually occurs in two components that are probably caused by separate mechanisms: (a) a rapidly reversible non–H^+-mediated perturbation, perhaps related to changes in E-C coupling and (b) a slower change that is probably mediated by H^+ and Pi. Reduction in central motor drive that occurs at the highest levels of the brain can also accompany fatigue, but this aspect is much less well studied, and the mechanisms have not been elucidated.

In prolonged endurance exercise, the depletion of skeletal muscle carbohydrate stores frequently occurs, and it appears that muscle glycogen depletion is an important factor in fatigue. Additionally, minimal levels of muscle glycogen metabolism may be important in maintaining essential Krebs cycle intermediates. Undoubtedly, other factors are involved because muscle glycogen depletion can exist without fatigue and vice versa. Disruption of muscle protein, particularly the E-C coupling complex, has been shown to be associated with LFF. This process may be mediated by elevated levels of reactive oxygen species (free radicals) or intracellular Ca^{2+}. Increased brain serotonin metabolism has also been implicated in central fatigue under these circumstances.

ENVIRONMENTAL CONSIDERATIONS: HEAT AND COLD

> **1.1.12-CES: Describe the effects of variation in environmental factors (e.g., temperature, humidity, altitude) for normal individuals and those with cardiovascular, pulmonary, and metabolic diseases.**

The prevailing thermal environment can profoundly change the physiological response to exercise and increase the risk of an environment-related disorder. In healthy individuals, a limited core temperature range (36.1 to 37.8°C) is maintained. With this narrow temperature range, an understanding of the interrelationships between thermal environment and exercise allows better management of risk for heat or cold disorders during exercise. The physiological response to heat and cold are different, and the disorders associated with these two stressors differ fundamentally. This chapter presents the interaction between the environment and exercise and disorders that may occur. See the ACSM position stands for detailed information about environmental stressors (2,3,5).

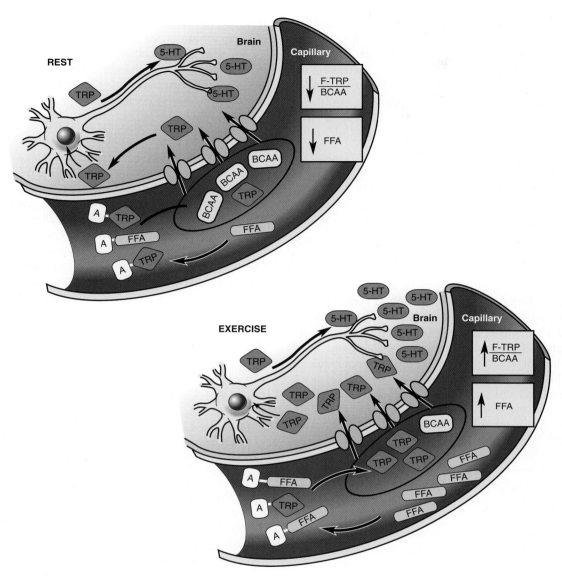

FIGURE 3-19. An illustration of the mechanisms involved in the control of brain serotonin synthesis and turnover at rest and during exercise. The well-known influence of these mechanisms on depression, sleepiness, mood, and pain make this a likely candidate for a center of fatigue. BCAA, branched chain amino acid; TRP, tryptophan; 5-HT, 5-hydroxytryptamine; FFA, free fatty acids.

HEAT STRESS

Heat stress is the combination of environmental conditions, metabolic rate, and clothing that increases core temperature. The traditional approach to the study and assessment of heat stress is to describe the balance that must be achieved between all sources of heat gain and heat loss. If a balance cannot be achieved, risk of excessive core temperature increases. A basic understanding of heat exchange is necessary to appreciate the interactions of environment, exercise, and clothing. The risk of a serious heat-related disorder is associated with the level of heat stress, and control of risk is based on maintaining health and managing exposure to heat stress (see Box 34-11).

Comprehensive risk reduction strategies to prevent heat related injury and illness include (a) scheduling activities to avoid extremely hot and humid conditions; (b) individual heat acclimatization with gradual increases in work stress for at least 10–14 days; (c) monitoring of participants performing physical activity for signs and symptoms of heat strain, because early recognition is key in preventing event severity; and (d) a careful monitoring of fluid replacement strategies (2,3).

HEAT BALANCE

The major source of heat gain is internal heat generated by energy metabolism. Approximately 25% of metabolic energy expenditure is actually translated to mechanical work during locomotion (i.e., walking, biking); the remaining 75% is released as heat in contracting muscles. As the metabolic rate increases to meet increasing demands of exercise, the rate of internal heat generation also increases. The rate of energy expenditure can be estimated using tables or equations (3). An average man (73 kg) walking on a level surface at 1.6 m·s⁻¹ (3.5 mph) has a metabolic rate of about 350 W.

SWEAT EVAPORATIVE COOLING

The major avenue of heat loss is evaporation of sweat from the skin surface. Evaporative cooling by secreting water onto the skin surface through the eccrine sweat glands is one response to heat stress. As water absorbs heat from the skin, it changes from liquid to vapor. Surrounding air carries the vapor away. Because the heat of vaporization is quite high, small amounts of sweat remove relatively large amounts of heat. Specifically, the evaporation of 0.5 L of sweat per hour is sufficient to remove the 350 W of excess heat in the preceding walking example.

If sufficient volumes of sweat are produced quickly enough and evaporation is not impeded, thermal balance is maintained and core temperature does not increase. However, this scenario may not occur for several reasons. First, there are physiological limits to sweat evaporation. In the short term, it is not reasonable to expect a sustained sweat rate of more than 1 L·h⁻¹. In the long term (several hours), the rate of evaporation may be reduced by dehydration (2).

The physiological limit to volume of sweat produced varies by state of acclimation, by aerobic fitness, and genetically among individuals (2,3). Acclimation (also known as acclimatization) is a physiological adjustment that occurs naturally in conjunction with repeated exposures to exercise performed in a different environment. Acclimation to a heat environment increases rate of sweating, shortens onset time, and conserves sodium. Resulting benefits include reduced cardiovascular strain and lower core temperature for the same level of heat stress. Most improvement occurs over the initial 3 to 5 days, with smaller additional improvements over the subsequent 2 to 7 days (3). As a rule, 1 day of acclimation is lost for every 3 days away from exercise in heat stress, or in the case of illness, 1 day is lost per day of illness. Aerobic fitness is the single best indicator of a person's ability to tolerate heat stress.

Second, the physical limits to rate of evaporative cooling are caused by environmental conditions and clothing (2,3). The primary drive for evaporative cooling is the difference in water vapor pressures on the skin and in the air. If the difference is small, the rate of evaporative cooling decreases; if the difference is large, the evaporation rate can be sufficient to balance even high rates of metabolic heat production. Water vapor pressure on the skin is relatively constant. The vapor pressure of water in air is the primary source of differences in environmental con-

tribution to heat stress. It is for this reason that humidity is an important factor in heat stress. Air movement also modifies the rate of evaporative cooling. If air movement is 2 to 3 m·s⁻¹ (4–6 mph), the maximum rate of evaporative cooling is achieved; higher speeds do not appreciably increase evaporative cooling (46).

CLOTHING

Clothing further restricts the maximum rate of evaporative cooling. Clothing between skin and the environment decreases the possibility of evaporation caused by the absorption of sweat or the prevention of vapor passage (3,46). Under some circumstances, the effect of clothing is negligible. For example, if the air is very dry (low humidity) or if the metabolic rate is low, the rate of sweat evaporation through clothing is sufficient to allow adequate cooling. The resistance of clothing to sweat evaporation depends on surface area covered, nature of the fabric, number of layers, and construction of the ensemble. The following are important to minimize the effect of clothing:

- The covered surface area should be as small as is reasonable.
- The fabric should be lightweight open weave or other material that freely allows water vapor to pass through.
- Trapped air spaces from multiple layers should be minimized.
- The construction should be loose, with openings to allow easy movement of air around and through the clothing.

At the other extreme is clothing that covers most of the body; is impermeable to water vapor (e.g., plastic or rubber rain clothing); and is tightly fitting around openings for arms, legs, and head. Little evaporative cooling can occur in a person wearing this type of clothing.

CONVECTION AND RADIATION

Other factors that modify overall heat stress are convection and radiation. When the air temperature is greater than skin temperature (nominally 35°C or 95°F), heat is added by convection. Conversely, when air temperature is lower than 35°C, some heat is lost by convection. The rate of convection is enhanced by air movement and reduced by clothing insulation. Whereas infrared radiation from the sun and warm or hot surfaces increase heat stress, cool surfaces reduce heat stress. Clothing insulation reduces rate of heat flow (in either direction) by radiation. Convection and radiation combined usually account for less than 20% of either heat gain or heat loss during exercise.

PHYSIOLOGICAL RESPONSE

The physiological response to heat stress is reflected in body temperature, HR, and sweating. Metabolic heat increases the temperature of working muscles, and circulating blood transports heat to the central organs, causing an increase in core temperature. Additional blood flow carries excess heat to the skin. To move heat from working muscles to the skin, cardiac output increases and blood flow is shunted from the splanchnic and renal circulation.

HEAT-RELATED DISORDERS

The normal and acceptable response to heat stress includes elevated core temperature, increased HR, and water loss caused by sweating. Left unchecked, however, these responses may lead to heat-related disorders and decrements in psychomotor and cognitive performance. The disorders of particular importance during exercise are the following:

- Heat cramps
- Heat syncope
- Dehydration

- Heat exhaustion
- Heat stroke

Box 3-1 lists these disorders and describes signs, symptoms, and first aid. It is important for exercise professionals to understand these features of heat disorders. Preventive measures are described next.

HEAT CRAMPS AND SYNCOPE

Heat cramps are most likely to occur during or after sustained exercise with profuse sweating. Cramps usually appear in fatigued calf or abdominal muscles. Heat syncope may result from dehydration or excessive pooling of blood in peripheral vascular beds. The consequent hypotension may cause familiar blackout symptoms. Recovery is relatively quick, and most people are generally aware of the occurrence. In addition to adequate hydration and maintaining salt balance, risk of syncope can be reduced by avoiding prolonged standing or rapid transition to standing.

BOX 3-1 HEAT-RELATED DISORDERS, INCLUDING SYMPTOMS, SIGNS, AND FIRST AID

Disorder	Symptoms	Signs	First Aid
Heat cramps	Painful muscle cramps, especially in abdominal or fatigued muscles	Incapacitating pain in voluntary muscles	Rest in cool environment Drink salted water (0.5% salt solution) Massage muscles
Heat syncope	Blurred vision (gray out) Fainting (brief blackout)	Brief fainting or near fainting Normal temperature	Lie on back in cool environment Drink water
Dehydration	No early symptoms Fatigue, weakness Dry mouth	Loss of work capacity Increased response time	Fluid and salt replacement
Heat exhaustion	Fatigue Weakness Blurred vision Dizziness, headache	High pulse rate Profuse sweating Low blood pressure Insecure gait Pale face Collapse Body temperature normal to slightly increased	Lie flat on back in cool environment Drink water Loosen clothing
Heat stroke	Chills Restlessness Irritability	Red face Euphoria Shivering Disorientation Erratic behavior Collapse Unconsciousness Convulsions Body temperature >40°C (104°F)	Immediate, aggressive, effective cooling Transport to the hospital

DEHYDRATION AND HEAT EXHAUSTION

Dehydration and heat exhaustion are most likely to occur in unacclimated people and in those who do not drink enough or ignore early warning signs. In competitive sports, a 5% loss of body weight is not unusual (2). Losses greater than 1.5% should be followed by a period of recovery and rehydration. The ACSM Position Stand on Exercise and Fluid Replacement (2) provides comprehensive guidelines for fluid replacement to sustain appropriate hydration during physical activity.

HEAT STROKE

Heat stroke is a medical emergency, and the least suspicion that it may be present justifies an immediate and aggressive response. The risk of heat stroke is greatest among those who abuse alcohol or drugs, who are highly motivated and ignore symptoms of heat exhaustion, who are heat intolerant (i.e., do not acclimate), or who have poor physical fitness.

COLD STRESS

Cold stress is the combination of environment, metabolic rate, and clothing that results in heat loss from the core as a whole or from local areas (5,45). The physiological and/or psychological consequences of cold stress are referred to as cold strain (5). Cold-related disorders include hypothermia and varying degrees of local tissue damage (5). Again, control of cold stress is accomplished through comprehensive management of risk factors. Specifically, the ACSM recommends the use of a risk management strategy that "a) identifies/assesses the cold hazards; b) identifies/assesses contributing factors for cold-weather injuries; c) develops controls to mitigate cold stress/strain; d) implements controls into formal plans; and e) utilizes administrative oversight to ensure controls are enforced and modified." For detailed advice on these parameters, the reader should start with the ACSM Position Stand on Prevention of Cold Injuries during Exercise (5).

HEAT BALANCE

Similar to heat stress, cold stress is described as an imbalance between heat gained from metabolism and heat lost to the environment by convection, radiation, evaporation, and conduction (5). The problem, however, is net loss rather than net gain.

The sole source of heat gain during cold stress is metabolic heat released during muscular work along with basal biological processes. As exercise demands increase, the rate of heat gain from metabolism increases. If the rate of metabolic heat decreases because of fatigue or changes in demand, a disorder is more likely (5,45). Re-

search on the effect of cold exposure on metabolism and substrate use during exercise has produced inconsistent findings (45). Future research must control the variety of factors that may exert influence on metabolism and substrate use in the cold, including duration and intensity of exercise imposed, training (fitness) status and cold acclimatization of the subjects, duration and intensity of resting pre-exercise cold exposure to cold conditions, duration and intensity of cold exposure during exercise, and the insulating effects of clothing (45).

HEAT LOSS

Heat is lost primarily by convection resulting from the difference between skin and ambient temperature (5). The rate of convection increases with air movement from wind (see Box 34-12) or motion through the air (e.g., cycling or running). Sitting or lying on a cold, solid surface may cause heat loss by conduction. Cyclic exercise and rest in which heat accumulates and the person sweats under clothing may be associated with heat loss through evaporation. Additional loss by radiant heat flow to colder surfaces is also possible.

CLOTHING

Proper clothing is the primary mechanism for achieving thermal balance during cold stress (5,45). The amount of insulation that clothing affords is described in units called *clo*. A wool business suit has an insulating value of approximately 1 clo. Generally, each quarter inch of clothing adds 1 clo of insulation. Figure 3-20 illustrates the relations among air temperature, metabolic rate, and clothing in maintaining thermal balance (5). The insulating quality of clothing decreases precipitously when it becomes wet.

Sometimes clothing is sufficient to protect from hypothermia, but exposed skin is still at risk for excessive local cooling. The major method of heat loss is convection, but conduction via contact with cold objects can also occur. Adequate heating from circulating blood may

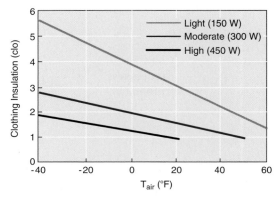

FIGURE 3-20. Relationship between air temperature and adequate clothing insulation for three levels of exercise. W, Watts

not be available because of reductions in peripheral blood flow (vasoconstriction) that naturally occur as a mechanism for heat conservation.

COLD-RELATED DISORDERS

Normal physiological response to cold stress is directed toward heat conservation, decreasing peripheral circulation, and increasing metabolic rate. These mechanisms, however, are not adequate for most cold stress, and behavioral thermal regulation is crucial for preventing cold-related disorders. Cold-related disorders can be systemic or local. Box 3-2 is a list of some common cold-related disorders along with symptoms, signs, and steps for first aid (5).

SYSTEMIC COLD

The systemic cold disorder is hypothermia. Mild cases are marked by shivering and cold sensation in the extremities. Progression is associated with unstable cardiac function followed by CNS depression. Mild cases can be addressed by simple first aid, but moderate to severe hypothermia requires medical attention. As previously stated, hypothermia is best prevented by employing a comprehensive risk management strategy as detailed in the ACSM position stand (5).

LOCAL DISORDERS

Acute local disorders are associated with local tissue freezing (frostbite) or cooling (frost nip and trench foot). Frostbite can occur only when ambient temperature is less than −1°C (30°F): it is marked by actual crystallization of water in tissue and subsequent destruction of cells. Because of the risk of further complications, significant cases of frostbite should be referred to medical personnel. Frost nip and trench foot are skin disorders that result from extreme cooling of the skin and underlying tissue, but without actual freezing of water in the tissue. The distinguishing characteristic between frost nip and trench foot is the presence of damp clothing that has accelerated heat loss. Predisposing factors for cold injuries and frostbite include the environmental, mechanical, physiological, and psychological domains (5).

SUMMARY

Environmental stressors such as heat and cold can significantly affect exercise and can be dangerous if uncontrolled. Adequate preventive precautions for both heat and cold are possible and should be known by exercise professionals. Situations that require medical attention are fairly common, and immediate referral of such problems is important.

BOX 3-2 COLD-RELATED DISORDERS, INCLUDING SYMPTOMS, SIGNS, AND FIRST AID

Disorder	Symptoms	Signs	First Aid
Hypothermia	Chills Fatigue or drowsiness Pain in the extremities	Euphoria Slurred speech Slow, weak pulse Shivering Collapse or unconsciousness Body core temperature ≤35°C (95°F)	Move to warm area and remove wet clothing Modest external warming Drink warm fluids containing carbohydrates Transport to the hospital
Frostbite	Burning sensation at first Coldness, numbness, tingling	Skin color white or grayish yellow to reddish violet to black Blisters Response to touch depends on depth of freezing	Move to warm area and remove wet clothing External warming (e.g., warm water) Drink warm fluids containing carbohydrates if conscious Treat as a burn; do not rub affected area Transport to the hospital
Frost nip	Possible itching or pain	Skin turns white	Similar to that for frostbite
Trench foot	Severe pain Tingling, itching	Edema Blisters Response to touch depends on depth of cooling	Similar to that for frostbite

EXERCISE AND THE ENVIRONMENT: ALTITUDE AND AIR POLLUTION

> **1.7.16-HFS: Knowledge of special precautions and modifications of exercise programming for participation at altitude, different ambient temperatures, humidity, and environmental pollution.**

The condition of ambient air, which is inhaled into the lungs for respiratory gas exchange, has great importance for exercise capacity, physiological performance, and general health. This section discusses two main characteristics of ambient air: density, which changes with altitude, and contaminants, generally referred to as air pollution. It is necessary to be aware of hazards because exposure to altitude and polluted air can have profound effects on physical performance and can cause serious illnesses, even in well-trained individuals.

HIGH TERRESTRIAL ALTITUDE

Considerable evidence indicates that altitude training in preparation for competition at altitude is beneficial; therefore, many athletes spend considerable resources training at altitude. However, the value of this training for increasing performance at sea level is controversial. The lack of consensus may be attributed to differences in duration of exposure to altitude, elevations of training, initial fitness levels, and lack of a control group (25). Recent studies indicate that under specific conditions, intermittent altitude exposure may have some beneficial effects for sea-level performance (49,65). In this section, physiological responses that occur at altitudes up to 3,000 m (11,800 feet) are discussed. Above 3,000 m, the negative effects of prolonged exposure to hypoxia outweigh any positive training effects (47).

PHYSIOLOGICAL RESPONSES

The amount of oxygen bound to hemoglobin in RBCs depends on the partial pressure of oxygen in the inspired air (P_{IO_2}). P_{IO_2} decreases as a result of declines in barometric pressure with increasing altitude at a constant oxygen percentage (Table 3-4). There is a decrease in the arterial

oxygen saturation (Pa_{O_2}) with the decline in P_{IO_2} and, thus, in the amount of oxygen available. Acute exposure to reduced oxygen saturation triggers several compensatory mechanisms to increase oxygen transfer to tissue. After these acute reactions, acclimation occurs with more fundamental adaptations.

ACUTE PHYSIOLOGICAL RESPONSES

One of the most significant physiological compensatory reactions during acute exposure above 1,200 m is increased pulmonary ventilation, or **hypoxic ventilatory response**, at rest and during exercise. Chemoreceptors in arterial blood vessels are stimulated, and signals are sent to the brain to increase ventilation. The increase in pulmonary ventilation is primarily associated with an increase in tidal volume, but with prolonged exposure or higher altitude, breathing frequency also increases. Hyperventilation substantially increases the arterial oxygen saturation. Increased ventilation also leads to washout of carbon dioxide in the blood. Therefore, uncompensated respiratory alkalosis (higher pH) may develop. This respiratory alkalosis can cause a left shift of the oxygen–hemoglobin dissociation curve, resulting in higher arterial oxygen saturation, a second compensatory mechanism. Finally, early in exposure to altitude, reduced oxygen pressure is compensated for by small increases in cardiac output. This is primarily due to an increased HR, which occurs because SV is constant or even slightly reduced at rest and during submaximal and maximal exercise.

Despite acute responses that compensate for lower oxygen tension at altitude, arterial oxygen saturation is decreased (Fig. 3-21). The magnitude of desaturation is directly related to altitude and exercise intensity. The primary pulmonary factor leading to increasing desaturation with increasing exercise intensity is limited alveolar end capillary diffusion. The result is an almost linear decrease

TABLE 3-4. BAROMETRIC PRESSURE FOR A STANDARD ATMOSPHERE AND INSPIRED PARTIAL OXYGEN PRESSURE FOR FIVE ALTITUDES, ACCOUNTING FOR THE PRESSURE OF WATER VAPOR IN THE LUNGS (47 mm Hg)

ALTITUDE (m)	BAROMETRIC PRESSURE (mm Hg)	INSPIRED OXYGEN PRESSURE (mm Hg)
0	760	149
1500	627	123
2000	596	115
2500	627	107
3000	522	100

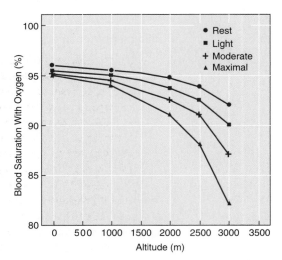

FIGURE 3-21. Effect of altitude and exercise levels on arterial oxygen saturation.

of maximal oxygen uptake at a ratio of 10% per 1,000 m altitude above 1,500 m (33). Because the oxygen uptake required by a fixed submaximal workload is not affected by altitude, the result is a higher relative exercise intensity for any given workload. Because of the nonlinear relationship between relative intensity (percentage of maximal oxygen uptake) and endurance time, the magnitude of the performance decrement at altitude is not constant but varies in proportion to the duration of the activity. Therefore, the longer the running distance, the larger the relative decrement (33).

Muscular strength and muscular endurance seem unaffected during acute exposure to altitude. However, subtle neuropsychological effects associated with acute mountain sickness (AMS) can occur at altitudes of 3,000 m within 6 hours of exposure. Above 4,500 m, the deterioration in most mental functions may be considerable, although variations between individuals are large (19). These neuropsychological effects may, in turn, affect muscular strength and endurance.

HIGH-ALTITUDE ILLNESS

Exposure to high altitude can lead to a number of illnesses that vary in seriousness. The speed of ascent and the absolute altitude are primary determinants of the incidence of altitude illness. Those exercising in or exposed to altitude (athletes and coaches) should anticipate the hazards and prepare through prevention and recognition of symptoms.

ACUTE MOUNTAIN SICKNESS

Acute mountain sickness is characterized by severe headache and often accompanied by nausea, vomiting, decreased appetite, weariness, and sleep disturbances (41,51). AMS begins 6 to 12 hours after arrival, usually peaks on the second or third day, and disappears on the fourth or fifth day. AMS normally appears above 2,500 m, and the frequency of AMS increases with altitude and rate of ascent. Generally, above 3,000 m, 24 hours of acclimation should be acquired for every 300-m altitude gain (41). Although AMS is self-limiting, persistence of symptoms may require medical treatment. If AMS is not at least partially resolved within 2 to 3 days, descent is the only effective treatment. Supplemental oxygen and pharmacological treatment (acetazolamide, furosemide, and analgesics) may be necessary for severe cases.

HIGH-ALTITUDE PULMONARY EDEMA

High-altitude pulmonary edema (HAPE) is considered a progression in the severity of AMS, associated with pulmonary edema (41). The onset may be subtle. Signs and symptoms include dyspnea, fatigue, chest pain, tachycardia, coughing, and cyanosis of the lips and extremities.

As HAPE progresses, affected individuals may cough frothy or blood-tinged sputum (51). This complication can be fatal if not treated promptly. Children and young adults are at higher risk of developing HAPE than adults, and immediate medical attention is necessary. Evacuation to a lower altitude is essential. Individuals with a history of HAPE appear to be particularly susceptible to subsequent bouts upon return to high altitudes.

HIGH-ALTITUDE CEREBRAL EDEMA

High-altitude cerebral edema (HACE) may develop when the rate of ascent is too fast. The signs and symptoms of HACE include severe headache, fatigue, vomiting, nausea, ataxia, and changes of mental status (51). The incidence of HACE is low (1%), but it can be fatal if untreated. In cases of symptoms of cerebral edema, direct medical care with immediate evacuation to a low altitude and supplemental oxygen is recommended (41).

PREVENTING ALTITUDE SICKNESS

Acute mountain sickness can be prevented by adjusting the amount and rate of ascent. Options include an interrupted ascent with time (days) to acclimate at successive altitudes before reaching the final elevation or limiting daily gain in altitude to 300 m or less. Initially, unacclimated subjects should avoid vigorous exercise. Adequate hydration and a high-carbohydrate diet may aid prevention. Acetazolamide is the only drug for altitude sickness approved by the U.S. Food and Drug Administration (FDA). Because acetazolamide may affect exercise performance, it is contraindicated when training at high altitudes. Prophylactic administration of acetazolamide may be effective (51).

AIR POLLUTION

Air pollution can also affect exercise performance and health. Although nature contributes to pollution through ozone (O_3) from lightning, dust, sulfuric oxides from volcanic activity, and other natural pollutants, modern industrialization has exacerbated the problem. Because of the severity of pollution in many areas, organizers of sporting events and exercisers are frequently confronted with problems related to exercising in polluted air. Both large sporting events and daily activity are performed in major cities, which are generally the sites with the highest pollution levels. Also, with indoor training and sports events, the infiltration of outdoor air pollution may be significant. Furthermore, the indoor environment may actually add to the problem with indoor air pollutants emitted by the occupants, activities, and building materials.

There are two major groups or types of pollutants: primary and secondary. **Primary pollutants** are directly attributable to a source of pollution, such as carbon monoxide

(CO), sulfur oxides, nitrogen oxides, hydrocarbons, and particulates (dust, smoke, and soot). **Secondary pollutants** result from an interaction of the environment (sunlight, moisture, other pollutants) with primary pollutants. These include O_3, aldehydes, sulfuric acid (H_2SO_4), and peroxyacetyl nitrate (PAN). City air commonly contains both primary and secondary pollutants.

GENERAL EFFECTOR MECHANISMS

The effect of pollutants is partly related to level of penetration. This "dosage" is determined by exposure time, concentration of pollutant in inspired air, ventilation rate and volume, temperature and humidity of inspired air, and route of inspiration (the nose versus the mouth). Pollution primarily affects the respiratory tract. This tract provides a large surface area for contact by the pollutant. The mucous membranes of the nose effectively remove large particles and highly soluble gases (e.g., 99.9% of inhaled SO_2), preventing them from affecting deeper airways and lung tissue. However, smaller particles and agents with low solubility easily pass through this barrier. During exercise, when mouth breathing plays an important role, this air filtration is less efficient, and more pollutants reach the lungs, traverse the diffusion surface, and enter the blood and body tissues. Pollutants can have several effects on the body's tissues, including the following:

- Irritation of the airways, which may lead to bronchoconstriction, hence increased airway resistance
- Reduction of alveolar diffusion capacity
- Reduction of oxygen transport capacity

Other effects of pollutants that can indirectly affect exercise performance are irritation of eyes (PAN and formaldehyde) and skin. Short-term effects of exposure to pollutants rather than long-term effects of exposure are discussed in this section.

OUTDOOR POLLUTION

Geographical distribution of outdoor pollution is strongly related to industry and population density. Automobiles, trucks, buses, aircrafts, industrial sources, and combustion of fossil fuels are major sources of CO, sulfur and nitrogen oxides, hydrocarbons, and particles. Areas with equal production of pollutants do not necessarily have equally polluted air, or smog, because climate and topography play major roles. River and mountain valleys generally have greater smog levels than hilltops and plains. High temperature and humidity typically promote photochemical smog with associated high O_3 levels. For example, in the Los Angeles area, photochemical smog, trapped by summer winds blowing toward the surrounding mountains, is a common phenomenon (43). Low temperature with a concomitant increase in fuel consumption for heating and high humidity (fog, rain) promote a different type of fog, in which high sulfur oxide

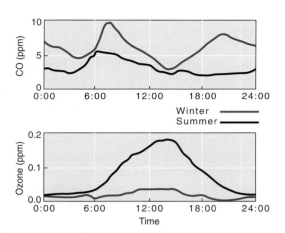

FIGURE 3-22. Daily and seasonal fluctuations in CO and ozone concentrations in the Los Angeles area. (Adapted with permission from McCafferty W. *Air Pollution and Athletic Performance.* Springfield (IL): Charles C Thomas; 1981.)

concentrations combined with particulate matter are converted into sulfuric acid (acid rain) and sulfates. The most famous fog of this type is the London fog, which produced a large number of deaths in 1952 (4,000 in a 4-day period). Such fog can be persistent when temperature inversion occurs, a condition brought about by little wind and a layer of cool polluted air trapped beneath a layer of warmer air.

PREVENTION

Avoidance of exposure is the primary method for preventing acute and long-term adverse effects of outdoor pollutants. Timing and selection of optimal location for exercise and moderating intensity and duration are key factors (15). Knowledge of daily and seasonal patterns

TABLE 3-5. NATIONAL AMBIENT AIR QUALITY STANDARDS AS PROVIDED BY THE ENVIRONMENTAL PROTECTION AGENCY

	TIME PERIOD	
POLLUTANT	FOR AVERAGING	STANDARD LIMIT LEVEL
Carbon monoxide	8 h	9 ppm
	1 h	35 ppm
Ozone	1 h	0.12 ppm
	8 h	0.08 ppm
Nitrogen dioxide (NO_2)	AAM	0.053 ppm
Sulfur dioxide (SO_2)	AAM	80 $\mu g \cdot m^{-3}$
	24 h	365 $\mu g \cdot m^{-3}$
Particulates (PM-2.5)	AAM	15 $\mu g \cdot m^{-3}$
($\leq$2.5-μ diameter)	24 h	65 $\mu g \cdot m^{-3}$
Particulates (PM-10)	AAM	50 $\mu g \cdot m^{-3}$
($\leq$10-micron diameter)	24 h	150 $\mu g \cdot m^{-3}$

AAM, annual arithmetic mean.

For pollutants with high hourly or daily fluctuations, longer duration averages and short-term peak level limits are provided. The numbers correspond to a pollution standards index (PSI) of 100.

TABLE 3-6. POLLUTANT STANDARDS INDEX AND IMPLICATIONS FOR SHORT-TERM HEALTH EFFECTS

INDEX VALUE	PSI DESCRIPTOR	GENERAL HEALTH EFFECTS	CAUTIONARY STATEMENTS
Up to 50	Good	None for the general population	None required
51–100	Moderate	Few or none for the general population	None required
101–200	Unhealthful	Mild aggravation of symptoms among susceptible people, with irritation symptoms in the healthy population	People with existing heart or respiratory ailments should reduce physical exertion and outdoor activity; the general population should reduce vigorous outdoor activity
201–300	Very unhealthful	Significant aggravation of symptoms and decreased exercise tolerance in people with heart or lung disease; widespread symptoms in the healthy population	Elderly and people with heart or lung disease should stay indoors and reduce physical activity; general population should avoid vigorous outdoor activity
>300	Hazardous	Early onset of certain diseases in addition to significant aggravation of symptoms and decreased exercise tolerance in healthy people At PSI levels greater than 400, premature death of ill and elderly people may result Healthy people have adverse symptoms that affect normal activity	Elderly and people with diseases should stay indoors and avoid physical exertion At PSI levels greater than 400, the general population should avoid outdoor activity All people should remain indoors, keeping windows and doors closed, and minimize physical exertion.

PSI, pollution standards index. Also see Table 34–8.

and fluctuations (Fig. 3-22) is important when planning an event involving high-intensity exercise. Avoiding periods and areas with heavy traffic can minimize CO exposure. Summer and early autumn afternoons can be unfavorable because of high O_3 exposure.

Information on air pollution can be acquired from local meteorological authorities, many of which provide a pollutant standards index (PSI) developed by the U.S. Environmental Protection Agency (EPA). The PSI converts measured pollutant concentration to a number on a scale from 0 to 500. The critical number is 100, which corresponds to the threshold established under the Clean Air Act (Table 3-5) (24). A PSI greater than 100 indicates pollution in an unhealthful range. PSI places maximum emphasis on acute health effects (24 hours or less), rather than chronic effects, making it useful for exercise planning. It does not incorporate interactions between pollutants. Table 3-6 has information on the PSI (24).

The important factors for controlling exposure to indoor pollution include selecting an optimal location for air intake, using low-emission building materials, regularly cleaning and use of low-dust floor coverings, clean ventilation and air conditioning systems, and sufficiently high fresh-air ventilation rate. More specifically, exercise centers and fitness facilities require higher ventilation rates than offices and living quarters. A CO_2 concentration limit of 1,000 ppm at an outdoor concentration of 350 ppm is often used as an indicator of adequate ventilation. At that level, 80% of the users are satisfied with air quality. A level of 650 ppm CO_2 is needed to increase satisfaction to 90% (24). Indoor exercise areas should maintain the lowest CO_2 concentration practically possible.

SUMMARY

The environmental effects of altitude and air pollution can affect exercise and athletic performance. Physiological adaptation or maladaptation (in the case of altitude sickness or exposure to air pollution) is often a factor in fitness, exercise, and training programs. Although some effects of altitude can be overcome with chronic adaptations to training at altitude, prevention of harmful effects of pollution is often a function of avoiding and minimizing exposure.

REFERENCES

1. Allen GM, Gandevia SC, McKenzie DK. Reliability of measurements of muscle strength and voluntary activation using twitch interpolation. *Muscle Nerve.* 1995;18:593–600.
2. **American College of Sports Medicine. ACSM position stand on exercise and fluid replacement.** *Med Sci Sports Exerc.* 2007;39: 377–90.
3. **American College of Sports Medicine. ACSM position stand on exertional heat illness during training and competition.** *Med Sci Sport Exerc.* 2007;39:556–72.
4. **American College of Sports Medicine.** *Guidelines for Exercise Testing and Prescription.* 8th ed. Baltimore: Lippincott Williams & Wilkins; 2009.
5. **American College of Sports Medicine. ACSM position stand on prevention of cold injuries during exercise.** *Med Sci Sports Exerc.* 2006;38:2012–29.
6. **American College of Sports Medicine. ACSM position stand on exercise and hypertension.** *Med Sci Sports Exerc.* 2004;36:533–53.
7. Atkins JM, Matthews OA, Blomqvist CG, et al. Incidence of arrhythmias induced by isometric and dynamic exercise. *Br Heart J.* 1976;38:465–71.
8. Bassett DR, Howley ET. Limiting factors for maximum oxygen uptake and determinants of endurance performance. *Med Sci Sports Exerc.* 2000;32:70–84.
9. Berstrom M, Hultman E. Energy cost and fatigue during intermittent electrical stimulation of human skeletal muscle. *J Appl Physiol.* 1988;65:1500.

10. Bigland-Ritchie B, Furbush BW. Fatigue of intermittent submaximal voluntary contractions: central and peripheral factors. *J Appl Physiol*. 1986;61:421–9.

11. Bigland-Ritchie B, Rice CL, Garland SJ, et al. Task-dependent factors in fatigue of human voluntary contractions. In: Gandevia SC, Enoka RM, McComas AJ, et al., editors. *Fatigue: Neural and Muscular Mechanisms*. New York: Plenum; 1995. p. 361–80.

12. Bruce RA, Kusumi F, Hosmer D. Maximal oxygen intake and nomographic assessment of functional aerobic impairment in cardiovascular disease. *Am Heart J*. 1973;85:546–62.

13. Byrd SK, McCutcheon LJ, Hodgson DR, et al. Altered sarcoplasmic reticulum function after high-intensity exercise. *J Appl Physiol*. 1989;67:2072.

14. Byrne NM, Hills AP, Hunter GR, et al. Metabolic equivalent: one size does not fit all. *J Appl Physiol*. 2005;99:1112–9.

15. Cedaro R. Environmental factors and exercise performance: a review, II. *Air Pollution Excel*. 1992;8:161–6.

16. Concu A, Marcello C. Stroke volume response to progressive exercise in athletes engaged in different types of training. *Eur J Appl Physiol*. 1993;66:11–7.

17. Coyle EF, Jeukendrup AE, Wagonmakers AJM, Saris WHM. Fatty acid oxidation is directly regulated by carbohydrate metabolism during exercise. *Am J Physiol*. 1997;273:E268.

18. Coyle EF, Gonzalez-Alonso J. Cardiovascular drift during prolonged exercise: new perspectives. *Exerc Sport Sci Rev*. 2001;29:88–92.

19. Cudaback DD. Four-km altitude effects on performance and health. *Pub Astronom Soc Pac*. 1984;96:463–77.

20. Davis JM, Bailey SP. Possible mechanisms of central nervous system fatigue during exercise. *Med Sci Sports Exerc*. 1997;29:45–57.

21. diPrampero P, Boutellier U, Pietsch P. Oxygen deficit and stores at onset of muscular exercise in humans. *J Appl Physiol*. 1983;55:146.

22. Edgerton VR, Roy RR, Gregor RJ, et al. Muscle fiber activation and recruitment. In Knuttgen HG, Vogel JA, Poortmans S, eds. *Biochemistry of Exercise*. Champaign (IL): Human Kinetics; 1983. p. 31–49.

23. Enoka RM, Stuart DG. Neurobiology of muscle fatigue. *J Appl Physiol*. 1992;72:1631–48.

24. Environmental Protection Agency. Public information provided on the World Wide Web server: http://www.epa.gov. Accessed 10/14/08.

25. Favier R, Spielvogel H, Desplanches D, et al. Training in hypoxia vs. training in normoxia in high-altitude natives. *J Appl Physiol*. 1995;78:2286–93.

26. Fitts RH. Cellular mechanisms of muscle fatigue. *Physiol Rev*. 1994;74:49.

27. Fitts RH. Cellular, molecular, and metabolic basis of muscle fatigue. In: Rowell LB, Shephard JT, editors. *Handbook of Physiology: Section 12: Regulation and Integration of Multiple Systems*. New York: Oxford University; 1996.

28. Fleck SJ. Cardiovascular responses to strength training. In: Komi P, editor. Strength and power in sports. *The Encyclopaedia of Sports Medicine*. 2nd ed. Oxford (UK): Blackwell Scientific; 2003. p. 387–408.

29. Franklin BA. Diagnostic and functional exercise testing: test selection and interpretation. *J Cardiovasc Nurs*. 1995;10:8–29.

30. Franklin BA. Exercise testing, training and arm ergometry. *Sports Med*. 1985;2:100–19.

31. Franklin BA. Pitfalls in estimating aerobic capacity from exercise time or workload. *Appl Cardiol*. 1986;14:25–6.

32. Fry AC, Allemeier CA, Staron RS. Correlation between percentage fiber type area and myosin heavy chain content in human skeletal muscle. *Eur J Appl Physiol*. 1994;68:246–51.

33. Fulco CS. Maximal and submaximal exercise performance at altitude. *Aviat Space Environ Med*. 1998;69:793–801.

34. Gaesser G, Brooks G. Metabolic bases of excess post-exercise oxygen consumption: a review. *Med Sci Sports Exerc*. 1984;16:29.

35. Garner SH, Sutton JR, Burse RL, et al. Operation Everest II: neuromuscular performance under conditions of extreme simulated altitude. *J Appl Physiol*. 1990;68:1167–72.

36. Gaskill SE, Ruby BC, Walker AJ, at al. Validity and reliability of combining three methods to determine ventilatory threshold. *Med Sci Sports Exerc*. 2001;33:1841–8.

37. Gladden LB. Lactate metabolism: a new paradigm for the third millennium. *J Physiol*. 2004;558:5–30.

38. Godt RE, Nosek TM. Changes of intracellular milieu with fatigue or hypoxia depress contraction of skinned rabbit skeletal and cardiac muscle. *J Physiol*. 1989;412:155.

39. Gollnick P. Metabolism of substrates: energy substrate metabolism during exercise and as modified by training. *Fed Proc*. 1985;44:353.

40. Gollnick P, RiedyM, Quintinskie J, Bertocci L. Differences in metabolic potential of skeletal muscle fibres and their significance for metabolic control. *J Exp Biol*. 1985;115:191.

41. Hamilton AJ, Cymerman A, Black P. High altitude cerebral edema. *Neurosurgery*. 1986;19:841–9.

42. Harms CA, McClaran SR, Nickele GA, et al. Exercise induced arterial hypoxemia in healthy young women. *J Physiol*. 1998;507:619–28.

43. Haymes EM, Welss CL. *Environment and Human Performance*. Champaign (IL): Human Kinetics; 1986.

44. Hester RL, Choi J. Blood flow control during exercise: role for the venular epithelium. *Exerc Sport Sci Rev*. 2002;30:147–51.

45. Jett DM, Adams KJ, Stamford BA. Cold exposure and exercise metabolism. *Sports Med*. 2006;36:643–56.

46. Kamon E, Avellini BD. Wind speed limits to work under hot environments for clothed men. *J Appl Physiol*. 1979;46:340–9.

47. Kayser B. Nutrition and energetics of exercise at altitude: theory and possible practical implications. *Sports Med*. 1994;17:309–23.

48. Kitamura K, Jorgenson CR, Gobel FL, et al. Hemodynamic correlates of myocardial oxygen consumption during up-right exercise. *J Appl Physiol*. 1972;32:516–22.

49. Levine BD, Stray-Gundersen J. A practical approach to altitude training. *Int J Sports Med*. 1992;13:S209–12.

50. Lind AR, McNichol GW. Muscular factors which determine the cardiovascular responses to sustained and rhythmic exercise. *Can Med Assoc J*. 1967;96:706–15.

51. Malconian MK, Rock PB. Medical problems related to altitude. In: Pandolf KB, Swaka MN, Gonzalez RR, editors. *Human Performance Physiology and Environmental Medicine at Terrestrial Extremes*. Indianapolis: Benchmark; 1988.

52. Metzger JM, Fitts RH. Fatigue from high and low frequency muscle stimulation: role of sarcolemma action potentials. *Exp Neurol*. 1986;93:320.

53. Metzger JM, Fitts RH. Role of intracellular pH in muscle fatigue. *J Appl Physiol*. 1987;62:1392.

54. Mitchell JH, Payne FC, Saltin B, et al. The role of muscle mass in the cardiovascular response to static contractions. *J Physiol*. 1980;309:45–54.

55. Nelson RR, Gobel FL, Jorgensen CR, et al. Hemodynamic predictors of myocardial oxygen consumption during static and dynamic exercise. *Circulation*. 1974;50:1179–89.

56. Newsholme E. The control of fuel utilization by muscle during exercise and starvation. *Diabetes*. 1979;28(Suppl 1):1.

57. Porszasz J, Casaburi R, Somfay A, et al. A treadmill ramp protocol using simultaneous changes in speed and grade. *Med Sci Sports Exerc*. 2003;35:1596–603.

58. Powers SK, Martin D, Dodd S. Exercise induced hypoxemia in elite endurance athletes: incidence causes and impact on VO₂ max. *Sports Med*. 1993;16:14–22.

59. Powers S, Howley E, Cox R. A differential catecholamine response during prolonged exercise and passive heating. *Med Sci Sports Exerc*. 1982;14:435.

60. Powers S, Howley E, Cox R. Ventilatory and metabolic reactions to heat stress during prolonged exercise. *J Sports Med*. 1982;22:32.

61. Powers S, Dodd S, Beadle R. Oxygen uptake kinetics in trained athletes differing in $\dot{V}O_{2max}$. *Eur J Appl Physiol*. 1985;54:306.

62. Powers S, Riley W, Howley E. Comparison of fat metabolism between trained men and women during prolonged aerobic work. *Res Q Exerc Sport*. 1980;51:427.

63. Richardsen RS, Noyszewsky EA, Leogh JS, Wagner PD. Lactate efflux from exercising human skeletal muscle: role of intracellular P_{O2}. *J Appl Physiol*. 1998;85:627.

64. Robergs RA, Giasvand F, Parker D. Biochemistry of exercise-induced metabolic acidosis. *Am J Physiol Regul Integr Comp Physiol*. 2004;287:502–16.

65. Rodriguez FA, Casa H, Casa M, et al. Intermittent hypobaric hypoxia stimulates erythropoiesis and improves aerobic capacity. *Med Sci Sports Exerc*. 1999;31:264–8.

66. Schwade J, Blomqvist CG, Shapiro W. A comparison of the response to arm and leg work in patients with ischemic heart disease. *Am Heart J*. 1977;94:203–8.

67. Sjogaard G. Role of exercise-induced potassium fluxes underlying muscle fatigue: a brief review. *Can J Physiol Pharmacol*. 1990;69:238.

68. Staron RS, Karapondo DL, Kraemer WJ, et al. Skeletal muscle adaptations during the early phase of heavy-resistance training in men and women. *J Appl Physiol*. 1994;76:1247–55.

69. Thompson LV, Balog EM, Fitts RH. Muscle fatigue in frog semitendinosus: role of intracellular pH. *Am J Physio.l* 1992;263:C1507.

70. Thompson LV, Fitts RH. Muscle fatigue in the frog semitendinosus: role of high energy phosphates and P(I). *Am J Physiol*. 1992;263:C803.

71. Westing SH, Cresswell AG, Thorstensson A. Muscle activation during maximal voluntary eccentric and concentric knee extension. *Eur J Appl Physiol*. 1991;62:104–8.

72. Wilkie DR. Muscular fatigue: effects of hydrogen ions and inorganic phosphate. *Fed Proc*. 1986;45:2921.

SELECTED REFERENCES FOR FURTHER READING

Ainsworth BE, Haskell WL, Whitt MC, et al. Compendium of physical activities: an update of activity codes and MET intensities. *Med Sci Sports Exerc*. 2000;32:5498–5516.

Astrand PO, Rodahl K, Dahl HA, Stromme SB. *Textbook of Work Physiology: Physiological Basis of Exercise*. Champaign (IL): Human Kinetics; 2003.

Baechle TR, Earle RW, editors. *Essentials of Strength and Conditioning*. Champaign (IL): Human Kinetics; 2000.

Brooks G, Fahey T, Baldwin K. *Exercise Physiology: Human Bioenergetics and Its Applications*. 4th ed. Boston: McGraw Hill; 2005.

Fleck SJ, Kraemer WJ. *Designing Resistance Training Programs*. Champaign (IL): Human Kinetics; 2004.

Gleeson M, Maughan RJ. *The Biochemical Basis of Sports Performance*. Lavallette (NJ): Oxford University Press; 2004.

Hargreaves M, Spriet L, editors. *Exercise Metabolism*. 2nd ed. Champaign (IL): Human Kinetics; 2006.

Hoffman J. *Physiological Aspects of Sport Training and Performance*. Champaign (IL): Human Kinetics; 2002.

Komi PV, editor. *Strength and Power in Sport*. Malden (MA): Blackwell Science; 2003.

Kraemer WJ, Hakkinen K, editors. *Strength Training for Sport*. Malden (MA): Blackwell Science; 2002.

Maud PJ, Foster C, editors. *Physiological Assessment of Human Fitness*. Champaign (IL): Human Kinetics; 2006.

Nieman, DC. *Exercise Testing and Prescription*. 6th ed. Boston (MA): McGraw Hill; 2007.

Noakes T. *Lore of Running*. Champaign (IL): Human Kinetics; 2003.

Plowman SA, Smith DL. *Exercise Physiology—For Health, Fitness, and Performance*. San Francisco: Benjamin Cummings; 2003.

Powers SK, Howley ET. *Exercise Physiology—Theory and Application to Fitness and Performance*. 6th ed. Boston: McGraw Hill; 2007.

Saltin B, Boushel R, Secher N, Mitchell J, editors. *Exercise and Circulation in Health and Disease*. Champaign, IL: Human Kinetics; 2000.

Shephard RJ, Astrand PO, editors. *Endurance in Sport*. Malden (MA): Blackwell Science; 1992.

Skinner JS, editor. *Exercise Testing and Exercise Prescription for Special Cases: Theoretical Basis and Clinical Application*. 3rd ed. Philadelphia: Lippincott Williams & Wilkins; 2005.

Whiting WC, Zernicke RF. *Biomechanics of Musculoskeletal Injury*. Champaign (IL): Human Kinetics; 1998.

INTERNET RESOURCES

- Accuweather: http://www.accuweather.com
- American Academy of Pediatrics: http://www.aap.org
- American Association of Cardiovascular and Pulmonary Rehabilitation (AACVPR): http://www.aacvpr.org
- American Cancer Society: http://www.cancer.org
- American College of Sports Medicine: http://www.acsm.org
- American Diabetes Association: http://www.diabetes.org
- American Heart Association: http://www.americanheart.org
- American Medical Association: http://www.ama-assn.org
- Coalition for a Healthy and Active America (CHAA): http://www.chaausa.org
- The Cooper Institute: http://www.cooperinstitute.org
- Gatorade Sports Science Institute: http://www.gssiweb.com
- Healthy People 2010: http://www.healthypeople.gov
- International Society for Aging and Physical Activity (ISAPA): http://www.isapa.org
- National Athletic Trainers' Association: http://www.nata.org
- The National Center on Physical Activity and Disability (NCPAD): http://www.ncpad.org
- National Heart, Lung, and Blood Institute: http://www.nhlbi.nih.gov
- National Heart, Lung, and Blood Institute: Clinical Guidelines on the Identification, Evaluation, and Treatment of Overweight and Obesity in Adults: http://www.nhlbi.nih.gov/guidelines/obesity/ob_home.htm
- National Heart, Lung, and Blood Institute Healthy People 2010 Gateway: http://hp2010.nhlbihin.net
- The National Institute for Occupational Safety and Health (NIOSH): http://www.cdc.gov/niosh
- National Institute on Aging: http://www.nia.nih.gov
- National Institutes of Health: http://www.nih.gov
- National Osteoporosis Foundation: http://www.nof.org
- National Strength and Conditioning Association (NSCA): http://www.nsca-lift.org
- Nutrition Navigator: http://www.navigator.tufts.edu
- Sportscience: http://www.sportsci.org
- StrongWomen.com: http://www.strongwomen.com
- United States Department of Health and Human Services: http://www.-os.dhhs.gov
- The Weather Channel: http://www.weather.com

A basic knowledge of nutrition principles is essential for individuals working with physically active individuals. This chapter presents fundamental information regarding the macronutrients (i.e., carbohydrate, protein, fat), highlights selected vitamins and minerals with specific regard for physical activity and human performance, and provides a basis for estimating energy requirements. Nutritional considerations for athletic performance and exercise are incorporated throughout the chapter.

> > > KEY TERMS

Aerobic: Requirement of or presence of oxygen to sustain biological process such as β-oxidation.

Adequate intake (AI): The recommended average daily intake level based on observed or experimentally determined approximations or estimates of nutrient intake by a group (or groups) of apparently healthy people that are assumed to be adequate—used when an RDA cannot be determined.

Acceptable macronutrient distribution range (AMDR): Represents a range of intakes for a particular macronutrient associated with reduced risk of chronic diseases while providing adequate intake of essential nutrients.

Anaerobic: Living or biological processes that occur in the absence of oxygen.

Antioxidants: Dietary components present in small concentrations, such as vitamins C and E, which prevent or reduce the extent of oxidative damage of cellular components such as DNA and cell membranes by scavenging free radicals.

Dietary reference intake (DRI): A set of reference values for specific nutrients that expands upon the former recommended dietary allowances (RDA), which includes the estimated average requirement (EAR), RDA, adequate intake (AI), and tolerable upper intake level (UL).

Essential amino acid (EAA): Amino acids required for maintaining proper growth and development that are not synthesized in the body and therefore must be consumed in the diet. EAAs are also referred to as indispensible amino acids.

Essential nutrient: Essential nutrient refers to any nutrient, such as essential amino acids and fatty acids, necessary for normal body functions that is not synthesized in the body and must be consumed in the diet.

Estimated average requirement (EAR): Average daily nutrient intake level estimated to meet the requirement for half of the healthy individuals of a particular gender or life stage.

Gluconeogenesis: Endogenous production of new glucose from nonglucose carbon precursors, such as amino acids, lactate, pyruvate, and glycerol, which occurs primarily in the liver and, to a lesser extent, the kidney.

Glycemic index: The rate at which ingestion of a food or food component, such as carbohydrate, increases blood glucose in comparison to a reference food, white bread in particular.

Glycogenolysis: The release of glucose from liver and muscle glycogen to produce new glucose in the liver that is able to be circulated throughout the body or utilized for energy production in skeletal muscle in response to elevated glucagon and epinephrine levels.

Glycolysis: The conversion of glucose to high-energy molecules (adenosine triphosphate and high-energy electron donors) as sources of cellular energy from aerobic and anaerobic metabolism.

Macronutrients: Organic energy-providing nutrients, which include carbohydrate, fat, and protein, consumed in large quantities in the diet.

Micronutrients: Organic and inorganic nutrients including vitamins and minerals, respectively, which are consumed and/or required in much lower amounts in comparison to the macronutrients.

Nonessential amino acids (NEAA): Often referred to as dispensable amino acids, these amino acids are synthesized in the body and therefore not essential to the diet.

Recommended dietary allowance (RDA): Average daily dietary nutrient intake level sufficient to meet the nutrient requirement of nearly all healthy individuals of a particular gender and life stage.

Tolerable upper intake level (UL): The highest average daily nutrient intake level not likely to pose any risk of adverse health effects to almost all individuals in the general population. The potential risk for adverse effects may increase as intakes exceed the UL.

NUTRITION BASICS: THE MAJOR NUTRIENTS

There are two major classes of nutrients critical to the understanding of human nutrition: macronutrients and micronutrients. Each class of nutrients has an important role in optimizing growth, development, and health status. These nutrients are also vital for physical performance regardless of an individual's training status. The macronutrients, carbohydrate, protein, and fat, are organic compounds that contain carbon, hydrogen, and oxygen. Protein is unique given it also contains nitrogen as a component of its constituent amino acids. The macronutrients provide energy (i.e., kilocalories), and the respective energy contents of these nutrients are listed in Table 4-1. Micronutrients include vitamins and minerals and are required in much lower quantities than the macronutrients. In addition, micronutrients do not provide energy. Nonetheless, vitamins and minerals are critical to proper growth and metabolism. A list of major vitamins and minerals is provided in Tables 4-2 and 4-3, respectively.

The proper blend of nutrients is necessary for normal growth and development, as well as maintenance of health. The Food and Nutrition Board of the National Academy of Sciences Research Council periodically issues a set of reference values known as the dietary reference intakes (DRIs), which include the recommended dietary allowance (RDA), adequate intake (AI), tolerable upper intake level (UL), and the estimated average requirement (EAR) of each macro- and micronutrient necessary to meet the nutritional needs of nearly all healthy people (5). The following sections review the roles of

macronutrients and selected nutrients with consideration for the level of nutrient intake necessary for healthy adults.

 1.8.1-HFS: Knowledge of the role of carbohydrates, fats, and proteins as fuels for aerobic and anaerobic metabolism.

1.8.11-HFS: Knowledge of the number of kilocalories in 1 g of carbohydrate, fat, protein, and alcohol.

CARBOHYDRATE

Carbohydrate, glucose specifically, is the preferred fuel source for the body and the nervous system, in particular. As an energy source, carbohydrate provides 4 kilocalories per gram (Table 4-1). Carbohydrates are classified by the number of sugar molecules they contain and can be divided into either simple or complex carbohydrates. Simple carbohydrates refer to either a monosaccharide (i.e., one sugar molecule) or a disaccharide (i.e., two sugar molecules). The most common forms of monosaccharides include glucose, fructose, and galactose. The most common disaccharides include sucrose, lactose, and maltose. Sucrose, more commonly referred to as table sugar, is composed of glucose and fructose and found primarily in sugar cane, honey, and maple syrup. Lactose is composed of glucose and galactose and is the sugar most commonly found in milk. Lastly, maltose, a disaccharide composed of two glucose molecules, is a byproduct of complex carbohydrate digestion, starches in particular, and is frequently present in a variety of sport nutrition products.

Complex carbohydrates consist of three or more monosaccharides linked together. Depending on chain length, complex carbohydrates are referred to as either oligosaccharides or as polysaccharides. Oligosaccharides are between 3 and 10 monosaccharides in length and are found naturally in foods such as legumes, onions, and bananas. Polysaccharides are complex carbohydrates greater than 10 monosaccharides in length. The most common polysaccharides are glycogen and starch. Glycogen, the storage form of glucose in humans, consists of

TABLE 4-1. MACRONUTRIENT AND ENERGY CONTENT

MACRONUTRIENT	ENERGY (kcal · g^{-1})
Carbohydrate	4
Protein	4
Fat	9
Alcohol	7

TABLE 4-2. MICRONUTRIENTS: VITAMINS

VITAMIN	MAJOR FUNCTION	DIETARY SOURCES	RECOMMENDED INTAKE (ADULTS)
Fat Soluble			
A	Maintenance of skin, bone, teeth, growth, and vision	Carrots, broccoli, spinach, eggs, cheese, and milk	700–900 $\mu g \cdot d^{-1}$
D	Maintenance and growth of bones	Milk, egg yolk, tuna, and salmon	5–15 $\mu g \cdot d^{-1}$ [a]
E	Antioxidant	Vegetable oils, whole grains, green leafy vegetables	15 $mg \cdot d^{-1}$
K	Blood clotting	Green leafy vegetables, cabbage, and milk	90–120 $\mu g \cdot d^{-1}$ [a]
Water Soluble			
B_1 (thiamin)	Energy production	Breads, pasta, pork, oysters	1.1–1.2 $mg \cdot d^{-1}$
B_2 (riboflavin)	Energy production	Milk, meat, cereals, pasta, dark green vegetables	1.1–1.3 $mg \cdot d^{-1}$
B_3 (niacin)	Energy production	Poultry, meat, tuna, cereal, pasta, bread, nuts, legumes	14–16 mg $NE \cdot d^{-1}$ [b]
B_6 (pyridoxine)	Protein and fat metabolism	Avocados, green beans, spinach, cereals, bread	1.3–1.7 $mg \cdot d^{-1}$
B_{12} (cobalamine)	Red blood cell formation	Meat, fish, milk, eggs	2.4 $\mu g \cdot d^{-1}$
Folic acid	DNA synthesis, red blood cell formation	Dark green leafy vegetables, fortified cereals, wheat germ, oranges, bananas	400 $\mu g \cdot d^{-1}$
Pantothenic acid	Macronutrient metabolism, hormone synthesis	Cereals, bread, nuts, eggs, dark green vegetables	5 $\mu g \cdot d^{-1}$ [a]
C (ascorbic acid)	Antioxidant, maintenance of bones, teeth, collagen	Citrus fruits, melons, strawberries, tomatoes, green peppers, potatoes	75–90 $mg \cdot d^{-1}$
Biotin	Fatty acid synthesis, energy production	Egg yolk, green leafy vegetables	30 $\mu g \cdot d^{-1}$ [a]

[a]Adequate intakes.

[b]NE, niacin equivalents.

numerous branched-chains of glucose molecules stored in both the liver and skeletal muscle. When necessary, glycogen is easily broken down under conditions where glucose is needed. In particular, glycogen becomes the major source of glucose for the exercising muscle during prolonged endurance exercise events. The role of glycogen is discussed in greater detail later in this chapter. Starches, the primary storage of carbohydrates in plants, are composed of either amylose, which consists of straight chains of glucose molecules or amylopectin, which is made up of branched-chain glucose molecules. These starches are found in various food sources such as vegetables, legumes, wheat, and barley.

Fiber is another type of complex carbohydrate. Fibers are not digested in the human body and therefore are not absorbed. However, fiber consumption can have beneficial effects on health, including improved gastrointestinal health, glucose homeostasis, and enhanced satiety. In addition, fiber consumption has been linked to reduced cardiovascular disease risk by lowering hypertension and

TABLE 4-3. MICRONUTRIENTS: SPORTS-RELATED MINERALS

MINERAL	MAJOR FUNCTION	DIETARY SOURCES	RECOMMENDED INTAKE (ADULTS)
Major Minerals			
Calcium	Growth, bone and teeth formation, nerve impulses	Dairy, dark green vegetables, sardines, clams	1,000–1,200 $mg \cdot d^{-1}$
Sodium[b]	Body water and acid–base balance, nerve function	Abundant in most foods	1,500 $mg \cdot d^{-1}$ [a]
Potassium[b]	Body water and acid–base balance, nerve function	Meat, milk, fruits, vegetables, cereals, legumes	4,700 $mg \cdot d^{-1}$ [a]
Chloride[b]	Acid–base balance	Table salt, seafood, meets, eggs, milk	2,300 $mg \cdot d^{-1}$ [a]
Phosphorous	Bone and teeth formation, acid–base balance	Dairy, meat, fish, poultry, nuts, grains	700 $mg \cdot d^{-1}$
Trace Minerals			
Iron	Component of hemoglobin and enzymes	Meats, eggs, legumes, grains, dark green vegetables	8–18 $mg \cdot d^{-1}$
Chromium	Glucose and energy metabolism	Fats, meats, cereals	25–35 $\mu g \cdot d^{-1}$ [a]
Zinc	Component of enzymes	Milk, shellfish, wheat bran	8–11 $mg \cdot d^{-1}$

[a]Adequate intakes.

[b]Electrolytes.

improving plasma cholesterol. Fiber has also been associated with reduced risk of cancer. Currently, the DRI for fiber is 25 and 38 g per day for adult men and women, respectively (5).

Fibers are classified based upon their solubility in water. Water-soluble and water-insoluble fibers are present in varying amounts in all plant sources. Insoluble fibers are derived from the cell walls of plants and include cellulose, hemicellulose, and lignins. Insoluble fibers are most commonly found in vegetables such as broccoli, carrots, green beans, celery, and potato skins. In addition, insoluble fibers are found in whole wheat, wheat bran, and flax seed lignins. Insoluble fibers increase bulk, soften stool, and shorten intestinal transit time. In contrast, soluble fibers undergo a metabolic processing via fermentation by bacteria in the large intestine. The end product of this bacterial fermentation is gas and short-chain fatty acids, which can be absorbed. Soluble fibers, such as pectins, gums, and certain hemicelluloses, can be found within plant cells. Dietary sources of soluble fibers include oats, apples, and beans. These soluble fibers, along with psyllium, have been shown to be beneficial in reducing blood cholesterol levels.

Carbohydrate Digestion and Absorption

Digestion and absorption of carbohydrates is a well-choreographed series of events that occur in the mouth, stomach, small intestine, and large intestine, along with a number of essential secretory organs. Ultimately dietary carbohydrates are broken down into monosaccharides; the sugar molecules are then transported across the intestine into the blood, where they are distributed to all tissues in the body. Not all carbohydrates are digested and absorbed at the same rate within the intestine. The rate at which carbohydrate is absorbed and causes a rise in blood glucose level is known as the glycemic response.

Glycemic Response and Glycemic Index

The glycemic response relates to the rate at which carbohydrates are digested and absorbed, what extent they raise blood glucose, and for how long blood glucose remains elevated. This varies upon the type and amount of carbohydrate ingested, as well as the other nutrients with which the carbohydrate is consumed. Simple sugars, starches, and refined (i.e., fiber has been removed) carbohydrates typically cause a greater glycemic response as reflected by a more rapid rise in blood glucose following their consumption. Unrefined carbohydrates, which contain fiber, take longer to be digested and absorbed and therefore cause a lower glycemic response. Protein and fat, when consumed in conjunction with carbohydrates, can decrease the rate of carbohydrate digestion and absorption and subsequent appearance of glucose in blood.

The glycemic response of a specific food is calculated by its glycemic index. Glycemic index is a ranking of how a food affects blood glucose in comparison to an equal amount of a reference carbohydrate such as white bread or glucose. The reference food is assigned a value of 100 and test foods are expressed relative to the test value. Foods with glycemic indexes greater than or equal to 70 are considered high glycemic foods, whereas foods with an index less than 55 are considered low glycemic foods. Although the glycemic index can provide information regarding food sources effects on blood glucose, the glycemic index does not predict the impact of consuming these foods as a part of a mixed meal. In addition, the role of the glycemic index with specific regard to glycogen replenishment after exercise continues to be debated (12).

Carbohydrate Metabolism

In general, carbohydrates produce energy in the form of adenosine triphosphate (ATP) through aerobic metabolism. Complete (i.e., aerobic) metabolism of one molecule of glucose yields 38 ATP. The basic formula to describe this process is

$$C_6H_{12}O_6 + 6O_2 \Rightarrow 6CO_2 + 6H_2O + 38ATP$$

The following sections provide a brief overview of carbohydrate metabolism and energy production.

Glycolysis

Glycolysis is the first stage of glucose metabolism, which consists of a series of reactions involving highly regulated enzymes. Depending upon oxygen availability, glycolysis can be considered aerobic or anaerobic. In the presence of oxygen, pyruvate is converted to acetyl-CoA within the mitochondria, beginning the first stage of aerobic metabolism. However, when oxygen is limited, acetyl-CoA is not formed, and pyruvate is converted to lactate. Lactate is a metabolic waste product of anaerobic glucose metabolism.

Citric Acid Cycle and Electron Transport Chain

During aerobic metabolism of glucose, acetyl-CoA produced from pyruvate within the mitochondria enters a series of reactions known as the citric acid cycle. During these reactions, the citric acid cycle generates two ATP molecules for each pyruvate formed from one glucose molecule. In addition, this process generates high-energy electrons via reduced cofactors, which are transported to the final stage of aerobic glucose metabolism, the electron transport chain.

The electron transport chain is the final step in aerobic glucose metabolism. It involves a series of molecules, mostly proteins, associated with the inner mitochondrial membrane, which accepts the high-energy electrons shuttled to the mitochondria produced via glycolysis and the citric acid cycle and passes them down the chain of molecules until they are combined with oxygen and water. During the passing of the electrons, the energy is conserved

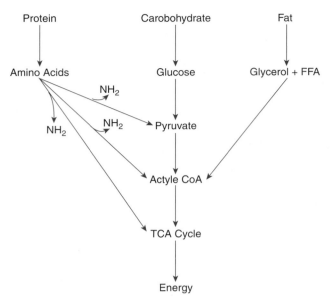

FIGURE 4-1. Integrated macronutrient metabolism.

and used to generate ATP. The citric acid cycle and the electron transport chain are essential to all energy-producing processes in the body. Utilization of the macronutrients for fuel is highly integrated, with the citric acid cycle being the primary point of convergence (Fig. 4-1).

Gluconeogenesis and Glycogenolysis: The Maintenance of Blood Glucose

In conditions where blood glucose levels are low, such as fasting or low carbohydrate intake, many of the reactions of glycolysis are reversed to produce new blood glucose. The production of new glucose is referred to as gluconeogenesis. This process occurs primarily in the liver. The major substrates for gluconeogenesis are lactate, selected amino acids (i.e., alanine), and glycerol. Gluconeogenesis is highly regulated, mostly through the action of hormones such as insulin and glucagon.

Another source of glucose for the body is glycogen stored in the liver and muscle. Liver glycogenolysis supplies new blood glucose, whereas muscle glycogen is a source of glucose exclusive to the muscle. As glycogen stores decrease, adipose tissue is degraded, providing fatty acids as an alternative fuel and glycerol for the synthesis of glucose via gluconeogenesis. During an overnight fast, gluconeogenesis and glycogenolysis work synergistically to maintain blood glucose. However, after approximately 30 hours of fasting, liver glycogen is depleted; therefore gluconeogenesis becomes the only source of new blood glucose.

Hormones and the Regulation of Blood Glucose

The regulation of blood glucose is mainly regulated via two key pancreatic hormones, insulin and glucagon.

Insulin is released in response to an increase in blood glucose; it stimulates glucose uptake into cells and promotes glucose storage as glycogen in the liver. In muscle, insulin promotes glucose uptake for energy production and stimulates glycogen synthesis for energy storage in the muscle. The major role of insulin is to maintain glucose homeostasis by decreasing blood glucose levels after a meal containing carbohydrates.

In the fasted state, blood glucose levels begin to decline. Low blood glucose levels stimulate the release of the glucagon, which stimulates gluconeogenesis and glycogenolysis in the liver to increase blood glucose. In addition to glucagon, the hormone epinephrine also promotes glucose production under conditions of increased energy demand. Overall, the role of glucagon and epinephrine are to increase blood glucose, whereas the primary action of insulin is to decrease blood glucose levels.

Recommended Carbohydrate Intake

On average, carbohydrate intake provides approximately 40% to 60% of the total energy intake in the American diet. Recommendations regarding carbohydrate intake for maintaining and promoting health are presented here.

Carbohydrate Dietary Reference Intakes

Carbohydrates are not a required nutrient per se given the body's ability to produce glucose via gluconeogenesis. However, carbohydrates provide an important source of energy for not only for the central nervous system but also the exercising muscle. In addition, diets high in fiber have been shown to confer health benefits. Therefore, the current DRIs suggest an RDA for total carbohydrate intake, an acceptable macronutrient distribution range (AMDR) for carbohydrates, and an AI for fiber. There is no UL for carbohydrates.

The current RDA for carbohydrates is based on the minimum amount of glucose required by the central nervous system: 130 g per day for both children and adults. This equates to approximately 25% of the energy in a 2,000 kilocalorie diet. The AMDR for carbohydrate intake for a healthy diet ranges from 45% and 65% of total energy. The source of carbohydrates come from complex unrefined carbohydrates with no more than 25% of the total energy derived from refined carbohydrates and less than 10% from simple sugars. The absolute intake of carbohydrate (i.e., grams per day) will differ between individuals based upon total energy needs. To calculate energy intake, please refer to Table 4-4. Once an estimated energy requirement has been determined, multiply total kilocalories by the percentage of carbohydrate intake to estimate carbohydrate kilocalories. Divide this estimate of carbohydrate kilocalories by 4 kilocalories per gram of carbohydrate to determine grams of carbohydrate. As previously discussed, the AI for fiber is 38 and 25 g per day for adult men and women, respectively.

TABLE 4-4. CALCULATING ESTIMATED ENERGY REQUIREMENTS (ERR)[a]

	DETERMINATION OF PHYSICAL ACTIVITY LEVEL (PAL)			
ACTIVITY LEVEL	BOYS 3–18 YR	GIRLS 3–18 YR	MEN ≥ 19 YR	WOMEN ≥ 19 YR
Sedentary	1.00	1.00	1.00	1.00
Low active	1.13	1.16	1.11	1.12
Active	1.26	1.31	1.25	1.27
Very active	1.42	1.56	1.48	1.45
AGE GROUP	EER PREDICTION EQUATIONS[b]			
Boys 9–18 yr	EER = 88.5 − (61.9 × Age in yr) + PAL [(26.7 × Weight in kg) + (903 × Height in m)] + 25			
Girls 9–18 yr	EER = 135.5 − (30.8 × Age in yr) + PAL [(10.0 × Weight in kg) + (934 × Height in m)] + 25			
Men ≥ 19 yr	ERR = 662 − (9.53 × Age in yr) + PAL [(15.91 × Weight in kg) + (539.6 × Height in m)]			
Women ≥ 19 yr	ERR = 354 − (6.91 × Age in yr) + PAL [(9.36 × Weight in kg) + (726 × Height in m)]			

[a]Referenced from the 2005 dietary reference intakes (DRIs).

[b]These equations are based on energy required for weight maintenance in normal-weight individuals.

Although the recommendation for dietary fiber intake will remain the same for all athletes, carbohydrate intakes should approximate 6–10 g·kg^{-1} for endurance athletes (8,15). This amount of carbohydrate should be consumed throughout training and competition to replenish and maintain adequate muscle glycogen stores for endurance performance. Depending on the athlete (i.e., age, sex, height, weight, and training status), the recommended intake of carbohydrate will range from approximately 50%–65% of the total kilocalorie intake.

In conclusion, the DRIs recommend that a healthy diet contain carbohydrates in the aforementioned amounts. Americans can meet these requirements by consuming a diet high in whole grains, fruits and vegetables. More so, the healthy American diet should be low in added simple sugars and refined carbohydrates such as those seen in soft drinks, bakery products, and candy.

FAT

Fat, or lipid, is the most energy-dense macronutrient. Fats provide 9 kilocalories per gram—more than twice the energy content of both carbohydrate and protein (Table 4-1). The most recognizable forms of fats in the diet are oils, butter, high-fat dairy products, and animal products. Although a negative perception often exists with regard to consumption of fat because of its implications in the development of cardiovascular disease, some sources of dietary fats such as avocados, nuts, and certain oils confer many health benefits.

Fat is stored in the body in large amounts in adipose tissue. These fat stores represent a large energy reservoir utilized during resting conditions, certain modes of exercise, and during energy-restricted states (i.e., weight-loss diets). In addition to being a source of energy, fat serves many vital roles in the human body such as insulating and protecting vital organs. Fats are also are an integral component of cell membranes and necessary for the production of steroid hormones such as testosterone and estrogen.

The primary fats in both food and in the body are in the form of triglycerides and cholesterol. Depending on their chemical structure, fats are classified as either saturated or unsaturated fatty acids (which include mono- and polyunsaturated fatty acids). Unsaturated fatty acids differ from saturated fatty acids: some carbons are not saturated with hydrogen and therefore contain carbon–carbon double bonds. Unsaturated fatty acids are classified by the number of double bonds in the carbon chain, which can either be monounsaturated (one double bond) or polyunsaturated (more than one) fatty acids. The most common dietary monounsaturated fatty acid, oleic acid, is found primarily in olive and canola oil. Linoleic acid, found in corn, safflower, and soybean oils, is the most common polyunsaturated fatty acid in the diet.

Dietary fat provides the essential fatty acids (EFAs), linoleic and linolenic acids. The most common ω-3 fatty acids are alpha-linolenic acid, eicosapentaenoic acid (EPA), and docasahexaenoic acid (DHA), found in vegetable and fish oils. Linoleic acid, present in corn and safflower oil, and arachidonic acid, found in meat and fish, are the most common ω-6 fatty acids. These EFAs are required for growth, for healthy skin, and for producing elements of the immune system. Although the body requires only small amounts of EFA (2% to 3% of total energy), obtaining sufficient amounts may require consuming a diet containing at least 10% of total energy from fat because the proportion of fatty acids in the diet is small.

The properties of unsaturated fatty acids are also affected by the position of the hydrogen atoms around the carbon–carbon double bond. In general, most unsaturated fatty acids have both hydrogen atoms on the same side of the double bond, referred to as a cis configuration. Other unsaturated fatty acids with hydrogen atoms on opposing sides of the double bond are in the trans configuration, more commonly referred to as trans fatty acids. Trans fatty acids are less commonly found in naturally occurring foods. However, through a process known as hydrogenation, unsaturated fatty acids are altered from the cis to the trans configurations and become more saturated. Trans fatty acids have been shown to be deleterious to health by increasing the risk of coronary artery disease (CAD) by negatively influencing blood cholesterol. Although no DRI has been set for trans fatty acids per se, it is now recommended that total intake not exceed approximately 3% of total energy intake.

Cholesterol is a waxy, fat-like substance found in foods of animal origin. It is found in the membranes of all cells and performs a number of essential anatomical and physiological functions; it is necessary for bile acid and steroid hormone formation. It is not found in plants or plant products. Cholesterol, produced by the liver, is transported in the blood by distinct particles containing both lipids and proteins (i.e., lipoproteins). There are three major classes of lipoproteins: (a) low-density lipoproteins (LDL), (b) high-density lipoproteins (HDL), and (c) very-low-density lipoproteins (VLDL). In general, the liver produces sufficient amounts of cholesterol to meet requirements. Therefore, dietary consumption is unnecessary. However, cholesterol is found in many food sources. Thus, recommendations regarding dietary cholesterol intake suggest consuming no more than 300 mg per day. Although monitoring cholesterol intake is important, dietary saturated and trans fatty acids have a more substantial negative impact on blood cholesterol, a risk factor for CAD. For more information regarding cholesterol and its influence on CAD, please refer to the Adult Panel Treatment III issued by the National Cholesterol Education Program (9).

Fat Digestion and Absorption

The majority of fat digestion occurs in the small intestine. In the presence of fat, the small intestine releases cholecystokinin, or CCK, a hormone that signals the release of bile acid from the gallbladder. Bile acids "emulsify" dietary fat in the small intestine so there is effective mixing with the fat-digesting enzymes in the small intestine, ultimately leaving triglycerides and diglycerides to monoglycerides, fatty acids, and glycerol for absorption.

Short- and medium-chain fatty acids, along with glycerol, can be taken up directly by the intestine and enter the blood. Monoglycerides and long-chain fatty acids, however, are repackaged into micelles that are absorbed by the small intestine. In the intestinal cells, the micelles are repackaged into chylomicrons (i.e., lipoproteins) and released into the lymphatic system for eventual entry into the blood stream.

The lipoproteins, with the exception of the chylomicron, are produced in the liver for the transport of triglycerides and cholesterol through the blood. VLDLs are a major carrier of triglycerides. LDLs are principally composed of cholesterol. The cholesterol transported by LDLs may be deposited in the arterial walls, contributing to atherosclerosis. The smallest group of lipoproteins, the HDLs, appears to be protective by carrying cholesterol to

the liver for breakdown and excretion. Therefore, individuals with high levels of HDL, low levels of LDL, low total cholesterol, and low total cholesterol/HDL cholesterol ratio carry the lowest risk of CAD. The impact of the type of fat consumed (saturated vs. unsaturated vs. trans fatty acids) on blood lipid levels occurs through changes in the metabolism of these lipoproteins. Dietary modifications (i.e., reduced total, saturated, and trans fat), along with regular exercise, have been shown to favorably impact lipoprotein profiles.

Fat and Energy Metabolism

During periods of excess energy intake, the body stores excess calories as fat in adipose tissue. Calories from dietary fat have the most efficient and direct route to storage when energy intake is higher than energy expenditure (i.e., energy surplus). During times of energy deficit (i.e., fasting) the body can utilize dietary fat to produce energy. During endurance exercise, the body also utilizes stored fat as an energy source.

Defining Fat Intake

Fats are vital for numerous roles in the body, including energy production, structural components of cell membranes, and the production of steroid hormones. In addition, fats are necessary in the diet for the absorption of fat-soluble vitamins and the essential fatty acids. Similar to carbohydrates and unlike protein, fats can be synthesized from endogenous nonfat precursors, which reduce their necessity in the diet. In general, American diets are composed of approximately 33% fat, more than enough to meet daily requirements for the EFAs and to allow for absorption of fat-soluble vitamins. Recommendations for a healthy diet include limiting certain fat intakes and increasing complex, unrefined carbohydrate and fiber.

Fat DRIs

There is no RDA for fat. However, the DRIs do include an AI and AMDR for essential fatty acids along with an AMDR for total fat intake. There are no specific guidelines for saturated fats, cholesterol, and trans fats. However, recommendations suggest that their intake be limited. More specifically, saturated fat intake should no more than 10% of the total energy intake and cholesterol should be less than 300 mg per day. In addition, trans fat should be no more than 2.6% of the total energy intake. For linoleic acid, an EFA, the AI is 17 and 12 g per day for men and women, respectively. The AI for alpha-linolenic acid is 1.6 g per day for men and 1.1 g per day for women. The AMDR for linoleic acid is between 5% and 10% of total energy intake, whereas the AMDR for alpha-linolenic acid is between 0.6% and 1.2% of total energy intake.

The AMDR for total fat intake is between 20% and 35% of the total energy intake. Diets providing fat in excess of 35% of total energy intake are likely high in calories and saturated fats. On the other hand, diets providing fat intake of less than 20% of the total energy intake increase the risk of certain fat-soluble vitamin deficiencies and negative alterations in lipoprotein and blood triglyceride levels. To estimate dietary fat intake, calculate energy intake as shown in Table 4-4. Once an estimated energy requirement has been determined, multiply total kilocalories by the percentage of fat intake and divide by 9 kilocalories per gram of fat.

PROTEIN

Of the macronutrients, protein is unique because of the nitrogen (N) content of its constituent amino acids. Similar to carbohydrate, protein provides 4 kilocalories per gram (Table 4-1). When proteins are oxidized for energy purposes or when dietary intake exceeds recommended amounts, CO_2 and water are produced, whereas the N component is (a) incorporated into urea and eliminated from the body in urine or (b) used in the synthesis of dispensable amino acids and other nitrogen-containing compounds in the body. Proteins are considered a required and vital nutrient that serves both structural and functional roles in the body. In addition to serving as structural components of muscle, bone, tendons, and ligaments, proteins function as enzymes critical in energy-producing reactions, hormones that regulate metabolism, transporters of other critical nutrients, and as an energy source in energy-deprived conditions. The latter function is the least desirable for this particular macronutrient.

Both dietary and body proteins are composed of amino acids, which are classified as either essential (indispensable) or nonessential (dispensable). Nonessential amino acids (NEAAs) are amino acids that can be made by the body, whereas essential amino acids (EAAs) cannot be synthesized in the body and therefore must be consumed in the diet. A list of the EAAs and NEAAs is shown in Table 4-5. All amino acids are needed to maintain optimal protein utilization in the body such that health, growth and development, and tissue maintenance and repair are promoted. The branched-chain amino acids (BCAA: leucine, isoleucine, valine) are a unique class of essential amino acids used almost exclusively by skeletal muscle.

Sources of Dietary Protein and Protein Quality

Protein is abundant in meat and dairy products and is found in significant levels in cereals, grains, nuts, and legumes. In addition, certain fruits (i.e., apples, blueberries, and apricots) and vegetables (i.e., green beans and asparagus) contain small amounts of protein. Protein quality is determined by both the amino acid content and the digestibility of the protein. Proteins derived from plant foods are approximately 85% digestible; those in a mixed diet of meat products and refined carbohydrates

TABLE 4-5. CLASSIFICATION OF AMINO ACIDS

Essential (Indispensable) Amino Acids (EAA)
Isoleucine
Leucine
Lysine
Methionine
Phenylalanine
Threonine
Tryptophane
Valine
Histidine

Nonessential (Dispensable) Amino Acids (NEAA)
Alanine
Arginine
Aspartic acid
Asparagine
Glutamic acid
Glutamine
Glycine
Proline
Serine

Branched-Chain Amino Acids (BCAA)
Isoleucine
Leucine
Valine

are approximately 95% digestible. Protein quality also considers the "completeness" of the dietary protein.

Complete, or high quality proteins, contain all of the EAAs. Plant proteins are generally classified as incomplete and considered to be of less quality than animal proteins. Plants do contain all of the amino acids, but in lower amounts than animal proteins. Thus, one needs to eat more of a plant protein source to obtain adequate amounts of the amino acids, particularly the EAAs. In some cases, one must consume more than one source of plant protein to obtain a sufficient amount of the EAA. Grains tend to lack lysine, for example, and legumes tend to lack methionine. Consuming both plant protein sources simultaneously allow for complementary amino acid combinations (such as soybeans and rice, wheat bread and peanut butter, pinto beans and corn tortillas) so that sufficient amounts of EAAs are derived from the diet. The latter point is important for individuals adhering to a vegan diet plan (11).

Protein Digestion, Absorption, and Utilization

Protein digestion begins in the stomach and completed in the intestine. Amino acids resulting form dietary protein degradation are absorbed in the intestine. Once amino acids have been absorbed, they become available to the body. Collectively, amino acids reside in various amino acid pools, from which they can be used for (a) maintenance, synthesis, or repair of body proteins, (b) synthesis of other nitrogen-containing compounds, and (c) energy production.

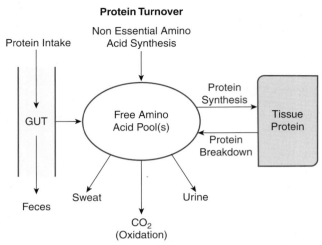

FIGURE 4-2. General representation of protein turnover.

Protein Turnover

Body proteins and amino acids are in a constant state of flux, referred to as protein turnover. Protein turnover encompasses both the synthesis of new body proteins and the breakdown of existing proteins. Amino acids derived from dietary sources and from endogenous breakdown of body proteins are utilized to maintain protein turnover (Fig. 4-2). The rate of protein turnover varies between proteins and is specific to their individual function. Intricate cycling of amino acids and body proteins is important for growth, maintenance, and repair of body tissues and for adaptation to different conditions.

Recommended Protein Intake and the DRIs

The RDA for protein for adults remains at 0.8 g of protein per kilogram body weight, or approximately 0.4 g of protein per pound; the DRIs for protein range approximately from 0.7 to 1.5 g per kilogram (or about 0.3 to 0.7 g per pound). The DRIs are based on the concept that there is a range of protein intakes for optimal protein utilization that span 10% to 35% of the total calories provided by the diet.

 1.8.8-HFS: Knowledge of the USDA My Pyramid and Dietary Guidelines for Americans.

To calculate protein intake using the AMDR, refer to Table 4-4 and follow the same steps previously described for carbohydrates. A diet for which protein provides 10% of the total energy intake will meet the RDA but is considered a relatively low-protein diet based upon normal protein consumption in the United States. The upper end of the AMDR for protein can be considered a high-protein diet. Although protein intakes at the upper end of the AMDR raise concerns regarding kidney damage, dehydration, and increased urinary calcium excretion, these concerns do not apply to healthy individuals with normal

renal function (13). Following recommendations put forth by My Pyramid (Fig. 4-3) will help ensure the appropriate blend of protein sources necessary for a healthy diet.

In brief, individuals should consume a variety of proteins with smaller and larger intakes of animal and plant proteins, respectively. Animal sources include lean meats, poultry, fish, eggs, and low-fat milk products, whereas vegetable sources include soy, whole grains, legumes, and vegetables.

Protein Intake for Physically Active Individuals

Protein metabolism during and following exercise is affected by gender, age, exercise intensity and duration, carbohydrate availability, type of exercise, and energy intake. The current RDA is 0.8 $g \cdot kg^{-1}$ body weight and does not consider the unique needs of routinely active individuals and competitive athletes. The 2005 DRIs provides a range of protein intakes (~10%–35% of total energy intake) necessary for most populations.

The noted increase in protein oxidation during endurance exercise, coupled with nitrogen balance studies, serves as the basis for recommending increased protein intakes to aid the body in recovery from habitual endurance training. Nitrogen balance studies suggested that the dietary protein intake necessary to support nitrogen balance in endurance athletes ranges from 1.2 to 1.4 $g \cdot kg^{-1} \cdot d^{-1}$ (16). Resistance exercise is thought to increase protein needs to a greater extent than endurance exercise because additional amino acids, as well as sufficient energy, are needed in excess of the requirement to support muscle growth. This is particularly true at the initiation of strength training because the most significant gains in muscle size will occur in the early period. Individuals who have habitually engaged in resistance training may not require as much protein because of more efficient protein utilization (14). The recommended protein intakes for strength-trained athletes range approximately from 1.4 to 1.7 $g \cdot kg^{-1} \cdot d^{-1}$.

ALCOHOL

Although not a macronutrient per se, alcohol (i.e., ethanol) does provide 7 kilocalories per gram (Table 4-1). Alcohol is readily absorbed by simple diffusion along the gastrointestinal tract, with the majority of absorption occurring in the small intestine. Rapid absorption of alcohol is responsible for its deleterious effects on mental and physical function. Body weight, gender, the type of alcohol, rate at which an alcoholic beverage is consumed, and the consumption with other foods determine blood alcohol levels. The majority of alcohol is metabolized by the liver. The remainder is lost in urine or exhaled. Excess alcohol consumption can cause acute alcohol intoxication, malnutrition, and chronic diseases, liver damage in particular. However, moderate consumption (i.e., one and two

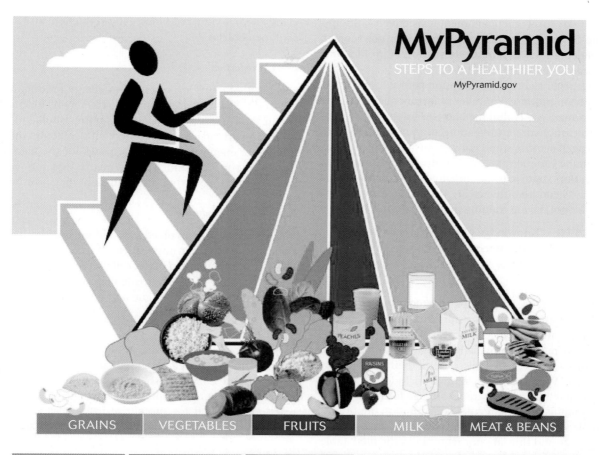

MyPyramid
STEPS TO A HEALTHIER YOU
MyPyramid.gov

GRAINS	VEGETABLES	FRUITS	MILK	MEAT & BEANS

GRAINS	VEGETABLES	FRUITS	MILK	MEAT & BEANS
Make half your grains whole	Vary your veggies	Focus on fruits	Get your calcium-rich foods	Go lean with protein
Eat at least 3 oz. of whole-grain cereals, breads, crackers, rice, or pasta every day	Eat more dark-green veggies like broccoli, spinach, and other dark leafy greens	Eat a variety of fruit	Go low-fat or fat-free when you choose milk, yogurt, and other milk products	Choose low-fat or lean meats and poultry
1 oz. is about 1 slice of bread, about 1 cup of breakfast cereal, or ½ cup of cooked rice, cereal, or pasta	Eat more orange vegetables like carrots and sweetpotatoes	Choose fresh, frozen, canned, or dried fruit	If you don't or can't consume milk, choose lactose-free products or other calcium sources such as fortified foods and beverages	Bake it, broil it, or grill it
	Eat more dry beans and peas like pinto beans, kidney beans, and lentils	Go easy on fruit juices		Vary your protein routine — choose more fish, beans, peas, nuts, and seeds

For a 2,000-calorie diet, you need the amounts below from each food group. To find the amounts that are right for you, go to MyPyramid.gov.

Eat 6 oz. every day	Eat 2½ cups every day	Eat 2 cups every day	Get 3 cups every day; for kids aged 2 to 8, it's 2	Eat 5½ oz. every day

Find your balance between food and physical activity
- Be sure to stay within your daily calorie needs.
- Be physically active for at least 30 minutes most days of the week.
- About 60 minutes a day of physical activity may be needed to prevent weight gain.
- For sustaining weight loss, at least 60 to 90 minutes a day of physical activity may be required.
- Children and teenagers should be physically active for 60 minutes every day, or most days.

Know the limits on fats, sugars, and salt (sodium)
- Make most of your fat sources from fish, nuts, and vegetable oils.
- Limit solid fats like butter, margarine, shortening, and lard, as well as foods that contain these.
- Check the Nutrition Facts label to keep saturated fats, trans fats, and sodium low.
- Choose food and beverages low in added sugars. Added sugars contribute calories with few, if any, nutrients.

MyPyramid.gov
STEPS TO A HEALTHIER YOU

U.S. Department of Agriculture
Center for Nutrition Policy and Promotion
April 2005
CNPP-15

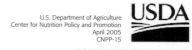

FIGURE 4-3. My Pyramid: steps to a healthier you.

drinks per day for women and men, respectively) of some alcoholic beverages, in particular red wine, may confer health benefits such as improved lipoprotein profiles and reduced cardiovascular disease risk.

The effects of alcohol consumption persist for up to 48 hours and compromise a number of factors related to athletic performance. Alcohol metabolism by the liver interferes with carbohydrate utilization, ultimately interfering with glycogen synthesis and glucose metabolism. In addition, immune function, recovery from exercise or injury, and hydration status can be impaired with alcohol consumption. Therefore, athletes are discouraged from consuming alcohol during training or competition (3,8).

 1.8.6-HFS: Knowledge of the difference between fat-soluble and water-soluble vitamins.

VITAMINS

Vitamins are vital organic compounds not synthesized by the body and are essential for optimal growth, development, and the maintenance of health. These nutrients are required and must be provided in small amounts in the diet. Vitamins are classified based upon their solubility in water or fat. Water-soluble vitamins include the B vitamins and vitamin C. There are no storage forms of water-soluble vitamins, making regular consumption important. Fat-soluble vitamins A, D, E and K, however, are stored in adipose tissue and thus are not required in the diet. Table 4-2 provides a comprehensive list of the water- and fat-soluble vitamins, their primary function, dietary sources, and respective requirements for adults. An overview of this information with specific regard for exercise and physical performance is provided here.

Function of Vitamins

Each vitamin, be it water- or fat-soluble, has a unique role and, in some cases, works synergistically with other vitamins to contribute to health and well-being. Vitamins serve as promoters and regulators of many reactions in the body, including energy-producing reactions (thiamin, riboflavin, niacin, B6, B12, biotin, and pantothenic acid). More specifically, the B vitamins, along with biotin and pantothenic acid, act as coenzymes that bind to enzymes to promote their activity and assure proper function in the metabolism of the macronutrients. Other important roles of vitamins include aiding in the visual processes (vitamin A), blood coagulation (vitamin K), and protection of cells from oxidative damage (antioxidants; vitamins E and C). Table 4-2 summarizes the major functions of these vitamins.

B Complex Vitamins

The B complex vitamins include thiamin, riboflavin, niacin, B6, B12, biotin, pantothenic acid, and folate. These vitamins can be further classified as having roles in energy production, red blood cell production, and amino acid metabolism.

Energy Production

Several B vitamins are essential to energy production by the body. These include thiamin, riboflavin, niacin, B6, biotin, and pantothenic acid. Thiamin, riboflavin, and niacin in particular are associated with cofactors that are integral to energy-producing pathways for the macronutrients. Biotin, B6, and B12 are coenzymes for various carboxylases involved in macronutrient metabolism.

Red Blood Cell Production

Folate and B12 are involved in red blood cell production. Deficiencies of either nutrient can lead to anemia. Given the critical role that red blood cells serve in oxygen delivery throughout the body, inadequate intake of folate or B12 is associated with fatigue and compromised athletic performance.

Amino Acid Metabolism

Vitamin B6 is required for amino acid metabolism. B6 is part of several enzyme systems that are involved in nitrogen metabolism. Therefore, this nutrient is essential to reactions required for protein utilization as a fuel and synthesis of nitrogen-containing compounds in the body.

Vitamin C

Vitamin C supplementation is popular, given this nutrient's roles in supporting the immune system and the healing process. Consumption of vitamin C (i.e., food source or supplement) can simultaneously facilitate iron absorption. Vitamin C is also a powerful antioxidant.

Fat-Soluble Vitamins

The fat-soluble vitamins (A, D, E, and K) are stored in body lipids. As a result, these nutrients can be toxic if taken in excess. The respective roles of these nutrients are given in Table 4-2. Of the fat-soluble vitamins, only vitamin E has a role specific to exercise and human performance as an antioxidant.

Antioxidants

Vitamin E acts as an antioxidant by protecting the polyunsaturated fatty acids in cell membranes from oxidative damage (1,2). This protective action helps maintain the integrity of cell membranes.

Dietary Sources of Vitamins

The presence of vitamins in foods is ubiquitous. Most foods contain some, if not many, of the vitamins (Table 4-2). For example, the B vitamins can be found in grains, meat, and fish. Vitamins A, E, and K are found in large amounts in leafy green vegetables. Vitamin C can be found in large amounts in citrus fruits. Dairy products are good sources of vitamins A and D. Another source of vitamins in the diet is fortified foods. Fortification is the process of adding nutrients to foods to increase nutrient intake and have a beneficial effect by preventing deficiencies. Folic acid fortification, which was mandated by the U.S. Food and Drug Administration (FDA) in 1998 in an attempt to reduce serious birth defects (i.e., neural tube defects), is the most recent example of nutrient fortification. Overall, the goal of the fortification program is to provide adequate nutrients for a beneficial effect without increasing the risk of vitamin toxicity.

MINERALS

Minerals are needed for numerous metabolic reactions and physiologic processes (Table 4-3). Major minerals are found in the body in amounts greater than 5 g, whereas trace minerals are needed in lesser amounts, less than 5 g. Major minerals include calcium, phosphorus, potassium, magnesium, sulfur, sodium, and chloride. Iron, zinc, copper, iodine, and chromium are common trace minerals that are also needed for normal body functions. Mineral salts, or electrolytes, such as sodium and chloride, are dissolved in water in the body. Water balance and electrolyte balance are closely linked. The most noted functions of sodium, chloride, and potassium are as electrolytes involved in the regulation of water balance by the body. The major mineral, calcium, and the trace mineral, iron, are highlighted here.

 1.8.9-HFS: Knowledge of the importance of calcium and iron in women's health.

Calcium

Calcium is required for healthy bones and teeth, muscle contraction, nerve transmission, and blood clotting. The role of calcium in bone formation is well known (10). Low intakes of dietary calcium result in calcium removal from the bone to maintain normal body processes. If low calcium intakes persist, bone turnover is compromised and bone mass is reduced. Routine exercise, particularly weight-bearing exercise, enhances calcium utilization and maintenance of bone mass (10,19). Although it is important for men to consume adequate calcium, women appear to be at particular risk for poor calcium intakes that may ultimately increase risk for osteoporosis later in life. The current RDA for calcium is 1,300 mg daily for young men and women aged 13–25 years. This amount of calcium, in combination with routine physical activity or exercise, will promote attainment of peak bone mass, which may reduce risk for or postpone the onset of osteoporosis later in life (18).

Iron

Iron is one of the most highly regarded trace minerals given its role as a component of the oxygen-carrying proteins, hemoglobin and myoglobin. Because hemoglobin carries oxygen in the body and myoglobin aids in oxygen delivery in the muscle, iron is important for aerobic metabolism and endurance exercise performance. Iron is also a constituent of several of the enzymes that constitute the electron transport chain. Therefore, iron has an essential role in energy production by the body.

Maintaining iron reserves by consistently consuming adequate amounts of iron is important for support of aerobic metabolism and energy production. When iron intake is compromised and iron stores are sufficiently reduced, iron deficiency anemia results. Females are particularly susceptible to iron deficiency anemia. Other risk populations includes female athletes, adolescent girls, athletes with low body weight, and those individuals who do not consume red meat. Iron requirements are set at 15 and 18 mg/day for males and females, respectively (6).

The diet provides two different types of iron: heme and nonheme. Heme iron, derived mostly from hemoglobin and myoglobin, is found mainly in animal products. Nonheme iron is found mainly in plant products. Heme and nonheme iron are absorbed differently. Heme iron is readily absorbed by the small intestine and is more highly bioavailable than nonheme iron. About 25% of heme iron is typically absorbed from the diet, whereas only 16.8% of nonheme iron is absorbed. Absorption of heme iron is not influenced by other dietary factors, whereas nonheme iron absorption is improved with ingestion of vitamin C. Good sources of heme iron include animal products, whereas nonheme iron is provided in dark, leafy vegetables, beans, and raisins.

Vitamin and Mineral Supplementation

Individuals who restrict their total energy intake or consume a diet with limited dietary variety are at risk for insufficient vitamin and mineral intakes. These individuals would benefit from a multivitamin mineral supplement that provides the recommended amounts of these micronutrients. Consumption of multiple vitamin or mineral supplements should be discouraged given the potential for toxicities or altered metabolism of other vitamins and minerals. Routine consumption of a variety of nutritious foods among the basic food groups practically ensures adequate intakes of vitamins and minerals.

DIETARY GUIDELINES FOR AMERICANS

The 2005 dietary guidelines for Americans are science-based directives aimed at promoting health and reducing risk for chronic diseases through diet and physical activity. The foundation for the dietary guidelines is that nutrient needs should be met predominantly by eating foods. Key recommendations for the general population address the following areas: adequate nutrients within calorie needs, weight management, physical activity, food groups to encourage fats, carbohydrates, sodium, potassium, alcoholic beverages, and food safety. In brief, the dietary guidelines describe a healthy diet as one that emphasizes whole grains, fruits, vegetables, and fat-free or low-fat milk and milk products; includes lean meats, fish, poultry, eggs, beans, and nuts; and is low in saturated fats, trans fats, cholesterol, salt (sodium), and added sugars. The complete recommendations contained in the report, as well as additional directives for various populations (i.e., children, older adults), can be found at http://www.health.gov/dietaryguidelines/.

The USDA food guide pyramid (Fig. 4-3) was developed to provide the consumer with direction regarding food choices and menu planning that are consistent with the dietary guidelines. The food guide pyramid is an illustrated translation of the dietary guidelines into consumer-friendly recommendations that consider physical activity in concert with appropriate food choices to meet nutrient needs. The food guide pyramid is a resource that can be used to assist people with making smart choices from each food group, finding balance between food and physical activity, maximizing the nutrition from calories, and staying within daily calorie needs.

WATER BALANCE

Approximately two thirds of a person's body weight is water. Water serves a number of functions in the body. These include carrying nutrients and waste products; maintaining the integrity of proteins and glycogen; participating in metabolic reactions; providing a medium for the nutrients; maintaining blood volume, blood pressure, and body temperature; and acting as a lubricant. Although imbalances in body water can occur (i.e., dehydration), the body is efficient in restoring water balance by regulating water intake and excretion with various mechanisms.

Water, or fluid, balance consists of water intake and water excretion. In healthy individuals, thirst controls water intake. Although thirst sensation can fall behind the body's water needs, most individuals are able to stay adequately hydrated. Sources of water to the body are liquids, foods, and metabolic water. These sources can provide approximately 1.4 to 3.0 L of water daily.

Water losses from the body are primarily controlled by the kidney, which responds to various hormones. Water is lost from the body as excretory products (i.e., urine and feces) and sweat and through respiration. Cumulative water losses on a daily basis approximate 1.4 to 3.0 L. Antidiuretic hormone, or ADH, is released from the brain when the blood volume or blood pressure is too low, stimulating kidney resorption of water. When body water losses are increased, the associated decrease in blood volume and blood pressure elicits the release of aldosterone, which causes sodium and water retention by the kidneys. Water balance is maintained when fluid intake from foods, liquids, and metabolism equals losses from the kidneys, skin, lungs, and feces.

Water needs are variable and are dependent on the foods and individual eats, the environment (i.e., heat and humidity), and activity level. The AI for total water is 3.7 and 2.7 $L \cdot day^{-1}$ for men and women, respectively. This recommendation is based on average intakes because a wide range of water intakes can prevent dehydration (7).

> **1.8.7-HFS: Knowledge of the importance of maintaining normal hydration before, during, and after exercise.**

GENERAL CONSIDERATIONS FOR ATHLETIC PERFORMANCE AND EXERCISE

Trained athletes and individuals who routinely exercise have increased energy and therefore macronutrient needs. These individuals should pay special attention to carbohydrate and protein intakes. Dietary carbohydrate should provide 6–8 $g \cdot kg^{-1} \cdot day^{-1}$ to maintain, as well as replenish, the body's glycogen stores. Protein intake of approximately 1.2–1.7 $g \cdot kg^{-1}$ is needed to maintain, build, and repair tissue on a daily basis. Fat intake should be adequate to provide the essential fatty acids and fat-soluble vitamins. In addition, dietary fat is an important energy source for weight maintenance. Active individuals should consume adequate food and fluid before, during, and after exercise to support maintenance of blood glucose levels during exercise, optimize exercise performance, and support recovery, respectively.

As long as athletes meet their energy needs to maintain body weight by consuming a varied and balanced diet, vitamin and mineral supplementation is not necessary. Micronutrient supplementation may be necessary for athletes who restrict energy intake, routinely eliminate one or more food groups from their diet, or habitually consume unbalanced diets of low micronutrient content.

Hydration status cannot be overemphasized. Athletes should be well-hydrated before exercise. Genuine effort should be made drink enough fluid during and after exercise to balance fluid losses (17). Consumption of sports beverages containing carbohydrates and electrolytes before, during, and after exercise can provide fuel for muscles and decrease risk of dehydration.

SUMMARY

The chapter provides an overview of basic nutrition principles for the health fitness professional. The intent is to provide a foundation for application of essential nutrition information to the health and well-being of healthy, physically active adults. Recommendations are made with regard to appropriate food choices to balance energy intake with expenditure while acquiring essential nutrients from the diet. Basic nutrition concepts are consistent with the current 2005 dietary guidelines for Americans, and where appropriate, considerations in support of exercise and athletic performance are provided.

REFERENCES

1. Bruno RS, Leonard SW, Park SI, Zhao Y, and Traber MG. Human vitamin E requirements assessed with the use of apples fortified with deuterium-labeled alpha-tocopheryl acetate. *Am J Clin Nutr*. 2006; 83:299–304.

2. Bruno RS, Traber, MG. Vitamin E biokinetics, oxidative stress, and cigarette smoking. *Pathophysiology*. 2006;13:143–9.

3. Burke L. *Practical Sports Nutrition*. Champaign (IL): Human Kinetics; 2007.

4. *Dietary Reference Intakes for Calcium, Phosphorous, Magnesium, Vitamin D, and Fluoride*. Washington (DC): National Academies Press; 1997.

5. *Dietary Reference Intakes for Energy, Carbohydrate, Fiber, Fat, Fatty Acids, Cholesterol, Protein, and Amino Acids*. Washington (DC): National Academies Press; 2005. p. 1331.

6. *Dietary Reference Intakes for Vitamin A, Vitamin K, Arsenic, Boron, Chromium, Copper, Iodine, Iron, Manganese, Molybdenum, Nickel, Silicon, Vanadium, and Zinc*. Washington (DC): National Academies Press; 2001.

7. *Dietary Reference Intakes for Water, Potassium, Sodium, Chloride, and Sulfate*. Washington (DC): National Academies Press; 2004.

8. *Sports Nutrition: A Practice Manual for Professionals*. 4th ed. Chicago: American Dietetic Association; 2006. p. 547.

9. Executive summary of the third report of the National Cholesterol Education Program (NCEP) Expert Panel on Detection, Evaluation, and Treatment of High Blood Cholesterol in Adults (Adult Treatment Panel III). *JAMA*. 2001;285:2486–97.

10. Heaney RP, Weaver CM. Newer perspectives on calcium nutrition and bone quality. *J Am Coll Nutr*. 2005;24:574S–81S.

11. Larson-Meyer D. *Vegetarian Sports Nutrition*. Champaign (IL): Human Kinetics; 2007.

12. Manore MM. Using glycemic index to improve athletic performance. In: *GSSI Sports Science News (Web series)*, 2004. www.gssiweb.com. Accessed on 10/13/08.

13. Martin WF, Armstrong LE, Rodriguez NR. Dietary protein intake and renal function. *Nutr Metab (Lond)*. 2005;2:25.

14. Phillips SM, Hartman JW, Wilkinson SB. Dietary protein to support anabolism with resistance exercise in young men. *J Am Coll Nutr*. 2005;24:134S–9S.

15. Position of the American Dietetic Association, Dietitians of Canada, and the American College of Sports Medicine: nutrition and athletic performance. *Med Sci Sports Exerc*. 2000;32(12):2130–45.

16. Rodriguez NR, Vislocky LM, Gaine PC. Dietary protein, endurance exercise, and human skeletal–muscle protein turnover. *Curr Opin Clin Nutr Metab Care*. 2007;10:40–5.

17. Sawka MN, Burke LM, Eichner ER, Maughan RJ, Montain SJ, Stachenfeld NS. American College of Sports Medicine position stand on exercise and fluid replacement. *Med Sci Sports Exerc*. 2007;39:377–90.

18. Specker B, Vukovich M. Evidence for an interaction between exercise and nutrition for improved bone health during growth. *Med Sport Sci*. 2007;51:50–63.

19. Specker BL. Evidence for an interaction between calcium intake and physical activity on changes in bone mineral density. *J Bone Miner Res*. 1996;11:1539–44.

SELECTED REFERENCES FOR FURTHER READING

Clark, N. *Nancy Clark's Sports Nutrition Guidebook*. 4th ed. Champaign (IL): Human Kinetics; 2008.

Clinical Sports Nutrition. 3rd. ed. Australia: McGraw Hill; 2006.

INTERNET RESOURCES

- Dietary Guidelines for Americans: http://www.health.gov/dietaryguidelines/
- U.S. Department of Agriculture: http://www.mypyramid.gov/

Lifespan Effects of Aging and Deconditioning

THE IMPACT OF AGING

> **1.1.35-HFS: Knowledge of the effect of the aging process on the musculoskeletal and cardiovascular structure and function at rest, during exercise, and during recovery.**

Differences exist within individuals of the same chronologic age because of physiologic aging and response to exercise stimuli (7). Complex issues arise when attempting to distinguish the aging effects on an individual's physiologic functions whether they are due to deconditioning and/or disease (7). Now, more consideration is being given to the changes in functional ability of the elderly and the contributions of the aging process versus inactivity to these changes as life span continues to increase (57). Growth and development, maturation, and degeneration are the inevitable processes involved in biologic aging. Healthcare professionals often use intervention strategies that functionally categorize individuals based solely on chronologic age. Table 5-1 lists these chronologic stages of aging. However, caution is warranted because individual distinctions in activity level, aging, environment, and disease confound making generalizations with regard to health, fitness, and functional status. The purpose of this chapter is to identify the effects of aging and deconditioning on the systems most relevant to exercise testing and prescription (see GETP8 Chapter 18).

FUNCTIONAL CAPACITY

The period from infancy through adolescence is characterized by dramatic increases in stature, body mass, and motor control. Maximal work capacity is directly related to fat-free mass (FFM), age, and sex, and indirectly related to percent body fat in healthy children (66). However, maximal work relative to FFM (W_{max}/FFM) is significantly related to age and sex, but not FFM. From early adulthood onward, there is a general decline in physical work capacity, which is matched with a concurrent loss in FFM. In older adults, the decline in FFM does not fully determine the observed loss in capacities for short-term and long-term work (55,112). Thus, throughout the lifespan, the ability to effectively perform extended (aerobic) and short-term (anaerobic) work is notably related to FFM in addition to numerous other physiologic factors.

Aerobic capacity, assessed by maximal oxygen uptake ($\dot{V}O_{2max}$), appears to remain constant throughout childhood when expressed relative to body mass ($mL \cdot kg^{-1} \cdot min^{-1}$) (98). However, absolute aerobic capacity ($L \cdot min^{-1}$) is lower in children as a result of less FFM. Thus, any absolute workload will result in a greater relative work stress (% of peak load) in children compared with adults. Although children exhibit similar relative aerobic capacities as adults, during weight-bearing exercise, such as walking and running, they display significantly lower movement efficiency because of shorter stride lengths and lower ventilatory efficiency related to requirements for greater air exchange at any given level of exercise (185).

During adulthood, a steady age-related decline in $\dot{V}O_{2max}$ has been observed, with the losses averaging about 1% per year between 25 and 75 years (about 5 mL $O_2 \cdot kg^{-1} \cdot min^{-1}$ with each decade of aging) (82,156). In

> > > **KEY TERMS**

Anaerobic capacity: The ability of the anaerobic energy systems to produce energy during short-term maximal effort exercise (65).

Deconditioning: A partial or complete reversal of physiologic adaptations to exercise, resulting from a significant reduction or cessation of exercise (122).

Detraining: The process that occurs after the cessation of training in which adaptations to exercise are gradually reduced or lost (76,124,165).

Muscle atrophy: Reduction in muscle size from disuse.

TABLE 5-1. STAGES OF AGING

Neonatal	Birth to 3 weeks
Infancy	3 weeks to 1 year
Childhood	
Early	1–6 years
Middle	7–10 years
Later	Prepubertal
Puberty	Girls 9–15 years
	Boys 12–16 years
Adolescence	Up to 6 years after puberty
Adulthood	
Early	20–29 years
Middle	30–44 years
Later	45–64 years
Senescence	
Elderly	65–74 years
Older elderly	75–84 years
Very old	85 years and older

fact, it has been suggested that the apparent loss of $\dot{V}O_{2max}$ may begin as early as age 12 years, perhaps related to decreased levels of physical activity (150). The degree to which this decline occurs, and the time point at which the decline commences, are significantly affected by amount and intensity of physical activity. The decline in $\dot{V}O_{2max}$ parallels reduced maximum work capacity and is attributed to decreased maximal cardiac output and reduced arterial-venous oxygen difference (a-v DO_2) as well as a loss of skeletal muscle mass (64,90). Reductions in a-v DO_2 have been related to reduced levels of arterial oxygen saturation, increases in subcutaneous adipose, diminished perfusion of skeletal muscle, and reductions in levels of aerobic enzymes (151). The decline in aerobic capacity in sedentary men and women is almost twice that of persons who remain physically active (94). Exercise training has been shown to reverse the decreased energy efficiency (increased energy cost of exercise) that is associated with the aging process and contributes to decreases in aerobic capacity (191). In addition to physical limitations resulting from sedentary lifestyles, loss of coordination, lack of familiarity of required skills, and disabling diseases such as arthritis and obesity may also play a role in limiting $\dot{V}O_{2max}$ (54,77).

Ironically, anaerobic capacity in children has not been well documented, although their activity patterns are exemplified by short-term anaerobic activities (9). Anaerobic power is lower in children than adults in both absolute power and when corrected for body mass as a consequence of differences in adenosine triphosphate (ATP), creatine phosphate (CP), and muscle glycogen, ATPase, creatine kinase, phosphorylase, phosphofructokinase, and other factors (65). Motivation and neuromuscular coordination also factor into diminished anaerobic capacity in children. Both sexes maintain a plateau in

anaerobic capacity through about age 35 years, at which time it begins to decline.

By age 65 years, anaerobic capacity declines to essentially the level of late childhood. However, maximal power output for 30 seconds is highly associated (r = 0.84) with lean thigh volume, and high-intensity training significantly increases (+12.5%) peak power output in older persons aged 60 to 70 years (111,112). The aged anaerobic system does not work as quickly to produce energy, and when lactic acid is produced, it is not cleared as quickly. The probable reasons for the decline in the anaerobic system is the loss of mass in large muscles and the decrease in the size and number of glycolytic fast-twitch fibers, which are known to rely more on glycolysis. Intramuscular blood flow is also lower in older people, which contributes to a slower recovery and lactate removal rate. Even in power-trained or endurance-trained master's athletes, anaerobic power declines 50% by age 75 years (162).

CARDIOVASCULAR SYSTEM

> **1.1.34-HFS: Knowledge of and the ability to describe the changes that occur in maturation from childhood to adulthood for the following: skeletal muscle, bone structure, reaction time, coordination, heat and cold tolerance, maximal oxygen consumption, strength, flexibility, body composition, resting and maximal heart rate, and resting and maximal blood pressure.**

Heart

Although maximal cardiac output increases with growth in children, at any given level of submaximal work, cardiac output is somewhat lower in children than adults primarily because of lower stroke volume (SV) (51,142). Lower sympathetic stimulation of the heart in children compared with adults has been suggested as a cause for the smaller SV (177). However, during modest submaximal exercise, increases in SV do not seem to be related to aging. This phenomenon is a result of the Frank-Starling mechanism to compensate for a reduced number of pacemaker cells and impaired adrenergic chronotropic function (100,174). In boys, SV is higher and heart rate (HR) lower than in girls at given absolute submaximal work rates (177).

Numerous physiologic changes to the heart transpire with aging. It is imperative to differentiate between these normal biologic changes and underlying pathologies that exist in cardiovascular disease. The aging heart shows decreases in intracellular transportation and pacemaker cells as well as sensitivity to β-receptor, baroreceptor, and chemoreceptor stimulation. Furthermore, interstitial fibrosis within the myocardium and calcification of the heart's connective tissue skeleton results in collagen crosslinking and elasticity loss. The heart's function is attenuated by an increase in arterial stiffness, systolic blood pressure (SBP), and left ventricular afterload and hypertrophy. Further changes in the left ventricle result in extended diastolic relaxation (34,56).

Maximal cardiac output in a 65-year-old person is 10% to 30% less than in a young adult. Decreases in both maximal HR and maximal SV contribute to decreased maximal cardiac output of older adults. By contrast, in the period immediately after high-intensity exercise, HR recovery, return of oxygen uptake to baseline, and muscular power recovery occur faster in children than in young adults and adults (14,70,194).

Several studies over the past 25 years have shown that resting cardiac output and SV decrease with age (141,147). Results suggest resting cardiac output decreases about 1% per year, from a mean of 6.5 L per minute in the third decade to a mean of 3.9 L per minute in the ninth decade. From 25 to 85 years resting SV decreases 30%, from 85 mL to 60 mL (147). However, in subjects who have been carefully screened for coronary artery disease, investigators have demonstrated that overall left ventricular function, using resting ejection fraction as an index, does not decline between 25 and 80 years (141). Estimates of volume made by echocardiography and radionuclide scintigraphy demonstrate resting SV also does not decline with age. Because resting HR is also not age related, these data suggest that resting cardiac output does not decline with age in healthy individuals.

Heart Rate

In children, HR is often high at rest (80–100 bpm), apparently as a result of reduced SV relative to body size (153). This reduced SV generally vanishes with growth and increased levels of physical activity, thus it is not age specific. In combination with an increase in the oxygen-carrying capacity of the blood secondary to hemoglobin increases that occur through the late teens, resting HR decreases to approximately 65 to 75 bpm by adulthood.

Resting HR is relatively unchanged throughout adulthood. However, maximal attainable HR declines proportionally with age (predicted maximum HR = 220 – age) (35). A decrease in myocardial sensitivity to catecholamines and the effect of prolonged diastolic filling appear to be responsible for this decline in maximal HR. In addition, as aging occurs through adulthood, a greater HR response to a given submaximal exercise intensity is observed (153). A decrease of 5 to 10 bpm per decade for peak HR also occurs. For those who train, this reduction in peak HR can be offset somewhat by increases in end-diastolic volume and stroke volume, which help to reduce the negative effects on peak cardiac output. As a result, recovery HR remains higher, and recovery takes longer after maximal exercise as one ages (162).

Blood Vessels

Vascular stiffness occurs with aging and is the result of worn elastin and changes in collagenous properties in the arterial walls. As a result, peripheral vascular resistance increases with age. The capillary-to-muscle-fiber ratio also becomes lower with age, further reducing peripheral blood flow (163). Loss of plasticity of the aorta impedes pulsatile ejection, which delays the arteries in accepting SV. In turn, this results in an increase in SBP and mean arterial pressure (11,162).

PULMONARY SYSTEM

> **1.1.34-HFS: Knowledge of and the ability to describe the changes that occur in maturation from childhood to adulthood for the following: skeletal muscle, bone structure, reaction time, coordination, heat and cold tolerance, maximal oxygen consumption, strength, flexibility, body composition, resting and maximal heart rate, and resting and maximal blood pressure.**

Thoracic wall compliance decreases with age, and the ability to expand the chest cavity becomes limited (11). This is particularly evident by age 65 years. Starting in adulthood, a progressive decrease occurs in both maximal expiratory flow and lung volume reserve with aging. Residual volume increases by 30% to 35%, and vital capacity decreases by 40% to 50% by age 70 years (145), possibly because of a loss of elastic recoil of the lungs (153). Furthermore, during exertion, increased ventilation is accomplished via greater frequency of breathing rather than depth of breathing in adulthood. The overall net effect is a 20% increase in the work of respiratory muscles (42). Despite these changes, respiratory function does not limit exercise capacity or the ability to benefit from exercise training unless lung function is severely impaired. However, because of the increased work imposed on the respiratory muscles, elderly individuals may report breathing discomfort owing to the increased ventilatory demand caused by physical exertion, despite having normal cardiopulmonary function (85).

MUSCULOSKELETAL SYSTEM

Muscle

The number and proportion of muscle fiber types are predetermined at birth and classified by pH sensitivity of myofibrillar ATPase (39,164). Type I slow-twitch fibers are more resistant than type II fast-twitch fibers to atrophy until the seventh decade. Hence, the percentage of type I fibers increases because of the atrophy and degeneration of type II fibers. The selective loss of type II fibers, however, may be more a function of disuse given that activity patterns suggest that less muscle contraction against resistance occurs from adulthood to senescence.

The loss of skeletal muscle mass is common with the aging process and has been termed **sarcopenia** (39). Declines in muscle fiber number and area, motor unit size and recruitment, innervation, capillarization, protein synthesis, and growth factor alterations are to some degree responsible for sarcopenia (17,115). Sarcopenia limits muscle function with 25% of maximal force–generating capacity lost by the age of 65 years and as much as 40% over a lifetime (8,152,154). Whereas the decline in muscle strength in men and women is primarily the result of muscle mass losses, neural factors are responsible for additional functional decrements (4). The dual myopathic and neuropathic etiology of sarcopenia is characterized by changes that result in functional limitations in gait and activities of daily living (13,16,116) and increased risk of accidental falls (39). Additionally, sarcopenia impairs thermoregulation, metabolism, and glucose sensitivity (115). There exists some agreement, however, that sarcopenia is primarily a result of diminishing stimulus secondary to sedentary lifestyles (35). Furthermore, changes in the architecture of muscle (pennation angle, muscle thickness, fascicle length) may be additional factors worthy of consideration in muscle function (99). The evidence is unequivocal that exercise training (cardiovascular and resistance) can help to attenuate these aging processes.

Body Composition

Approximately one third of the population of the United States is obese and one sixth of teenagers (12–19 years) are overweight, escalating the risk of chronic disease (130). Body fat percentages are independent of sex in prepubescent children but are highly influenced by genetics as well as environmental factors. Acceptable body fat percentages for prepubescent children are between 10% and 15% (123). Sex differences begin to show during puberty and extend through adulthood with acceptable limits of 20% in men and 30% in women. Distribution of body fat is sex specific from the third to seventh decade. Whereas women tend to exhibit greater increases in internal body fat after age 45 years, men accumulate greater subcutaneous fat. The previously discussed losses in FFM with aging have been associated with decreases in basal metabolic rate of approximately 5% per decade throughout adulthood, which in turn is a contributing factor along with genetics in fat gain (26). An accumulating body of

knowledge points to lifestyle changes, including decreased physical activity, as the underlying culprit in the changes in body composition (decreased FFM and increased fat mass [FM]) with aging. In elderly subjects, increased levels of body fat contribute to slower gait speed and functional limitations (169). Exercise training plays an important role in the maintenance of FFM and FM as one ages.

Bone

Bone, or *osseous tissue,* is continuously remodeling as a result of osteoblastic (formation) and osteoclastic (reabsorption) activity (35,150). This dynamic, efficacious process of remodeling acts as a source of stored bone and calcium and is a result of the ever-changing mechanical stresses placed on the body as individuals pass through the various stages of life (35). Genetics plays a major role in prepubescent bone maturation and is highly correlated to the loading factor imposed by the muscle mass in accordance with Wolff's law (186). Bone growth during childhood presents two primary problems because the epiphysis is not united with the bone shaft. First, overuse can result in epiphysitis during this growth period. Second, fracture may pass through the epiphyseal plate, sometimes leading to abnormal growth (153). Children exposed to various weight-bearing activities exhibit positive bone growth responses (187). Peak bone mass is posited to occur by the end of the second decade of life, although others claim that bone can continue to mature up to age 30 years (35).

Senescence generally occurs at the beginning of the sixth decade and is characterized by predominant osteoclastic activity, or "uncoupling." As a result, decreases in bone density manifested by decreases in calcium regulatory mechanisms, hormone levels, and metabolic activity occur (150). Lifestyle factors, such as physical activity level, calcium intake, and nutritional status, play a major role as well, making it difficult to determine the intrinsic contribution of aging itself on bone loss (128,150). The loss of muscle mass with aging has been associated with reductions in bone mineral density (BMD) (59). The rate of bone loss is site specific (e.g., the calcaneus shows significant bone loss earlier than other bones). Women tend to begin losing bone mass between 30 and 35 years of age at a rate of 0.75% to 1.0% per year (150). Bone loss in men generally commences between 50 to 55 years of age at an initial rate of 0.4% per year. In addition, women lose 36 g of BMD per decade compared with $30 \text{ g} \cdot \text{decade}^{-1}$ in men. By age 80 years, the trend has reversed somewhat. Men have shown a 55% decrease from their peak bone mineral content, and women only drop 40%. This is at least partially responsible for the 1.5-cm height loss that occurs for every 30 years past the fifth decade of life (35). This marked reduction of bone loss precipitates normal and pathologic fractures causing increased morbidity and mortality (75). Thus, clinical osteoporosis exposes a vulnerability to accommodate bone health and is a precursor to disability (128).

Joints and Flexibility

Joint flexibility, required to produce fluid and efficient motion of the body, is commonly compromised with aging. Specifically, tendons and ligaments often lose elasticity leading to decreases in joint mobility (10). This progressive loss of flexibility, resulting from several factors, including disease, deterioration of joint structures, and progressive degeneration of collagen fibers, begins during young adulthood. Increased incidence of knee and back problems from osteoarthritis has been observed beginning with middle age and progressing through old age (153). Degeneration of joints, especially the spine, is often found in elderly persons. Along with loss of strength, loss of flexibility plays a significant role in increase risk of falls and other injuries. Particularly, decreased ankle flexibility has a direct link with risk of falls as a result of diminished balance and functional ability (117). The rate of deterioration accelerates beyond age 65 years, but few specific findings are available for this age group. Exercise training and range of motion exercise helps to maintain and/or increase flexibility as aging occurs.

NERVOUS SYSTEM

Infants and very young children undergo intensive learning to develop motor skills for function and performance. The central nervous system (CNS) is recognized as the predominant center for determining the outcomes of this learning. The learning process includes the integration of movement patterns that minimize physiologic cost, asymmetry, and variability of body segment coordination (88). The resulting improvement in economy of movement may decrease oxygen consumption at submaximal velocities. This improvement may also enhance reaction time, which decreases by about 15% by age 70 years as compared with early adulthood (50).

Detrimental changes in neurotransmitters, nerve conduction velocities, and fine motor control are all indicative of normal CNS aging (148). The increased incidence of sensory deficits, particularly hearing and vision, and higher thresholds of perception for many stimuli may be related to the 35% to 40% increase in falls by persons older than age 60 years (129,155).

IMMUNE SYSTEM

Aging and environmental factors (e.g., pollutants, electromagnetism, environmental tobacco smoke) are responsible to varying degrees for decreased immune system function (153). From peak immune system activity around puberty, an overall decline of 5% to 30% over a normal lifespan is expected, with some functional indices decreasing to 5% to 10% of early adulthood function. The major reason for the immune system loss is a falloff of suppressor T-cell function, which leads to an inability to fight pathogens (35). The end result is reduced resistance to pathogens and increased incidence of both tumors and autoimmune disorders.

RENAL FUNCTION, FLUID REGULATION, AND THERMOREGULATION

> **1.1.34-HFS: Knowledge of and the ability to describe the changes that occur in maturation from childhood to adulthood for the following: skeletal muscle, bone structure, reaction time, coordination, heat and cold tolerance, maximal oxygen consumption, strength, flexibility, body composition, resting and maximal heart rate, and resting and maximal blood pressure.**

Renal function declines approximately 30% to 50% between ages 30 and 70 years (153). Along with this decline, acid-based control, glucose tolerance, and drug clearance decrease. A general reduction in total cellular water occurs with aging, with a decline of 10% to 50% in total body water compared with cellular water levels in early adults.

The primary maturational characteristics related to exercise in heat occur in late puberty or early adulthood. Before that time, children have a consistently lower sweat rate characterized by lower absolute and relative sweat volumes along with a higher core temperature required to start sweating. Thus, children tend to rely more on radiation and convection for heat dissipation than adults. The composition of children's sweat also differs, particularly in regard to chloride, which is lower in children than adults (52,118). Aging is also associated with attenuated skin blood flow, which may contribute to a reduced ability to thermoregulate. Furthermore, the effects of aging predispose older individuals to rapidly dehydrate. This may become particularly important during exercise through evaporative water loss and perspiration (95). In addition, many older adults take a variety of medications that may further confound hydration levels, placing further limitations on thermoregulation.

Children have a greater ratio of surface area to mass than adults, which enhances convective and radiant heat transfer between skin and the environment, making tolerance to cold more difficult (96). However, it has been suggested that other factors that occur with aging, such as thermogenic and vasoconstrictive responses, may also limit thermoregulation to cold in children. Beyond childhood, it has been demonstrated that the ability to regulate core temperature is negatively affected by aging (21,173,192).

SUMMARY

Growth, development, maturation, and degeneration have profound effects on the body's capability to respond

TABLE 5-2. SYSTEM CHANGES

	NEONATAL INFANCY	CHILDHOOD	ADOLESCENCE	ADULTHOOD	SENESCENCE
Cardiovascular System					
Cardiac output		↑	↑	↔	↔
Stroke volume		↑	↑	↔	↓
HR_{max}		↑	↔	↓	↓
$\dot{V}O_{2max}$		↑	↑	↓	↓
Pulmonary System					
Vital capacity	↑	↑	↑	↓	↓
Musculoskeletal System					
Bone mineral density	↑	↑	↑	↔	↓
Muscle mass	↑	↑	↑	↑	↓
Anaerobic capacity		↑	↑	↑	↓
Flexibility		↑	↑	↓	↓
% Body fat		↑	↑	↑	↔
Nervous System					
Motor control	↑	↑	↑	↔	↓
Immune System					
Immune system function		↑	↑	↔	↓

↑ = increases; ↔ = no change; ↓ = decreases.

to the external stresses placed on it through exercise. Lifestyle factors associated with aging make it difficult to distinguish between degeneration attributable to normal physiologic aging and alterations in habitual physical activity. Gerontologic investigations reveal that reduction of activity is predictive of lifespan and attributable at least partly to altered neurotransmission in dopamine activity (78). Table 5-2 highlights selected age-related changes. The interrelationships between biologic aging and physical activity warrant further investigation.

IMPACT OF DECONDITIONING

Reductions in physical activity affect almost everyone; therefore, a health/fitness professional must understand musculoskeletal adaptations to reduced physical activity so that changes in functional ability can be predicted. The appropriate exercise and/or physical activity would then be prescribed after disuse or in the rehabilitation process not only of elite or weekend athletes but also of diseased, disabled, and aging populations. Deconditioning can result from detraining, bed rest, casting, use of crutches, paralysis, aging, or even exposure to microgravity during space flight (Table 5-3). The following section is a brief description of each of the modes of deconditioning that have yielded information regarding the effects of inactivity on the musculoskeletal system.

MODES OF DECONDITIONING

Decreased muscle activity is defined as a reduction in intensity or in amount of regularly performed daily activity by a muscle or muscle group. Detraining (returning to a sedentary lifestyle after formalized exercise training)

does not suggest the same adaptive response as a sedentary individual would have with 1 month of bed rest. For example, bed rest for 1 month, which constitutes a dramatic change in the daily amount of muscle activity, even for a previously sedentary individual, causes greater skeletal muscle atrophy than for an individual who ceases resistance training for the same period but continues daily physical activity (69,71). Thus, the magnitude of the adaptive response to decreased activity depends on relative change in an individual's muscle use, which may be caused by injury, illness, or cessation of exercise program. Table 5-3 indicates noted changes in the various modes used to study deconditioning.

Detraining

Detraining in athletes often occurs during the off-season or because of an injury when normal training routines are interrupted. Detraining is most often observed in previously sedentary individuals who exercise for several weeks or months and then discontinue the practice.

Bed Rest

> **1.1.2-CES: Describe the physiologic effects of bed rest and discuss the appropriate physical activities that might be used to counteract these changes.**

Periods of bed rest, in the clinical setting, are usually associated with some underlying disease, so differentiating musculoskeletal changes caused by inactivity versus disease process is often difficult. However, bed-resting healthy individuals has been used as an experimental model of muscle unloading to rule out disease complications and has yielded results similar to casting or the use of crutches (20,21,43,47,60,71,102,135,146,160,190).

TABLE 5-3. TYPES OF DECONDITIONING

TYPE	NOTED CHANGES	REFERENCES
Detraining	Muscle atrophy	72
	Decrease in muscle size	68
	Decrease in fiber numbers	176
	Capillaries undamaged	136
	Fiber type reverts to composition before training	165
Bed rest	Muscle atrophy (greater than in exercising individuals)	165
	Considerable atrophy of fast- and slow-twitch fibers	71
	No change in myonuclear number per mm of fiber length	131
Casting	Decrease in strength attributed to neural factors if short term	40
	Severe atrophy if muscles in shortened position	61, 134
	Neuromuscular transmission defects	63
Crutches	Reduction of strength by 20% in non–weight-bearing limb	137
	No changes in contralateral weight-bearing muscle	31, 137
Paralysis	Reduced mitochondrial content	31, 114
	Poor fatigue resistance	114
	Fast-twitch fibers greater atrophy after 6 months	31
	Proportion of type II B increases, and type II A decreases	31
	Actomyosin ATPase activity not elevated	114
	Exercise activities generally limited to motor units above spinal cord injury	83
	Activities of daily living improved by strength and conditioning	84
	Atrophy of 50% or more after 6 months of injury	30, 31
Space Flight	Muscle atrophy	37
	Muscle strength decreases	48, 103
	Greater loss in fast-twitch than slow-twitch fibers	37
	Bone loss to 12%	184
	Reduced $\dot{V}O_{2max}$	106
	Decreased work capacity and fatigued earlier	37
	Exercise counteracts harmful effects	37

Casting

A cast characteristically places a joint in a fixed position with the objective of immobilizing injured tissue or bone. When a cast is used, the muscle activity not only decreases, but also fixes the joint position in which the muscles are held at a relatively constant length. A cast brace is specifically designed with materials that can be used in the treatment of fractures in order for an individual to return to earlier activity and early joint motion (166), which would lead to better recovery (121,133,170).

Crutches

The use of crutches may or may not be associated with casting. Although a lower limb in a cast often requires crutches, minor injuries (sprains and strains) may not require casting but may require non–weight bearing. Human lower-limb suspension via the use of crutches has also been used as an experimental technique to study adaptations to unloading (46,68,136,140).

Paralysis

Many diseases and spinal cord injuries (SCIs) can lead to partial or total paralysis. Automobile accidents, sports (football, diving, and gymnastics), and gunshot wounds have been reported as the most common causes of SCIs (62). Although it is often difficult to distinguish how a disease process interacts with muscle disuse to produce functional changes, SCIs are unique in that affected muscles may still be innervated yet receive no input from higher nervous centers. Thus, muscles are innervated by intact motor neurons but are seldom activated except during spasm (30,31,33,45,72,73,114,167).

Space Flight

In 2004, the president announced the United States would send astronauts back to the moon by 2020 then on to the planet Mars, shortly afterward. This announcement initiated funding that has led to more research into zero-gravity environments. On a limited basis, researchers have been able to scientifically study the body's response to muscle unloading in the unique microgravity environment of outer space (2,189). However, with minimum flights and small numbers of crew members who repeat space missions, reproducibility of results has been difficult (36). Therefore, simulations of microgravity have been used and involve lower-limb suspension, water immersion, and head-down tilt protocols (1,5,138). Ongoing investigations are using exercise as a means to reduce the effects of prolonged exposure to microgravity.

EFFECTS ON BONE

> **1.1.34-HFS: Knowledge of and the ability to describe the changes that occur in maturation from childhood to adulthood for the following: skeletal muscle, bone structure, reaction time, coordination, heat and cold tolerance, maximal oxygen consumption, strength, flexibility, body composition, resting and maximal heart rate, and resting and maximal blood pressure.**

Exercise that promotes skeletal loading induces a compensatory adaptation in the structure and functional integrity of bone (see Chapter 39). The processes underlying the adaptive mechanisms of bone to loading represent a complex interaction of endocrine and musculoskeletal systems. Exercise serves as a stimulus for skeletal adaptation that includes the maintenance or addition of bone mass. Conversely, inactivity—as in bed rest because of injury or partly caused by inactivity associated with aging—reduces bone mass by adversely affecting calcium metabolism and the bone formation process.

Bone formation may be described as a dynamic lifelong process. As such, bone health has been studied in young and old subjects under conditions of short-term immobilization, prolonged bed rest, exposure to microgravity associated with space flight, and clinical conditions such as paralysis. Although results from studies are similar, comparisons across subject populations regarding bone loss and genesis are made difficult by underlying pathologies.

Depending on the length of enforced inactivity as well as underlying pathologies, recovery of lost bone or osteogenesis may be protracted. Healthcare practitioners need to know that extended periods of deconditioning and disuse not only result in bone loss but also compromise future bone health by increasing the patient's susceptibility to fracture and promoting early-onset osteoporosis.

The discussion that follows includes information from studies aimed at revealing the effects of inactivity, bed rest, and immobilization on bone mass and calcium metabolism in adult humans. Evidence of changes in bone mass and structural integrity has been inferred from radiologic measurements. Assays of endocrine regulators indicative of calcium absorption from the gut and deposition of calcium in bone are used in conjunction with urinary and fecal excretion of calcium to reveal the role of calcium metabolism in bone health. Several review articles offer additional detail (23,24,49,178).

Bone Mineral Density

Whereas removal of the exercise stimulus has been shown to reverse gains in lumbar spine BMD in postmenopausal women (38,81), reducing the level of activity in habitually active middle-aged persons was associated with significant losses of bone mineral content in trabecular bone (119). Similarly, elderly patients who must drastically reduce their level of activity because of hip fractures show significant decreases in BMD in the unaffected hip up to 13 months after the fracture (110). Alfredson et al. (6) reported that male athletes who underwent Achilles tendon surgery showed significant calcaneal bone loss on the surgically repaired side compared with the noninjured side at 52 weeks after surgery with no signs of bone recovery.

Transient bone mass changes, as a consequence of seasonal loads versus no load associated with the off-season, have been reported in female collegiate gymnasts (161) and male ice hockey players (126). A recent investigation revealed greater BMD in premenarcheal gymnasts compared with inactive control subjects (125), owing to speculation that the active subjects' more robust skeletal architecture provides protection later in life. Contrary to the notion that above-average BMD early in life protects individuals in the later years, Magnusson et al. (110) reported that young adult soccer players with above-average BMD experienced a gradual decline in bone mass over the years, with follow-up observations at age 70 years revealing no significant differences in bone mass between the former soccer players and control subjects.

Over the short term, however, Valdimarsson et al. (180) reported that female college soccer players had greater bone mass in the trochanter than age-matched controls nearly a decade after retiring from competition. Similarly, Nordstrom et al. (127) found a wide range of male athletes to have greater trochanter bone mass than controls at 3 and 5 years postcompetition. Although the loss of bone mass in previously active individuals is subject to decline over time as a result of disuse, it may be only in later years that any bone accrual that results from sports participation is truly negated. Additional study is needed to determine if highly active elderly persons present significantly different bone mass profiles than their less active counterparts.

In the absence of mechanical stress produced by weight-bearing activity, bed rest negatively affects the homeostatic mechanisms that underlie bone health. Without weight-bearing activity, calcium balance is disturbed, and, ultimately, bone mass is lost (93).

Calcium Balance

To preserve bone mass, a balance must exist between resorption of existing bone and the formation of new bone. Prolonged inactivity, such as bed rest, is known to upset this balance, resulting in excessive resorption of calcium from bone, as manifested in elevated levels of serum calcium or hypercalcemia and a concurrent increase in urinary and fecal calcium (104). During periods of increased resorption, serum, urinary, and fecal levels of calcium fluctuate in response to hormonal regulation and decreased absorption of calcium from the intestines. Within weeks of inactivity, negative calcium balance has been observed in healthy persons subjected to bed rest (104), persons experiencing weightlessness (158), and individuals with SCIs (25).

Hormonal regulation of calcium metabolism, although altered during periods of bed rest, plays a less prominent role in the maintenance of bone mass than the influences of mechanical load. That is, reduction in mechanical load or stress appears to trigger an ordered response of bone resorption and endocrine activity, including the regulation of calcium absorption from the gut by 1,25 dihydroxyvitamin D (1,25-D) (159). Whereas the other prominent calcium regulator, parathyroid hormone (PTH), is unchanged or decreases slightly during periods of negative calcium balance in healthy subjects experiencing bed rest, 1,25-D decreases or does not change (104,144,181,195). Conversely, during the acute phase, individuals with SCIs who are immobilized show low PTH and 1,25-D levels (25).

Bone Mass

Site-specific losses in BMD of 1% to 2% per month have been reported based on animal models, microgravity experienced by astronauts, and as a result of bed rest (15,29,87,105). The rate and, ultimately, the amount of bone loss may be tied to health status. Based on ultrasound calcaneal measures, healthy men lost approximately 0.017% to 0.11% of bone mass per week during a 120-day bed-rest study. Persons with SCIs, however, lose as much as 33% of calcaneus bone volume within 6 months of the injury (25). It appears that the effect of SCI on bone loss is even more pronounced in women with SCI who are postmenopausal (157).

Susceptibility to bone loss increases as a function of the proximity to mechanical load and type of bone. LeBlanc et al. (105) observed a 10% loss in BMD in the calcaneus compared with 4% at the femoral neck and spine; however, no significant reduction in bone mass occurred in the radius of the forearm after 17 weeks of bed rest. During periods of unloading, trabecular bone, lying inside cortical bone, with its high surface-to-volume area, is targeted by bone-absorbing osteoclasts. Under conditions of disuse, trabecular bone loss is greatest at load-bearing sites (e.g., proximal tibia) and occurs more rapidly than cortical bone loss (105,193).

Biochemical markers of bone turnover are used extensively in bed-rest studies to assess the metabolic activity of bone. A recent study of healthy male subjects, subjected to 120 days of bed rest, showed increased bone resorption by day 7 and a decrease in bone formation by day 50 (79). Other investigators have also reported excessive bone resorption in healthy subjects during disuse (183,195), as well as in paraplegic subjects (120). However, Palle et al. (132) reported only transient changes in bone resorption

early in the course of bed rest, with values returning to baseline by the fourth and final month of the study. It appears that the bone loss may be explained as a disproportionate increase in osteoclast cell activity (101). Moreover, osteoclast activity is noticeably localized in the lower body (e.g., calcaneus, tibia), ultimately compromising the structural components (e.g., matrix, collagen) of bone and increasing the risk of fracture.

An uncoupling of the bone resorption and formation process is evidenced by the fact that biochemical markers of bone formation do not increase during unloading. Investigators have reported that biochemical markers of bone resorption remain elevated for weeks upon resumption of activity (107,179,181). Thus, individuals with a history of bone loss who subsequently undergo forced unloading are particularly vulnerable to injury caused by fracture as they regain their mobility.

Remobilization: Can Lost Bone Be Regained?

The timeline for regaining bone lost caused by disuse has been studied in animals and humans. Jaworski and Uhthoff (86) evaluated the osteogenic activity of old and young dogs after immobilization of the forelimbs for 32 weeks. At 28 weeks into remobilization, there was a 40% and 70% recovery of bone mass in old and young dogs, respectively. Significant deficits in bone mass were still apparent in horses who remobilized for 8 weeks after 7 weeks of disuse (182). In contrast, the restoration of bone architecture in young rats after 3 weeks of hind-limb immobilization was nearly complete after several weeks of exercise (28). Similarly, Kaneps et al. (92) found the cancellous and cortical mechanical properties of immobilized forelimbs in dogs to be significantly less than controls at 16 weeks. However, at 32 weeks, including 16 weeks of treadmill running, no significant difference between immobilized and control limbs was observed.

Although limited, recovery of bone mass and the associated architectural integrity in humans is protracted, with evidence that deficits can persist indefinitely. Bone mineral deficits induced by multiple space flights could still be observed in astronauts 5 years later (175). Similarly, lumbar and femoral neck bone mass lost during 17 weeks of bed rest was not regained in healthy subjects after 6 months of normal remobilization (105). Lower-extremity bone density (calcaneus and proximal tibia), however, was regained in this study sample. Although tibial bone mass may take 1 to 1.5 years to recover after periods of non–weight-bearing associated with hip surgery (105), permanent losses in BMD were reported in the lower limbs and spines of men who suffered tibial fractures 9 years earlier (80).

Implications and Considerations

After immobilization, the bone restoration process may be particularly difficult in certain populations (elderly, those with SCIs). Depending on baseline levels and the amount of bone loss, elderly individuals may be at greater risk of fracture after immobilization. Similarly, men older than age 60 years and postmenopausal women may be predisposed to accelerated bone loss, a condition that may exacerbate bone loss during immobilization. As such, an intervention strategy might be used that includes brief periods of assisted mobility during forced inactivity followed by remobilization at the earliest possible time. Thus, it would appear that retrieval of lost bone following periods of disuse is difficult at best even under loading conditions. However, the administration of insulinlike growth factor-1 (IGF-1) has been shown to promote osteogenesis during periods of unloading (27) and loading (109) in animal models, whereas human trials have been limited to special populations (e.g., children deficient in growth hormone). Perhaps IGF-1 will be a promising intervention in the fight to regain bone mass in humans.

Considering that bone mass restoration is outpaced by muscle strength, practitioners must be careful not to induce fracture by overly aggressive exercise programs. Clearly, the individual may possess normal strength while having bone that is close to the fracture threshold. A conservative approach—including range-of-motion exercises, a gradual overload of balance and stability challenges, site-specific muscle strengthening (Box 4-1) as supported by clinical evaluations and bone scans—is recommended.

Summary

Exercise that promotes skeletal loading stimulates compensatory adaptations, resulting in structural changes and healthier bones. Inactivity, regardless of the reason, is detrimental to maintaining bone health. It is difficult to distinguish between effects of normal physiologic aging and alterations in exercise and physical activity patterns. Transient bone mass changes have been observed in athletes, persons with mobility issues, and individuals experiencing unloading for brief periods. Bone loss is greatest at distal points of loading and areas associated with pos-

tural integrity and mobility (e.g., vertebra, hip). Accelerated bone loss is associated with age, menopause, space flight, SCI, and extended periods of unloading. Although hormonal regulation of calcium balance is altered during periods of inactivity, the most salient feature of bone health is the influence of mechanical loading. Recovery of lost bone is at best protracted with evidence that deficits can persist indefinitely. Depending on baseline levels and amount of bone loss, practitioners must be careful not to rush rehabilitation because the risk of fracture is increased after immobilization.

EFFECTS ON SKELETAL MUSCLE

> **1.1.34-HFS: Knowledge of and the ability to describe the changes that occur in maturation from childhood to adulthood for the following: skeletal muscle, bone structure, reaction time, coordination, heat and cold tolerance, maximal oxygen consumption, strength, flexibility, body composition, resting and maximal heart rate, and resting and maximal blood pressure.**

Morphologic Consequences

Regardless of the method of unloading (Table 5-3), the predominant adaptive response to decreased use is skeletal muscle atrophy (30,72). Atrophy is the process whereby muscle size is reduced, almost exclusively because of reductions in the contractile proteins actin and myosin (113). Specifically, in the absence of contractile activity or disuse, proteolytic and synthetic systems are altered, probably by specific signaling pathways, which in turn promote ubiquitination and the expression of specific atrophy genes (12,89).

For the first several weeks of disuse, atrophy is almost linearly related to duration and extent of unloading and differs among muscles depending on function. Generally, atrophy is most severe in the muscles involved in weight bearing and postural control; extensor muscles are typically more severely affected than flexor muscles

---

BOX 4-1   **GUIDELINES FOR EXERCISE PROFESSIONALS WORKING WITH SEVERELY DETRAINED OR BED-RESTED INDIVIDUALS***

- Emphasize strength training of back and lower-limb postural muscle groups:
  - Back extensors
  - Quadriceps
  - Hip extensors
  - Ankle plantarflexors (soleus and gastrocnemius)
- Start with low-intensity training
  - To accommodate potential neuromuscular deficits
  - To minimize potential for muscle damage

- Use gradual, progressive overload
- Be aware of increased risk of bone fracture
  - Particularly in estrogen-deficient women and the elderly
  - Even after muscle strength has returned to normal
- Incorporate training for postural stability and dynamic balance

(31,68,102). Likewise, it has recently been shown that the atrophic response of thigh adductor muscles to unloading is intermediate to that of extensor and flexor muscles (21,68). Of particular concern are muscles of the thigh and calf. These are critical in normal walking and show marked atrophy in non–weight-bearing conditions (31,74).

In lower mammals, fiber-type composition may influence the atrophic response to unloading; however, this has not been demonstrated in humans (30). Human skeletal muscle generally does not present the clear segmentation of fiber type found in lower mammals (143).

Fast subtypes, unlike fast versus slow fibers, appear to show transformation with several months of unloading or after detraining (31,69,165). Type IIB fibers in human muscle appear to serve as the default expression of the fast myosin gene. These transformations do not markedly alter energy demand of contraction, unlike slow to fast fiber movement. This is because of a greater difference in actomyosin adenosine triphosphatase (ATPase) activity between slow and fast fibers than between fast subtypes (32).

Metabolic Consequences

The influence of unloading on metabolic characteristics of human skeletal muscle has received less attention than atrophy and reduced strength. Whereas homogenates of muscle biopsies show decreased concentrations of enzyme markers of aerobic oxidative capacity after unloading, anaerobic enzymes of energy supply do not seem to change (19,71). Reduced enzymes associated with aerobic capacity may reflect preferential loss of contractile protein with unloading; that is, aerobic oxidative enzyme content per fiber volume may not change, and the anaerobic enzyme content may actually increase (31,113). Nonetheless, fiber atrophy results in lower total mitochondrial content, so unloading compromises absolute muscular endurance (19,44,168). This also suggests that relative muscular endurance is not significantly affected by unloading (19). However, preferential loss of contractile protein requires the remaining muscle to work against greater absolute load. This work is accomplished with reduced total capacity for aerobic–oxidative energy supply because mitochondrial content is lower.

Strength and Local Muscular Endurance

Unloading reduces muscular strength, regardless of the type of action or movement performed or the method of strength expression (3,18,19,21,47,60,69,102). Strength reduction is nearly linearly related to the duration of unloading and extent of muscle atrophy for the first few weeks. Atrophy accounts for a large part but not all of decreased force production, suggesting the ability to activate muscle is also compromised by unloading (discussed later). This is interesting because marked force reduction during eccentric, isometric, and slow-speed

concentric muscle contraction is believed to be controlled by some neural inhibitory mechanisms (46,188). However, the relative decline in strength is comparable across speeds and types of muscle actions, so increased inhibition is not responsible for reduced voluntary activation, or if it is, the reduction is uniform across speeds and types of muscle actions (18,22,46,47).

The lack of shape change in the force–velocity relationship with short-term unloading may suggest that muscle fiber type composition is not altered. However, as transformation to a faster muscle occurs with long-term extreme unloading, an increased ability to maintain force as speed increases during concentric actions should be evident (67). This finding has been reported after long-term space flight (48). However, 120 days of unloading of otherwise healthy individuals did not alter relative rise time during surface electrical stimulation of the triceps surae muscle group, suggesting that myofibrillar actomyosin ATPase activity is not altered by 3 months of disuse (97). Likewise, time to peak tension for a twitch of tibialis anterior muscle has been reported comparable between SCI patients and healthy control subjects, suggesting that long-term unloading does not markedly alter calcium kinetics (167). Comparable twitch mechanics in SCI patients and healthy controls may be interpreted to imply that fiber-type composition of muscle and, thereby, myofibrillar actomyosin ATPase activity is not altered by SCI (31,32,114). Thus, a muscle appears faster in chronic SCI patients than control subjects, yet is comparable to those of healthy individuals for myofibrillar actomyosin ATPase activity and mechanical function.

The magnitude of strength reduction is also specific to muscle group, with weight-bearing muscles most affected. For knee extensors, the decline in strength averages about 0.6% per day. In contrast, the first dorsal interosseus hand muscle is relatively resistant to adaptation after 3 to 5 weeks of immobilization (20,58).

Muscular endurance associated with disuse has not been widely studied. One recent report suggests that after 4 weeks of casting of the elbow flexors, endurance time was paradoxically increased in female but not male subjects. Furthermore, the electromyography (EMG) activity during the endurance test was altered in the female subjects. The EMG was associated with intermittent motor unit activity instead of the continuous activity typically observed. This suggests that motor unit activation patterns are altered after disuse, at least in women (149). The ability to maintain force over repeat contractions is not altered within 6 months of SCI but is markedly compromised in chronic SCI patients (30,72,167).

Neuromuscular Consequences

Decreased strength with reduced use has consistently been shown to be greater than that explained by muscle atrophy (136). An exception to this concept has been reported after short-term space flight. Muscle strength decreases in proportionately similar amounts, or perhaps less than fiber size, after 5 or 11 days of unloading (about 15% versus 20%) (48,102). This implies increased ability to recruit muscle or greater specific tension (force per unit muscle size). Neither has been reported in studies of unloading at normal gravity (21,43,71,91). Thus, neuromuscular impairment may occur after unloading.

Electromyographic studies demonstrate that maximal firing rate and maximal integrated EMG activity are decreased and periods of silent EMG activity appear during maximal voluntary contractions after unloading (91). The ability to recruit high-threshold motor units also seems to be compromised (61). The greater relative decline in strength than in size suggests that more muscle may be used to perform a given submaximal task. This has recently been reported using magnetic resonance imaging (MRI), supporting EMG analyses in which greater numbers of motor units are required to develop submaximal force (21,22,136,137).

The exercise professional should account for these neuromuscular adaptations to unloading in exercise prescriptions for subjects recovering from reduced muscular activity. Submaximal loads that were once easily borne require more absolute muscle involvement. In addition, individuals may not have visible muscle atrophy but may be particularly weak because of irregularities in motor control. Thus, although caution should be taken when training an older person following disuse, recent studies indicate that significant gains in strength, rate of contraction, and muscle size are accrued after several months of training following periods of disuse (171,172).

Vulnerability of Muscle Damage

Unloading lower-limb skeletal muscle for 5 weeks has demonstrated increased vulnerability to eccentric exercise-induced dysfunction and muscle injury (137). MRI obtained 3 days after eccentric exercise demonstrated muscle damage over the unloaded cross-sectional area, but none was evident in the contralateral weight-bearing limb.

These results have practical importance to the exercise professional. Dysfunction and injury during reloading may be sufficient to prolong recovery. In the previous study, 10 days after the eccentric exercise, strength remained reduced by 20% (before unloading). Low-intensity exercise should be used with care initially during renewal of walking to minimize muscle dysfunction and injury.

Increased vulnerability to exercise-induced muscle injury has also been reported in elderly individuals (113). Whether this is caused by aging, low physical activity, or both is not known, but when starting an exercise program for an elderly person, it is important to be cautious.

Possible Countermeasures

Few data exist regarding the efficacy of various countermeasures designed to prevent muscle atrophy and dysfunction or to enhance recovery during disuse. Endurance activity enhances fatigue resistance of skeletal muscle during unloading. Electrical stimulation of tibialis anterior muscle for 45 minutes to 2 hours/day in complete SCI patients evoked a marked increase in ability to maintain force during contraction. This response is partly attributed to increased muscle fiber aerobic–oxidative enzyme content (114,167). Resistancelike exercise (high-force intermittent stimulation) in patients with SCIs or ladder climbing in hindlimb–suspended rats has been shown to increase muscle size (45), the former to near preinjury levels. One recent report using only four subjects suggests that wearing a Penguin antigravity suit for 10 hours a day and performing resistance exercise for 15 minutes each hour can prevent muscle atrophy associated with bed rest (131). A more practical approach to offsetting the muscle-wasting effects of disuse comes from the work of Rittweger et al., who found that subjects who engaged in flywheel resistive exercise lost significantly less power and recovered power significantly faster than control subjects (139).

Although neuromuscular dysfunction cannot be attributable solely to disuse in elderly patients, it is clear that resistance exercise induces gains in strength, muscle mass, and functional mobility (41,53,176). Thus, as a countermeasure to the loss of muscle associated with disuse, resistance exercise is a means to recovery for most individuals.

RETRAINING

Short-term retraining after detraining appears to return muscle strength and size to those of the previously trained state (165). However, less deconditioning appears to exist than expected in previously trained individuals during detraining in the previously mentioned study, and there is more rapid adaptation after resuming training than expected. In a 30-year follow-up of the Dallas bedrest study, a 6-month endurance training program reversed the age-related decline in aerobic power that was attributed to peripheral adaptation. However, no subject reached the same $\dot{V}O_{2max}$ as in the initial test (108).

Summary

Muscles atrophy regardless of the method of unloading (decreased training, bed rest, space flight), resulting in decreased strength and possible dysfunction and muscle injury. Therefore, individuals need to continue with activities that increase strength and are weight-bearing.

REFERENCES

1. Adams GR. Human unilateral lower limb suspension as a model for spaceflight effects on skeletal muscle. *J Appl Physiol*. 2002; 93: 1563–5.

2. Adams GR, Caiozzo VJ, Baldwin KM. Skeletal muscle unweighting: spaceflight and ground-based models. *J Appl Physiol*. 2003; 95:2185–201.

3. Adams GR, Hather BM, Dudley GA. Effect of short-term unweighting on human skeletal muscle strength and size. *Aviat Space Environ Med*. 1994;65:1116–21.

4. Akima H, Kano Y, Enomoto Y. Muscle function in 164 men and women aged 20–84 yr. *Med Sci Sports Exerc*. 2001;33:220–6.

5. Akima H, Kuno S, Suzuki Y, Gunji A, Fukunaga T. Effects of 20 days of bed rest on physiological cross-sectional area of human thigh and leg muscles evaluated by magnetic resonance imaging. *J Gravit Physiol*. 1997;4:S14–21.

6. Alfredson H, Nordstrom P, Lorentzon R. Prolonged progressive calcaneal bone loss despite early weightbearing rehabilitation in patients surgically treated for Achilles tendinosis. *Calcif Tissue Int*. 1998;62:166–71.

7. American College of Sports Medicine. *ACSM's Guidelines for Exercise Testing and Prescription*. 8th ed. Philadelphia: Lippincott Williams & Wilkins; 2009.

8. Aoyahi Y, Shephard RJ. Aging and muscle function. *Sports Med*. 1992;14:376–396.

9. Armstrong N, Welsman JR, Williams C. Longitudinal changes in young people's short-term power output. *Med Sci Sports Exerc*. 2000;32:1140–5.

10. Arnesen SM, Lawson MA. Age-related changes in focal adhesions lead to altered cell behavior in tendon fibroblasts. *Mech Ageing Develop*. 2006;127:726–32.

11. Babb TG. Mechanical ventilatory constraints in aging, lung disease, and obesity: perspectives and a brief review. *Med Sci Sports Exerc*. 1999;31:S12–22.

12. Bajotto G, Shimomura Y. Determinants of disuse-induced skeletal muscle atrophy: exercise and nutrition countermeasures to prevent protein loss. *J Nutr Sci Vitaminol*. 2006;52:233–47.

13. Bales CW, Ritchie CS. Sarcopenia, weight loss, and nutritional frailty in the elderly. *Ann Rev Nutr*. 2002;22:309–23.

14. Baraldi E, Cooper DM, Zanconato S, Armon Y. Heart rate recovery from 1 minute of exercise in children and adults. *Pediatr Res*. 1991;29:575–9.

15. Barou O, Valentin D, Vico L, Tirode C, Barbier A, Alexandre C, Lafage-Proust MH. High-resolution three-dimensional micro-computed tomography detects bone loss and changes in trabecular architecture early: comparison with DEXA and bone histomorphometry in a rat model of disuse osteoporosis. *Invest Radiol*. 2002;37:40–6.

16. Bemben MG. *The Physiology of Aging*. ACSM Current Comment, 2001.

17. Bemben MG, Miccalip GA. Strength and power relationships as a function of age. *J Strength Cond Res*. 1999;13:330–8.

18. Berg HE, Dudley GA, Haggmark T, Ohlsen H, Tesch PA. Effects of lower limb unloading on skeletal muscle mass and function in humans. *J Appl Physiol*. 1991;70:1882–5.

19. Berg HE, Dudley GA, Hather BM, Tesch PA. Work capacity and metabolic and morphologic characteristics of the human quadriceps muscle in response to unloading. *Clin Physiol*. 1993;13:337–47.

20. Berg HE, Eiken O, Miklavcic L, Mekjavic IB. Hip, thigh and calf muscle atrophy and bone loss after 5-week bedrest inactivity. *Eur J Appl Physiol*. 2007;99:283–9.

21. Berg HE, Larsson L, Tesch PA. Lower limb skeletal muscle function after 6 weeks of bedrest. *J Appl Physiol*. 1996;82:182–8.

22. Berg HE, Tesch PA. Changes in muscle function in response to 10 days of lower limb unloading in humans. *Acta Physiol Scand*. 1996;157:63–70.

23. Bikle DD, Halloran BP. The response of bone to unloading. *J Bone Miner Metab*. 1999;17:233–44.

24. Bloomfield SA. Changes in musculoskeletal structure and function with prolonged bed rest. *Med Sci Sports Exerc*. 1997;29: 197–206.

25. Bloomfield SA, Mysiw WJ, Jackson RD. Bone mass and endocrine adaptations to training in spinal cord injured individuals. *Bone*. 1996;19:61–8.

26. Bosy-Westphal A, Eichhorn C, Kutzner D, Illner K, Heller M, Muller MJ. The age-related decline in resting energy expenditure in humans is due to the loss of fat-free mass and to alterations in its metabolically active components. *J Nutr*. 2003;133:2356–62.

27. Boudignon BM, Bikle DD, Kurimoto P, et al. Insulin-like growth factor I stimulates recovery of bone lost after a period of skeletal unloading. *J Appl Physiol*. 2007;103:125–31.

28. Bourrin S, Palle S, Genty C, Alexandre C. Physical exercise during remobilization restores normal bone trabecular network after tail suspension-induced osteopenia in young rats. *J Bone Miner Res*. 1995;10: 820–8.

29. Carmeliet G, Vico L, Bouillon R. Space flight: a challenge for normal bone homeostasis. *Crit Rev Eukaryot Gene Expr*. 2001;11:131–44.

30. Castro MJ, Apple DF Jr, Hillegass EA, Dudley GA. Influence of complete spinal cord injury on skeletal muscle morphology within six months of injury. *Eur J Appl Physiol*. 1999;80:373–8.

31. Castro MJ, Apple DF Jr, Rogers S, Dudley GA. Influence of complete spinal cord injury on skeletal muscle mechanics within six months of injury. *Eur J Appl Physiol*. 2000;81:128–31.

32. Castro MJ, Apple DF Jr, Rogers S, Dudley GA. Muscle fiber-type specific Ca2+ actomyosin ATPase activity after complete spinal cord injury. *Muscle Nerve*. 2000;23:119–21.

33. Castro MJ, Apple DF Jr, Staron RS, Campos GE, Dudley GA. Influence of complete spinal cord injury on skeletal muscle within six months of injury. *J Appl Physiol*. 1999;86:350–8.

34. Cheitlin MD. Cardiovascular physiology—changes with aging. *Am J Geriatr Cardiol*. 2003;12:9–13.

35. Christiansen JL, Grzybowski JM. *Biology of Aging*. New York: McGraw-Hill; 1999.

36. Convertino VA. Insight into mechanisms of reduced orthostatic performance after exposure to microgravity: comparison of ground-based and space flight data. *J Gravit Physiol*. 1998;5:P85–8.

37. Convertino VA. Planning strategies for development of effective exercise and nutrition countermeasures for long-duration space flight. *Nutrition*. 2002;18:880–8.

38. Dalsky G, Stocke KS, Ehsani AA, Slatopolsky E, Lee WC, Birge SJ Jr. Weight-bearing exercise training and lumbar bone mineral content in postmenopausal women. *Ann Intern Med*. 1988;108: 824–8.

39. Deschenes MR. Effects of aging on muscle fiber type and size. *Sports Med*. 2004;34(12):809–24.

40. Deschenes MR, Giles JA, McCoy RW, Volek JS, Gomez AL, Kraemer WJ. Neural factors account for strength decrements observed after short-term muscle unloading. *Am J Physiol Regul Integr Comp Physiol*. 2001;282:578–83.

41. deVos NJ, Singh NA, Ross DA, Stavrinos TM, Orr R, Fiatarone Singh MA. Optimal load for increasing muscle power during explosive resistance training in older adults. *J Gerontol A Biol Sci Med Sci*. 2005;60:638–47.

42. DeVries HA, Adams GM. Comparison of exercise responses in old and young men. *J Gerontol*. 1972;27:344–8.

43. Duchateau J. Bed rest induces neural and contractile adaptations in triceps surae. *Med Sci Sports Exerc*. 1995;27:1581–9.

44. Duchateau J, Hainaut K. Effects of immobilization on contractile properties, recruitment and firing rates of human motor units. *J Physiol*. 1990;422:55–65.

45. Dudley GA, Castro MJ, Rogers S, Apple DF Jr. A simple means of increasing muscle size after SCI: a pilot study. *Eur J Appl Physiol*. 1999;80:394–6.

46. Dudley GA, Duvoisin MR, Adams GR, Meyer RA, Belew AH, Buchanan P. Adaptations to unilateral lower limb suspension in humans. *Aviat Space Environ Med*. 1992;63:678–83.

47. Dudley GA, Duvoisin MR, Convertino VA, Buchanan P. Alterations of the in vivo torque-velocity relationship of human skeletal muscle following 30 days exposure to simulated microgravity. *Aviat Space Environ Med.* 1989;60:659–63.

48. Edgerton VR, Zhou MY, Ohira Y, et al. Human fiber size and enzymatic properties after 5 and 11 days of spaceflight. *J Appl Physiol.* 1995;78:1733–9.

49. Ehrlich PJ, Lanyon LE. Mechanical strain and bone cell function: a review. *Osteoporos Int.* 2002;13:688–700.

50. Elia EA. Exercise and the elderly. *Clin Sports Med.* 1991;10:141–55.

51. Falk B, Bar-Or O, McDougall JD. Aldosterone and prolactin response to exercise in the heat in circumpubertal boys. *J Appl Physiol.* 1991;71:1741–5.

52. Falk B, Bar-Or O, Smolander J, Frost G. Response to rest and exercise in the cold: effects of age and aerobic fitness. *J Appl Phyisol.* 1994;76:72–8.

53. Fiatarone MA, Marks EC, Ryan ND, Meredith CN, Lipsitz LA, Evans WJ. High-intensity strength training in nonagenarians: effects on skeletal muscle. *JAMA.* 1990;263:3029–34.

54. Fitzgerald PL. Exercise for the elderly. *Med Clin North Am.* 1995;69:189–96.

55. Flegg FL, Morrell CH, Bos AG, Brant LF, Talbot LA, Wright JG, Lakkatta EG. Accelerated longitudinal decline of aerobic capacity in healthy older adults. *Circulation.* 2005;112:674–82.

56. Franklin SS. Hypertension in older people: part 1. *J Clin Hypertens.* 2006;8:444–9.

57. Freedman VA, Martin LG. Contribution of chronic conditions to aggregate changes in old-age functioning. *Am J Pub Health.* 2000;90:1755–60.

58. Fuglevand AJ, Bilodeau M, Enoka RM. Short-term immobilization has a minimal effect on the strength and fatigability of a human hand muscle. *J Appl Physiol.* 1995;78:847–55.

59. Gentil P, Lima RM, Jaco do Oliveira R, Pereira RW, Rels VM. Association between femoral neck bone density and lower limb fat-free mass in postmenopausal women. *J Clin Densitom.* 2007;10:174–8.

60. Gogia PP, Schneider VS, LeBlanc AD, Krebs J, Kasson C, Pientok C. Bed rest effect on extremity muscle torque in healthy men. *Arch Phys Med Rehabil.* 1988;69:1030–2.

61. Goldspink DF, Morton AJ, Loughna P, Goldspink G. The effect of hypokinesia and hypodynamia on protein turnover and the growth of four skeletal muscles of the rat. *Pflugers Arch.* 1986;407:333–40.

62. Gordon T, Mao J. Muscle atrophy and procedures for training after spinal cord injury. *Phys Ther.* 1994;74:50–60.

63. Grana EA, Chiou-Tan F, Jaweed M. Endplate dysfunction in healthy muscle following a period of disuse. *Muscle Nerve.* 1996;19:989–93.

64. Granath A, Johnson B, Strandell T. Circulation in healthy old men studied by right heart catheterization at rest and during exercise in a supine and sitting position. *Acta Med Scand.* 1964;176:425–46.

65. Green S. A definitive and systems view of anaerobic capacity. *Eur J Appl Physiol.* 2004;69:168–73.

66. Gulmans VA, de Meer K, Binhorst RA, Helders PJ, Saris WH. Reference values for maximum work capacity in relation to body composition in healthy Dutch children. *Eur Respir J.* 1997;10:94–7.

67. Harris RT, Dudley GA. Factors limiting force during slow, shortening actions of the quadriceps femoris muscle group in vivo. *Acta Physiol Scand.* 1994;152:63–71.

68. Hather BM, Adams GR, Tesch PA, Dudley GA. Skeletal muscle responses to lower limb suspension in humans. *J Appl Physiol.* 1992;72:1493–8.

69. Hather BM, Tesch PA, Buchanan P, Dudley GA. Influence of eccentric actions on skeletal muscle adaptations to resistance training. *Acta Physiol Scand.* 1991;143:177–85.

70. Heberstreet H, Mimura KI, Bar-Or O. Recovery of muscle power after high intensity short-term exercise: comparing boys and men. *J Appl Physiol.* 1993;74:2875–80.

71. Hikida RS, Gollnick PD, Dudley GA, Convertino VA, Buchanan P. Structural and metabolic characteristics of human skeletal muscle following 30 days of simulated microgravity. *Aviat Space Environ Med.* 1989;60:664.

72. Hillegass EA, Dudley GA. Surface electrical stimulation of skeletal muscle after spinal cord injury. *Spinal Cord.* 1999;37:251–7.

73. Ho C, Wuermser L, Priebe M, Chiodo A, Scelza W, Kirshblum S. Spinal cord injury medicine: epidemiology and classification. *Arch Phys Med Rehabil.* 2007;88: S49–54.

74. Hodges P, Holm AK, Hansson T, Holm S. Rapid atrophy of the lumbar multifidus follows experimental disc or nerve root injury. *Spine.* 2006;31:2926–33.

75. Hofbauer LC, Brueck CC, Shanahan CM, Schoppet M, Dobnig H. Vascular calcification and osteoporosis—from clinical observation towards molecular understanding. *Osteoporos Int.* 2007;18:251–9.

76. Houston ME, Froese EA, Valeriote SP, Green HJ, Ranney DA. Muscle performance, morphology and metabolic capacity during strength training and detraining: a one leg model. *Eur J Appl Physiol.* 1983;51:25–35.

77. Ike RW, Lampman RM, Castor CW. Arthritis and aerobic exercise. *Phys Sportsmed.* 1989;17:128–39.

78. Ingram DK. Age-related decline in physical activity: generalization to nonhumans. *Med Sci Sports Exerc.* 2000;32:1623–9.

79. Inoue M, Tanaka H, Moriwake T, Oka M, Sekiguchi C, Seino Y. Altered biochemical markers of bone turnover in humans during 120 days of bed rest. *Bone.* 2000;26:281–6.

80. Ito M, Matsumoto T, Enomoto H, et al. Effect of nonweight bearing on tibial bone density measured by QCT in patients with hip surgery. *J Bone Miner Metab.* 1999;17:45–50.

81. Iwamoto J, Takeda T, Ichimura S. Effect of exercise training and detraining on bone mineral density in postmenopausal women with osteoporosis. *J Orthop Sci.* 2001;6:128–32.

82. Jackson AS, Wier LT, Ayers GW, Beard EF, Stuteville JE, Blair SN. Changes in aerobic power of women ages 20–64 yr. *Med Sci Sports Exerc.* 1996;28:844–91.

83. Jacobs PL, Mahoney ET. Peak exercise capacity of electrically induced ambulation in persons with paraplegia. *Med Sci Sports Exerc.* 2002;34:1551–6.

84. Jacobs PL, Nash MS, Rusinowski JW. Circuit training provides cardiorespiratory and strength benefits in persons with paraplegia. *Med Sci Sports Exerc.* 2001;33:711–7.

85. Janssens JP. Aging of the respiratory system: impact on pulmonary function tests and adaptation to exertion. *Clin Chest Med.* 2005;26:469–84.

86. Jaworski ZF, Uhthoff HK. Reversibility of nontraumatic disuse osteoporosis during its active phase. *Bone.* 1986;7:431–9.

87. Jee WS, Wronski TJ, Morey ER, Kimmel DB. Effects of spaceflight on trabecular bone in rats. *Am J Physiol.* 1983;244:310–4.

88. Jeng SF, Lliao HF, Lai JS, Hou JW. Optimization of walking in children. *Med Sci Sports Exerc.* 1997;29:370–6.

89. Judge AR, Koncarevic A, Hunter RB, Liou HC, Jackman RW, Kandarian SC. Role for IkappaBalpha, but not c-Rel, in skeletal muscle atrophy. *Am J Physiol Cell Physiol.* 2007;292:C372–82.

90. Julius S, Amery A, Whitlock LS, Conway J. Influence of age on the hemodynamic response to exercise. *Circulation.* 1967;36:222–30.

91. Kandarin SC, Boushel RC, Schulte LM. Elevated interstitial fluid volume in rat soleus muscles by hindlimb unweighting. *J Appl Physiol.* 1991;71:910–4.

92. Kaneps AJ, Stover SM, Lane NE. Changes in canine cortical and cancellous bone mechanical properties following immobilization and remobilization with exercise. *Bone.* 1997;5:419–23.

93. Karlsson MK. Does exercise during growth prevent fractures in later life? *Med Sport Sci.* 2007;51:121–36.

94. Kasch FW, Boyer JL, VanCamp SP, Verity LS, Wallace J. The effect of physical activity and inactivity on aerobic power in older men (a longitudinal study). *Phys Sportsmed.* 1990;18:73–83.

95. Kenney WL. Control of heat-induced vasodilatation in relation to age. *Eur J Appl Physiol.* 1988;57:120–5.

96. Kenney WL, Tankersley CG, Newswanger DL, Hyde DE, Puhl SM, Turner NL. Age and hypohydration independently influence the peripheral vascular response to heat stress. *J Appl Physiol.* 1990;68: 1902–8.

97. Koryak Y. Contractile properties of the human triceps surae muscle during simulated weightlessness. *Eur J Appl Physiol.* 1995;70:344–50.

98. Krahenbuhl GS, Skinner JS, Kohrt WM. Development aspects of maximal aerobic power in children. *Exerc Sport Sci Rev.* 1985;13: 503–38.

99. Kubo K, Kanehisa H, Azuma K, Ishizu M, Kuno S, Okada M, Fukunaga T. Muscle architecture characteristics in women aged 20–79 years. *Med Sci Sports Exerc.* 2003;35:39–44.

100. Lakatta EG. Cardiovascular regulatory mechanisms in advanced age. *Physiol Rev.* 1993;73:413–67.

101. Laugier P, Novikov V, Elmann-Larsen B, Berger G. Quantitative ultrasound imaging of the calcaneus: precision and variations during 120-day bed rest. *Calcif Tissue Int.* 2000;66:16–21.

102. LeBlanc A, Gogia P, Schneider V, Krebs J, Schonfeld E, Evans H. Calf muscle area and strength changes after five weeks of horizontal bed rest. *Am J Sports Med.* 1988;16:624–9.

103. LeBlanc A, Rowe R, Schneider V, Evans H, Hedrick T. Regional muscle loss after short duration spaceflight. *Aviat Space Environ Med.* 1995;66:1151–4.

104. LeBlanc A, Schneider V, Spector E, et al. Calcium absorption, endogenous excretion, and endocrine changes during and after long-term bed rest. *Bone.* 1995;16:301S–4S.

105. LeBlanc A, Schneider VS, Evans HJ, Engelbretson DA, Krebs JM. Bone mineral loss and recovery after 17 weeks of bed rest. *J Bone Miner Res.* 1990;5:843–50.

106. Levine BD, Lane LD, Watenpaugh DE, Gaffney FA, Buckey JC, Blomqvist CG. Maximal exercise performance after adaptation to microgravity. *J Appl Physiol.* 1996;81:686–94.

107. Lueken SA, Arnaud SB, Taylor AK, Baylink DJ. Changes in markers of bone formation and resorption in a bed rest model of weightlessness. *J Bone Miner Res.* 1993;8:1433–8.

108. McGuire DK, Levine BD, Williamson JW, Snell PJ, Blomqvist CG, Saltin B, Mitchell JH. A 30 year follow-up of the Dallas bedrest and training study: II. Effect of age on cardiovascular adaptation to exercise training. *Circulation.* 2001;104:1358–66.

109. Machwate M, Zerath E, Holy X, Pastoureau P, Marie PJ. Insulin-like growth factor-I increases trabecular bone formation and osteoblastic cell proliferation in unloaded rats. *Endocrinology.* 1994;134:1031–8.

110. Magnusson HI, Linden C, Obrant KJ, Johnell O, Karlsson MK. Bone mass changes in weight loaded and unloaded skeletal regions following a fracture of the hip. *Calcif Tissue Int.* 2001;69:78–83.

111. Makrides L, Heighenhauser GJ, Jones NL. High-intensity endurance training in 20–30 and 60–70 yr-old healthy men. *J Appl Physiol.* 1990;69:1792–8.

112. Makrides L, Heigenhauser GJ, McCartney N, Jones NL. Maximal short term exercise capacity in healthy subjects aged 15–70 years. *Clin Sci.* 1985;69:197–205.

113. Manfredi TG, Fielding RA, O'Reilly KP, Meredith CN, Lee HY, Evans WJ. Plasma creatine kinase activity and exercise-induced muscle damage in older men. *Med Sci Sports Exerc.* 1991;23:1028–34.

114. Martin TP, Stein RB, Hoeppner PH, Reid DC. Influence of electrical stimulation on the morphological and metabolic properties of paralyzed muscle. *J Appl Physiol.* 1992;72:1401–6.

115. Mazzeo RS. Exercise and the older adult. ACSM Current Comment, 2000.

116. Melton LJ, Khosia S, Crowson CS. Epidemiology of sarcopenia. *J Am Geriatr Soc.* 2000;48:625–30.

117. Menz HB, Morris ME, Lord SR. Foot and ankle characteristics associated with impaired balance and functional ability in older people. *J Gerontol A Biol Sci Med Sci.* 2005;60:1546–52.

118. Meyer F, Bar-Or O, MacDougall D, Heigenhauser GJ. Drink composition and electrolyte balance of children exercising in the heat. *Med Sci Sports Exerc.* 1995;27:882–7.

119. Michel BA, Lane NE, Bloch DA, Jones HH, Fries JF. Effect of changes in weight-bearing exercise on lumbar bone mass after age fifty. *Ann Med.* 1991;23: 397–401.

120. Minaire P, Neunier P, Edouard C, Bernard J, Courpron P, Bourret J. Quantitative histological data on disuse osteoporosis: comparison with biological data. *Calcif Tissue Res.* 1974;17:57–73.

121. Mohtadi N. Injured limbs recover better with early mobilization and functional bracing than with cast immobilization. *J Bone Joint Surg Am.* 2005;87:1167.

122. Mujika I, Sabino S. Muscular characteristics of detraining in humans. *Med Sci Sports Exerc.* 2001;33:1297–303.

123. Müller MJ, Grund A, Kraus H. Determinants of fat mass in prepubertal children. *Br J Nutr.* 2002;88:545–54.

124. Narici MV, Roi GS, Landoni L, Minetti AE, Cerretelli P. Changes in force, cross-sectional area and neural activation during strength training and detraining of the human quadriceps. *Eur J Appl Physiol.* 1989;59:310–9.

125. Nichols-Richardson SM, Modlesky CM, O'Connor PJ, Lewis RD. Premenarcheal gymnasts possess higher bone mineral density than controls. *Med Sci Sports Exerc.* 2000;32:63–9.

126. Nordström A, Olsson T, Nordström P. Bone gained from physical activity and lost through detraining: a longitudinal study in young males. *Osteoporos Int.* 2004;16:835–41.

127. Nordström A, Olsson T, Nordström P. Sustained benefits from previous physical activity on bone mineral density in males. *J Clin Endocrinol Metab.* 2006;91:2600–4.

128. O'Flaherty EJ. Modeling normal aging bone loss, with consideration of bone loss in osteoporosis. *Toxicol Sci.* 2000;55:171–88.

129. Ogawa T, Spina RJ, Martin WH, Kohrt WM, Schechtman KB, Holloszy JO, Ehsani AA. Effects of aging, sex, and physical training on cardiovascular responses to exercise. *Circulation.* 1992;86:494–503.

130. Ogden CL, Yanovski SZ, Carroll MD, Flegal KM. The epidemiology of obesity. *Gastroenterology.* 2007;132:2087–102.

131. Ohira Y, Yoshinaga T, Ohara M, et al. Myonuclear domain and myosin phenotype in human soleus after bed rest with or without loading. *J Appl Physiol.* 1999;87:1776–85.

132. Palle S, Vico L, Bourrin S, Alexandre C. Bone tissue response to four-month antiorthostatic bed rest: a bone histomorphometric study. *Calcif Tissue Int.* 1992;51:189–94.

133. Pathare NC, Stevens JE, Walter GA, et al. Deficit in human muscle strength with cast immobilization: contribution of inorganic phosphate. *Eur J Appl Physiol.* 2006;98:71–8.

134. Pattullo MC, Cotter MA, Cameron NE, Barry JA. Effects of lengthened immobilization on functional and histochemical properties of rabbit tibialis anterior muscle. *Exp Physiol.* 1992;77:433–42.

135. Pawelczyk JA, Zuckerman JH, Blomqvist CG, Levine BD. Regulation of muscle sympathetic nerve activity after bed rest deconditioning. *Am J Physiol Heart Circ Physiol.* 2001;280:H2230–9.

136. Ploutz-Snyder LL, Tesch PA, Crittenden DJ, Dudley GA. Effect of unweighting on skeletal muscle use during exercise. *J Appl Physiol.* 1995;79:168–75.

137. Ploutz-Snyder LL, Tesch PA, Hather BM, Dudley GA. Vulnerability to dysfunction and muscle injury after unloading. *Arch Phys Med Rehabil.* 1996;77:773–7.

138. Prisk GK. Physiology of a microgravity environment: invited review: microgravity and the lung. *J Appl Physiol.* 2000;89:385–96.

139. Rittweger J, Felsenberg D, Maganaris C, Ferretti JL. Vertical jump performance after 90 days bed rest with and without flywheel resistive exercise, including a 180 days follow-up. *Eur J Appl Physiol.* 2007;100:427–36.

140. Rittwenger J, Winwood K, Seynnes O, et al. Bone loss from the human distal tibia epiphysis during 24 days of unilateral lower limb suspension. *J Physiol.* 2006;577(Pt 1):331–7.

141. Rodeheffer RJ, Gerstenblith G, Becker LC, Fleg JL, Weisfeldt ML, Lakatta EG. Exercise cardiac output is maintained with advancing age in healthy human subjects: cardiac dilation and increased stroke volume compensate for a diminished heart rate. *Circulation.* 1984;69:203–13.

142. Rowland T, Popowski B, Ferrone L. Cardiac responses to maximal upright exercise in healthy boys and men. *Med Sci Sports Exerc.* 1997;29:1146–51.

143. Roy RR, Baldwin KM, Edgerton VR. The plasticity of skeletal muscle effects of neuromuscular activity. *Exerc Sports Sci Rev.* 1991;19: 269–312.

144. Ruml LA, Dubois SK, Roberts ML, Pak CY. Prevention of hypercalciuria and stone-forming propensity during prolonged bedrest by alendronate. *J Bone Miner Res.* 1995;10:655–62.

145. Schneider EL, Rowe JW. *Biology of Aging.* San Diego (CA): Academic Press; 1990.

146. Schneider SM. Bed rest and orthostatic-hypotensive intolerance. In: Greenleaf JE, editor. *Deconditioning and Reconditioning.* Boca Raton (FL): CRC Press; 2004. p. 137–156.

147. Schulman SP, Lakatta EG, Fleg JL, Lakatta L, Becker LC, Gerstenblith G. Age related decline in left ventricular filling at rest and exercise. *Am J Physiol.* 1992;263:H1932–8.

148. Schut L. Motor system changes in the aging brain: what is normal and what is not. *Geriatrics.* 1998;53:S16–9.

149. Semmler JG, Kutzscher DV, Enoka RM. Gender differences in the fatigability of human skeletal muscle. *J Neurophysiol.* 1999;82: 3590–3.

150. Shephard RJ. *Aging, Physical Activity and Health.* Champaign (IL): Human Kinetics, 1997.

151. Shephard RJ. Age and physical work capacity. *Exp Aging Res.* 1999; 25:331–43.

152. Shephard RJ. *Body Composition in Biological Anthropology.* London: Cambridge University; 1991.

153. Shephard RJ. Physiologic changes over the years. In: *ACSM's Resource Manual for Guidelines for Exercise Testing and Prescription.* 2nd ed. Philadelphia: Lea & Febiger; 1993.

154. Shephard RJ, Montelpare W, Plyley M, McCracken D, Goode RC. Handgrip dynamometry, Cybex measurements and lean mass as markers of the ageing of muscle. *Br J Sports Med.* 1991;25:204–8.

155. Shock NW. Physiological aspects of aging in man. *Ann Rev Physiol.* 1961;23:97–122.

156. Shvartz E, Reibold RC. Aerobic fitness norms for males and females aged 6 to 75 years: a review. *Aviat Space Environ Med.* 1990;61:3–11.

157. Slade JM, Bickel CS, Modlesky CM, Majumdar S, Dudley GA. Trabecular bone is more deteriorated in spinal cord injured versus estrogen-free postmenopausal women. *Osteoporos Int.* 2004;16:263–72.

158. Smith SM, Wastney ME, Morukov BV, et al. Calcium metabolism before, during, and after a 3-mo spaceflight: kinetic and biochemical changes. *Am J Physiol.* 1999;277:R1–10.

159. Smith SM, Wastney ME, O'Brien KO, et al. Bone markers, calcium metabolism, and calcium kinetics during extended-duration space flight on the Mir space station. *J Bone Miner Res.* 2004;20:208–18.

160. Smorawinski J, Nazasr K, Kaciuba-Uscilko H, et al. Effects of 3-day bed rest on physiological responses to graded exercise in athletes and sedentary men. *J Appl Physiol.* 2001;91:249–57.

161. Snow CM, Williams DP, LaRiviere J, Fuchs RK, Robinson TL. Bone gains and losses follow seasonal training and detraining in gymnasts. *Calcif Tissue Int.* 2001;69:7–12.

162. Spirduso WW. *Physical Dimensions of Aging.* Champaign (IL): Human Kinetics; 2005.

163. Spina RJ. Cardiovascular adaptations to endurance exercise training in older men and women. *Exerc Sport Sci Rev.* 1999;27:317–32.

164. Staron RS. The classification of human skeletal muscle fiber types. *J Strength Cond Res.* 1997;11:67.

165. Staron RS, Leonardi MJ, Karapondo DL, Malicky ES, Flakel JE, Hagerman FC, Hikida RS. Strength and skeletal muscle adaptations in heavy-resistance-trained women after detraining and retraining. *J Appl Physiol.* 1991;70:631–40.

166. *Stedman's Medical Dictionary for the Health Professions and Nursing.* 5th ed. Philadelphia: Lippincott Williams & Wilkins; 2005.

167. Stein RB, Gordon T, Jefferson J, Sharfenberger A, Yang JF, deZepetnek JT, Belanger M. Optimal stimulation of paralyzed muscle after human spinal cord injury. *J Appl Physiol.* 1992;72:1393–400.

168. Stein TP, Wade CE. Metabolic consequences of muscle disuse atrophy. *J Nutr.* 2005;135:1824S–8S.

169. Sternfeld B, Ngo L, Satariano WA. Associations of body composition with physical performance and self-reported functional limitation in elderly men and women. *Am J Epidemiol.* 2002;156:110–21.

170. Stevens JE, Walter GA, Okereke E, et al. Muscle adaptations with immobilization and rehabilitation after ankle fracture. *Med Sci Sports Exerc.* 2004;36:1695–701.

171. Suetta C, Aagaard P, Magnusson SP, et al. Muscle size, neuromuscular activation, and rapid force characteristics in elderly men and women: effects of unilateral long-term disuse due to hiposteoarthritis. *J Appl Physiol.* 2007;102:942–8.

172. Suetta C, Aagaard P, Rosted A, Jakobsen AK, Duus B, Kjaer M, Magnusson SP. Training-induced changes in muscle CSA, muscle strength, EMG, and rate of force development in elderly subjects after long-term unilateral disuse. *J Appl Physiol.* 2004;97:1954–61.

173. Tankersley CG, Smolander J, Kenney WL, Fortney SM. Sweating and skin blood flow during exercise: effects of age and maximal oxygen uptake. *J Appl Physiol.* 1991;71:236–42.

174. Tate CA, Hyek MF, Taffett GE. Mechanisms for the responses of cardiac muscle to physical activity. *Med Sci Sports Exerc.* 1994;26: 561–7.

175. Tilton FE, Degioanni JJ, Schneider VS. Long-term follow-up of Skylab bone demineralization. *Aviat Space Environ Med.* 1980;51: 1209–13.

176. Tseng BS, Marsh DR, Hamilton MT, Booth FW. Strength and aerobic training attenuate muscle wasting and improve resistance to the development of disability with aging [special issue]. *J Gerontol* 1995;50A:113–9.

177. Turley KR, Wilmore JH. Cardiovascular responses to submaximal exercise in 7–9 year-old boys and girls. *Med Sci Sports Exerc.* 1997;29:824–32.

178. Uebelhart D, Demiaux-Domenech B, Roth M, Chantraine A. Bone metabolism in spinal cord injured individuals and in others who have prolonged immobilisation: a review. *Paraplegia.* 1995; 33:669–73.

179. Uebelhart D, Bernard J, Hartmann DJ, et al. Modifications of bone and connective tissue after orthostatic bedrest. *Osteoporos Int.* 2000;11:59–67.

180. Valdimarsson O, Alborg HG, Düppe H, Nyquist F, Karlsson M. Reduced training is associated with increased loss of BMD. *J Bone Miner Res.* 2005;20:906–12.

181. Van der Wiel HE, Lips P, Nauta J, Netelenbos JC, Hazenberg GJ. Biochemical parameters of bone turnover during ten days of bed rest and subsequent mobilization. *Bone Miner.* 1991;13: 123–29.

182. van Harreveld PD, Lillich JD, Kawcak CE, Turner AS, Norrdin RW. Effects of immobilization followed by remobilization on mineral density, histomorphometric features, and formation of the bones of the metacarpophalangeal joint in horses. *Am J Vet Res.* 2002;2:276–81.

183. Vico L, Chappard D, Alexandre C, et al. Effects of a 120 day period of bed rest on bone mass and bone cell activities in man: attempts at countermeasure. *Bone Miner.* 1987;2:383–94.

184. Vico L, Collet P, Guignandon A, Lafage-Proust MH, Thomas T, Rehaillia M, Alexandre C. Effects of long-term microgravity exposure on cancellous and cortical weight-bearing bones of cosmonauts. *Lancet.* 2000;355:1607–11.

185. Walker JL, Murray TD, Jackson AS, Morrow JR Jr, Michaud TJ. The energy cost of horizontal walking and running in adolescents. *Med Sci Sports Exerc.* 1999;31:311–22.

186. Wang J, Horlick M, Thornton JC. Correlations between skeletal muscle mass and bone mass in children 6–18 years: influences of sex, ethnicity, and pubertal status. *Growth Dev Aging.* 1999;63: 99–109.

187. Wang Q, Alen M, Nicholson P, Suominen H, Koistinen A, Kröger H, Cheng S. Weight-bearing, muscle loading and bone mineral accrual in pubertal girls—a 2-year longitudinal study. *Bone.* 2007;40:1196–202.

188. Westing SH, Seger H, Thorstensson A. Effects of electrical stimulation on eccentric and concentric torque-velocity relationships during knee extension in man. *Acta Physiol Scand.* 1990;140: 17–22.

189. Widrick JJ, Romatowski JG, Norenberg KM, et al. Functional properties of slow and fast gastrocnemius muscle fibers after a 17-day spaceflight. *J Appl Physiol.* 2001;90:2203–11.

190. Wilson TE, Shibasaki M, Cui J, Levine BD, Crandall CG. Effects of 14 days of head-down tilt bed rest on cutaneous vasoconstrictor responses in humans. *J Appl Physiol.* 2003;94:2113–8.

191. Woo JS, Derleth C, Stratton JR, Levy WC. The influence of age, gender, and training on exercise efficiency. *J Am Coll Cardiol.* 2006; 47(5):1049–57.

192. Young A. Effects of aging on human cold tolerance. *Exp Aging Res.* 1991;17:205–13.

193. Young DR, Niklowitz WJ, Brown RJ, Jee WS. Immobilization-associated osteoporosis in primates. *Bone.* 1986;7:109–17.

194. Zancanato S, Cooper DM, Armon Y. Oxygen cost and oxygen uptake dynamics and recovery with 1 minute of exercise in children and adults. *J Appl Physiol.* 1991;71:993–8.

195. Zerwekh JE, Ruml LA, Gottchalk F, Pak CY. The effects of twelve weeks of bed rest on bone histology, biochemical markers of bone turnover, and calcium homeostasis in eleven normal subjects. *J Bone Miner Res.* 1998;13:1594–601.

SELECTED REFERENCES FOR FURTHER READING

Christiansen JL, Grzybowski JM: *Biology of Aging.* New York: McGraw-Hill; 1999.

Shephard RJ: *Aging, Physical Activity and Health.* Champaign (IL): Human Kinetics; 1997.

Spirduso WW, Francis KL, MacRae PG: *Physical Dimensions of Aging.* Champaign (IL): Human Kinetics; 2005.

INTERNET RESOURCES

- ISAPA: International Society for Aging and Physical Activity: www.isapa.org
- National Institute on Aging: www.nia.nih.gov
- NCPAD: National Center on Physical Activity and Disability: www.ncpad.org
- Tufts University Health & Nutrition Newsletter: http://healthletter.tufts.edu
- WebMD: www.webmd.com

Pathophysiology and Treatment of Cardiovascular Disease

The World Health Organization estimates that cardiovascular disease (CVD) kills 16.7 million people worldwide each year and that it will account for five times more deaths than HIV/AIDS in low- and middle-income countries. In the United States, CVD kills more people than cancer, respiratory diseases, accidents and diabetes mellitus combined, and was the underlying cause of 36.3% of all deaths in 2004 and a contributing factor in 58% of all deaths that year. Almost 2,400 Americans die each day from CVD, an average of one death every 36 seconds. An estimated 79,400,000 American adults have one or more types of CVD, which will generate over $430 billion in direct and indirect healthcare costs (46).

This chapter will discuss the outcomes and manifestations of specific CVDs, the physiologic process of atherosclerosis, and treatments of CVDs, including pharmacologic, surgical, and lifestyle interventions. Furthermore, the role of cardiovascular risk factors in CVD will be presented as well as the goals of risk factor modification strategies.

ATHEROSCLEROSIS

> **1.2.1-CES: Summarize the atherosclerotic process, including current hypotheses regarding onset and rate of progression and/or regression.**

> **1.2.6-CES: Describe the lipoprotein classifications, and define their relationship to atherosclerosis.**

> **1.2.4-HFS: Knowledge to define the following terms: total cholesterol (TC), high-density lipoprotein cholesterol (HDL-C), TC/HDL-C ratio, low-density lipoprotein cholesterol (LDL-C), triglycerides, hypertension, and atherosclerosis.**

> **1.2.7-HFS: Knowledge of the atherosclerotic process, the factors involved in its genesis and progression, and the potential role of exercise in treatment.**

> **2.2.2 HFS: Knowledge of the pathophysiology of myocardial ischemia and infarction.**

Our understanding of atherosclerosis has evolved over the past several decades, and the disease is no longer viewed as a passive deposition of cholesterol in the arterial wall causing progressive arterial stenosis and ultimately creating an occlusive thrombus. Today we recognize that atherosclerosis is an active process involving molecular signals that produce altered cellular behavior as well as endothelial dysfunction and a subsequent inflammatory response (32). Although lipid deposition is a fundamental part of the atherosclerotic process, interactions among bloodborne molecules and intrinsic cells of

> > > KEY TERMS

Acute myocardial infarction: The death of myocardial tissue resulting from prolonged ischemia.

Angina pectoris: Chest pain or discomfort that is caused by myocardial ischemia.

Cardiovascular disease: Class of diseases that affect the heart or circulatory system.

Ischemia: A state of oxygen deprivation that is due to impaired blood flow.

Morbidity: The rate of incidence of a particular disease.

Mortality: The number of deaths in a given time or place.

Peripheral arterial disease: Condition in which blood flow through noncoronary arterial beds is inhibited.

Sudden cardiac death: An instant, unexpected death that results from the abrupt loss of heart function.

Thrombosis: The formation or presence of a fibrin clot in a blood vessel.

the arterial wall are now recognized as important contributors to the pathogenesis of this disease.

We often consider atherosclerosis in chronologic phases, although the disease is far more complicated than this simplistic perspective suggests. Initiation of the process typically occurs in childhood. The lesion progresses to form a fatty streak, typically during young adulthood through middle age. Ultimately, the lesion matures to form a complex fibrous plaque that may produce symptoms or complications such as myocardial infarction, sudden cardiac death, or stroke, typically as a result of an occlusive thrombus. The rate at which an individual lesion progresses through these stages is related to the presence of classic and emerging risk factors.

Initiation of the atherosclerotic process begins with injury of the endothelial lining of the arterial wall, stemming from several possible causes, including carbon monoxide or other tobacco-related irritants, hypertension, low-density lipoprotein cholesterol (LDL-C), and homocysteine. For reasons that are still unclear, normal endothelial function is not restored by the inherent repair mechanisms (27). Platelets adhere to the damaged arterial wall, aggregate, and become activated, secreting growth factors and vasoconstrictive substances, such as thromboxane A2.

LDL-C passes through the endothelial monolayer at the site of injury and undergoes the process of oxidation. Oxidized phospholipids such as LDL-C can elicit the expression of vascular adhesion molecules on the surface of the endothelial cells, promoting the adhesion of peripheral blood monocytes to the area of injury. Furthermore, constituents of oxidized LDL-C can stimulate the expression of chemoattractant cytokines, such as MCP-1, which encourage migration of monocytes into the subendothelial space (32). Activated platelets induce an inflammatory reaction in cells of the vascular wall (42), which induces endothelial activation and secretion of chemoattractants, further promoting monocyte recruitment (11,20,49,58). Upon moving into the arterial wall, monocytes are transformed into macrophages and collect the subintimal LDL-C, further augmenting the oxidative and subsequent inflammatory processes. At this point of development, the lesion consists primarily of foam cells (i.e., engorged macrophages), as well as T- and B-lymphocytes and mast cells (19). It is referred to as a *fatty streak*, reflecting its appearance and composition (Fig. 6-1).

Lipid accumulation during this phase may be slowed or reversed through the cardioprotective effects of high-density lipoprotein cholesterol (HDL-C). HDL-C uses the reverse cholesterol transport mechanism to remove cholesterol from engorged macrophages and carry it out of the subendothelial space to be excreted (55). In addition, HDL holds antioxidant enzymes that may mitigate inflammation as well as the endothelial expression of vascular adhesion molecules that augment atherosclerotic progression (2,32).

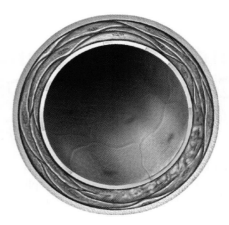

FIGURE 6-1. Disease progression of atherosclerosis: fatty streak. (Asset provided by Anatomical Chart Co.)

With continued maturation, a fatty streak progresses to a more fibrous plaque (Fig. 6-2). Specific cells in and around the lesion are affected by signaling mechanisms from platelets, monocytes, and endothelial cells that result in growth and proliferation (36). Fibroblasts and smooth muscle cells (SMCs) migrate to the intima from the media layer of the blood vessel (34). SMCs create the primary components of the complex extracellular matrix, including collagens, elastin, and glycosaminoglycans. In the intima, expression of these molecules gives rise to the characteristic structure of atherosclerotic plaque, including a rigid fibrous cap (31,51). Beneath this cap lies one or more lipid cores, which typically contain macrophage foam cells, inflammatory molecules, SMCs, calcium, dead cells, and acellular debris.

It was previously believed that atherosclerotic lesions would progress to occlusive stenoses that ultimately resulted in an ischemic event. It is now understood that compensatory arterial enlargement (i.e., remodeling) allows for considerable atherosclerotic development without substantial lumenal occlusion (50) and that the majority of adverse cardiovascular events are the result of

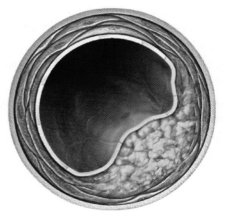

FIGURE 6-2. Disease progression of atherosclerosis: fibrous plaque. (Asset provided by Anatomical Chart Co.)

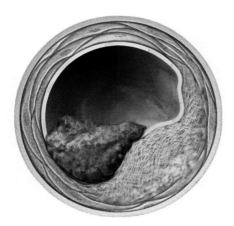

FIGURE 6-3. Disease progression of atherosclerosis: complicated lesion with blood clot. (Asset provided by Anatomical Chart Co.)

plaque erosion or rupture with subsequent thrombus development (Fig. 6-3). Physical disruption of the lesion exposes blood coagulation factors to prothrombotic stimuli that reside in the core of the plaque. The ensuing blood clot may dissolve; it may become dislodged from the arterial wall and substantially occlude a downstream artery; or it may be incorporated into the rapidly growing lesion. Plaques that are most vulnerable to rupture tend to have a large lipid core with reduced collagen content, a thinned fibrous cap, and pronounced outward remodeling of the arterial wall (52). Atherothrombotic events also depend on the thrombogenic properties of the blood (33), and the risk of ischemic events is associated with elevated coagulation activity and decreased fibrinolytic capacity (48,56).

OUTCOMES AND MANIFESTATIONS OF CARDIOVASCULAR DISEASE AND THE UNIQUE PATHOPHYSIOLOGIES RESPECTIVE TO EACH CONDITION

> **1.2.2-CES: Compare and contrast the differences between typical, atypical, and vasospastic angina and how these may differ in specific subgroups.**

> **2.2.3-HFS: Knowledge of the pathophysiology of stroke, hypertension, and hyperlipidemia.**

HYPERTENSION

Hypertension is defined as having systolic blood pressure (SBP) 140 mm Hg or diastolic blood pressure (DBP) 90 mm Hg or higher, or taking antihypertensive medication. The most commonly diagnosed cardiovascular disease, hypertension affects an estimated one of every three American adults, or approximately 72,000,000 people (15). Age-adjusted prevalence of hypertension is greater in men than in women, and African Americans have

higher prevalence than other ethnic groups (46). The number of deaths from hypertension rose 56.4% from 1994 to 2004 (1). Elevated blood pressure increases risk of heart failure (24), end-stage renal disease (35), myocardial infarction (15), and stroke (15), and is associated with reduced overall life expectancy (17).

In general, hypertension causes a constriction of peripheral arteries so that blood flow is hindered, increasing workload of the heart. In a relatively small number of diagnosed cases of hypertension, the elevated blood pressure is caused by another abnormality, such as renal disorders or congenital narrowing of particular arteries. However, 90% to 95% of all cases of high blood pressure are "essential," or "primary" hypertension. That is, there is no known cause for the elevated blood pressure.

CORONARY HEART DISEASE

Coronary heart disease (CHD) is the manifestation of advanced atherosclerotic progression in one or more coronary arteries. CHD is the single largest killer of American men and women, causing one of every five deaths in the United States in 2004 (46). Common sequelae of CHD include angina pectoris, myocardial infarction, and sudden cardiac death.

Angina pectoris is referred pain resulting from myocardial ischemia. The pain is often described as substernal pressure, heaviness, or burning that is sometimes accompanied by dyspnea. Chronic stable angina pectoris is typically elicited by physical or emotional stress and is relieved by rest or nitrate medication. Unstable angina pectoris does not share the predictability of chronic stable angina and may present itself with no provocation. Unstable angina may result from coronary vasospasm or transient occlusion and is relieved by spontaneous arterial relaxation and/or thrombolysis. Vasospastic or Prinzmetal angina is caused by focal coronary artery vasospasm, typically at the site of or adjacent to a fixed stenosis. Animal experiments suggest that coronary vasospasm is caused primarily by vascular smooth muscle hypercontraction and not by local endothelial dysfunction. The molecular mechanism(s) of this smooth muscle cell abnormality remains unclear.

HEART FAILURE

Heart failure (HF) is a chronic, degenerative condition in which the ability of one or both ventricles to fill with (diastolic failure) or eject (systolic failure) blood is impaired (see Table 6-1 for disease classification). Primarily a condition of the elderly, incidence of HF is increasing, and more Medicare dollars are spent for the diagnosis and treatment of HF than for any other diagnosis (37). Principal manifestations of HF include dyspnea, fatigue, exercise intolerance, and fluid retention. HF may be caused by any number of conditions that damage the

TABLE 6-1. CLASSIFICATION OF HEART FAILURE (24)

STAGE	DEFINITION
A	At high risk for HF but without structural heart disease or symptoms of HF
B	Structural heart disease but without signs or symptoms of HF
C	Structural heart disease with prior or current symptoms of HF
D	Refractory HF requiring specialized interventions

HF, heart failure.

TABLE 6-2. FONTAINE'S CLASSIFICATION OF PERIPHERAL ARTERIAL DISEASE

STAGE	CLINICAL FINDING
I	Asymptomatic
IIa	Mild claudication
IIb	Moderate-severe claudication
III	Ischemic rest pain
IV	Ulceration or gangrene

heart, including cardiomyopathies, coronary heart disease, or established risk factors for cardiovascular disease, such as smoking, obesity, hypertension, high cholesterol, and diabetes mellitus (24). Most patients experience symptoms that result from an impairment of left ventricular myocardial function and exhibit both systolic and diastolic abnormalities (24). Ventricular dysfunction in HF typically progresses, resulting in a change in the structure of the ventricle such that it becomes more spherical. This "cardiac remodeling" increases hemodynamic stress on the chamber walls and may increase regurgitant blood flow through the mitral valve, further exacerbating the remodeling process. Activation of neurohormonal systems also contributes to cardiac remodeling. Patients with HF have elevated catecholamines, cytokines, aldosterone, and angiotensin II. These hormonal changes may increase hemodynamic stress and have direct toxic effects on cardiac myocytes, as well as stimulate myocardial fibrosis, resulting in the further alteration of cardiac geometry and depressed function of the heart (24).

STROKE

Stroke is one of the leading causes of death and long-term disability in America (1,46). It is described as the loss of brain function subsequent to the interruption of blood flow. This may occur because of hemorrhage or obstruction, typically by an occlusive thrombus or embolism. Depending on the hemisphere of the brain that is affected, stroke patients may experience hemiplegia, altered coordination, vertigo, memory loss, problems with speech or vision, and behavioral changes.

Approximately 87% of all strokes are ischemic in nature rather than hemorrhagic (46), and transient ischemic attacks (TIA) are particularly predictive of a stroke. The risk of stroke is 3% to 17% within the first 90 days after a TIA; approximately 15% of all strokes are preceded by a TIA (18). The pathogenic mechanism of TIA is similar to ischemic stroke, but the transient attack is defined by neurologic symptoms that last <24 hours (47). Patients with TIA and stroke have a high prevalence of asymptomatic coronary disease (13,14,45), so strategies for the prevention of ischemic stroke include modi-

fying cardiovascular risk factors, such as dyslipidemia, hypertension, obesity, smoking, and physical inactivity. Furthermore, individuals with atrial fibrillation, women who are pregnant or within 6 weeks postpartum, and postmenopausal women are at greater risk of stroke than their age- and sex-matched counterparts (4,28,59).

PERIPHERAL ARTERIAL DISEASE

Peripheral arterial disease (PAD) refers to a series of disorders in which blood flow through noncoronary arterial beds is inhibited (see Table 6-2 for disease classification). This condition most commonly affects the femoral, popliteal, tibial, iliac, abdominal aorta, renal, and mesenteric arteries. PAD affects an estimated 8 million Americans, including 12% to 20% of Americans aged 65 years and older (22). Despite the prevalence and significant morbidity and mortality associated with PAD, only 25% of those diagnosed are undergoing treatment (3).

Peripheral arterial disease is primarily caused by atherosclerosis and related thrombotic processes that may occlude the affected vessel and produce ischemia in downstream muscle tissue. Risk factors for PAD include age, obesity, sedentary lifestyle, dyslipidemia, hyperhomocysteinemia, hypertension, and especially smoking and diabetes mellitus. The classic manifestation of PAD is intermittent claudication: leg pain (e.g., cramping, burning) that predictably follows physical exertion and is relieved by rest. It should be noted, however, that only approximately 10% of PAD patients report having intermittent claudication, approximately 50% report some variety of leg symptoms, and 40% do not report leg pain (10,21). Peripheral arterial disease is associated with increased risk of other cardiovascular complications, such as myocardial infarction and stroke, and, left untreated, may lead to gangrene and amputation. Treatment of PAD includes risk factor modification, pharmacologic intervention, and possibly surgical revascularization.

SURGICAL TREATMENTS FOR CARDIOVASCULAR DISEASE

> **1.6.1-CES: Describe percutaneous coronary interventions (PCI) and peripheral interventions as an alternative to medical management or bypass surgery.**

In situations in which primary prevention strategies have been unsuccessful in decreasing or reversing the progression of cardiovascular disease, surgical intervention may be necessary to restore perfusion to the affected tissues. Revascularization techniques have advanced over the years and physicians now have a large arsenal of procedures, including some minimally invasive methods that require little or no convalescence.

Catheter-based interventions utilize a thin, flexible tube that is threaded through an artery from the groin or arm and into the occluded arteries. The catheter may then be used to perform a percutaneous coronary intervention such as an angioplasty, in which a small balloon is positioned over a lesion and expanded to push the vessel wall out (Fig. 6-4). One of the primary drawbacks of the balloon procedure is the risk of restenosis (53). To prevent restenosis, the angioplasty procedure commonly includes the use of a stent, a small metal tube that provides support to the opened vessel. Stents may be bare metal or drug coated, or carry time-released medicine (drug-eluting stent). A catheter may also be used to perform an atherectomy. A laser or rotating burr is used to break the lesion and thus remove the plaque from the artery. In some cases, a stent or balloon angioplasty is performed after the atherectomy.

The location or number of arterial blockages may necessitate the more invasive coronary artery bypass graft (CABG). A blood vessel (usually a saphenous vein, internal mammary, or radial artery) is surgically grafted to a coronary artery, bypassing an area that is narrowed as a result of advanced atherosclerosis. The conventional CABG procedure involves opening the chest with a sternum-splitting incision and stopping the heart, using a cardiopulmonary bypass pump to sustain circulation. Surgical advances have led to techniques in which a CABG can be completed without separating the sternum and/or without the use of a bypass pump, leading to shorter recovery times and improved operative mortality rates. Currently, this primarily occurs only in very-high-risk patients who are not acceptable candidates for traditional CABG (12,57).

CARDIOVASCULAR RISK FACTORS: ROLE IN DISEASE PROGRESSION, GOALS FOR RISK FACTOR MODIFICATION

> **1.2.5-CES:** Examine the role of lifestyle on cardiovascular risk factors, such as hypertension, blood lipids, glucose tolerance, and body weight.

> **1.2.15-CES:** Recognize the pathologic process that various risk factors contribute for the development of cardiac, pulmonary, and metabolic diseases (e.g., smoking, hypertension, abnormal blood lipid values, obesity, inactivity, sex, genetics, diabetes).

> **1.5.13-CES:** Recognized treatment goals and guidelines for dyslipidemia using the most recent National Cholesterol Education Program (NCEP) report and other relevant evidence-based guidelines.

> **1.5.12-HFS:** Recognize treatment goals and guidelines for hypertension using the most recent Joint National Committee on Prevention, Detection, Evaluation and Treatment of High Blood Pressure report and other relevant evidence-based guidelines.

> **1.2.5-HFS:** Knowledge of plasma cholesterol levels for adults as recommended by the National Cholesterol Education Program.

Although it is not possible to control for all CVD risk factors, such as age and family history, adopting a lifestyle that focuses on each of the controllable risk factors—and using medications in many cases—may positively affect cardiovascular morbidity and mortality. The American College of Sports Medicine positive risk factors for CVD that may be modified through lifestyle choices are

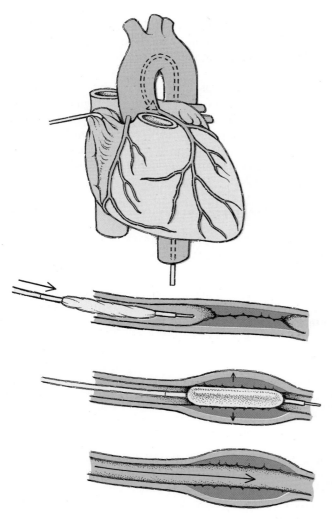

FIGURE 6-4. Percutaneous transluminal angioplasty. (Acknowledgment: Neil O. Hardy, Westpoint, CT.)

cigarette smoking, sedentary lifestyle, obesity, hypertension, dyslipidemia, and impaired fasting glucose. A recent study of a large cohort of healthy men estimated that >60% of all primary coronary events could be prevented with a healthy lifestyle (7), further supporting the well-established benefits of risk factor modification.

SMOKING

Cigarette smoke contains several thousand chemicals and at least 40 known carcinogens. Several constituents of smoke contribute to the initiation and progression of atherosclerosis. Absorbed through active smoking or through passive exposure, cigarette smoke damages endothelial cells, leads to acute increases in blood pressure, and increases platelet aggregation.

The smoking risk factor threshold is defined as current smoking habit or having quit within the previous 6 months or exposure to environmental tobacco smoke. Complete smoking cessation is the goal of this risk factor modification. Furthermore, patients should be urged to avoid any and all exposure to environmental tobacco smoke.

HYPERTENSION

High blood pressure (systolic blood pressure ≥140 mm Hg and/or diastolic pressure ≥90 mm Hg, *or* on antihypertensive medication) contributes to nearly all CVDs, as well as to renal failure, aneurysm, and eye damage.

It is recommended that all patients with elevated blood pressure initiate or maintain lifestyle modifications, including weight control, increased physical activity, and diet that is low in sodium and saturated fat (Table 6-3). Blood pressure–lowering medication is necessary for optimal control for many patients. The goal of blood pressure control is to reduce blood pressure to <140/90 mm Hg, or <130/80 if the patient has diabetes of chronic kidney disease. The Seventh Report of the Joint National Committee on Prevention, Detection, Evaluation and Treatment of High Blood Pressure (JNC 7) (8) points out that the risk of CVD doubles with each increment of 20/10 mm Hg higher than 115/75 and first introduced the classification of *prehypertensive*. The JNC 7 report recommends health-promoting lifestyle modifications even for patients whose blood pressure does not reach the threshold of hypertension.

DYSLIPIDEMIA

As previously discussed, cholesterol plays a significant role in atherogenesis. LDL-C plays a primary role in the initiation and progression of lesion development. Conversely, high serum concentration of HDL-C may slow or reverse atherosclerosis and is considered a negative risk factor. The most recent recommendations of the NCEP indicate that the goal of lipid management techniques is to keep LDL-C concentrations <100 mg/dL if triglycerides are ≥200 mg/dL, and all non-HDL-C should be <130 mg/dL (43). All individuals should be encouraged to reduce dietary intake of saturated fats, *trans*-fatty acids, and cholesterol, and to increase consumption of plant sterols, viscous fiber, and omega-3 fatty acids. Promotion of weight management and regular physical activity should accompany these dietary recommendations. For many patients, LDL-lowering medication is necessary. For patients with coronary heart disease, statin medications are considered mandatory, even if LDL-C is <100.

SEDENTARY LIFESTYLE

The positive effects of regular exercise on cardiovascular disease are diverse and well documented in the

TABLE 6-3. LIFESTYLE MODIFICATIONS TO MANAGE HYPERTENSION[*†] (8)

Modification	Recommendation	Approximate SBP Reduction
Weight reduction	Maintain normal body weight (BMI 18.5–24.9 kg/m^2)	5–20 mm Hg/10 kg weight loss
Adopt DASH eating plan	Consume a diet rich in fruits, vegetables, and lowfat dairy products with a reduced content of saturated and total fat.	8–14 mmHg
Dietary sodium reduction	Reduce dietary sodium intake to no more than 100 mmol per day (2.4 g sodium or 6 g sodium chloride).	2–8 mm Hg
Physical activity	Engage in regular aerobic physical activity, such as brisk walking (at least 30 min per day, most days of the week).	4–9 mm Hg
Moderation of alcohol consumption	Limit consumption to no more than 2 drinks (e.g., 1 oz or 30 mL ethanol; 24 oz beer, 10 oz wine, or 3 oz 80-proof whiskey) per day in most men and to no more than 1 drink per day in women and lighter-weight persons.	2–4 mm Hg

SBP, systolic blood pressure; BMI, body mass index; DASH, Dietary Approaches to Stop Hypertension.

[*]For overall cardiovascular risk reduction, stop smoking.

[†]The effects of implementing these modifications are dose and time dependent and could be greater for some individuals.

scientific literature. All individuals are encouraged to accumulate 30 to 60 minutes of moderate-intensity aerobic activity per day for a minimum of 5 days per week, but ideally as many as 7 days per week, supplemented by an increase in daily lifestyle activity. Resistance training should be done two or more days per week. A medical and physical activity history should be assessed before participation in an exercise program, and high-risk patients should be advised to participate in medically supervised programs.

OBESITY

Obesity is a major independent risk factor for numerous hypokinetic diseases, including CVD. Furthermore, excess body fat is closely related to the presence of other CVD risk factors. It is estimated that as much as 75% of hypertension may be attributed to obesity, although the mechanism for this relationship is not fully understood (30). Increased total body weight has a strong effect on lipoprotein metabolism, and is a determinant of decreased HDL-C, elevated triglycerides and LDL-C. Obesity also contributes to glucose tolerance, and may be responsible for $\geq$50% of the variance in insulin sensitivity (30). It should also be noted that fat distribution patterns are likely to mediate the effect of obesity on CVD risk. Abdominal fat, in particular, is highly correlated with insulin resistance and, thus, complications of CVD. The goal for weight management is to maintain a body mass index (BMI) of 18.5 to 24.9 kg/m^2, with a waist circumference (measured horizontally at the iliac crest) <40 inches for men and <35 inches for women. Weight maintenance and reduction should be accomplished with a healthy balance of regular exercise and caloric intake.

IMPAIRED FASTING GLUCOSE

Chronic hyperglycemia, a hallmark of diabetes mellitus, is associated with accelerated atherosclerosis (41) and may bring about neurologic and cardiovascular complications. Transgenic mouse models and human autopsy studies suggest that diabetes-induced hyperglycemia, independent from dyslipidemia that is common among this patient population, results in accelerated lesion formation (25,38,39,44). Elevations in blood glucose concentrations also promote monocyte recruitment and adherence to the endothelial monolayer by stimulating expression of endothelial adhesion molecules (5,9). Diabetes and elevated glucose concentrations are related to advanced atherosclerotic plaques and clinical outcomes, but it is unclear if these effects are direct or simply secondary to the accelerated lesion initiation (26). The goal of glucose control management strategies is to maintain glycosylated hemoglobin (HbA$_{1C}$) levels of <7%. Patients should initiate lifestyle changes and, as warranted, pharmacologic interventions.

PHARMACOLOGIC TREATMENT OF CARDIOVASCULAR DISEASE

> **1.5.3-CES: Recognize medications associated in the clinical setting, their indications for care, and their effects at rest and during exercise.**

> **1.5.1-HFS: Knowledge of common drugs from each of the following classes of medications, and describe the principal action and the effects on exercise testing and prescription, including antianginals; antihypertensives; antiarrhythmics; anticoagulants, bronchodilators; hypoglycemics; psychotropics; and vasodilators.**

Blood coagulation activity is elevated around a complicated atherosclerotic lesion and is responsible for most acute cardiovascular events. Thus, pharmacologic treatment of cardiovascular disease often includes drugs that prevent the development of an occlusive thrombus. Antiplatelet medications, such as aspirin and clopidogrel, interfere with platelet activation and/or aggregation, thus interfering with one of the initial steps of the coagulation process. Other common anticoagulant agents, such as warfarin and heparin, interfere with the coagulation cascade, either by preventing hepatic synthesis of vitamin K–dependent clotting factors or stimulating coagulation enzyme inhibitors.

Other common medications used in the treatment of CVD focus on controlling one or more risk factors. One of the key components of strategies for primary and secondary prevention of CVD is the control of hypertension. As such, several medications are available for the maintenance of healthy blood pressure, including diuretics, β-blockers, calcium channel blockers, angiotensin-converting enzyme (ACE) inhibitors, and angiotensin receptor blockers.

β-blockers (e.g., atenolol, propanolol, metaprolol) bind to β-adrenergic receptors, inhibiting the action of endogenous catecholamines. These drugs reduce the sympathetic effects of catecholamines on the heart and blood vessels, resulting in reduced heart rates and blood pressure, and decreasing myocardial oxygen demand.

Voltage-gated calcium channels, when stimulated in the heart and blood vessels, allow the influx of calcium into the cells, resulting in vasoconstriction and increased myocardial contractility. Calcium channel blockers (e.g., diltiazem, verapamil) inhibit stimulation of these voltage-regulated gates and promote vasodilation, decreased peripheral resistance, and cardiac output. However, calcium antagonists have negative inotropic effects and must be used with caution, if at all, in patients with CVD.

A diuretic (e.g., furosemide, thiazides, amiloride, spironolactone) is a medication that controls blood pressure by modulating the rate of urine excretion and, thus, plasma volume. The various classes of diuretic accomplish this in slightly different ways, such as inhibiting reabsorption of sodium in the kidney, promoting osmotic diuresis, or inhibiting vasopressin (antidiuretic hormone) or aldosterone. Although diuretics are often not tolerated as well as some of the newer classes of antihypertensive medications, recent evidence suggests diuretic therapy may be more effective at reducing blood pressure and preventing various forms of CVD (40).

The angiotensin-converting enzyme catalyzes the conversion of angiotensin I to angiotensin II, which is a potent vasoconstrictor. ACE inhibitors (e.g., enalapril, ramipril, lisinopril) block this reaction and the ensuing increase in blood pressure related to vessel constriction. ACE inhibitors may also impart secondary cardiovascular benefits. Angiotensin II stimulates expression of proinflammatory cytokines as well as vascular adhesion molecules on the surface of endothelial cells (6,29). Thus, ACE inhibitors may slow the rate of atherosclerotic initiation and progression. Furthermore, ACE inhibition may enhance the ability to dissolve fibrin blood clots, reducing risk of complications related to occlusive thrombi (60).

The effect of angiotensin II on blood pressure may also be minimized through the use of angiotensin receptor blockers (ARBs). Blockade of the angiotensin II receptor causes vasodilation and reduced secretion of aldosterone and vasopressin, ultimately reducing blood pressure and myocardial workload. ARBs (e.g., irbesartan, losartan, valsartan) are typically used in the treatment of hypertension and heart failure.

Control of blood cholesterol is another key focus of CVD treatment and prevention. Several medications are available that affect concentrations of total cholesterol, LDL-C, and/or HDL-C. Statins (e.g., simvastatin, lovastatin, atorvastatin) are the most popular cholesterol-lowering medication. They have few immediate side effects, are very effective at lowering LDL-C, and may increase HDL-C and lower triglyceride concentration. Statins inhibit hepatic synthesis of cholesterol and increase the number of LDL receptors on hepatocytes, enhancing the elimination of LDL from the blood. Resins (e.g., cholestyramine) bind to bile acids in the intestine, preventing their reabsorption and thereby increasing their excretion. The increased bile acid excretion promotes increased cholesterol metabolism. Resins decrease total cholesterol and LDL-C. Fibrates (e.g., gemfibrozil, fenofibrate) produce moderate decreases in blood concentrations of LDL-C and increases in HDL-C, but are extremely effective at lowering triglyceride (54). Some gastrointestinal side effects have been reported, and fibrates may interact with anticoagulant medication. Nicotinic acid (niacin) lowers serum levels of total cholesterol, LDL-C, very-low-density lipoprotein (VLDL), and triglycerides, and increases levels of HDL-C substantially. The mechanism of the antihyperlipidemic action of nicotinic acid is not well understood, but it is thought that the effect is mediated, in part, via decreases in the release of free fatty acids from adipose tissue and the rate of production of hepatic VLDL.

Other medications and nutritional supplements are commonly used in the treatment of CVD. Vasodilators such as nitroglycerin are used in tablet, spray, or transdermal patch form and relieve ischemia-related pain by dilating blood vessels. Antioxidant vitamins, such as vitamins E, C, and β-carotene, are thought to reduce the risk of cardiovascular disease by preventing the oxidation of LDL-C. The lack of data from well-designed clinical trials makes it premature to recommend dietary supplements to prevent CVD, but all patients should be encouraged to consume a diet rich in food sources of antioxidant and other cardioprotective nutrients, such as omega-3 fatty acids.

PATHOPHYSIOLOGY OF THE HEALING MYOCARDIUM

> **1.2.3-CES:** Describe the pathophysiology of the healing myocardium and the potential complications after acute myocardial infarction (remodeling, rupture).

It is estimated that 700,000 Americans will experience a new myocardial infarction (MI) in the coming year, and 500,000 more will have a recurrent attack (46). The healing process that follows an MI includes a series of changes in ventricular function, tissue composition, and regional deformation, as well as several possible complications.

In the first 4 to 6 hours following an MI, the myocardium experiences acute ischemia. The infarcted tissue loses the ability to generate force and is changed to a passive, viscoelastic body. The loss of systolic power is the primary functional change in this phase. Several hours later, inflammation and necrosis become the dominant pathologic processes. This phase of healing typically lasts approximately 7 days, although signs of necrosis may persist for several months (16). The infarcted area may expand, growing thinner and occupying greater endothelial surface area. This remodeling process, in which the chamber dilates and weakens, may exacerbate increases in ventricular wall stress. The healing infarct soon transitions to a phase in which collagen deposition rapidly increases, leading to increased myocardial stiffness, impaired filling, and potentially impaired systolic function. Eventually, systolic function improves because of a decline in stiffness despite continued increases in collagen content. The infarct "scar" shrinks in this final stage of healing to occupy a smaller percentage of the ventricular wall. Chamber dilation decreases, and wall-motion abnormalities partially resolve. Although the myocardium experiences dramatic improvements in structure and function, the tissue may never stabilize to the point that the healing process could be considered complete (23) (Box 6-1).

BOX 6-1	POTENTIAL WAYS A HEALING INFARCT MAY IMPAIR LEFT VENTRICULAR FUNCTION (23)

- Infarct may fail or rupture.
- Infarct bulging or stretching wastes energy generated by healthy myocardium.
- Infarct stiffness may limit diastolic function of healthy myocardium.
- Infarct expansion and cavity dilation may increase wall stress throughout the chamber.

- Coupling to the infarct may limit deformation of the adjacent myocardium.
- Material properties of the infarct determine pattern of ventricular remodeling and hypertrophy.

REFERENCES

1. *Incidence and Prevalence: 2006 Chart Book on Cardiovascular and Lung Diseases.* Bethesda (MD): National Heart, Lung, Blood Institute, 2006.
2. Barter PJ, Nicholls S, Rye KA, Anantharamaiah GM, Navab M, Fogelman AM. Antiinflammatory properties of HDL. *Circ Res.* 2004;95:764–72.
3. Becker GJ, McClenny TE, Kovacs ME, Raabe RD, Katzen BT. The importance of increasing public and physician awareness of peripheral arterial disease. *J Vasc Interv Radiol.* 2002;13:7–11.
4. Bonita R. Epidemiology of stroke. *Lancet.* 1992;339:342–4.
5. Booth G, Stalker TJ, Lefer AM, Scalia R. Mechanisms of amelioration of glucose-induced endothelial dysfunction following inhibition of protein kinase C in vivo. *Diabetes.* 2002;51:1556–64.
6. Chen XL, Tummala PE, Olbrych MT, Alexander RW, Medford RM. Angiotensin II induces monocyte chemoattractant protein-1 gene expression in rat vascular smooth muscle cells. *Circ Res.* 1998;83:952–9.
7. Chiuve SE, McCullough ML, Sacks FM, Rimm EB. Healthy lifestyle factors in the primary prevention of coronary heart disease among men: benefits among users and nonusers of lipid-lowering and antihypertensive medications. *Circulation.* 2006;114:160–7.
8. **Chobanian AV, Bakris GL, Black HR, et al. The Seventh Report of the Joint National Committee on Prevention, Detection, Evaluation, and Treatment of High Blood Pressure: the JNC 7 report.** *JAMA.* **2003;289:2560–72.**
9. Cipolletta C, Ryan KE, Hanna EV, Trimble ER. Activation of peripheral blood CD14+ monocytes occurs in diabetes. *Diabetes.* 2005;54:2779–86.
10. Criqui MH, Fronek A, Klauber MR, Barrett-Connor E, Gabriel S. The sensitivity, specificity, and predictive value of traditional clinical evaluation of peripheral arterial disease: results from noninvasive testing in a defined population. *Circulation.* 1985;71: 516–22.
11. Danese S, de la Motte C, Reyes BM, Sans M, Levine AD, Fiocchi C. Cutting edge: T cells trigger CD40-dependent platelet activation and granular RANTES release: a novel pathway for immune response amplification. *J Immunol.* 2004;172:2011–15.
12. Detter C, Reichenspurner H, Boehm DH, Thalhammer M, Raptis P, Schutz A, Reichart B. Minimally invasive direct coronary artery bypass grafting (MIDCAB) and off-pump coronary artery bypass grafting (OPCAB): two techniques for beating heart surgery. *Heart Surg Forum.* 2002;5:157–62.
13. Di Pasquale G, Andreoli A, Pinelli G, Grazi P, Manini G, Tognetti F, Testa C. Cerebral ischemia and asymptomatic coronary artery disease: a prospective study of 83 patients. *Stroke.* 1986;17:1098–101.
14. Di Pasquale G, Pinelli G, Grazi P, et al. Incidence of silent myocardial ischaemia in patients with cerebral ischaemia. *Eur Heart J.* 1988;9(Suppl N):104–7.
15. Fields LE, Burt VL, Cutler JA, Hughes J, Roccella EJ, Sorlie P. The burden of adult hypertension in the United States 1999 to 2000: a rising tide. *Hypertension.* 2004;44:398–404.
16. Fishbein MC, Maclean D, Maroko PR. The histopathologic evolution of myocardial infarction. *Chest.* 1978;73:843–9.

17. Franco OH, Peeters A, Bonneux L, de Laet C. Blood pressure in adulthood and life expectancy with cardiovascular disease in men and women: life course analysis. *Hypertension.* 2005;46:280–6.
18. Hankey GJ. Long-term outcome after ischaemic stroke/transient ischaemic attack. *Cerebrovasc Dis.* 2003;16(Suppl 1):14–9.
19. Hansson GK, Libby P, Schonbeck U, Yan ZQ. Innate and adaptive immunity in the pathogenesis of atherosclerosis. *Circ Res.* 2002;91: 281–291.
20. Henn V, Slupsky JR, Grafe M, Anagnostopoulos I, Forster R, Muller-Berghaus G, Kroczek RA. CD40 ligand on activated platelets triggers an inflammatory reaction of endothelial cells. *Nature.* 1998 391:591–4.
21. Hirsch AT, Criqui MH, Treat-Jacobson D, et al. Peripheral arterial disease detection, awareness, and treatment in primary care. *JAMA.* 2001;286:1317–14.
22. **Hirsch AT, Haskal ZJ, Hertzer NR, et al. ACC/AHA 2005 Practice Guidelines for the management of patients with peripheral arterial disease (lower extremity, renal, mesenteric, and abdominal aortic): a collaborative report from the American Association for Vascular Surgery/Society for Vascular Surgery, Society for Cardiovascular Angiography and Interventions, Society for Vascular Medicine and Biology, Society of Interventional Radiology, and the ACC/AHA Task Force on Practice Guidelines (Writing Committee to Develop Guidelines for the Management of Patients with Peripheral Arterial Disease): endorsed by the American Association of Cardiovascular and Pulmonary Rehabilitation; National Heart, Lung, and Blood Institute; Society for Vascular Nursing; TransAtlantic Inter-Society Consensus; and Vascular Disease Foundation.** *Circulation.* **2006;113:e463–654.**
23. Holmes JW, Borg TK, Covell JW. Structure and mechanics of healing myocardial infarcts. *Annu Rev Biomed Eng.* 2005;7:223–53.
24. **Hunt SA, Abraham WT, Chin MH, et al. ACC/AHA 2005 Guideline Update for the Diagnosis and Management of Chronic Heart Failure in the Adult: a report of the American College of Cardiology/American Heart Association Task Force on Practice Guidelines (Writing Committee to Update the 2001 Guidelines for the Evaluation and Management of Heart Failure): developed in collaboration with the American College of Chest Physicians and the International Society for Heart and Lung Transplantation: endorsed by the Heart Rhythm Society.** *Circulation.* **2005;112:e154–235.**
25. Jarvisalo MJ, Putto-Laurila A, Jartti L, Lehtimaki T, Solakivi T, Ronnemaa T, Raitakari OT. Carotid artery intima-media thickness in children with type 1 diabetes. *Diabetes.* 2002;51:493–8.
26. Kanter JE, Johansson F, LeBoeuf RC, Bornfeldt KE. Do glucose and lipids exert independent effects on atherosclerotic lesion initiation or progression to advanced plaques? *Circ Res.* 2007;100:769–81.
27. Karra R, Vemullapalli S, Dong C, et al. Molecular evidence for arterial repair in atherosclerosis. *Proc Natl Acad Sci U S A.* 2005;102: 16789–94.
28. Kittner SJ, Stern BJ, Feeser BR, et al. Pregnancy and the risk of stroke. *N Engl J Med.* 1996;335:768–74.
29. Kranzhofer R, Schmidt J, Pfeiffer CA, Hagl S, Libby P, Kubler W. Angiotensin induces inflammatory activation of human vascular smooth muscle cells. *Arterioscler Thromb Vasc Biol.* 1999;19:1623–9.

30. Krauss RM, Winston M, Fletcher BJ, Grundy SM. Obesity: impact on cardiovascular disease. *Circulation*.1998;98:1472–6.

31. Lafont A, Libby P. The smooth muscle cell: sinner or saint in restenosis and the acute coronary syndromes? *J Am Coll Cardiol*. 1998;32:283–5.

32. Libby P, Ridker P. Inflammation and atherothrombosis: from population biology and bench research to clinical practice. *J Am Coll Cardiol*. 2007;48:A33–46.

33. Libby P, Theroux P. Pathophysiology of coronary artery disease. *Circulation*. 2005;111:3481–8.

34. Libby P, Warner SJ, Salomon RN, Birinyi LK. Production of platelet-derived growth factor-like mitogen by smooth-muscle cells from human atheroma. *N Engl J Med*. 1988;318:1493–8.

35. Martinez-Maldono M. Hypertension in end-stage renal disease. *Kidney Int*. 1998;68:567–572.

36. Massberg S, Vogt F, Dickfeld T, Brand K, Page S, Gawaz M. Activated platelets trigger an inflammatory response and enhance migration of aortic smooth muscle cells. *Thromb Res*. 2003;110:187–94.

37. Massie BM, Shah NB. Evolving trends in the epidemiologic factors of heart failure: rationale for preventive strategies and comprehensive disease management. *Am Heart J*. 1997;133:703–12.

38. McGill HC Jr, McMahan CA, Malcom GT, Oalmann MC, Strong JP. Relation of glycohemoglobin and adiposity to atherosclerosis in youth. Pathobiological Determinants of Atherosclerosis in Youth (PDAY) Research Group. *Arterioscler Thromb Vasc Biol*. 1995;15: 431–40.

39. McGill HC Jr, McMahan CA, Zieske AW, Malcom GT, Tracy RE, Strong JP. Effects of nonlipid risk factors on atherosclerosis in youth with a favorable lipoprotein profile. *Circulation*. 2001;103:1546–50.

40. Moser M. Current recommendations for the treatment of hypertension: are they still valid? *J Hypertens Suppl*. 2002;20:S3–10.

41. Nathan DM, Cleary PA, Backlund JY, et al. Intensive diabetes treatment and cardiovascular disease in patients with type 1 diabetes. *N Engl J Med*. 2005;353:2643–53.

42. Pitsilos S, Hunt J, Mohler ER, et al. Platelet factor 4 localization in carotid atherosclerotic plaques: correlation with clinical parameters. *Thromb Haemost*. 2003;90:1112–20.

43. **National Cholesterol Education Program. Third Report of the National Cholesterol Education Program (NCEP) Expert Panel on Detection, Evaluation, and Treatment of High Blood Cholesterol in Adults (Adult Treatment Panel III). Bethesda (MD): National Heart, Lung, and Blood Institute: 2002; p. 279.**

44. Renard CB, Kramer F, Johansson F, et al. Diabetes and diabetes-associated lipid abnormalities have distinct effects on initiation and progression of atherosclerotic lesions. *J Clin Invest*. 2004;114: 659–668.

45. Rokey R, Rolak LA, Harati Y, Kutka N, Verani MS. Coronary artery disease in patients with cerebrovascular disease: a prospective study. *Ann Neurol*. 1984;16:50–3.

46. **Rosamond W, Flegal K, Friday G, et al. Heart disease and stroke statistics—2007 update: a report from the American Heart Association Statistics Committee and Stroke Statistics Subcommittee. *Circulation*. 2007;115:e69–171.**

47. Sacco RL, Adams R, Albers G, et al. Guidelines for prevention of stroke in patients with ischemic stroke or transient ischemic attack: a statement for healthcare professionals from the American Heart Association/American Stroke Association Council on Stroke: co-sponsored by the Council on Cardiovascular Radiology and Intervention: the American Academy of Neurology affirms the value of this guideline. *Circulation*. 2006;113:e409–49.

48. Salomaa V, Stinson V, Kark J, Folsom A, Davis C, Wu K. Association of fibrinolytic parameters with early atherosclerosis. The ARIC Study. Atherosclerosis Risk in Communities Study. *Circulation*. 1995;91:284–90.

49. Schober A, Manka D, von Hundelshausen P, et al. Deposition of platelet RANTES triggering monocyte recruitment requires P-selectin and is involved in neointima formation after arterial injury. *Circulation*. 2002;106:1523–9.

50. Schoenhagen P, Ziada KM, Kapadia SR, Crowe TD, Nissen SE, Tuzcu EM. Extent and direction of arterial remodeling in stable versus unstable coronary syndromes: an intravascular ultrasound study. *Circulation*. 2000;101:598–603.

51. Schwartz SM, Virmani R, Rosenfeld ME. The good smooth muscle cells in atherosclerosis. *Curr Atheroscler Rep*. 2000;2:422–9.

52. Shah PK. Insights into the molecular mechanisms of plaque rupture and thrombosis. *Indian Heart J*. 2005;57:21–30.

53. **Smith SC Jr., Dove JT, Jacobs AK, et al. ACC/AHA guidelines for percutaneous coronary intervention (revision of the 1993 PTCA guidelines)—executive summary: a report of the American College of Cardiology/American Heart Association task force on practice guidelines (committee to revise the 1993 guidelines for percutaneous transluminal coronary angioplasty) endorsed by the Society for Cardiac Angiography and Interventions. *Circulation*. 2001;103: 3019–41.**

54. Staels B, Dallongeville J, Auwerx J, Schoonjans K, Leitersdorf E, Fruchart JC. Mechanism of action of fibrates on lipid and lipoprotein metabolism. *Circulation*. 1998;98:2088–93.

55. Tall AR, Jiang X, Luo Y, Silver D. 1999 George Lyman Duff memorial lecture: lipid transfer proteins, HDL metabolism, and atherogenesis. *Arterioscler Thromb Vasc Biol*. 2000;20:1185–8.

56. Thompson S, Kienast J, Pyke S, Haverkate F, Van De Loo J. Hemostatic factors and the risk of myocardial infarction or sudden death in patients with angina pectoris. *New Engl J Med*. 1995;332:635–41.

57. Verma S, Fedak PW, Weisel RD, et al. Off-pump coronary artery bypass surgery: fundamentals for the clinical cardiologist. *Circulation*. 2004;109:1206–11.

58. von Hundelshausen P, Weber KS, Huo Y, Proudfoot AE, Nelson PJ, Ley K, Weber C. RANTES deposition by platelets triggers monocyte arrest on inflamed and atherosclerotic endothelium. *Circulation*. 2001;103:1772–7.

59. Wolf PA, Abbott RD, Kannel WB. Atrial fibrillation as an independent risk factor for stroke: the Framingham Study. *Stroke*. 1991; 22:983–8.

60. Wright R, Flapan A, Alberti K, Ludlam C, Fox K. Effects of captopril therapy on endogenous fibrinolysis in men with recent, uncomplicated myocardial infarction. *J Am Coll Cardiol*. 1994;24:67–73.

SELECTED REFERENCES FOR FURTHER READING

Libby P, Ridker P. Inflammation and atherothrombosis: from population biology and bench research to clinical practice. *Am Coll Cardio l*2007;48:A33–46.

Sanz J, Moreno PR, Fuster V. The year in atherothrombosis. *J Am Coll Cardiol* 2007;49:1740–1749,.

INTERNET RESOURCES

- American Heart Association: www.americanheart.org
- Centers for Disease Control—Heart Disease: www.cdc.gov/heartdisease/
- Mayo Clinic—Coronary Artery Disease: www.mayoclinic.com/health/coronary-artery-disease/DS00064
- National Heart, Lung, Blood Institute: www.nhlbi.nih.gov/

Pathophysiology and Treatment of Pulmonary Disease

Successful implementation of an exercise program in individuals with pulmonary disease can be a challenging task. The low exercise capacity extending from the type and severity of pulmonary disease affects the ability to perform any type of physical activity, including activities of daily living. Additionally, the severity of the physiologic aberration can be further amplified by physical activity. Dyspnea and fatigue initiate the perpetuating process of anxiety, activity avoidance, and progressive disability.

A basic understanding of disease pathophysiology, particularly in the context of the physiology of exercise, improves the efficacy and success of any exercise program for these patients. The design of the exercise program can be enhanced by recognizing disease features that can be used to individualize the program and optimize the individual exercise response. Through this knowledge base, elements key to the evaluation or assessment of the exercise response become more apparent, providing further direction to modifications that will enhance program design. Acquiring this knowledge base can be a large and complicated task, particularly if the diseases are approached in an individual manner. This task can be simplified by grouping diseases based on physiologic similarities. Four groups of diseases can be defined and named for their primary limitation: obstructive pulmonary disease, restrictive pulmonary disease, pulmonary vasculature disease, and disturbances in ventilatory control. The physiologic pattern associated with each category can be generally applied to all the diseases in the respective category.

This chapter provides an overview of the key pathophysiologic principles important to exercising individuals with chronic pulmonary disease. A categorical approach is used to convey these concepts. The more prevalent diseases are used to exemplify these concepts. Chapter 23 reviews assessment and limitations associated with pulmonary disease.

OBSTRUCTIVE PULMONARY DISEASE

Increased airway resistance is a major physiologic limitation in obstructive pulmonary disease. Generally, a reduced cross-sectional airway diameter attributable to

Asthma: A chronic inflammatory disease of the airways characterized by airflow limitation that is often reversible and usually associated with airway hyperresponsiveness.

Bronchiectasis: A pulmonary disease characterized by irreversible dilation of the distal bronchi, usually arising from acute or chronic bronchial infection.

Chronic bronchitis: A chronic obstructive pulmonary disease that primarily affects the conducting airways.

Emphysema: A chronic obstructive pulmonary disease that primarily involves enlargement of the airspaces.

Interstitial lung diseases (ILD): A group of restrictive pulmonary diseases involving pathology primarily confined to the lung parenchyma.

Obstructive pulmonary disease: A category of diseases of the pulmonary system characterized by airflow limitation that is not fully reversible; also termed *chronic obstructive pulmonary disease.*

Pulmonary hypertension: A category of pulmonary diseases characterized by an elevation of arterial pressure and vascular resistance in the pulmonary circulation.

Restrictive pulmonary disease: A category of pulmonary diseases in which the underlying pathologic process involved with each disease interferes with normal lung expansion.

structural or dynamic changes in the airway accounts for the increase in airway resistance. Structural airway abnormalities are chronic, specified by disease processes, and usually related to disease severity. Dynamic changes are variable and precipitated by acute stimuli, such as physical activity, stress, or acute illness. Clinically, airway resistance can be attributed to both processes, particularly in exercising individuals. Regardless of the causation, the common endpoint for high airway resistance is air trapping and lung hyperinflation (31,83).

CHRONIC OBSTRUCTIVE PULMONARY DISEASE

> **1.2.7-CES: Describe the resting and exercise cardiorespiratory and metabolic responses in those with pulmonary disease.**

> **1.2.15-CES: Recognize the pathologic process that various risk factors contribute for the development of cardiac, pulmonary, and metabolic diseases (e.g., smoking, hypertension, abnormal blood lipid values, obesity, inactivity, sex, genetics, diabetes).**

Chronic obstructive pulmonary disease (COPD) is characterized by progressive airflow limitation that is not fully reversible and associated with an abnormal inflammatory response of the lung to noxious particles or gases (93). It is a leading but underrecognized cause of morbidity and mortality, and a major healthcare cost. The global prevalence increases with age and is more than 10% in those aged 40 years or more (40). It is now the fourth leading cause of death, accounting for 4.8% of all deaths worldwide, and is projected to become the third leading cause of death by 2020 (54). In the European Union in 2000, COPD accounted for 56% (about 38.7 billion Euros) of the total direct costs of respiratory disease (53). In the United States in 2004, the direct costs of COPD were $20.9 billion, and the indirect costs totaled $16.3 billion (1).

The pathologic features of COPD are chronic bronchitis, emphysema, and obstructive bronchiolitis (small airway disease) (3). Chronic bronchitis is the inflammation and eventual scarring of the large airways. It is defined as the presence of cough and sputum production for at least 3 months in each of two consecutive years (3,93). Emphysema, on the other hand, is the permanent enlargement of airspaces distal to the terminal bronchiole accompanied by destruction of alveolar walls. Increased numbers of alveolar macrophages, neutrophils and cytoxic T lymphocytes (predominately CD8+), and the release of multiple inflammatory mediators (such as lipids, chemokines, cytokines, growth factors) are characteristic of emphysema. Proteases with activity against elastin are likely to be responsible for generating emphysema. An inherited deficiency of the most well-known antiprotease, α_1-antitrypsin, is a significant risk factor

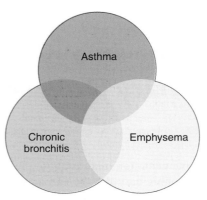

FIGURE 7-1. The interrelationship between asthma, chronic bronchitis, and emphysema depicted as a Venn diagram. (Adapted from Standards for the diagnosis and care of patients with chronic obstructive pulmonary disease. American Thoracic Society. *Am J Respir Crit Care Med.* 1995;152:S77–121.)

for early development of emphysema, although this deficiency explains <3% of all cases (5). From a practical perspective, it is usually difficult to separate chronic bronchitis and emphysema, and these conditions frequently coexist.

The relationship between COPD and asthma has been debated for many years (12,13,99). The classic definition for asthma is airflow limitation that is often reversible and usually associated with airway hyperresponsiveness (37). One perspective considers chronic bronchitis, emphysema, and asthma as mutually exclusive diseases, sometimes manifesting overlapping features (Fig. 7-1). A more recent version of this diagram eloquently presented by Soriano et al. (101) proportionally modified the boundaries based on disease incidence both in the U.S. and U.K. An alternative perspective, which was proposed in 1961 and debated recently (10,49), claims that asthma, chronic bronchitis, and emphysema should not be considered as separate diseases but as different expressions of one disease entity (Fig. 7-2). This perspective, which later became termed the *Dutch hypothesis* (92), seems to be driven by the high degree of variability seen in the manner in which these three diseases manifest clinically. For now, the general consensus is that COPD refers to chronic bronchitis and emphysema alone. Partially reversible airflow obstruction is the primary physiologic abnormality of COPD. The reversible component to the airflow obstruction seen in COPD may sometimes be linked to the coexistence of asthma (3,11).

Treatment and Exercise Considerations

> **1.1.14-CES: Identify normal and abnormal respiratory responses during rest and exercise as assessed during a pulmonary function test (i.e., FVC, MVV, FEV$_{1.0}$, flow volume loop).**

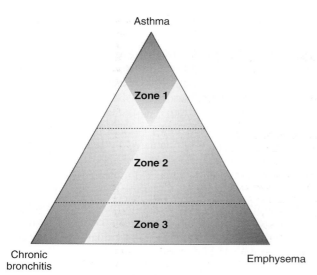

FIGURE 7-2. The Dutch Hypothesis: one disease (i.e., chronic obstructive pulmonary disease [COPD]) with three different manifestations (i.e., asthma, chronic bronchitis, and emphysema). Overlap largely accounts for the variability often seen clinically with COPD, with the extent of variability viewed as a continuum (*graded regions*) extending from the limits of this spectrum (*darkened corners*). The variable manifestations of COPD are also a function of the extent of airflow obstruction (zones 1, 2, and 3 defined as reversible, partially reversible, and irreversible airflow, respectively). (Adapted from Postma DS, Boezen HM. Rationale for the Dutch hypothesis: allergy and airway hyperresponsiveness as genetic factors and their interaction with environment in the development of asthma and COPD. *Chest.* 2004;126:96S–104S.)

> **1.2.7-CES: Describe the resting and exercise cardiorespiratory and metabolic responses in those with pulmonary disease.**

> **1.2.15-CES: Recognize the pathologic process that various risk factors contribute for the development of cardiac, pulmonary, and metabolic diseases (e.g., smoking, hypertension, abnormal blood lipid values, obesity, inactivity, sex, genetics, diabetes).**

> **1.5.3-CES: Recognize medications associated in the clinical setting, their indications for care, and their effects at rest and during exercise (i.e., β-blockers, nitrates, calcium channel blockers, digitalis, diuretics, vasodilators, anitarrhythmic agents, bronchodilators, antilipemics, psychotropics, nicotine, antihistamines, over-the-counter [OTC] cold medications, thyroid medications, alcohol, hypoglycemic agents, blood modifiers, pentoxifylline, antigout medications, and anorexiants/diet pills).**

> **1.10.6-CES: Risk stratify individuals with cardiovascular, pulmonary, and metabolic diseases, using appropriate risk-stratification methods and understanding the prognostic indicators for high-risk individuals.**

> **1.5.1-HFS: Knowledge of common drugs from each of the following classes of medications and describe the principal action and the effects on exercise testing and prescription, including antianginals, antihypertensives, antiarrhythmics, anticoagulants, bronchodilators, hypoglycemics, psychotropics, and vasodilators.**

> **3.2.1-HFS: Knowledge of pulmonary risk factors or conditions that may require consultation with medical personnel before testing or training, including asthma, exercise-induced asthma/bronchospasm, extreme breathlessness at rest or during exercise, bronchitis, and emphysema.**

A variety of factors interact to cause exercise intolerance in patients with COPD (79,84). Such factors include structural and functional changes in ventilatory mechanics, gas exchange abnormalities, peripheral muscle dysfunction, cardiovascular limitations, and intolerable dyspnea and limb discomfort (see also Chapter 23). Obliteration of alveolar walls along with the degradation of alveolar and parenchymal elastin in COPD causes marked reductions in elastic recoil and airway tethering, both of which predispose the airway to premature collapse when intrathoracic pressure is increased during active expiration. The result is incomplete lung emptying, which results in dynamic lung hyperinflation. Dynamic hyperinflation results in a substantial increase in the work of breathing because of mechanical inefficiency of the inspiratory muscles and the increased load presented to the lungs and chest wall at higher thoracic volumes. Increased inward recoil of the chest wall in combination with dynamic airway collapse often results in air trapping, and a significant amount of work may be required to overcome the intrinsic load during inspiration. In severe COPD, the mechanical inefficiency and respiratory muscle load during maximal exercise may lead to hypoventilation. The resultant hypercapnia and hypoxemia lead to decreased systemic oxygen delivery and reduced pH, both of which stimulate ventilatory drive and compromise peripheral skeletal muscle function, contributing to the sensations of dyspnea and limb discomfort.

The severity of COPD influences treatment selection and exercise prescription. Multiple classification schemas have been proposed to describe disease severity. The most recent, known as the GOLD (Global Initiative for Chronic Obstructive Lung Disease) guidelines (93), recommends spirometric classification (Table 7-1). A post-bronchodilator FEV_1/FVC ratio <0.70 indicates airflow limitation that is not fully reversible (93). Using a fixed ratio, however, may result in overdiagnosis of COPD in elderly patients with mild disease because aging affects lung volumes (41). Hence, FEV_1 values should be compared with age-related, postbronchodilator reference values (Table 7-1) (93). This latter recommendation is

TABLE 7-1. GOLD GUIDELINES FOR CHRONIC OBSTRUCTIVE PULMONARY DISEASE DIAGNOSIS AND STAGING

STAGE[a]	PREDICTED FEV$_1$[b]	SYMPTOM	SEVERITY
I	≥80%	± Symptoms	Mild
II	50%–79%	± Symptoms	Moderate
III	30%–49%	± Symptoms	Severe
IV	<30% or <50% with chronic respiratory failure	± Symptoms	Very severe

FEV$_1$, forced expiratory volume in 1 second; FVC, forced vital capacity.

[a]For stages I through IV, the FEV$_1$/FVC ratio needs to be <70%.

[b]FEV$_1$ values are based on postbronchodilator measurements.

Adapted from Rabe KF Hurd S, Anzueto A, et al. Global strategy for the diagnosis, management, and prevention of chronic obstructive pulmonary disease—2006 update. *Am J Respir Crit Care Med.* 2007;175:1222–32.

consistent with American Thoracic Society/European Respiratory Society (ATS/ERS) guidelines (22).

A limitation of spirometric classification is that it does not represent the complex clinical consequences of COPD. Accordingly, the BODE index was developed as a way to assesses the systemic as well as the respiratory manifestations of COPD (21). The BODE index is a multidimensional scale that assigns points based on the results of four measures: nutritional status, measured using the body-mass index (B); airflow obstruction (O), measured as a percentage of the predicted FEV$_1$ (74); dyspnea (D), assessed with the modified Medical Research Council scale (56); and exercise capacity (E), measured as the best of two 6-minute walk tests performed at least 30 minutes apart (2). The variables are graded 0 to 3 (0 or 1 for body mass index) and summed to give a total score between 0 and 10 (Table 7-2). The BODE index is much better at predicting mortality than spirometry data alone (21), with higher scores indicating a greater risk of death. In addition, the BODE index captures the beneficial effects induced by pulmonary rehabilitation (24).

COPD lung damage is irreversible, but a patient's quality of life can be improved with appropriate treatment. Smoking cessation is an important goal to slow the progression of COPD (6). Before starting an exercise program, it is important to maximize pulmonary function

TABLE 7-2. BODE INDEX

VARIABLE	POINTS ON BODE INDEX			
	0	1	2	3
FEV$_1$ (% predicted)	≥65	50–64	36–49	≤35
Distance walked in 6 min (m)	≥350	250–349	150–249	≤149
MMRC dyspnea scale	0–1	2	3	4
BMI	>21	≤21		

BODE, body-mass index, airflow obstruction, dyspnea, and exercise capacity; FEV$_1$, forced expiratory volume in 1 second; MMRC scale, Modified Medical Research Council scale; BMI, body mass index.

Adapted from Celli BR, Cote CG, Marin JM, et al: The body-mass index, airflow obstruction, dyspnea, and exercise capacity index in chronic obstructive pulmonary disease. *N Engl J Med.* 2004;350:1005–12.

by pharmacotherapy (79). The principal bronchodilator treatments are β$_2$-adrenoreceptor agonists (e.g., formoterol, salbutamol/albuterol), anticholinergics (e.g., ipratropium, oxitropium, tiotropium), and methylxanthines (e.g., aminophylline, theophylline) (22,93). All categories of bronchodilators have been shown to increase exercise tolerance in COPD, without necessarily producing significant changes in FEV$_1$. The beneficial effect of bronchodilators may be mediated by reduced airway resistance, increased airflow, and enhanced lung emptying. Such changes would be expected to decrease dynamic hyperinflation, thereby leading to a reduction in dyspnea (19). Combining bronchodilators may improve efficacy and decrease the risk of side effects compared with increasing the dose of a single bronchodilator (95). Regular treatment with long-acting bronchodilators is often more effective and convenient than short-acting bronchodilators (93). Inhaled glucocorticosteroids should be added to the treatment of symptomatic patients with an FEV$_1$ <50% of predicted (i.e., GOLD stage III and IV) and repeated exacerbations (93). Chronic treatment with oral glucocorticosteroids has no proven benefit in COPD and is associated with a high risk of serious adverse side effects (93).

After pharmacotherapy, the need for oxygen therapy should be assessed. Hypoxemia is determined by the diffusion capacity of the lungs, the ability of the lung to match alveolar ventilation to the appropriate metabolic rate, and the ability to direct pulmonary blood flow to those alveoli that are adequately ventilated. As COPD progresses, derangements in all three of these components contribute significantly to the hypoxemia and hypercapnia observed during exercise, and contribute substantially to exercise limitation in this patient population. Long-term oxygen therapy (15 hours or more per day) should be initiated if arterial oxygen tension is <55 mm Hg or oxyhemoglobin saturation is <88% while breathing room air (93). These same guidelines apply when considering supplemental oxygen during exercise (3,79). Interestingly, supplemental oxygen often increases exercise tolerance in nonhypoxemic patients—patients who would not normally meet the criteria for supplemental oxygen (16,28,30,82). The improvement in exercise tolerance with oxygen therapy may be due, in part, to a reduction in ventilatory drive consequent to a reduction in the carotid bodies' responses to hypoxemia and hydrogen ions. This, in turn, allows more time to exhale between breaths and, hence, reduce dynamic hyperinflation, resulting in reduced exertional dyspnea (19). In hypoxemic patients, exercise tolerance may also be improved through an increase in cardiac function or an increase in oxygen delivery to the working muscles (57,84).

ASTHMA

> **1.2.7-CES: Describe the resting and exercise cardiorespiratory and metabolic responses in those with pulmonary disease.**

> **1.2.15-CES: Recognize the pathologic process that various risk factors contribute for the development of cardiac, pulmonary, and metabolic diseases (e.g., smoking, hypertension, abnormal blood lipid values, obesity, inactivity, sex, genetics, diabetes).**

> **1.10.6-CES: Risk stratify individuals with cardiovascular, pulmonary, and metabolic diseases, using appropriate risk-stratification methods and understanding the prognostic indicators for high-risk individuals.**

> **3.2.1-HFS: Knowledge of pulmonary risk factors or conditions that may require consultation with medical personnel before testing or training, including asthma, exercise-induced asthma/bronchospasm, extreme breathlessness at rest or during exercise, bronchitis, and emphysema.**

Asthma is a chronic inflammatory disorder of the airways that is characterized by airway hyperresponsiveness, airflow obstruction that is often reversible, and respiratory symptoms, including recurrent episodes of wheezing, dyspnea, chest tightness, and coughing (37). It affects approximately 300 million people worldwide (63). The global prevalence ranges from 1% to 18% of the population, and its prevalence is increasing, especially among children (63). It is the twenty-fifth leading cause of disability-adjusted life years lost annually, accounting for 1% of the total global disease burden (63). It accounts for about 1 in every 250 deaths worldwide (63). The social and economic consequences are considerable, both in terms of direct medical costs (such as hospital admissions and medication costs) and indirect nonmedical costs (such as time lost from work and premature death) (63).

A consistent feature of asthma is airway inflammation (37). Activation of several inflammatory cells (e.g., mast cells, eosinophils, T lymphocytes, natural killer cells) leads to the release of various chemical mediators (e.g., chemokines, cysteinyl leukotrienes, cytokines, histamine, nitric oxide, prostaglandin D_2), which contribute to the persistence of inflammation (15). Chronic airway inflammation inevitably leads to morphologic changes to both the airway smooth muscle and the respiratory epithelium, often described as airway remodeling (32). Increased deposition of collagen and proteoglycans under the basement membrane and other layers of the airway wall results in fibrosis. Airway smooth muscle increases in mass by hypertrophy and hyperplasia, and bronchial blood vessels increase in size and number (angiogenesis). These structural changes result in thickening of the airway wall that may result in relatively irreversible narrowing of the airways. Mucous gland enlargement and goblet cell differentiation result in mucous hypersecretion, which predisposes the individual to distal airway plugging. This development, in combination with an increased surface tension through disruption of surfactant function, leads to atelectasis (closure of peripheral lung units). Atelectasis results in a reduced functional lung volume and hypoxia through a mismatch between ventilation and perfusion.

Risk factors that trigger airway inflammation are important to recognize and avoid if possible (37). Allergens (such as house dust mites, furred animals, cockroaches, pollens, fungi, molds, and yeasts) increase the risk of airway inflammation. Occupational asthma has been associated with more than 300 substances, including plastic resin, wood dust, certain metals, and plant-animal biologic products. Latex sensitivity is increasingly prevalent in healthcare workers and must be taken into consideration in the rehabilitation environment. Outdoor air pollutants (such as particulates, tobacco smoke, sulphur dioxide, nitrogen oxide, and ozone) and indoor air pollutants (such as carbon monoxide, nitric oxide, and nitrogen dioxide) are known to trigger airway inflammation. Drugs (such as aspirin and β-blockers) are also common risk factors in susceptible individuals. Exercise is a cause of bronchoconstriction in approximately 90% of people with asthma, and for some it is the only cause. Water loss and cooling of the airways by increased ventilation during exercise are likely involved in the pathogenesis of exercise-induced bronchoconstriction (36).

Traditionally, asthma severity has been classified into four categories: intermittent, mild persistent, moderate persistent, or severe persistent (Box 7-1). Although this classification schema may be useful at the initial assessment of an individual, it cannot guide treatment decisions or predict an individual's response to treatment. For these reasons, the most recent guidelines by the World Health Organization (WHO)'s Global Initiative for Asthma (GINA) (37) recommend a classification system by level of control: controlled, partly controlled, uncontrolled, or exacerbation. This system is based on clinical features of asthma, including daytime and nocturnal symptoms, functional limitations, reliever treatment, lung function abnormalities, and exacerbations (Table 7-3). An individual's level of asthma control can be used to guide treatment selection.

Treatment and Exercise Considerations

> **1.1.14-CES: Identify normal and abnormal respiratory responses during rest and exercise as assessed during a pulmonary function test (i.e., FVC, MVV, $FEV_{1.0}$, flow volume loop).**

> **1.2.7-CES: Describe the resting and exercise cardiorespiratory and metabolic responses in those with pulmonary disease.**

> **1.2.15-CES: Recognize the pathologic process that various risk factors contribute for the development of cardiac, pulmonary, and metabolic diseases (e.g., smoking, hypertension, abnormal blood lipid values, obesity, inactivity, sex, genetics, diabetes).**

BOX 7-1   CLASSIFICATION OF ASTHMA SEVERITY BY CLINICAL FEATURES BEFORE TREATMENT

INTERMITTENT

Symptoms <1 per week

Brief exacerbations

Nocturnal symptoms ≤2 per month

    FEV_1 or PEF ≥80% predicted

    PEF or FEV_1 variability <20%

MILD PERSISTENT

Symptoms >1 per week but <1 per day

Exacerbations may affect activity and sleep

Nocturnal symptoms >2 per month

    FEV_1 or PEF 60%–80% predicted

    PEF or FEV_1 variability <20%–30%

MODERATE PERSISTENT

Symptoms daily

Exacerbations may affect activity and sleep

Nocturnal symptoms >1 per week

Daily use of inhaled short-acting β_2-agonist

    FEV_1 or PEF 60%–80% predicted

    PEF or FEV_1 variability >30%

SEVERE PERSISTENT

Symptoms daily

Frequent exacerbations

Frequent nocturnal asthma symptoms

Limitation of physical activities

    FEV_1 or PEF ≤60% predicted

    PEF or FEV_1 variability >30%

Adapted from Global Initiative for Asthma (GINA). *Global Strategy for Asthma Management and Prevention.* 2006 (37); PEF = peak expiratory flow

> **1.3.33-CES: Recognition of the value of heart and lung sounds in the assessment of patients with cardiovascular and/or pulmonary disease.**

> **1.5.3-CES: Recognize medications associated in the clinical setting, their indications for care, and their effects at rest and during exercise (i.e., β-blockers, nitrates, calcium channel blockers, digitalis, diuretics, vasodilators, anitarrhythmic agents, bronchodilators, antilipemics, psychotropics, nicotine, antihistamines, over-the-counter (OTC) cold medications, thyroid medications, alcohol, hypoglycemic agents, blood modifiers, pentoxifylline, antigout medications, and anorexiants/ diet pills).**

> **1.5.1-HFS: Knowledge of common drugs from each of the following classes of medications and describe the principal action and the effects on exercise testing and prescription, including antianginals, antihypertensives, antiarrhythmics, anticoagulants, bronchodilators, hypoglycemics, psychotropics, and vasodilators.**

A correct diagnosis of asthma is important if appropriate treatment is to be given. A diagnosis is often made by using a combination of an individual's medical history, symptoms, and pulmonary function. An increase in FEV_1 of at least 12% (or 200 mL) 15 minutes after inhalation of a short-acting β_2-agonist indicates reversible airflow limitation consistent with asthma (37,91). In addition,

TABLE 7-3. LEVELS OF ASTHMA CONTROL

CHARACTERISTIC	CONTROLLED (ALL OF THE FOLLOWING)	PARTLY CONTROLLED (ANY MEASURE PRESENT IN ANY WEEK)	UNCONTROLLED
Daytime symptoms	None (≤2 per week)	≥2 per week	
Limitations of activities	None	Any	Three or more features of partly controlled asthma present in any week
Nocturnal symptoms/awakening	None	Any	
Need for reliever/rescue treatment	None (≤2 per week)	≥2 per week	
Lung function (PEF or FEV_1)	Normal	<80% predicted or personal best (if known)	
Exacerbations	None	≥1 per year	One in any week

PEF, peak expiratory flow; FEV_1, forced expiratory volume in 1 second.

Adapted from Global Initiative for Asthma (GINA). *Global Strategy for Asthma Management and Prevention.* 2006.

asthma is suspected if peak expiratory flow (PEF) increases by at least 20% (or 60 L·min^{-1}) after inhalation of a bronchodilator or there is day-to-day variation in PEF of at least 20% (or 10% with twice daily readings) (37). In individuals with symptoms consistent with asthma, but with normal lung function, measurements of airway responsiveness to methacholine, histamine, mannitol, or exercise may help establish a diagnosis of asthma (23). The test results are usually expressed as a dose of the agonist that gives rise to a specific (often 20%) reduction in FEV$_1$. Noninvasive markers of airway inflammation, such as hypertonic saline-induced sputum for eosinophilic or neutrophilic inflammation, may be useful. Exhaled nitric oxide has been suggested as a noninvasive marker of airway inflammation, but this measure is nonspecific for asthma. Skin tests with allergens or measurement of specific IgE in serum may be used to detect the presence of allergies and can increase the diagnosis of asthma and help to identify risk factors that cause asthma symptoms.

Exercise-induced bronchoconstriction should be suspected in individuals with symptoms of wheezing, dyspnea, or cough after exercise. A firm diagnosis of exercise-induced bronchoconstriction is based on a decline in FEV$_1$ from baseline of at least 10% within 30 minutes after exercise (25,88). Running for 6 to 8 minutes at an intensity >80% of predicted maximum heart rate is usually recommended, but rapid incremental protocols (8–12 min) can also be diagnostic (25,88). Inhalation of dry cold air during exercise markedly increases the test's sensitivity while maintaining a high degree of specificity (25,88).

Differential diagnoses of asthma require some consideration. Cough-variant asthma is a condition in which cough is the predominant or sole symptom (26). Postviral hyperreactive airways syndrome has an asthmalike presentation that occurs after a viral illness. *Cardiac asthma* refers to the wheezing associated with congestive heart failure. It is caused by airway compression that is a consequence of pulmonary edema, causing signs and symptoms that mimic asthma.

Gastroesophageal reflux disease (GERD)—that is, the backflow of stomach contents into the esophagus—is a common cause of cough and is nearly three times as prevalent in patients with asthma compared with the general population (44). Acid in the distal esophagus can, via a vagally mediated reflex, provoke bronchoconstriction and airway hypersensitivity. It is diagnosed by symptom disappearance with antireflux treatment, which involves dietary and lifestyle changes, acid suppression therapy (H$_2$-receptor antagonist or proton pump inhibitor), and prokinetic therapy. Exercise can potentially induce gastroesophageal reflux in susceptible individuals through increases in intra-abdominal pressure and intrathoracic pressure. Rigorous exercise does not need to be avoided in individuals manifesting GERD, but measures should be implemented to minimize the severity of reflux. Nonpharmacologic interventions include maintaining head elevation at a minimum of 30 degrees while exercising and avoiding stomach overdistention with food or fluids before exercise.

A common differential diagnosis or coexisting factor to asthma is vocal cord dysfunction (VCD). VCD is characterized by abnormal adduction of the vocal cords, usually during inspiration, resulting in variable airway obstruction and symptoms mimicking asthma. VCD may arise from an alteration in the autonomic balance between the glottis and central control areas, with potential aggravation from direct laryngeal insult, laryngeal hyperresponsiveness, and psychological factors (7). Many people with VCD are wrongly diagnosed with asthma and suffer morbidity from unnecessary treatment, such as high-dose glucocorticosteroid and bronchodilator use. The true population figures for exercise-induced VCD are unclear, but the estimated incidence in people with refractory asthma may be as much as 30%, with VCD the single cause of dyspnea in about one third and coexisting asthma in two thirds of these individuals (78). It is typically a condition of younger women, and rhinosinus conditions and GERD are often associated with this entity. The current gold standard for diagnosis rests with visualization of the vocal cords by laryngoscopy while the patient is symptomatic. Laryngoscopy is not practical, however, when VCD occurs only during exercise. Spirometry may be useful in about one fifth of asymptomatic patients, with flattening/truncation of the inspiratory limb (i.e., ratio of expiratory to inspiratory flows at 50% of FVC <1.0) confirming the presence of a variable extrathoracic obstruction (91). Exercise-induced VCD is often accompanied by inspiratory stridor over the larynx and inspiratory flow oscillations ("sawtooth" pattern) during the exercise (43). This contrasts with exercise-induced asthma, in which wheezing is heard over the thorax and airflow obstruction usually occurs after exercise and during expiration. Treatment of VCD typically involves speech therapy, breathing techniques, pharmacologic management of associated factors (asthma, rhinosinus conditions, and GERD), and psychological counseling.

Interruption of the inflammatory pathways is pivotal to asthma treatment (37). Inflammatory control is achieved primarily through inhaled glucocorticosteroids, although uncontrolled asthma may also require extra controller options, such as a long-acting β$_2$-agonist (formoterol, salmeterol), a leukotriene modifier (montelukast, pranlukast, zafirlukast, zileuton), or sustained release theophylline. Inhaled rapid-acting β$_2$-agonists (fenoterol, metaproterenol, pirbuterol, salbutamol/albuterol, terbutaline) are effective reliever treatments that should be used as needed. Alternative reliever treatments include inhaled anticholinergics (ipratropium bromide, oxitropium bromide), short-acting oral β$_2$-agonists, and short-acting theophylline (aminophylline). In individuals with severe allergic asthma who are uncontrolled on glucocorticosteroids, anti-IgE treatment with omalizumab injections has been shown to reduce symptoms, decrease the need for reliever medications, and produce fewer exacerbations (20,37).

Side effects associated with β_2-agonist therapy require some consideration because the cardiovascular side effects—such as tachycardia, palpitations, tachyarrhythmias, tremors, and headache—could potentially compromise exercise responses. Many of the β_2-agonist preparations are not entirely selective for bronchial tissue in that β_1-adrenergic receptors in the heart can also be stimulated (17). Levalbuterol was developed as a selective β_2-agonist, having less direct effect on β_1-receptors in the heart and fewer cardiac side effects. Another consideration is that with prolonged use of short- and long-acting β_2-agonists, there may be a decline in the protection against asthma via desensitization of the β_2 receptor, a phenomenon known as tachyphylaxis (17). To minimize this tolerance effect, β_2-agonists should be used only intermittently, either as a reliever or before exercise (37).

In people with exercise-induced bronchoconstriction, inhalation of a rapid-acting β_2-agonist 15 minutes before exercise provides full protection for 2 to 3 hours (51). Long-acting β_2-agonists have the same effect for 10–12 h, but must be taken at least 30 min before exercise (51). Inhalation of a cromone (disodium cromoglycate or nedocromil) 15 minutes before exercise offers partial protection against exercise-induced bronchoconstriction for 1 to 2 hours, whereas combining these drugs prolongs the protection to 4 hours (51). Similarly, inhaled glucocorticosteroids, methylxanthines, and leukotriene modifiers offer partial protection against exercise-induced bronchoconstriction (51). The World Anti-doping Agency (WADA) prohibits oral/inhaled glucocorticosteroids and β_2-agonists, and if used by athletes in international competition, a therapeutic use exemption is required before participation in the event (www.wada-ama.org/en/). Several nonpharmacologic interventions aimed at reducing the severity of exercise-induced bronchoconstriction have been proposed. A warm-up, which may or may not elicit exercise-induced asthma, can be effective in decreasing the severity and duration of exercise-induced bronchoconstriction triggered by a subsequent exercise bout (69). Incorporating a warm-down after exercise also appears to be beneficial. Dietary modifications, such as antioxidant (105) or fish oil (72) supplementation and salt restriction (73), may also be useful in decreasing the severity of exercise-induced bronchoconstriction. Prophylactic measures that may minimize the deleterious effect of cold environmental conditions on airway function include nasal breathing during low-intensity activities, covering the mouth and nose with a scarf or mask, avoiding exercise during the early morning or evening, and exercising indoors when possible.

BRONCHIECTASIS

> **1.2.7-CES: Describe the resting and exercise cardiorespiratory and metabolic responses in those with pulmonary disease.**

> **1.2.15-CES: Recognize the pathologic process that various risk factors contribute for the development of cardiac, pulmonary, and metabolic diseases (e.g., smoking, hypertension, abnormal blood lipid values, obesity, inactivity, sex, genetics, diabetes).**

> **1.3.33-CES: Recognition of the value of heart and lung sounds in the assessment of patients with cardiovascular and/or pulmonary disease.**

Bronchiectasis is a condition characterized by irreversible airway dilation, usually arising from acute or chronic bronchial infection (9). Airway inflammation and inadequate host defense mechanisms are the dominant features of the disease. The cause of bronchiectasis is unknown in most cases, but genetic disorders, such as cystic fibrosis, are most likely in younger patients, whereas pulmonary tuberculosis, whooping cough, and measles are common causes in developing countries (47). The prevalence and economic burden of bronchiectasis are substantial. Between 1999 and 2001, at least 110,000 patients in the U.S. received treatment at an annual medical-care expenditure of $630 million (108).

The clinical features of bronchiectasis usually include chronic cough that produces purulent sputum with or without blood (hemoptysis), dyspnea, rhinosinusitis, fatigue, and lung crackles that are often bibasal (47). Differentiating between a diagnosis of bronchiectasis and chronic bronchitis can be challenging because both entities are characterized by daily sputum production and dyspnea. Furthermore, many patients with COPD have associated bronchiectasis (90). High-resolution computed tomography (CT) scanning of the chest is the gold standard for diagnosis of bronchiectasis (68). Spirometry usually reveals moderate airflow obstruction, although a restrictive defect may also be noted in patients with advanced disease and extensive parenchymal destruction. Airway hyperresponsiveness to histamine challenge is also a common finding.

Treatment and Exercise Considerations

> **1.5.3-CES: Recognize medications associated in the clinical setting, their indications for care, and their effects at rest and during exercise (i.e., β-blockers, nitrates, calcium channel blockers, digitalis, diuretics, vasodilators, anitarrhythmic agents, bronchodilators, antilipemics, psychotropics, nicotine, antihistamines, over-the-counter (OTC) cold medications, thyroid medications, alcohol, hypoglycemic agents, blood modifiers, pentoxifylline, antigout medications, and anorexiants/diet pills).**

> **1.5.1-HFS: Knowledge of common drugs from each of the following classes of medications and describe the principal action and the effects on exercise testing and prescription, including antianginals, antihypertensives, antiarrhythmics, anticoagulants, bronchodilators, hypoglycemics; psychotropics, and vasodilators.**

The aims of treatment are to inhibit or abolish the underlying host deficiency, relieve bronchoconstriction, control airway inflammation, and improve clearance of secretions. Regular treatment with systemic antibiotics may produce small benefits in reducing sputum volume and purulence, reducing colonizing microbes in sputum, improving exacerbations and symptoms, and reducing airway inflammation (29). In patients with airflow obstruction or hyperresponsiveness, therapy with bronchodilators may be useful (98). Oral glucocorticosteroids may provide some benefit by reducing the volume of sputum and improving lung function, but the evidence is insufficient to justify regular use (48). A reduction in sputum volume has also been found with indomethacin, a nonsteroidal anti-inflammatory drug (104). Mucolytic drugs alter the properties of sputum to make it easier to clear. One such drug, bromhexine, has been shown to reduce sputum production as well as the difficulty associated with sputum clearance (85). Recombinant human deoxyribonuclease (rhDNase) does not provide significant benefit in patients with noncystic fibrosis bronchiectasis, but does assist sputum clearance and improve spirometry in patients with bronchiectasis associated with cystic fibrosis (98). Agents that increase the osmolality of lung mucus, such as dry-powder mannitol and hypertonic saline, have also been shown to improve airway clearance (109).

Chest physiotherapy is often used to enhance airway clearance. A variety of manual and mechanical interventions have been used, including chest wall percussion and vibration, postural and autogenic drainage, mechanically assisted cough, forced expiration ("huffing"), positive expiratory pressure, and airway oscillation. Although such interventions are considered to be mainstays in the treatment of bronchiectasis, they offer only a modest benefit in increasing airway clearance, and the long-term effectiveness of these interventions is unknown (66). Theoretically, chest physiotherapy before exercise may improve exercise quality if mucous plugging impedes the distal lung unit from participation in gas exchange and promotes air trapping. Exercise training *per se* does not appear to increase the clearance of sputum, but may be effective in improving exercise tolerance (77).

NONOBSTRUCTIVE LUNG DISEASES

RESTRICTIVE PULMONARY DISEASE

> **1.1.14-CES: Identify normal and abnormal respiratory responses during rest and exercise as assessed during a pulmonary function test (i.e., FVC, MVV, FEV$_{1.0}$, flow volume loop).**

> **1.2.7-CES: Describe the resting and exercise cardiorespiratory and metabolic responses in those with pulmonary disease.**

> **1.2.15-CES: Recognize the pathologic process that various risk factors contribute for the development of cardiac, pulmonary, and metabolic diseases (e.g., smoking, hypertension, abnormal blood lipid values, obesity, inactivity, sex, genetics, diabetes).**

The **restrictive pulmonary disease** category encompasses many diseases (64). The overall incidence for these diseases is low compared with that for obstructive lung disease. The pathogenesis, pathology, natural history, and treatment are rather variable for the diseases in this group (80). One commonality exists among this variability: abnormal lung mechanics. The pathologic process involved with each disease interferes with the ability for normal lung expansion (80). The mechanisms responsible for the abnormal lung mechanics can be divided into the three groups depicted in Fig. 7-3, and they include diseases that involve the lung parenchyma, pleura, and thoracic cage.

Relative to the restrictive pulmonary disease category, there has been very little investigation into the exercise physiology of this category, particularly as it applies to the **interstitial lung diseases (ILDs)** (42,59–61). Recently, some authors have argued for the usefulness of exercise testing in the evaluation of at least some restrictive pulmonary diseases (62). This argument probably relates to the low incidence of this group of diseases, particularly when evaluating a specific ILD. Because of the different pathophysiologic features, it is probably not accurate to extrapolate observations on exercise response identified in a specific cohort to all of the lung diseases because there are likely to be multiple disease-specific variances.

Few generalities can be made for this category of diseases. Whether anatomic involvement is intraparenchymal or extraparenchymal, the volume of air entering the lung is restricted (64). The extent of restriction is usually proportional to disease severity. To meet criteria using pulmonary function testing (PFT), a reduction in the total lung capacity (TLC) must be evident, with severity defined by the vital capacity (VC) measurement (91). Early disease may show as its only abnormality an isolated reduction in functional residual capacity (FRC) and residual volume (RV). The diffusing capacity is usually low, even with early disease. Investigators have shown that one of the earliest objective pulmonary function measurements for the disease is exercise-induced hypoxemia (42,59–61).

Flow limitation is usually not a problem with these diseases, unless complicating features develop (64). Lung fibrosis leading to traction bronchiectasis or the coexistence of COPD extending from tobacco use illustrates complicating features that can occur. Some restrictive lung diseases are classically characterized by a combination of lung restriction and lung obstruction as part of the pathology (64). The diseases typically associated with both processes include sarcoidosis, hypersensitivity pneumonitis, and eosinophilic granuloma (a disease

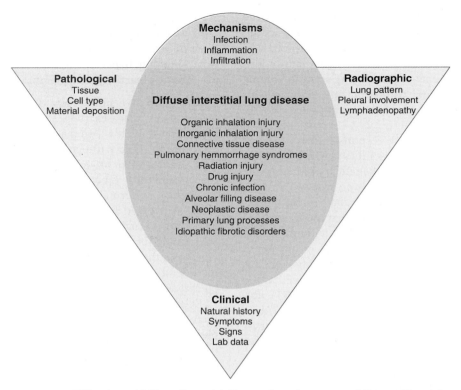

FIGURE 7-3. Diffuse interstitial lung disease (*circle*) comprises a large group of diseases. The etiology for these diseases (*lower circle*) can be linked to three basic mechanisms of injury (*upper circle*). Multiple factors are used to characterize each of these diseases. These factors can be simplified by grouping into pathologic, radiographic, and clinical differences (*corners of triangle*). This diagram is used to illustrate the complexity of features to consider when diagnosing diseases within this category and the high degree of overlap seen in the characteristics that describe each disease. (Adapted from Nield M, Arora A, Dracup K, et al. Comparison of breathing patterns during exercise in patients with obstructive and restrictive ventilatory abnormalities. *J Rehabil Res Dev.* 2003;40:407–14.)

within the spectrum of histiocytosis X, which involves a proliferation of the Langerhans histiocytes) (64).

The exercise-induced hypoxemia primarily extends from mismatch between ventilation and perfusion (42, 59–62). This ventilation-perfusion mismatch occurs because of an increase in dead-space ventilation. Increased dead-space ventilation extends from a disproportionate rise in the ventilatory rate during exercise, leading to rapid shallow breathing. Respiratory rates will often exceed 50 breaths per minute. The work limitation usually extends from a low breathing reserve. A reduced capillary bed surface area accentuates the dead-space ventilation. This surface area reduction can occur either in the form of pathologic disruption of the capillary bed (seen with ILD) or impairment in capillary bed recruitment through the secondary development of **pulmonary hypertension** (potentially seen with all of the restrictive pulmonary diseases). Even though the diffusing capacity is abnormal, hypoxemia does not usually result from a diffusion defect because of the high oxygen diffusion rates. Only with a high level of exercise or with alveolar proteinosis can a diffusion defect account for the hypoxia.

Relative to the obstructive pulmonary disease category, there has been very little investigation of exercise rehabilitation effects in restrictive pulmonary disease. This phe-

nomenon is largely attributed to the low incidence for all restrictive pulmonary diseases, particularly when comparing them with obstructive pulmonary diseases. Furthermore, it is probably not entirely accurate to extrapolate physiologic responses to exercise rehabilitation observed in one restrictive pulmonary disease and apply it to an unrelated restrictive pulmonary disease that has a different pathologic process.

Interstitial Lung Disease

The first group of restrictive pulmonary diseases involves pathology primarily confined to the lung parenchyma (Fig. 7-3) (64). Under normal conditions, the lung interstitium is a potential space that exists between the basement membrane of the alveolar epithelium and capillary epithelium. The matrix or stroma contains collagen and noncollagenous proteins along with a sporadic number of macrophages, fibroblasts, and myofibroblasts. With ILD, the interstitial stroma consists of a higher percentage of protein material, and the cellularity is often increased. Further magnifying the problem, the pathology is often not limited to the interstitium, and there is involvement of the alveoli and terminal bronchi. The lungs become stiff and noncompliant, lending to the

BOX 7-2   DIFFUSE LUNG DISEASES OUTLINED BY PATHOGENESIS

ORGANIC INHALATION INJURY
Farmer's lung

Bird fancier's lung

INORGANIC INHALATION INJURY
Asbestosis

Silicosis

Berylliosis

Talc

CONNECTIVE TISSUE DISEASE
Rheumatoid arthritis

Scleraderma

Sjogren syndrome

Systemic lupus erythematosus

PULMONARY HEMORRHAGE SYNDROMES
Wegener syndrome

Goodpasture disease

Vasculitis

PHYSICAL AGENTS
Radiation

Oxygen

Mechanical ventilation

DRUG INJURY
Methotrexate

Bleomycin

Paraquat

Cocaine

CHRONIC INFECTION
Virus

Fungus

Mycobacterial disease

Parasites

ALVEOLAR FILLING DISEASE
Alveolar proteinosis

Amyloidosis

Microlithiasis

NEOPLASTIC DISEASE
Pulmonary lymphoma

Bronchoalveolar cell carcinoma

Lymphangitic carcinomatosis

PRIMARY LUNG PROCESSES
Sarcoidosis

Eosinophilic granuloma

Amyloidosis

Lymphangioleiomyomatosis

IDIOPATHIC FIBROTIC DISEASES, INCLUDING USUAL INTERSTITIAL PNEUMONITIS
Desquamative interstitial pneumonitis

Fibrosing alveolitis

Bronchiolitis obliterans with organizing pneumonia

Lymphocytic interstitial pneumonia

restrictive physiology and diffusion abnormality often seen with this disease. Different natural histories are encountered for each of the ILDs, influencing disease acuity and severity as well as the exercise potential (Box 7-2).

Multiple classifications have been proposed for the ILDs. Classification schemes, however, are subject to change because the pathogenesis is not clearly understood for many of these diseases, and many questions remain unanswered. This phenomenon is largely responsible for the multiple revisions seen with disease nomenclature. The classification scheme used in this chapter (Fig. 7-3) is structured to enhance clinical practicality. With this approach, the ILDs are grouped into categories based on the most recognized feature causing disease.

Three primary pathologic features are fundamental to this classification schematization. These features include either an infiltrating, inflammatory, or infectious process. Diseases categorized as infiltrating show deposition of a dominant substance within the interstitium, such as amyloid or tumor (64). Cardiogenic pulmonary edema is arbitrarily included as an infiltrating process because water is displaced into the interstitium by hydrostatic forces within the pulmonary vasculature. Diseases categorized as inflammatory include those processes well recognized as having inflammatory mediators propagating the pathogenesis. Noncardiogenic pulmonary edema, or adult respiratory distress syndrome, is arbitrarily assigned to this category because inflammatory mediators are well recognized as the primary mediator of disease. The infectious category includes processes whereby microorganisms are known to be involved (64).

Remember, this categorization scheme is used here to simplify the approach to ILD. Not only does it help with disease organization, but it also has clinical utility by simplifying the differential diagnosis for this large and diverse group of diseases. In actuality, most diseases within this group manifest overlapping characteristics and mechanisms of injury, which lends to the inherent complexity of this disease group.

Treatment and Exercise Considerations

> **1.1.14-CES: Identify normal and abnormal respiratory responses during rest and exercise as assessed during a pulmonary function test (i.e., FVC, MVV, FEV$_{1.0}$, flow volume loop).**

> **1.2.7-CES: Describe the resting and exercise cardiorespiratory and metabolic responses in those with pulmonary disease.**

Mechanical limitations directly result from forces generated by the pathology and usually parallel disease severity (64). Impaired lung expansion translates to a reduced lung volume and lung capacity. The ILDs are characteristically associated with a loss of lung elasticity. PFT criteria for lung restriction require a reduced TLC, with a normal ratio of FEV$_1$ to VC (91). Early disease may only show abnormality after exhalation, including an isolated reduction in the functional residual capacity and residual volume measurements (FRC, RV) (64).

The diffusion capacity measured during the PFT is usually low with restrictive disease (64). This abnormality reflects impaired gas diffusion through the alveolar and capillary interface. This diffusion abnormality usually does not translate into clinically significant hypoxemia because there is adequate pulmonary capillary transit time to allow complete diffusion equilibrium of the oxygen molecules. The one exception to this rule is exercise (64). Hypoxemia extending directly from an impaired diffusion rate can be seen when individuals with ILD exercise (42,59–62).

The restrictive pulmonary diseases extrinsic to the lung parenchyma can be viewed either as an intrapleural or extrapleural process (64). Intrapleural processes can be viewed by physical properties creating the abnormal pleural characteristics. Pneumothorax occurs when there is a collection of air within the pleural space. When liquid accumulates within the pleural space, it is referred to as a *pleural effusion*. There are many causes of pleural effusions, including renal disease, heart failure, pneumonia, and malignancy. Infiltration of a solid substance into the pleural space occurs with certain fibrotic processes and malignancy. The last group of restrictive pulmonary diseases includes extrapleural pleural processes that affect muscle strength or function of the diaphragm or thoracic cage (64). Any process that results in an increase in the intra-abdominal

pressure will inhibit diaphragmatic function. Exercises performed with a recumbent body position will have the same impact on diaphragmatic excursion. Neuromuscular diseases affect the ventilatory muscle strength. Thoracic deformities and poor posture interfere with the proper function of thoracic cage to operate as a bellows (64).

Physiologic responses to exercise extend directly from the impaired lung inhalation (42,59–62,80). Ventilatory rate increases to compensate for the low lung volume. The rate can exceed 50 breaths per minute, frequently approaching the ventilatory threshold or maximum voluntary ventilation (MVV) for that individual. MVV is determined by the lung disease severity, regardless of the disease category. The result is reduced work efficiency and reduced exercise endurance (80).

Pulmonary vascular abnormalities are often found with restrictive pulmonary disease (64). These vascular abnormalities are usually associated with advanced lung disease. Pulmonary hypertension can result from either vascular bed destruction, seen with many fibrotic lung processes, or from a high pulmonary vascular tone, which can occur with chronic hypoxic states. Exercise limitations associated with pulmonary hypertension are discussed in the next section of this chapter.

Airflow limitation is not usually routinely encountered in restrictive lung disease (64). By contrast, increased lung elastic recoil can enhance expiratory flow. The exception to this rule is the development of traction bronchiectasis with advanced pulmonary fibrosis. Forces generated by the fibrotic process create a tethering effect on the adjacent bronchi, distorting their conformation. As with primary bronchiectasis, mucociliary clearance is affected, creating a secondary obstructive component. Sometimes the primary pathologic process is characterized by both lung restriction and lung obstruction. Diseases in this group include sarcoidosis, hypersensitivity pneumonitis, and eosinophilic granuloma. Because of the frequency of COPD with tobacco inhalation, individuals who smoke and develop a restrictive lung process often have COPD as a comorbid problem.

DISORDERS IN THE PULMONARY VASCULATURE

> **1.2.7-CES: Describe the resting and exercise cardiorespiratory and metabolic responses in those with pulmonary disease.**

> **1.2.15-CES: Recognize the pathologic process that various risk factors contribute for the development of cardiac, pulmonary, and metabolic diseases (e.g., smoking, hypertension, abnormal blood lipid values, obesity, inactivity, sex, genetics, diabetes).**

> **1.10.6-CES: Risk stratify individuals with cardiovascular, pulmonary, and metabolic diseases, using appropriate risk-stratification methods and understanding the prognostic indicators for high-risk individuals.**

BOX 7-3   WHO CLASSIFICATION OF THE CAUSE OF PULMONARY HYPERTENSION

Pulmonary arterial hypertension

Pulmonary venous hypertension

Extending from respiratory disease/hypoxia

Extending from thromboembolic disease

Extending from disease directly affecting pulmonary vasculature

Adapted from Galie N, Torbicki A, Barst R, et al. Guidelines on diagnosis and treatment of pulmonary arterial hypertension. *Eur Heart J.* 2004;25:2243–78.

The healthy pulmonary vasculature is a low-pressure system with a low resistance to flow. Pulmonary hypertension is a rare condition characterized by an elevation of the arterial pressure and vascular resistance in the pulmonary circulation, eventually resulting in right-heart failure (70). Pulmonary hypertension has a multifactorial pathophysiology, with vasoconstriction, vascular remodeling, and thrombosis all contributing to the increased pulmonary vascular resistance. Pulmonary arterial hypertension (PAH) is distinguished from other forms of pulmonary hypertension that can occur as a consequence of left-heart disease, pulmonary diseases/hypoxia (such as COPD, interstitial lung disease, hypoventilation disorders, or residence at high altitude), thromboembolic disease, or disorders directly affecting the pulmonary vasculature (such as sarcoidosis) (Box 7-3). PAH is classified into subgroups (33). Idiopathic PAH—that is, PAH with no obvious cause—is a rare condition affecting about 2 to 5 per million per year. Familial PAH involves genetic transmission of PAH and accounts for <10% of patients with PAH. Associated PAH is pulmonary hypertension associated with various risk factors or conditions, including connective tissue diseases (such as scleroderma or lupus erythematosus), congenital heart disease, portal hypertension, HIV infection, and drugs/toxins (such as appetite suppressants, cocaine, or amphetamines). Other subgroups include PAH associated with significant venous or capillary involvement and persistent pulmonary hypertension of the newborn.

A firm diagnosis of PAH requires the placement of a right-heart catheter. Using this approach, PAH is defined as a mean pulmonary artery pressure >25 mm Hg at rest or at least 30 mm Hg during exercise, with a mean pulmonary capillary wedge pressure and left ventricular end diastolic pressure of <15 mm Hg (33,67). Severity of pulmonary hypertension is determined using the WHO functional classification, which is an adaptation of the New York Heart Association (NYHA) classification for congestive heart failure (Box 7-4). Establishment of the correct diagnosis and the specific classification can influence the treatment a patient receives (8,33,67).

Treatment and Exercise Considerations

> **1.2.7-CES: Describe the resting and exercise cardiorespiratory and metabolic responses in those with pulmonary disease.**

> **1.5.3-CES: Recognize medications associated in the clinical setting, their indications for care, and their effects at rest and during exercise (i.e., β-blockers, nitrates, calcium channel blockers, digitalis, diuretics, vasodilators, anitarrhythmic agents, bronchodilators, antilipemics, psychotropics, nicotine, antihistamines, over-the-counter (OTC) cold medications, thyroid medications, alcohol, hypoglycemic agents, blood modifiers, pentoxifylline, antigout medications, and anorexiants/diet pills).**

> **1.2.2-HFS: Knowledge of the cardiovascular, pulmonary, metabolic, and musculoskeletal risk factors that may require further evaluation by medical or allied health professionals before participation in physical activity.**

> **1.5.1-HFS: Knowledge of common drugs from each of the following classes of medications and describe the principal action and the effects on exercise testing and prescription, including antianginals, antihypertensives, antiarrhythmics, anticoagulants, bronchodilators, hypoglycemics, psychotropics, and vasodilators.**

BOX 7-4   WHO CLASSIFICATION OF THE SEVERITY OF ILLNESS FOR PULMONARY HYPERTENSION

Class I	Asymptomatic, no physical limitations
Class II	Mild limitations with physical activity
Class III	Marked limitation with physical activity
	No discomfort at rest
Class IV	Unable to perform any physical activity
	Symptomatic at rest
	Right-heart failure

Adapted from Galie N, Torbicki A, Barst R, et al. Guidelines on diagnosis and treatment of pulmonary arterial hypertension. *Eur Heart J.* 2004;25:2243–78.

Dyspnea, especially when exercising, is the primary symptom of pulmonary hypertension (102). Other symptoms that can develop as the condition gets worse include fatigue, angina, syncope, edema, tachycardia, palpitations, and cough. Dyspnea can be attributed to an increased ventilatory response to exercise, resulting from mismatch between ventilation and perfusion that leads to an elevated ratio of dead-space volume to tidal volume. A second mechanism for the increased ventilatory response to exercise is increased hydrogen ion and carbon dioxide production resulting from early lactic acidosis. A third mechanism is arterial hypoxemia owing to a reduced functional capillary bed and an abnormally rapid transit time of red blood cells through the pulmonary capillary bed, shortening the time available for diffusion equilibration. Another important cause of arterial hypoxemia is right-to-left shunt through a patent foramen ovale (103), which is a congenital communication between the right and left aorta. In patients with a patent foramen ovale and abnormally high pulmonary vascular resistance, exercise-induced increases in venous return cause right atrial pressure to rise. When right atrial exceeds left atrial pressure, venous return can flow from the right to the left atrium, diverting deoxygenated, acidemic, and carbon-dioxide–rich blood to the systemic arterial circulation. This stimulates arterial chemoreceptors so that ventilation is increased in proportion to the shunted hydrogen ion and carbon dioxide load. Fatigue associated with pulmonary hypertension may also limit exercise tolerance. The fatigue may be attributed to blunted cardiac output during exercise because pulmonary vasoconstriction reduces the delivery of blood to the left atrium. In addition, the reduction in oxygen delivery consequent to arterial hypoxemia results in an increased rate of anaerobic glycolysis, early lactic acidosis, and impaired contractility of working muscles.

Treatments for pulmonary hypertension include supportive therapy (chronic oxygen supplementation, anticoagulants, and diuretics) and a combination of disease-targeted therapies (calcium-channel blockers, prostaglandins, endothelin-receptor antagonists, and phosphodiesterase type 5 inhibitors) (8,33,70). Such treatments have been shown to improve symptoms, exercise tolerance, quality of life, and possibly survival (8,33,70). Surgical treatments for severely ill patients include the creation of a right-to-left interatrial shunt (atrial septostomy), removal of clot formation from the pulmonary arteries (thromboendarterectomy), and lung/heart-transplantation (27,33,70). Exercise in patients with pulmonary hypertension is controversial (8). Theoretically, an increase in cardiac output resulting in elevation of pulmonary arterial pressure and pulmonary vascular resistance may predispose to right ventricular decompensation and circulatory collapse. Results from a 2006 study, however, suggest that closely monitored aerobic exercise training is safe and can improve exercise capacity, peak oxygen consumption, quality of life, and functional status in patients with severe pulmonary hypertension (71). Blood pressure and heart rate should be monitored closely throughout exercise and the exercise stopped if the patient develops chest pain, lightheadedness, or palpitations (79). Resistance training should be avoided because of the increased risk of syncope and circulatory collapse with elevated intrathoracic pressure (79).

DISTURBANCES IN VENTILATORY CONTROL

HYPERVENTILATION DISORDERS

> **1.1.11-HFS: Knowledge of the following cardiorespiratory terms: ischemia, angina pectoris, tachycardia, bradycardia, arrhythmia, myocardial infarction, claudication, dyspnea, and hyperventilation.**

> **1.2.7-CES: Describe the resting and exercise cardiorespiratory and metabolic responses in those with pulmonary disease.**

> **1.2.15-CES: Recognize the pathologic process that various risk factors contribute for the development of cardiac, pulmonary, and metabolic diseases (e.g., smoking, hypertension, abnormal blood lipid values, obesity, inactivity, sex, genetics, diabetes).**

Hyperventilation, characterized as a reduced partial pressure of carbon dioxide in arterial blood (hypocapnia), is the result of alveolar ventilation that is excessive in relation to metabolically produced carbon dioxide. To compensate for the metabolic acidosis and minimize the fall in arterial blood and central chemoreceptor pH that would otherwise occur, ventilation is increased until the partial pressure of arterial carbon dioxide is reduced to a new lower set point. Examples of metabolically induced hyperventilation include excessive ingestion of acid (ethanol, methanol, aspirin), poorly controlled diabetes mellitus (diabetic ketoacidosis), hypoglycemia, chronic renal failure, renal tubular acidosis, or the result of use of carbonic anhydrase inhibitor drugs (acetazolamide). The consequence of metabolic acidosis before exercise is a marked elevation in the ventilatory requirement to perform a given work rate. Consequently, the sensation of dyspnea is high, and, in patients with other pulmonary diseases, ventilation may encroach on the breathing reserve, resulting in premature curtailment of exercise (100).

Chronic "idiopathic" hyperventilation is defined as sustained hypocapnia at rest and during exercise with no other apparent pathologies (34,45,46). The etiology of idiopathic hyperventilation is controversial (34). Behavioral factors, such as stress and anxiety, are often assumed to be involved, but these factors may be absent or secondary to hyperventilation. Psychosomatic disorders have also been implicated because many such individuals have a high incidence of depression and phobias. An increase in progesterone during the luteal phase of the menstrual cycle, and particularly during pregnancy, results in hyperventilation through the combined effect of progesterone and estrogen on the central and peripheral chemoreceptors. This effect of sex hormones on ventilation may explain why the incidence of idiopathic hyperventilation is higher in women. Regardless of etiology, many individuals with idiopathic hyperventilation are compromised in activities of daily living and quality of life because of symptoms such as chest pain, dyspnea, lightheadedness, and paresthesia.

HYPOVENTILATION DISORDERS

> **1.2.7-CES: Describe the resting and exercise cardiorespiratory and metabolic responses in those with pulmonary disease.**

> **1.2.15-CES: Recognize the pathologic process that various risk factors contribute for the development of cardiac, pulmonary, and metabolic diseases (e.g., smoking, hypertension, abnormal blood lipid values, obesity, inactivity, sex, genetics, diabetes).**

Hypoventilation is characterized by an elevated partial pressure of carbon dioxide in arterial blood (hypercapnia). It overlaps with other pulmonary disease categories, particularly when the disease is severe. For example, severe COPD may elicit hypoventilation because of decreased responsiveness to hypoxia and hypercapnia, increased ventilation-perfusion mismatch leading to increased dead-space ventilation, and abnormal respiratory muscle function owing to fatigue and muscular disadvantage from hyperinflation. Patients with hypoventilation can develop clinically significant hypoxemia, which aggravates the clinical manifestations of hypoventilation. Two hypoventilation disorders—obesity hypoventilation syndrome and obstructive sleep apnea-hypopnea syndrome—require consideration.

Obesity hypoventilation syndrome is defined as obesity (body mass index >30 kg$\cdot$m^{-2}) in combination with awake hypercapnia (arterial partial pressure of carbon dioxide >45 mm Hg) without any other known causes of hypoventilation (86). Historically, the disorder was referred to as Pickwickian syndrome. The mechanisms responsible for obesity hypoventilation syndrome are not clearly defined, but may result from complex relationships between deranged respiratory mechanics, abnormalities in central ventilatory control, sleep-disordered breathing, and neurohormonal impairments. Many individuals with the disorder also have obstructive sleep apnea-hypopnea syndrome, which is the frequent complete (apnea) or partial (hypopnea) cessation of airflow during sleep resulting in hypercapnia and arterial hypoxemia (86). Obstructive sleep apnea-hypopnea syndrome occurs as a result of upper-airway collapse that is often associated with excess fat. The symptoms of both disorders include extreme daytime drowsiness (hypersomnolence), fatigue, mood disorders, and nocturnal or morning headaches. Left untreated, individuals may be at increased risk of pulmonary hypertension, right ventricular hypertrophy (cor pulmonale), cardiac ischemia, arrhythmias, and stroke.

Treatment and Exercise Considerations

Patients with hypoventilation disorders can be treated successfully using noninvasive positive-pressure ventilation via a nasal mask (86). Bilevel intermittent positive airway pressure (BiPAP) is used to treat obesity hypoventilation syndrome, whereas nocturnal continuous positive airway pressure (CPAP) is used to treat obstructive sleep apnea-hypopnea syndrome. Such interventions are effective means of maintaining upper airway patency, eliminating apneas and hypopneas, correcting daytime hypercapnia, and alleviating symptoms. Weight loss and exercise are also effective treatments for reversing the respiratory complications of obesity (86,89). Multiple factors associated with obesity may have considerable impact on exercise (89). Obese individuals require extra energy to move heavy legs during cycling or a large body mass while walking. The extra O_2 needed to perform external work results in a greater than normal cardiopulmonary response. The added mass on the chest wall and the increased pressure in the abdomen increases the load on the inspiratory muscles. The increased abdominal pressure may impair diaphragmatic excursion during inspiration, reducing the vital capacity. Expiratory reserve volume (ERV) is reduced in obese individuals because of a decrease in FRC. The reductions in ERV and FRC can result in atelectasis and hypoxemia at rest. Arterial oxygenation usually improves during exercise because lung inflations re-expand the atelectic lung units. The respiratory complications that are associated with obesity are accentuated in the supine position. Therefore, exercise in a recumbent position should be minimized in these individuals.

PULMONARY REHABILITATION

Pulmonary rehabilitation is defined as an evidence-based, multidisciplinary, and comprehensive intervention for patients with chronic respiratory disease who are symptomatic and often have decreased daily life activities (79). The components of pulmonary rehabilitation are outlined in Box 7-5 and should be prescribed depending on the individual needs of the patient.

The goal of pulmonary rehabilitation is not to improve lung function, but rather to reverse the systemic consequences of the disease (79,106). For example, peripheral muscle weakness is common in patients with chronic pulmonary disease and, at the level of the muscle, this weakness is associated with reduced capillarization, a shift from type I to type IIa fibers, reduced oxidative

BOX 7-5   COMPONENTS OF PULMONARY REHABILITATION PROGRAM

PATIENT ASSESSMENT

Pulmonary function

Symptoms (dyspnea and fatigue)

Activity levels

Exercise capacity

Weight and body composition

Respiratory and limb muscle function

Quality of life

EXERCISE TRAINING

Endurance and strength training of lower and upper extremities

Flexibility and balance training

Respiratory muscle training

NUTRITIONAL INTERVENTION

Calorie supplementation

Fat loss through exercise

EDUCATION AND SELF-MANAGEMENT

Knowledge of disease

Breathing techniques

Energy conservation and pacing techniques

Secretion clearance techniques

Prevention of exacerbations

Treatment (medication, oxygen, and surgery)

Bronchial hygiene

Irritant avoidance

Leisure, travel, and sexuality

End-of-life planning

PHARMACOLOGIC INTERVENTION (ANABOLIC STEROIDS, GROWTH HORMONE)

Psychosocial support

Smoking cessation

Stress management

Relaxation training

Patient and family support groups

Adapted from Nici L, Donner C, Wouters E, et al. American Thoracic Society/European Respiratory Society statement on pulmonary rehabilitation. *Am J Respir Crit Care Med.* 2006;173:1390–413.

enzyme activities, and increased concentrations of glycolytic enzymes (4). The consequences of such alterations are twofold. First, metabolic acidosis is encountered at low work rates, resulting in an increased drive to breathe and dynamic hyperinflation that increases the work of breathing. Second, the peripheral muscles are more susceptible to fatigue, resulting in task failure and early exercise termination. The exercise training component of pulmonary rehabilitation aims at reversing these systemic consequences (79,106). The benefits resulting from pulmonary rehabilitation are shown in Box 7-6.

Patients with COPD make up the largest proportion of those referred for pulmonary rehabilitation, and most of the research has been conducted in this area. Treatable comorbidities, however, are common to all chronic pulmonary diseases, and treatment strategies have been applied to an increasingly wide range of pulmonary conditions, including asthma (94), bronchiectasis (77), cystic fibrosis (87), restrictive pulmonary disease (75), and pulmonary hypertension (71). Pulmonary rehabilitation has also been successfully used in the preparation and selection of patients for surgical treatments such as lung transplantation and lung volume reduction surgery

BOX 7-6   BENEFITS OF PULMONARY REHABILITATION

Improved quality of life

Improved psychological well-being (cognitive functioning, anxiety, depression, self-esteem)

Improved symptoms (dyspnea)

Increased functional status

Increased participation in everyday activities

Reduced healthcare costs

Adapted from Ries AL, Bauldoff GS, Carlin BW, et al. Pulmonary rehabilitation. Joint ACCP/AACVPR evidence-based clinical practice guidelines. *Chest.* 2007;131:4S–42S.

(97). Furthermore, rehabilitation after surgery is beneficial because the improved lung function after the surgery facilitates exercise at higher intensity.

EXERCISE TRAINING

Exercise training is the cornerstone of pulmonary rehabilitation and, when optimally delivered, produces the greatest improvements in exercise tolerance (79,96,106). The optimal duration of the exercise program has not been clearly defined. Physiologic changes can occur within just a few weeks, but longer training programs produce larger and more sustained effects. Patients should perform at least three supervised sessions per week, although two supervised sessions per week in combination with one or more unsupervised sessions at home may be acceptable. The benefits of exercise training tend to decline gradually over time. Benefits of health status, however, appear better preserved than exercise tolerance and may still be identified up to 2 years after the intervention. The role of maintenance programs after the initial training is uncertain, but evidence to date suggests only a modest effect of such programs on long-term benefits. Guidelines for the general prescription of exercise training are outlined in Chapter 28 and for those with pulmonary disease in Chapter 36.

ADJUNCTIVE THERAPIES

As indicated in previous sections, bronchodilator and oxygen therapy in the acute setting can improve exercise tolerance in patients with airflow limitation. More recent evidence suggests that both strategies can enhance the effects of pulmonary rehabilitation, probably by enabling patients to exercise at higher intensities for longer durations (18,81,96).

Another adjunctive therapy that may benefit selected patients with pulmonary disease is noninvasive positive-pressure ventilation (79,96). Noninvasive ventilation during an acute bout of exercise can reduce dyspnea and increase exercise tolerance, potentially by reducing the load on the respiratory muscles (50,110). More recent evidence suggests that exercise training with noninvasive ventilation in patients with severe disease can improve exercise tolerance through increasing training intensity and duration. An alternative way to reduce the load on the respiratory muscles is to breathe a low-density gas mixture, such as 79% helium, 21% oxygen (heliox). Heliox has been shown to be beneficial in reducing dynamic hyperinflation, relieving symptoms, and improving exercise tolerance in patients with chronic pulmonary disease (30,52,58). In addition, breathing a combined mixture of heliox and hyperoxia has additive effects on improving exercise tolerance (30,52,58).

Respiratory muscle training may enhance the effects of aerobic exercise on overall exercise tolerance, particularly in patients with reduced inspiratory muscle strength (35,55,65). The most commonly used training modalities are flow resistive breathing, pressure threshold loading, and voluntary isocapnic hyperpnea. Each of these modalities can increase respiratory muscle function, reduce dyspnea, and improve exercise tolerance in patients with obstructive pulmonary disease. Additional breathing techniques that may be effective in alleviating symptoms of dyspnea in patients with obstructive pulmonary disease include forward leaning and active expiration against pursed lips (38). Diaphragmatic breathing—that is, the conscious expansion of the abdominal wall during diaphragmatic inspiration—is not recommended because it increases the work of breathing and reduces the mechanical efficiency of breathing (39).

An adjunctive therapy that may be beneficial in patients who are bed bound or suffering from extreme peripheral muscle weakness is neuromuscular electrical stimulation (14,76,107,111). Transcutaneous stimulation of the nerve roots supplying the limb locomotor muscles has been shown to improve muscle strength and endurance, symptoms, and exercise tolerance in patients with moderate-to-severe pulmonary disease. The advantages of the technique are that it is safe, well tolerated, and relatively inexpensive; it can be implemented at home; and it may help to prevent functional decline during exacerbations.

SUMMARY

Exercise in patients with chronic pulmonary disease can be performed regardless of the illness severity. Pulmonary rehabilitation principles should be used as the framework for the exercise prescription, but disease-specific principles should also be incorporated. Disease-specific principles can be easily identified with a basic understanding of lung pathophysiology as it relates to pattern recognition for each of the disease categories. These principles also facilitate identification of the proper therapeutic interventions. Incorporating modifications based on the patient's response to exercise can further individualize the exercise program.

REFERENCES

1. American Lung Association. *Trends in Chronic Bronchitis and Emphysema: Morbidity and Mortality.* 2006.
2. American Thoracic Society. Guidelines for the six-minute walk test. *Am J Respir Crit Care Med.* 2002;166:111–7.
3. American Thoracic Society. Standards for the diagnosis and care of patients with chronic obstructive pulmonary disease. *Am J Respir Crit Care Med.* 1995;152:s77–121.
4. American Thoracic Society/European Respiratory Society. Skeletal muscle dysfunction in chronic obstructive pulmonary disease. *Am J Respir Crit Care Med.* 1999;159:s1–40.
5. American Thoracic Society/European Respiratory Society. Standards for the diagnosis and management of individuals with

alpha-1 antitrypsin deficiency. *Am J Respir Crit Care Med.* 2003;168: 818–900.

6. Anthonisen NR, Connett JE, Kiley JP, et al. Effects of smoking intervention and the use of an inhaled anticholinergic bronchodilator on the rate of decline of FEV1. The lung health study. *JAMA.* 1994; 272:1497–505.

7. Ayres JG, Gabbott PL. Vocal cord dysfunction and laryngeal hyperresponsiveness: a function of altered autonomic balance? *Thorax.* 2002;57:284–5.

8. Badesch DB, Abman SH, Ahearn GS, et al. Medical therapy for pulmonary arterial hypertension: ACCP evidence-based clinical practice guidelines. *Chest.* 2004;126:35s–62s.

9. Barker AF. Bronchiectasis. *N Engl J Med.* 2002;346:1383–93.

10. Barnes PJ. Against the Dutch hypothesis: asthma and chronic obstructive pulmonary disease are distinct diseases. *Am J Respir Crit Care Med.* 2006;174:240–243; discussion 243–4.

11. Barnes PJ. Asthma guidelines: recommendations versus reality. *Respir Med.* 2004;98 suppl A:S1–7.

12. Barnes PJ. Mechanisms in COPD: differences from asthma. *Chest.* 2000;117:10s–4s.

13. Bleecker ER. Similarities and differences in asthma and COPD: the Dutch hypothesis. *Chest.* 2004;126:93s–95s; discussion 159s–61s.

14. Bourjeily-Habr G, Rochester CL, Palermo F, Snyder P, Mohsenin V. Randomised controlled trial of transcutaneous electrical muscle stimulation of the lower extremities in patients with chronic obstructive pulmonary disease. *Thorax.* 2002;57:1045–9.

15. Bousquet J, Jeffery PK, Busse WW, Johnson M, Vignola AM. Asthma: from bronchoconstriction to airways inflammation and remodeling. *Am J Respir Crit Care Med.* 2000;161:1720–45.

16. Bradley JM, O'Neill B. Short-term ambulatory oxygen for chronic obstructive pulmonary disease. *Cochrane Database Syst Rev.* 2005; cd004356.

17. Broadley KJ. Beta-adrenoceptor responses of the airways: for better or worse? *Eur J Pharmacol.* 2006;533:15–27.

18. Casaburi R, Kukafka D, Cooper CB, Witek TJ Jr, Kesten S. Improvement in exercise tolerance with the combination of tiotropium and pulmonary rehabilitation in patients with COPD. *Chest.* 2005;127:809–17.

19. Casaburi R, Porszasz J. Reduction of hyperinflation by pharmacologic and other interventions. *Proc Am Thorac Soc.* 2006; 3:185–9.

20. Cates CJ, Jefferson TO, Bara AI, Rowe BH. Vaccines for preventing influenza in people with asthma. *Cochrane Database Syst Rev.* 2004;cd000364.

21. Celli BR, Cote CG, Marin JM, et al. The body-mass index, airflow obstruction, dyspnea, and exercise capacity index in chronic obstructive pulmonary disease. *N Engl J Med.* 2004;350:1005–12.

22. Celli BR, MacNee W. Standards for the diagnosis and treatment of patients with COPD: a summary of the ATS/ERS position paper. *Eur Respir J.* 2004;23:932–46.

23. Cockcroft DW. Bronchoprovocation methods: direct challenges. *Clin Rev Allergy Immunol.* 2003;24:19–26.

24. Cote CG, Celli BR. Pulmonary rehabilitation and the BODE index in COPD. *Eur Respir J.* 2005;26:630–6.

25. Crapo RO, Casaburi R, Coates AL, et al. Guidelines for methacholine and exercise challenge testing. *Am J Respir Crit Care Med.* 2000;161:309–29.

26. Dicpinigaitis PV. Chronic cough due to asthma: ACCP evidence-based clinical practice guidelines. *Chest.* 2006;129:75s–9s.

27. **Doyle RL, McCrory D, Channick RN, Simonneau G, Conte J. Surgical treatments/interventions for pulmonary arterial hypertension: ACCP evidence-based clinical practice guidelines. *Chest.* 2004; 126:63s–71s.**

28. Emtner M, Porszasz J, Burns M, Somfay A, Casaburi R. Benefits of supplemental oxygen in exercise training in nonhypoxemic chronic obstructive pulmonary disease patients. *Am J Respir Crit Care Med.* 2003;168:1034–42.

29. Evans DJ, Bara AI, Greenstone M. Prolonged antibiotics for purulent bronchiectasis in children and adults. *Cochrane Database Syst Rev.* 2007;cd001392.

30. Eves ND, Petersen SR, Haykowsky MJ, Wong EY, Jones RL. Heliumhyperoxia, exercise, and respiratory mechanics in chronic obstructive pulmonary disease. *Am J Respir Crit Care Med.* 2006;174: 763–71.

31. Ferguson GT. Why does the lung hyperinflate? *Proc Am Thorac Soc.* 2006;3:176–9.

32. Fixman ED, Stewart A, Martin JG. Basic mechanisms of development of airway structural changes in asthma. *Eur Respir J.* 2007;29: 379–89.

33. **Galie N, Torbicki A, Barst R, et al. Guidelines on diagnosis and treatment of pulmonary arterial hypertension. The task force on diagnosis and treatment of pulmonary arterial hypertension of the European Society of Cardiology. *Eur Heart J.* 2004;25:2243–78.**

34. Gardner WN. The pathophysiology of hyperventilation disorders. *Chest.* 1996;109:516–34.

35. Geddes EL, Reid WD, Crowe J, O'Brien K, Brooks D. Inspiratory muscle training in adults with chronic obstructive pulmonary disease: a systematic review. *Respir Med.* 2005;99:1440–58.

36. Gilbert IA, McFadden ER Jr. Airway cooling and rewarming: the second reaction sequence in exercise-induced asthma. *J Clin Invest.* 1992;90:699–704.

37. Global Initiative for Asthma. Global Strategy for Asthma Management and Prevention, 2006. Pp. 1–92. www.ginasthma.com/guidelinelist.asp. Accessed on 10/08/08.

38. Gosselink R. Breathing techniques in patients with chronic obstructive pulmonary disease. *Chronic Respir Dis.* 2004;1:163–72.

39. Gosselink RA, Wagenaar RC, Rijswijk H, Sargeant AJ, Decramer ML. Diaphragmatic breathing reduces efficiency of breathing in patients with chronic obstructive pulmonary disease. *Am J Respir Crit Care Med.* 1995;151:1136–42.

40. Halbert RJ, Natoli JL, Gano A, Badamgarav E, Buist AS, Mannino DM. Global burden of COPD: systematic review and meta-analysis. *Eur Respir J.* 2006;28:523–32.

41. Hardie JA, Buist AS, Vollmer WM, Ellingsen I, Bakke PS, Morkve O. Risk of over-diagnosis of COPD in asymptomatic elderly neversmokers. *Eur Respir J.* 2002;20:1117–22.

42. Harris-Eze AO, Sridhar G, Clemens RE, Zintel TA, Gallagher CG, Marciniuk DD. Role of hypoxemia and pulmonary mechanics in exercise limitation in interstitial lung disease. *Am J Respir Crit Care Med.* 1996;154:994–1001.

43. Haverkamp HC, Miller JD, Rodman J, et al. Extrathoracic obstruction and hypoxemia occurring during exercise in a competitive female cyclist. *Chest.* 2002;124:1602–5.

44. Irwin RS. Chronic cough due to gastroesophageal reflux disease: ACCP evidence-based clinical practice guidelines. *Chest.* 2006;129: 80s–94s.

45. Jack S, Rossiter HB, Pearson MG, Ward SA, Warburton CJ, Whipp BJ. Ventilatory responses to inhaled carbon dioxide, hypoxia, and exercise in idiopathic hyperventilation. *Am J Respir Crit Care Med.* 2004;170:118–25.

46. Jack S, Rossiter HB, Warburton CJ, Whipp BJ. Behavioral influences and physiological indices of ventilatory control in subjects with idiopathic hyperventilation. *Behav Modif.* 2003;27:637–52.

47. King P, Holdsworth S, Freezer N, Holmes P. Bronchiectasis. *Intern Med J.* 2006;36:729–37.

48. Kolbe J, Wells A, Ram FS. Inhaled steroids for bronchiectasis. *Cochrane Database Syst Rev.* 2000;cd000996.

49. Kraft M. Asthma and chronic obstructive pulmonary disease exhibit common origins in any country! *Am J Respir Crit Care Med.* 2006;174:238–40; discussion 243–44.

50. Kyroussis D, Polkey MI, Hamnegard CH, Mills GH, Green M, Moxham J. Respiratory muscle activity in patients with COPD walking to exhaustion with and without pressure support. *Eur Respir J.* 2000;15:649–55.

51. Larsson K, Carlsem K-H, Bonini S. Anti-asthma drugs: treatment of athletes and exercise-induced bronchoconstriction. *Eur Respir Mono.* 2005;33:73–88.

52. Laude EA, Duffy NC, Baveystock C, et al. The effect of helium and oxygen on exercise performance in chronic obstructive pulmonary disease: a randomized crossover trial. *Am J Respir Crit Care Med.* 2006;173:865–70.

53. Loddenkemper R, Gibson GJ, Sibille Y. *European Lung White Book.* Sheffield: European Respiratory Society, 2003.

54. Lopez AD, Shibuya K, Rao C, et al. Chronic obstructive pulmonary disease: current burden and future projections. *Eur Respir J.* 2006;27:397–412.

55. Lotters F, Van Tol B, Kwakkel G, Gosselink R. Effects of controlled inspiratory muscle training in patients with COPD: a meta-analysis. *Eur Respir J.* 2002;20:570–7.

56. Mahler DA, Wells CK. Evaluation of clinical methods for rating dyspnea. *Chest.* 1988;93:580–6.

57. Maltais F, Simon M, Jobin J, Desmeules M, Sullivan MJ, Belanger M, Leblanc P. Effects of oxygen on lower limb blood flow and O2 uptake during exercise in COPD. *Med Sci Sports Exerc.* 2001;33:916–22.

58. Marciniuk DD, Butcher SJ, Reid JK, et al. The effects of helium-hyperoxia on 6-minute walking distance in chronic obstructive pulmonary disease—a randomized, controlled trial. *Chest.* 2007;131:1659–65.

59. Marciniuk DD, Sridhar G, Clemens RE, Zintel TA, Gallagher CG. Lung volumes and expiratory flow limitation during exercise in interstitial lung disease. *J Appl Physiol.* 1994;77:963–73.

60. Marciniuk DD, Watts RE, Gallagher CG. Dead space loading and exercise limitation in patients with interstitial lung disease. *Chest.* 1994;105:183–9.

61. Markovitz GH, Cooper CB. Exercise and interstitial lung disease. *Curr Opin Pulm Med.* 1998;4:272–80.

62. Mascolo MC, Truwit JD. Role of exercise evaluation in restrictive lung disease: new insights between March 2001 and February 2003. *Curr Opin Pulm Med.* 2003;9:408–10.

63. Masoli M, Fabian D, Holt S, Beasley R. The global burden of asthma: executive summary of the GINA dissemination committee report. *Allergy.* 2004;59:469–78.

64. Mason RJ, Broaddus C, Murray JF, Nadel JA. Part III: Clinical respiratory medicine. In: *Murray and Nadel's Textbook of Respiratory Medicine,* 4th ed. New York: Elsevier, 2005.

65. McConnell AK, Romer LM. Dyspnoea in health and obstructive pulmonary disease: the role of respiratory muscle function and training. *Sports Med.* 2004;34:117–32.

66. McCool FD, Rosen MJ. Nonpharmacologic airway clearance therapies: ACCP evidence-based clinical practice guidelines. *Chest.* 2006;129:250s–9s.

67. McGoon M, Gutterman D, Steen V, et al. Screening, early detection, and diagnosis of pulmonary arterial hypertension: ACCP evidence-based clinical practice guidelines. *Chest.* 2004;126:14s–34s.

68. McGuinnes, G, Naidich DP. CT of airways disease and bronchiectasis. *Radiol Clin North Am.* 2002;40:1–19.

69. McKenzie DC, McLuckie SL, Stirling DR. The protective effects of continuous and interval exercise in athletes with exercise-induced asthma. *Med Sci Sports Exerc.* 1994;26:951–6.

70. McLaughlin VV, McGoon MD. Pulmonary arterial hypertension. *Circulation.* 2006;114:1417–31.

71. Mereles D, Ehlken N, Kreuscher S, et al. Exercise and respiratory training improve exercise capacity and quality of life in patients with severe chronic pulmonary hypertension. *Circulation.* 2006;114:1482–9.

72. Mickleborough TD, Lindley MR, Ionescu AA, Fly AD. Protective effect of fish oil supplementation on exercise-induced bronchoconstriction in asthma. *Chest.* 2006;129:39–49.

73. Mickleborough TD, Lindley MR, Ray S. Dietary salt, airway inflammation, and diffusion capacity in exercise-induced asthma. *Med Sci Sports Exerc.* 2005;37:904–14.

74. Miller MR, Hankinson J, Brusasco V, et al. Standardisation of spirometry. *Eur Respir J.* 2005;26:319–38.

75. Naji NA, Connor MC, Donnelly SC, McDonnell TJ. Effectiveness of pulmonary rehabilitation in restrictive lung disease. *J Cardiopulm Rehabil.* 2006;26:237–43.

76. Neder JA, Sword D, Ward SA, MacKay E, Cochrane LM, Clark C.J. Home based neuromuscular electrical stimulation as a new rehabilitative strategy for severely disabled patients with chronic obstructive pulmonary disease (COPD). *Thorax.* 2002;57:333–7.

77. Newall C, Stockley RA, Hill SL. Exercise training and inspiratory muscle training in patients with bronchiectasis. *Thorax.* 2005; 60:943–8.

78. Newman KB, Mason UG 3rd, Schmaling KB. Clinical features of vocal cord dysfunction. *Am J Respir Crit Care Med.* 1995;152: 1382–1386.

79. **Nici L, Donner C, Wouters E, et al. American Thoracic Society/European Respiratory Society statement on pulmonary rehabilitation.** *Am J Respir Crit Care Med.* **2006;173:1390–413.**

80. Nield M, Arora A, Dracup K, Hoo GW, Cooper CB. Comparison of breathing patterns during exercise in patients with obstructive and restrictive ventilatory abnormalities. *J Rehabil Res.* 2003;40:407–14.

81. Nonoyama M, Brooks D, Lacasse Y, Guyatt G, Goldstein R. Oxygen therapy during exercise training in chronic obstructive pulmonary disease. *Cochrane Database Syst. Rev.* 2007;cd005372.

82. O'Donnell DE, D'arsigny C, Webb KA. Effects of hyperoxia on ventilatory limitation during exercise in advanced chronic obstructive pulmonary disease. *Am J Respir Crit Care Med.* 2001;163:892–8.

83. O'Donnell DE. Hyperinflation, dyspnea, and exercise intolerance in chronic obstructive pulmonary disease. *Proc Am Thorac Soc.* 2006;3: 180–4.

84. O'Donnell DE. Ventilatory limitations in chronic obstructive pulmonary disease. *Med Sci Sports Exerc.* 2001;33:s647–55.

85. Olivieri D, Ciaccia A, Marangio E, Marsico S, Todisco T, Del Vita M. Role of bromhexine in exacerbations of bronchiectasis: double-blind randomized multicenter study versus placebo. *Respiration.* 1991;58:117–21.

86. Olson AL, Zwillich C. The obesity hypoventilation syndrome. *Am J Med.* 2005;118:948–56.

87. Orenstein DM, Franklin BA, Doershuk CF, et al. Exercise conditioning and cardiopulmonary fitness in cystic fibrosis: the effects of a three-month supervised running program. *Chest.* 1981;80:392–8.

88. Palange P, Ward SA, Carlsen KH, et al. Recommendations on the use of exercise testing in clinical practice. *Eur Respir J.* 2007;29: 185–209.

89. Parameswaran K, Todd DC, Soth M. Altered respiratory physiology in obesity. *Can Respir J.* 2006;13:203–10.

90. Patel IS, Vlahos I, Wilkinson TM, et al. Bronchiectasis, exacerbation indices, and inflammation in chronic obstructive pulmonary disease. *Am J Respir Crit Care Med.* 2004;170:400–7.

91. Pellegrino R, Viegi G, Brusasco V, et al. Interpretative strategies for lung function tests. *Eur Respir J.* 2005;26:948–68.

92. Postma DS, Boezen HM. Rationale for the Dutch hypothesis: allergy and airway hyperresponsiveness as genetic factors and their interaction with environment in the development of asthma and COPD. *Chest.* 2004;126:96s–104s; discussion 159s–61s.

93. Rabe KF, Hurd S, Anzueto A, et al. Global strategy for the diagnosis, management, and prevention of chronic obstructive pulmonary disease—2006 update. *Am J Respir Crit Care Med.* 2007;176: 532–55.

94. Ram FS, Robinson SM, Black PN, Picot J. Physical training for asthma. *Cochrane Database Syst Rev.* 2005;cd001116.

95. Rennard SI, Stoner JA. Challenges and opportunities for combination therapy in chronic obstructive pulmonary disease. *Proc Am Thorac Soc.* 2005;2:391–3; discussion 394–5.

96. **Ries AL, Bauldoff GS, Carlin BW, et al. Pulmonary rehabilitation: joint ACCP/AACVPR evidence-based clinical practice guidelines.** *Chest.* **2007;131:4s–42s.**

97. Ries AL, Make BJ, Lee SM, et al. The effects of pulmonary rehabilitation in the national emphysema treatment trial. *Chest.* 2005;128:3799–809.

98. **Rosen MJ. Chronic cough due to bronchiectasis: ACCP evidence-based clinical practice guidelines. *Chest.* 2006;129: 122s–31s.**

99. Sciurba FC. Physiologic similarities and differences between COPD and asthma. *Chest.* 2004;126:117s–124s; discussion 159s–61s.

100. Shea SA, Andres LP, Shannon DC, Banzett RB. Ventilatory responses to exercise in humans lacking ventilatory chemosensitivity. *J Physiol.* 1993;468:623–40.

101. Soriano JB, Davis KJ, Coleman B, Visick G, Mannino D, Pride NB. The proportional Venn diagram of obstructive lung disease: two approximations from the United States and the United Kingdom. *Chest.* 2003;124:474–81.

102. Sun XG, Hansen JE, Oudiz RJ, Wasserman K. Exercise pathophysiology in patients with primary pulmonary hypertension. *Circulation.* 2001;104:429–35.

103. Sun XG, Hansen JE, Oudiz RJ, Wasserman K. Gas exchange detection of exercise-induced right-to-left shunt in patients with primary pulmonary hypertension. *Circulation.* 2002;105:54–60.

104. Tamaoki J, Chiyotani A, Kobayashi K, Sakai N, Kanemura T, Takizawa T. Effect of indomethacin on bronchorrhea in patients with chronic bronchitis, diffuse panbronchiolitis, or bronchiectasis. *Am Rev Respir Dis.* 1992;145:548–52.

105. Tecklenburg SL, Mickleborough TD, Fly AD, Bai Y, Stager JM. Ascorbic acid supplementation attenuates exercise-induced bronchoconstriction in patients with asthma. *Respir Med.* 2007;101: 1770–8.

106. Troosters T, Casaburi R, Gosselink R, Decramer M. Pulmonary rehabilitation in chronic obstructive pulmonary disease. *Am J Respir Crit Care Med.* 2005;172:19–38.

107. Vivodtzev I, Pepin JL, Vottero G, Mayer V, Porsin B, Levy P, Wuyam B. Improvement in quadriceps strength and dyspnea in daily tasks after 1 month of electrical stimulation in severely deconditioned and malnourished COPD. *Chest.* 2006;129:1540–8.

108. Weycker D, Edelsberg J. Prevalence and economic burden of bronchiectasis. *Clin Pulm Med.* 2005;14:205–9.

109. Wills P, Greenstone M. Inhaled hyperosmolar agents for bronchiectasis. *Cochrane Database Syst Rev.* 2006;cd002996.

110. Wrigge H, Golisch W, Zinserling J, Sydow M, Almeling G, Burchardi H. Proportional assist versus pressure support ventilation: effects on breathing pattern and respiratory work of patients with chronic obstructive pulmonary disease. *Intensive Care Med.* 1999; 25:790–8.

111. Zanotti E, Felicetti G, Maini M, Fracchia C. Peripheral muscle strength training in bed-bound patients with COPD receiving mechanical ventilation: effect of electrical stimulation. *Chest.* 2003; 124:292–6.

SELECTED REFERENCES FOR FURTHER READING

American Thoracic Society/European Respiratory Society Statement on Pulmonary Rehabilitation. *Am J Respir Crit Care Med.* 2006;173: 1390–413.

Durstine JL, Moore GE, editors. *ACSM's Exercise Management for Persons with Chronic Diseases and Disabilities.* 2nd ed. Philadelphia: Lippincott, Williams & Wilkins; 2003.

Ehrman JK, Gordon PM, Visich PS, Keteyian SJ. *Clinical Exercise Physiology.* Champaign (IL): Human Kinetics; 2nd edition, 2008.

LeMura LM, von Duvillard SP, editors. *Clinical Exercise Physiology: Application and Physiological Principles.* Philadelphia: Lippincott, Williams & Wilkins; 2004.

Ries AL, Bauldoff GS, Carlin BW, et al. Pulmonary rehabilitation. Joint ACCP/AACVPR evidence-based clinical practice guidelines. *Chest.* 2007;131:4S–42S.

INTERNET RESOURCES

- American Thoracic Society statements: www.thoracic.org/sections/publications/statements/index.html
- American Thoracic Society Best of the Web Reviews: www.thoracic.org/sections/clinical-information/best-of-the-web/reviews.html
- American Thoracic Society/European Respiratory Society COPD Guidelines: www.ersnet.org/lrPresentations/copd/files/main/index.html
- eMedicine: www.emedicine.com/med/PULMONOLOGY.htm
- Global Initiative for Asthma (GINA): www.ginasthma.org/
- Global Initiative for Obstructive Lung Disease (GOLD): www.goldcopd.com
- MedlinePlus: www.nlm.nih.gov/medlineplus/lungsandbreathing.html
- Pulmonary Hypertension Association (PHA): www.phassociation.org

CHAPTER 8

Pathophysiology and Treatment of Metabolic Disease

Diabetes contributes to elevated rates of morbidity and mortality by increasing the risk of cardiovascular disease, kidney failure, and other chronic metabolic conditions. Diabetes is a complex heterogeneous disease that requires the management of serum glucose levels, lipids parameters, blood pressure, and thrombotic factors. Intensive lifestyle modification of increased physical activity and adaptation of a heart-healthy diet is usually a first line of therapy for patients with type 2 diabetes. Regular exercise reduces body weight and fat mass; improves insulin sensitivity, blood pressure control, and lipid profiles; and reduces cardiovascular risk. This chapter will define the types of diabetes, describe risk factors for diabetes, provide information on the metabolic syndrome, and focus on the effects of regular exercise and physical activity on glucose metabolism and the metabolic syndrome. The importance of exercise and physical activity on risk factors for diabetes such as central obesity, insulin resistance, hypertension, hypertriglyceridemia, and associated metabolic abnormalities will be further elucidated. Finally, the role of oral antidiabetic drugs in maintaining normal glycemia as diabetes progresses will be discussed.

DESCRIPTION OF NORMAL GLUCOSE METABOLISM AND TYPE 1, TYPE 2, AND GESTATIONAL DIABETES

According to the most recent 2007 standards of the American Diabetes Association (ADA) (2), a normal fasting plasma glucose (FPG) concentration is defined as <100 mg $\cdot$ dL^{-1} (5.6 mmol $\cdot$ L^{-1}). Hyperglycemia that does not meet the criteria for type 2 diabetes is classified as either impaired fasting glucose (IFG), defined as FPG = 100 to 125 mg $\cdot$ dL^{-1} (5.6–6.9 mmol $\cdot$ L^{-1}), or impaired glucose tolerance (IGT), defined as a 2-hour plasma glucose = 140 to 199 mg $\cdot$ dL^{-1} (7.8–11.0 mmol $\cdot$ L^{-1}). The ADA also terms both IFG and IGT as *prediabetes,* as both of these conditions are risk factors for diabetes and cardiovascular disease (CVD).

Three criteria are used for the diagnosis of diabetes (Table 8-1) (2). These criteria must be confirmed on a subsequent day unless unequivocal symptoms of hyperglycemia are present. The FPG is the preferred diagnostic test for diabetes, whereas the use of hemoglobin A$_{1C}$ values is not recommended in the diagnosis of diabetes. In addition, the use of the 75-g oral glucose tolerance test (OGTT) is not recommended for routine clinical use unless a patient with IFG or suspected diabetes (e.g., a women with a history of gestational diabetes [GDM]) needs to be further evaluated. Screening for diabetes is recommended for adults older than 45 years, especially for those who are classified as overweight and obese by a body mass index (BMI) (25 kg $\cdot$ m^{-2} (2). Other conditions with a rationale for asymptomatic individuals to be tested for diabetes include individuals with additional risk factors described below.

Type 1 diabetes, an immune-mediated disease, is characterized by β-cell destruction, which usually leads to absolute insulin deficiency. Serologic markers of

TABLE 8-1. CRITERIA FOR THE DIAGNOSIS OF DIABETES

1. Symptoms of diabetes and a casual plasma glucose $\geq$200 mg/dL^{-1} (11.1 mmol/L^{-1}). Causal is defined as any time of day without regard to time since last meal. The classic symptoms of diabetes include polyuria, polydipsia, and unexplained weight loss.
   OR
2. FPG $\geq$126 mg/dL^{-1} (7.0 mmol/L^{-1}). Fasting is defined as no caloric intake for at least 8 hours.
   OR
3. 2-hour plasma glucose $\geq$200 mg/dL^{-1} (11.1 mmol/L^{-1}) during an OGTT. The test should be performed according to the World Health Organization, using a glucose load containing the equivalent of 75 g anhydrous glucose dissolved in water.

FPG, fasting plasma glucose; OGTT, oral glucose tolerance test.

pancreatic destruction, such as islet cell autoantibodies, insulin autoantibodies, glutamic acid decarboxylase, and human leukocyte antigens, may be present upon diagnosis and support the autoimmune nature of this disease (3). The rate of β-cell destruction varies widely and is typically slow in infants and fast in adults (1). This type of diabetes accounts for only 5% to 10% of all cases of diabetes and is characterized by islet cell autoantibodies, autoantibodies to insulin, autoantibodies to glutamic acid decarboxylase (GAD$_{65}$), and autoantibodies to the tyrosine phosphatases IA-2 and IA-2-β, any of which are present in 85% to 90% of individuals when hyperglycemia is discovered (1). Patients may present with ketoacidosis or have modest fasting hyperglycemia that can quickly change to severe hyperglycemia and/or ketoacidosis. Ketoacidosis occurs when a high level of ketones (β-hydroxybutyrate, acetoacetate) are produced as a by-product of fatty acid metabolism. In type 1 diabetes, the combination of deficient insulin and increased counterregulatory hormones (e.g., catecholamines, cortisol, glucagons) results in excessive ketone production and metabolic acidosis (1). Adults with type 1 diabetes may not present with ketoacidosis for many years because they maintain some β-cell function. Type 1 diabetes has many genetic predispositions and likely environmental influences. Patients are rarely obese, but obesity is possible in type 1 diabetes. Patients with type 1 diabetes are also at risk to develop other autoimmune disorders such as Graves disease, Hashimoto thyroiditis, Addison disease, vitiligo, celiac sprue, autoimmune hepatitis, myasthenia gravis, and pernicious anemia. Other forms of type 1 diabetes, which are more rare, have no known etiology (idiopathic diabetes). This type 1 is strongly inherited, and patients are mainly of African or Asian descent.

Type 2 diabetes is characterized predominantly by insulin resistance with relative insulin deficiency and can progress to an insulin secretory defect with insulin resistance. Insulin resistance is defined as a reduction in glucose disposal rate elicited by a given insulin concentration

(24). This type of diabetes occurs in approximately 90% to 95% of cases of diabetes. Specific etiologies are not known, and there are many different causes of type 2 diabetes, but autoimmune destruction of the β-cell does not occur. Many individuals with type 2 diabetes go undiagnosed because hyperglycemia develops gradually, and there are no classic symptoms. Most type 2 patients are obese and/or have central obesity and are at risk for the development of micro- and macrovascular complications. Type 2 diabetes can occur in children and adolescents, likely as a result of obesity and reduced physical activity.

GDM is any degree of carbohydrate intolerance of variable severity with onset or first recognition during pregnancy (1). Recommendations for screening in pregnancy utilize a risk factor analysis and possibly an OGTT. Risk factors for GDM include marked obesity, personal history of GDM or delivery of a previous large-for-gestation-age infant, glycosuria, polycystic ovary syndrome, or a strong family history of diabetes (1). Central adiposity by high waist-to-hip ratio (88), as well as African-American and Hispanic race (4), are also associated with the development of GDM. Women with a history of GDM are at an increased risk for the development of type 2 diabetes mellitus (2,39,57). There are many other types of diabetes, including maturity-onset diabetes of the young (MODY), which is associated with genetic defects in β-cell function, or diabetes caused by genetic defects in insulin action, drugs or chemical-induced diabetes, endocrinopathies, infections, immune-mediated diabetes, and other genetic syndromes that are associated with diabetes. Examples of these types of diabetes are provided in greater detail elsewhere (1).

DEVELOPMENT, RISK FACTORS, AND COMORBIDITIES FOR DIABETES

Obese individuals, particularly those with visceral fat accumulation, are more likely to develop type 2 diabetes. Increased body fat mass is associated with higher levels of inflammatory adipocyte cytokines (adipokines). Inflammation not only plays an important role in atherosclerosis but also in the development of diabetes and its microvascular complications. Factors that augment inflammation in patients with type 2 diabetes include increased oxidative stress, hyperglycemia, and the formation of advanced glycation end products (65,67,86). Prospective studies indicate an association between physical activity and the development of type 2 diabetes (49,53,54). In a population-based prospective study that directly measured activity by maximal exercise test, men in the low-fitness group had a 1.9-fold risk for IGT, and the risk for the development of type 2 diabetes was 3.7-fold higher in men in the low-fitness group compared with men in the high-fitness group (82). These associations persist even after adjustment for age, parental history of diabetes, alcohol consumption, and cigarette smoking (82). Thus, it appears physical fitness may be a major factor to reduce the development of type 2 diabetes.

Risk factors for diabetes include age ≥45 years; BMI ≥25 kg·m^{-2}; habitual physical inactivity; having a first-degree relative with diabetes; being a member of a high-risk ethnic population, such as African American, Latino, Native American, Asian American, or Pacific Islander; delivering a baby weighing >9 lb or having been diagnosed with GDM; and having polycystic ovary syndrome (2). Additional risk factors include hypertension (≥140/90 mm Hg), low HDL cholesterol (<35 mg·dL^{-1} or 0.90 mmol·L^{-1}), high triglyceride level (>250 mg·dL^{-1} or 2.82 mmol·L^{-1}), previous diagnosis of IGT or IFG, other clinical conditions associated with insulin resistance, and a history of vascular disease (2). The National Heart, Lung, and Blood Institute (61) also classifies central obesity (waist circumference as a surrogate for visceral fat) with BMI level as a risk factor for type 2 diabetes. For example, a waist circumference of 40 inches in men and ≥35 inches in women with BMIs in the overweight category (25–29.9 kg·m^{-2}) are at a high risk. This increases to extremely high risk at BMI levels of extreme obesity (≥40 kg·m^{-2}) (61). A sedentary lifestyle is an important and modifiable risk factor for type 2 diabetes with a 30% to 50% risk reduction associated with a physically active, compared with a sedentary, lifestyle (75).

Insulin resistance, a primary defect in patients with type 2 diabetes, affects all of the normal metabolic actions of insulin, including glucose transport, hexokinase activity, glycogen synthesis, and glucose oxidation. Skeletal muscle is the primary site of glucose disposal under insulin-stimulated conditions. In response to insulin binding, insulin receptors on skeletal muscle cells undergo autophosphorylation on tyrosine residues, leading to activation of the receptor tyrosine kinase and subsequent tyrosine phosphorylation of insulin receptor substrate-1 (IRS-1) (33). IRS-1 in turn associates with the regulatory subunit of phosphatidylinositol 3-kinase, which is necessary for mediating insulin's metabolic effects, including glucose transporter 4 (GLUT4) translocation, disposing of glucose, and increasing the activity of glycogen synthase and hexokinase (33). Impaired glucose clearance from the circulation by skeletal muscle and adipose tissue, and to a lesser degree an increase in the production of glucose by hepatocytes and portal adipocytes, are key aspects of the metabolic dysfunction that are associated with insulin resistance and impaired insulin secretion. Patients with diabetes often have multiple comorbid CVD risk factors, including dyslipidemia and hypertension.

DEVELOPMENT AND RISK FACTORS FOR OTHER METABOLIC CONDITIONS

 1.2.8-CES: Describe the influence of exercise on cardiovascular, pulmonary, and metabolic risk factors.

METABOLIC SYNDROME

Syndrome X, now known as metabolic syndrome, was first introduced by Reaven (69) as a disorder characterized by impaired glucose tolerance, dyslipidemia, and hypertension, which were associated with increased risk of type 2 diabetes and CVD. The primary underlying mechanism for the syndrome was attributed to insulin resistance at the level of the skeletal muscle. In 2001, the Third Report of the National Cholesterol Education Program (NCEP) Expert Panel on Detection, Evaluation, and Treatment of High Blood Cholesterol in Adults (Adult Treatment Panel III) (ATP III) (62) called attention to the importance of the metabolic syndrome. The World Health Organization (WHO) also selected criteria to define the metabolic syndrome (85). More recently, the International Diabetes Federation (IDF), which reflects the ATP III and WHO definitions, created their definition of the metabolic syndrome. These definitions of the metabolic syndrome are presented in Table 8-2 (31).

In addition to the similar criteria among the three groups (ATP III, WHO, and IDF), the ATP III discusses the presence of prothrombotic and proinflammatory states as part of the metabolic syndrome. These components associated with the metabolic syndrome include inflammation (23,51,56,60,66), intimal-medial wall thickness of the carotid arteries (56), and coagulation markers (23,66). Participants in NHANES III (National Health and Nutrition Examination Survey) with the metabolic syndrome according to ATP III criteria had elevated C-reactive protein (CRP) concentrations and higher fibrinogen concentrations and white blood cell (WBC) counts than those adults without the metabolic syndrome (23). Furthermore, physically active individuals with the metabolic syndrome had lower levels of CRP, WBC counts, and fibrinogen levels, as well as other adipokines, including serum amyloid-A, interleukin-6, and tumor necrosis factor-α (TNFα) levels than sedentary individuals with the metabolic syndrome (66). Consistent with this, lean mass, visceral fat area, and plasma-soluble TNF receptor 1 concentration (sTNFR1) are independently related to the severity of metabolic syndrome (i.e., the number of components) in postmenopausal women (87). These studies suggest that inflammation is a risk factor for the presence of the metabolic syndrome.

Several teams have investigated the WHO and ATP III definitions of the metabolic syndrome in different populations to see if they concur and if they differ in relation to mortality (30,55,74,80). In a study of more than 1,500 patients with type 2 diabetes, 78% fulfilled the ATP III criteria and 81% met the WHO criteria, indicating a good agreement between the two definitions of the metabolic syndrome (55). In the Cardiovascular Health Study, there was an 80% concordance in classifying the participants (74). In a sample of approximately 400 obese adults, the

TABLE 8-2. ADULT TREATMENT PANEL III (ATPIII), (3) WORLD HEALTH ORGANIZATION (WHO), AND INTERNATIONAL DIABETES FEDERATION (5) CRITERIA FOR THE METABOLIC SYNDROME

	ATP III (3 or more criteria below)	WHO INSULIN RESISTANCE (impaired glucose tolerance, impaired fasting glucose or type 2 diabetes, +2 or more criteria below)	INTERNATIONAL DIABETES FEDERATION (central obesity plus any two of remaining four criteria)
Central obesity/obesity	Abdominal obesity: waist circumference >102 cm in men and >88 cm in women	Abdominal obesity: waist to hip ratio >0.90 in men and >0.85 in women and/or BMI >30 kg·m^{-2}	Waist circumference ≥94 cm for Europid men and ≥80 cm for Europid women, with ethnicity specific values for other groups
Lipid	Hypertriglyceridemia: ≥150 mg·dL^{-1}	Hypertriglyceridemia: ≥150 mg·dL^{-1}	Hypertriglyceridemia: ≥150 mg·dL^{-1}
	Low HDL cholesterol: <40 mg·dL^{-1} in men and <50 mg·dL^{-1} in women	Low HDL cholesterol: <35 mg·dL^{-1} in men and <39 mg·dL^{-1} in women	Low HDL cholesterol: <40 mg·dL^{-1} in men and <50 mg·dL^{-1} in women or specific treatment for this lipid abnormality
Blood pressure	High blood pressure: ≥130/85 mm Hg	High blood pressure: ≥140/90 mm Hg and/or antihypertensive medication	High blood pressure ≥130/85 mm Hg or treatment of previously diagnosed hypertension
Glucose	High fasting glucose: ≥110 mg·dL^{-1}	Impaired glucose regulation or type 2 diabetes	High fasting glucose: ≥100 mg·dL^{-1} or previously diagnosed type 2 diabetes
		Insulin resistance (under hyperinsulinemic euglycemic conditions, glucose uptake below lowest quartile for background population under investigation)	
Microalbuminuria		Urine albumin excretion rate: ≥20 μg·min^{-1} or albumin:creatinine ratio ≥30 mg·g^{-1} units throughout chapter have been in the form of mg·g^{-1}–except here?	

HDL, high-density lipoprotein.

prevalence of the metabolic syndrome was higher in those defined by WHO than the ATP III criteria (80). Of approximately 2,800 participants in the San Antonio Heart Study, one fourth met both WHO and ATP III criteria for the metabolic syndrome, with an additional one fourth of adults meeting only one of the criteria (30). Furthermore, both definitions were predictive of all-cause and cardiovascular mortality, but the ATP III definition was slightly more predictive in lower-risk adults in the San Antonio Heart Study (30). Finally, the metabolic syndrome defined by ATP III and not by WHO was an independent predictor of coronary or cerebrovascular events (74), suggesting that the ATP III criteria may be especially useful in this regard. In a recent review of prospective studies between 1998 and 2004, Ford (22) concluded that the population-attributable fraction for the metabolic syndrome is approximately 6% to 7% for all-cause mortality, 12% to 17% for CVD, and 30% to 52% for diabetes.

A 2005 report provides a critical view of the definition, pathogenesis, and utility of the metabolic syndrome (35). This review of the American Diabetes Association and the European Association for the Study of Diabetes concludes that clinicians should evaluate and treat all CVD risk factors without regard to whether the patient meets the criteria for diagnosis of the metabolic syndrome. Another 2005 review provides an examination of the mechanisms underlying the metabolic syndrome and the management of the metabolic syndrome (19).

There is some evidence to suggest that a low cardiorespiratory fitness is associated with increased clustering of metabolic abnormalities of the metabolic syndrome (84). Additionally, a follow-up of healthy men and men with the metabolic syndrome showed that a low cardiorespiratory fitness was a risk factor for premature mortality (37). In another study (21), the age and smoking-adjusted prevalence of the metabolic syndrome in women was highest (19.0%) in those with the lowest cardiorespiratory fitness and decreased across quintiles of increasing fitness levels. The significance of cardiorespiratory fitness in the metabolic syndrome is that fitness levels attenuate the effect of the metabolic syndrome on all-cause and cardiovascular disease mortality (38).

Several studies have examined the amount of physical activity that is associated with a reduction in the prevalence of the metabolic syndrome. Men who engage in >1 hour/week but <3 hours/week of moderate-intensity leisure-time physical activity are 60% more likely to have the metabolic syndrome (using a modified definition of the

WHO) than those who participate in (3 hours/week) (46). In young adults from the Bogalusa Heart study, the Caucasian and African-American women who were moderately active compared with physically inactive women had significantly less risk of having three risk factors of the metabolic syndrome (25). Finally, leisure-time physical activity levels determined by questionnaire are inversely associated with the prevalence of the metabolic syndrome in Caucasian, African-American, and Native-American women (32).

ROLE OF EXERCISE/PHYSICAL ACTIVITY AND BODY WEIGHT ON DIABETES

TYPE 2 DIABETES

Significant progress has been made toward an understanding of the molecular basis underlying the beneficial effects of exercise training in stimulating the entry of glucose into tissue responsive to insulin action (33,89). Accordingly, it is well accepted that regular physical exercise offers an effective therapeutic intervention to improve insulin action in skeletal muscle and adipose tissue in insulin-resistant individuals. Chronic exercise results in numerous physiologic and cellular adaptations that favor sustained improvement in insulin action (Fig. 8-1) (33,89).

The link between physical inactivity and insulin resistance was first noted in migrant populations who experienced dramatic increases in the incidence of type 2 diabetes after exposure to a more modern, westernized environment that was quite different from their traditional lifestyles. Hunter-gatherer societies exhibit only a 1% to 2% prevalence of diabetes compared with a much higher prevalence rate in industrialized nations (18,58). In addition, Japanese migrants living in Hawaii had an elevated risk of diabetes compared with their counterparts living in Hiroshima (40). Likewise, Pima Indians in rural Mexico living a traditional Pima Indian lifestyle have markedly lower rates of diabetes compared with the Arizona Pimas consuming a westernized diet and maintaining a sedentary lifestyle (68). The difference in the prevalence of diabetes in these populations despite the similarity in genetic background can directly be attributed to changes in lifestyle behavior, in particular the level of habitual physical activity.

Further evidence to support the hypothesis that physical inactivity plays a significant role in the increased incidence of diabetes is provided by observational and retrospective studies (26,53,54). Data from the University of Pennsylvania Alumni Study document a 6% lower risk of diabetes for each 500 kcal/week of self-reported

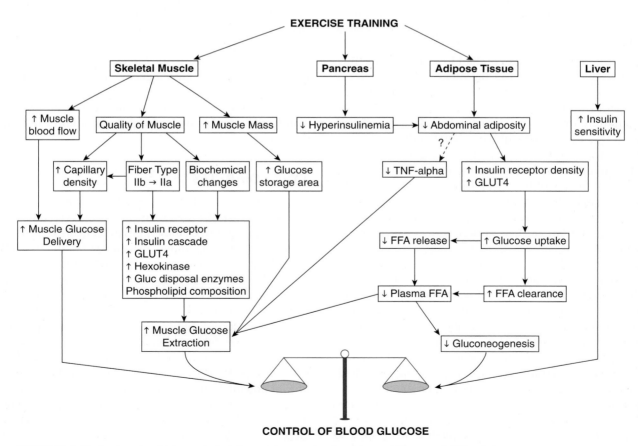

FIGURE 8-1. Mechanisms by which exercise training may improve insulin action and the control of blood glucose.

leisure-time physical activity (26). In the Physician Health Studies (53,54), the risk of diabetes was approximately 35% less for women who reported vigorous exercise at least once per week; men who exercise vigorously five or more times per week showed a 42% reduction in the age-adjusted risk of diabetes compared with those who exercised less than once per week, suggesting a dose-response relationship between increased physical activity and diabetes risk.

Prospective studies also document the beneficial effects that maintaining an active lifestyle plays in reducing the incidence of diabetes, quantified either by self-report (27,28,83) or directly by maximal exercise treadmill testing (47,50,81). The Nurses Health Study showed that brisk walking for at least 2.5 hours/week was associated with a 25% reduction in diabetes over an 8-year follow-up period (28). Data from the Women's Health Study demonstrated that participants who reported walking 2 to 3 hours/week were 34% less likely to develop diabetes than women who reported no exercise (83). Furthermore, participants enrolled in the Women's Health Initiative Observational Study stratified to the lowest quartile of total energy and walking energy expenditure had a 22% and 18% higher risk of developing diabetes compared with women in the highest quartiles of energy expenditures (27). Thus, there is strong evidence of a graded inverse association between levels of self-reported physical activity and incident diabetes over long follow-up periods. Middle-aged Finnish men in the lowest quartile of cardiorespiratory fitness (peak VO_2 <25.8 $mL \cdot kg^{-1} \cdot min^{-1}$) were more than four times as likely to develop diabetes as men in the highest two quartiles of fitness (peak VO_2 >31.1 $mL \cdot kg^{-1} \cdot min^{-1}$) (50). At the Cooper Institute for Aerobics Research, a 6-year longitudinal study demonstrated that men in the low-fitness group (the least fit 20% of the cohort) at the time of enrollment had risk for impaired fasting glucose and diabetes compared with those in the highest fitness group (the most fit 40% of the cohort) (81). These studies support the hypothesis that a sedentary lifestyle and low cardiorespiratory fitness play a significant role in the progression from normal glucose tolerance to type 2 diabetes.

Randomized clinical trials in high-risk populations with impaired glycemic control also provide evidence to support the hypothesis that implementation of a lifestyle behavior that incorporates an increase in leisure-time physical activity can prevent or postpone the development of type 2 diabetes (41,64,77). Chinese men encouraged to increase their daily physical activity (i.e., either 30 minutes of mild-intensity activity, 20 minutes of moderate-intensity activity, 10 minutes of strenuous activity, or 5 minutes of very strenuous exercise) were 46% less likely to develop diabetes than a control group over a 6-year period (64). During a mean follow-up of 3 to 4 years in the Finnish and U.S. Diabetes Prevention Studies,

the progression to frank diabetes was 60% lower for men and women with impaired glucose tolerance assigned to an intense lifestyle intervention that included regular physical activity (approximately 150 minutes/week of moderate- to vigorous-intensity activities), modest weight loss, and healthier dietary habits compared with glucose-intolerant men and women in the control group (41,77). Thus, there remains little doubt that incorporating physical activity into the lifestyle of high-risk individuals is a critical modification to reduce the worsening of glucose metabolism.

Intervention studies demonstrate that structured and supervised training regimens that utilize either aerobic or resistive training have positive effects on insulin sensitivity and glucose homeostasis in individuals with IGT and type 2 diabetes. Chronic training leads to improvements in glucose tolerance, the insulin response to glucose, and insulin sensitivity of as much as 30% (with insulin sensitivity measured via euglycemic-hyperinsulinemic or hyperglycemic clamps) (10,11,29,34,70–72). Exercise training reduces the glycosylated hemoglobin (HbA_{1c}) concentration in type 2 diabetic patients (6), indicating improved glycemic control. A meta-analysis of 14 randomized clinical trials indicates a 0.74-percentage-points reduction in HbA_{1c} after moderate-intensity exercise training in type 2 diabetics with no change in a control group (6). High-intensity resistance training interventions were also very effective in reducing HbA_{1c} in patients with type 2 diabetes with absolute change of as much as 1.2% (7,17).

In summary, there is an extensive body of observational and experimental evidence supporting the hypothesis that an active lifestyle prevents the dysregulation in glucose homeostasis and substantially delays the progression from a state of impaired glycemic control to frank diabetes.

TYPE 1 DIABETES

Patients with type 1 diabetes should be encouraged to perform regular exercise similar to normal and type 2 diabetic individuals because of the long-term benefits of physical activity in improving known risk factors for atherosclerosis and cardiovascular disease. Physical activity has been linked in prospective epidemiologic studies to reduced cardiovascular mortality in type 1 diabetes mellitus (59). During a 6-year follow-up period, patients with type 1 diabetes in the lowest quintile of reported baseline physical activity had a sixfold and fourfold higher mortality rate in men and women respectively, compared with the quintile with the highest physical activity level even after controlling for potential confounding variables, such as age, body mass index, insulin dose, cigarette smoking, and alcohol drinking (59). Because diabetes is associated with an increased risk of macrovascular disease, the benefit of exercise is hypothesized to derive from the antiatherogenic effects on lipid and lipoprotein metabolism (3,44). In fact, a randomized controlled clinical trial in patients with type 1 diabetes showed that 12 to 16 weeks of aerobic exercise training at 60% to 80% VO_2 peak produced favorable changes in lipid, lipoprotein, and apolipoprotein levels. The level of aerobic activity was inversely associated triglyceride levels and directly associated with the apo A-I/apo B ratio, even after controlling for adiposity and glycemic control (44). Unfortunately, unlike patients with type 2 diabetes, exercise training studies fail to show an independent effect of physical activity on improving glycemic control as measured by HbA_{1c} in patients with type 1 diabetes (3). In summary, the benefits of exercise training in patients with type 1 diabetes are the improvements in lipid and lipoprotein profiles, which reduce the risk of CVD in patients encouraged to perform regular aerobic-type exercise.

PHARMACOLOGIC AND MEDICAL TREATMENT OF DIABETES

TYPE 2 DIABETES

The pathogenesis of type 2 diabetes involves peripheral and hepatic insulin resistance, and impaired or abnormal insulin and glucagon secretion from the pancreas. Hyperglycemia gradually develops as a result of the decrease in insulin sensitivity, the abnormal metabolic adaptation of a decrease in glucose uptake in peripheral tissue, and an increase glucose output from the liver (33,89). Diabetes is a complex chronic disease that requires adequate management of hyperglycemia and other comorbid physiologic dysfunctions, such as dyslipidemia, high blood pressure, and elevated thrombotic factors—conditions that are highly associated with insulin resistance. Therefore, achieving metabolic control via tight monitoring of glycosylated hemoglobin, fasting, and postprandial glucose is clinically important to decrease the risk of cardiovascular disease in diabetic patients (2) as well as many other diabetes-related complications (Box 8-1).

The results of United Kingdom Prospective Diabetes Study (UKPDS), a randomized multicenter clinical trial, provided the knowledge and standard for clinical practice with the primary goal of maintaining glycosylated hemoglobin concentrations between 6.5% and 7.0% (2,78,79). The maintenance of HbA_{1c} to near normoglycemia with intensified treatment in the form of oral antidiabetic agents, insulin, or in combination therapy significantly reduced the development of micro- and macrovascular complications associated with diabetes (8,42). Because of the beneficial effects of improved insulin sensitivity, improved glucose tolerance, and reduction in the risk of cardiovascular complications, the first line of therapy for patients with newly diagnosed type 2 diabetes is the implementation of an intensive lifestyle modification of increased physical activity and adaptation of heart-healthy diet (2,8). A common recommendation is to eventually reduce body weight by 5% to 10% because the majority of patients that present with diabetes are overweight or obese. Unfortunately, the compliance with such intense programs over the long term tends to be difficult. The UKPDS demonstrates that only 25% of the patients were able to maintain the optimal HbA_{1c} levels of <7% after 9 years without an oral agent or insulin (79). Glycemic control frequently deteriorates with conventional therapies as diabetes progresses, despite the initial drop in HbA_{1c}. Therefore, the need may arise to use oral antidiabetic agents in combination therapy to aggressively maintain glycemic control to as near normal as possible. However, the use of oral agents in this aggressive manner can only maintain adequate HbA_{1c} levels for an estimated period of approximately 10 years, after which many patients may require insulin therapy (8).

BOX 8-1   DIABETES-RELATED COMPLICATIONS (3)

- Coronary heart disease death rates in adults with diabetes are two to four times higher than in adults without diabetes.
- Stroke risk is two to four times higher among adults with diabetes.
- Hypertension is present in about 73% of adults with diabetes.
- Retinopathy is the leading cause of new cases of blindness among adults 20 to 74 years old.
- Nephropathy: Diabetes is a leading cause of end-stage renal disease, accounting for 43% of new cases.

- Neuropathy: About 65% of people with type 1 or type 2 diabetes have mild to severe forms of nervous system damage involving peripheral motor sensory nerves and autonomic nerves.
- Severe forms of diabetic nerve disease are a major contributing cause of lower-extremity amputations; more than 60% of nontraumatic lower-limb amputations in the United States occur among people with diabetes.

There are currently three groups of oral antidiabetic drugs according to their principle mode of action: (a) those that increase insulin secretion (insulin secretagogues); (b) those that delay the rate of carbohydrates digestion and absorption (α-glucosidase inhibitors); and (c) those with direct effects on insulin-responsive tissue (insulin sensitizers).

Insulin secretagogues, such as sulfonylureas and glinides, lower circulating blood glucose by enhancing pancreatic insulin secretion (8,42). However, because the hypoglycemic effect of this class of drugs is attributable to increased insulin secretion, its effectiveness is highly dependent on adequate β-cell function. Fasting glucose levels decrease with these drugs by 2 to 4 $mmol \cdot L^{-1}$ with an accompanying decrease in HbA_{1c} of one to two percentage points (8,42).

α-Glucosidase inhibitors, such as acrabose, miglitol, and voglibose, reduce the rate of digestion of carbohydrates in the proximal small intestine, primarily lowering postprandial glucose concentrations as they inhibit intestinal α-glucosidase enzymes. The chance of causing hypoglycemia is very minimal in this class of drugs because of their mode of action. However, α-glucosidase inhibitors generally reduce HbA_{1c} by 0.5 to 1.0, depending on the dosage on the drug. In addition, α-glucosidase typically reduces postprandial glucose concentrations by 1 to 4 $mmol \cdot L^{-1}$, thereby resulting in significant reduction the incremental area under the postprandial glucose curve (8,42).

The insulin sensitizers are attractive oral agents for therapy in patients with type 2 diabetes because peripheral insulin resistance is a primary defect in these individuals. Metformin, the therapy of choice for overweight and obese type 2 patients, improves insulin action in skeletal muscle and hepatic tissue. However, because metformin does not increase insulin release, the presence of insulin is crucial for its effectiveness. The principal modes of action are to decrease hepatic glucose output by reducing gluconeogenesis, decrease hepatic extraction of gluconeogenic substrates, decrease hepatic glycogenolysis, and enhance insulin-stimulated glucose uptake in skeletal muscle (8,42). Metformin, the only biguanide currently available for clinical use, typically reduces fasting glucose by 2 to 4 $mmol \cdot L^{-1}$ with corresponding decreases in HbA_{1c} of one to two percentage points. Thiazolidinediones (TZDs), such as pioglitazone, are also insulin sensitizers that improve whole-body insulin sensitivity via multiple actions on gene regulation (8,42). TZD treatments effectively control glycemia by altering cellular mechanisms in tissues, such as muscle, adipose tissue, and liver, thereby improving insulin action. The metabolic effects observed in skeletal muscle tissue include increases in glucose uptake, glycolysis, glucose oxidation, and inconsistent changes in glycogenesis. The metabolic effects observed in adipose tissue include increased glucose uptake, fatty acid uptake, lipogenesis,

and preadipocyte differentiation. The metabolic effects observed in the liver include decreased gluconeogenesis, glycogenolysis, and increased lipogenesis and glucose uptake. TZD agents reduce HbA_{1c} approximately 0.5 to 1.5 percentage points.

Insulin is usually the last line of treatment and is reserved for those patients who fail to respond adequately to a combination of orals agents, whose glycemic control continues to deteriorate despite adequate drug combinations, and for whom safety and efficacy considerations favors its use as the drug of choice, such as in cases of pregnancy or severe hepatic and renal impairments (2,8,42). Inability to achieve adequate glycemic control with combinations of oral therapies probably indicates that the natural history of the disease has progressed to a state of severe β-cell failure, and a switch to insulin therapy is usually recommended (42). An insulin pump can be used to manage some patients with type 2 diabetes and gestational diabetes. Management of GDM focuses on similar interventions that are commonly recommended in type 2 diabetes; however, insulin therapy can be initiated when glucose control is not achieved and reduces serious perinatal complications (9). Insulin administered by syringe is injected into subcutaneous tissue using a rotation of sites, including the abdomen (fastest absorption rate), upper arms, lateral thigh, and buttocks. Continuous Subcutaneous Insulin Infusion (CSII) is subcutaneously delivered only in the abdominal area. Insulin administered by syringe can be rapid acting (peak action: 0.5–1.0 hour), short acting (peak action: 2–3 hours), intermediate acting (peak action: 4–10 hours), or long acting (peak action: sustained for 20–24 hours). A mixed dose of different types of insulin produces a more normal glucose response and is used most commonly. Usually, rapid-acting insulin is used with CSII.

In summary, irrespective of the treatment modality, any intervention is likely to improve the probability that a patient will experience better long-term glycemic control, decrease the risk of development of macro- and microvascular complications, and decrease the risk of cardiovascular disease. This is especially true when the diagnosis of diabetes is detected early, when the metabolic abnormalities usually associated with this chronic disease are less severe.

TYPE 1 DIABETES

Type 1 diabetes mellitus is associated with long-term complications of the eyes, kidneys, and peripheral and autonomic nervous system (2). Diabetes-related complications are listed in Box 8-1. In addition, type 1 diabetes is associated with a 10-fold increase in CVD as compared with aged-matched nondiabetic individuals (45). Because hyperglycemia appears to play a significant role in the pathophysiology of these complications, the need to achieve glycemic control to near-normal blood glucose and glycosylated hemoglobin concentrations as safely possible without inducing hypoglycemia with insulin therapy is crucial for long-term clinical benefits (2). The Diabetes Control and Complication Trial (DCCT) was designed to assess whether intensive insulin therapy (at least three insulin injections per day or continuous infusion of insulin with an external pump with at least four blood measurements of glucose per day) would reduce the risk of macro- and microvascular complications compared with conventional therapy (one or two insulin injections per day with one urine or blood glucose test per day). The desired goal for the intensive therapy was to maintain blood glucose and glycosylated hemoglobin to as close to normal range as possible, whereas conventional therapy had no glucose goal except to prevent symptoms of hyperglycemia and hypoglycemia (13). At the end of the 6.5 years of the DCCT, mean glycosylated hemoglobin was 7.2% in the intensive therapy group versus 9% in the conventional therapy group. Subsequently, intensive insulin therapy reduced the risk of development and progression of microvascular and neuropathic complications by 35% and 76% respectively (12) and decreased progression of intima-media thickness, a sensitive marker for coronary and cerebral vascular disease in patients with type 1 diabetes (15). The DCCT/Epidemiology of Diabetes Interventions and Complications Research Group also demonstrated that intensive therapy to maintain near-normal glycosylated hemoglobin concentrations has beneficial effects on long-term complications associated with type 1 diabetes (14,16). The risk of progressive retinopathy and nephropathy remained lower in the intensive versus the conventional treatment group 4 years after the completion of the DCCT trials (14). Seventeen-year follow-up showed reduced risk of cardiovascular events by 42%, and the risk of severe clinical events—such as nonfatal myocardial infarction, stroke, or death from CVD—was reduced by 57% in the intensive treatment group (16). In summary, intensive therapy implemented early to achieve glycemic control to as near normal as possible without the possibility of hypoglycemia is beneficial in patients with type 1 diabetes to reduce the short- and long-term macro- and microvascular complications associated with this disease (2).

SUMMARY

The clinical importance of physical activity in diabetes is underscored by studies that indicate that a low level of physical fitness is associated with increased risk of all-cause and CVD mortality (20,48,73,82). Men who improve their physical fitness reduce their mortality risk by approximately 44% (5). In addition, both avoiding obesity and beginning moderately vigorous sports activity are separately associated with lower death rates from all causes and from CVD, and with reductions in the incidence of

coronary events in middle-aged and older men and postmenopausal women (36,43,52,63). Maintenance of a healthy lifestyle by not being overweight, not smoking, exercising moderately or vigorously 30 minutes/day, and eating a healthy diet results in more than an 80% reduction in the incidence of coronary events (76). Therefore, increased physical activity is an effective treatment for the significant health benefits in diabetes and other metabolic conditions.

REFERENCES

1. American Diabetes Association. Clinical Practice Recommendations: Diagnosis and classification of diabetes mellitus. *Diabetes Care.* 2007;30:S42–S47.
2. American Diabetes Association. Clinical Practice Recommendations: Standards of medical care in diabetes. *Diabetes Care.* 2007; 230:S4–S41.
3. American Diabetes Association. Physical activity/exercise and diabetes. *Diabetes Care.* 2004;27(suppl 1):S58–S62.
4. Berkowitz GS, Lapinski RH, Wein R, Lee D. Race/ethnicity and other risk factors for gestational diabetes. *Am J Epidemiol.* 1992; 135:965–973.
5. Blair SN, Kohl HW, Barlow CE, et al. Changes in physical fitness and all-cause mortality: a prospective study of healthy and unhealthy men. *JAMA.* 1995;273:1093–1098.
6. Boule NG, Haddad E, Kenny G, Wells GA, Sigal RJ. Effects of exercise on glycemic control and body mass in type 2 diabetes mellitus: a meta-analysis of controlled clinical trials. *JAMA.* 2001;286(10): 1218–1227.
7. Castaneda C, Layne JE, Muboz-Orians L, et al. A randomized controlled trial of resistance exercise training to improve glycemic control in older adults with type 2 diabetes. *Diabetes Care.* 2002; 25(12):2335–2341.
8. Cohen A, Horton ES. Progress in the treatment of type 2 diabetes: new pharmacologic approaches to improve glycemic control. *Curr Med Res Opin.* 2007;23(4):905–917.
9. Crowther CA, Hiller JE, Moss JR, et al. Effect of treatment of gestational diabetes mellitus on pregnancy outcomes. *N Engl J Med.* 2005;352:2477–2486.
10. Dengel DR, Hagberg JM, Pratley RE, Rogus EM, Goldberg AP. Improvements in blood pressure, glucose metabolism, and lipoprotein lipids after aerobic exercise plus weight loss in obese, hypertensive middle-aged men. *Metabolism.* 1998;47:1075–1082.
11. Dengel DR, Pratley RE, Hagberg JM, Rogus EM, Goldberg AP. Distinct effects of aerobic exercise training and weight loss on glucose homeostasis in obese sedentary men. *J Appl Physiol.* 1996;81: 318–325.
12. Diabetes Control and Complications Trial. Effect of intensive diabetes management on macrovascular disease and risk factors in the Diabetes Control and Complications Trial. *Am J Cardiol.* 1995;75: 894–903.
13. Diabetes Control and Complications Trial. The effects of intensive treatment of diabetes on the development and progression of long-term complications in insulin-dependent diabetes. *N Engl J Med.* 1993;329:977–986.
14. The Diabetes Control and Complications Trial/Epidemiology of Diabetes Interventions and Complications Research Group. Retinopathy and nephropathy in patients with type 1 diabetes four years after a trial of intensive therapy. *N Engl J Med.* 2000; 342:381–389.
15. The Diabetes Control and Complications Trial/Epidemiology of Diabetes Interventions and Complications Research Group. Intensive diabetes therapy and carotid intima-media thickness in type 1 diabetes mellitus. *N Engl J Med.* 2003;348:2294–2303.

16. The Diabetes Control and Complications Trial/Epidemiology of Diabetes Interventions and Complications (DCCT/EDIC) Study Research Group. Intensive diabetes treatment and cardiovascular disease in patients with type 1 diabetes. *N Engl J Med.* 2005;353: 2643–2653.

17. Dunstan DW, Daly RM, Owen N, et al. High-intensity resistance training improves glycemic control in older patients with type 2 diabetes. *Diabetes Care.* 2002;25(10):1729–1736.

18. Eaton SB, Konner M, Shostak M. Stone agers in the fast lane: chronic degenerative diseases in evolutionary perspective. *Am J Med.* 1988;84:739–749.

19. Eckel RH, Grundy SM, Zimmet PZ. The metabolic syndrome. *Lancet.* 2005;1415–1428.

20. Ekelund LG, Haskell WL, Johnson JL, et al. Physical fitness as a predictor of cardiovascular mortality in asymptomatic North American men. The Lipid Research Clinics Mortality Follow-up Study. *N Engl J Med.* 1998;319:1379–1384.

21. Farrell SW, Cheng YJ, Blair SN. Prevalence of the metabolic syndrome across cardiorespiratory fitness levels in women. *Obes Res.* 2004;12:824–830.

22. Ford ES. Risks for all-cause mortality, cardiovascular disease, and diabetes associated with the metabolic syndrome: a summary of the evidence. *Diabetes Care.* 2005;28:1769–1778.

23. Ford ES. The metabolic syndrome and C-reactive protein, fibrinogen, and leukocyte count: findings from the Third National Health and Nutrition Examination Survey. *Atherosclerosis.* 2003;168:351–358.

24. Godsland IF, Stevenson JC. Insulin resistance: syndrome or tendency? *Lancet.* 1995;346:100–103.

25. Gustat JS, Srinivasan J, Elkasabany A, Berenson GS. Relation of self-rated measures of physical activity to multiple risk factors of insulin resistance syndrome in young adults: the Bogalusa Heart Study. *J Clin Epidemiol.* 2002;55:997–1006.

26. Helmrich SP, Ragland DR, Leung RW, Paffenbarger RS. Physical activity and reduced occurrence of non-insulin-dependent diabetes mellitus. *N Engl J Med.* 1991;325:147–152.

27. Hsia J, Wu L, Allen C, et al. Physical activity and diabetes risk in postmenopausal women. *Am J Prev Med.* 2005;28:19–25.

28. Hu FB, Sigal RJ, Rich-Edwards JW, et al. Walking compared with vigorous physical activity and risk of type 2 diabetes in women: a prospective study. *JAMA.* 1999;282:1433–1439.

29. Hughes VA, Fiatarone MA, Fielding RA, et al. Exercise increases muscle GLUT-4 levels and insulin action in subjects with impaired glucose tolerance. *Am J Physiol.* 1993;264:E855–E862.

30. Hunt KJ, Resendez RG, Williams K, Haffner SM, Stern MP. San Antonio Heart Study. National Cholesterol Education Program versus World Health Organization metabolic syndrome in relation to all-cause and cardiovascular mortality in the San Antonio Heart Study. *Circulation.* 2004;100:1251–1257.

31. International Diabetes Federation. The IDF consensus worldwide definition of the metabolic syndrome. www.idf.org/webdata/docs/Metac_syndrome_def.pdf. Accessed April 3, 2008.

32. Irwin ML, Ainsworth BE, Mayer-Davis EJ, Addy CL, Pate RR, Durstine JL. Physical activity and the metabolic syndrome in a tri-ethnic sample of women. *Obes Res.* 2002;10:1030–1037.

33. Ivy JL, Zderic TW, Fogt DL. Prevention and treatment of non-insulin dependent diabetes mellitus. *Exerc Sports Sci Rev.* 1999;27: 1–35.

34. Joseph LJO, Farrell PA, Davey SL, Evans WJ, Campbell WW. Effect of resistance training with or without chromium picolinate supplementation on glucose metabolism in older men and women. *Metabolism.* 1999;48:546–553.

35. Kahn R, Buse J, Ferrannini E, Stern M. The metabolic syndrome: time for a critical appraisal. Joint statement from the American Diabetes Association and the European Association for the Study of Diabetes. *Diabetes Care.* 2005;28:2289–2304.

36. Kanaya AM, Vittinghoff E, Shlipak MG, et al. Association of total and central obesity with mortality in postmenopausal women with coronary heart disease. *Am J Epidemiol.* 2003;158:1161–1170.

37. Katzmarzyk PT, Church TS, Blair SN. Cardiorespiratory fitness attenuates the effects of the metabolic syndrome on all-cause and cardiovascular disease mortality in men. *Arch Intern Med.* 2004;164: 1092–1097.

38. Katzmarzyk PT, Church TS, Janssen I, Ross R, Blair SN. Metabolic syndrome, obesity, and mortality. *Diabetes Care.* 2005;28:391–397.

39. Kaufmann RC, Schleyhahn FT, Huffman DG, Amankwah KS. Gestational diabetes diagnostic criteria: long-term maternal follow-up. *Am J Obstet Gynecol.* 1995;172:621–625.

40. Kawate R, Yamakido M, Nishimoto Y, Bennett PH, Hamman RF, Knowler WC. Diabetes mellitus and its vascular complications in Japanese migrants on the island of Hawaii. *Diabetes Care.* 1979;2: 161–170.

41. Knowler WC, Barrett-Connor E, Fowler SE, et al. Reduction in the incidence of type 2 diabetes with lifestyle intervention or metformin. *N Engl J Med.* 2002;346:393–403.

42. Krentz AJ, Bailey CJ. Oral antidiabetic agents: current role in type 2 diabetes mellitus. *Drugs.* 2005;65(3):385–411.

43. Kushi LH, Fee RM, Folsom AR, Mink PJ, Anderson KE, Sellers TA. Physical activity and mortality in postmenopausal women. *JAMA.* 1997;277:1287–1292.

44. Laaksonen DE, Atalay M, Niskanen LK, et al. Aerobic exercise and the lipid profile in type 1 diabetic men: a randomized controlled trial. *Med Sci Sports Exerc.* 2000;32:1541–1548.

45. Laing SP, Swerdlow AJ, Slater SD, et al. Mortality from heart disease in a cohort of 23,000 patients with insulin-treated diabetes. *Diabetologia.* 2003:46:760–765.

46. Lakka TA, Laaksonen DE, Lakka HM, et al. Sedentary lifestyle, poor cardiorespiratory fitness, and the metabolic syndrome. *Med Sci Sports Exerc.* 2003;35:1279–1286.

47. LaMonte MJ, Blair SN, Church TS. Physical activity and diabetes prevention. *J Appl Physiol.* 2005;99:1205–1213.

48. Lie H, Mundal R, Erikssen J. Coronary risk factors and incidence of coronary death in relation to physical fitness: seven-year follow-up study of middle-aged and elderly men. *Eur Heart J.* 1985;6: 147–157.

49. Lipton RB, Liao Y, Cao G, Cooper RS, McGee D. Determinants of incident non-insulin-dependent diabetes mellitus among blacks and whites in a national sample. The NHANES I Epidemiologic Follow-Up Study. *Am J Epidemiol.* 1993;138:826–839.

50. Lynch J, Helmrich SP, Lakka TA, et al. Moderately intense physical activities and high levels of cardiorespiratory fitness reduce the risk of non-insulin-dependent diabetes mellitus in middle-aged men. *Arch Intern Med.* 1996;156:1307–1314.

51. Malik S, Wong ND, Franklin S, Pio J, Fairchild C, Chen R. Cardiovascular disease in U.S. patients with metabolic syndrome, diabetes, and elevated C-reactive protein. *Diabetes Care.* 2005;28: 690–693.

52. Manson JE, Hu FB, Rich-Edwards JW, et al. A prospective study of walking as compared with vigorous exercise in the prevention of coronary heart disease in women. *N Engl J Med.* 1999;341:650–658.

53. Manson JE, Nathan DM, Krolewski AS, Stampfer MJ, Willett WC, Hennekens CH. A prospective study of exercise and incidence of diabetes among US male physicians. *JAMA.* 1992;268:63–67.

54. Manson JE, Rimm EB, Stampfer MJ, Colditz GA, Willett WC, Krolewski AS. Physical activity and incidence of non-insulin-dependent diabetes mellitus in women. *Lancet.* 1991;338:774–778.

55. Marchesini G, Forlani G, Cerrelli F, et al. WHO and ATPIII proposals for the definition of the metabolic syndrome in patients with type 2 diabetes. *Diabet Med.* 2004;21:383–387.

56. McNeill AM, Rosamond WD, Girman CJ, et al. Prevalence of coronary heart disease and carotid arterial thickening in patients with the metabolic syndrome (the ARIC Study). *Am J Cardiol.* 2004;94: 1249–1254.

57. Metzger BE, Cho NH, Roston SM, Radvany R. Pre-pregnancy weight and antepartum insulin secretion predict glucose tolerance five years after gestational diabetes mellitus. *Diabetes Care.* 1993;16:1598–1605.

58. Mokdad AH, Ford ES, Bowman BA, et al. Prevalence of obesity, diabetes, and obesity-related health risk factors. *JAMA.* 2003;289: 76–79.

59. Moy CS, Songer TJ, Laporte RE, et al. Insulin-dependent diabetes mellitus, physical activity, and death. *Am J Epidemiol.* 1993;137:74–81.

60. Nakanishi N, Shiraishi T, Wada M. C-reactive protein concentration is more strongly related to metabolic syndrome in women than in men: the Minoh Study. *Circ J.* 2005;69:386–391.

61. **National Heart, Lung, and Blood Institute. Clinical Guidelines on the identification, evaluation and treatment of overweight and obesity in adults: the evidence report. National Institutes of Health.** *Obes Res.* **1998;6 Suppl 2:51S–209S.**

62. **National Institutes of Health.** *Third Report of the National Cholesterol Education Program Expert Panel on Detection, Evaluation, and Treatment of High Blood Cholesterol in Adults (Adult Treatment Panel III).* **Bethesda (MD): National Institutes of Health; 2001. NIH Publication 01-3670.**

63. Paffenbarger RS, Hyde RT, Wing AL, Lee IM, Jung DL, Kampert JB. The association of changes in physical-activity level and other lifestyle characteristics with mortality among men. *N Engl J Med.* 1993;328:538–545.

64. Pan XR, Li GW, Hu YH, et al. Effects of diet and exercise in preventing NIDDM in people with impaired glucose tolerance: the Da Quing IGT and Diabetes Study. *Diabetes Care.* 1997;20:537–544.

65. Pennathur S, Heinecke JW. Mechanisms of oxidative stress in diabetes: implications for the pathogenesis of vascular disease and antioxidant therapy. *Front Biosci.* 2004;9:565–574.

66. Pitsavos C, Panagiotakos DB, Chrysohoou C, Kavouras S, Stefanadis C. The associations between physical activity, inflammation, and coagulation markers, in people with metabolic syndrome: the ATTICA study. *Eur J Cardiovasc Prev Rehabil.* 2005;12:151–158.

67. Pradhan AD, Ridker PM. Do atherosclerosis and type 2 diabetes share a common inflammatory basis? *Eur Heart J.* 2002;23:831–834.

68. Ravussin E, Valencia ME, Esparza J, Bennett PH, Schulz LO. Effects of a traditional lifestyle on obesity in Pima Indians. *Diabetes Care.* 1994;17:1067–1074.

69. Reaven GM. Role of insulin resistance in human disease. *Diabetes.* 1988;37:1595–1607.

70. Ryan AS, Hurlbut DE, Lott ME, et al. Improved insulin action after resistive training in insulin resistant older men and women. *J Am Geriatr Soc.* 2001;49:247–253.

71. Ryan AS, Nicklas BJ, Berman DM. Aerobic exercise is necessary to induce improvements in glucose utilization with moderate weight loss in obese postmenopausal women. *Obes Res.* 2006;14(6):1064–1072.

72. Ryan AS, Pratley RE, Goldberg AP, Elahi D. Increased insulin sensitivity in post-menopausal women following resistive training and weight loss. *J Gerontol.* 1996;51A(5):M199–M205.

73. Sandvik L, Erikssen J, Thaulow E, Erikssen G, Mundal R, Rodahl K. Physical fitness as a predictor of mortality among healthy, middle-aged Norwegian men. *N Engl J Med.* 1993;328:533–537.

74. Scuteri A, Najjar SS, Morrell CH, Lakatta EG. The metabolic syndrome in older individuals: prevalence and prediction of cardiovascular events: the cardiovascular health study. *Diabetes Care.* 2005; 28:882–887.

75. Skerrett PJ, Manson JE. Reduction in risk of coronary heart disease and diabetes. In: Ruderman N, Devlin JT, Schenider SH, Kriska A, editors. *Handbook of Exercise in Diabetes.* Alexandria (VA): American Diabetes Association; 2002.

76. Stampfer MJ, Hu FB, Manson JE, Rimm EB, Willett WC. Primary prevention of coronary heart disease in women through diet and lifestyle. *N Engl J Med.* 2000;343:16–22.

77. Tuomilehto J, Lindstrom J, Eriksson JG, et al. Preventions of type 2 diabetes mellitus by changes in lifestyle among subjects with impaired glucose tolerance. *N Engl J Med.* 2001;344:1343–1350.

78. UK Prospective Diabetes Study (UKPDS) Group. Effect of intensive blood-glucose control with metformin on complications in overweight patients with type 2 diabetes (UKPDS 34). *Lancet.* 1998;352: 854–865.

79. UK Prospective Diabetes Study (UKPDS) Group. Intensive blood-glucose control with sulphonylureas or insulin compared with conventional treatment and risk of complications in patients with type 2 diabetes. *Lancet.* 1998;352:837–853.

80. Vidal J, Morinigo R, Codocceo VH, Casamitjana R, Pellitero S, Gomis R. The importance of diagnostic criteria in the association between the metabolic syndrome and cardiovascular disease in obese subjects. *Int J Obes Relat Metab Disord.* 2005;29(6): 668–674.

81. Wei M, Gibbons LW, Mitchell TL, Kampert JB, Lee CD, Blair SN. The association between cardiorespiratory fitness and impaired fasting and type 2 diabetes mellitus in men. *Ann Intern Med.* 1999;130:89–96.

82. Wei M, Kampert JB, Barlow CE, et al. Relationship between low cardiorespiratory fitness and mortality in normal-weight, overweight, and obese men. *JAMA.* 1999;282:1547–1553.

83. Weinstein AR, Sesso HD, Lee IM, et al. Relationship of physical activity vs. body mass index with type 2 diabetes in women. *JAMA.* 2004;292:1188–1194.

84. Whaley MH, Kampert JB, Kohl HW, Blair SN. Physical fitness and clustering of risk factors associated with the metabolic syndrome. *Med Sci Sports Exerc.* 1999;31:287–293.

85. **World Health Organization. Definition, diagnosis and classification of diabetes mellitus and its complications: report of a WHO Consultation. Part 1: diagnosis and classification of diabetes mellitus.** *World Health Organization,* **1999.**

86. Yan SF, Ramasamy R, Naka Y, Schmidt AM. Glycation, inflammation, and RAGE: a scaffold for the macrovascular complications of diabetes and beyond. *Circ Res.* 2003;93:1159–1169.

87. You T, Ryan AS, Nicklas BJ. The metabolic syndrome in obese postmenopausal women: relationship to body composition, visceral fat and inflammation. *J Clin Endocrinol Metab.* 2004;89: 5517–5522.

88. Zhang S, Folsom AR, Glack JM, Liu K. Body fat distribution before pregnancy and gestational diabetes: findings from coronary artery risk development in young adults (CARDIA) study. *BMJ.* 1995;311: 1139–1140.

89. Zierath JR. Invited review: exercise training induced changes in insulin signaling in skeletal muscle. *J Appl Physiol.* 2002;93: 773–781.

SELECTED REFERENCES FOR FURTHER READING

American College of Sports Medicine. Exercise and Type 2 Diabetes Position stand. *Med Sci Sports Exerc,* 2002;34:1345–60.

American College of Sports Medicine ACSM; Exercise Management for Persons with Chronic Disease and Disabilities. 2nd Ed. Champaign, Il: Human Kinetics; 2003.

Ruderman N., Deoless J, Schneider S, Krishna A, eds: Handbook of Excercise of Diabetes. 2nd Ed. Alexandria, VA: American Diabites Association; 2001.

INTERNET RESOURCES

- www.eatright.org
- www.diabeteseducator.org
- www.nhlbi.nih.gov/suidelines/obesiy/ob_home.htm
- www.guideline.gov

Psychopathology

DEFINING MENTAL ILLNESS

> **1.9.7-HFS: Knowledge of signs and symptoms of mental health states (e.g., anxiety, depression, eating disorders) that may necessitate referral to a medical or mental health professional.**

Disturbances in psychological functioning are commonly encountered by exercise professionals working with patients. Some disorders are more common in certain patient populations. Understanding and identifying mental disorders is important because of their effects on exercise participation and overall health and well-being. For example, population studies consistently show that persons who have more depressive symptoms are less likely to be physically active (10). Furthermore, there are numerous studies demonstrating that individuals with more depressive symptoms are likely to develop chronic diseases, e.g.,

cardiovascular disease, compared with those who have fewer symptoms (14). Also, when individuals have chronic disease and depressive symptoms, they are more likely to have worse outcomes compared with those with chronic disease and few depressive symptoms (28).

Mental health and mental illness are considered part of a continuum of mental functioning. Mental health involves being able to engage in useful work, join in productive relationships with others, and be able to cope with change and adversity. Disruptions in mental health are likely to occur in most people at least once in their lifetime. These disruptions can be transient or chronic and can range from mild to severe. Some may require referral to treatment by a specialist or to a support group, or they may resolve over time (28). In this chapter, the most common mental health problems that are likely to be encountered by the exercise professional will be discussed. Terminology established by the most recent Surgeon

> > > KEY TERMS

Anorexia nervosa: An eating disorder that involves intake of calories that is insufficient to maintain normal height and body weight for age.

Binge-eating disorder: An eating disorder that involves recurrent binge-eating episodes at least 2 days per week over 6 months, without compensatory behaviors to prevent weight gain.

Bipolar disorder: A disorder of mood that involves periods of depressive symptoms and mania.

Bulimia disorder: An eating disorder that involves recurrent binge-eating episodes and purging or compensatory behaviors to prevent weight gain.

Generalized anxiety disorder (GAD): A type of anxiety disorder that is characterized by chronic, exaggerated worry that is more extreme than expected for the actual situation.

Major depressive disorder (MDD): A mood disorder that is characterized by depressed mood or loss of

interest or pleasure most of the day, nearly every day, for at least 2 weeks; weight loss or weight gain; insomnia or hypersomnia; psychomotor retardation or agitation; fatigue; feelings of worthless or guilt; inability to think; and recurrent thoughts of death.

Panic attacks: A type of anxiety disorder that is characterized by sudden feeling of loss of control or fear, including heart palpitations, sweating, difficulty breathing, chest pain, dizziness, or gastrointestinal distress.

Substance abuse: A type of substance-use disorder that is characterized by repeated substance use that results in impairment in functioning or distress.

Substance dependence: A type of substance-use disorder that is characterized by cognitive, behavioral, and physiologic symptoms that are the result of continued substance use despite problems.

General's Report on Mental Health that differentiates *mental health problems* and *mental illness* will be used. Also, criteria for diagnosis for mental disorders established by the fourth edition of the American Psychiatric Association in the *Diagnostic and Statistical Manual of Mental Disorders* (DSM-IV) will be the basis for describing symptoms (1). Discussion will be limited to disorders described in DSM-IV.

Mental illness refers to mental disorders that are diagnosable and involve alterations in thinking, mood, or behavior or some combination of these and that are associated with impaired functioning. **Mental health problems** are those signs and symptoms that are not of a sufficient level of severity and duration that they can be diagnosed (28). Each type of mental health problem or mental disorder, including signs and symptoms, methods of assessment, effective treatments, and considerations for referral will be described. It is important that exercise professionals understand that effective treatments for most mental illnesses and mental health problems are available, and are able to recognize symptoms of mental health problems so individuals can be referred to appropriate treatment resources.

RECOGNIZING STRESS: SYMPTOMS, ASSESSMENT, TREATMENT, AND REFERRAL

Psychological stress is something everyone experiences to varying degrees. The causes of stress may be specific life events, such as the death of a loved one or the loss of a job, or acute or chronic illness. Stress may be caused by less identifiable triggers, such as daily hassles, difficult work, or maladaptive coping strategies. Symptoms of stress often overlap those of depression and anxiety disorders (Box 9-1).

Physical symptoms of acute stress include autonomic nervous system activation, such as elevated heart rate and blood pressure. Prolonged stress may impair the immune system, resulting in susceptibility to illness. In addition, persons experiencing high levels of stress often report higher pain ratings and feelings of anger and irritability.

BOX 9-1   SYMPTOMS OF STRESS (7)

Symptoms of stress are often similar to symptoms of depression and anxiety and include:

- Difficulty sleeping and fatigue
- Muscle tension and soreness
- Changes in appetite
- Headaches or gastrointestinal problems
- Irritability

They may be at increased risk for injury. High levels of stress may negatively influence health behaviors, including smoking, exercise, diet, and medication (8).

Formal assessment of stress typically involves the administration of questionnaires to measure an individual's experience and appraisal of stressful life events. A reliable and valid questionnaire that is commonly used to measure an individual's perception of stress is the Perceived Stress Scale (7). This instrument quantifies the degree to which individuals appraise their lives as unpredictable, uncontrollable, and overloaded.

Interventions for stress often include social support networks, including family and friends, self-help groups (which could include general group therapy, relaxation, or meditation), or support groups for specific issues. In addition, assisting individuals in developing problem-focused coping skills can enable them to identify solutions to their problems and enhance feelings of controllability, thereby reducing the risk of developing other serious mental or physical disorders (14). More formal interventions, including psychotherapy or biofeedback training, may be needed to help individuals develop appropriate coping strategies.

Exercise professionals should be able to recognize when stress is negatively affecting a patient's daily functioning or is causing health problems. Many people find relief from stress by participating in exercise, and exercise professionals can work with their patients to determine the most appropriate types of activities for meeting fitness goals and reducing stress.

RECOGNIZING DEPRESSION: SYMPTOMS, ASSESSMENT, TREATMENT, AND REFERRAL

> **1.9.7-HFS: Knowledge of signs and symptoms of mental health states (e.g., anxiety, depression, eating disorders) that may necessitate referral to a medical or mental health professional.**

> **1.9.5-CES: Recognize observable signs and symptoms of anxiety or depressive symptoms and the need for a psychiatric referral.**

The burden of depressive disorders is significant. According to the Global Burden of Disease Study conducted by the World Health Organization, major depression ranks second behind ischemic heart disease in the significance of disease burden worldwide (20). The lifetime prevalence of all mood disorders, including **major depressive disorder**, is 20.8% (18).

Depression occurs twice as often in women as men, and the sex differences are seen as early as adolescence (1). However, depression affects both men and women of all age groups, ethnicities, and socioeconomic categories (1). Certain populations may be at increased risk for

BOX 9-2   SYMPTOMS OF MAJOR DEPRESSIVE DISORDER (MDD) (1)

Symptoms of depression include the following:

- Persistent feelings of sadness or irritability
- Loss of interest in previously enjoyed activities
- Feelings of guilt, worthless, or helplessness
- Fatigue or decreased energy
- Difficulty thinking or concentrating
- Sleep disturbances, including insomnia or over-sleeping
- Changes in appetite and/or weight gain or loss
- Psychomotor agitation or retardation
- Thoughts of death or suicide

depression, including women in the perinatal or menopausal periods, individuals who have experienced a stressful life event, and people with certain medical conditions, including heart disease and diabetes (14). Depression can be triggered by negative life events, such as the loss of a spouse or a job, or it can be triggered by physiologic and biologic factors, such as having an acute or chronic disease like cancer (12). Family and genetic factors, biologic factors, and cognitive factors all appear to play a causal role in the development of depressive disorders (28). Depressive disorders are diagnosed according to clinical criteria such as the DSM-IV (1) (Box 9-2).

Mood disorders also include **bipolar disorder**, which is characterized by periods of both depression and mania. Symptoms of mania include extreme elation or irritability, increased energy and decreased need for sleep, grandiose ideas, inflated self-esteem, distractibility, physical agitation, and poor judgment or inappropriate behavior.

Questionnaires such as the Beck Depression Inventory (BDI) (3,4) and Center for Epidemiological Studies Depression Scale (CES-D) (23) are commonly used to assess symptoms of depression. Self-report instruments assess the frequency and/or severity of symptomatology and commonly include items relating to emotional, cognitive, and/or physical symptoms of depression. Although questionnaires can give a good indication of presence of depressive symptoms, depressive disorders should only be diagnosed by a physician using criteria set forth by resources such as DSM-IV (1). Consultation with a psychiatrist, psychologist, or physician is important to rule out any other potential causes of symptoms, such as medication or illness, and to develop an appropriate treatment plan.

Effective treatments for depression are available, but many individuals do not seek treatment or receive inadequate treatment. Treatment of depression depends on type and severity of symptoms and patient preference. Effective treatments include classes of antidepressant medications, such as selective serotonin reuptake inhibitors (SSRIs), tricyclic antidepressants (TCAs), and monoamine oxidase inhibitors (MAOIs). Newer antidepressant medications that act on the neurotransmitter systems (e.g., serotonin, norepinephrine, and/or dopamine) generally have fewer side effects than TCAs or MAOIs (2,29). Antidepressant pharmacotherapy takes several weeks before symptoms begin to decrease, and often the dosage must be adjusted for optimal therapeutic effect. Psychotherapy has also been found to be effective in managing depression and may include cognitive behavioral therapy and interpersonal psychotherapy (2). Psychotherapy may be used alone or in combination with antidepressant medication to treat depression. In cases of severe depression or when depression persists despite treatment, electroconvulsive therapy (ECT) may be used and has been found to be effective (2). Regardless of the treatment modality, it is important that patients are regularly assessed throughout the course of treatment to ensure remission of depressive symptoms (25). For individuals who do not respond to the initial course of treatment, it may be necessary to use a combination of treatments, change medication dose, or switch treatment modalities. This process often requires long-term follow-up and continued treatment (13).

Exercise professionals working with individuals who are receiving antidepressant treatment should be aware of the type of medication and any potential somatic or cardiac effects (12). Although most antidepressant medications should not affect response to exercise, some medication side effects, such as weight change or sleep disturbances, may be relevant to exercise participation. In addition, research suggests that exercise may be useful in reducing depressive symptoms and can be recommended as an adjunctive therapy (22); thus, patients should inform their mental health providers of their exercise participation.

If untreated depression is suspected, individuals can be referred to several community resources that are able to provide diagnostic and treatment services (Box 9-3).

BOX 9-3   TREATMENT RESOURCES FOR MENTAL HEALTH

First-line resources for local mental health services include:

- Mental health practitioners, including psychiatrists, psychologists, social workers, or mental health counselors
- Family practice physicians
- Community mental health centers
- Hospital psychiatry departments and outpatient clinics
- Family service, social agencies, religious organizations, and clergy

An exercise professional may encounter someone who expresses such hopelessness or depression to the degree that suicidal risk is suspected (17). It may be necessary to directly inquire if a person is thinking about suicide. Simply by asking "You seem pretty down. Have you had any recent thoughts of harming yourself?" can be a good gauge of suicidal threat. People will usually respond honestly, which allows the opportunity to gauge the seriousness of such thoughts. Immediate action is needed if a person communicates planned harmful or suicidal intentions. If the person is not under the care of mental health provider, he or she can be referred to a local suicide or crisis center or be taken directly to a hospital emergency room. It is important to make sure that the person is accompanied to the treatment center and that the person is not left alone until professional help is available. The National Hopeline Network (1-800-SUICIDE) is a 24-hour hotline that connects individuals to trained counselors at a local crisis center.

RECOGNIZING ANXIETY: SYMPTOMS, ASSESSMENT, TREATMENT, AND REFERRAL

> **1.9.7-HFS: Knowledge of signs and symptoms of mental health states (e.g., anxiety, depression, eating disorders) that may necessitate referral to a medical or mental health professional.**

> **1.9.5-CES: Recognize observable signs and symptoms of anxiety or depressive symptoms and the need for a psychiatric referral.**

The most prevalent of the mental disorders are anxiety disorders with an estimated lifetime prevalence of approximately 28.8% (18). As with depression, women are twice as likely as men to suffer from anxiety disorders. In contrast to the feelings of fear that people experience during a stressful event, anxiety disorders are characterized by chronic symptoms that may worsen if left untreated (Box 9-4). Types of anxiety disorders include panic disorder, specific phobias, generalized anxiety disorder, obsessive-compulsive disorder, posttraumatic

| BOX 9-4 | SYMPTOMS OF ANXIETY (1) |

Common symptoms of anxiety disorders include the following:

- Intense worry, fear, or dread
- Difficulty sleeping
- Sympathetic nervous system activation with physical symptoms, such as dry mouth, increased heart rate, sweating, trembling, agitation, or gastrointestinal distress

stress disorder, and social anxiety disorder. The disorders are diagnosed according to DSM-IV symptom profile and etiology (1).

Panic attacks are characterized by the sudden experience of intense feelings of fear or loss of control. Symptoms include palpitations, sweating, difficulty breathing, chest pain, dizziness, and gastrointestinal distress. The attacks have an abrupt onset and peak within 10 to 15 minutes, but during that time individuals often feel as if they are having a heart attack, dying, or "going crazy."

Specific phobias are anxiety disorders in which individuals experience intense fear and avoidance around objects or situations that present no actual danger. In some individuals, exposure to the object may induce a panic attack. Depending on the phobia, the disorder may or may not interfere with daily functioning.

Generalized anxiety disorder (GAD) is characterized by chronic, exaggerated worry and anxiety. An individual with GAD may worry over everyday situations, but the concerns are constant and more extreme than the situation actually presents. Symptoms often include difficulty concentrating and irritability, as well as physical symptoms such as fatigue, headaches, muscle aches and tension, gastrointestinal distress, trembling, and sweating.

Obsessive-compulsive disorder (OCD) involves the experience of disturbing and irrational thoughts (obsessions) and the need to engage in repeated behaviors or rituals (compulsions) to prevent or relieve the anxiety. Individuals with OCD usually recognize that their thoughts and behaviors are senseless, but they are controlled by the troubling thoughts and the urgent need to engage in rituals. Rituals often involve counting, checking, or washing and may significantly interfere with daily functioning.

Posttraumatic stress disorder (PTSD) develops after experiencing or witnessing an intense, terrifying event, such as a violent attack, serious accident, natural disaster, or abuse. Symptoms include repeated disturbing thoughts of the trauma, nightmares, sleep disturbances, emotional detachment, irritability, and exaggerated startle response. Persons with PTSD may also experience sudden flashbacks of the event and avoid trigger situations that cause memories of the incident. The disorder usually begins within 3 months of the event but may not develop until years later.

Social anxiety disorder is also known as social phobia. This disorder is characterized by intense anxiety and self-consciousness during normal social situations. Individuals with this disorder have a persistent, excessive fear of being watched and evaluated by others and worry of being embarrassed or humiliated. Social anxiety disorder can be specific to certain situations such as speaking or eating in public or be generalized to any social setting.

As with depressive disorders, questionnaires are commonly used to assess symptoms of anxiety. Self-report instruments such as the State/Trait Anxiety Inventory

(STAI) typically assess the frequency and/or intensity of symptoms, including emotional, cognitive, and/or physical domains (27). Although questionnaires can give a good indication of presence of symptoms of anxiety, they typically do not categorize symptoms to indicate type of anxiety disorder (i.e., social phobia, generalized anxiety disorder, etc.). Thus, the presence of anxiety disorders can only be determined by trained professionals using standard diagnostic criteria (1). Referral to a psychiatrist, psychologist, or physician is important to develop an appropriate treatment plan, which may include psychotherapy and/or medication.

Common medications for anxiety include antidepressants, benzodiazepines, and β-blockers. SSRI antidepressant medications are often prescribed for panic disorder, OCD, PTSD, and social phobia; however, this class of medications takes several weeks to achieve full therapeutic effect and is not useful for acute anxiety symptom relief. Benzodiazepines quickly reduce anxiety symptoms and are commonly used in the treatment of panic disorder, social phobia, and GAD. However, people develop tolerance to benzodiazepines and may become dependent on them; symptom rebound may also occur when medication is discontinued. β-blockers, typically used to treat heart conditions, may be indicated when an anxiety-provoking event is anticipated to minimize physical symptoms (11).

Targeted psychotherapy is often indicated for anxiety disorders (16). Cognitive behavioral therapy (CBT) has been found to be particularly useful for treatment of panic disorder and social phobia. Exposure therapy, a type of behavioral therapy, is often used to treat specific phobias, OCD, and PTSD. This technique involves exposing individuals to the feared object or situation in a safe environment so that individuals can practice controlling their anxiety and responding in more appropriate and productive ways (21). Relaxation training, including breathing exercises and biofeedback, may also be used as a component of anxiety treatment. Treatment plans for an anxiety disorder should also include evaluation and treatment of comorbid mental disorders, because depression, substance abuse, or other anxiety disorders often occur concomitantly (1).

If a person exhibits symptoms of anxiety, he or she can be referred to the same community mental health resources that treat depression. However, mental health professionals with specialized training in CBT and anxiety treatment may provide the most comprehensive treatment options. Additionally, self-help groups are often particularly helpful for people with anxiety disorders, as people find it comforting to share experiences with people who can understand their concerns and problems.

As with antidepressant medications, exercise professionals working with individuals who are receiving antianxiety medication should be aware of the type of medication and any potential side effects. Some types of medication may affect the sympathetic nervous system response to exercise so that heart rate or blood pressure may not increase as expected (9). As with depressive symptoms, research suggests that exercise may be useful in reducing symptoms of stress and anxiety (22). Although individuals with panic disorder may avoid participating in exercise for fear of inducing a panic attack, the attacks are not more likely to occur during physical activity than during other daily activities (6). By understanding a person's individual concerns, exercise professionals can work to create a safe and comfortable environment by minimizing potential exposure to anxiety-inducing situations.

RECOGNIZING EATING DISORDERS: SYMPTOMS, ASSESSMENT, TREATMENT, AND REFERRAL

> **1.9.7-HFS: Knowledge of signs and symptoms of mental health states (e.g., anxiety, depression, eating disorders) that may necessitate referral to a medical or mental health professional.**

Disordered eating comprises a spectrum of behavioral, cognitive, and emotional symptoms involving disturbances in eating and body image. Eating disorders are diagnosed according to standard criteria and include the disorders of anorexia nervosa, bulimia nervosa, and binge-eating disorders (1). Eating disorders are more common in women than in men, and disorders often develop in adolescence or young adulthood. Because eating disorders can cause significant health problems and even death, early recognition and treatment is critical. Symptoms of eating disorders are presented in Box 9-5.

Anorexia nervosa is characterized by insufficient caloric intake to sustain body weight, below normal weight for age and height, intense fear of becoming fat,

---

BOX 9-5	**SYMPTOMS OF EATING DISORDERS (1)**

Symptoms of eating disorders include the following:

- Extreme eating patterns, including restriction and overeating
- Body weight loss or gain
- Purging behaviors, including vomiting, laxative use, or excessive exercise
- Unusual eating behaviors, including preferences or phobias of certain foods and obsessive rituals
- Excessive weighing or avoidance of weighing
- Distorted body image, low self-esteem, or feelings of guilt and self-disgust

distorted body image, and disturbances in menstrual cycles in women. Health complications of this disorder include osteoporosis and muscle atrophy, electrolyte imbalances, and cardiac arrhythmias, sometimes resulting in death (19).

Bulimia nervosa involves episodes of binge eating, or consuming large amounts of food within a discrete period of time and purging, or compensatory behaviors to prevent weight gain, such as self-induced vomiting, use of diuretics or laxatives, fasting, and excessive exercise. Individuals with this disorder are often of normal body weight but may express intense body dissatisfaction and desire to lose weight. Health consequences of bulimia nervosa include gastrointestinal disturbances, electrolyte imbalances, esophageal ruptures, pancreatitis, and erosion of tooth enamel (26).

Binge-eating disorder involves recurrent binge eating-episodes, at least 2 days per week over 6 months, without compensatory behaviors to prevent weight gain. The episodes often involve eating more rapidly than usual, feeling uncomfortably full, eating when not hungry, eating alone, and feelings of guilt or disgust (5).

Symptoms of eating disorders are often readily recognizable to outside observers. However, determining the extent of the problem is often difficult, as individuals with eating disorders are often very good at hiding their behaviors and resist intervention. Professional assessment of eating disorders involves multiple components: (a) medical evaluation to assess body weight and health problems; (b) psychological evaluation to assess the severity of the eating disorder and presence of comorbid mental disorders; and (c) nutritional consultation to evaluate current eating habits.

Treatment is also a multifaceted process that often involves a team of healthcare professionals, including physicians, psychologists or counselors, and nutritionists. Several eating disorders are often treated in an inpatient setting so that weight can stabilized and medical conditions can be treated. Psychotherapy is an important component of treatment to reduce inappropriate eating behaviors and explore psychological issues such as body image, self-esteem, and interpersonal relationships. Nutritionists and exercise professionals can play an important role on the intervention team to regulate energy balance through appropriate caloric intake and energy expenditure. Finally, SSRI medications may be helpful in the treatment of some eating disorders (15).

Exercise professionals can play an important role in recognizing symptoms of eating disorders and referring individuals to treatment. When working with patients who have eating disorders, care should be taken to monitor energy balance and to modify exercise prescriptions to accommodate any medical problems. Furthermore, the exercise professional should use sensitivity when weighing or conducting body composition measurements, and communicate appropriate messages to protect body image and self-esteem.

RECOGNIZING ALCOHOL AND DRUG ABUSE: SYMPTOMS, ASSESSMENT, TREATMENT, AND REFERRAL

Substance-use disorders include any disorders related to problems associated with the use of alcohol, drugs of abuse, prescribed or over-the-counter medications, and toxins. Substance-use disorders include substance abuse and substance dependence (28).

Substance abuse refers to a condition in which repeated substance use results in significant adverse effects that produce distress or impairment in functioning. Use of the substance may interfere with role obligations, occur in hazardous situations, and result in legal, interpersonal, or social problems (1).

Substance dependence is characterized by cognitive, behavioral, and physiologic symptoms that result when an individual continues substance use despite problems. Specific symptoms of substance dependence include tolerance to the substance, such that more is needed to achieve the desired effect, and withdrawal symptoms in the absence of the substance. Additional symptoms characterizing substance dependence include the inability to control use of the substance, the use of more than intended, obligation neglect, significant time spent using or recovering from effects of the substance, and continued use despite psychological or health problems.

Professional assessment of substance-use disorders is critical to ensure the safety of the individual and to implement appropriate treatment. Substance abuse commonly occurs with other mental disorders, such as depression, and treatment may involve a combination of individual therapy, group therapy, and/or medication (24). Local hospitals and substance-abuse centers can provide medical and psychological evaluation and treatment in inpatient or outpatient settings.

Exercise professionals are most likely to recognize symptoms of substance use during acute intoxication or when the patient reports questionable behaviors, such as recurrent bingeing or blackouts (30). Written food diaries used in nutrition counseling may also provide evidence of substance abuse. Often, individuals with drug or alcohol problems may deny a problem and resist treatment; however, they may be open to receiving referrals if the information is presented in a professional and caring manner.

SUMMARY

Mental disorders are common problems affecting people of all ages and backgrounds. If recognized, mental health problems can be effectively managed, with significant improvement in psychological functioning, physical health, and quality of life. In most cases, exercise is a useful adjunctive therapy to the treatment of mental disorders and may be effective in preventing symptoms of disorders, such as anxiety and depression. Exercise professionals should be able to recognize symptoms of mental disorders and refer patients to appropriate community resources for treatment.

REFERENCES

1. American Psychiatric Association. *Diagnostic and Statistical Manual of Mental Disorders, Fourth Edition.* 4th ed. Washington (DC): American Psychiatric Association; 1994.
2. **American Psychiatric Association. Practice guideline for the treatment of patients with major depressive disorder (revision).** *Am J Psychiatry.* **2000;157(4 Suppl):1–45.**
3. Beck AT, Steer RA, Garbin MG. Psychometric properties of the Beck Depression Inventory: twenty-five years of evaluation. *Clin Psych Rev.* 1988;8:77–100.
4. Beck AT, Ward CH, Mendelson M, Mock J, Ergaugh J. An inventory for measuring depression. *Arch Gen Psychiatry.* 1961;4:561–57.
5. Brownley KA, Berkman ND, Sedway JA, Lohr KN, Bulik CM. Binge eating disorder treatment: a systematic review of randomized controlled trials. *Int J Eat Disord.* 2007;40(4):337–348.
6. Cameron OG, Hudson CJ. Influence of exercise on anxiety level in patients with anxiety disorders. *Psychosomatics.* 1986;27(10): 720–723.
7. Cohen S, Kamarck T, Mermelstein R. A global measure of perceived stress. *J Health Soc Behav.* 1983;24(4):385–396.
8. Cohen S, Schwartz JE, Bromet EJ, Parkinson DK. Mental health, stress, and poor health behaviors in two community samples. *Prev Med.* 1991;20(2):306–315.
9. Davidson JR. Pharmacologic treatment of acute and chronic stress following trauma: 2006. *J Clin Psychiatry.* 2006;67 (Suppl 2):34–39.
10. Dunn AL, Trivedi MH, O'Neal HA. Physical activity dose-response effects on outcomes of depression and anxiety. *Med Sci Sports Exerc.* 2001;33(6 Suppl):S587–S597.
11. Elliott HW, Reifler B. Social anxiety disorder: a guide for primary care physicians. *N C Med J.* 2000;61(3):176–178.
12. Evans DL, Charney DS, Lewis L, et al. Mood disorders in the medically ill: scientific review and recommendations. *Biol Psychiatry.* 2005;58(3):175–189.
13. Fava M. Augmentation and combination strategies in treatment-resistant depression. *J Clin Psychiatry.* 1992;62(Suppl 18):4–11.
14. Fenton WS, Stover ES. Mood disorders: cardiovascular and diabetes comorbidity. *Curr Opin Psychiatry.* 2006;19(4):421–427.
15. Hainer V, Kabrnova K, Aldhoon B, Kunesova M, Wagenknecht M. Serotonin and norepinephrine reuptake inhibition and eating behavior. *Ann N Y Acad Sci.* 2006;1083:252–269.
16. Hunot V, Churchill R, Silva DE, Lima M, Teixeira V. Psychological therapies for generalised anxiety disorder. *Cochrane Database Syst Rev.* 2007;1: Art. No.: CD001848. DOI: 10.1002/14651858. CD001848. pub4.
17. Jacobs DG, Brewer ML. Application of The APA Practice Guidelines on Suicide to Clinical Practice. *CNS.Spectr.* 2006;11(6):447–454.
18. Kessler RC, Berglund P, Demler O, et al. Lifetime prevalence and age-of-onset distributions of DSM-IV disorders in the National Comorbidity Survey Replication. *Arch Gen Psychiatry.* 2005;62(6): 593–602.
19. Morris J, Twaddle S. Anorexia nervosa. *BMJ.* 2007;334(7599): 894–898.
20. Murray CJ, Lopez AD. Alternative projections of mortality and disability by cause 1990–2020: Global Burden of Disease Study. *Lancet.* 1997;349(9064):1498–1504.
21. Norton PJ, Price EC. A meta-analytic review of adult cognitive-behavioral treatment outcome across the anxiety disorders. *J Nerv Ment Dis.* 2007;195(6):521–531.
22. Otto MW, Church TS, Craft LL, Greer TL, Smits JA, Trivedi MH. Exercise for mood and anxiety disorders. *J Clin Psychiatry.* 2007;68(5): 669–676.
23. Radloff LS. The CES-D Scale: a self-report depression scale for research in the general population. *Appl Psychol Meas.* 1977;1: 385–401.
24. Riggs PD, Mikulich-Gilbertson SK, Davies RD, Lohman M, Klein C, Stover SK. A randomized controlled trial of fluoxetine and cognitive behavioral therapy in adolescents with major depression, behavior problems, and substance use disorders. *Arch Pediatr Adolesc Med.* 2007;161(11):1026–1034.
25. **Rush AJ, Kraemer HC, Sackeim HA., et al. Report by the ACNP Task Force on Response and Remission in Major Depressive Disorder. Neuropsychopharmacology. 2006;31(9):1841–1853.**
26. Shapiro JR, Berkman ND, Brownley KA, et al. Bulimia nervosa treatment: a systematic review of randomized controlled trials. *Int J Eat Disord.* 2007;40(4):321–336.
27. Spielberger CD, Gorsuch RL, Lushene R. Manual for the State-Trait Anxiety Inventory (Self-Evaluation Questionnaire). Palo Alto (CA): Consulting Psychologists Press; 1970.
28. **U.S. Department of Health and Human Services. *Mental Health: A Report of the Surgeon General.* Rockville (MD): U.S. Department of Health and Human Services, Substance Abuse and Mental Health Services Administration, Center for Mental Health Services, National Institutes of Health, National Institute of Mental Health; 1999.**
29. Williams JW Jr, Mulrow CD, Chiquette E, et al. A systematic review of newer pharmacotherapies for depression in adults: evidence report summary. *Ann Intern Med.* 2000;132(9):743–756.
30. Zeigler DW, Wang CC, Yoast RA, et al. The neurocognitive effects of alcohol on adolescents and college students. *Prev Med.* 2005;40(1): 23–32.

SELECTED REFERENCES FOR FURTHER READING

Brownell KD, Fairburn CG. *Eating Disorders and Obesity: A Comprehensive Handbook.* New York: Guilford Press; 1995.

Davis M, Eshelman ER, McKay M. *The Relaxation & Stress Reduction Workbook.* 5th ed. Oakland (CA): New Harbinger Publications, Inc.; 2000.

Morey B, Mueser KT. *The Family Intervention Guide to Mental Illness: Recognizing Symptoms and Getting Treatment.* Oakland (CA): New Harbinger Publications, Inc.; 2007.

Sapolsky RM. *Why Zebras Don't Get Ulcers.* 3rd ed. New York: Henry Holt and Company; 2004.

Wood JC. *Getting Help: The Complete & Authoritative Guide to Self-Assessment & Treatment of Mental Health Problems.* Oakland (CA): New Harbinger Publications, Inc.; 2007.

INTERNET RESOURCES

- Anxiety Disorders Association of America: www.adaa.org (information about anxiety disorders, effective treatments, referral)
- Depression and Bipolar Support Alliance: www.dbsalliance.org (information on depression and local treatment resources)
- Mind Garden: http://www.mindgarden.com/ (publisher of psychological assessments and instruments)
- National Association of Anorexia Nervosa and Associated Disorders: www.anad.org (information about anxiety disorders and local treatment services)
- National Drug and Alcohol Treatment Referral Routing Service: http://findtreatment.samhsa.gov (information about local substance-abuse treatment services)
- National Eating Disorders Association: http://nationaleatingdisorders.org (information about eating disorders, effective treatments, referral)
- National Institute of Mental Health: www.nimh.nih.gov (information about all disorders, effective treatments, referral)
- www.depression-screening.org (site to assess symptoms of depression and resources for effective treatments)

Health Appraisal, Risk Assessment, and Safety of Exercise

ANN SWANK, PhD, FACSM, *Section Editor*

> **1.2.2-HFS: Knowledge of cardiovascular, pulmonary, metabolic, and musculoskeletal risk factors that may require further evaluation by medical or allied health professionals before participation in physical activity.**

> **1.2.6-HFS: Knowledge of the risk-factor thresholds for ACSM risk stratification, which includes genetic and lifestyle factors related to the development of CVD.**

> **1.3.3-HFS: Knowledge of the value of a medical clearance before exercise participation.**

> **1.3.4-HFS: Knowledge of and the ability to perform risk stratification and its implications toward medical clearance before administration of an exercise test or participation in an exercise program.**

> **1.3.6-HFS: Knowledge of the limitations of informed consent and medical clearance before exercise testing exercise testing.**

> **1.3.23-HFS: Ability to identify individuals for whom physician supervision is recommended during maximal and submaximal exercise testing.**

> **1.3.6-CES: Identify individuals for whom physician supervision is recommended during maximal and submaximal exercise testing.**

> **1.10.6-CES: Risk stratify individuals with cardiovascular, pulmonary, and metabolic diseases, using appropriate risk-stratification methods and understanding the prognostic indicators for high-risk individuals.**

It is clear that a physically active lifestyle reduces the risk of several major chronic diseases. Regular physical activity has been shown to be beneficial in the primary prevention of cardiovascular disease (CVD), stroke, diabetes, and some cancers (22). Given the high prevalence of a sedentary lifestyle (13), there is little doubt that considerable public health benefit would accrue if inactive individuals became more active.

The many health-related benefits, as well as the responsible physiologic mechanisms, of a physically active lifestyle are well documented. However, it is essential to realize that to be most effective, regular exercise must be combined with other positive lifestyle interventions and, when applicable, with appropriate medical therapy. Furthermore, although exercise is extremely safe for most individuals, it is

> > > KEY TERMS

AHA/ACSM Health/Fitness Facility Preparticipation Screening Questionnaire: Slightly more complex than the Physical Activity Readiness Questionnaire, this questionnaire was designed for fitness professionals to help assess readiness of starting a physical activity program; developed jointly by the American Heart Association and the American College of Sports Medicine (see GETP8, Fig. 2.2).

Medical screening examination: A thorough medical examination performed by a healthcare professional, often a physician, to assess readiness of starting a physical activity program; often the need of obtaining a medical screening examination is identified during

the preparticipation health screening and risk assessment (see GETP8, Chapter 3).

Physical Activity Readiness Questionnaire (PAR-Q): A widely used and simple prescreening health-assessment questionnaire developed by the British Columbia Ministry of Health for assessing readiness of starting a physical activity program (see GETP8, Fig. 2.1).

Preparticipation health screening and risk assessments: Standardized tools for identifying existing medical conditions with the goal of assessing the risks associated with starting a new exercise program or performing an exercise test (see GETP8, Figs. 2.3 and 2.4).

prudent to take certain precautions to optimize the benefit-to-risk ratio. The two most common risks associated with starting a new physical activity program or performing an exercise test are sudden cardiac events and orthopedic injury. The risks associated with physical activity and exercise testing are detailed in Chapter 1 of ACSM's Guidelines for Exercise Testing and Prescription (GETP8).

To ensure an optimal benefit-to-risk ratio, exercise professionals should incorporate some form of health appraisal before performing fitness testing or initiating an exercise program. Although Chapter 2 of the GETP8 provides a thorough description of proper **preparticipation health screening and risk stratification**, the intent of this current chapter is to provide a general overview of the process, as well as address medical conditions that demand special consideration. The purpose of the preparticipation health screening is to provide information relevant to the safety of fitness testing or beginning exercise training and to identify known diseases and risk factors for CVD so that appropriate lifestyle interventions can be initiated. Furthermore, it is important to identify additional factors that require special consideration when developing an appropriate exercise prescription and programming that optimize adherence, minimize risks, and maximize benefits. The purposes of the preparticipation health screen include the following:

- Identification and exclusion of individuals with medical contraindications to exercise testing (see GETP8, Chapter 3)
- Identification of individuals who should undergo a medical evaluation and exercise testing before starting an exercise program because of increased risk for disease because of age, symptoms, or risk factors (see GETP8, Figures 2.3 and 2.4)
- Identification of persons with clinically significant disease who should participate in medically supervised exercise programs
- Identification of individuals with other special needs

The precise nature and extent of the appraisal should be determined by the age, sex, and perceived health-status characteristics of the participants, as well as the available economic, personnel, and equipment resources. Most prospective participants in exercise programs conducted in nonmedical settings are sedentary individuals who consider themselves "generally healthy" and whose goals are to improve their fitness and well-being, reduce weight, and reduce risk of chronic disease. For such individuals, the primary safety goal of a preparticipation health appraisal is to identify individuals who should receive further medical evaluation to determine whether there are contraindications to exercise testing or training or whether referral to a medically supervised exercise program is necessary.

Health appraisals can range from a short questionnaire to interviews and sophisticated computerized evaluations. Also, many appraisals include common screening measurements including height and weight, waist circumference, percent body fat, blood pressure (BP), and blood testing (serum lipids and glucose). Specifics of these screening items are addressed in detail in Chapter 3 (Tables 3.1–3.3) and Chapter 4 (Tables 4.1–4.6) of the GETP8. The most common method of prescreening health assessment is the use of standardized forms, and several standardized forms are available that can be used to risk stratify individuals. Standardized forms should be viewed as a minimal standard for entry into a new exercise program. In general, these forms are aimed at identifying individuals at moderate to high risk who should receive medical advice before beginning or increasing their level of physical activity. Two of the more reputable standardized forms are the **Physical Activity Readiness Questionnaire (PAR-Q)** and AHA/ACSM (American Heart Association/American College of Sports Medicine) Health/Fitness Facility Preparticipation Screening Questionnaire. The PAR-Q is well developed and has been used and tested extensively (20). It is designed to be used when a person wants to begin a program of light to moderate physical activity. One of the benefits of the PAR-Q is simplicity, so much so that in some circumstances in which there is no alternative, the PAR-Q can be self-administered by the participant. The **AHA/ACSM Health/Fitness Facility Preparticipation Screening Questionnaire** is designed to be completed when the participant registers at a health or fitness facility or program (9) (see GETP8, Fig. 2.2). This form is slightly more complex than the PAR-Q and uses history, symptoms, and risk factors (including age) to assess the need for physician evaluation before beginning a new exercise program. This form was specifically designed for prescreening in health and fitness facilities. It can be completed in a few minutes, identifies moderate- and high-risk individuals, documents the results of the screening, educates the consumer and staff, and encourages appropriate use of the healthcare system. The use of the PAR-Q and AHA/ACSM Health/Fitness Facility Preparticipation Screening Questionnaire are explained in detail, and sample forms are provided in Chapter 2 of GETP8. Both of these forms have limitations and should only be interpreted by qualified staff, who should always document the results. Again, it needs to be emphasized that many sedentary individuals can safely begin a light- to moderate-intensity physical activity program without the need for extensive medical screening.

No form or set of guidelines for preparticipation screening can cover all situations. Furthermore, the use of forms such as the PAR-Q can only identify those who are at high risk; they do not differentiate between those at low and moderate risk. Additionally, most forms do not make recommendations based on intensity of the proposed exercise program. The ACSM's recommendations for medical examinations and exercise testing before participation in a new exercise program both stratify individuals into categories of low, moderate, and high risk and combine this with proposed exercise intensity to assess need of medical evaluation before the start of a new exercise program.

Although a variety of risks are associated with exercise participation, the most important is the precipitation of major cardiac events, such as a myocardial infarction or sudden cardiac death. Several studies clearly demonstrate that the transiently increased risk of cardiac arrest occurring during vigorous exercise results largely from the presence of preexisting cardiac abnormalities, particularly CVD. The importance of identifying individuals at high risk of CVD or demonstrating symptoms associated with CVD cannot be overstated for ensuring the safe participation in a physical activity program. Thus, it is critically important for exercise professionals to have a good understanding of the medical history, signs, and symptoms that require evaluation by a physician before a patient starts a new physical activity program. Important medical history includes any heart conditions, such as heart attack, cardiac catheterization, abnormal rhythms, valve disease, or congenital conditions. As described in GETP8, Table 2-3, the common CVD risk factors are all deserving of attention and include age, impaired fasting glucose, sedentary lifestyle, obesity, high cholesterol, smoking, hypertension, and family history of CVD. Important signs and symptoms (see GETP8, Table 2-2) include any form of chest discomfort or unreasonable shortness of breath with exertion, dizziness, fainting, blackouts, or cramping or burning in the legs. Limitations attributable to bone or joint issues or previous injuries should also be addressed. This is a brief overview of the medical history, signs, and symptoms that should raise concern in the exercise professional and are usually associated with referral for physician clearance. Both the ACSM (GETP8) and the AHA (11) provide guidance on when a medical referral is recommended. It should also be noted that detection of elevated BP, cholesterol, or glucose should also trigger a medical referral (7,15,16). Prescreening forms have been recommended as a minimum preexercise screening standard for entry into a light- to moderate-intensity physical activity program. After an individual has been provided with medical clearance to participate in an exercise program (as a recommended follow-up to either the AHA/ACSM Health/Fitness Facility Preparticipation Screening Questionnaire or a more comprehensive health appraisal), it is important for the exercise professional to determine whether there are any additional health-related factors that require special consideration.

OVERVIEW OF THE MEDICAL SCREENING EXAMINATION

 1.3.16-CES: Evaluate medical history and physical examination findings as they relate to health appraisal and exercise testing.

1.3.2-HFS: Knowledge of the value of the health/medical history.

1.3.13-HFS: Ability to obtain a health history and risk appraisal that includes past and current medical history, family history of cardiac disease, orthopedic limitation, prescribed medications, activity patterns, nutritional habits, stress and anxiety levels, and smoking and alcohol use.

A **medical screening examination** to evaluate the risk of starting a new physical activity program can range in complexity from a simple clinical examination to extensive diagnostic testing, depending on the age, medical history, risk factors, and symptoms of the individual. At a minimum, the medical prescreening examination should include a detailed medical history and thorough physical examination. In obtaining the medical history, every effort should be made to acquire specific information about previous medical diagnoses, particularly those pertaining to cardiac and vascular disease, as well as the associated risk factors such as hypertension, diabetes, high cholesterol, tobacco use, and family history. Particular attention should also be given to reviewing past skeletal and muscular injuries and current physical limitations caused by either acute injury or chronic conditions such as arthritis or osteoporosis. A review of the individual's medications is an important part of the medical history to identify medical problems that may have been missed during the interview and also to identify any medications that may alter the exercise prescription. Although a review of symptoms should be standard part of the examination, any symptoms of chest discomfort or shortness of breath associated with exertion should be probed in detail.

If dictated by preliminary screening, a standard physical examination should be performed. These are performed for those at moderate risk who wish to participate in vigorous exercise or anyone at high risk wishing to perform any intensity exercise. There should be particular importance placed on the assessment of the cardiovascular and respiratory systems as well as the skeletal muscular system. BP and heart rate (HR) should be measured, and an auscultatory examination of the heart and lungs should be performed. Weight and height should be measured to classify the individual as normal weight, overweight, or obese, but also to assess the potential impact of excess weight on joint health. Joint mobility should be checked, as well as range of motion (ROM) and strength. A neurologic examination that includes a balance test should be administered. Examining the feet, looking for open wounds, is particularly important in elderly individuals and those with diabetes.

Based on the information obtained during the history and examination combined with the participant's exercise goals and in accordance with published recommendations, the examining physician may elect to order or perform more advanced diagnostic or screening tests. These include exercise stress test with or without nuclear imaging (technetium or thallium), radiographs, magnetic resonance imaging, or even cardiac catheterization if symptoms warrant. For more detailed information about the medical screening, refer to Chapter 3 of the GETP8.

COMMON RISK-STRATIFICATION SCHEMA AND THEIR USES

The use of national guidelines to stratify risk of adverse health events, usually cardiac, can be very useful. Common sources of risk-stratification schema include the National Cholesterol Education Program Expert Panel on Detection, Evaluation, and Treatment of High Blood Cholesterol in Adults (NCEP ATP III); the Seventh Report of the Joint National Committee on Prevention, Detection, Evaluation, and Treatment of High Blood Pressure (JNC 7); and the American Heart Association Scientific Statement on Exercise Standards for Testing and Training (11,15,16). Although these references serve as excellent resources for risk stratification, they can also serve as a point of confusion, both in terms of using different schema to define low, moderate, and high risk and by occasionally having different thresholds of risk for the same risk factor. These differences may be caused by several reasons, but the two most obvious are the dates when guidelines were produced and the specific focus of the individual guidelines. Even a 1- or 2-year gap between when different sets of guidelines were released allows for new information to evolve that may affect acceptable risk-factor thresholds. For example, the NCEP ATP III guidelines define hypertension as systolic BP of 140 mm Hg or greater, and although JNC 7 generally agrees with this threshold, it also suggests that systolic BP >130 mm Hg should be treated like hypertension in individuals with diabetes. This example is also a good illustration of how each set of guidelines has a specific focus, such as cholesterol or BP, that is addressed in great detail, but other important risk factors are only briefly mentioned or oversimplified. Although the treatment guidelines from respected national organizations may have small inconsistencies in content, they all put a premium on the value of screening for the most common risk factors and leave the decision to treat with medication or not up to the physician. Furthermore, they all recognize the value of exercise as part of the lifestyle changes for individuals with borderline abnormalities and as an adjunct treatment for those needing drug therapy.

MEDICAL CONDITIONS THAT COMPLICATE THE EXERCISE PRESCRIPTION

There are several issues that warrant special consideration when assessing the need for further screening before a patient begins a physical activity program. There are varieties of conditions that may affect the exercise prescription; a few of the more common ones are discussed here. However, a safe strategy when a complicating medical condition is present is to assure that the individual's healthcare provider is aware of the individual's desire to become physically active and that the provider has approved this change in behavior.

CARDIOVASCULAR DISEASE

> **2.2.1-HFS: Knowledge of cardiovascular risk factors or conditions that may require consultation with medical personnel before testing or training, including inappropriate changes of resting or exercise heart rate and blood pressure, new onset discomfort in chest, neck, shoulder, or arm, changes in the pattern of discomfort during rest or exercise, fainting or dizzy spells, and claudication.**

It is well documented that regular exercise has powerful benefits for both preventing and treating CVD. However, it is also well known that an acute bout of exercise, particularly in sedentary individuals, can precipitate a cardiac event in those with preexisting CVD. Thus, exercise prescription in individuals with CVD must be done with both physician approval and input (11). Often, individuals with CVD need to start their program under medically supervised conditions, and some individuals may never progress to unsupervised exercise. Although a good strategy for all sedentary individuals starting a new exercise program, it is especially important for individuals with CVD to start slowly and progress gradually in exercise intensity and duration. The recommended physical activity goal for patients with coronary and other vascular diseases is to progress to daily aerobic exercise sessions (i.e., 7 days a week, with 5 being the minimum frequency), incorporate a moderate intensity, with each session lasting between 30 to 60 minutes in duration. Furthermore, it is suggested that this standard aerobic program be supplemented with additional lifestyle activities as well as twice-a-week resistance training (21). All individuals with CVD who wish to start an exercise program must be taught the warning signs of acute cardiac events, such as chest pain, unreasonable shortness of breath, and tingling in jaw or left hand. For more detailed discussions related to exercise for individuals with CVD, see Chapter 9 of GETP8, Chapters 22, 30, and 35 of this Resource Manual, recommendations cited in *Circulation* (11,14,21) and *Stroke* (19), as well as Web sites for the American Heart Association (www.americanheart.org) and the American Association of Cardiovascular and Pulmonary Rehabilitation (www.aacvpr.org).

HYPERTENSION

 2.2.1-HFS: Knowledge of cardiovascular risk factors or conditions that may require consultation

with medical personnel before testing or training, including inappropriate changes of resting or exercise heart rate and blood pressure; new onset discomfort in chest, neck, shoulder, or arm; changes in the pattern of discomfort during rest or exercise; fainting or dizzy spells; and claudication.

As noted earlier in this chapter, hypertension is listed as a positive risk factor for heart disease. However, hypertension is unique in that it is also considered to be a cardiovascular disease (15) of its own accord, necessitating a risk stratification of *diseased* or *high risk* (Chapter 2, GETP8). It is therefore not simply a risk factor to tally or ignore if no other risk factors are present. Hypertension is an insidious disease wherein during the initial stages there are often no signs or symptoms, lending to its ominous nickname, "the silent killer." It is a pervasive disease with more than a billion people worldwide, including 50 million Americans, diagnosed as hypertensive (16). Hypertension is often present as an underlying disease process within diabetes, chronic obstructive pulmonary disease, renal failure, and ischemic stroke (16,19). Hence, when considering exercise testing procedures and designing exercise prescriptions for hypertensive patients, it is usually necessary to account for the impact of multiple disease processes. For more detailed discussions related to exercise for individuals with hypertension, see Chapter 10 in GETP8; the ACSM position stand on exercise and hypertension (4); recommendations cited in *JAMA* (16), *Circulation* (11,14,21), and *Stroke* (19); the American Society of Hypertension's Web site (www.ash-us.org); and the AHA and AACVPR Web sites mentioned previously.

CHRONIC OBSTRUCTIVE PULMONARY DISEASE

> **3.2.1-HFS: Knowledge of pulmonary risk factors or conditions that may require consultation with medical personnel before testing or training, including asthma, exercise–induced asthma/bronchospasm, extreme breathlessness at rest or during exercise, bronchitis, and emphysema.**

Chronic obstructive pulmonary disease (COPD) is a general term used to describe long-term illnesses of the respiratory system, including such diseases as asthma, chronic bronchitis, and emphysema. The risk stages have changed: stage 0 (at risk) has been eliminated because of insufficient evidence that those exhibiting symptoms (e.g., chronic cough with sputum) actually progress to more severe stages of COPD. The four classification stages have been renamed as follows: stage 1 (previously 0)—mild; stage 2 (previously 1)—moderate; stage 3 (previously 2)—severe; and stage 4 (previously 3)—very severe (12). (See GETP8, Table 3.4 for revised spirometric information and classification schemas for identifying

and managing pulmonary conditions.) Regular exercise is an important part of rehabilitation for chronic lung disease and can help improve endurance and feelings of dyspnea (1). In addition to using the standard dyspnea 1 to 4 rating scale used during exercise (Chapter 5, GETP 8), the Modified Medial Research Council Questionnaire for Assessing the Severity of Breathlessness created by the British Medical Research Council (MRC) is an excellent adjunct health prescreening tool (12). It consists of five short questions assessing which activity patterns bring on breathlessness, with the activity pattern ranging from simple activities of daily living to strenuous exercise. The MRC has a demonstrated relationship with other health-risk assessments as well as mortality predictive value (10,17).

As with most chronic diseases, it is important to have permission from the individual's healthcare provider before starting a program. Furthermore, it is likely that a respiratory therapist or other healthcare professional will have to be involved during the initial stages for individuals who have been sedentary for an extended period of time. This is another group that stands to benefit from starting slowly and progressing gradually in exercise intensity and duration. One important safety consideration when working with anyone with a breathing disorder is making sure the individual always has enough "rescue" medication available when exercising, particularly individuals with asthma. For more detailed discussion related to exercise for individuals with COPD, see Chapter 10 of GETP8; Chapters 23, 30, and 36 of this Resource Manual; and two Web sites: the Global Initiative for Chronic Obstructive Lung Disease (www.goldcopd.com) and the American Lung Association (www.lungusa.org).

DIABETES

> **4.2.1-HFS: Knowledge of metabolic risk factors or conditions that may require consultation with medical personnel before testing or training, including obesity, metabolic syndrome, thyroid disease, kidney disease, diabetes or glucose intolerance, and hypoglycemia.**

Diabetes is a strong and independent contributor to the risk of developing CVD. This excessive risk includes CVD, peripheral vascular disease, and congestive heart failure. Diabetes is a metabolic disease that requires specific diet and exercise therapy alone or in combination with prescribed medications. Regular physical activity greatly reduces both the risk of developing diabetes and the medical complications associated with diabetes. A minimum of 150 minutes of moderate to vigorous aerobic exercise per week coupled with resistance training is recommended, allowing no more than 2 consecutive days of no activity weekly (8). However, given the large CVD risk associated with having diabetes, the prescription of exercise for individuals with the disorder must be done with great thought and care (8,9). Additional long-term complications, such as retinopathy and autonomic neuropathy, must also be considered. Vigorous exercise may exacerbate retinal detachment, and autonomic neuropathy can decrease the diabetic patient's ability to thermoregulate and adjust to postural changes (8). Given these known risks, virtually every individual with diabetes who wants to start an exercise program needs to be referred to his or her primary care doctor for clearance, which includes a graded exercise test with electrocardiographic monitoring (8). It is important to not only assess risk based on history, symptoms, and stress test results, but also to evaluate glycemic control measures as glucose-related medication requirements are likely to change with participation in an exercise program.

Many individuals with diabetes are at risk for foot ulceration attributable to peripheral neuropathy, peripheral vascular disease, or other reasons. For these individuals, it may be advisable to limit their physical activity to non–weight-bearing exercises, such as swimming or bicycling, although the weight-loss potential of these activities versus weight-bearing activity may be reduced. Also, some acute issues related to blood sugar must be addressed when an individual with diabetes who is treated with insulin or a secretagogue starts a new exercise program. For example, for these individuals, blood sugar should be checked before and after each exercise session, and blood glucose levels <100 and >300 mg·dL^{-1} should preclude exercise. Those taking other antidiabetic medications may benefit from blood glucose assessment when beginning an exercise program but can reduce the frequency of monitoring if their blood glucose values are stable. Furthermore, hypoglycemia may occur hours after the exercise session if the individual is on exogenous insulin. For more details related to exercise and diabetes, see the position stand by the American College of Sports Medicine (2), Chapter 10 of GETP8, Chapters 24 and 37 of this Resource Manual, or the American Diabetes Association's (ADA) recommendations (7,8) (www.diabetes.org).

ELDERLY INDIVIDUALS

> **5.2.1-HFS: Knowledge of musculoskeletal risk factors or conditions that may require consultation with medical personnel before testing or training, including acute or chronic back pain, osteoarthritis, rheumatoid arthritis, osteoporosis, inflammation/pain, and low back pain.**

Special consideration must be made in elderly individuals (>65 years of age) when assessing the need for medical clearance before they start exercise programs, as well as in developing the exercise prescription (3,11). Several physiologic changes occur with aging, and they affect how elderly individuals respond to acute exercise and training. Maximal HR, left ventricular (LV) function, and

cardiac output decrease with age, and there is general loss of muscle mass. For more details regarding the physiologic response to aging, refer to Chapter 5 in this Resource Manual. The musculoskeletal changes are further complicated by compromised balance and mobility in elderly individuals. Given the concerns of comorbidities, the referral of elderly individuals to their primary care doctors for clearance is most often the prudent course of action. Furthermore, many elderly individuals will benefit from medically supervised exercise sessions, and although some may graduate to unsupervised sessions, many may not. For most elderly individuals who have been sedentary for an extended period, there needs to be an extended building-up period, in terms of both intensity and duration, as they begin a new exercise program. This building-up period could take weeks to months. Furthermore, given the high prevalence of functional limitations in this population, low-impact simple activities, such as walking or stationary biking, are recommended. Additional information about exercise testing and prescription is provided in Chapter 10 of GETP8, Chapters 26 and 41 of this Resource Manual, and the American College of Sports Medicine position stand (3). Furthermore, the National Institute of Aging (NIA), a division of the National Institutes of Health (NIH), and the American Association of Retired People (AARP) Web sites provide excellent public resources for exercise in elderly individuals (http://nihseniorhealth.com;www.arp.org/health/fitness).

ARTHRITIS

> **5.2.1-HFS: Knowledge of musculoskeletal risk factors or conditions that may require consultation with medical personnel before testing or training, including acute or chronic back pain, osteoarthritis, rheumatoid arthritis, osteoporosis, inflammation/pain, and low back pain.**

Regular exercise can reduce joint pain and stiffness and increase flexibility, muscle strength, cardiac fitness, and endurance in individuals with arthritis. It also helps with weight reduction and contributes to an improved sense of well-being. Exercise is considered by many to be one part of a comprehensive arthritis treatment plan. Individuals with arthritis should discuss exercise options with their doctors and other healthcare providers. A doctor may refer the patient to a physical therapist who can help design an appropriate exercise program and teach patients about pain relief methods, proper body mechanics, and joint protection. There are many types of arthritis. Experienced doctors, physical therapists, and occupational therapists can recommend exercises that are particularly helpful for specific types of arthritis. Doctors and therapists also know specific exercises for particularly painful joints. There may be exercises that are off limits for people with a particular type of arthritis or when the joints are swollen and inflamed. Many people with arthritis begin with easy, ROM exercises and low-impact aerobics. People with arthritis can participate in a variety of, but not all, exercise programs. The three types of exercise often cited as best for people with arthritis are ROM exercises (e.g., dance), resistance training, and aerobic exercises. Weight control can be important to people who have arthritis because extra weight puts extra pressure on many joints. Some studies show that aerobic exercise can reduce inflammation in some joints. For more details related to exercise and arthritis, refer to Chapter 10 of GETP8, Chapter 40 in this Resource Manual, and the Arthritis Foundation's Web site (www.arthritis.org).

OSTEOPOROSIS

> **5.2.1-HFS: Knowledge of musculoskeletal risk factors or conditions that may require consultation with medical personnel before testing or training, including acute or chronic back pain, osteoarthritis, rheumatoid arthritis, osteoporosis, inflammation/pain, and low back pain.**

Weight-bearing exercise and resistance training have an important role in both the prevention and treatment of osteoporosis (5). However, the diagnosis of osteoporosis has its own set of safety concerns, and the start of any new exercise in an individual with osteoporosis should not be undertaken without physician approval. Particular attention must be given to frail individuals, those who have had a fracture, and those who fall frequently. Certain movements (e.g., twisting of the spine, high-impact aerobics, and bending from the waist) should be avoided in individuals with osteoporosis. A primary concern in individuals with osteoporosis is avoiding fractures, and preventing falls is essential to this goal. Thus, when working with individuals with osteoporosis, helping prevent opportunities to fall should always be a top priority. For more detailed information, refer to Chapter 10 of GETP8, Chapter 39 in this Resource Manual, the American College of Sports Medicine position stand (5), and the National Osteoporosis Foundation Web site (www.nor.org).

SPECIAL SAFETY CONSIDERATIONS FOR RESISTANCE TRAINING

Numerous investigations in healthy adults and low-risk cardiac patients have reported few orthopedic complications or cardiovascular events associated with resistance training (18). The safety of resistance testing and training in moderate- to high-risk cardiac patients requires additional study. Contraindications to resistance training are similar to those used to assess readiness to start an aerobic exercise program. Contraindications to resistance training include unstable angina, uncontrolled hypertension, uncontrolled dysrhythmias, recent history of congestive heart failure that has not been evaluated and effectively treated, severe stenotic or regurgitant valvular disease, and hypertrophic cardiomyopathy. Because patients with myocardial ischemia or poor LV function may develop wall-motion abnormalities or serious ventricular arrhythmias during resistance training exertion, moderate to good LV function and cardiorespiratory fitness (>5 or 6 metabolic equivalents) without anginal symptoms or ischemic ST-segment depression have been suggested as additional prerequisites for participation in traditional resistance training programs, with cardiac medications maintained as clinically indicated.

Low- to moderate-risk cardiac patients who wish to initiate mild to moderate resistance training should first participate in a traditional aerobic exercise program for a minimum of 5 weeks (GETP8, Chapter 9). This period permits sufficient surveillance of the patient in a supervised setting and allows the cardiorespiratory and musculoskeletal adaptations that may reduce the potential for complications to occur (6).

A preliminary orientation should establish appropriate weight loads and instruct the participant on proper lifting techniques, ROM for each exercise, correct breathing patterns to avoid straining, and the Valsalva maneuver. Because systolic BP measurements taken by the standard cuff method immediately after resistance exercise may significantly underestimate true physiologic responses, such measurement is usually not recommended. For more details related to resistance training and health, see Chapters 7 and 9 in GETP8, Chapter 29 in this Resource Manual, Pollock et al. (18), and the American College of Sports Medicine's 2002 position stand on resistance training in adults (6).

SUMMARY

The purpose of preparticipation health screening is to provide information relevant to the safety of fitness testing or beginning exercise training to identify known diseases and risk factors for CVD so that appropriate lifestyle interventions can be initiated. Furthermore, it is important to identify additional factors that require special consideration when developing an appropriate exercise prescription and programming that optimize adherence, minimize risks, and maximize benefits. The precise nature and extent of the appraisal should be determined by the age, sex, and perceived health-status characteristics of the participants, as well as the available economic, personnel, and equipment resources. The primary safety goal of a preparticipation health appraisal is to identify individuals who should receive further medical evaluation to determine whether there are contraindications to exercise testing or training or whether referral to a medically supervised exercise program is necessary.

REFERENCES

1. American College of Chest Physicians. American Association of Cardiovascular and Pulmonary Rehabilitation. ACCP/AACVPR Pulmonary Rehabilitation Guidelines Panel: Pulmonary rehabilitation: Joint ACCP/AACVPR evidence-based guidelines [review]. *Chest.* 1997;112:1363–1396.

2. American College of Sports Medicine. Position stand: Exercise and type 2 diabetes. *Med Sci Sports Exerc.* 2000;32:1345–1360.

3. American College of Sports Medicine. Position stand: Exercise and physical activity for older adults [review]. *Med Sci Sports Exerc.* 1998;30:992–1008.

4. American College of Sports Medicine. Position stand: Exercise and hypertension. *Med Sci Sports Exerc.* 2004;36:533–553.

5. American College of Sports Medicine. Position stand: Physical activity and bone health. *Med Sci Sports Exerc.* 2004;36:1985–1996.

6. American College of Sports Medicine. Position stand: Progression models in resistance training for healthy adults. *Med Sci Sports Exerc.* 2002;34:364–380.

7. American Diabetes Association. Physical activity/exercise and diabetes mellitus. *Diabetes Care.* 2004;27(suppl 1):S58–S62.

8. American Diabetes Association. Position statement: Standards of Medical Care in Diabetes—2007. Part F: Physical activity. *Diabetes Care.* 2007;30(suppl 1):S4–S41.

9. Balady GJ, Chaitman B, Driscoll D, et al. Recommendations for cardiovascular screening, staffing, and emergency policies at health/fitness facilities. *Circulation.* 1998;97:2283–2293.

10. Bestall JC, Paul EA, Garrod R, Gamham R, Jones PW, Wedzicha JA. Usefulness of the Medical Research Council (MRC) dyspnoea scale as a measure of disability in patients with chronic obstructive pulmonary disease. *Thorax.* 1999;54:581–586.

11. Fletcher GF, Balady GJ, Amsterdam EA, et al. Exercise standards for testing and training: a statement for healthcare professionals from the American Heart Association. *Circulation.* 2001;104:1694–1740.

12. Global Initiative for Chronic Obstructive Lung Disease. Global strategy for the diagnosis, management, and prevention of chronic obstructive pulmonary disease. [cited 2007 Oct 1]. Available from: www.goldcopd.com.

13. Ham SA, Yore MM, Sapkota S, Kohl HW. Trends in physical activity during leisure-time: 35 states and District of Columbia, United States 1988–2002. *MMWR Morb Mortal Wkly Rep.* 2004;53:76–81.

14. Leon AS, Franklin BA, Costa F, et al. Cardiac rehabilitation and secondary prevention of coronary heart disease: an American Heart Association scientific statement from the Council on Clinical Cardiology and the Council on Nutrition, Physical Activity, and Metabolism in collaboration with the American Association of Cardiovascular and Pulmonary Rehabilitation. *Circulation.* 2005; 111:369–376.

15. National Cholesterol Education Program. Expert Panel on Detection, Evaluation, and Treatment of High Blood Cholesterol in Adults: Executive Summary of the Third Report of the National Cholesterol Education Program (NCEP) Expert Panel on Detection, Evaluation, and Treatment of High Blood Cholesterol in Adults (Adult Treatment Panel III). *JAMA.* 2001;285: 2486–2497.

16. National High Blood Pressure Education Program. The Seventh Report of the Joint National Committee on Detection, Evaluation, and Treatment of High Blood Pressure (JNC VII). *JAMA.* 2003;289: 2560–2572.

17. Nishimura K, Izumi GT, Tsukino M, Oga T. Dyspnea is a better predictor of 5-year survival than airway obstruction in patients with COPD. *Chest.* 2002;121:1434–1440.

18. Pollock ML, Franklin BF, Balady GF, et al. Resistance exercise in individuals with and without cardiovascular disease: benefits, rationale, safety and prescription. *Circulation.* 2000;101:828–833.

19. Sacco RL, Adams R, Albers G, et al. Guidelines for prevention of stroke in patients with ischemic stroke or transient ischemic attack: a statement for healthcare professionals from the American Heart Association/American Stroke Association Council on Stroke. *Stroke.* 2006;37:577–617.

20. Shephard RJ, Thomas S, Weller I. The Canadian home fitness test: 1991 update. *Sports Med.* 1991;11:358.

21. Smith SC, Allen J, Blair SN, et al. AHA/ACC guidelines for secondary prevention for patients with coronary and other atherosclerotic vascular disease: 2006 update. *Circulation.* 2006;113:2363–2372.

22. U.S. Department of Health and Human Services. *Physical Activity and Health: A Report of the Surgeon General, Atlanta, GA. U.S. Department of Health and Human Services, Centers for Disease Control and Prevention, National Center for Chronic Disease Prevention and Health Promotion.* Washington, D.C.: U.S. Government Printing Office; 1996.

SELECTED REFERENCES FOR FURTHER READING

American Association of Cardiovascular and Pulmonary Rehabilitation. *AAVCPR Cardiac Rehab Resource Manual.* Champaign (IL): Human Kinetics; 2006.

American Association of Cardiovascular and Pulmonary Rehabilitation. *Guidelines for Cardiac Rehabilitation and Secondly Prevention Programs.* 4th ed. Champaign (IL): Human Kinetics; 2004.

National Strength and Conditioning Association. *Essentials of Strength Training and Conditioning.* Champaign (IL): Human Kinetics; 2005.

INTERNET RESOURCES

- American Association of Cardiovascular and Pulmonary Rehabilitation (www.aacvpr.org)
- American Association of Retired People (AARP) (www.aarp.org/health/fitness)
- American Diabetes Association (www.diabetes.org)
- American Heart Association (www.americanheart.org)
- American Lung Association (www.lungusa.org)
- American Society of Hypertension (www.ash-us.org)
- Arthritis Foundation (www.arthritis.org)
- Global Initiative for Chronic Obstructive Lung Disease (www.goldcopd.com)
- National Institute of Aging (NIA) (http://nihseniorhealth.com)
- National Osteoporosis Foundation (www.nor.org)

In this chapter, we will examine the evidence linking physical inactivity and chronic disease and the evidence linking increased physical activity and reductions in risk for all-cause and cardiovascular mortality, cardiovascular disease, stroke, type 2 diabetes mellitus, hypertension, and cancer. We will contrast data on physical inactivity as a contributor to disease with physical activity as treatment for this condition and contrast the evidence supported by assessments of cardiorespiratory fitness with those of physical activity level.

The importance of regular movement to the maintenance of physical and mental health has recently drawn a focus to physical inactivity as a disease entity (16). An increasing volume of scientific evidence implicates physical inactivity as a major modifiable risk factor for several chronic diseases and premature mortality (18,57,99).

Given the high prevalence of physical inactivity observed in many developed and developing nations, the burden of physical inactivity on public health is substantial (15,24,88). This concept is not entirely new. For many years, investigators have considered moderate levels of physical activity as the "normal" condition and low to extremely low levels of physical activity as associated with higher risk for chronic diseases (54). It has become increasingly apparent in the interim that physical inactivity not only leads to an alarming increase in metabolic risk (102), but also results in a significant financial burden to the general population. However, this phenomenon is not restricted to technologically advanced countries. Even in developing countries, physical inactivity is a major risk factor for all-cause mortality and cardiovascular morbidity and mortality. For example, in China, where

> > > **KEY TERMS**

Confidence interval (CI): A range around a relative risk estimate that refers to the probability that the range includes the true value of the relative risk estimate.

Dose–response relationship: A relationship between two variables in which any increase or change in one variable is associated with a corresponding change in the other variable. A dose–response relationship does not have to be linear, but it can follow several patterns (e.g., curvilinear, quadratic).

Epidemiology: The study of the distribution and determinants of disease or injury.

Intervention study: A study in which subjects are assigned to undergo an intervention to test the strength of that intervention on previously selected outcome variables, such as cardiorespiratory fitness, serum levels of lipids or lipoproteins, parameters of insulin action, bone mineral density, muscle strength and endurance, or the like. The best intervention studies are those that randomly assign study subjects to treatment assignment, one of which is a null intervention assignment, or

control group, which are carried out in parallel. These are referred to as **randomized controlled clinical trials (RCT)** and carry the highest level of evidence relating an activity or intervention to prespecified outcomes.

Physical activity: A behavior that is any bodily movement produced by the contraction of skeletal muscles that substantially increases energy expenditure.

Physical inactivity: A behavioral state of not achieving, on a regular basis, a certain minimal common standard of physical activity.

Physical fitness: An attained set of attributes (i.e., cardiorespiratory endurance; flexibility; body composition; and skeletal muscle endurance, and strength) that relates to the ability to perform physical activity.

Relative risk (RR): The risk of disease or injury in one group compared with another group. The two groups usually differ in terms of one or more key factors (e.g., physical activity levels). RR is usually expressed as a risk ratio comparing incidence or prevalence rates among two groups.

underweight is a risk factor for all-cause mortality, physical inactivity remains a major risk marker (76). The purpose of this chapter is to review the current state of the evidence linking physical activity status to the risk of selected chronic diseases.

In October 2008 the federal government released 'The Physical Activity Guidelines for Americans'. (See Selected references for further reading.) This for the first time, provides a national government-sanctioned recommendation for physical activity for all ages. It was developed with the broader view that links physical inactivity to the development of many chronic diseases. There are also specific guidelines for those with disabilities, children and pregnant/post partum women. The Surgeon General's Report on Physical Activity and Health serves as a valuable resource of the body of literature available before 1996 (99). A report of the Institute of Medicine that briefly reviews physical activity and chronic disease is available (92), summarizing some of the new data available before October 2006.

IS PHYSICAL ACTIVITY OR PHYSICAL FITNESS THE APPROPRIATE ENDPOINT FOR STUDY?

> **1.7.27-HFS: Ability to differentiate between the amount of physical activity required for health benefits and/or fitness development.**

A question currently of interest to physical activity epidemiologists is whether physical activity or physical fitness best predicts the risk of chronic disease. Whereas **physical activity** is a behavior that is any bodily movement produced by the contraction of skeletal muscles that substantially increases energy expenditure, **physical fitness** is an attained set of attributes (i.e., cardiorespiratory endurance, flexibility, body composition, and skeletal muscle endurance and strength) that relates to the ability to perform physical activity (102). As noted subsequently, whereas physical fitness can be accurately and precisely measured, it is influenced by inherited factors (17) as well as by volitional increases in physical activity, and it is not readily assessable to measurement in large epidemiologic studies. In contrast, physical activity is harder to measure precisely, especially across the spectrum of intensities, using self-report survey tools that are commonly used in large prospective observational studies. Although physical fitness has several components, the majority of the studies discussed in this chapter have relied on an index of cardiorespiratory fitness in assessing relationships with chronic disease. However, since the previous version of this manual, there has begun to appear more extensive literature outlining intervention studies that directly test the relationship between physical activity and exercise and disease outcomes (22,102). Important areas of future research include the degree to

which other components of physical fitness, such as musculoskeletal fitness, and forms of exercise other than aerobic training, for instance resistance training and flexibility training, are associated with the risk of chronic diseases and intermediates of chronic disease risk. These intermediates include serum lipids, insulin sensitivity, blood pressure control, and inflammatory state.

Some reviews (11) and meta-analyses (113) conclude that both physical activity and cardiorespiratory fitness are related to the risk of coronary heart disease (CHD) and other health outcomes in a **dose–response relationship**. In other words, for any increase in physical activity or fitness, there was a corresponding reduction in the risk of chronic diseases and all-cause mortality. However, these data will not be conclusive until a prospective study can be performed.

Epidemiologic studies depend on indirect measures of physical activity and exercise, such as recall surveys (11), which are known to underestimate relatively low-intensity exercise. As evidence of this finding and probably for this reason, the relationships across categories of cardiorespiratory fitness are different than for physical activity. In general, the dose–response relationship across categories of cardiorespiratory fitness is steeper than the relationship across categories of physical activity. Thus, the finding that physical fitness may be a better predictor of health outcomes is to be expected because of the more objective and reliable nature of the measurements. Whatever the outcome of the continuing scientific discourse around the issue of physical activity versus physical fitness as predictors of chronic disease, it is clear that public health initiatives should target increasing physical activity levels of the population rather than increasing physical fitness (12). Through an increase in physical activity levels, there should be a consequent increase in physical fitness levels. Although from 30% to 50% of the variation in cardiorespiratory fitness levels can be explained by familial factors (genetic and shared lifestyle factors [17]), the most logical way to increase physical fitness levels is through an increase in physical activity. Recent studies have demonstrated that relatively modest levels of physical activity can result in measurable and significant increases in cardiorespiratory fitness (22). Some hypothesize that this phenomenon becomes more apparent as the mean level of physical activity and cardiorespiratory fitness in the general population continues to decline.

THE SCIENTIFIC EVIDENCE

 1.2.3-HFS: Knowledge of risk factors that may be favorably modified by physical activity habits.

This chapter has traditionally presented scientific evidence primarily from the field of physical activity epidemiology. With advancements in the field, some strong evidence from intervention studies and clinical trials can now also be included. **Epidemiology** is the study of the distribution and determinants of disease or injury, and physical activity epidemiologists place a particular emphasis on physical inactivity and poor physical fitness as risk factors for disease and injury. The studies described in this chapter use mainly observational prospective designs in which a group of people are evaluated for a given set of characteristics (age, sex, physical activity, physical fitness, obesity) and followed over time to describe the incidence of disease, injury, or mortality. In most studies, the incidence of chronic disease in two or more groups that differ from one another in their level of physical activity or fitness are compared with one another using a ratio called the **relative risk (RR)**. The confidence we have in the point estimate of the RR (i.e., the precision) is generally expressed as a 90% or 95% **confidence interval (CI)** around the RR. If the 95% CI crosses the value of 1, one would generally say that the RR is not statistically significant. For an in-depth description of the study designs used in epidemiology with reference to research in exercise science, readers are referred to the reviews of Heath (46) and Paffenbarger (82).

The idea that physically active individuals are generally healthier than their sedentary peers has been around for centuries; however, modern physical activity epidemiology arguably began with the classic studies of occupational physical activity and the incidence of CHD conducted by Jeremy Morris et al. in the 1950s. Briefly, these early studies demonstrated that men in physically demanding occupations (bus conductors and postmen) had lower incident CHD rates than men in less demanding occupations (bus drivers and office workers [81]). Over the subsequent 50 years, the field of physical activity epidemiology has progressed greatly by extending and expanding upon the work of Morris et al. (83).

PHYSICAL ACTIVITY AND ALL-CAUSE MORTALITY

Although the purpose of this chapter is to outline the relationships between physical activity levels and specific chronic diseases, it is useful to start with a discussion of all-cause mortality. Among the major causes of mortality in the United States are heart disease (27.2%), cancer (23.1%), stroke (6.3%), and diabetes mellitus (3.1%) (50). Thus, discussions of physical activity and all-cause mortality largely reflect the relationship between physical activity and these major chronic diseases. However, deaths caused by other causes such as suicide, homicide, infectious diseases, and accidents are included under the rubric of "all-cause mortality," so the results are diluted by these causes of death that are not linked with physical activity by a pathway of biologic plausibility.

For detailed reviews of the role of physical activity in averting premature mortality, readers are referred to two excellent reviews of the topic (68,69). Two classic studies are used here to illustrate the relationships between physical activity and cardiorespiratory fitness and all-cause mortality. First, the Aerobics Center Longitudinal Study (ACLS) is a prospective observational study of physical activity, physical fitness, and health outcomes among men and women receiving a preventive medical examination, including a graded exercise treadmill test, at the Cooper Clinic in Dallas, Texas. The results depicted in Figure 11-1 are from an analysis of approximately 10,000 men and 3,000 women followed for 8 years for all-cause mortality in relation to initial level (quintiles) of cardiorespiratory fitness (Fig. 11-1, top panel [13]). A salient inverse relationship between cardiorespiratory fitness and all-cause mortality was observed in both men and women. Men and women in the lowest fitness quintile were 3.44 (95% confidence interval [CI]: 2.05–5.77) and 4.65 (95% CI: 2.22–9.75) times more likely to die of any cause compared with men and women in the upper quintile, respectively. The greatest decrease in the risk of mortality occurred when moving between the first and second quintiles. Of interest, in a follow-up to this study, when men increased their fitness level, they decreased their cardiovascular risk, such that for every minute of increase in time to exhaustion on a treadmill test, the cardiovascular risk was decreased 8% (14). It was discovered that men could progress from the lowest quintile for fitness to the next (higher) quintile by participating in a program similar to the ACSM/AHA recommendations for physical activity for health, i.e., a minimum of to 30 minutes of moderate-intensity aerobic physical activity on 5 days each week or 20 minutes of vigorous-intensity aerobic activity on 3 days each week (45).

Second, the Harvard Alumni Study is a prospective observational study of approximately 17,000 men who attended Harvard University between 1916 and 1950. The results of a 16-year follow-up of physical activity levels and all-cause mortality revealed an inverse dose–response relationship between physical activity levels and all-cause mortality (Fig. 11-1, bottom panel [84]). Greater levels of physical activity were associated with a lower risk of death from all causes, and men who expended >2,000 kcal · week^{-1} (8,372 kJ · week^{-1}) of energy in physical activity had a 27% lower risk of mortality compared with men expending <2,000 kcal/week^{-1}. For an average person walking at 4 mph, approximately 400 kcal are expended each hour. Thus, an energy expenditure of 2,000 kcal can be accumulated in about 5 hours of brisk walking per week. A clear dose–response relationship between physical activity or physical fitness and all-cause mortality has been observed in these and many other studies.

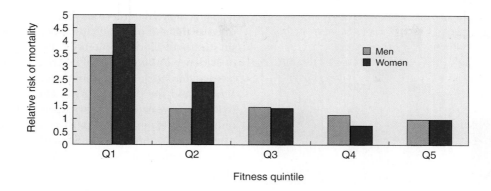

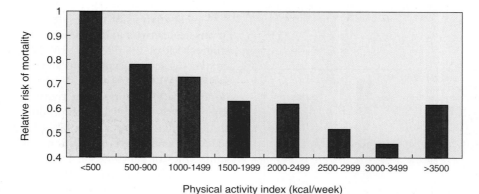

FIGURE 11-1. Relative risks of all-cause mortality across levels of cardiorespiratory fitness in the Aerobics Center Longitudinal Study (13) (*top panel*) and physical activity in the Harvard Alumni Study (84) (*bottom panel*).

CHANGES IN PHYSICAL ACTIVITY OR FITNESS AND ALL-CAUSE MORTALITY

Some of the strongest evidence for an effect of physical activity or physical fitness on mortality rates comes from studies of changes over time and their relationship with mortality. Although there is consistent evidence from intervention studies that increases in physical activity result in improvements in intermediate markers for chronic disease (27,31,56,70), it is much more difficult to demonstrate changes in actual risk of disease caused by changes in physical activity levels. A minimum requirement for these types of studies is an assessment of physical activity or fitness performed twice, separated by a significant period of time, along with a subsequent follow-up period for ascertainment of mortality.

Only eight published studies have related natural changes in physical activity or changes in physical fitness over time to changes in the risk of all-cause mortality (9,14,29,40,62,72,85,110). Figure 11-2 presents the results of studies that used comparable fitness or physical activity change groups. Participants who maintain persistently high physical activity or fitness levels over a period of time are less likely to die than those who maintain consistently low physical activity or fitness levels. Additionally, those who increase their level of physical activity or fitness over time have a decreased risk of mortality

compared with those who were consistently physically inactive or unfit. In general, a reduced risk of mortality is also observed in participants who decreased their physical activity over time compared with those who were persistently unfit. These results suggest that there are some short-term benefits of physical activity that may persist for a period of time after a change in physical activity levels. Given that physical activity and fitness were assessed at only two time points in these studies, it is impossible to determine when the changes actually occurred during the interval between the two measurements.

In addition to the studies presented in Figure 11-2, two other studies have examined the effects of changes in physical activity or fitness and all-cause mortality. Swedish women who decreased their physical activity levels over 6 years had approximately double (relative risk [RR] = 2.07) the risk of dying over a subsequent 20-year follow-up period compared with women who maintained consistent physical activity levels over the same time period (72). Finally, a study of changes in physical fitness over 7 to 10 years among men 20 to 60 years of age demonstrated an inverse relationship between changes in physical fitness and all-cause mortality, regardless of initial level of fitness (29). Taken together, all of the available studies show a consistently lower risk of all-cause mortality in people who maintain high levels of physical activity or physical fitness over a period of years compared with

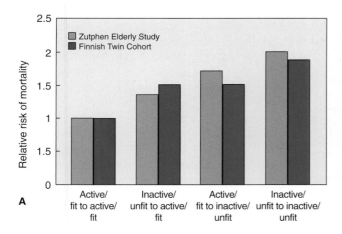

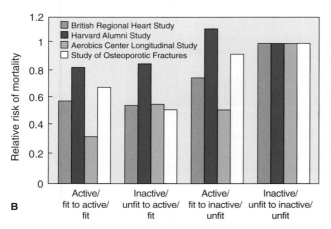

FIGURE 11-2. Changes in physical activity or cardiorespiratory fitness and relative risks of all-cause mortality. **A** presents the results of two studies that used the active/fit to active/fit group as the reference group; results in left bars are from the Zutphen Elderly Study (9), and results in right bars are from a Finnish twin cohort (62). **B** presents the results of four studies that used the inactive/unfit to inactive/unfit group as the reference group; results from left to right bars are from the British Regional Heart Study (110), results in red are from the Harvard Alumni Study (85), results in pink are from the Aerobics Center Longitudinal Study (14), and results in white are from the Study of Osteoporotic Fractures (40). The average time between successive measurements of physical activity or cardiorespiratory fitness ranged from approximately 6 years to 11 to 15 years.

those who decreased to or maintained low levels of physical activity or physical fitness over the same time period.

PHYSICAL ACTIVITY AND CARDIORESPIRATORY HEALTH

The most studied chronic disease in relation to physical activity and physical fitness is coronary heart disease (CHD), largely because CHD is a leading cause of death in many developed countries and there is biologic plausibility linking physical activity with CHD risk. Several excellent reviews and meta-analyses have been written on the topic of physical activity and CHD (8,60,89), and the

reader is referred to these and the general references identified at the end of this chapter. Beginning with the classic studies of Morris et al. in the 1950s (81), a large body of evidence linking physical inactivity to the risk of CHD has accumulated. The cardioprotective effects of physical activity and the proatherogenic effects of physical inactivity are now being acknowledged by the medical community. For example, the most recent guidelines for the primary prevention of cardiovascular disease and stroke from the American Heart Association emphasize regular, appropriate physical activity as an integral part of maintaining a healthy lifestyle, a cornerstone of primary through tertiary prevention (104).

A meta-analysis of the results from published studies of physical activity and CHD estimated a summary (four studies) RR of 1.4 (95% CI: 1.0–1.8) comparing sedentary versus active occupations and a summary (five studies) RR of 1.6 (95% CI: 1.3–1.8) for low versus high nonoccupational physical activity (8). The corresponding analysis for CHD death produced a summary (five studies) relative risk of 1.9 (95% CI: 1.6–2.2) comparing sedentary and active occupations and a summary (two studies) RR of 1.9 (95% CI: 1.0–3.4) for low versus high nonoccupational physical activity (8). A review of the rigorous principles of epidemiology as they relate to the relationship between physical inactivity and CHD suggests that physical inactivity is linked with CHD in a causal manner (82). As a result of this strong body of evidence, in 1992, the American Heart Association elevated physical inactivity to a major modifiable risk factor for cardiovascular disease (33). A more recent review supports the notion that the inverse relationship between physical activity and CHD is causal and that it follows a dose–response pattern (60). In other words, higher levels of physical activity result in an incrementally reduced risk of CHD. That being said, this relationship has yet to be proven rigorously in a prospective randomized study.

PHYSICAL ACTIVITY AND STROKE

Studies of physical activity and risk of stroke have produced interesting results. Table 11-1 presents the available prospective studies of physical activity or physical fitness and risk of stroke that reported estimates of RR (3,4,10,30,39,44,53,58,64,65,66,71,95,97,108). The trends reported in Table 11-1 are also supported by two case-control studies (48,96) that demonstrated significant associations between physical activity and stroke risk. In most studies, there is a trend toward an increased risk of stroke among those who are physically inactive, but an inverse dose–response relationship between physical activity levels and stroke risk is generally not found (60). It has been pointed out that whereas studies with more cases and a more detailed assessment of physical activity have found an inverse dose–response relationship between physical activity and stroke, studies with less

TABLE 11-1. RESULTS OF PROSPECTIVE LONGITUDINAL STUDIES OF PHYSICAL INACTIVITY OR PHYSICAL FITNESS AND RSK OF STROKE THAT PROVIDED RELATIVE RISK ESTIMATES

POPULATION	SAMPLE SIZE	STROKE CLASSIFICATION	ACTIVITY/FITNESS CLASSIFICATION	RR (95% CI)
Finnish women (97)	3,688	Incident stroke (ICD 430–437)	None vs some LTPA	1.30 (0.73–2.16)*
Finnish men (97)	3,978	Incident stroke (ICD 430–437)	None vs some LTPA	1.00 (0.65–1.62)*
Swedish men (44)	7,495	Total stroke mortality	PA score 1 vs scores 2–4	1.2 (0.8–1.8)
		Subarachnoid hemorrhage mortality	PA score 1 vs scores 2–4	1.8 (0.6–5.5)
		Intracerebral hemorrhage mortality	PA score 1 vs scores 2–4	1.1 (0.4–3.7)
		Cerebral infarction mortality	PA score 1 vs scores 2–4	1.2 (0.7–2.0)
		Unspecified stroke mortality	PA score 1 vs scores 2–4	1.2 (0.6–2.2)
Seventh-day Adventist men (71)	9,484	Stroke mortality	Low vs moderate PA	1.28 (1.00–1.64)
			Low vs high PA	1.06 (0.74–1.54)
British men (108)	7,630	Incident stroke (ICD 430–438)	None vs occasional PA	1.25 (0.59–2.50)
			None vs light PA	1.67 (0.77–5.00)
			None vs moderate PA	1.67 (0.67–5.00)
			None vs moderately vigorous PA	1.67 (0.63–5.00)
			None vs vigorous PA	5.00 (0.67–>10)
Asian American men (3)	7,530	Incident hemorrhagic stroke	Middle vs high tertile PA	2.2 (0.8–6.4)
			Low vs high tertile PA	3.7 (1.3–10.4)
		Incident thromboembolic stroke	*Nonsmokers*	
			Middle vs high tertile PA	1.7 (1.0–2.8)
			Low vs high tertile PA	1.8 (1.1–3.1)
			Smokers	
			Middle vs high tertile PA	0.6 (0.4–1.0)
			Low vs high tertile PA	1.2 (0.8–1.8)
Framingham Study men (58)	1,228	Incident stroke	Tertile 1 vs tertile 2 PA	2.44 (1.45–4.17)
			Tertile 1 vs tertile 3 PA	1.89 (1.19–2.94)
Framingham Study women (58)	1,676	Incident stroke	Tertile 1 vs tertile 2 PA	1.03 (0.68–1.56)
			Tertile 1 vs tertile 3 PA	0.83 (0.51–1.33)
U.S. white women (39)	1,473	Incident stroke	Moderate vs high LTPA	1.80 (0.52–6.22)
			Low vs high LTPA	3.13 (0.95–10.32)
		Incident nonhemorrhagic stroke	Moderate vs high LTPA	1.54 (0.44–5.42)
			Low vs high LTPA	2.89 (0.87–9.55)
U.S. white men (39)	1,285	Incident stroke	Moderate vs high LTPA	1.17 (0.61–2.27)
			Low vs high PA	1.24 (0.63–2.41)
		Incident nonhemorrhagic stroke	Moderate vs high LTPA	1.16 (0.58–2.32)
			Low vs high LTPA	1.10 (0.54–2.23)
U.S. black men and women (39)	771	Incident stroke	Moderate vs high LTPA	1.33 (0.63–2.79)
			Low vs high PA	1.33 (0.67–2.63)
		Incident nonhemorrhagic stroke	Moderate vs high LTPA	1.34 (0.61–2.94)
			Low vs high LTPA	1.43 (0.70–2.94)
Swedish men (95)	7,142	Stroke mortality	Sedentary vs moderate/high PA	1.12 (0.61–2.04)
Dutch men (10)	802	Stroke mortality (ICD 430–438)	Low vs middle tertile PA	1.54 (0.80–3.03)
			Low vs upper tertile PA	1.82 (0.79–4.17)
Harvard University alumni (66)	11,130	Incident stroke	<4,184 vs 4,184–8,367 kJ/wk PA	1.32 (1.02–1.69)
			<4,184 vs 8,368–12,548 kJ/wk PA	1.85 (1.32–2.63)
			<4,184 vs 12,549–16,736 kJ/wk PA	1.28 (0.87–1.89)
			<4,184 vs ≥16,736 kJ/wk PA	1.22 (0.88–1.72)
Reykjavik men (4)	4,484	Incident stroke (ICD 430–434,436)	None vs some PA after age 40	1.45 (0.99–2.13)
		Incident ischemic stroke	None vs some PA after age 40	1.61 (1.03–2.50)
ARIC study men and women (30)	14,575	Incident ischemic stroke	Low vs high quartile LTPA	1.12 (0.73–1.75)
U.S. male physicians (65)	21,823	Incident stroke	None vs vigorous PA 1 time/wk^{-1}	1.27 (0.97–1.64)
			None vs vigorous PA 2–4 times/wk^{-1}	1.25 (1.01–1.54)
			None vs vigorous PA 5 times/wk^{-1}	1.27 (0.97–1.64)

(continued)

TABLE 11-1. RESULTS OF PROSPECTIVE LONGITUDINAL STUDIES OF PHYSICAL INACTIVITY OR PHYSICAL FITNESS AND RSK OF STROKE THAT PROVIDED RELATIVE RISK ESTIMATES (*Continued*)

POPULATION	SAMPLE SIZE	STROKE CLASSIFICATION	ACTIVITY/FITNESS CLASSIFICATION	RR (95% CI)
		Incident ischemic stroke	None vs vigorous PA 1 time/wk^{-1}	1.18 (0.88–1.56)
			None vs vigorous PA 2–4 times/wk^{-1}	1.19 (0.93–1.49)
			None vs vigorous PA 5 times/·wk^{-1}	1.15 (0.86–1.52)
		Incident hemorrhagic stroke	None vs vigorous PA 1 time/wk^{-1}	1.69 (0.85–3.33)
			None vs vigorous PA 2–4 times/wk^{-1}	1.45 (0.86–2.44)
			None vs vigorous PA 5 times/wk^{-1}	1.82 (0.89–3.70)
U.S. female nurses (53)	72,488	Incident stroke	Quintile 1 vs 2 PA	1.02 (0.78–1.33)
			Quintile 1 vs 3 PA	1.22 (0.91–1.64)
			Quintile 1 vs 4 PA	1.35 (0.99–1.85)
			Quintile 1 vs 5 PA	1.52 (1.10–2.13)
		Incident ischemic stroke	Quintile 1 vs 2 PA	1.15 (0.81–1.61)
			Quintile 1 vs 3 PA	1.20 (0.84–1.72)
			Quintile 1 vs 4 PA	1.32 (0.90–1.92)
			Quintile 1 vs 5 PA	1.92 (1.25–3.03)
		Incident hemorrhagic stroke	Quintile 1 vs 2 PA	1.09 (0.62–1.89)
			Quintile 1 vs 3 PA	1.12 (0.63–2.00)
			Quintile 1 vs 4 PA	1.45 (0.76–2.78)
			Quintile 1 vs 5 PA	0.98 (0.55–1.72)
U.S. men (64)	16,877	Stroke mortality (ICD 430–438)	Low vs moderate aerobic fitness	2.70 (1.20–5.88)
			Low vs high aerobic fitness	3.13 (1.22–8.33)

*95% confidence interal calculated from 90% confiidence interval reported in study.

ARIC, Atherosclerosis Risk In Communities; CI, confiidence interval; ICD, International Classifiication of Diseases; PA, physical activity; LTPA, leisure-time physical activity; RR, relative ris

stringent designs have produced weaker results (7,48). Only one study has examined an objective measure of cardiorespiratory fitness in relation to the risk of mortality from stroke. A sample of 16,878 men from the ACLS was followed prospectively for 10 years to evaluate the relationship between baseline cardiorespiratory fitness level and stroke mortality. Men in the low-fitness category had 2.70 (95% CI: 1.20–5.88) and 3.13 (95% CI: 1.22–8.33) times the risk of developing a stroke during the follow-up period compared with men in the moderate- and high-fit categories, respectively (64). These results support the notion that studies that use more objective measures of physical activity or physical fitness may produce stronger results than those that use less objective measures. Conversely, physical inactivity appears to be a significant risk factor for stroke.

Because of methodologic constraints, most studies have reported relationships with total stroke incidence or mortality rather than examining ischemic or hemorrhagic stroke separately. Given the strong inverse relationship between physical activity and CHD, it seems logical that physical inactivity should be related to ischemic stroke because it shares the same underlying pathophysiologic mechanisms with ischemic heart disease (60). However, studies that examined the effects of physical activity on both ischemic and hemorrhagic stroke have found mixed results. For example, whereas data from the U.S. Nurses' Health Study demonstrated a significant inverse dose–response relationship between physical activity and both total stroke ($P = 0.005$) and ischemic stroke ($P = 0.003$) incidence, the trend for hemorrhagic stroke was less clear and not significant ($P = 0.88$) (53). On the other hand, results from the Physicians' Health Study demonstrated a significant inverse trend between physical activity and total stroke incidence ($P = 0.04$), and the relationships appeared stronger for hemorrhagic stroke than for ischemic stroke in subgroup analyses (65). Thus, there is a need for more research addressing the protective effects of physical activity, specifically on hemorrhagic versus ischemic stroke.

In summary, physical activity provides protection against stroke. It is unclear whether a dose–response or a threshold relationship exists, but better-designed studies tend to show stronger results. There is a need for more studies of physical activity, fitness, and stroke, particularly in women and minority groups, and for those who test hypotheses regarding dose–response issues.

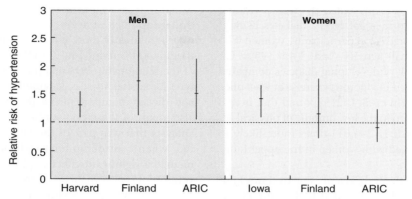

FIGURE 11-3. Relative risks of incident hypertension comparing low versus high physical activity levels in published studies. Data for Harvard alumni are from Paffenbarger et al. (86), Finnish men and women are from Haapanen et al. (43), Atherosclerosis Risk in Communities (ARIC) study men and women are from Pereira et al. (87), and from Folsom et al. for the Iowa women (34). Error bars denote 95% confidence intervals.

PHYSICAL ACTIVITY AND HYPERTENSION

Hypertension is a prevalent chronic disease in developed nations. For example, it is estimated that in 2000, approximately 50 million Americans had hypertension (2). Given the high prevalence of hypertension, it is interesting that there have been relatively few prospective studies of physical activity and incident hypertension (34,43,86,87). Figure 11-3 presents the risk ratios from available studies. The first epidemiologic investigation of physical activity levels and hypertension was published using data from 14,998 men from the Harvard Alumni Study who were followed prospectively for 6 to 10 years. The risk of developing hypertension was 1.30 (95% CI: 1.09–1.55) times higher in men expending <2000 kcal/week in physical activity versus those expending >2,000 kcal/week (86). Similarly, Iowa women with "low" physical activity levels were 1.43 (95% CI: 1.11–1.67) times more likely to develop hypertension compared with women with "high" physical activity levels over a 2-year follow-up period (34). Two more recent population-based studies that included both men and women as participants have also shown a protective effect of physical activity on the risk of hypertension (43,87) (Fig. 11-3). Thus, although there have been few prospective studies of hypertension risk, the results are consistent in showing a protective effect of physical activity in both men and women.

PHYSICAL ACTIVITY, TYPE 2 DIABETES, AND THE METABOLIC SYNDROME

Like many of the chronic diseases associated with modern living, type 2 or adult-onset diabetes mellitus is a multifactorial disease with no established single cause. Rather, a host of risk factors predisposes individuals to develop the disease. The traditional risk factors for type 2 diabetes include older age, obesity, a family history of diabetes, his-

tory of gestational diabetes, physical inactivity, and race or ethnicity (1). Whereas older age, a family history of diabetes, race or ethnicity, and a history of gestational diabetes are nonmodifiable risk factors, physical inactivity and obesity are modifiable risk factors, ones over which individuals have some control. There is consistent evidence that a physically active lifestyle provides protection against the development of type 2 diabetes, and the relationship follows a clear dose–response pattern. The results of available prospective studies of physical activity and incident type 2 diabetes are presented in Figure 11-4. Three of the major epidemiologic investigations of physical activity and type 2 diabetes are described below.

The Nurses' Health Study is a prospective cohort study of 121,700 U.S. female nurses aged 30 to 55 years, established

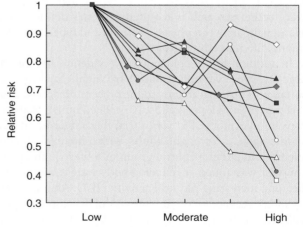

FIGURE 11-4. Results of longitudinal prospective studies of physical activity and incident type 2 diabetes. Physical activity levels are defined in the individual studies. Data are from Manson et al. (75) ◇ (women), Manson et al. (74) ◆ (men), Haapanen et al. (43) □ (women) ■ (men), Hu et al. (52) ▲ (men), Wannamethee et al. (109) △ (men), Helmrich et al. (47) ○ (men), Burchfiel et al. (20) • (men), and Hu et al. (51) – (men).

in 1976. Manson et al. (75) presented the results relating physical activity levels to incident type 2 diabetes using 8 years of follow-up data on 87,253 participants. Women who engaged in no physical activity had 1.45 (95% CI: 1.00–2.08) times the risk of developing diabetes compared with women who engaged in vigorous exercise at least once a week. More recently, Hu et al. (52) reported that over 8 years of follow-up, women in the low quintile of physical activity were 1.35 (95% CI: 1.12–1.61) times more likely to develop diabetes compared with women in the upper quintile of physical activity.

The Physicians' Health Study is a prospective, randomized, double-blind, placebo-controlled trial of the effects of low-dose aspirin and β-carotene on cardiovascular diseases and cancer. A total of 22,271 male physicians aged 40 to 84 years at entry in 1982 participated. Manson et al. (74) reported the results relating physical activity and incident type 2 diabetes after 5 years of follow-up. Similar to the results from the Nurses' Health Study, men who were physically inactive had 1.41 (95% CI: 1.10–1.79) times the risk of developing diabetes compared with men who engaged in vigorous activity at least once a week.

The Health Professionals' Follow-up Study started in 1986 when 51,529 male health professionals, including dentists, optometrists, pharmacists, podiatrists, osteopaths, and veterinarians, enrolled in the study. Hu et al. (51) reported the results for physical inactivity and incident diabetes in the 10-year follow-up of 37,918 of the men aged 40 to 75 years at baseline. Men in the low versus the high quintile were 1.61 (95% CI: 1.32–2.00) times more likely to develop diabetes.

Taken together, the available prospective studies indicate a protective effect for physical activity and type 2 diabetes. There is a dose–response relationship (Fig. 11-4) in which greater levels of physical activity result in a lower risk for the development of type 2 diabetes. However, further research is required to better delineate the relationship between physical activity and type 2 diabetes among different ethnic groups.

In addition to the epidemiologic evidence, two recent large-scale intervention studies have highlighted the importance of physical activity in the prevention of type 2 diabetes in high-risk people (59,107). The Finnish Diabetes Prevention Study (DPS) was a trial that randomized 522 middle-aged, overweight adults with impaired glucose tolerance to either a control group or a lifestyle intervention that was aimed at reducing body weight, improving diet, and increasing physical activity (107). After an average of 3.2 years of follow-up, the risk of developing type 2 diabetes was 58% lower in the lifestyle intervention compared with the control group. Similarly, the U.S. Diabetes Prevention Program (DPP) was an intervention that randomized 3,234 participants into one of three groups: (a) placebo control, (b) metformin drug therapy (850 mg twice daily), or (c) lifestyle-modification program. The lifestyle program in this study also reduced the risk of de-

veloping type 2 diabetes by 58% compared with the control group over an average of 2.8 years of follow-up and was significantly more effective than the metformin drug therapy (31% reduction in incidence) (59). Confounders of the relationship between physical activity and incident type 2 diabetes in at risk populations are the weight loss and dietary components of the interventions that were also a part of these two studies. However, in a secondary analysis that was part of the DPP, investigators observed that when controlling for weight loss and diet, there remained a significant effect of physical activity on the prevention of type 2 diabetes in their study population (61). Thus, the weighted evidence indicates that leading a healthy lifestyle, including being physically active, is an effective prevention strategy for type 2 diabetes.

PHYSICAL ACTIVITY AND CANCER

Cancer is a group of diseases characterized by the uncontrolled growth of abnormal cells. Given the wide range of possible cancer causes and potential anatomic sites, risk factors for specific cancers vary widely. Physical activity has the potential to influence cancer risk through several mechanisms, including improved circulation, ventilation, energy balance, immune surveillance, reduced oxidative damage and increased free radical buffering, and possibly improved DNA repair processes (106). Physical activity has been studied in relation to incident cancers at many sites; however, the available evidence for a protective effect is strongest for overall cancer risk and for cancers of the colon and breast, specifically. Other cancer sites that have been investigated in relation to physical activity include endometrial, ovarian, prostate, testicular, and lung; however, the evidence for a protective effect is less clear for these sites (106). Thus, reviewed here is the available evidence for a relationship between physical activity and cancers of the colon and breast.

A large body of evidence links a sedentary lifestyle to an increased risk of colon cancer. Men and women in sedentary occupations have an elevated risk of colon cancer, as do men and women who are physically inactive in their leisure time (101,103,106). However, a relationship between physical activity and rectal cancer has not been consistently observed. Whether physical activity differentially affects cancers of the ascending, transverse, or descending colon is an area for future investigation. It has been hypothesized that a lower risk of colon cancer may be conferred by a decreased transit time for fecal matter through the colon of physically active individuals, leading to decreased exposure of the susceptible regions of the intestinal wall to carcinogens.

Table 11-2 summarizes the available prospective studies of physical activity and incident breast cancer (5,19,21,25,26,35,37,67,73,78–80,93,94,100,105,114). There is now sufficient epidemiologic evidence that physical activity reduces the risk of breast cancer (36), and the

TABLE 11-2. RESULTS OF PROSPECTIVE LONGITUDINAL STUDIES OF PHYSICAL INACTIVITY OR PHYSICAL FITNESS AND RISK OF BREAST CANCER THAT PROVIDED RELATIVE RISK ESTIMATES

POPULATION	SAMPLE SIZE	ACTIVITY/FITNESS CLASSIFICATION	RR (95% CI)
U.S. college alumni (37)	5,398	College nonathletes vs athletes	1.86 (1.00–3.47)
U.S. women (5)	7,407	Little to no exercise vs much exercise	1.00 (0.60–1.60)
Framingham Heart Study women (26)	2,307	Low vs high quartile PA	1.60 (0.90–2.90)
Seventh-day Adventist women (35)	20,341	Low vs moderate exercise	1.46 (1.11–1.92)
Norwegian women (105)	25,624	Sedentary vs regular exercise	1.59 (1.05–2.38)
University of Pennsylvania alumni (100)	1,566	<2,092 vs ≥4186 kJ/wk PA	1.37 (0.88–2.17)
Iowa women (21)	1,806	Inactive vs moderate PA	2.00 (0.91–3.33)
U.S. female nurses (94)	104,468	<1 vs ≥7 h/wk moderate to vigorous PA	0.91 (0.67–1.25)
U.S. female nurses (93)	85,364	<1 vs ≥7 h/wk moderate to vigorous PA	1.22 (1.03–1.43)
Swedish women (79)	253,336	Sedentary vs high/very high occupational PA	1.30 (1.20–1.40)
Iowa women (78)	37,105	No moderate PA vs >4 times/wk	1.18 (0.98–1.41)
U.S. college alumni (114)	3,940	College nonathletes vs athletes	1.65 (1.20–2.28)
Finnish women (73)	30,548	<1 time/wk vs daily LTPA	0.99 (0.70–1.39)
U.S. women (67)	39,322	<840 vs ≥6,300 kJ/wk PA	1.49 (1.00–2.27)
U.S. women (19)	6,160	Consistently high vs low PA	1.72 (0.93–3.23)
Danish women (25)	2,924	<30 vs >90 min/day LTPA	1.32 (1.01–1.72)
Swedish twins (80)	9,539	Sedentary vs regular LTPA	1.67 (1.00–2.50)

CI, confidence interval; LTPA, leisure-time physical activity; PA, physical activity; RR, relative risk.

association follows a dose–response pattern (106). Two studies that illustrate the dose–response relation are outlined below.

A 10-year follow-up of 77,024 women from the Nurses' Health Study yielded valuable information on the dose–response relationship between physical activity and breast cancer risk (93). Compared with women accumulating <1 hour per week in moderate or vigorous physical activity, women who accumulated 1.0 to 1.9 hours, 2.0 to 3.9 hours, 4.0 to 6.9 hours, and 7.0 hours or more had 0.88 (95% CI: 0.79–0.98), 0.89 (95% CI: 0.81–0.99), 0.85 (95% CI: 0.77–0.94), and 0.82 (95% CI: 0.70–0.97) times the risk of incident breast cancer (P for trend = 0.04), respectively (93). Similarly, a 13.7-year follow-up of 25,625 Norwegian women also demonstrated a significant dose–response relationship between physical activity and incident breast cancer (105). Compared with women who were sedentary in their leisure time, women who were moderately active or regular exercisers had 0.93 (95% CI: 0.71–1.22) and 0.63 (95% CI: 0.42–0.95) times the risk of breast cancer, respectively (P for trend = 0.04). A similar trend was observed for occupational physical activity.

The biologically plausible mechanisms whereby physical activity may affect breast cancer risk include the alteration of menstrual cycle patterns and exposure to sex hormones, enhancement of immune function, better energy balance, and changes in insulin and insulinlike growth factors (49).

PHYSICAL ACTIVITY AND MORTALITY IN UNHEALTHY PARTICIPANTS

The majority of the prospective studies on physical activity or physical fitness and chronic diseases or mortality

have relied on asymptomatic or healthy participants at baseline to better quantify the relationships with incident disease. However, another area of interest is the effects of physical activity or fitness on mortality among those with existing chronic conditions. There are fewer prospective studies of this type; however, several examples are presented here. The prospective relationship between cardiorespiratory fitness and mortality was examined in healthy men and men with cardiovascular disease using 8.5-year follow-up data from the Lipid Research Clinics Study (28). The RRs of all-cause mortality for physical fitness (per 2 standard deviation lower treadmill time) in healthy men and men with cardiovascular disease were 1.8 (95% CI: 1.2–2.6) and 2.9 (95% CI: 1.7–4.9), respectively. These results support the notion that maintaining physical fitness is important for preventing premature mortality in healthy men and particularly in those with diagnosed cardiovascular disease.

The relationship between cardiorespiratory fitness and all-cause mortality was examined in men without hypertension (n = 15,726), with hypertension (n = 3,184), and without a history of hypertension but an elevated laboratory blood pressure measurement at baseline (white-coat hypertension; n = 3,257) in the ACLS (23). The RR of all-cause mortality in high-fit versus low-fit men was similar in the normotensives (RR = 0.50 [95% CI: 0.37–0.68]), hypertensives (RR = 0.42 [95% CI: 0.27–0.66]), and those with an elevated clinic blood pressure measurement (RR = 0.44 [95% CI: 0.29–0.68]). Similar results were also seen for cardiovascular disease mortality in all three groups (23). Similarly, Wei et al. (112) examined the relationship between cardiorespiratory fitness and mortality in men with type 2 diabetes (n = 1,263) in the ACLS. Compared with men in the low-fit group, men in the high-fit group had a RR of all-cause mortality of 0.48 (95% CI: 0.34–0.67) after adjustment for age, examination year, and traditional lifestyle and conventional risk factors. Thus, there is consistent evidence that physically fit men with existing chronic conditions such as cardiovascular disease, hypertension, or type 2 diabetes have a lower risk of mortality compared with men who are unfit. More research is required to confirm these findings in women and different ethnic groups.

MUSCULOSKELETAL FITNESS AND ALL-CAUSE MORTALITY

All of the studies of the relationship between physical fitness and mortality or incidence of chronic diseases described in this chapter to this point have been concerned with the effects of cardiorespiratory fitness. An important area for future research is the relation between other measures of musculoskeletal fitness and various health outcomes. Musculoskeletal fitness includes aspects of bone health, joint flexibility, and mus-

cular strength and endurance. Musculoskeletal fitness is related to health-related quality of life and mobility (111), and lower body function has been shown to be predictive of disability and death in elderly individuals (41,42). On the other hand, there is relatively little research on the effects of musculoskeletal fitness on the incidence of chronic diseases or premature mortality. There are apparently only eight studies that have examined the relationship between musculoskeletal fitness and mortality (6,32,38,55,63,77,90), and all but two (38,55) relied on an index of muscular strength (usually grip strength) only when examining the relationship with mortality. In general, higher levels of musculoskeletal fitness are associated with a lower risk of mortality; however, the nature of the relationship varies from indicator to indicator and from study to study (Table 11-3). More research on the relationships between other measures of musculoskeletal fitness and the incidence of chronic diseases and premature mortality is required. Studies that examine the effects of sex, ethnicity, and age on the relationships would be particularly timely.

TABLE 11-3. PROSPECTIVE LONGITUDINAL STUDIES OF MUSCULOSKELETAL FITNESS AND MORTALITY

POPULATION	SAMPLE SIZE	AGE RANGE (Y)	FOLLOW-UP LENGTH (Y)	INDICATORS OF MUSCULOSKELETAL FITNESS	RESULTS
American men and women (32)	9,105	20–82	14	Sit-ups, bench press, and leg press	Mortality rates were lower in men and women with moderate and high muscular fitness compared with those with low fitness
Canadian men and women (55)	8,116	20–69	13	Grip strength, sit-ups, push-ups, trunk flexibility	Sit-ups (men and women) and grip strength (men) inversely related to mortality
American men (77)	1,071	NR	17.5	Grip strength	Grip strength related to mortality in total sample and in men ≥60 y old in particular
Australian men and women (6)	1,464	70–84	6	Grip strength	Grip strength inversely relate to mortality in combined sample of men and women
Japanese-American men (91)	6,040	45–68	30	Grip strength	Grip strength inversely related to mortality within several body mass index categories
Danish men and women (98)	406	75	5	Knee extension and body extension strength	Knee extension strength inversely related to mortality in women only
Japanese men and women (38)	7,286	40–85	6.1	Grip strength, sit-ups, side step, vertical jump, trunk flexion	Grip strength, side step, and vertical jump inversely related to mortality in men only
Finnish men and women (63)	463	75 and 80	4.0–4.8	Grip strength and knee extension strength	Grip strength and knee extension strength inversely related to mortality in combined sample of men and women

NR, not reported.

SUMMARY

There is abundant evidence that physical activity and physical fitness levels are inversely associated with the risk of premature mortality and many chronic diseases, including CHD, stroke, hypertension, type 2 diabetes, and some cancers (particularly of the colon and breast). Furthermore, dose–response relationships have been observed in many studies that have used multiple physical activity or physical fitness categories, and better-designed studies tend to produce stronger results. It is also important to note that individuals can change their risk of chronic disease or premature mortality by changing their level of physical activity. This has been shown for many common maladies. These observations have several important public health implications. First, given the high prevalence of physical inactivity in many developed nations, the burden of sedentary living on healthcare associated with the treatment of chronic diseases is substantial. Second, measures of physical activity or physical fitness should be incorporated into assessing an individual's global risk of developing chronic diseases in the clinical setting. Third, the knowledge that increasing an individual's physical activity level results in a reduction in disease risk should be highlighted in public health campaigns designed to increase the physical activity levels of the population.

REFERENCES

1. Centers for Disease Control and Prevention: National diabetes fact sheet: General information and national estimates on diabetes in the United States, 2000. Centers for Disease Control and Prevention. U.S. Department of Health and Human Services (Ed.) Atlanta, GA; 2002.

2. NHLBI: Fact Book, Fiscal Year 2002 Bethesda (MD): National Heart Lung and Blood Institute, National Institutes of Health; 2003.

3. Abbott RD, Rodriguez BL, Burchfiel CM, Curb JD. Physical activity in older middle-aged men and reduced risk of stroke: the Honolulu Heart Program. *Am J Epidemiol.* 1994;139:881–893.

4. Agnarsson U, Thorgeirsson G, Sigvaldason H, Sigfusson N. Effects of leisure-time physical activity and ventilatory function on risk of stroke for men: the Reykjavik Study. *Ann Intern Med.* 1999;130:987–990.

5. Albanes D, Blair A, Taylor PH. Physical activity and risk of cancer in the NHANES I population. *Am J Public Health.* 1989;79:744–750.

6. Anstey KJ, Luszcz MA, Giles LC, Andrews GR. Demographic, health, cognitive, and sensory variables as predictors of mortality in very old adults. *Psychol Aging.* 2001;16:3–11.

7. Batty GD, Lee IM. Physical activity for preventing strokes. *BMJ.* 2002;325:350–351.

8. Berlin JA, Colditz GA. A meta-analysis of physical activity in the prevention of coronary heart disease. *Am J Epidemiol.* 1990;132:612–628.

9. Bijnen FC, Feskens EJ, Caspersen CJ, et al. Baseline and previous physical activity in relation to mortality in elderly men: the Zutphen Elderly Study. *Am J Epidemiol.* 1999;150:1289–1296.

10. Bijnen FCH, Caspersen CJ, Feskens EJM, et al. Physical activity and 10-year mortality from cardiovascular diseases and all causes: the Zutphen Elderly Study. *Arch Intern Med.* 1998;158:1499–1505.

11. Blair SN, Cheng Y, Holder JS. Is physical activity or physical fitness more important in defining health benefits? *Med Sci Sports Exerc.* 2001;33:S379–S399.

12. Blair SN, Jackson AS. Physical fitness and activity as separate heart disease risk factors: a meta-analysis. *Med Sci Sports Exerc.* 2001;33:762–764.

13. Blair SN, Kohl HW, Paffenbarger RS, et al. Physical fitness and all-cause mortality: a prospective study of healthy men and women. *JAMA.* 1989;262:2395–2401.

14. Blair SN, Kohl HW, Barlow CE, et al. Changes in physical fitness and all-cause mortality" a prospective study of healthy and unhealthy men. *JAMA.* 1995;273:1093–1098.

15. Booth FW, Chakravarthy MV. Physical activity and dietary intervention for chronic diseases: a quick fix after all? *J Appl Physiol.* 2006;100:1439–1440.

16. Booth FW, Lees SJ. Fundamental questions about genes, inactivity, and chronic diseases. *Physiol Genomics.* 2007;28:146–157.

17. Bouchard C, Daw EW, Rice T, et al. Familial resemblance for VO$_2$max in the sedentary state: the HERITAGE family study. *Med Sci Sports Exerc.* 1998;30:252–258.

18. Bouchard C, Shephard RJ, Stephens T. *Physical Activity, Fitness, and Health.* Champaign, (IL): Human Kinetics; 1994.

19. Breslow RA, Ballard-Barbash R, Munoz K, Graubard BI. Long-term recreational physical activity and breast cancer in the National Health and Nutrition Examination Survey I epidemiologic follow-up study. *Cancer Epidemiol Biomarkers Prev.* 2001;10:805–808.

20. Burchfiel CM, Sharp DS, Curb JD, et al. Physical activity and incidence of diabetes: the Honolulu Heart Program. *Am J Epidemiol.* 1995;141:360–368.

21. Cerhan JR, Chiu BCH, Wallace RB, et al. Physical activity, physical function, and the risk of breast cancer in a prospective study among elderly women. *J Gerontol.* 1998;53A:M251–M256.

22. Church TS, Earnest CP, Skinner JS, Blair SN. Effects of different doses of physical activity on cardiorespiratory fitness among sedentary, overweight or obese postmenopausal women with elevated blood pressure: a randomized controlled trial. *JAMA.* 2007;297:2081–2091.

23. Church TS, Kampert JB, Gibbons LW, et al. Usefulness of cardiorespiratory fitness as a predictor of all-cause and cardiovascular disease mortality in men with systemic hypertension. *Am J Cardiol.* 2001;88:651–656.

24. Colditz GA. Economic costs of obesity and inactivity. *Med Sci Sports Exerc.* 1999;31:S663–S667.

25. Dirx MJ, Voorrips LE, Goldbohm RA, van den Brandt PA. Baseline recreational physical activity, history of sports participation, and postmenopausal breast carcinoma risk in the Netherlands Cohort Study. *Cancer.* 2001;92:1638–1649.

26. Dorgan JF, Brown C, Barrett M, et al. Physical activity and risk of breast cancer in the Framingham Heart Study. *Am J Epidemiol.* 1994;139:662–669.

27. Durstine JL, Grandjean PW, Davis PG, et al. Blood lipid and lipoprotein adaptations to exercise: a quantitative analysis. *Sports Med.* 2001;31:1033–1062.

28. Ekelund LG, Haskell WL, Johnson JL, et al. Physical fitness as a predictor of cardiovascular mortality in asymptomatic North American men: The Lipid Research Clinics Mortality Follow-up Study. *N Engl J Med.* 1988;319:1379–1384.

29. Erikssen G, Liestol K, Bjornholt J, et al. Changes in physical fitness and changes in mortality. *Lancet.* 1998;352:759–762.

30. Evenson KR, Rosamond WD, Cai J, et al. Physical activity and ischemic stroke risk: the atherosclerosis risk in communities study. *Stroke.* 1999;30:1333–1339.

31. Fagard RH. Exercise characteristics and the blood pressure response to dynamic physical training. *Med Sci Sports Exerc.* 2001;33:S484–S492.

32. Fitzgerald SL, Barlow CE, Kampert JB, et al. Muscular fitness and all-cause mortality: prospective observations. *J Phys Act Health.* 2004;1(1) 7–18.

33. Fletcher GF, Blair AN, Blumenthal J, et al. Statement on exercise. Benefits and recommendations for physical activity programs for all Americans. A statement for health professionals by the Committee on Exercise and Cardiac Rehabilitation of the Council on Clinical Cardiology, American Heart Association. *Circulation.* 1992;86:340–344.

34. Folsom AR, Prineas RJ, Kaye SA, Munger RG. Incidence of hypertension and stroke in relation to body fat distribution and other risk factors in older women. *Stroke.* 1990;21:701–716.

35. Fraser GE, Shavlik DRF. Risk factors, lifetime risk, and age at onset of breast cancer. *Ann Epidemiol.* 1997;7:375–382.

36. Friedenreich CM, Thune I, Brinton LA, Albanes D. Epidemiologic issues related to the association between physical activity and breast cancer. *Cancer.* 1998;83:600–610.

37. Frisch RE, Wyshak G, Witschi J, et al. Lower lifetime occurrence of breast cancer and cancers of the reproductive system among former college athletes. *Int J Fertil.* 1987;32:217–225.

38. Fujita Y, Nakamura Y, Hiraoka J, et al. Physical-strength tests and mortality among visitors to health-promotion centers in Japan. *J Clin Epidemiol.* 1995;48:1349–1359.

39. Gillum RF, Mussolino ME, Ingram DD. Physical activity and stroke incidence in women and men: the NHANES I Epidemiologic Follow-up Study. *Am J Epidemiol.* 1996;143:860–869.

40. Gregg EW, Cauley JA, Stone K, et al. Relationship of changes in physical activity and mortality among older women. *JAMA.* 2003; 289:2379–2386.

41. Guralnik JM, Ferrucci L, Simonsick EM, et al. Lower-extremity function in persons over the age of 70 years as a predictor of subsequent disability. *N Engl J Med.* 1995;332:556–561.

42. Guralnik JM, Simonsick EM, Ferrucci L, et al. A short physical performance battery assessing lower extremity function: association with self-reported disability and prediction of mortality and nursing home admission. *J Gerontol.* 1994;49:M85–94.

43. Haapanen N, Miilunpalo S, Vuori I, Oja P, Pasanen M. Association of leisure time physical activity with the risk of coronary heart disease, hypertension and diabetes in middle-aged men and women. *Int J Epidemiol.* 1997;26:739–747.

44. Harmsen P, Rosengren A, Tsipogianni A, Wilhelmsen L. Risk factors for stroke in middle-aged men in Goteborg, Sweden. *Stroke.* 1990;21:223–229.

45. **Haskell WL, Lee IM, Pate RR, et al. Physical activity and public health: updated recommendation for adults from the American College of Sports Medicine and the American Heart Association. *Med Sci Sports Exerc.* 2007;39:1423–1434.**

46. Heath GW. Epidemiologic research: a primer for the clinical exercise physiologist. *Clin Exerc Physiol.* 2000;2:60–67.

47. Helmrich SP, Ragland DR, Leung RW, Paffenbarger RS. Physical activity and reduced occurrence of non-insulin-dependent diabetes mellitus. *N Engl J Med.* 1991;325:147–152.

48. Herman B, Schmitz PI, Leyten AC, et al. Multivariate logistic analysis of risk factors for stroke in Tilburg, The Netherlands. *Am J Epidemiol.* 1983;118:514–525.

49. Hoffman-Goetz L, Apter D, Demark-Wahnefried W, et al. Possible mechanisms mediating an association between physical activity and breast cancer. *Cancer.* 1998;83:621–628.

50. Hoyert DL, Arias E, Smith BL, Murphy SL, Kochanek KD. Deaths: final data for 1999. *Natl Vital Stat Rep* 49:2001.

51. Hu FB, Leitzmann MF, Stampfer MJ, et al. Physical activity and television watching in relation to risk for type 2 diabetes mellitus in men. *Arch Intern Med.* 2001;161:1542–1548.

52. Hu FB, Sigal RJ, Rich-Edwards JW, et al. Walking compared with vigorous physical activity and risk of type 2 diabetes in women: a prospective study. *JAMA.* 1999;282:1433–1439.

53. Hu FB, Stampfer MJ, Colditz GA, et al. Physical activity and risk of stroke in women. *JAMA.* 2000;283:2961–2967.

54. Kannel WB. Habitual level of physical activity and risk of coronary heart disease: the Framingham study. *Can Med Assoc J.* 1967;96: 811–812.

55. Katzmarzyk PT, Craig CL. Musculoskeletal fitness and risk of mortality. *Med Sci Sports Exerc.* 2002;34:740–744.

56. Kelley DE, Goodpaster BH. Effects of exercise on glucose homeostasis in type 2 diabetes mellitus. *Med Sci Sports Exerc.* 2001;33: S495–S501.

57. Kesaniemi YK, Danforth E, Jensen MD, et al. Dose-response issues concerning physical activity and health: an evidence-based symposium. *Med Sci Sports Exerc.* 2001;33:S351–S358.

58. Kiely DK, Wolf PA, Cupples LA, Beiser AS, Kannel WB. Physical activity and stroke risk: the Framingham Study. *Am J Epidemiol.* 1994;140:608–620.

59. Knowler WC, Barrett-Connor E, Fowler SE, et al. Reduction in the incidence of type 2 diabetes with lifestyle intervention or metformin. *N Engl J Med.* 2002;346:393–403.

60. Kohl HW. Physical activity and cardiovascular disease: evidence for a dose response. *Med Sci Sports Exerc.* 2001;33:S472–S483.

61. Kriska AM, Edelstein SL, Hamman RF, et al. Physical activity in individuals at risk for diabetes: Diabetes Prevention Program. *Med Sci Sports Exerc.* 2006;38:826–832.

62. Kujala UM, Kaprio J, Koskenvuo M. Modifiable risk factors as predictors of all-cause mortality: the roles of genetics and childhood environment. *Am J Epidemiol.* 2002;156:985–993.

63. Laukkanen P, Heikkinen E, Kauppinen M. Muscle strength and mobility as predictors of survival in 75–84-year-old people. *Ageing* 1995;24:468–473.

64. Lee CD, Blair SN. Cardiorespiratory fitness and stroke mortality in men. *Med Sci Sports Exerc.* 2002;34:592–595.

65. Lee I-M, Hennekens CH, Berger K, et al. Exercise and risk of stroke in male physicians. *Stroke.* 1999;30:1–6.

66. Lee I-M, Paffenbarger RS. Physical activity and stroke incidence: the Harvard Alumni Health Study. *Stroke.* 1998;29:2049–2054.

67. Lee I-M, Rexrode KM, Cook NR, Hennekens CH, Burin JE. Physical activity and breast cancer risk: the Women's Health Study (United States). *Cancer Causes Control.* 2001;12:137–145.

68. Lee, IM, Paffenbarger RS. Do physical activity and physical fitness avert premature mortality? *Exerc Sport Sci Rev.* 1996;24: 135–171.

69. Lee IM, Skerrett PJ. Physical activity and all-cause mortality: what is the dose–response relation? *Med Sci Sports Exerc.* 2001; 33:S459–S471.

70. Leon AS, Sanchez OA. Response of blood lipids to exercise training alone or combined with dietary intervention. *Med Sci Sports Exerc.* 2001;33:S502–S515.

71. Lindsted KD, Tonstad S, Kuzma JW. Self-report of physical activity and patterns of mortality in seventh-day Adventist men. *J Clin Epidemiol.* 1991;44:355–364.

72. Lissner L, Bengtsson C, Bjorkelund C, Wedel H. Physical activity levels and changes in relation to longevity: a prospective study of Swedish women. *Am J Epidemiol.* 1996;143:54–62.

73. Luoto R, Latikka P, Pukkala E, Hakulinen T, Vihko V. The effect of physical activity on breast cancer risk: a cohort study of 30,548 women. *Eur J Epidemiol.* 2000;16:973–980.

74. Manson JE, Nathan DM, Krolewski AS, et al. A prospective study of exercise and incidence of diabetes among US male physicians. *JAMA.* 1992;268:63–67.

75. Manson JE, Rimm EB, Stampfer MJ, et al. Physical activity and incidence of non-insulin-dependent diabetes mellitus in women. *Lancet.* 1991;338:774–778.

76. Matthews CE, Jurj AL, Shu XO, et al. Influence of exercise, walking, cycling, and overall nonexercise physical activity on mortality in Chinese women. *Am J Epidemiol.* 2007;165:1343–1350.

77. Metter EJ, Talbot LA, Schrager M, Conwit R. Skeletal muscle strength as a predictor of all-cause mortality in healthy men. *J Gerontol B Biol Sci Med Sci.* 2002;57:B359–B365.

78. Moore DB, Folsom AR, Mink PJ, et al. Physical activity and incidence of postmenopausal breast cancer. *Epidemiology.* 2000;11: 292–296.

79. Moradi T, Adami HO, Bergstrom R, et al. Occupational physical activity and risk for breast cancer in a nationwide cohort study in Sweden. *Cancer Causes Control*. 1999;10:423–430.

80. Moradi T, Adami HO, Ekbom A, et al. Physical activity and risk for breast cancer a prospective cohort study among Swedish twins. *Int J Cancer*. 2002;100:76–81.

81. Morris JN, Heady JA, Raffle PAB, Roberts CG, Parks JW. Coronary heart-disease and physical activity of work. *Lancet*. 1953; 1053–1057, 1111–1120.

82. Paffenbarger RS. Contributions of epidemiology to exercise science and cardiovascular health. *Med Sci Sports Exerc*. 1988;20: 426–438.

83. Paffenbarger RS, Blair SN, Lee IM. A history of physical activity, cardiovascular health and longevity: the scientific contributions of Jeremy N Morris, DSc, DPH, FRCP. *Int J Epidemiol*. 2001;30: 1184–1192.

84. Paffenbarger RS, Hyde RT, Wing AL, Hsieh CC. Physical activity, all-cause mortality, and longevity of college alumni. *N Engl J Med*. 1986;314:605–613.

85. Paffenbarger RS, Hyde RT, Wing AL, et al. The association of changes in physical-activity level and other lifestyle characteristics with mortality among men. *N Engl J Med*. 1993;328:538–545.

86. Paffenbarger RS, WingAL, Hyde RT, Jung DL. Physical activity and incidence of hypertension in college alumni. *Am J Epidemiol*. 1983;117:245–257.

87. Pereira MA, Folsom AR, McGovern PG, et al. Physical activity and incident hypertension in black and white adults: the Atherosclerosis Risk in Communities Study. *Prev Med*. 1999;28: 304–312.

88. Powell KE, Blair SN. The public health burdens of sedentary living habits: theoretical but realistic estimates. *Med Sci Sports Exerc*. 1994;26:851–856.

89. Powell KE, Thompson PD, Caspersen CJ, Kendrick JS. Physical activity and incidence of coronary heart disease. *Ann Rev Public Health*. 1987;8:253–287.

90. Rantanen T, Harris T, Leveille SG, et al. Muscle strength and body mass index as long-term predictors of mortality in initially healthy men. *J Gerontol A Biol Sci Med Sci*. 2000;55:M168–73.

91. Rantanen T, Masaki K, Foley S, et al. Grip strength changes over 27 yr in Japanese-American men. *J Appl Physiol*. 1998;85: 2047–2053.

92. Report of the Institute of Medicine, the National Academy of Sciences. *Adequacy of Evidence for Physical Activity Guidelines Development*. Washington, DC: National Academies Press; 2007.

93. Rockhill B, Willett WC, Hunter DJ, et al. A prospective study of recreational physical activity and breast cancer risk. *Arch Intern Med*. 1999;159:2290–2296.

94. Rockhill B, Willett WC, Hunter DJ, et al. Physical activity and breast cancer risk in a cohort of young women. *J Natl Cancer Inst*. 1998;90:1155–1160.

95. Rosengren A, Wilhelmsen L. Physical activity protects against coronary death and deaths from all causes in middle-aged men: evidence from a 20-year follow-up of the primary prevention study in Goteborg. *Ann Epidemiol*. 1997;7:69–75.

96. Sacco RL, Gan R, Boden-Albala B, et al. Leisure-time physical activity and ischemic stroke risk: the Northern Manhattan Stroke Study. *Stroke*. 1998;29:380–387.

97. Salonen JT, Puska P, Tuomilehto J. Physical activity and risk of myocardial infarction, cerebral stroke and death: a longitudinal study in Eastern Finland. *Am J Epidemiol*. 1982;115:526–537.

98. Schroll M, Avlund K, Davidsen M. Predictors of five-year functional ability in a longitudinal survey of men and women aged 75 to 80: the 1914 population in Glostrup, Denmark. *Aging (Milano)*. 1997;9:143–152.

99. United States Department of Health and Human Services. *Physical Activity and Health: A Report of the Surgeon General*: Department of Health and Human Services, Centers for Disease Control and Prevention, National Center for Chronic Disease Prevention and Health Promotion, 1996.

100. Sesso HD, Paffenbarger RS, Lee IM. Physical activity and breast cancer risk in the College Alumni Health Study (United States). *Cancer Causes Control*. 1998;9:433–439.

101. Shephard RJ, Futcher R. Physical activity and cancer: How may protection be maximized? *Crit Rev Oncog*. 1997;8:219–272.

102. Slentz CA, Houmard JA, Kraus WE. Modest exercise prevents the progressive disease associated with physical inactivity. *Exerc Sport Sci Rev*. 2007;35:18–23.

103. Sternfeld B. Cancer and the protective effect of physical activity: the epidemiological evidence. *Med Sci Sports Exerc*. 1992;24:1195–1209.

104. Thompson PD, Buchner D, Piña IL, et al. Exercise and physical activity in the prevention and treatment of atherosclerotic cardiovascular disease. A statement from the Council on Clinical Cardiology and the Council on Nutrition, Physical Activity and Metabolism. *Circulation*. 2003;107:3109–3116.

105. Thune I, Brenn T, Lund E, Gaard M. Physical activity and the risk of breast cancer. *N Engl J Med*. 1997;336:1269–1275.

106. Thune I, Furberg AS. Physical activity and cancer risk: dose-response and cancer, all sites and site-specific. *Med Sci Sports Exerc*. 2001;33:S530–S550.

107. Tuomilehto J, Lindstrom J, Eriksson JG, et al. Prevention of type 2 diabetes mellitus by changes in lifestyle among subjects with impaired glucose tolerance. *N Engl J Med*. 2001;344:1343–1350.

108. Wannamethee G, Shaper AG. Physical activity and stroke in British middle aged men. *BMJ*. 1992;304:597–601.

109. Wannamethee S, Shaper AG, Alberti KG. Physical activity, metabolic factors, and the incidence of coronary heart disease and type 2 diabetes. *Arch Intern Med*. 2000;160:2108–2116.

110. Wannamethee SG, Shaper AG, Walker M. Changes in physical activity, mortality, and incidence of coronary heart disease in older men. *Lancet*. 1998;351:1603–1608.

111. Warburton DE, Gledhill N, Quinney A. Musculoskeletal fitness and health. *Can J Appl Physiol*. 2001;26:217–237.

112. Wei M, Gibbons LW, Kampert JB, Nichaman MZ, Blair SN. Low cardiorespiratory fitness and physical inactivity as predictors of mortality in men with type 2 diabetes. *Ann Intern Med*. 2000;132: 605–611.

113. Williams PT. Physical fitness and activity as separate heart disease risk factors: a meta-analysis. *Med Sci Sports Exerc*. 2001;33:754–761.

114. Wyshak G, Frisch RE. Breast cancer among former college athletes compared to non-athletes: a 15-year follow-up. *Br J Cancer*. 2000; 82:726–730.

SELECTED REFERENCES FOR FURTHER READING

Blair SN, Kohl HW, Barlow CE, Paffenbarger RS Jr, Gibbons LW, Macera CA. Changes in physical fitness and all-cause mortality: a prospective study of healthy and unhealthy men. *JAMA*. 1995;273: 1093–1098,.

Blair SN, Kohl HW, Paffenbarger RS Jr, Clark DG, Cooper KH, Gibbons LW. Physical fitness and all-cause mortality: a prospective study of healthy men and women. *JAMA*. 1989;262:2395–2401.

Kohl HW 3rd. Physical activity and cardiovascular disease: evidence for a dose response. *Med Sci Sports Exerc*. 2001;33:S472–S483.

Paffenbarger RS Jr, Blair SN, Lee IM. A history of physical activity, cardiovascular health and longevity: the scientific contributions of Jeremy N Morris, DSc, DPH, FRCP. *Int J Epidemiol*. 2001;30: 1184–1192.

Paffenbarger RS Jr, Hyde RT, Wing AL, Hsieh CC. Physical activity, all-cause mortality, and longevity of college alumni. N Engl J Med. 1986;314:605–613.

Physical Activity Guidelines Advisory Committee. Physical Activity Guidelines Advisory Committee Report, 2008. Washington, DC: U.S. Department of Health and Human Services, 2008.

Thune I, Furberg AS. Physical activity and cancer risk: dose-response and cancer, all sites and site-specific. *Med Sci Sports Exerc.* 2001; 33:S530–S550.

Whaley MH, Blair SN. Physical activity, physical fitness and coronary heart disease. *J Cardiovascular Risk.* 1995;2:289–295.

INTERNET RESOURCES

- Health Canada Physical Activity Unit: www.hc-sc.gc.ca/hppb/fitness/about.html
- National Center for Disease Prevention and Health Promotion, Nutrition and Physical Activity: www.cdc.gov/nccdphp/dnpa/physical/index.htm
- National Coalition for Promoting Physical Activity: www.ncppa.org/physactfactsheets.asp
- United States Department of Health & Human Services: http://aspe.hhs.gov/health/reports/physicalactivity/
- World Health Organization: www.who.int/ hpr/ physactiv/ index.shtml

Assessment of Physical Activity

Physical activity has been defined as bodily movement generated by skeletal muscles resulting in energy expenditure (15). The physical activity portion of energy expenditure can be further divided into spontaneous activities, including nonexercise activity thermogenesis (NEAT), such as fidgeting or work-related walking, and voluntary physical activity. Voluntary physical activity includes activities of daily living and those that require amounts of energy above that necessary to perform activities of daily living (47). It is this component of physical activity that varies most among individuals (43).

The benefits of a physically active lifestyle are widely known (42,63). The American College of Sports Medicine (ACSM) physical activity recommendations have evolved over time (5,6,7,22,42). Early recommendations focused on higher-intensity physical activities to achieve significant or maximal improvements in physical fitness. Since the mid-1990s, however, the emphasis has shifted toward getting individuals to participate in moderate-intensity lifestyle physical activities to improve health. This change in emphasis was brought about by the realization that moderate-intensity lifestyle physical activities can contribute to health in a similar fashion to structured exercise programs (20). Given the health implications of physical activity, it is important to assess the type, frequency, and intensity of physical activities. Specific reasons to measure physical activity include the ability to

investigate the direct relationship between physical activity and disease endpoints, as well as the indirect relationship with disease through the effects of activity on diet or body weight (45). Additional reasons include being able to study physical activity patterns, determinants, and barriers in different groups and to evaluate physical activity interventions (3,65,66).

Various **subjective methods** and **objective methods** can be used to measure physical activity. When using subjective methods, such as questionnaires or diaries, the physical activity assessment is based on the individual's perception of his or her level of activity. With objective methods, physical activity assessment is determined by an instrument, and the individual's interpretation and perception of physical activity are not taken into account.

Several of the advantages and disadvantages of using subjective and objective methods of assessment are listed in Table 12-1. The main advantage of using subjective measures, such as questionnaires or diaries, is the ability to administer the assessment relatively inexpensively to many individuals in a short amount of time. Disadvantages of subjective assessment include inaccurate recall that results in the over- or underreporting of physical activity and the inability to accurately capture all types of physical activity (e.g., moderate, lifestyle, occupational). Unlike subjective assessment methods, recall error is not an issue for objective methods, such as **pedometers**,

TABLE 12-1. ADVANTAGES AND DISADVANTAGES OF SUBJECTIVE AND OBJECTIVE PHYSICAL ACTIVITY MEASURES

SUBJECTIVE		OBJECTIVE	
ADVANTAGES	DISADVANTAGES	ADVANTAGES	DISADVANTAGES
Relatively inexpensive	Inaccurate recall	Not subject to recall error	Specific types of activity not assessed (e.g., water sports, arm exercise, inclined walking)
Easy to administer	Fails to accurately capture all types of activity (e.g., moderate, lifestyle, and occupational activity)	Small and lightweight	Extraneous variables may affect results
Data collected for many individuals	Not recommended for children younger than age 10 years	Unobtrusive	Usually more expensive than questionnaires
Can be ascertained with a few questions			

accelerometers, and **heart rate monitors**. These objective monitors, for the most part, are small, lightweight, and unobtrusive. The disadvantages of this type of assessment include the expense, the inability to assess specific types of activities, and the potential effect of extraneous factors on the physical activity assessment results.

Regardless of the technique, because of day-to-day and seasonal variation, the method should reflect physical activity participation on the weekends and weekdays as well as each season of the year (39). It is also important to use a reliable and valid evaluation method. A reliable method is reproducible, giving the same results for a given amount of physical activity. A valid method is one that accurately measures what it is intended to measure. Establishing validity of a physical activity measure is difficult because no true gold standard of physical activity exists (61). Methods of energy expenditure (i.e., doubly labeled water, indirect and direct calorimetry) are often used to validate physical activity assessments. These measures are not gold standards for physical activity validation because physical activity encompasses movement, and energy expenditure takes into account movement and body mass (39). In addition, doubly labeled water and indirect calorimetry, although serving as good criteria for measurement of energy expenditure, provide no information on the types of activities performed or the context in which these activities are performed. Given these limitations, validity is indirectly established by comparing results with other physical activity measures as well as physiologic variables. To determine if a physical activity assessment tool is reliable, the reproducibility should be examined with a test–retest period of 2 to 4 weeks. This period is sufficiently short that behaviors should not change, but it is long enough that the initial administration is not influencing the second test (65). The following sections describe various valid and reliable subjective and objective methods of physical activity assessment as well as the various criteria to consider when deciding on the appropriate method to use.

SUBJECTIVE ASSESSMENT: SELF-REPORT MEASURES OF PHYSICAL ACTIVITY

Subjective physical activity measurements include questionnaires and diaries. The complexity of the questionnaire can vary from a single, physical activity–related question to a more thorough, detailed account regarding physical activity patterns (23,31,43,49,66). Even though a single-item questionnaire cannot provide a complete account of one's physical activity, it may be an adequate measure for classifying individuals into crude activity categories. A more comprehensive questionnaire takes into account the type of activity, how frequently it is performed over a certain time period, and the duration and intensity of the activity session (43). A physical activity diary can also range in complexity from one that has participants record every activity every minute of the day to those that have participants record activities in 4-hour periods and can be as general as including only the intensity of the activity. One example is the ACTIVITYGRAM, a component of the FITNESSGRAM assessment (70). Children are asked to record their activities in 30-minute time blocks for this component. However, this may be further divided into 15-minute intervals, depending on whether the activity was performed "all of the time" (given credit for entire 30 minutes) during the 30-minute segment or "some of the time" (given credit for 15 minutes). Other examples of popular questionnaires and diaries are found in resources by Montoye et al. (39), Periera et al. (43), and Kriska and Caspersen (32). The following sections describe questionnaires and diaries as well as several advantages and disadvantages to using each (Table 12-2).

QUESTIONNAIRES

A physical activity questionnaire usually can be administered quickly and inexpensively, is reliable, and does not cause a person's normal daily activity habits to change

TABLE 12-2. SUBJECTIVE MEASUREMENT OF PHYSICAL ACTIVITY

	ADVANTAGES	DISADVANTAGES
Diary	• Suitable for large populations • Little expense • No observer or interviewer • Collected in many subjects at the same time • Specific activities and patterns can be recorded	• Large amount of data to process, increasing the time and expense • Participants' cooperation and motivation required • Longer collection period can result in less accurate data • Need to record throughout the year to get typical physical activity
Questionnaire	• Suitable for large populations • Specific activities can be recorded • Patterns of behavior not affected • Total energy expenditure may be estimated • Applicable to wide age range	• Inaccurate recall • May be burdensome • Must be age appropriate • Interviewer may be necessary for accuracy • Limited use with younger children (younger than age 10 years)

(35). This type of instrument does not provide an absolute measurement of energy expenditure, but it allows energy expenditure to be estimated and for individuals to be ranked from least to most active (31). As soon as a person's relative activity level is known, it is possible to examine the associations between physical activity and various disease endpoints, such as heart disease, diabetes, various types of cancer, and obesity (31).

Self-report measures, such as questionnaires, can be used by various age groups and may be modified based on the study purpose or population (31,51,71). When using a questionnaire to assess physical activity in young children, a proxy report (e.g., time spent playing outside [50]) can be used. Assessing physical activity level in women is an example of the importance of questionnaire modification based on the population. According to national data from 2000, women were almost 7% less active than men (8). This discrepancy may be partly attributable to the nature of the physical activity questions asked by national surveys rather than women's actual activity levels. Some women may spend a large part of their day involved in household, family, and transportation activities, which are not captured by national survey questions (2).

Limitations of questionnaires include recall bias, individuals' problems with accurately recalling information, and differing recollection based on factors such as the person's age and disease status. Sedentary and high-intensity activities are the most reliably recalled using self-reported methods (28,49,51). Difficulties remembering and accurately recording moderate physical activities, especially lifestyle activities, offer another challenge to using questionnaires to assess physical activity. Finally, individuals may feel compelled to give socially desirable answers to physical activity questions when responding directly to an interviewer. Overall, the evidence suggests that adults tend to overestimate their physical activity levels (51).

DIARIES

Collecting physical activity information with a diary allows for data collection from many participants at the same time and eliminates the expense associated with an interviewer or observer. With this method of assessment, specific activities are usually recorded on the diary; therefore, physical activity patterns can be determined. Given that participants are asked to record their activities throughout the day, it is important that they are cooperative and willing to perform the task accurately. Recording all activities can be quite tedious. Therefore, keeping a diary over long periods of time can result in inaccurate data collection. Three days of diary collection—2 weekdays and 1 weekend day—are adequate to accurately assess physical activity patterns (13). The short, 3-day assessment time frame limits participant burden.

A limitation to using a diary is the time and expense it takes to process large amounts of data. In addition, the diary process should be completed at various times (seasons) throughout the year to help ensure that regular activity patterns are being ascertained. For example, in some areas of the country, physical activity levels are higher in the summer than in the winter (44).

SUMMARIZING DATA

> **1.1.5-CES: Identify the metabolic equivalent (MET) requirements of various occupational, household, sport/exercise, and leisure-time activities.**

After the data have been collected with a diary or questionnaire, they can be summarized in several different ways. Ways to express physical activity summary scores include time, metabolic equivalents (METs), and kilocalories (kcals) (43). Figure 12-1 illustrates three potential ways to derive a physical activity summary score (43). The most basic way is to calculate total time spent in physical activity. This is done by multiplying the number of sessions per week of the activity by the time spent performing the activity each session. A second calculation weighs the time spent in the activity by an estimated metabolic cost of each activity (MET). A MET is an estimate of intensity based on the ratio of working metabolic rate to resting metabolic rate. One MET is equivalent to oxygen uptake of $3.5 \text{ mL} \cdot \text{kg}^{-1} \cdot \text{min}^{-1}$ and represents energy expended at rest; an activity that expends eight times

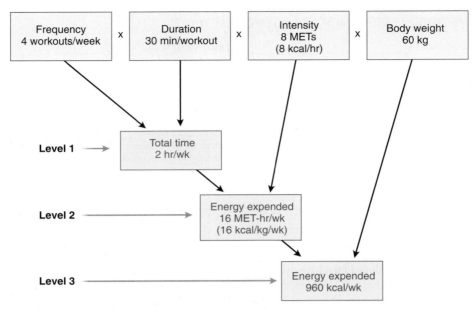

FIGURE 12-1. Ways to summarize physical activity data. Modified with permission from Kriska AM, Caspersen CJ. A collection of physical activity questionnaires for health related research. *Med Sci Sports Exerc.* 1997;29(6 Suppl):S7.

the resting energy expenditure, such as running, is 8 METs. The Compendium of Physical Activities compiled by Ainsworth et al. is a popular resource for obtaining MET values for a wide range of physical activities (1,3,4). An example of a calculation using METs (Fig. 12-1) follows. An individual reported running four times a week for 30 minutes a session. As shown at level 1 in the figure, this equates to 2 hours a week spent running. Multiplying the total time spent in running by its MET value, or 8 METs, results in an estimated energy expended from running of 16 MET-hr $\cdot$ wk^{-1} (level 2; Fig. 12-1). Finally, if the individual's body weight is known, one can calculate the kilocalories per week expended in physical activity. The results from this calculation are provided at level 3 (Fig. 12-1). For an individual weighing 60 kg, this equates to 960 kcal $\cdot$ wk^{-1}. Assumptions made when using these calculations include (a) MET values are representative of the way an activity is performed, regardless of the skill level of the individual or pace of the activity, and (b) the metabolic cost of performing activities (in METs) is constant among individuals, regardless of body weight (43).

OBJECTIVE ASSESSMENT: DIRECT MEASUREMENT OF PHYSICAL ACTIVITY

Physical activity monitors, such as pedometers, accelerometers, and heart rate (HR) monitors, provide objective estimates of one's physical activity. Other objective measures of physical activity and energy expenditure—such as direct observation, doubly labeled water, and indirect calorimetry—are often used to estimate physical activity level; however, these costly methods may not al-

ways be practical with large groups of individuals. Direct observation is primarily used for physical activity assessment in children over short periods of time. Examples of direct observation systems include the System for Observing Play and Leisure Activity in Youth (SOPLAY) and the Children's Activity Rating Scale (CARS) (38,46). Total energy expenditure measures, such as doubly labeled water, are limited because they do not allow for the determination of physical activity patterns (10). Different activity combinations or patterns (e.g., a small amount of strenuous activity versus a larger amount of moderate-intensity activity) can result in the same amount of energy expenditure (39). Many energy expenditure methods do not provide accurate estimates of absolute amount of physical activity (51).

Accelerometers and pedometers can accurately determine baseline and small changes in activity level (61). The cost of the instruments makes these measures potentially more expensive to administer than questionnaires. Unlike questionnaires, they are not subject to recall bias or inaccurate recall by participants. Physical activity monitors are also relatively easy to use, and participant language and reading ability are not issues. However, the monitors are designed to record ambulatory activity and cannot be worn while performing water activities. Therefore, they may not accurately detect movement from activities such as bicycling, weightlifting, or swimming (10). Monitors appear to provide reasonable measures of ambulatory activity (39). Several methods of objective assessment of physical activity as well as the advantages and disadvantages of each are described below and listed in Table 12-3.

TABLE 12-3. OBJECTIVE MEASUREMENT OF PHYSICAL ACTIVITY

	ADVANTAGES	DISADVANTAGES
Pedometer	• Instrument low to moderate expense • Small and lightweight • Unobtrusive • With proper instruction, is easy to use and provides immediate feedback	• Detects only ambulatory activity • Cannot determine type, intensity, or pattern of activity • Cannot detect changes in terrain • Cannot be worn in the water • Can be worn on shoe or ankle during cycling
Accelerometer	• Total energy expenditure may be estimated • Applicable to wide age range • Enjoyable with respect to amount of information provided	• Detects only ambulatory activity • Cannot detect changes in terrain • Cannot be worn in the water or when cycling • Expense of instrument and hardware or software to process data • Cannot determine type of activity • Requires a computer to process and report data
Heart rate monitor	• Physiologic marker • Can record and store heart rate data over an extended period of time • Can detect different intensities of activity	• Influenced by factors not related to physical activity participation • Cannot determine type of activity • Hard to detect low-intensity activities • Time and cost of processing data

PEDOMETERS

Pedometers detect vertical accelerations of the body and record a "step" when vertical acceleration exceeds a threshold value (69). These monitors are small and relatively inexpensive but do not provide information as extensive as accelerometers. Some pedometers have proven to be quite accurate for recording the number of steps taken and distance walked at various walking paces (9,19,52). Pedometers are more reliable for faster walking (4.0 vs. 2–3.0 mph) and running paces compared with slower ones (8,69). It has been shown that a pedometer records a higher number of steps for walking compared with running for the same distance (9). This finding is not surprising given that the stride length is shorter when walking compared with running. The accuracy of the pedometer does not appear to differ based on the type of walking or running surface (9,69). Welk et al. (69) extended the pedometer research to compare step counts with energy expenditure estimated from self-reported physical activities. They found that the relationship between pedometer step counts and energy expended in moderate-intensity activities was stronger than the relationship with energy expended in vigorous activities (69). Finally, some pedometers express energy expenditure in kilocalories; however, these functions have not been as well validated as actual step counting. Hence, researchers recommend reporting pedometer data as "steps", because that is the most direct expression of what the pedometer measures (48,62).

For certain groups, special types of pedometers are needed. A problem with pedometers that have a horizontal spring-suspended lever arm to register steps is that they are much less sensitive if they are tilted away from the vertical plane. Thus, in obese adults, pedometers may fail to record steps at slow walking speeds if the belt is tilted. However, a new type of pedometer with a piezoelectric accelerometer mechanism (New Lifestyles NL-2000) overcomes this problem and is thus a good choice for monitoring ambulatory activity in obese individuals (18). Another problem with waist-mounted pedometers is that they are not sensitive enough to detect steps taken in frail, older individuals who walk with a slow, shuffling gait. In this population, a comfortable, lightweight ankle-mounted device called the Stepwatch 3 (Cyma Corporation, Seattle, WA) will record steps with a high level of accuracy, even at 1.0 mile per hour (27).

Limitations to using a pedometer for physical activity assessment include the insensitivity to changes in walking speed and the inability of most pedometers to determine intensity or duration of the activity being performed (39). Even though the pedometer does not give a complete picture of physical activity patterns, step count results are related to physical activity assessments from various accelerometers, which provide a more thorough pattern of activity (10,36). Therefore, a pedometer is a practical and accurate means of assessing physical activity (11,59).

ACCELEROMETERS

Accelerometers can be worn on the trunk or limbs and measure movement based on acceleration and deceleration of the body. These measurements are proportional to muscular forces (39). Given this principle, most results from accelerometers are in proportion to energy expenditure and are used to ascertain the time, frequency, and duration of physical activity performed at various intensities (2,39). These types of activity patterns cannot be determined from other methods of energy expenditure, such as doubly labeled water (10).

Single plane accelerometers, such as the Caltrac (Muscle Dynamics, Torrence, CA) accelerometer and Acti-Graphs (formerly known as CSA; MTI Health Services, Ft. Walton Beach, FL), measure movement in the vertical plane. Triaxial monitors, such as the Tritrac-R3D (Hemokinetics Inc., Madison, WI), measure movement in the vertical, horizontal, and mediolateral planes (21).

Advantages of the accelerometer include its small size and ability to record data over long periods of time (e.g., several days or weeks) as well as the ability to download data and to segment physical activity periods (25). To reduce the expense of using this type of device, the same accelerometer can be worn repeatedly by different participants. When using one monitor worn at different times for multiple participants, only small amounts of data can be collected at one time (61).

This type of objective assessment requires more time and resources than a pedometer because technical expertise, hardware, and software are needed to calibrate, input, download, and analyze data (60,61). Single-plane accelerometers may not accurately detect movement from activities such as bicycling, weightlifting, or swimming (10). In addition, when worn on the hip, certain accelerometers may not accurately identify activity level on other areas of the body (67). None are able to detect increased activity level resulting from upper-body movement, carrying a load, or variations in the surface (e.g., climbing uphill) (25). Given the limitation of type of movement detected, Swartz et al. had participants wear monitors on the hip and wrist simultaneously and determined that the extra monitor slightly increased the accuracy of estimating the energy expenditure necessary to perform various physical activities (56). The small increases in accuracy reported with the additional monitor need to be weighed against the time, cost, and effectiveness of an additional monitor (56).

An additional limitation of this mode of measuring physical activity is the potential to misclassify one's activity levels. The accelerometer equations that estimate energy expenditure are typically derived from specific laboratory activities; therefore, they may not be applicable to free-living situations (19). For instance, accelerometer equations derived from treadmill walking and jogging have been shown to predict the energy cost of those activities quite accurately. However, when these same equations are applied to lifestyle activities, such as gardening and housework, they tend to over- or underestimate the actual energy cost (10,67). Thus, the relationship between treadmill walking or running measured in a laboratory with an accelerometer and indirect calorimetry is stronger than that reported for moderate lifestyle activities (67).

Several investigators have developed accelerometer equations that are based on moderate-intensity lifestyle activities, including housework, yard work, and occupational tasks (25,56). These equations are generally more accurate for moderate-intensity lifestyle activities, but they tend to overpredict sedentary and light activities and to underpredict vigorous sports. For this reason, Crouter et al. (17) developed a new two-regression model that examines the variability in accelerometer counts and uses this to determine whether an individual is performing (a) intermittent lifestyle activities or (b) dynamic, rhythmic locomotion, such as walking or jogging. It then uses either a walk/jog regression or an intermittent lifestyle regression to predict the energy cost from the mean accelerometer counts. The Crouter two-regression approach may provide a more accurate estimate of energy expenditure across a wide range of physical activities (17). However, this study has yet to be replicated at the time of this writing.

According to Welk et al., accelerometers give the most objective and detailed physical activity data for research purposes (67). Overall, accelerometers provide a useful measure of physical activity, but they are less accurate than other devices for determining total energy expenditure (25,67). In the future, it may be possible to improve estimations of physical activity by supplementing accelerometer data with questionnaire data. In addition, researchers are seeking to improve upon the accuracy of accelerometers by developing more sophisticated mathematic algorithms to convert acceleration data into energy expenditure (25,67).

HEART RATE MONITORING

> **1.1.26-HFS: Knowledge of the response of the following variables to acute static and dynamic exercise: heart rate, stroke volume, cardiac output, pulmonary ventilation, tidal volume, respiratory rate, and arteriovenous oxygen difference.**

Heart rate is linearly related to $\dot{V}O_2$; therefore, HR monitoring is another reasonable method of physical activity assessment (21). Other physiologic variables, such as cardiac output, pulmonary ventilation, tidal volume, respiratory rate, and arteriovenous oxygen difference also increase with increasing $\dot{V}O_2$ but are more difficult to measure. Thus, HR is one of the most practical physiologically based ways to estimate energy expenditure in the field (39). HR monitoring is "low cost, noninvasive and able to give information of the pattern of physical activity" (55). As with accelerometers, HR recorders can store data, which allows for the estimation of frequency, duration, and intensity of physical activity for days and weeks. Strath et al. reported a correlation of 0.87 when comparing the relationship between energy expenditure for lifestyle activities measured with indirect calorimetry and estimates from HR monitoring (55). This correlation is stronger than those reported between energy expenditure measured with indirect calorimetry and accelerometers for lifestyle activities (54).

Strath et al. (54) suggested that when subjects wear an accelerometer and a HR monitor simultaneously, energy expenditure estimation and classification of time spent in light, moderate, and hard activity were more accurate. Further research needs to be conducted, but it appears that HR monitors with additional types of activity assessment may be effective means of assessing physical activity (39,54).

> **1.1.12-CES: Describe the effects of variation in environmental factors (e.g., temperature, humidity, altitude) for normal individuals and those with cardiovascular, pulmonary, and metabolic diseases.**

A limitation to using HR monitors to assess physical activity is that factors such as ambient temperature, humidity, and high altitude will increase the HR response to exercise. In addition, emotional state, hydration status, type of contraction (static versus dynamic), and the amount of muscle mass recruited will affect HR, independent of physical activity level (39). In addition, the HR response to a given physical activity challenge is highly individual, and to maximize accuracy, individualized HR-energy cost calibrations must be performed, which is time consuming. Finally, the specific type of activity cannot be determined, and low-intensity activities are hard to detect.

OTHER POTENTIAL METHODS

There are several other types of technologically advanced objective measures, such as task-specific monitoring sensors and the global positioning system (GPS), which may be helpful for improving physical activity assessment in the future. Eventually, it may be possible to have sensors located on clothing and accessories that can monitor physiologic responses, such as HR and respiration, and transmit the information to a computer (24). This information, along with that provided by a wearable digital camera that can provide pictures of the day's activities, could give an accurate, objective account of an individual's physical activities throughout the day (24). GPS is a satellite-based navigational system that uses signal information between satellites and receivers, worn by individuals, to ascertain the velocity and duration of displacement (24). Research studies to date support the ability of GPS to provide accurate assessments of speed, ranging from slow walking to fast running, as well as other biomechanical parameters (53,57). Currently, there are relatively inexpensive ($100) GPS units available that are lightweight; can be worn on the wrist; and provide speed, distance, and pace information while walking or running. However, GPS units cannot be used for stationary exercise and may be unable to be used indoors. As these methods continue to become more feasible and their cost is reduced, they have the potential to expand our ability to accurately assess physical activity.

CHOOSING A METHOD

Various types of subjective and objective physical activity assessments have been described. There are several criteria to consider when choosing an assessment method. These criteria include the purpose of the assessment, cost, characteristics of the population being assessed, and the endpoints being evaluated. The method chosen should be valid and reproducible in a representative population (45). There are also additional considerations, such as the assessment time frame and method of administration, that should be taken into account when administering questionnaires.

PURPOSE

Regardless of your health or fitness profession, at least one of the tools described in this chapter can help you achieve the purpose of assessing physical activity. For example, if you are a health and fitness specialist in a fitness center, are working with a new participant, and would like to assess his or her past physical activity habits, you may want to use a past-year assessment tool, such as the Modifiable Activity Questionnaire (43). This type of questionnaire allows you to determine the frequency and duration of an individual's specific activities performed over the past year to ascertain his or her usual physical activity habits. Knowing an individual's physical activity patterns is also helpful in developing an appropriate exercise program. If your purpose is monitoring a participant's physical activity level or change in physical activity level, you could use an objective measure or an activity log. If ambulatory activity is primarily being performed, then a participant could wear a pedometer and record the number of steps taken. For this method to be effective, the baseline number of steps the participant takes should be established. Then the monitor should be worn continuously or at various intervals over time to evaluate the maintenance or change in physical activity. If the activities primarily involve weight training, it is important to use a log that includes the exercise performed, the amount of weight lifted, and the number of sets and repetitions performed. For monitoring general activity, logs can be completed by participants through the Internet at no cost. An example of this type of log can be found at the following site: http://www.presidentschallenge.org/activity_log/track_progress.aspx. Versions of this log can either be printed out and completed or completed online. This type of log allows participants to record the type of physical activity as well as intensity and duration. Alternatively, there is an option for recording the number of pedometer steps taken each day.

COST

With all these measures, it is necessary to weigh the cost of assessment against the quality of data obtained. More expensive techniques usually provide more precise data. Self-report methods to assess physical activity typically involve low to moderate costs, mostly for printing and data processing. Higher costs with diary administration relate to the large amounts of data to process. Interviewer-administered questionnaire expenses are predominantly attributable to personnel costs. The cost of using physical activity monitors depends on the expense associated with the instrument. Pedometers (~$10 to $40, with some combination models costing as much as $70) are less expensive than accelerometers ($300–$450) and HR monitors ($200–$1,000). Data-storage capabilities with accelerometers and HR monitors also result in the additional cost of downloading, preparing, and analyzing the data.

CLINICAL POPULATION

As discussed previously, there are issues with accurately measuring moderate and lifestyle physical activities and physical activity in women. Therefore, it is crucial that methods used to assess physical activity levels accurately capture these types of activities. Similar issues exist when assessing physical activity in various minority ethnic or racial groups. It is important to determine the activities that contribute most to energy expenditure in the study population (30). For some minority groups, the activities include occupational activities, transportation, household chores, and caretaking, rather than sports and high-intensity leisure activities (30). Therefore, physical activity assessment tools should validly and reliably measure physical activity common to the population under study.

Age should also be a consideration, especially in questionnaire administration. This method may not be appropriate for children younger than age 10 years old. For older individuals, it has been suggested that effective questionnaire administration should involve an interviewer. This mode of administration is important to clarify questions individuals may have. The type of domains assessed should be age appropriate (i.e., in older adults, activities such as walking, light to moderate housework, and yard work should be the focus of the assessment), and recall time frames should be short (39). Older adults also tend to handle short, specific questions involving specific activities and periods (e.g., minutes spent in an activity, times per week an activity is done) better than general, open-ended questions (39). If using an objective measure, pedometers may be as effective for assessing energy expenditure as accelerometers in older individuals if the activities predominantly involve walking rather than jogging, running, and upper-body motion. These instruments also appear to be appropriate in children (68).

ENDPOINTS

The endpoint being evaluated is also an important consideration when choosing a method to assess physical ac-

tivity. For example, measuring lifetime patterns of physical activity may be important when examining the relationships between cancer and bone health (37,40,64). If the focus of the study is to establish a dose–response relationship with a health-related endpoint, a questionnaire, accelerometer, or HR monitor that allows for physical activity pattern determination is necessary. Finally, if the study goal is to determine the effectiveness of a physical activity intervention, comparing pre- and postintervention data from questionnaires with shorter time frames (e.g., past week or 3-day diary) or physical activity monitors should be appropriate. Exceptions to using a monitor include the evaluation of interventions that involve strength training or another type of nonambulatory activity not accurately assessed with a monitor.

CONSIDERATIONS FOR QUESTIONNAIRE AND DIARY USE

Time Frames

Time frames used when assessing physical activity vary from a diary that segments the day and has participants record their activities in 15-minute intervals to questionnaires that ask about lifetime physical activity. The time frame assessed depends on the population and endpoint of interest to the researcher.

Shorter time frames are the easiest to recall; however, they may not give an accurate picture of typical physical activity patterns. There are certain endpoints that rely on recent physical activity to accurately predict risk because it may affect the outcome more than the history of physical activity. This is reflected in studies by Blair et al. and Paffenbarger et al. that demonstrated that changes in physical activity or fitness levels predict mortality risk (12,41). For example, a person may be unfit at one point in time, but if her fitness level improves, her mortality risk is lower than someone who remained unfit. One's relatively recent physical activity level, rather than one's physical activity history, was related to mortality. Questionnaires that cover shorter periods of time, however, may not provide an adequate representation of a person's normal activity level (e.g., during bad weather, assessment of activities from the past week or past month may substantially underestimate one's activity level for the remainder of the year) (35). Physical activities performed over the past year may not be remembered as accurately, but they do provide a more complete physical activity profile. Lifetime physical activity may be important to assess for its relationship to certain types of cancer as well as bone health (37,40,64). Although this time frame might be the most difficult to recall accurately, several studies have reported reasonable reliability results for long-term physical activity recall (16,33,34). In addition, researchers have examined the validity of long-term recall (i.e., 10–15 years) and have found results comparable to that of questionnaires with shorter recall time frames (14,29,68).

Administration Techniques

Questionnaires are administered in a variety of ways. Questionnaires that are interviewer administered (either in person or over the telephone) take more time and are more costly than those that are self-administered. This method allows participants to clarify any issues and uncertainties about the questions, thereby reducing response errors.

Self-administered questionnaires are inexpensive and provide information comparable to that from interviewer-administered questionnaires (26). Using this method of administration, the questionnaire can either be given to participants or sent to them through the mail. These questionnaires can be easily administered to large groups of individuals in a short amount of time.

More recent advances in technology have made the Internet a viable means of questionnaire administration. With the popularity and widespread availability of computers and Internet access, this may be a cost-effective way to monitor activity levels. Potential uses include online questionnaire administration and continuous monitoring of physical activity (e.g., online physical activity diaries). Further validation is needed for this potentially valuable method of recording and tracking physical activity behaviors.

SUMMARY

It is important to use a valid and reliable method that is appropriate for the population as well as the study endpoint. The advantages and disadvantages of each type of subjective and objective physical assessment have been introduced. Given these strengths and weaknesses, a combination of physical activity assessment methods may provide the most accurate estimate of physical activity. This combination approach to assessment has not been widely examined (40). However, based on the conclusion of various reports regarding the assessment of physical activity, using more than one method of ascertainment should increase the accuracy of the measurement (29,53,59,60,61). Treuth recently recommended that additional research should focus on applying different combinations of assessment techniques to larger samples as well as various age groups and special populations (58).

REFERENCES

1. Ainsworth BE. The compendium of physical activities. *The President's Council on Physical Fitness and Sports Research Digest Series.* 2003;4(2):1–8.
2. Ainsworth BE. Issues in the assessment of physical activity in women. *Res Q Exerc Sport.* 2000;71(2 Suppl):S37–42.
3. Ainsworth BE, Haskell WL, Leon AS, et al. Compendium of physical activities: classification of energy costs of human physical activities. In: *ACSM's Resource Manual for Guidelines for Exercise Testing and Prescription.* Philadelphia: Lippincott Williams & Wilkins; 2005. p. 667–698.
4. Ainsworth BE, Haskell WL, Whitt MC, et al. Compendium of physical activities: an update of activity codes and MET intensities. *Med Sci Sports Exerc.* 2000;32(9 Suppl):S498–516.
5. American College of Sports Medicine. Position Stand. The recommended quantity and quality of exercise for developing and maintaining fitness in healthy adults. *Med Sci Sports.* 1978;10(3):vii–x.
6. American College of Sports Medicine. Position Stand. The recommended quantity and quality of exercise for developing and maintaining cardiorespiratory and muscular fitness in healthy adults. *Med Sci Sports Exerc.* 1990;22(2):265–74.
7. American College of Sports Medicine. Position Stand. The recommended quantity and quality of exercise for developing and maintaining cardiorespiratory and muscular fitness, and flexibility in healthy adults. *Med Sci Sports Exerc.* 1998;30:975–991.
8. Barnes PM, Schoenborn CA. Physical activity among adults: United States, 2000. *Adv Data* (from Vital and Health Statistics of the CDC) 2003;333:1–23.
9. Bassett DR Jr, Ainsworth BE, Leggett SR, et al. Accuracy of five electronic pedometers for measuring distance walked. *Med Sci Sports Exerc.* 1996;28(8):1071–1077.
10. Bassett DR Jr, Ainsworth BE, Swartz AM, et al. Validity of four motion sensors in measuring moderate intensity physical activity. *Med Sci Sports Exerc.* 2000;32(9 Suppl):S471–480.
11. Bassett DR Jr, Strath SJ. Use of pedometers to assess physical activity. In Welk GJ, editor. *Physical Activity Assessments for Health-Related Research.* Champaign (IL): Human Kinetics; 2002. p. 213–225.
12. Blair SN, Kohl HW III, Barlow CE, et al. Changes in physical fitness and all-cause mortality: a prospective study of healthy and unhealthy men. *JAMA.* 1995;273(14):1093–1098.
13. Bouchard C, Tremblay A, Leblanc C, et al. A method to assess energy expenditure in children and adults. *Am J Clin Nutr.* 1983;37(3):461–467.
14. Bowles HR, FitzGerald SJ, Morrow JR, Jackson AW. Construct validity of self-reported historical physical activity. *Res Q Exerc Sport.* 2007;78(2):24–31.
15. Caspersen CJ, Powell KE, Christenson GM. Physical activity, exercise, and physical fitness: definitions and distinctions for health-related research. *Public Health Rep.* 1985;100(2):126–131.
16. Chasan-Taber L, Erickson JB, McBride JW, et al. Reproducibility of a self-administered lifetime physical activity questionnaire among female college alumnae. *Am J Epidemiol.* 2002;155(3):282–289.
17. Crouter SE, Clowers KG, Bassett DR Jr. A novel method for using accelerometer data to predict energy expenditure. *J Appl Physiol.* 2006;100(4):1324–1331.
18. Crouter SE, Schneider PL, Bassett DR Jr. Spring-levered versus piezo-electric pedometer accuracy in overweight and obese adults. *Med Sci Sports Exerc.* 2005;37(10):1673–1679.
19. Crouter SE, Schneider PL, Karabulut M, Bassett DR Jr. Validity of 10 electronic pedometers for measuring steps, distance, and energy cost. *Med Sci Sports Exerc.* 2003;35(8):1455–1460.
20. Dunn AL, Marcus BH, Kampert JB, et al. Comparison of lifestyle and structured interventions to increase physical activity and cardiorespiratory fitness: a randomized trial. *JAMA.* 1999;281(4):327–334.
21. Freedson PS, Miller K. Objective monitoring of physical activity using motion sensors and heart rate. *Res Q Exerc Sport.* 2000;71(2):S21–29.
22. Haskell WL, Lee IM, Pate RR, et al. Physical activity and public health: updated recommendation for adults from the American College of Sports Medicine and the American Heart Association. *Med Sci Sports Exerc.* 2007;39:1423–1434.
23. Haskell WL, Taylor HL, Wood PD, et al. Strenuous physical activity, treadmill exercise test performance and plasma high-density lipoprotein cholesterol. The Lipid Research Clinics Program Prevalence Study. *Circulation.* 1980;62(4 Pt 2):IV53–61.
24. Healey J. Future possibilities in electronic monitoring of physical activity. *Res Q Exerc Sport.* 2000;71(2 Suppl):S137–145.

25. Hendelman D, Miller K, Baggett C, Debold E, Freedson P. Validity of accelerometry for the assessment of moderate intensity physical activity in the field. *Med Sci Sports Exerc*. 2000;32(9 Suppl):S442–449.

26. Jacobs DRJ, Ainsworth BE, Hartman TJ, Leon AS. A simultaneous evaluation of 10 commonly used physical activity questionnaires. *Med Sci Sports Exerc*. 1993;25(1):81–91.

27. Karabulut M, Crouter SE, Bassett DR Jr. Comparison of two waist-mounted and two ankle-mounted electronic pedometers. *Eur J Appl Physiol*. 2005;95(4):335–343.

28. Kimsey CD, Ham SA, Macera CA, et al. Reliability of moderate and vigorous physical activity questions in the Behavioral Risk Factor Surveillance System (BRFSS) [abst]. *Med Sci Sports Exerc*. 2003; 35(5 Suppl):S114.

29. Kohl HW III, Kampert JB, Måasse LC, et al. The accuracy of historical physical activity recall among middle- aged women and men [abs]. *Med Sci Sports Exerc*. 1997;29(5 Suppl):S242.

30. Kriska AM. Ethnic and cultural issues in assessing physical activity. *Res Q Exerc Sport*. 2000;71(2 Suppl):S47–53.

31. Kriska AM, Bennett PH. An epidemiological perspective of the relationship between physical activity and NIDDM: from activity assessment to intervention. *Diabetes Metab Rev*. 1992;8(4):355–372.

32. Kriska AM, Caspersen CJ. Introduction to a collection of physical activity questionnaires. *Med Sci Sports Exerc*. 1997;29(6 Suppl):S5–S9.

33. Kriska AM, Knowler WC, LaPorte RE, et al. Development of questionnaire to examine relationship of physical activity and diabetes in Pima Indians. *Diabetes Care*. 1990;13(4):401–411.

34. Kriska AM, Sandler RB, Cauley JA, et al. The assessment of historical physical activity and its relation to adult bone parameters. *Am J Epidemiol*. 1988;127(5):1053–1063.

35. LaPorte RE, Montoye HJ, Caspersen CJ. Assessment of physical activity in epidemiologic research: problems and prospects. *Public Health Rep*. 1985;100(2):131–146.

36. Leenders NYJM, Sherman WM, Nagaraja HN. Comparisons of four methods of estimating physical activity in adult women. *Med Sci Sports Exerc*. 2000;32(7):1320–1326.

37. Matthews CE, Shu XO, Jin F, et al. Lifetime physical activity and breast cancer risk in the Shanghai Breast Cancer Study. *Br J Cancer*. 2000;84(7):994–1001.

38. McKenzie TL, Marshall SJ, Sallis JF, Conway TL. Leisure-time physical activity in school environments: an observational study using SOPLAY. *Prev Med*. 2000;30(1):70–77.

39. Montoye HJ, Kemper HCG, Saris WHM, Washburn RA. *Measuring Physical Activity and Energy Expenditure*. Champaign (IL): Human Kinetics; 1996. 191 p.

40. Nieves JW, Grisso JA, Kelsey JL. A case-control study of hip fracture: evaluation of selected dietary variables and teenage physical activity. *Osteoporos Int*. 1992;2(3):122–127.

41. Paffenbarger RS Jr, Hyde RT, Wing AL, et al. The association of changes in physical-activity level and other lifestyle characteristics with mortality among men. *N Engl J Med*. 1993;328(8):538–545.

42. **Pate RR, Pratt M, Blair SN, et al. Physical activity and public health: a recommendation from the Centers for Disease Control and Prevention and the American College of Sports Medicine. *JAMA*. 1995;273(5):402–407.**

43. Pereira MA, FitzGerald SJ, Gregg EW, et al. A collection of physical activity questionnaires for health-related research. *Med Sci Sports Exerc*. 1997:29(6 Suppl):S1–205.

44. Pivarnik JM, Reeves MJ, Rafferty AP. Seasonal variation in adult leisure-time physical activity. *Med Sci Sports Exerc*. 2003;35(6): 1004–1008.

45. Pols MA, Peeters PH, Kemper HC, Grobbee DE. Methodological aspects of physical activity assessment in epidemiological studies. *Eur J Epidemiol*. 1998;14(1):63–70.

46. Puhl J, Greaves K, Hoyt M, Baranowski T. Children's Activity Rating Scale (CARS): description and calibration. *Res Q Exerc*. 1990;61(1): 26–36.

47. Ravussin E, Swinburn BA. Pathophysiology of obesity. *Lancet*. 1992;340(8816):404–408.

48. Rowlands AV, Eston RG, Ingledew EK. Measurement of physical activity in children with particular reference to the use of heart rate and pedometry. *Sports Med*. 1997;24(4):258–272.

49. Sallis JF, Haskell WL, Wood PD, et al. Physical activity assessment methodology in the Five-City Project. *Am J Epidemiol*. 1985;121(1): 91–106.

50. Sallis JF, Nader PR, Broyles SL, et al. Correlates of physical activity at home in Mexican-American and Anglo-American preschool children. *Health Psychol*. 1993;12(5):390–398.

51. Sallis JF, Saelens BE. Assessment of physical activity by self-report: status, limitations, and future directions. *Res Q Exerc Sport*. 2000; 71(2 Suppl):S1–14.

52. Schneider PL, Crouter SE, Lukajic O, Bassett DR Jr. Accuracy and reliability of 10 pedometers for measuring steps over a 400-m walk. *Med Sci Sports Exerc*. 2003;35(10):1779–1784.

53. Schutz Y, Herren R. Assessment of speed of human locomotion using a differential satellite global positioning system. *Med Sci Sports Exerc*. 2000;32(3):642–646.

54. Strath SJ, Bassett DR Jr, Thompson DL, Swartz AM. Validity of the simultaneous heart rate-motion sensor technique for measuring energy expenditure. *Med Sci Sports Exerc*. 2002;34(5):888–894.

55. Strath SJ, Swartz AM, Bassett DR Jr., et al. Evaluation of heart rate as a method for assessing moderate intensity physical activity. *Med Sci Sports Exerc*. 2000;32(9 Suppl):S465–470.

56. Swartz AM, Strath SJ, Bassett DR Jr, et al. Estimation of energy expenditure using CSA accelerometers at hip and wrist sites. *Med Sci Sports Exerc*. 2000;32(9 Suppl):S450–456.

57. Terrier P, Ladetto Q, Merminod B, Schutz Y. High-precision satellite positioning system as a new tool to study the biomechanics of human locomotion. *J Biomech*. 2000;33(12):1717–1722.

58. Treuth MS. Applying multiple methods to improve the accuracy of activity assessments. In: Welk GJ, editor. *Physical Activity Assessments for Health-Related Research*. Champaign (IL): Human Kinetics; 2002. p. 213–225.

59. Tudor-Locke CE. Taking steps toward increased physical activity: using pedometers to measure and motivate. *The President's Council on Physical Fitness and Sports Research Digest Series*. 2002;3(17): 1–8.

60. Tudor-Locke C, Ainsworth BE, Thompson RW, Matthews CE. Comparison of pedometer and accelerometer measures of free-living physical activity. *Med Sci Sports Exerc*. 2002;34(12):2045–2051.

61. Tudor-Locke CE, Myers AM. Challenges and opportunities for measuring physical activity in sedentary adults. *Sports Med*. 2001; 31(2):91–100.

62. Tudor-Locke CE, Myers AM. Methodological considerations for researchers and practitioners using pedometers to measure physical (ambulatory) activity. *Res Q Exerc Sport*. 2001;72(1):1–12.

63. **U.S. Department of Health and Human Services. *Physical Activity and Health: A Report of the Surgeon General*. Atlanta: U.S. Department of Health and Human Services, Centers for Disease Control and Prevention, National Center for Chronic Disease Prevention and Health Promotion; 1996.**

64. Vuillemin A, Guillemin F, Jouanny P, et al. Differential influence of physical activity on lumbar spine and femoral neck bone mineral density in the elderly population. *J Gerontol A Biol Sci Med Sci*. 2001;56(6):B248–253.

65. Washburn RA, Heath GW, Jackson AW. Reliability and validity issues concerning large-scale surveillance of physical activity. *Res Q Exerc Sport*. 2000;71(2 Suppl):S104–113.

66. Weiss TW, Slater CH, Green LW, et al. The validity of single-item, self-assessment questions as measures of adult physical activity. *J Clin Epidemiol*. 1990;43(11):1123–1129.

67. Welk GJ, Blair SN, Wood K, et al. A comparative evaluation of three accelerometry-based physical activity monitors. *Med Sci Sports Exerc*. 2000;32(9 Suppl):S489–497.

68. Welk GJ, Corbin CB, Dale D. Measurement issues in the assessment of physical activity in children. *Res Q Exerc Sport*. 2000;71(2 Suppl):S59–73.

69. Welk GJ, Differding JA, Thompson RW, et al. The utility of the Digi-walker step counter to assess daily physical activity patterns. *Med Sci Sports Exerc*. 2000;32(9 Suppl):S481–488.

70. Welk GJ, Morrow JR. Physical activity assessments. In: Meredith MD, Welk GJ, editors. *The Fitnessgram Test Administration Manual*. Champaign(IL): Human Kinetics; 1999. p. 55–65.

71. Winters-Hart CS, Brach JS, Storti KL, Kriska AM. Validity of a questionnaire to assess historical leisure physical activity in post-menopausal women. *Med Sci Sports Exerc*. 2003;36(12): 2082–2087.

SELECTED REFERENCES FOR FURTHER READING

Lee I-M, Blair S, Manson J, Pafferbarger RS. Physical Activity and Health: Epidemiologic Methods and Studies. USA: Oxford University Press; 2008.

Measurement of Physical Activity: The Cooper Institute Conference Series. Proceedings from the 9th Measurement and Evaluation Symposium. *Res Q Exerc Sport*. 2000;71(suppl 2).

Montoye HJ, Kemper HCG, Saris WHM, Washburn RA. *Measuring Physical Activity and Energy Expenditure*. Champaign (IL): Human Kinetics; 1996.

National Center for Health Statistics. *Assessing Physical Fitness and Physical Activity in Population-Based Surveys*. Drury TF, ed. DHHS Pub. No. (PHS) 89-1253. Public Health Service. Washington, D.C: U.S. Government Printing Office; 1989.

Pereira MA, FitzGerald SJ, Gregg EW, et al. A collection of physical activity questionnaires for health related research. *Med Sci Sports Exerc*. 1997;29(6):S1–205.

Welk GJ, editor. *Physical Activity Assessments for Health-Related Research*. Champaign (IL): Human Kinetics; 2002.

INTERNET RESOURCES

- Centers for Disease Control and Prevention: Nutrition and Physical Activity: www.cdc.gov/nccdphp/dnpa/
- The Cooper Institute: www.cooperinst.org
- PACE Projects: www.paceproject.org
- The President's Challenge: www.presidentschallenge.org/activity_log/track_progress.aspx
- USC PRC Reports and Tools: http://prevention.sph.sc.edu/tools/index.htm

13

Nutritional Status and Chronic Diseases

Compelling evidence proves that lifestyle changes such as dietary improvements, increased physical activity, and behavior modification can prevent or delay major chronic diseases, including cardiovascular disease (CVD), obesity, diabetes, and osteoporosis. Importantly, recent research (108) confirms that the effects of dietary and other lifestyle changes may be additive. At the same time that clinical and population studies have supported the importance of diet, the effects of nutrients and foods on genome stability, imprinting, expression, and viability have also correlated with dietary factors at the molecular level that lead to prevention of chronic diseases (130). Largely because of this emerging evidence, a paradigm shift in healthcare approaches has occurred toward early and aggressive prevention strategies. Accordingly, a greater proportion of the population will need behavioral strategies for lifestyle changes that positively affect chronic metabolic disease risk. Thus, the purpose of this chapter is to examine the relationship of diet and nutrition to chronic disease and to encourage healthcare professionals to promote healthier lifestyles.

Chronic metabolic diseases are often interrelated. For example, obesity is associated with the comorbidities of CVD, diabetes, and hypertension, all of which are characterized by increased morbidity and mortality risk from insulin resistance and its consequences (37). Increased levels of circulating free fatty acids from excess stored fat, particularly intra-abdominal, appear to contribute to insulin resistance, although the mechanisms are still debated (120). A related condition known as metabolic syndrome encompasses most of these chronic conditions (52,97).

> **1.8.2-HFS: Knowledge of the following terms: obesity, overweight, percent fat, BMI, lean body mass, anorexia nervosa, bulimia, metabolic syndrome, and body fat distribution.**

> > > KEY TERMS

Antioxidants: Dietary components such as vitamins C and E, selenium, carotenoids, and other phytochemicals (chemicals from plants with antioxidant or hormonelike actions) that can protect DNA and cell membranes against oxidative damage from carcinogens.

Body mass index (BMI): Body weight (in kg) divided by height^2 (in meters) is an expression used to evaluate weight in the context of the distribution of mass over an individual's height (39).

Cholesterol: A steroid alcohol present in human cells and blood that regulates membrane fluidity and functions as a precursor molecule in metabolism. As a constituent of LDL-C, it contributes to plaque formation in arteries, and recommendations concerning maximal blood levels have been made as part of the National Cholesterol Education Program (NCEP [86]).

Glycemic index: The increase in blood sugar after ingestion of a food or food component compared with the increase after ingestion of glucose, which is assigned an index of 100, with foods being assigned higher and lower relative values. The glycemic response varies with the type of sugar, other food components, amount of carbohydrate, nature of the starch, and cooking or food processing.

Glycemic load: A value for each food that combines both the quality and quantity of carbohydrate to predict blood glucose responses to different types and amounts of food: (GI x the amount of carbohydrate) divided by 100.

High-density lipoprotein cholesterol (HDL-C): Compound that transports body cholesterol to other lipoproteins for disposal, contains a high proportion of phospholipids (30%) and protein (45%–50%), and generally decreases the risk of coronary artery disease (86).

Impaired fasting glucose (IFG): A prediabetic condition in which the fasting blood sugar is elevated ($100-125$ mg $\cdot$ dL^{-1}) after an overnight fast (6).

Impaired glucose tolerance (IGT): A prediabetic condition in which the blood sugar level is elevated (140 to 199 mg $\cdot$ dL^{-1}) after a 2-hour glucose tolerance test (6).

Interesterified fats: The latest modified (stearic acid-rich) fats created by manufacturers to replace unhealthy trans fats in commercial food products. This newer fat may raise blood glucose and depress insulin action in humans similarly to trans fat (131).

Low-density lipoprotein cholesterol (LDL-C): Substance that is taken up by receptor and scavenger pathways in blood vessels, contains a high proportion of cholesterol (45%), and generally increases the risk of coronary artery disease (86).

Metabolic syndrome: A cluster of metabolic conditions, including obesity, impaired fasting glucose, elevated triglycerides, low levels of HDL-C, and hypertension, usually characterized by insulin resistance and a high risk of developing CVD or diabetes (52).

Monounsaturated fats: Fatty acids with one double bond between the carbon atoms, prevalent in olive oil, canola oil, and high oleic acid oils. These fats are neutral or only slightly increase serum LDL-C levels.

Obesity: As defined by the National Institutes of Health, a body mass index of greater than 30 kg $\cdot$ m^{-2}.

Omega-3 fatty acids: Fatty acids with the first double bond between carbon atoms located between the third and fourth carbon, including alpha linolenic acid (ALA) and the three series such as eicosapentaenoic acid (EPA) and docosahexenoic acid (DHA). These fats decrease the risk of CVD and are prevalent in fish and flaxseed, walnut, canola, and soybean oils (86).

Omega-6 fatty acids: Fatty acids with the first double bond between carbon atoms located between the

sixth and seventh carbons, which are converted to hormonelike substances called eicosanoids. Sources of omega-6 fatty acids are corn, safflower, peanut, cottonseed, soybean, sesame, rapeseed, borage, and primrose oils (86).

Osteoporosis: A condition characterized by microarchitectural deterioration of bone tissue leading to decreased bone mass and increased bone fragility.

Overweight: As defined by the National Institutes of Health, a body mass index of 25 to 29.9 kg $\cdot$ m^{-2}.

Polyunsaturated fats: Fatty acids with two or more double bonds between carbon atoms. These fats decrease serum low-density lipoprotein cholesterol levels. Foods with a high percentage of polyunsaturated fats include corn, safflower, peanut, cottonseed, soybean, fish, walnut, and flaxseed oils (86).

Prediabetes: The intermediate metabolic state between normal blood glucose levels (<100 mg $\cdot$ dL^{-1}) and diagnosed diabetes (≥126 mg $\cdot$ dL^{-1}), which can include impaired glucose tolerance (IGT), impaired fasting glucose (IFG), or a combination of both conditions. Individuals with prediabetes are considered to be at risk for developing type 2 diabetes (6).

Prehypertensive: Systolic blood pressure of 120 to 139 mm Hg or a diastolic blood pressure of 80 to 89 mm Hg (30).

Saturated fats: Fatty acids with single bonds between the carbons atoms. These fats increase serum low-density lipoprotein cholesterol levels and are prevalent in animal fats; butter; meats; milk fat; cheeses; and tropical oils, such as palm, coconut, and palm kernel oil (86).

Trans fats: Fatty acids with a rearrangement of the bond between some of the carbon atoms to a form rarely found in natural foods. The change occurs because of processing such as the hydrogenation (the addition of hydrogen to change texture and improve shelf life). Foods containing these fats include margarine, shortening, processed foods, and commercially baked or fried foods (86).

> **1.8.17-HFS: Ability to describe the health implications of variations in body-fat distribution patterns and the significance of the waist-to-hip ratio.**

The National Cholesterol Education Program criteria (52) for the metabolic syndrome (or the "dysmetabolic syndrome") include any three of the following: large waist circumference >102 cm or 40 inches in men and >88 cm or 35 inches in women, high triglycerides (≥150 mg $\cdot$ dL^{-1}), low-serum high-density lipoprotein cholesterol (HDL-C) levels (<40 mg $\cdot$ dL^{-1} for men and <50 mg $\cdot$ dL^{-1}

for women), high blood pressure (BP; systolic ≥130 mm Hg or diastolic ≥85 mm Hg), and fasting plasma glucose concentration ≥100 mg $\cdot$ dL^{-1}. It is estimated that 47 million American adults, more than 25% of the population, meet three or more of these criteria, thereby increasing their risk for CVD and type 2 diabetes (123). Abdominal obesity is the most common, followed by decreased HDL-C levels, hypertension, and elevated plasma triglycerides, as stated in the AHA-NHLBI Scientific Statement about diagnosing and managing this syndrome (52). The risk for disease increases as the number of these characteristics accumulates, warranting the need for early intervention.

The prospective Insulin Resistance Atherosclerosis Study (94) found that the best predictor for developing the metabolic syndrome in adults without diabetes was waist circumference. The authors concluded that abdominal obesity may precede the development of other metabolic syndrome components. However, the existence of this syndrome is currently controversial, with some arguing that it cannot be considered a "real" syndrome in a strict sense because, at present, no unifying mechanism explains it (129). Its definitions vary as well, with differing criteria for waist circumference (International Diabetes Foundation), blood pressure (World Health Organization [WHO]), and HDL-C levels (WHO). In fact, adults may arguably fare better in managing their disease risk when each metabolic component that is present is simply treated separately rather than focusing on treating the syndrome as a whole. In other research, the development of insulin resistance in young adulthood was strongly predicted from childhood adiposity and serum insulin levels and from being the offspring of a parent with type 2 diabetes, underscoring the need to address excess weight gain in children to manage metabolic risk factors (96,126,127).

Unfortunately, there is also no agreement about the optimal diet for preventing and treating chronic metabolic diseases, but recommendations from professional organizations and government institutes or agencies provide evidence-based guidelines, such as the guidelines for diabetes, obesity, and CVD given in Table 13-1. The American Dietetic Association (9) advocates the terminology *medical nutrition therapy (MNT)* for the nutritional diagnostic, therapeutic, and counseling services to accomplish the following:

- Effectively treat and manage disease conditions
- Reduce or eliminate the need for prescription drug use
- Help reduce complications in patients with disease
- Improve patients' overall health and quality of life

The MNT recommendations for obesity, diabetes, and CVD specify dietary proportions of macronutrients: carbohydrate, fat, and protein. The average diet in the United States for individuals older than 20 years currently consists of 34% kcal from total fat, 49% kcal from carbohydrates, 15% to 16% kcal from protein, and 2% to 3% of kcal from alcohol (80). When a diet low in one macronutrient is promoted, other macronutrients are concomitantly increased at a given energy level; for example, a low-carbohydrate diet usually results in a higher fat and protein dietary intake (117). Therefore, frequent monitoring of fasting lipid panels may be indicated for persons at risk of chronic disease who choose a low-carbohydrate diet (7). Usually slight to moderate changes in macronutrient proportions have little effect on the short-term health parameters, such as serum lipids, but deleterious, long-term health effects are often unknown.

The greatest similarities across national diet recommendations (Table 13-1) for obesity, hypertension, CVD, and diabetes are the recommendations to maintain a healthy weight and to consume total dietary fat of approximately 30% kcal. The National Cholesterol Education Program (NCEP) Therapeutic Lifestyle Changes (TLC) recommends a dietary fat intake of 25% to 35% of daily kcals (86). The specified purpose of the TLC diet is for prevention and treatment of obesity, metabolic syndrome, and CVD. Although recommendations for specific diet components vary with disease risk, a healthy weight is a primary step toward decreasing chronic disease risk. All calorie-restricted diets can be balanced to result in weight loss, regardless of their composition, but some diets meet nutrition needs with less health risk and should be the preferred choice for health professionals. A reasonable guide is the Institute of Medicine/National Academy of Sciences' 2002 recommendation of acceptable macronutrient ranges of 20% to 35% fat, 45% to 65% carbohydrate, and 10% to 35% protein (61).

CARDIOVASCULAR DISEASE AND DIET

> **1.8.1-CES: Describe and discuss dietary considerations for cardiovascular and pulmonary diseases, chronic heart failure, and diabetes that are recommended to minimize disease progression and optimize disease management.**

> **1.2.8-HFS: Knowledge of how lifestyle factors, including nutrition and physical activity, influence lipid and lipoprotein profiles.**

Cardiovascular diseases leading to heart attacks and strokes are the leading cause of death and disability in the United States and worldwide (26,101). The World Health Organization currently attributes one third of all global deaths to CVD. This ongoing and increasing health problem underscores the need to improve our communication of improved diet and lifestyle interventions. Disease progression occurs over a lifetime, and dietary changes must be maintained to be effective. Public health and clinical approaches alone have limitations. Therefore, the American Heart Association's guide (101) for improving cardiovascular health at the community level advocates for concomitant and parallel public health and clinical approaches. They identify public health problems, including limited access to screening; limited long-term and effective strategies for diet and physical activity changes; poor identification of healthy food choices at grocery stores and restaurants; and lack of safe, attractive sites for physical activity in many communities. Clinical settings provide a complementary focus on individuals with high disease risk, but diet counseling and nutrition education are often inadequate and highly variable (101). Diverse

TABLE 13-1. MEDICAL NUTRITION THERAPY FOR OBESITY/METABOLIC SYNDROME, HYPERTENSION, CARDIOVASCULAR DISEASE, AND DIABETES

DIAGNOSTIC CRITERIA AND RISK FACTORS	NUTRITION AND LIFESTYLE RECOMMENDATIONS	THERAPEUTIC OBJECTIVES	PRACTICE GUIDELINES (REFERENCES)
Obesity/Metabolic Syndrome Criteria for metabolic syndrome include any three of the following: Waist circumference: Men >102 cm (>40 in) Women >88 cm (>35 in) BP: ≥130/≥85 mm Hg Trig: ≥150 mg·dL⁻¹ HDL-C: men <40 mg·dL⁻¹, women <50 mg·dL⁻¹ FPG: ≥100 mg·dL⁻¹ Other risk factors: BMI ≥30, sleep apnea, elevated CRP levels Hyperinsulinemia and insulin resistance may also be present	**Low Calorie Step I Diet and Referral to Dietitian** (for individuals at lower risk) 500–1,000 kcal·d⁻¹ reduction, ≤30% fat, 8–10% SFA, <300 mg cholesterol ~2.4 g Na, 1,000–1,500 mg Ca, 20–30 g fiber **TLC Diet and Referral to Dietitian** (for individuals at higher risk) Establish appropriate kcal Rx 50–60% CHO ~15% protein 25–35% total fat <7% SFA, <200 mg cholesterol **[same in Step II Diet]** PUFA (up to 10% of total kcals) MUFA (up to 20% of total kcals) 10–25 g viscous (soluble) fiber 2 g plant stanols/sterols **Weight reduction and long-term control** 1–2 pounds loss/wk and gradually reach healthy BMI (<30 initially, then <25) **Increase physical activity** (~200 Kcal/d) **Smoking cessation**	1) Reasonable weight loss of 5%–10%, maintain healthy BMI, prevent weight gain 2) Primary: ↓LDL-C to ↓CHD risk Secondary: recognize and treat metabolic syndrome for further risk reduction Optimal BMI range: 18.5–24.9 Target total cholesterol: <200 mg·dL⁻¹ Target TG: <150 mg·dL⁻¹ Target LDL-C: <100 mg·dL⁻¹ Target HDL-C: ≥40 (men), ≥50 (women) mg·dL⁻¹ Target BP: <130/<85 mm Hg Target FPG: <100 mg·dL⁻¹	NHLBI, NIH–Classification of Overweight and Obesity, Weight Loss Goals, and Low-Calorie Step I & Step II Diets (39) NCEP ATP III–Metabolic Syndrome Criteria and Therapeutic Lifestyle Changes (86) www.nhlbi.nih.gov/guidelines/obesity/ www.nhlbi.nih.gov/guidelines/cholesterol/ www.surgeongeneral.gov/topics/obesity
Hypertension BP classification: Normal: <120/80 mm Hg Pre-HTN: 120–139/ 80–89 mm Hg Stage 1 HTN: 140–159/ 90–99 mm Hg Stage 2 HTN: ≥160/ ≥100 mm Hg *Risk of CVD, beginning at 115 75 mm Hg, doubles with each increment of 20/10 mm Hg	**DASH Diet and Referral to Dietitian** Establish appropriate kcal Rx ≤2,400 mg Na, <30% total fat Limit alcohol: men ≤2 drinks/d, women ≤1 drink/d Reduce dietary sodium and red meat intake Increase dietary calcium, magnesium, potassium, and fiber via fruits, vegetables, whole grains, reduced fat dairy, and lean protein Include fish, nuts, seeds, and dry beans weekly Choose plant fats and oils. **Achieve and maintain healthy body weight** **Increase physical activity** **Smoking cessation**	1) Prevent progression to HTN in prehypertensive population 2) Decrease CVD complications and reduce cardiovascular and renal morbidity and mortality in hypertensive population Optimal BP: <120/<80 mm Hg Goal of tx: BP <130/<80 mm Hg(for patients with diabetes or chronic kidney disease) Goal of tx: BP <140/<90 mmHg (for patients with HTN)	NHLBI, NIH–Prevention, Detection, Evaluation, and Treatment of High Blood Pressure and Dash Eating Plan (138) www.nhlbi.nih.gov/guidelines/hypertension/ www.nhlbi.nih.gov/health/public/heart/hbp/dash/index/htm
Cardiovascular Disease Abnormal Blood Lipid Profile: Total cholesterol: ≥200 mg·dL⁻¹ Triglyceride: ≥150 mg·dL⁻¹ LDL-C: ≥100 mg·dL⁻¹ HDL-C: men <40 mg·dL⁻¹, women <50 mg·dL⁻¹	**AHA Dietary Guidelines and Referral to Dietitian** Establish appropriate kcal Rx <6 g NaCl (<2,400 mg Na) <30% total fat, limit TFAs **[AHA populationwide recommendations for individuals at lower risk]** <10% SFA, <300 mg cholesterol **[AHA MNT for individuals at higher risk]** <7% SFA, <200 mg cholesterol	1) Reduce CVD risk, morbidity, and mortality by preventing or reducing the development of atherosclerotic disease and stroke 2) For overweight/obese patients, ↓ weight by 10% in 1st year of therapy Target total cholesterol: <160 mg·dL⁻¹ (optimal) Total cholesterol: 160–199 mg·dL⁻¹ (low-risk profile) Target LDL-C: <100 mg·dL⁻¹ if ≥2 CHD risk factors	AHA Dietary Guidelines, Revision 2002 (11) AHA Dietary Guidelines, 2000 (70) www.americanheart.org

(continued)

TABLE 13-1. MEDICAL NUTRITION THERAPY FOR OBESITY/METABOLIC SYNDROME, HYPERTENSION, CARDIOVASCULAR DISEASE, AND DIABETES (*Continued*)

DIAGNOSTIC CRITERIA AND RISK FACTORS	NUTRITION AND LIFESTYLE RECOMMENDATIONS	THERAPEUTIC OBJECTIVES	PRACTICE GUIDELINES (REFERENCES)
Other major CVD risk factors include: Obesity, inactive lifestyle, atherogenic diet Elevated BP, blood glucose, and homocysteine levels Hyperinsulinemia and insulin resistance may also be present	Limit alcohol: men ≤2 drinks/d, women ≤1drink/d Limit high-caloric/low-nutrient dense foods and beverages Increase intake of antioxidants, omega fatty acids, and fiber via variety of fruits, vegetables, whole grains, reduced fat dairy, fish, legumes, nuts, plant fats and oils **Achieve and maintain healthy body weight** **Increase physical activity: 30 minutes daily of** moderate intensity exercise using large muscle groups (i.e., walking or swimming) **Smoking cessation**	Target HDL-C: >40 (men), >50 (women) mg·dL^{-1} Goal BP: <140/<90 or <130/<85 mm Hg for patients with renal insufficiency, heart failure, or <130/<80 mm Hg for patients with diabetes	
Diabetes *Normoglycemia:* FPG <100 mg·dL^{-1} 2-h PG <140 mg·dL^{-1} *IFG (Impaired Fasting Glucose):* FPG ≥100 and <126 mg·dL^{-1} *IGT (Impaired Glucose Tolerance):* 2-h PG ≥140 and <200 mg·dL^{-1} *Diabetes:* FPG ≥126 mg·dL^{-1} 2-h PG ≥200 mg·dL^{-1} Casual PG ≥200 mg·dL^{-1} (symptoms present)	**ADA Dietary Guidelines and Referral to Dietitian** Establish appropriate kcal Rx CHO and MUFA together should provide 60%–70% total kcal 15%–20% protein <30% total fat, minimize TFAs <10% SFA, <300 mg cholesterol if LDL-C <100 mg·dL^{-1} <7% SFA, <200 mg cholesterol if LDL-C ≥100 mg·dL^{-1} Limit alcohol: men ≤2 drinks/d, Women ≤1drink/d *Appropriate Rxs may integrate any of the following established regimens: Low Calorie Step I or Step II, TLC, DASH, AHA, or Mediterranean diets **Goals of MNT and Self- Management Education:** • Attain and maintain recommended metabolic outcomes, including glucose, A$_{1c}$, LDL-C, HDL-C, TG levels; BP; and body weight • Modify nutrient intake and lifestyle as appropriate for the prevention and treatment of obesity, dyslipidemia, HTN, CVD, depression, and nephropathy. • Structured, intensive lifestyle programs involving participant education, individualized counseling, regular physical activity, and SMBG. • Smoking cessation	1) Diabetes prevention: ↓risk by encouraging physical activity and food choices that facilitate moderate weight loss (5%–7%) or at least prevent weight gain 2) Prevent and treat chronic complications and comorbidities of diabetes Target HbA$_{1c}$: <7.0% Target FPG: 80–120 mg·dL^{-1} Target bedtime BG: 100–140 mg·dL^{-1} Target BP: <130/80 mm Hg Target blood lipids (mg·dL^{-1}): TG <150 LDL <100 HDL ≥40 (Men), ≥50 (Women) Target Microalbumin: <30 μg·mg^{-1} creatinine	American Diabetes Association: Clinical Practice Guidelines (6,7,8) American Dietetic Association: Nutrition Practice Guidelines at www.eatright.org www.diabetes.org

AHA, American Heart Association; ATP III, Adult Treatment Panel III; BG, blood glucose; BMI, body mass index; BP, blood pressure; Ca, calcium; CHD, coronary heart disease; CHO, carbohydrate; CRP, C-reactive protein; CVD, cardiovascular disease; FPG, fasting plasma glucose; IFG, impaired fasting glucose; IGT, impaired glucose tolerance; HDL-C, high density lipoprotein cholesterol; HTN, hypertension; LDL-C, low density lipoprotein cholesterol; MNT, medical nutrition therapy; MUFA, mono-unsaturated fatty acid; Na, sodium; NaCl, sodium chloride; NCEP, National Cholesterol Education Program; NIH, National Institutes of Health; NHLBI, National Heart Lung and Blood Institute; PG, Plasma glucose; PUFA, polyunsaturated fatty acid; Rx, prescription; SFA, saturated fatty acid; SMBG, ; TFA, trans fatty acid; TG, triglycerides; TLC, ; Trig, triglyceride; Tx, treatment.

Table used by permission of Loredo G and Herzog H, Division of Medical Nutrition and Center for Nutrition and Metabolic Disorders. Department of Internal Medicine. University of Nevada School of Medicine, Reno, NV. 2004.

and interdisciplinary diet and lifestyle changes are required to address the CVD risk.

CORONARY HEART DISEASE

> **1.2.4-HFS: Knowledge to define the following terms: total cholesterol (TC), high-density lipoprotein cholesterol (HDL-C), TC/HDL-C ratio, low-density lipoprotein cholesterol (LDL-C), triglycerides, hypertension, and atherosclerosis.**

> **1.2.5-HFS: Knowledge of plasma cholesterol levels for adults as recommended by the National Cholesterol Education Program.**

Coronary heart disease (CHD) includes the development of atherosclerosis with the potential negative outcome of clot formation, resulting in a myocardial infarction (MI) or heart attack (see Chapter 6). Risk factors for CHD include an abnormal lipid profile, obesity, inactive lifestyle, atherogenic diet, elevated blood glucose and homocysteine levels, and hyperinsulinemia and insulin resistance, among others (11). The preferred lipid profile, recommended by the National Cholesterol Education Program and others, includes a total cholesterol of 200 mg·dL^{-1} or less with a target of 160 mg·dL^{-1} with high CHD risk, triglycerides 150 mg·dL^{-1} or less, LDL-C 100 mg·dL^{-1} or less, and an HDL-C equal to or greater than 40 for women and 50 for men (11,70,86).

The primary dietary factors that prevent atherosclerotic lesions and abnormally elevated serum lipid levels include diets moderate or low in saturated fat and cholesterol, decreased trans fatty acids, increased omega-3 fatty acids, and shifted sources of fat to more monounsaturated fats (11,70,86) (Table 13-1). Vitamins decrease cardiovascular risk if patients consume an adequate food intake of antioxidants and dietary vitamins (B$_{12}$, B$_6$, folate) to maintain normal serum homocysteine levels. In addition, the recommended intake of fruits, vegetables, breads, cereals, nuts, seeds, and other plant foods provides fiber, plant sterols, and phytochemicals, such as flavonoids, that decrease cardiovascular risk. A variety of other foods and food components, such as alcohol and soy protein, have been investigated to decrease cardiovascular risk (86). Similar dietary factors that are important for CVD risk decrease clot formation (e.g., regular consumption of fish sources containing high concentrations of omega-3 fatty acids and alcohol intake). Also, a habitual high-fat diet may increase the activity of the blood clotting factor VII and increase cardiovascular risk (26).

Fats and Cholesterol

Saturated and Unsaturated

Saturated fatty acids, cholesterol, and high-fat diets are strongly associated with increased risk of CHD in susceptible persons (11,71). Changes in dietary cholesterol can

dramatically alter serum LDL-C in a select segment of the population. Genetic explanations, such as apoprotein E and E4 variants, have been explored, but the results have been variable and remain unclear (86). Egg yolks are a rich source of cholesterol, but are low in saturated fatty acids. The role of eggs has been controversial, but current approaches emphasize limiting dietary intake to achieve 200 to 300 mg per day of dietary cholesterol (no more than 100 mg per 1,000 kcals [71,86]). For reference, there is approximately 190 mg per large egg.

Dietary saturated fat can be decreased by changing total fat intake to moderate- (<30% kcal) or low-fat (20% kcal) levels while altering the sources and types of fat to increase monounsaturated and polyunsaturated fat intakes. Saturated fatty acids that need reduction include those with the greatest effect on increasing serum cholesterol and LDL-C: myristic and palmitic acids found in dairy products and meat (66) and trans fatty acids found in margarine, processed foods, and commercially baked or fried foods containing hydrogenated oils (65). The primary dietary monounsaturated fatty acid is oleic (abundant in olive and canola oils and nuts), whereas linoleic (abundant in soybean and sunflower oils) is the comparable polyunsaturated one (70).

Exactly how dietary fat intake should be modified to lower cardiovascular risk remains controversial. For example, in 2006, the results were published from a large-scale, randomized controlled trial of 48,835 postmenopausal women ages 50 to 79 years, of diverse backgrounds and ethnicities, who participated in the Women's Health Initiative Dietary Modification Trial (60). Intensive behavior modification in group and individual sessions was implemented to attempt to reduce total fat intake to 20% of calories and increase intakes of vegetables and fruits to five servings per day and grains to at least six daily servings in the intervention group (19,541 women). The comparison group (29,294 women) received diet-related education materials only. Over a mean of 8.1 years, the dietary intervention did not significantly reduce the risk of CHD, stroke, or CVD and achieved only modest effects on CVD risk factors, although a trend toward greater reductions in CHD risk was observed in women with lower intakes of saturated fat or trans fat or higher intakes of vegetables and fruits. At the time participants were enrolled (1993–1998), though, far less was known about the health benefits of omega-3 and other fats, and intake of all types of fats declined as a result of the intervention, making definitive conclusions based on these findings problematic.

Likely, dietary changes to lower LDL-C levels and cardiovascular risk involve more than a simple alteration in fat intake, though. By way of example, a randomized clinical trial compared LDL-C changes from a low-fat diet (consistent with former American Heart Association Step I guidelines that advocated avoiding saturated fat and cholesterol) to a low-fat diet incorporating considerably more vegetables, legumes, and whole grains, as per the

2000 American Heart Association revised guidelines (47). After 4 weeks in 120 hypercholesterolemic, but otherwise healthy, adults ages 30 to 65, the inclusion of more nutrient-dense plant-based foods resulted in a greater total and LDL-C-lowering effect of a low-fat diet. Along a similar vein, associations of dietary fat and specific types of fat with risk of CHD among 78,778 women in the Nurses' Health Study initially free of CVD and diabetes in 1980 were studied, the finding being an inverse association between polyunsaturated fat intake and CHD risk, particularly in overweight or younger women (92). In addition, a greater trans fat intake was associated with a higher risk, especially in younger women.

Omega-3 Fatty Acids

> **1.5.4-CES: Recognize the use of herbal and nutritional supplements, over-the-counter (OTC) medications, homeopathic remedies, and other alternative therapies often used by patients with chronic diseases.**

> **1.8.14-HFS: Knowledge of common nutritional ergogenic aids, the purported mechanism of action, and any risk and/or benefits (e.g., carbohydrates, protein/amino acids, vitamins, minerals, herbal products, creatine, steroids, caffeine.**

Omega-3 fatty acids exert a cardioprotective effect and reduce CHD risk by reducing elevated triglyceride levels, inhibiting platelet aggregation and formation of blood clots, lowering BP, preventing plaque formation, and promoting the health of the vascular epithelium in the coronary arteries (54). Omega-3 fatty acids are found in plant foods (flaxseed, canola oil, soybean oil, walnuts, mustard seed oil, and some leafy vegetables) as alpha linolenic acid (ALA) and in cold-water fish as the eicosanoids (eicosapentaenoic acid [EPA] and docosahexanoic acid [DHA]). About 10% of the ALA that is consumed is converted in the body to EPA and DHA, depending on the presence of omega-6 fatty acids that compete for the same enzymes.

The evidence for benefits of omega-3 fatty acids from the diet and supplements has been mixed (72), but a recent meta-analysis supports a strong association between a lower CHD risk and higher intake of fish (145). The meta-analysis consisted of 228,864 adult participants from 14 cohort and five case-control studies in which fish was consumed on a regular basis in the experimental group while the comparison group consumed little or no fish. Overall, fish consumption was associated with a 20% reduction in the risk of fatal CHD and a 10% reduction in total CHD, both hypothesized to be related to omega-3 fatty acid intake. In addition, a systematic review of prospective cohort studies found that high-risk populations had the most benefit from fish consumption, with an average of 1.5 to 2.0 oz of fish per day being associated with a 50% reduction in CHD death (78). More-

over, a secondary prevention trial, Diet and Reinfarction Trial (DART), found a 2-year, 29% decrease in mortality for survivors of a first MI in individuals consuming fatty fish two times per week (23). Supplemental omega-3 fatty acids have similar benefits as fish consumption to reduce CVD mortality, stroke, and all-cause mortality (49,77,121). The largest supplement trial included 11,324 patients who were survivors of MIs (49,77). The fish oil supplement group had a 20% reduction in total mortality, a 30% reduction in cardiovascular death, and a 45% decrease in sudden death 3.5 years after supplementation began. A more recent systematic review of prospective cohort studies, however, suggested that the benefits of fish oil are likely stronger in the secondary prevention of cardiovascular problems than primary (141).

Current AHA guidelines recommend at least two servings of fish (preferably oily varieties, such as tuna, salmon, and mackerel) per week for adult, nonpregnant or nursing patients without documented CHD (72). For patients with documented CHD, the recommendation is to consume a diet rich in ALA and 1 g of EPA and DHA per day, preferably from fish, but an omega-3 fatty acid supplement may be needed to meet this level. The use of supplements requires review by the patient's physician. Patients who use omega-3 fatty acids to lower triglyceride levels are recommended to take 2 to 4 g of EPA and DHA under their physician's care (72). The American Diabetes Association guidelines also recommend supplemental omega-3 fatty acids for patients with diabetes and severe hypertriglyceridemia, but recommend concomitant monitoring for potential increases in LDL-C (7).

Trans Fatty Acids

Trans fatty acids behave similarly to saturated fat in many ways, such as increasing LDL-C level. However, they are even more destructive than saturated fat because they also lower HDL-C level (145) and are associated with an increased risk of CHD (92). The Food and Drug Administration (FDA) instituted a requirement that food labels have the content of trans fatty acids listed starting in 2006, but there is insufficient information regarding the effects of various intake levels to establish a Daily Reference Value for them. A more recent concern is the substitution of interesterifed for trans varieties in commercial food products. This newer altered fat has preliminarily been shown to also negatively affect blood lipid levels and insulin action in humans more than saturated ones (131), but more research is clearly needed to assess their full health impact.

Recommended Diets

Patients who are at high risk of CHD or with diagnosed CHD can benefit from a nutrition plan that is consistent with the AHA Dietary Guidelines, including Step I and Step II diets (11,70) or the NCEP ATP III guidelines that use the TLC diet (86). The TLC diet is comparable to the Step II AHA diet except that the range of calories from fat is greater to accommodate evidence that CHD risk can be reduced with a variety of dietary patterns (Table 13-1). The Step II AHA and the TLC diets have the lower saturated fat recommendation of 7% versus 10% on Step I and the lower cholesterol recommendation of 200 mg·day^{-1} versus 300 mg·day^{-1}. A meta-analysis of 37 studies (148) found that the stricter Step II or TLC diets versus the Step I reduced total serum cholesterol by 15% versus 10% and LDL-C by 16% versus 12%, but both diets reduced triglycerides by 8%. One caveat was that whereas the Step I diet maintained HDL-C levels, the Step II and TLC diets led HDL-C to decrease by 7%. Thus, the AHA recommends the Step II diet for individuals who have CHD or who have not met the LDL-C goals with Step I (11).

Low-fat diets have an additional positive benefit when they contribute to weight loss, but the diet should be coupled with activity recommendations to maintain or improve the serum HDL-C level. Obesity decreases HDL-C levels as well, so the net effect of weight loss, when coupled with increased activity, is to improve cardiovascular health by decreasing LDL-C and increasing or maintaining HDL-C (86).

The Mediterranean diet may be useful for individuals who prefer a moderate fat intake with more added monounsaturated fats than the AHA or TLC diets (105,134). The Mediterranean diet also has positive cardiovascular benefits and approximates the Step I AHA diet with higher levels of monounsaturated fatty acids, such as oleic acid and polyunsaturated ALA. The traditional Mediterranean diet is composed of higher amounts of fruits, vegetables, bread and other cereals, potatoes, poultry, beans, nuts, fish, grains, dairy products, and moderate amounts of alcohol as well as olive oil. Given that it contains little red meat, this diet is also naturally low in saturated fat and high in monounsaturated fat (mainly from olive oil), complex carbohydrates, fiber, beta carotene, vitamin C, and tocopherols.

In the CARDIO2000 study, hypercholesterolemic participants who were taking statins were placed in control and diet groups (105). The Mediterranean diet group ate fruits, vegetables, dairy products, potatoes, and bread and used olive oil in cooking on a daily basis. Fish, poultry, and eggs, olives, and legumes were consumed two to three times per week. Red meat was only consumed one to two times per month, and wine was drunk in moderation (one to two glasses per day). Participants adhering to the Mediterranean diet had a 17% greater reduction in coronary event risk compared with those who did not adopt it. These results demonstrate the potential benefit of dietary interventions combined with statin therapy.

A population-based study examined the effects of the Mediterranean diet on total mortality, cardiac mortality, and cancer mortality in 22,043 adults in Greece (134). The median follow-up was 44 months, and adherence to the Mediterranean diet positively correlated with a reduction in total mortality, as well as death caused by coronary artery disease or cancer. Interestingly, the individual food groups contributing to the Mediterranean diet did not have a significant effect on total mortality unless they were integrated together into a diet.

A secondary prevention trial, the Lyon Diet Heart Study, with subjects who had a history of an initial MI, incorporated the Mediterranean diet with increased levels of ALA from fortified margarine, monounsaturates with olive oil, and polyunsaturated omega-6 fatty acids with rapeseed oil (32). The participants following the Mediterranean-style diet had 50% to 70% lower risk of recurrent heart disease with risk reductions of the same size as those typically associated with statin drug therapy. This multifactorial dietary intervention study demonstrated a positive effect of decreasing the ratio of omega-6 to omega-3 fatty acids to 4:1 versus the typical Western diet ratio of 14–20:1. In accordance, updated dietary guidelines from January 2006 for secondary prevention of cardiovascular events in individuals with known CVD were issued based on a review of all studies up to the prior year (81). They reiterated that lowering saturated fat intake appears to reduce morbidity in such individuals and further advised the addition of Mediterranean dietary habits and increased omega-3 fats for individuals with a prior myocardial infarction.

Vitamins

 1.5.4-CES: Recognize the use of herbal and nutritional supplements, over-the-counter (OTC) medications, homeopathic remedies, and other alternative therapies often used by patients with chronic diseases.

 1.8.6-HFS: Knowledge of the difference between fat-soluble and water-soluble vitamins.

Antioxidants

Food sources of antioxidant vitamins, instead of supplements, are advised because of the positive potential health effects of other associated food components such as flavones (a healthy phytochemical; see Table 13-2 for others). Epidemiologic studies of vitamin supplementation with antioxidant vitamins, particularly vitamins C, E, and A, as well as beta-carotene, have supported their possible role in reducing cardiovascular risk, but recent randomized, placebo-controlled trial results challenged the benefits for vitamins A and E and beta-carotene supplementation. Over a 5-year period, the Heart Protection Collaborative Group (56) studied the effects of supplementation with vitamins E and C and beta-carotene versus placebo on mortality and coronary events. There were no significant differences in any parameters for the 20,536 adults other than increased blood vitamin concentrations. The investigators reviewed the results for

TABLE 13-2. EXAMPLES OF PHYTOCHEMICAL RICH FOODS

PHYTOCHEMICAL	FOOD SOURCES
Ascorbic acid	Citrus, leafy green vegetables, broccoli, tomatoes, strawberries, melons
Beta-carotene	Carrots, sweet potatoes, pumpkin, winter squash, cantaloupe, mango, papaya
Coumarin	Citrus
d-Limonene	Oil from peel of citrus fruit
Ellagic acid	Blueberries, strawberries
Isothiocyanates, indole-3-carbinol	Cruciferous vegetables
Lutein	Green vegetables
Lycopene	Tomatoes
Organosulfur compounds	Onions, garlic, leeks, chives
Quercetin	Red wine, tea
Selenium	Plant foods from high-selenium soil
Vitamin E	Vegetable oils, whole grains

their 6,000 patients with diabetes and the results for 7,000 patients with no evidence of CHD before randomization and found no evidence of benefit from vitamin supplementation.

These results are in agreement with the Age-Related Eye Diseases (ARED) placebo-controlled trial of the same vitamins in 4,500 older adults without any recent cardiovascular events (2). Similarly, the Primary Prevention Project (31) studied the effects of vitamin E and the alpha-tocopherol beta-carotene (4) by investigating low-dose vitamin E and beta-carotene supplementation, with results indicating no significant differences in CHD outcomes. Likewise, natural vitamin E as opposed to synthetic products produced no significant difference for CHD (55). Finally, a recent meta-analysis also concluded that there was no evidence of a protective effect of antioxidant or B vitamin supplements against the progression of atherosclerosis, thus providing a mechanistic explanation for the lack of effect of such supplements on clinical cardiovascular events (18). Thus, despite previously encouraging results from nonrandomized, observational studies and small clinical trials, the preponderance of evidence from well-designed, large studies and meta-analyses of multiple studies found that there was no clear evidence of CHD benefits for antioxidant supplementation.

Homocysteine

Elevated serum homocysteine levels are a CHD risk factor that may be related to other risk factors rather than being an independent one (137). Homocysteine, a highly reactive sulfur-containing amino acid, has been thought to be damaging to health because of toxic effects that damage endothelial cells, increase cholesterol oxidation, modify apolipoproteins, promote platelet adhesion and aggregation, scavenge nitric oxide, and inhibit vascular motility. Homocysteine decreases nitric oxide, the smooth muscle relaxant in the arterial wall that decreases the tendency of platelets to aggregate and adhere to the vascular endothelium. Increased serum homocysteine is

most often caused by a combination of a genetic variant of an enzyme in its metabolism or suboptimal nutritional status for folate and vitamins B_{12} and B_6. The conversion of the amino acid methionine to homocysteine is limited when adequate folic acid is available, and its conversion to less toxic compounds is promoted when vitamin B_6 is available. B_{12} is another cofactor in the metabolism of this substance, and it interacts with folic acid or substitutes for folic acid in some cases (58).

A meta-analysis by Wald et al. (140) concluded that lowering homocysteine levels by 3 μmol$\cdot$L^{-1} from current levels (through increased folic acid intake) would reduce the risk of ischemic heart disease by 16% and stroke by 24%. Data from the Nurses' Health Study showed that folate and vitamin B_6 from the diet and supplements protected against CHD (112). Increased serum homocysteine levels have been associated with obesity in children in relation to folate intake and to hyperinsulinemia with insulin resistance (46). However, a recent meta-analysis examining the effects of folate supplementation failed to show a reduced risk of CVD or all-cause mortality among participants with prior history of vascular disease who supplemented with enough folate to lower homocysteine (16).

Plant Sources

> **1.5.4-CES: Recognize the use of herbal and nutritional supplements, over-the-counter (OTC) medications, homeopathic remedies, and other alternative therapies often used by patients with chronic diseases.**

Plant sources combined in a dietary plan, the Portfolio, have produced significant reductions in LDL-C compared with the traditional TLC diet and statin cholesterol-lowering drugs (62). The diet consists of 1 oz of almonds; 2 g of plant sterols from enriched margarine; 35 g of soy protein; and 15 g of viscous fiber from sources such as oats, barley, eggplant, and okra. A study of 25 hyperlipidemic patients showed a 35% reduction of LDL-C after 2 weeks of consuming the prepared diet compared with a

12% LDL-C reduction for those consuming the TLC diet (62). The benefit of these plant sources individually has been identified, and their inclusion is advocated in the TLC diet.

Fiber and Plant Sterols

Recommendations for dietary changes to decrease serum cholesterol include a greater intake of dietary fiber and plant sterols. The TLC diet recommends a total of 20 to 30 g of fiber each day (86). Soluble fiber increases the excretion of cholesterol in the bile, and an intake of 10 to 25 $g \cdot day^{-1}$ is suggested. To increase intake of soluble fiber, include or increase servings of fruits (especially those with high pectin content, such as apples, strawberries, and citrus), vegetables, oats, oat bran, and beans. The remainder of daily fiber intake is insoluble fiber that is not digested, adds bulk to the stool, and contributes to correcting diarrhea and constipation. Wheat bran is a good source of insoluble fiber (86).

The plant kingdom contains several sterols that differ from cholesterol because of their ethyl or methyl groups or unsaturation in the side chain. The major plant sterols—itosterol, stigmasterol, and campesterol—can be present in Western diets in amounts almost equal to dietary cholesterol. Sitosterol, the most prominent dietary sterol, with the saturated stanol derivative sitostanol, reduces the absorption of cholesterol and decreases blood cholesterol level. In 1999, several companies began marketing margarine, salad dressings, and other products containing either stanols or sterols made from soy and corn. An intake of 2 to 3 g per day or about 2 to 3 servings a day of products containing plant stanols and sterols decreased both dietary and biliary cholesterol absorption. Serum cholesterol levels decreased by 10%, and LDL-C decreased by 13% (25).

More recently, other studies suggested that elevated levels of plant sterols in the blood may actually cause CHD rather than preventing it. To study this, researchers evaluated the association between plant sterols and CHD in a cohort of 1,242 subjects older than 65 years participating in the Longitudinal Aging Study, Amsterdam (40). However, concentrations of sitosterol, campesterol, brassicasterol, and stigmasterol plant sterols (and their ratios to cholesterol) were found to be slightly but significantly lower in patients with CHD. Moreover, high plasma concentrations of sitosterol were associated with a markedly reduced risk for CHD. Thus, these data suggest that plant sterols could have neutral or even protective effects on development of CHD, a finding that needs to be confirmed in intervention trials. Sitosterols and a sterol precursor, squalene, are present in both monounsaturated and polyunsaturated vegetable oils and, thus, may be responsible for some of the variable cholesterol-lowering effects found in studies using these products. The levels of these sterols may also explain differences in study results with various sources and degrees of refinement of olive oil (73,98).

Flavonoids

Flavonoids are another type of phytochemical (Table 13-2) or chemically varied compound present in fruits, vegetables, nuts, and seeds that have been inversely linked with CHD, cancer, and other health problems. In the Zutphen Elderly Study (57), the Seven Countries Study (63), and a cohort study in Finland (68), people with low intakes of flavonoids had a higher death rate from CHD than did those who consumed more flavonoids. The amounts of foods rich in flavonoids, such as intake of about 5 to 6 cups of tea per day, that have been effective in these studies are at levels greater than usual dietary intake.

The major flavonoid categories are flavones (apple skins, berries, broccoli, celery, cranberries, grapes, lettuce, olives, onions, parsley), catechins (red wine, tea), flavanones (citrus fruits, citrus peel), isoflavones (soy), and anthocyanins (berries, cherries, red wine, grapes, tea). Subdivisions of flavonoids include quercetin glucoside in onions and quercetin rutinoside in tea. Some flavonoids have toxic effects (gastrointestinal or allergic), especially if taken in large amounts (89). Additionally, flavonoids have antioxidant properties. For example, the phenolic substances in red wine inhibit oxidation of human LDL-C. Flavonoids have also been shown to inhibit the aggregation and adhesion of platelets in the blood, which may be another way they lower the risk of CHD. Isoflavones in soy foods have been reported to lower plasma cholesterol level and to have effects similar to estrogen (89).

Although dietary flavonols and flavones, subgroups of flavonoids, have been suggested to decrease the risk of CHD, a recent prospective evaluation of their intake done using food-frequency questionnaires from the Nurses' Health Study reported no association between flavonol or flavone intake and risk of nonfatal myocardial infarction or fatal CHD (74). However, a weak reduction in risk for CHD death was found for a higher intake of kaempferol, an individual flavonol found primarily in broccoli and tea. Conversely, a recent prospective study examining 34,489 postmenopausal women in the Iowa Women's Health Study free of CVD also utilized food-frequency questionnaires (84). Although the researchers found no association between flavonoid intake and stroke mortality, individual flavonoid-rich foods were associated with significant mortality reduction from CHD and CVD: added bran (lower risk of mortality from stroke and CVD); apples, pears, and red wine (CHD and CVD); grapefruit (CHD); strawberries (CVD); and chocolate (CVD). These results suggest that dietary intakes of specific flavanones, anthocyanidins, and certain foods rich in flavonoids may be associated with reduced risk of death as a result of CHD, CVD, and all causes.

Soy Protein

The FDA approved the CVD health claim for soy protein, noting that when it is included in a low-fat and low-cholesterol diet, soy protein can lower total blood cholesterol and LDL-C levels (about 5% with 25 g·day^{-1}) without adversely affecting HDL-C levels (38). The FDA stated, "In order to claim the health effects of soy, a product must contain 6.25 g of soy protein or more, be low fat (less than 3 g), be low in saturated fat (less than 1 g) and low in cholesterol (less than 20 mg)." Food sources of soy protein (serving size and grams of protein) include soybeans (1/2 cup = 30 g), soy flour (1/2 cup = 15 g), textured soy protein (1 cup dry = 12 g), soy milk (1/2 cup = 3 g), tofu (1/2 cup = 20 g), and tempeh (1/2 cup = 16 g), but soy sauce and soy oil do not contain protein (139).

Soy isoflavones, fiber, phytic acid, and saponins in combination with soy protein are probably involved in this lipid-lowering effect, although soy protein was identified as the active component rather than isoflavones, fiber, phytic acid, or saponins (11,38). However, recent meta-regression analyses showed a dose-response relation between soy protein and isoflavone supplementation and net changes in serum lipids (111). Soy protein supplementation reduces serum lipids among adults with or without hypercholesterolemia; therefore, replacing foods high in saturated fat, trans fat, and cholesterol with soy protein will likely have a beneficial effect on coronary risk factors. The American Heart Association advocates a greater intake of soy products to enhance cardiovascular and overall health because of these products' high content of polyunsaturated fats, fiber, vitamins, and minerals and low content of saturated fat (114).

Alcohol

> **1.5.4-CES Recognize the use of herbal and nutritional supplements, over-the-counter (OTC) medications, homeopathic remedies, and other alternative therapies often used by patients with chronic diseases.**

The AHA's Dietary Guidelines: Revision 2000 (70) concluded that moderate alcohol consumption (one drink per day for women and two drinks a day for men) reduces the overall risk of CHD, but the basis for the protective effect of alcohol remains unclear. Alcohol consumption beginning in middle age (ages 35 to 69 years) might suffice for cardioprotective effects while averting much of the risk of accidents and cancer associated with drinking alcohol (67,132). The phenolic compounds in red wine contribute to a greater coronary risk reduction than other alcohol sources, but other wines, beer, and spirits also reduce CHD risk. Alcohol has potentially negative consequences for patients with diabetes, hypertension, cancer risk, and liver disease, however. Additional recommendations for alcohol consumption suggest that abstainers should not be encouraged to begin consuming alcohol

for its purported health benefits and that medications need to be reviewed by drinkers' physicians for potential interactions (50,100).

HYPERTENSION

> **1.2.4-HFS: Knowledge to define the following terms: total cholesterol (TC), high-density lipoprotein cholesterol (HDL-C), TC/HDL-C ratio, low-density lipoprotein cholesterol (LDL-C), triglycerides, hypertension, and atherosclerosis.**

Hypertension is the third leading cause of death in the world, with more than 1 billion individuals worldwide affected and approximately 65 million adults (~25% of individuals ages 18 and older) in the United States (26). High BP increases the risk of MI, heart failure, stroke, and kidney disease. Kottke et al. (69) identified high BP as a symptom of the "lifestyle syndrome," a cluster of conditions and diseases that result from consuming too many calories and too much saturated fat, sodium, and alcohol; not balancing intake with physical activity; and using tobacco. Obesity is a major risk factor for hypertension that is addressed later in this chapter. Unfortunately, current knowledge about the prevention and treatment of hypertension with lifestyle changes and other effective early interventions has not been adequately translated to the public and to high-risk individuals. For example, Greenlund et al. (51) found that more than one third of individuals with established stroke (secondary to elevated BP levels) did not receive advice from a healthcare professional on dietary or exercise changes that would benefit health and prevent stroke recurrence.

The Seventh Report of the Joint National Committee on Prevention, Detection, Evaluation, and Treatment of High Blood Pressure (30) established the optimal BP as a systolic BP of 115 mm Hg and a diastolic of 75 with the need to begin treatment when the patient has a systolic BP of 120 to 139 mm Hg or a diastolic BP of 80 to 89. This prehypertensive state initially requires health-promoting lifestyle modifications, rather than medications, to prevent CVD. This report also reiterates that in individuals older than age 50, systolic BP readings greater than 140 mm Hg indicate a greater risk for CVD than elevations in diastolic BP. Moreover, starting with a BP of 115/75 mm Hg, CVD risk doubles for each increment of 20/10 mm Hg, and even individuals with normal BP levels at the age of 55 have a 90% lifetime risk of developing hypertension, which demonstrates that it is a widespread health problem.

For children, especially those with a higher risk of hypertension because of obesity, prevention is an ideal intervention. In the Bogalusa Heart Study (125,126), hypertension and obesity in parents and relatives increased the risk of the child's development of hypertension. The prevalence of increased BP in elementary schoolchildren indicated that a high systolic BP was 4.5 times and an elevated diastolic 2.4 times more likely among obese children. Figueroa-Colon et al. (42) found that 20% to 30% of obese children ages 5 to 11 years from a high-risk population had hypertension. Recommendations related to dietary minerals to positively influence hypertension include limiting daily sodium intake to <1,500 mg (<4 g salt) and increasing intake of food sources of calcium, magnesium, and potassium (30,86). The response to dietary sodium may vary with the degree of adiposity in children and adolescents. Obese adolescents who changed from a high- to a low-salt diet had a significantly larger decrease in BP compared with an insignificant change among nonobese adolescents in one study (113).

The preponderance of a benefit from increasing minerals comes from potassium (144). Healthy food choices to provide the preferred mineral balance include an intake of five or more servings of fruits and vegetables, six or more servings of grains, and two to four servings of low-fat dairy products daily (30). The effect of dietary modifications varies among individuals because of genetic factors, age, medications, and other host factors. Two recent systematic reviews of the effects of reductions in dietary sodium or salt found minimal effects for normal and hypertensive patients, particularly of Caucasian ethnicity, but greater benefits for Asians and African Americans (64), including maintenance of a lower BP after antihypertensive drugs were discontinued (59). In addition, it appears that African Americans are particularly sensitive to the BP-lowering effects of reduced salt intake, increased potassium intake, and the DASH diet (12).

Benefits of Comprehensive Diet Changes

Changes encompassing several dietary factors have lowered BP in hypertensive and normotensive individuals with systolic BPs of <160 and diastolic BPs of 80 to 95 mm Hg. Following the lifestyle modifications to manage hypertension (30) resulted in decreases in systolic BP of 5 to 20 mm Hg per 10 kg of weight loss; 8 to 14 mm Hg for adopting the DASH diet high in fruits and vegetables; 2 to 8 mm Hg for dietary sodium restriction; 4 to 9 mm Hg for 30 min·day^{-1} of physical activity; and 2 to 4 mm Hg for moderate alcohol consumption. In particular, the DASH diet significantly reduced systolic and diastolic BP by 5.5 and 3.0 mm Hg more than a control diet followed by participants who were normotensive (13). In participants with hypertension, following this diet without a specific salt restriction still reduced systolic and diastolic BP by 11.4 and 5.5 mm Hg more, respectively, than the control diet. The DASH diet was lower in fat and higher in vegetables, fruits, and low-fat dairy foods, and included whole grains, poultry, fish, and nuts. The diet was also rich in calcium, magnesium, and potassium. The control group had a diet composition typical of the average individual in the United States (low in fruits, vegetables, and dairy products, with an average

fat content). The addition of a lower salt intake (1,500 mg·day^{-1}) resulted in a reduction in mean systolic BP of 7.1 mm Hg for participants without hypertension and 11.5 mm Hg in anyone with it (13,115,138).

As further evidence of the importance of dietary interventions, the PREMIER Collaborative Research Group (108) compared the implementation of three interventions in a population of 810 adults at four clinical centers: (a) "established" (a behavioral intervention that implemented established recommendations), (b) "established" + DASH diet, and (c) advice only. Both the established and the established + DASH diet interventions resulted in significant weight reduction, improved fitness, and lower sodium intake. Decreases in the prevalence of hypertension and increases in optimal BP were highly significant for the "established" + DASH intervention only.

Similarly, two independent systematic reviews of randomized, controlled trials (with 8 or more weeks follow-up and patients with a BP of at least 140/85 mm Hg) directly compared lifestyle, drug, and other interventions and concluded that in the short term, lifestyle treatment, including a healthier diet, may be effective at reducing blood pressure for some individuals and may reduce, delay, or remove the need for long-term drug therapy in others (35,87). In fact, in the more recent of the two (35), robust effects were found for improved diet, aerobic exercise, alcohol and sodium restriction, and fish oil supplements, with mean reductions in systolic blood pressure of 5.0, 4.6, 3.8, 3.6, and 2.3 mm Hg, respectively, and corresponding reductions in diastolic blood pressure, although supplements of potassium, magnesium, or calcium were unimportant.

However, Folsom et al. (43) recently studied whether a greater concordance with the DASH diet (using food-frequency data) is associated with reduced incidence of self-reported hypertension and mortality from CVD in 20,993 women (initially aged 55 to 69 years) followed from 1986 through 2002. In this case, a greater concordance with DASH guidelines was not independently associated with lesser hypertension or a reduced cardiovascular mortality, suggesting that a very high concordance, as achieved in the DASH trials, may be necessary to achieve measurable benefits from this diet. In most cases, combining lifestyle interventions results in additive effects and important implications for counseling patients.

OBESITY AND DIET

> **1.8.2-CES: Compare and contrast dietary practices used for weight reduction and address the benefits, risks, and scientific support for each practice. Examples of dietary practices are high protein/low carbohydrate diets, Mediterranean diet, and low-fat diets such as the American Heart Association recommended diet.**

1.8.1-CES: Describe the hypotheses related to diet, weight gain, and weight loss.

1.2.8-HFS: Knowledge of how lifestyle factors, including nutrition and physical activity, influence lipid and lipoprotein profiles.

1.8.2-HFS: Knowledge of the following terms: obesity, overweight, percent fat, BMI, lean body mass, anorexia nervosa, bulimia, metabolic syndrome, and body fat distribution.

1.8.3-HFS: Knowledge of the relationship between body composition and health.

1.8.4-HFS: Knowledge of the effects of diet, exercise, and behavior modification as methods for modifying body composition.

1.8.5-HFS: Knowledge of the importance of an adequate daily energy intake for healthy weight management.

1.8.10-HFS: Knowledge of the myths and consequences associated with inappropriate weight-loss methods (e.g., fad diets, dietary supplements, overexercising, starvation diets).

1.8.16-HFS: Knowledge of the NIH Consensus statement regarding health risks of obesity, Nutrition for Physical Fitness Position Paper of the American Dietetic Association, and the ACSM Position Stand on proper and improper weight-loss programs.

Obesity is a chronic, multifactorial problem caused by some factors over which the individual has no control (e.g., genetics, sex, age, developmental stages) and others that can be modified, such as weight loss, dietary choices, physical activity, medications, environmental contributions, and social considerations. The increased prevalence of obesity in the United States largely reflects a change in lifestyle patterns influenced by an overabundance of food choices, large portion sizes, and fast foods; industrialization, technology, and conveniences, which decrease opportunities and motivation for physical activity; and a decline in cigarette smoking (103,107,122). Approximately 14% of American adults are completely sedentary, and 38% spend insufficient time doing physical activity (107).

The prevalence of obesity and overweight in the United States has increased dramatically, with obesity (body mass index [BMI] ≥30) increasing from 13.4% in 1960 to 32.2% in 2004 among adults (91). Additionally, the incidence of severe obesity (BMI ≥35 with comorbidities or BMI ≥40) based on U.S. 2003 to 2004 population data is 2.8% for men and 6.9% for women, concentrated more heavily in ethnic minority groups like African American and Hispanic. Poor diet coupled with physical inactivity is the second leading cause of preventable death, underscoring the depth of this major public health challenge (3,85). Allison et al. (4) reported approximately 300,000 deaths from overweight and obesity in 1999. Mokdad et al. (85) then used the hazard ratios of that study along with the CDC's 1999 and 2000 NHANES data (27) to estimate that 400,000 U.S. deaths in 2000 were attributable to having a poor diet and being inactive, both lifestyles that contribute to excessive fat weight gain.

Obesity-associated diseases that increase morbidity include CHD, hypertension, stroke, sleep apnea, type 2 diabetes, and certain types of cancer (i.e., endometrial, breast, prostate, and colon [39,107]). The risks of obesity on health begin during pregnancy and extend throughout childhood into adulthood. Some of the obstetric and gynecologic risks include menstrual abnormalities, polycystic ovary syndrome, and shoulder dystopia in childbirth. Orthopedic problems are a common health consequence of obesity; for example, 30% to 50% of children with slipped capital epiphyses and bilateral slipped capital epiphyses in one study were obese (36). Likewise, Blount disease (i.e., severe bowing of the legs) is greatly increased by childhood obesity. Adult musculoskeletal problems may include increased joint pain and back pain (21). Obesity also stimulates biliary excretion of cholesterol that increases the likelihood of gallstone formation, leading childhood and adult obesity to be associated with up to 33% of the cases of gallstones (1,15).

The impact of childhood obesity on the progression of the metabolic syndrome in adulthood is alarming. Pinhas-Hamiel et al. (104) estimated that about one third of diabetes cases diagnosed in 10- to 19-year-old children and young adults was associated with obesity. A review of dyslipemias in adults aged 27 to 31 years who were previously Bogalusa Heart Study participants reported that adult hyperinsulinemia was 12.6 times more likely in individuals who had been obese children (45). In another study, adults who had been overweight adolescents had a 2.4-times increase in prevalence of total cholesterol values above 240 mg·dL^{-1}, a threefold increase in LDL-C values above 160 mg·dL^{-1}, and eight times the incidence of low HDL-C levels (below 35 mg·day^{-1}) (98). Modest weight loss of 5% to 15% of body weight has beneficial effects on serum triglycerides, total cholesterol, BP, degenerative joint disease, gynecologic problems, insulin sensitivity, and glucose control and may lead to improvement or resolution of other comorbidities in both children and adults (33). In overweight adults with type 2 diabetes, a recent meta-analysis examining the effectiveness of lifestyle and behavioral weight-loss interventions revealed that multicomponent interventions, including very-low- or low-calorie diets, may hold promise for achieving longer-term weight loss and greater health benefits, particularly when combined with intense physical activity (90).

The 1998 Behavioral Risk Factor Surveillance Survey found that about one third of U.S. adults were trying to lose weight and another third were trying to maintain weight at any one time (118). In 2002, an updated version of that survey showed that estimate to have risen to 48% of women (but only 34% of men) being on a weight-loss diet in the previous 12-month period (143). Many types of weight-loss and weight-management programs are available, including balanced deficit diets, very-low-calorie diets, gastric bypass surgery, and pharmacotherapy. It has been estimated that ≥$30 billion to ≥$50 billion dollars is spent annually on weight-loss gimmicks and remedies (93). However, fewer than one fourth of dieters chose to combine caloric restriction with levels of physical activity (300 or more minutes per week) recommended in the 2005 dietary guidelines by the U.S. Department of Health and Human Services and U.S. Department of Agriculture (143).

Even with programs that result in weight loss, the results are often short term, and regaining weight is a significant problem for most individuals who initially lose weight. The key to sustaining weight loss is to adopt permanent diet and physical activity changes. A more conservative means for achieving healthy body weight recommended by the American Dietetic Association's guidelines includes adoption of a healthful eating style with an energy intake that does not exceed expenditure (10). By way of example, individuals tracked by the National Weight Control Registry (147) (who have to lose at least 10% of their initial body weight and keep it off for a minimum of a year to qualify, although they have lost 33 kg on average and kept the weight off for more than 5 years) have certain behaviors in common. Most Registry members were found to rely heavily on high levels of daily physical activity (60 minutes per day on average); eat low-calorie, low-fat foods; eat breakfast regularly; self-monitor body weight; and maintain a consistent eating pattern across weekdays and weekends.

OSTEOPOROSIS

 1.8.9-HFS: Knowledge of the importance of calcium and iron in women's health.

Osteoporosis contributed to more than 2 million fractures in the United States in 2005, and by 2025, annual fractures are projected to rise by almost 50%, most rapidly increasing for individuals 65 to 74 years of age (increase >87%) and nearly 175% for Hispanic and other subpopulations (22). American women aged 50 years and older have an incidence of osteoporosis affecting 13% to 18% of women with early decreases in porosity. Osteopenia, is present in another 37% to 50% of women with early decreases in porosity (76). Although the incidence is less in men, men older than 65 years have approximately 30% of the hip fractures. Peak bone mass is usually achieved by age 30 years for both men and women.

The risk factors for osteoporosis include genetics, diet, activity, lifestyle, hormone status, medication use, and some diseases (Box 13-1) (88). Genetic and environmental factors contribute to poor bone mass acquisition during adolescence and accelerated bone loss in perimenopausal women and men in the sixth decade and older. Contributing factors for reduced bone mass include hormone deficiencies, such as estrogen; inadequate calcium and vitamin D intake; tobacco and alcohol abuse; decreased physical activity; comorbidities, such as renal failure, hyperparathyroidism, and athletic amenorrhea; and medication effects, such as chronic steroid use. A follow-up of the Nurses' Health Study found that whereas women with diets high in calcium and vitamin D tended to use more multivitamin, calcium, and estrogen supplements, women with the lowest intakes were more likely to smoke and consume alcohol (41).

Another compounding dietary factor may be excessive intake of phosphorus and possibly caffeine. For example,

BOX 13-1	**RISK FACTORS FOR OSTEOPOROSIS (5,88)**
Female sex	High caffeine intake
Petite body frame	High carbonated soda intake
White or Asian ancestry	Excessive alcohol use
Sedentary lifestyle or immobilization	Low body weight
Family history of osteoporosis	Anorexia nervosa
Nulliparity	Premenopausal amenorrhea (>1 yr)
Increasing age	Smoking
Lifelong low calcium intake	Postmenopausal status
Impaired calcium absorption	Long-term use of certain drugs
High protein intake	Renal disease
Vitamin A supplementation >3 mg/d	Bariatric surgery

in a recent study, bone mineral density was measured at the spine and three hip sites in 1,413 women and 1,125 men in the Framingham Osteoporosis Study (135), and intake of colas and other soft drinks was determined using a food-frequency questionnaire. The researchers found that although total phosphorus intake was not significantly higher in daily cola consumers than nonconsumers, the calcium-to-phosphorus ratios were lower in female cola drinkers. Thus, it appears that intake of cola, particularly caffeinated ones, but not other carbonated soft drinks, is associated with low bone mass in women.

CALCIUM BALANCE AND VITAMIN D

> **1.5.4-CES: Recognize the use of herbal and nutritional supplements, over-the-counter (OTC) medications, homeopathic remedies, and other alternative therapies often used by patients with chronic diseases.**

The FDA allowed a bone health claim for calcium-rich foods, and the National Institutes of Health Consensus Development Panel stated that a prolonged high calcium intake decreases osteoporosis (88). A high calcium intake does not protect a person against bone loss caused by hormone changes, physical activity, or other causes but does prevent osteoporosis caused by low calcium intake. Calcium supplementation in bone remodeling studies has shown an assimilation of additional calcium to increase bone density by about 2%, but density does not continue to increase, and losses occur after supplementation ends (17,119).

A systematic review of 15 randomized, controlled trials with 1,806 participants evaluated the use of calcium supplements versus usual dietary intake with placebo for at least 1 year (119). The review confirmed that the percent change from baseline was 2.05% for total body bone density. There were smaller increases for bone density for the lumbar spine (1.66%), hip (1.60%), and distal radius (1.91%). The data for a reduction in vertebral fractures showed a trend, but the nonvertebral fracture effects were inconclusive. Peacock et al. (99) investigated the effects of supplementation with 750 mg $\cdot$ day^{-1} of calcium and 15 μg oral 25-hydroxyvitamin D on hip bone density in men and women age 60 years or older over a 4-year trial. The calcium group lost 1% in bone density, the placebo group lost 3%, and the vitamin D group lost 2.7%. Feskanich et al. (41) reported a lower risk of hip fracture with a higher calcium intake when there was a concurrent high intake of vitamin D. They confirmed the lack of a relationship between risk of fractures and calcium intake, but concluded that adequate vitamin D was associated with a lower occurrence of osteoporotic hip fractures. Likewise, a 2005 meta-analysis of randomized controlled trials conducted by Bischoff-Ferrari et al. (17) reached similar conclusions: in their analysis, oral vitamin D supplementation of 700 to 800 IU $\cdot$ day^{-1} appeared to lower the risk of hip and any nonvertebral fractures in ambulatory or institu-

tionalized elderly persons, although 400 IU $\cdot$ day^{-1} appeared insufficient for fracture prevention. Decreased risk of fractures has been consistently shown for women who have higher milk or dairy food intake at age 30 years or younger but not necessarily for women older than age 50 years (142). However, another meta-analysis, focused on the need for additional calcium and designed to extend the findings of Bischoff-Ferrari et al., suggested that oral vitamin D appears to reduce the risk of hip fractures only when calcium supplementation is added (19).

Even after full skeletal growth is completed, the body loses calcium every day that must be replaced. The National Academy of Sciences recommends 1,000 to 1,200 mg $\cdot$ day^{-1} of calcium for adult men and women (128). Calcium supplements from unrefined oyster shell, bone meal, coral calcium, or dolomite without the United States Pharmacopeia (USP) symbol may contain higher levels of lead or other toxic metals and should be avoided, especially during pregnancy. Calcium from food and supplements is absorbed best when taken several times a day in amounts of 500 mg or less. Calcium carbonate is absorbed best when taken with food; calcium citrate can be taken at any time (128).

Vitamin D, phosphorus, magnesium, zinc, boron, and fluoride are nutrients that are important for bone growth and maintenance, but they neither have to be consumed with calcium for absorption nor require supplementation unless the diet is inadequate in these nutrients. Vitamin D increases calcium absorption in the gastrointestinal tract, and an adequate vitamin D intake reduces nonvertebral fracture rates (110). Vitamin D intake (1 μg cholecalciferol = 40 IU vitamin D) recommendations increase with age (5 μg $\cdot$ day^{-1} for those ages 19–0 years; 10 μg $\cdot$ day^{-1} for ages 51–70 years; and 15 μg $\cdot$ day^{-1} for anyone older than age 70 years) because of changes in absorption and utilization; a fourfold decrease in skin synthesis of vitamin D; and decreased exposure to sunlight, particularly in the winter (128). Nutrient needs and osteoporosis may be affected by medications such as glucocorticoids, anticonvulsants, long-term heparin therapy, and excessive thyroxine therapy (5).

Dietary factors may alter calcium balance by decreasing calcium bioavailability or increasing urinary calcium excretion. Foods high in oxalates (e.g., spinach, rhubarb, almonds) or in phytates (e.g., legumes and wheat bran) contain calcium that is unavailable for absorption and may bind with calcium in the gut to reduce absorption. Dietary advice includes eating calcium-rich foods before or several hours after foods with phytates and oxalates or compensate for their reduced absorption with a higher calcium intake for the day. Protein, alcohol, and sodium may increase calcium excretion through the kidneys (128). Protein intakes of 2 g $\cdot$ kg^{-1} of body weight used by some athletes have the potential to decrease calcium balance. Alcohol also has a negative impact on osteoblast function, and lower sodium diets have also been shown to reduce the loss of calcium in the urine (24).

OTHER FACTORS AND OSTEOPOROSIS

> **1.8.3-HFS: Knowledge of the relationship between body composition and health.**

> **1.8.10-HFS: Knowledge of the myths and consequences associated with inappropriate weight-loss methods (e.g., fad diets, dietary supplements, overexercising, starvation diets).**

> **1.8.15-HFS: Knowledge of nutritional factors related to the female athlete triad syndrome (i.e., eating disorders, menstrual cycle abnormalities, and osteoporosis).**

Although some observational studies have found a relationship between increased hip fracture and excessive supplemental use of vitamin A (82,83), others have not. In the Nurses' Health Study (41), vitamin A intake of $1.5 \text{ mg} \cdot \text{day}^{-1}$ or more retinol (most common form of vitamin A) was associated with a relative risk of 1.64 for hip fracture, and 21% of subjects exceeded $3 \text{ mg} \cdot \text{day}^{-1}$. On the other hand, the association between fasting serum retinyl esters and bone mineral density were examined in NHANES III (14), and although the prevalence of high fasting serum retinyl esters concentration and low bone mineral density were both substantial, no significant associations between them was found. More recently, serum retinyl esters were not found to be elevated in postmenopausal women despite intakes of total vitamin A that were nearly double the recommended amount (102). However, retinyl ester concentration (percentage of total vitamin A) was marginally associated with osteoporosis and should be further investigated before firm conclusions are reached.

Finally, eating disorders and the inability to maintain body mass promote osteoporosis. In addition to the impact of body mass, low-calorie diets, and particularly, low-carbohydrate diets that promote ketosis, have the potential to leach cationic minerals, such as calcium, from the bones (20). Patients who have recovered from anorexia nervosa require many years to improve their bone density, but may never have complete recovery (88). Along similar lines, female athletes with disordered eating and amenorrhea may develop low bone mineral density (the "female athlete triad") (48), although elite athletes with adequate calorie, vitamin, and mineral intake are two to three times less likely to experience thinning bones compared with similarly aged, nonathletic premenopausal women (133).

DIABETES

> **1.8.3-HFS: Knowledge of the relationship between body composition and health.**

> **1.8.5-HFS: Knowledge of the importance of an adequate daily energy intake for healthy weight management.**

> **1.8.17-HFS: Ability to describe the health implications of variations in body fat distribution patterns and the significance of the waist-to-hip ratio.**

Diabetes is a major cause of mortality and morbidity, with 224,092 deaths in 2002 attributable to diabetes in the United States alone, making it the sixth leading cause of death (albeit a likely underreported one) (29). In 2005, updated estimates of 20.8 million Americans with diabetes were released, with almost one third of them (6.2 million) still undiagnosed. Another 54 million Americans who have impaired glucose tolerance (IGT) and/or impaired fasting glucose (IFG) levels are at risk of developing diabetes. Moreover, the worldwide incidence of diabetes between 2000 and 2030 is projected to more than double from 171 million to 366 million (146). Prediabetes has also become a concern in the pediatric population. Conditions of hyperinsulinemia and impaired glucose have been directly related to overweight and obesity in children and adolescents (79).

Diabetes results from impairment of insulin secretion and defects in insulin action that likely occur simultaneously (6,44). Autoimmune processes with an absolute deficiency of insulin secretion characterize the less common type 1 diabetes, but insulin resistance and an inadequate insulin secretion characterize the more prevalent type 2. Acute symptoms include hyperglycemia with polyuria, polydipsia, weight loss, sometimes polyphagia, and often blurred vision. Chronic hyperglycemia may lead to retarded growth and to increased incidence of infections. An asymptomatic period and impaired glucose tolerance with slightly abnormal blood glucose level (i.e., IFG) and potential organ changes without clinical symptoms may precede overt symptoms. The incidence of retinopathy, peripheral neuropathy, foot ulcers, lower-limb amputation, gastroparesis, sexual dysfunction, peripheral vascular disease, MI, hyperlipidemia, periodontal disease, cerebrovascular disease, hypertension, and psychological dysfunction are well known to increase with a history of diabetes, particularly when blood glucose levels are not well controlled (29).

Symptoms associated with insulin resistance include acanthosis nigricans (dark, thickened skin at the back of the neck or under the breasts), hypertension, dyslipidemia, and polycystic ovarian syndrome. The visible presence of acanthosis nigricans correlated with higher insulin needs in a study of newly diagnosed type 2 diabetes (75). The study found 36.1% of the 216 patients with newly diagnosed type 2 diabetes and 54% of patients with a BMI of 30 or higher manifested the skin changes.

Type 2 diabetes has many different contributing causes, but obesity, especially abdominal distribution, may increase insulin resistance and contribute to diabetes development when coupled with genetic predisposition (family history, high-risk ethnic group), increasing age (steep increase after age 45 years), and a lack of physical activity (28). Other risk factors for diabetes include previously identified IFG or IGT, history of gestational diabetes mellitus or delivery of a baby weighing more than 9 lbs, hypertension ($\geq$140/90 mm Hg in adults), HDL-C of 35 mg $\cdot$ dL^{-1} or less or a triglyceride level of 250 mg $\cdot$ dL^{-1} or more, polycystic ovary syndrome, and a history of vascular disease (6,44).

Nutrient intake, both specific macronutrients and micronutrients, has not been widely linked to the development of diabetes, but in at least one study, higher consumption of sugar-sweetened beverages was associated with a greater weight gain and an increased risk for development of type 2 diabetes in women, possibly by providing excessive calories and large amounts of rapidly absorbable sugars (116). Moreover, in individuals at high risk for developing diabetes, a deficiency of vitamin D has been found to increase the risk of its onset in many observational studies (106). Type 2 diabetes has also been increasing in children and adolescents with combinations of risk factors, especially increasing rates of excessive weight and obesity. Screening for diabetes in high-risk groups has been recommended as a cost-effective practice to allow for implementation of prevention strategies.

LIFESTYLE MODIFICATION

> **1.8.1-CES: Describe and discuss dietary considerations for cardiovascular and pulmonary diseases, chronic heart failure, and diabetes that are recommended to minimize disease progression and optimize disease management.**

> **1.8.4-HFS: Knowledge of the effects of diet, exercise, and behavior modification as methods for modifying body composition.**

> **1.8.14-HFS: Knowledge of common nutritional ergogenic aids, the purported mechanism of action, and any risk and/or benefits (e.g., carbohydrates, protein/amino acids, vitamins, minerals, herbal products, creatine, steroids, caffeine.**

Several large, well-designed, randomized controlled studies have supported the value of lifestyle changes that include diet and physical activity to prevent diabetes in high-risk persons (34,95,136) (also see Chapter 37). Tuomilehto et al. (136) found that intensive individualized diet and exercise instruction had a 58% relative reduction in the incidence of diabetes compared with brief diet and exercise counseling in 522 middle-aged men with IGT and obesity (mean BMI, 31 kg $\cdot$ m^{-2}). The average follow-up time was 3.2 years. Halting the progression toward diabetes was strongly associated with the subject's ability to accomplish one of the following goals: 5% weight reduction, fat intake <30% of calories, saturated

fat <10% of calories, fiber intake of 15 g per 1,000 kcal or more, and exercise more than 150 minutes·week^{-1}. Another study—the Da Qing, China study of 520 normal-weight participants over 6 years—found significant reductions in diabetes for a diet group (31%), exercise group (46%), and diet plus exercise (42%) (95). Overall, the lifestyle intervention groups lost 3.4 kg more than the control subjects in the first year. Thus, this study underlines the value of lifestyle changes, especially exercise, for leaner subjects.

Similarly, in the United States, the Diabetes Prevention Program (34) (DPP) results supported the value of intensive diet and exercise interventions (58% relative reduction in progression to diabetes) compared with metformin (31% relative reduction in progression to diabetes) or placebo medication interventions with standard diet and exercise. The 3,234 ethnically and racially diverse subjects at high risk for type 2 diabetes development, with a mean age of 51 years, were followed for weight and glucose intolerance for an average of 2.8 years. The weight-reduction goal of a loss of more than 7% of initial weight at 6 months was met by 38% of the lifestyle change group. The exercise goal of more than 150 min·week^{-1} was maintained by 74% of the lifestyle change group. Over 3.2 years of follow-up, results from 1,079 DPP "lifestyle arm" participants were recently analyzed, and it was determined that for every kilogram of weight loss, they experienced an average 16% reduction in risk after adjustment for changes in diet and activity (53). Both lower percentage of calorie intake from fat and increased physical activity predicted weight loss, but increased physical activity was critical for sustained weight loss. In addition, for the 495 participants not meeting the weight-loss goal at end of the first year of the DPP trial, achievement of physical activity goals still resulted in a 44% lower diabetes incidence.

The battle over whether weight loss or physical activity is more important in preventing diabetes continues, though. By way of example, a recent study of 68,097 female nurses conducted by Rana et al. (109) attempted to determine the relative contribution of adiposity and physical inactivity to the development of type 2 diabetes. In this prospective study, researchers estimated adiposity using body mass index (BMI) and waist circumference measurements, and physical activity was assessed through average hours of moderate or vigorous exercise and computation of a MET (metabolic equivalent) score. During 16 years of follow-up (from 1986 to 2002), diabetes risk in these nurses increased progressively with increasing BMI and waist circumference and with decreasing physical activity levels. Compared with lean (BMI<25 kg $\cdot$ m^{-2}), physically active (exercise $\geq$21.8 MET h·week^{-1}) women, the relative risks of type 2 diabetes were 16.75 for their obese (BMI $\geq$30 kg $\cdot$ m^{-2}) and inactive (exercise<2.1 MET h·week^{-1}) counterparts; 10.74 for active, obese women; and 2.08 for lean, but inactive women. Both waist circumference and physical activity were independent predictors of type 2 diabetes, but the association for waist circumference was substantially stronger, leading the investigators to conclude that the magnitude of risk for diabetes contributed by obesity may be much greater than for physical inactivity.

There remains no doubt, however, that lifestyle interventions to prevent type 2 diabetes are effective and are recommended for all patients with prediabetes and possibly anyone meeting the criteria for metabolic syndrome (28,136). Management of diabetes itself includes balancing diet, exercise, and medications to achieve treatment goals associated with diabetes (117). Total carbohydrate intake is the dietary component that is the most important determinant of blood sugars. However, contrary to popular belief, studies have shown that simple or complex carbohydrates yield similar glycemic responses, and there is considerable variability in the results. Thus, presently no evidence-based research conclusion supports improving blood sugar control with the use of the glycemic index, although low-glycemic index foods that are rich in fiber and other important nutrients and intake of a lower glycemic load are encouraged (7,117). The American Diabetes Association's Nutrition Recommendations and Interventions for Diabetes Position Statement (7) suggests that people with type 2 diabetes can substitute carbohydrates with monounsaturated fats to reduce postprandial glycemia and triglyceridemia (117). A liberal intake of monounsaturated fat can promote weight gain, so this substitution should only be advised when carbohydrate calories are replaced by fat calories. Saturated fats should be limited to 7% to 10% of total daily energy intake, and total fat intake should be <30% of total calories with minimal intake of trans fats. Cholesterol should be <200 mg·day^{-1} if the LDL-C level is above 100 mg·dL^{-1}. Two or more servings of fish are recommended to provide heart-healthy fats. Protein intake is also a concern in the setting of diabetes because of the potential of promoting nephropathy. If renal function is normal, a protein intake of 15% to 20% of total daily energy intake is acceptable, but at this time, high-protein diets are not recommended for diabetic individuals (7).

Microalbuminuria, or small amounts of albumin in the urine, is the first evidence of damage to the kidneys (44). Ethnicity appears to be a primary determinant in the incidence of kidney disease for people with type 2 diabetes as it develops in 40% to 50% of Native Americans, 20% to 30% of African Americans and Latinos, and 10% of Caucasians with type 2 diabetes. High-protein diets cause hyperfiltration in the kidneys and may potentially contribute to kidney failure for high-risk individuals. The American Diabetes Association (7) currently recommends protein intakes of 0.8 to 1.0 g·kg^{-1} of body weight·day^{-1} for prevention of kidney disease and 0.8 g·kg^{-1} of good quality protein or about 10% of kcals for management of overt kidney disease.

A primary principle of diabetes management is the relationship of medication dosage, selection, and timing to dietary intake (especially carbohydrates) and physical activity (8). Patient preferences and lifestyle can be incorporated into a plan that typically focuses on consistency of dietary intake and exercise patterns balanced with medications. A recent meta-analysis conducted by Snowling and Hopkins (124) showed that all forms of exercise training (aerobic, resistance, or both) produce small benefits in overall blood glucose control for type 2 diabetic individuals similar to dietary, drug, and insulin treatments. Combined training was generally superior to aerobic or resistance training alone, though. Therefore, individuals who are willing to become educated and monitor themselves can increase their diet and physical activity options.

SUMMARY

Prevention of chronic disease with dietary interventions is one tool in the arsenal of lifestyle changes that combine to effectively improve disease risk. Dietary treatment of the diet-related chronic diseases—CVD, obesity, diabetes, and osteoporosis—improves morbidity, mortality, and quality of life. Prevention efforts for at-risk youth also need to be increased if the potential benefits of healthy lifestyles are to be realized for the population as a whole.

REFERENCES

1. Acalovschi MV, Blendea D, Pascu M, et al. Risk of asymptomatic and symptomatic gallstones in moderately obese women: a longitudinal follow-up study. *Am J Gastroenterol*. 1997;92(1):127–131.
2. Age-Related Eye Disease Study Research Group. A randomized, placebo-controlled, clinical trial of high-dose supplementation with vitamins C and E and beta carotene for age-related cataract and vision loss: AREDS report no. 9. *Arch Ophthalmol*. 2001; 119(10):1439–1452.
3. Allison DB, Fontaine KR, Manson JE, et al. Annual deaths attributable to obesity in the United States. *JAMA*. 1999;282(16): 1530–1538.
4. The Alpha-Tocopherol, Beta Carotene Cancer Prevention Study Group. The effect of vitamin E and beta carotene on the incidence of lung cancer and other cancers in male smokers. *N Engl J Med*. 1994;330(15):1029–1035.
5. American College of Obstetricians and Gynecologists. ACOG Practice Bulletin. Clinical management guidelines for obstetrician-gynecologists: osteoporosis. *Obstet Gynecol*. 2004;103(1):203–26.
6. American Diabetes Association. Diagnosis and classification of diabetes mellitus. *Diabetes Care*. 2006;29(Suppl 1):S43–48.
7. American Diabetes Association. Nutrition recommendations and interventions for diabetes: a position statement of the American Diabetes Association. *Diabetes Care*. 2007;30(Suppl 1):S48–65.
8. American Diabetes Association. Physical activity/exercise and diabetes mellitus: position statement. *Diabetes Care*. 2003;26(Suppl 1): S73–77.
9. American Dietetic Association. Position of the American Dietetic Association: Integration of medical nutrition therapy and pharmacotherapy. *J Am Diet Assoc*. 2003;103(10):1363–1370.
10. American Dietetic Association. Position of the American Dietetic Association: Weight management. *J Am Diet Assoc*. 2002;102(8): 1145–1155.

11. American Heart Association Science Advisory and Coordinating Committee. Guidelines for primary prevention of cardiovascular disease and stroke: 2002 update. *Circulation.* 2002;106(3): 388–391.

12. Appel LJ, Brands MW, Daniels SR, et al. Dietary approaches to prevent and treat hypertension: a scientific statement from the American Heart Association. *Hypertension.* 2006;47(2):296–308.

13. **Appel LJ, Moore TJ, Obarzanek E, et al. A clinical trial of the effects of dietary patterns on blood pressure. DASH Collaborative Research Group. *N Engl J Med.* 1997;336(16):1117–1124.**

14. Ballew C, Galuska D, Gillespie C. High serum retinyl esters are not associated with reduced bone mineral density in the Third National Health and Nutrition Examination Survey, 1988–1994. *J Bone Miner Res.* 2001;16(12):2306–2312.

15. Barlow SE, Dietz WH. Obesity evaluation and treatment: expert committee recommendations. *Pediatrics.* 1998;102(3):E29.

16. Bazzano LA, Reynolds K, Holder KN, He J. Effect of folic acid supplementation on risk of cardiovascular diseases: a meta-analysis of randomized controlled trials. *JAMA.* 2006;296(22):2720–2726.

17. Bischoff-Ferrari HA, Willett WC, Wong JB, et al. Fracture prevention with vitamin D supplementation: a meta-analysis of randomized controlled trials. *JAMA.* 2005;293(18):2257–2264.

18. Bleys J, Miller ER, Pastor-Barriuso R, et al. Vitamin-mineral supplementation and the progression of atherosclerosis: a meta-analysis of randomized controlled trials. *Am J Clin Nutr.* 2006;84(4):880–887.

19. Boonen S, Lips P, Bouillon R, et al. Need for additional calcium to reduce the risk of hip fracture with vitamin D supplementation: evidence from a comparative metaanalysis of randomized controlled trials. *J Clin Endocrinol Metab.* 2007;92(4):1415–1423.

20. Bray GA. Low-carbohydrate diets and realities of weight loss. *JAMA.* 2003;289(14):1853–1855.

21. Brown WJ, Dobson AJ, Mishra G. What is a healthy weight for middle aged women? *Int J Obes Relat Metab Disord.* 1998;22(6): 520–528.

22. Burge R, Dawson-Hughes B, Solomon DH, et al. Incidence and economic burden of osteoporosis-related fractures in the United States, 2005–2025. *J Bone Miner Res.* 2007;22(3):465–475.

23. Burr ML, Fehily AM, Gilbert JF, et al. Effects of changes in fat, fish, and fibre intakes on death and myocardial reinfarction: diet and reinfarction trial (DART). *Lancet.* 1989;2(8666):757–761.

24. Carbone LD, Barrow KD, Bush AJ, et al. Effects of a low sodium diet on bone metabolism. *J Bone Miner Metab.* 2005;23(6):506–513.

25. Carter NB. Plant stanol ester: review of cholesterol-lowering efficacy and implications for coronary heart disease risk reduction. *Prev Cardiol.* 2000;3(3):121–130.

26. **Centers for Disease Control and Prevention National Center for Health Statistics. Health, United States, 2006: Hypertension, Table 69 [Internet]. Atlanta (GA): Centers for Disease Control and Prevention; [cited 2007 Aug 14]. Available from: www.cdc.gov/nchs/ data/hus/hus06.pdf#069**

27. **Centers for Disease Control and Prevention National Center for Health Statistics. National Health Interview Survey [Internet]. Atlanta (GA): Centers for Disease Control and Prevention; [cited 2007 Aug 15]. Available from: www/cdc.gov/nchs/about/ major/ dvs/mortdata.htm**

28. **Centers for Disease Control and Prevention Primary Prevention Working Group. Primary prevention of type 2 diabetes mellitus by lifestyle intervention: implications for health policy. *Ann Intern Med.* 2004;140(11):951–957.**

29. **Centers for Disease Control and Prevention. National diabetes fact sheet: general information and national estimates on diabetes in the United States, 2005. Atlanta (GA): U.S. Department of Health and Human Services, Centers for Disease Control and Prevention; 2005. 10 p.**

30. **Chobanian AV, Bakris GL, Black HR, et al. The seventh report of the joint national committee on prevention, detection, evaluation, and treatment of high blood pressure: JNC 7 report. *JAMA.* 2003; 289(19): 2560–2572.**

31. Collaborative Group of the Primary Prevention Project (PPP). Low-dose aspirin and vitamin E in people at cardiovascular risk: a randomized trial in general practice. *Lancet.* 2001;357(9250): 89–95.

32. de Lorgeril M, Salen P, Martin JL, et al. Mediterranean diet, traditional risk factors, and the rate of cardiovascular complications after myocardial infarction: final report of the Lyon Diet Heart Study. *Circulation.* 1999;99(6):779–785.

33. Deitel M. How much weight loss is sufficient to overcome major comorbidities? *Obes Surg.* 2001;11(6):659.

34. Diabetes Prevention Program Research Group. Reduction in the incidence of type 2 diabetes with lifestyle intervention or metformin. *N Engl J Med.* 2002;346(6):393–403.

35. Dickinson HO, Mason JM, Nicolson DJ, et al. Lifestyle interventions to reduce raised blood pressure: a systematic review of randomized controlled trials. *J Hypertens.* 2006;24(2):215–233.

36. Dietz WH. Health consequences of obesity in youth: childhood predictors of adult disease. *Pediatrics.* 1998;101(3 Suppl):518–525.

37. **Einhorn D, Reaven GM, Cobin RH, et al. American College of Endocrinology: Position statement on the insulin resistance syndrome. *Endocrinol Pract.* 2003;9(3):237–252.**

38. Erdman JW Jr. Soy protein and cardiovascular disease. *Circulation.* 2000;102(20):2555–2559.

39. **Expert Panel on the Identification, Evaluation, and Treatment of Overweight in Adults. Clinical guidelines on the identification, evaluation, and treatment of overweight and obesity in adults; the evidence report. Washington, DC: National Heart, Lung, and Blood Institute Obesity Education Initiative; 1998. 228 p.**

40. Fassbender K, Lutjohann D, Dik MG, et al. Moderately elevated plant sterol levels are associated with reduced cardiovascular risk—The LASA study. *Atherosclerosis.* 2008;196(1):283–288.

41. Feskanich D, Willett WC, Colditz GA. Calcium, vitamin D, milk consumption, and hip fractures: a prospective study among postmenopausal women. *Am J Clin Nutr.* 2003;77(2):504–511.

42. Figueroa-Colon R, Franklin FA, Lee JY, et al. Prevalence of obesity with increased blood pressure in elementary school-aged children. *South Med J.* 1997;90(8):806–813.

43. Folsom AR, Parker ED, Harnack LJ. Degree of concordance with DASH diet guidelines and incidence of hypertension and fatal cardiovascular disease. *Am J Hypertens.* 2007;20(3):225–232.

44. Franz M, Bantle J, Beebe C, et al. Standards of medical care in diabetes. *Diabetes Care.* 2004;27(Suppl 1):S15–35.

45. Freedman DS, Dietz WH, Srinivasan SR, Berenson GS. The relation of overweight to cardiovascular risk factors among children and adolescents: the Bogalusa Heart Study. *Pediatrics.* 1999;103(6): 1175–1182.

46. Gallistl S, Sudi K, Mangge H, et al. Insulin is an independent correlate of plasma homocysteine levels in obese children and adolescents. *Diabetes Care.* 2000;23(9):1348–1352.

47. Gardner CD, Coulston A, Chatterjee L, et al. The effect of a plant-based diet on plasma lipids in hypercholesterolemic adults: a randomized trial. *Ann Intern Med.* 2005;142(9):725–733.

48. Gibson JH, Mitchell A, Harries MG, Reeve J. Nutritional and exercise-related determinants of bone density in elite female runners. *Osteoporos Int.* 2004;15(8):611–618.

49. GISSI-Prevenzione investigators. Dietary supplementation with n-3 polyunsaturated fatty acids and vitamin E after myocardial infarction: results of the GISSI-Prevenzione trial. *Lancet.* 1999; 354(9177): 447–455.

50. Goldberg IJ, Mosca L, Piano MR, Fisher EA. Wine and your heart: a science advisory for healthcare professionals from the Nutrition Committee, Council on Epidemiology and Prevention, and Council on Cardiovascular Nursing of the American Heart Association. *Circulation.* 2001;103(3):472–475.

51. Greenlund KJ, Giles WH, Keenan NL, et al. Physician advice, patient actions, and health-related quality of life in secondary prevention of stroke through diet and exercise. *Stroke.* 2002;33(2): 565–570.

52. Grundy SM, Cleeman JI, Daniels SR, et al. Diagnosis and management of the metabolic syndrome: an American Heart Association/National Heart, Lung, and Blood Institute Scientific Statement. *Circulation*. 2005;112(17):2735–2752.

53. Hamman RF, Wing RR, Edelstein SL, et al. Effect of weight loss with lifestyle intervention on risk of diabetes. *Diabetes Care*. 2006;29(9):2102–2107.

54. Harper CR, Jacobson TA. The fats of life: the role of omega-3 fatty acids in the prevention of coronary heart disease. *Arch Intern Med*. 2001;161(18):2185–2192.

55. The Heart Outcomes Prevention Evaluation Study Investigators. Vitamin E supplementation and cardiovascular events in high-risk patients. *N Engl J Med*. 2000;342(3):154–160.

56. Heart Protection Study Collaborative Group. MRC/BHF Heart Protection Study of antioxidant vitamin supplementation in 20,536 high-risk individuals: a randomised placebo-controlled trial. *Lancet*. 2002;360(9326):23–33.

57. Hertog MG, Feskens EJ, Hollman PC, et al. Dietary antioxidant flavonoids and risk of coronary heart disease: the Zutphen Elderly Study. *Lancet*. 1993;342(8878):1007–1011.

58. Homocysteine Lowering Trialists' Collaboration. Lowering blood homocysteine with folic acid based supplements: meta-analysis of randomised trials. *BMJ*. 1998;316(7135):894–898.

59. Hooper L, Bartlett C, Davey SG, Ebrahim S. Advice to reduce dietary salt for prevention of cardiovascular disease. *Cochrane Database Syst Rev*. 2004;(1):CD003656.

60. Howard BV, Van Horn L, Hsia J, et al. Low-fat dietary pattern and risk of cardiovascular disease: the Women's Health Initiative Randomized Controlled Dietary Modification Trial. *JAMA*. 2006; 295(6):655–666.

61. Institute of Medicine, National Academy of Sciences. *Dietary Reference Intakes Energy, Carbohydrate, Fiber, Fat, Fatty Acids, Cholesterol, protein and Amino Acids*. Washington (DC): National Academy of Sciences; 2002. 1,357 p.

62. Jenkins DJ, Kendall CW, Marchie A, et al. The effect of combining plant sterols, soy protein, viscous fibers, and almonds in treating hypercholesterolemia. *Metabolism*. 2003;52(11):1478–1483.

63. Joshipura KJ, Hu FB, Manson JE, et al. The effect of fruit and vegetable intake on risk for coronary heart disease. *Ann Intern Med*. 2001;134(12):1106–1114.

64. Jurgens G, Graudal NA. Effects of low sodium diet versus high sodium diet on blood pressure, renin, aldosterone, catecholamines, cholesterols, and triglyceride. *Cochrane Database Syst Rev*. 2004;(1):CD004022.

65. Katan MB. Trans fatty acids and plasma lipoproteins. *Nutr Rev*. 2000;58(6):188–191.

66. Katan MB, Zock PL, Mensink RP. Dietary oils, serum lipoproteins, and coronary heart disease. *Am J Clin Nutr*. 1995;61(6 Suppl):1368S–1373S.

67. Klatsky AL, Armstrong MA, Friedman GD. Red wine, white wine, liquor, beer, and risk for coronary artery disease hospitalization. *Am J Cardiol*. 1997;80(4):416–420.

68. Knekt P, Jarvinen R, Reunanen A, Maatela J. Flavonoid intake and coronary mortality in Finland: a cohort study. *BMJ*. 1996; 312(7029):478–481.

69. Kottke TE, Stroebel RJ, Hoffman RS. JNC 7—it's more than high blood pressure. *JAMA*. 2003;289(19):2573–2575.

70. Krauss RM, Eckel RH, Howard B, et al. AHA Dietary Guidelines: revision 2000: A statement for healthcare professionals from the Nutrition Committee of the American Heart Association. *Circulation*. 2000;102(18):2284–2299.

71. Kris-Etherton PM, Daniels SR, Eckel RH, et al. Summary of the scientific conference on dietary fatty acids and cardiovascular health: conference summary from the nutrition committee of the American Heart Association. *Circulation*. 2001;103(7):1034–1039.

72. Kris-Etherton PM, Harris WS, Appel LJ. Fish consumption, fish oil, omega-3 fatty acids, and cardiovascular disease. *Circulation*. 2002; 106(21):2747–2757.

73. Lichtenstein AH, Deckelbaum RJ. Stanol/sterol ester-containing foods and blood cholesterol levels. *Circulation*. 2001;103(8):1177–1179.

74. Lin J, Rexrode KM, Hu F, et al. Dietary intakes of flavonols and flavones and coronary heart disease in US women. *Am J Epidemiol*. 2007;165(11):1305–1313.

75. Litonjua P, Pinero-Pilona A, Aviles-Santa L, Raskin P. Prevalence of acanthosis nigricans in newly-diagnosed type 2 diabetes. *Endocrinol Pract*. 2004;10(2):101–106.

76. Looker AC, Wahner HW, Dunn WL, et al. Updated data on proximal femur bone mineral levels of US adults. *Osteoporos Int*. 1998;8(5):468–489.

77. Marchioli R, Barzi F, Bomba E, et al. Early protection against sudden death by n-3 polyunsaturated fatty acids after myocardial infarction: time-course analysis of the results of the Gruppo Italiano per lo Studio della Sopravvivenza nell'Infarto Miocardico (GISSI)-Prevenzione. *Circulation*. 2002;105(16):1897–1903.

78. Marckmann P, Gronbaek M. Fish consumption and coronary heart disease mortality: a systematic review of prospective cohort studies. *Eur J Clin Nutr*. 1999;53(8):585–590.

79. McCance DR, Pettitt DJ, Hanson RL, et al. Glucose, insulin concentrations and obesity in childhood and adolescence as predictors of NIDDM. *Diabetologia*. 1994;37(6):617–623.

80. McDowell MA, Briefel RR, Alaimo K, et al. *Energy and Macronutrient Intakes of Persons Ages 2 Months and Over in the United States: Third National Health and Nutrition Examination Survey, Phase 1, 1988–91*. Hyattsville, MD: National Center for Health Statistics, Division of Health Examination Statistics; 1994. 24 p.

81. Mead A, Atkinson G, Albin D, et al. Dietetic guidelines on food and nutrition in the secondary prevention of cardiovascular disease—evidence from systematic reviews of randomized controlled trials (second update, January 2006). *J Hum Nutr Diet*. 2006; 19(6):401–419.

82. Melhus H, Michaelsson K, Kindmark A, et al. Excessive dietary intake of vitamin A is associated with reduced bone mineral density and increased risk for hip fracture. *Ann Intern Med*. 1998; 129(10):770–778.

83. Michaelsson K, Lithell H, Vessby B, Melhus H. Serum retinol levels and the risk of fracture. *N Engl J Med*. 2003;348(4):287–294.

84. Mink PJ, Scrafford CG, Barraj LM, et al. Flavonoid intake and cardiovascular disease mortality: a prospective study in postmenopausal women. *Am J Clin Nutr*. 2007;85(3):895–909.

85. Mokdad AH, Marks JS, Stroup DF, Gerberding JL. Actual causes of death in the United States, 2000. *JAMA*. 2004;291(10):1238–1245.

86. National Cholesterol Education Program Expert Panel on Detection, Evaluation and Treatment of High Blood Cholesterol in Adults (Adult Treatment Panel III). Third Report of the National Cholesterol Education Program (NCEP) Expert Panel on Detection, Evaluation, and Treatment of High Blood Cholesterol in Adults (Adult Treatment Panel III) final report. *Circulation*. 2002;106(25): 3143–3421.

87. Nicolson DJ, Dickinson HO, Campbell F, Mason JM. Lifestyle interventions or drugs for patients with essential hypertension: a systematic review. *J Hypertens*. 2004;22(11):2043–2048.

88. NIH Consensus Development Panel on Osteoporosis Prevention, Diagnosis and Therapy. Osteoporosis prevention, diagnosis, and therapy. *JAMA*. 2001;285(6):785–795.

89. Nijveldt RJ, van Nood E, van Hoorn DE, et al. Flavonoids: a review of probable mechanisms of action and potential applications. *Am J Clin Nutr*. 2001;74(4):418–425.

90. Norris SL, Zhang X, Avenell A, et al. Long-term effectiveness of lifestyle and behavioral weight loss interventions in adults with type 2 diabetes: a meta-analysis. *Am J Med*. 2004;117(10):762–774.

91. Ogden CL, Carroll MD, Curtin LR, et al. Prevalence of overweight and obesity in the United States, 1999–2004. *JAMA*. 2006;295(13):1549–1555.

92. Oh K, Hu FB, Manson JE, et al. Dietary fat intake and risk of coronary heart disease in women: 20 years of follow-up of the nurses' health study. *Am J Epidemiol*. 2005;161(7):672–679.

93. The painful business of losing weight. *Economist*. 1997;344(8032): 45–47.

94. Palaniappan L, Carnethon MR, Wang Y, et al. Predictors of the incident metabolic syndrome in adults: the Insulin Resistance Atherosclerosis Study. *Diabetes Care*. 2004;27(3):788–793.

95. Pan XR, Li GW, Hu YH, et al. Effects of diet and exercise in preventing NIDDM in people with impaired glucose tolerance: the Da Qing IGT and Diabetes Study. *Diabetes Care*. 1997;20(4):537–544.

96. Pankow JS, Jacobs DR Jr., Steinberger J, et al. Insulin resistance and cardiovascular disease risk factors in children of parents with the insulin resistance (metabolic) syndrome. *Diabetes Care*. 2004;27(3):775–780.

97. **Park YW, Zhu S, Palaniappan L, et al. The metabolic syndrome: prevalence and associated risk factor findings in the US population from the Third National Health and Nutrition Examination Survey, 1988–1994. *Arch Intern Med*. 2003;163(4):427–436.**

98. Patel S. Sitosterolaemia: dietary cholesterol absorption. *Lancet*. 2001;358(Suppl):S63.

99. Peacock M, Liu G, Carey M, et al. Effect of calcium or 25 OH vitamin D3 dietary supplementation on bone loss at the hip in men and women over the age of 60. *J Clin Endocrinol Metab*. 2000; 85(9):3011–3019.

100. Pearson TA. Alcohol and heart disease. *Circulation*. 1996;94(11): 3023–3025.

101. **Pearson TA, Bazzarre TL, Daniels SR, et al. American Heart Association guide for improving cardiovascular health at the community level: a statement for public health practitioners, healthcare providers, and health policy makers from the American Heart Association Expert Panel on Population and Prevention Science. *Circulation*. 2003;107(4):645–651.**

102. Penniston KL, Weng N, Binkley N, Tanumihardjo SA. Serum retinyl esters are not elevated in postmenopausal women with and without osteoporosis whose preformed vitamin A intakes are high. *Am J Clin Nutr*. 2006;84(6):1350–1356.

103. Pi-Sunyer FX. The fattening of America. *JAMA*. 1994;272(3): 238–239.

104. Pinhas-Hamiel O, Dolan LM, Daniels SR, et al. Increased incidence of non-insulin-dependent diabetes mellitus among adolescents. *J Pediatr*. 1996;128(5):608–615.

105. Pitsavos C, Panagiotakos DB, Chrysohoou C, et al. The effect of Mediterranean diet on the risk of the development of acute coronary syndromes in hypercholesterolemic people: a case-control study (CARDIO2000). *Coron Artery Dis*. 2002;13(5):295–300.

106. Pittas AG, Lau J, Hu FB, Dawson-Hughes B. The role of vitamin D and calcium in type 2 diabetes: a systematic review and meta-analysis. *J Clin Endocrinol Metab*. 2007;92(6):2017–2029.

107. Plodkowski RA, St Jeor ST. Medical nutrition therapy for the treatment of obesity. *Endocrinol Metab Clin North Am*. 2003;32(4): 935–965.

108. PREMIER Collaborative Research Group. Effects of comprehensive lifestyle modification on blood pressure control: main results of the PREMIER clinical trial. *JAMA*. 2003;289(16):2083–2093.

109. Rana JS, Li TY, Manson JE, Hu FB. Adiposity compared with physical inactivity and risk of type 2 diabetes in women. *Diabetes Care*. 2007;30(1):53–58.

110. Reid IR. The roles of calcium and vitamin D in the prevention of osteoporosis. *Endocrinol Metab Clin North Am*. 1998;27(2): 389–398.

111. Reynolds K, Chin A, Lees KA, et al. A meta-analysis of the effect of soy protein supplementation on serum lipids. *Am J Cardiol*. 2006;98(5):633–640.

112. Rimm EB, Willett WC, Hu FB, et al. Folate and vitamin B6 from diet and supplements in relation to risk of coronary heart disease among women. *JAMA*. 1998;279(5):359–364.

113. Rocchini AP, Key J, Bondie D, et al. The effect of weight loss on the sensitivity of blood pressure to sodium in obese adolescents. *N Engl J Med*. 1989;321(9):580–585.

114. **Sacks FM, Lichtenstein A, Van Horn L, et al. Soy protein, isoflavones, and cardiovascular health: an American Heart Association Science Advisory for professionals from the Nutrition Committee. *Circulation*. 2006;113(7):1034–1044.**

115. Sacks FM, Svetkey LP, Vollmer WM, et al. Effects on blood pressure of reduced dietary sodium and the Dietary Approaches to Stop Hypertension (DASH) diet. DASH-Sodium Collaborative Research Group. *N Engl J Med*. 2001;344(1):3–10.

116. Schulze MB, Manson JE, Ludwig DS, et al. Sugar-sweetened beverages, weight gain, and incidence of type 2 diabetes in young and middle-aged women. *JAMA*. 2004;292(8):927–934.

117. Scott B, Perumean-Chaney S, St. Jeor S. Relationship of body mass index to energy density and diet composition in a free-living population. *Topics in Clinical Nutrition*. 2002;17(4):38–46.

118. Serdula MK, Mokdad AH, Williamson DF, et al. Prevalence of attempting weight loss and strategies for controlling weight. *JAMA*. 1999;282(14):1353–1358.

119. Shea B, Wells G, Cranney A, et al. Calcium supplementation on bone loss in postmenopausal women. *Cochrane Database Syst Rev*. 2004;(1):CD004526.

120. Shulman GI. Cellular mechanisms of insulin resistance. *J Clin Invest*. 2000;106(2):171–176.

121. Singh RB, Niaz MA, Sharma JP, et al. Randomized, double-blind, placebo-controlled trial of fish oil and mustard oil in patients with suspected acute myocardial infarction: the Indian experiment of infarct survival—4. *Cardiovasc Drugs Ther*. 1997;11(3):485–491.

122. Smiciklas-Wright H, Mitchell DC, Mickle SJ, et al. Foods commonly eaten in the United States, 1989–1991 and 1994–1996: are portion sizes changing? *J Am Diet Assoc*. 2003;103(1):41–47.

123. Smith SC Jr. Multiple risk factors for cardiovascular disease and diabetes mellitus. *Am J Med*. 2007;120(3 Suppl 1):S3–S11.

124. Snowling NJ, Hopkins WG. Effects of different modes of exercise training on glucose control and risk factors for complications in type 2 diabetic patients: a meta-analysis. *Diabetes Care*. 2006;29(11): 2518–2527.

125. Srinivasan SR, Bao W, Wattigney WA, Berenson GS. Adolescent overweight is associated with adult overweight and related multiple cardiovascular risk factors: the Bogalusa Heart Study. *Metabolism*. 1996;45(2):235–240.

126. Srinivasan SR, Frontini MG, Berenson GS. Longitudinal changes in risk variables of insulin resistance syndrome from childhood to young adulthood in offspring of parents with type 2 diabetes: the Bogalusa Heart Study. *Metabolism*. 2003;52(4):443–450.

127. Srinivasan SR, Myers L, Berenson GS. Predictability of childhood adiposity and insulin for developing insulin resistance syndrome (syndrome X) in young adulthood: the Bogalusa Heart Study. *Diabetes*. 2002;51(1):204–209.

128. **Standing Committee on the Scientific Evaluation of Dietary Reference Intakes, Food and Nutrition Board. Dietary reference intakes for calcium, phosphorus, magnesium, vitamin D, and fluoride. Washington (DC): Institute of Medicine, National Academy of Science; 2000. 448 p.**

129. Stolar M. Metabolic syndrome: controversial but useful. *Cleve Clin J Med*. 2007;74(3):199–202, 205–208.

130. Stover PJ. Nutritional genomics. *Physiol Genom*. 2004;16(2): 161–165.

131. Sundram K, Karupaiah T, Hayes KC. Stearic acid-rich interesterified fat and trans-rich fat raise the LDL/HDL ratio and plasma glucose relative to palm olein in humans. *Nutr Metab (Lond)*. 2007;4:3.

132. Thun MJ, Peto R, Lopez AD, et al. Alcohol consumption and mortality among middle-aged and elderly U.S. adults. *N Engl J Med*. 1997;337(24):1705–1714.

133. Torstveit MK, Sundgot-Borgen J. Low bone mineral density is two to three times more prevalent in non-athletic premenopausal women than in elite athletes: a comprehensive controlled study. *Br J Sports Med*. 2005;39(5):282–287; discussion 287.

134. Trichopoulou A, Costacou T, Bamia C, Trichopoulos D. Adherence to a Mediterranean diet and survival in a Greek population. *N Engl J Med.* 2003;348(26):2599–2608.

135. Tucker KL, Morita K, Qiao N, et al. Colas, but not other carbonated beverages, are associated with low bone mineral density in older women: the Framingham Osteoporosis Study. *Am J Clin Nutr.* 2006;84(4):936–942.

136. Tuomilehto J, Lindstrom J, Eriksson JG, et al. Prevention of type 2 diabetes mellitus by changes in lifestyle among subjects with impaired glucose tolerance. *N Engl J Med.* 2001;344(18):1343–1350.

137. Ueland PM, Refsum H, Beresford SA, Vollset SE. The controversy over homocysteine and cardiovascular risk. *Am J Clin Nutr.* 2000;72(2):324–332.

138. U.S. Department of Health and Human Services. *Your Guide to Lowering Your Blood Pressure with DASH.* Bethesda (MD): National Heart, Lung, and Blood Institute Information Center; 2006. 56 p.

139. U.S. National Agricultural Library. Nutrient Data laboratory [Internet]. Washington (DC): US Department of Agriculture, Agricultural Research Service; [cited 2007 Aug 15]. Available from: www.nal.usda.gov/fnic/foodcomp/search

140. Wald DS, Law M, Morris JK. Homocysteine and cardiovascular disease: evidence on causality from a meta-analysis. *BMJ.* 2002;325(7374):1202–1208.

141. Wang C, Harris WS, Chung M, et al. n-3 Fatty acids from fish or fish-oil supplements, but not alpha-linolenic acid, benefit cardiovascular disease outcomes in primary- and secondary-prevention studies: a systematic review. *Am J Clin Nutr.* 2006;84(1):5–17.

142. Weinsier RL, Krumdieck CL. Dairy foods and bone health: examination of the evidence. *Am J Clin Nutr.* 2000;72(3):681–689.

143. Weiss EC, Galuska DA, Khan LK, Serdula MK. Weight-control practices among U.S. adults, 2001–2002. *Am J Prev Med.* 2006; 31(1):18–24.

144. Whelton PK, He J, Cutler JA, et al. Effects of oral potassium on blood pressure: meta-analysis of randomized controlled clinical trials. *JAMA.* 1997;277(20):1624–1632.

145. Whelton SP, He J, Whelton PK, Muntner P. Meta-analysis of observational studies on fish intake and coronary heart disease. *Am J Cardiol.* 2004;93(9):1119–1123.

146. Wild S, Roglic G, Green A, Sicree R, King H. Global prevalence of diabetes: estimates for the year 2000 and projections for 2030. *Diabetes Care.* 2004;27(5):1047–1053.

147. Wing RR, Phelan S. Long-term weight loss maintenance. *Am J Clin Nutr.* 2005;82(1 Suppl):222S–2225S.

148. Yu-Poth S, Zhao G, Etherton T, et al. Effects of the National Cholesterol Education Program's Step I and Step II dietary intervention programs on cardiovascular disease risk factors: a meta-analysis. *Am J Clin Nutr.* 1999;69(4):632–646.

SELECTED REFERENCES FOR FURTHER READING

American Diabetes Association. Nutrition recommendations and interventions for diabetes: a position statement of the American Diabetes Association. *Diabetes Care.* 2007;30(Suppl 1):S48–65.

American Diabetes Association. Physical activity/exercise and diabetes mellitus: position statement. *Diabetes Care.* 2003;26(Suppl 1): S73–77.

Appel LJ, Brands MW, Daniels SR, et al. Dietary approaches to prevent and treat hypertension: a scientific statement from the American Heart Association. *Hypertension.* 2006;47(2):296–308.

National Cholesterol Education Program Expert Panel. Executive summary of the third report of the National Cholesterol Education Program (NCEP) Expert Panel on Detection, Evaluation, and Treatment of High Blood Cholesterol in Adults (Adult Treatment Panel III). *JAMA.* 2001;285(25):785–795.

NIH Consensus Development Panel on Osteoporosis Prevention, Diagnosis and Therapy. Osteoporosis prevention, diagnosis, and therapy. *JAMA.* 2001;285(19):785–795.

U.S. Department of Health and Human Services. *Your Guide to Lowering Your Blood Pressure with DASH.* Bethesda (MD): National Heart, Lung, and Blood Institute Information Center; 2006. 56 p.

Whelton SP, He J, Whelton PK, and Muntner P. Meta-analysis of observational studies on fish intake and coronary heart disease. *Am J Cardiol.* 2004;93(9):1119–1123.

INTERNET RESOURCES

- American Diabetes Association. Nutrition and Recipes: www.diabetes.org/nutrition-and-recipes/nutrition/overview.jsp
- American Dietetic Association. Food and Nutrition Information: www.eatright.org/cps/rde/xchg/ada/hs.xsl/nutrition.html
- American Heart Association. Healthy Lifestyle: www.americanheart.org/presenter.jhtml?identifier=1200009
- American Obesity Organization. Obesity Treatment: www.obesity.org/treatment/weight.shtml
- Centers for Disease Control and Prevention. National Center for Chronic Disease Prevention and Health Promotion. Nutrition and Physical Activity: www.cdc.gov/nccdphp/publications/aag/dnpa.htm
- Centers for Disease Control and Prevention. Preventing Obesity and Chronic Diseases Through Good Nutrition and Physical Activity: www.cdc.gov/nccdphp/publications/factsheets/Prevention/obesity.htm
- National Cholesterol Education Program. Third Report of the Expert Panel on Detection, Evaluation, and Treatment of High Blood Cholesterol in Adults (Adult Treatment Panel III): www.nhlbi.nih.gov/guidelines/cholesterol

Accurate **dietary assessment** is a challenge because of the day-to-day variation in the type and amount of foods and beverages people consume, the difficulty in describing and recalling these items, and the difficulty in estimating portion size. Furthermore, the lack of a single "best" method or gold standard to measure diet, the cost and amount of time to collect and process the data, and the need to translate the data to meaningful feedback using nutrient and food databases are hurdles that must be overcome (15). Despite these challenges, dietary assessment can provide worthwhile information if the assessment is conducted with the appropriate tool and both the interviewer and patient understand the level of detail required to accurately assess intake.

The objectives of this chapter are to (a) explain the steps and purpose of dietary assessment; (b) identify the strengths and weaknesses of the various dietary assessment tools, including when each should be used; and (c) discuss the analysis and evaluation of dietary intake, and how to provide beneficial feedback to patients. Practical tips are provided to illustrate main concepts. It should be noted that exercise professionals should consult state laws regarding providing nutritional counseling to patients.

THE STEPS OF DIETARY ASSESSMENT

Conducting a dietary assessment to estimate intake involves (a) identifying the purpose of the dietary assessment, (b) selecting the appropriate diet assessment tool, (c) obtaining the dietary intake data from the individual, (d) analyzing the dietary intake data, (e) evaluating the diet, and (f) providing useful feedback. Each of these steps is described in detail in this chapter.

IDENTIFYING THE PURPOSE OF DIETARY ASSESSMENT

A dietary assessment is performed to evaluate the quality and quantity of foods and beverages consumed by individuals. It is one of several indicators of nutritional

Diet history: A type of dietary assessment that uses a combination of several diet assessment methods to provide a detailed assessment of health habits and usual eating patterns.

Diet record: A diary-type of dietary assessment that provides details about all foods and beverages consumed over a defined period of time.

Dietary assessment: The use of any of a variety of methods to describe or quantify intake of foods and beverages in humans.

Dietary reference intakes: Science-based recommendations for intake of nutrients that consider risk of dietary deficiencies, protection against chronic diseases, and adverse dietary health risks. Three types of dietary reference intakes are published by the U.S. government: Recommended Dietary Allowance, Adequate Intake, and Tolerable Upper Intake Level.

Food frequency questionnaire: A type of dietary assessment that is designed to measure general dietary patterns over a defined period of time. Food frequency questionnaires have two parts, which are a defined food list of interest and a frequency response section for reporting how often each food of interest is eaten.

Observation: A type of dietary assessment in which a trained observer records all foods, beverages, and amounts consumed by an individual or group during mealtime.

24-hour recall: A type of dietary assessment method that relies on a person's recall and reporting of food and beverage intake in a defined (usually prior) day.

status, which also include anthropometrics, biochemical data, and clinical data (11). Dietary assessment may be conducted to evaluate an individual's intake in a counseling setting or for research purposes. Many of the diet assessment tools may be used for both purposes; however, this chapter focuses on individual dietary assessment.

The benefits to assessing an individual's diet include the ability to identify food consumption patterns, inadequate or excessive intakes of certain foods or food groups, and issues related to portion size. An individual may seek a diet assessment for several reasons: to assist with a weight-loss program; to learn how to lower fat intake, decrease calories, or increase fruit and vegetable consumption; to improve overall diet; or to optimize dietary intake for athletic performance. In addition, when the diet assessment is used as a part of counseling, the individual may become more aware of his or her intake habits, and this information can be a useful teaching tool.

SELECTING THE APPROPRIATE DIETARY ASSESSMENT TOOL

Dietary assessment methods include **diet records**, **24-hour recall**, **food frequency questionnaires (FFQs)**, **diet history**, and **observation**. Each of these methods have strengths and weaknesses, so selection of the appropriate dietary assessment tool depends on whether the information collected will be for an individual or group, and the reason for the assessment. Understanding the strengths and weaknesses of the tools used in each step of the dietary assessment process helps ensure that the most appropriate method is used. Certain types of dietary assessment tools may not be appropriate for use with children, persons with memory problems, persons with low literacy levels, or visual or hearing impaired individuals. This section begins with the methods most likely to be used for assessing individual dietary intake in a fitness setting and concludes with the tools used less commonly. A brief description of each tool, how it should be administered, and its strengths and weaknesses are discussed. The sections that follow provide specific information on analyzing the dietary intake data, evaluating the diet, and providing useful feedback to the patient.

Diet Records

Diet records are based on the report of actual intake over a specific number of days, typically 3 to 4 days and not more than 7 days. When selecting days, it is ideal to include at least one weekend day. The individual records all foods and beverages consumed for a predetermined number of days, with specific details and portion sizes (15). The data are then coded and averaged over the number of days collected. The respondent may also be encouraged to write down information about where, when, and with whom the foods were eaten. This method may be used with nonliterate populations by using tape recorders to record intake.

It is critical to remember that one day of intake does not provide an accurate assessment of usual dietary intake. The number of days of intake necessary to assess an individual's intake varies by the nutrient. Collecting more than 1 day of intake allows estimations of the within-person error, which can assist in determining the number of days to estimate true intake (20). The number of days necessary to estimate usual intake of energy and the macronutrients ranges from 3 to 10 days (2); to estimate many of the micronutrients requires even more days.

The strengths of the diet record are that it provides quantitatively accurate information for the time that the diet record is kept, and that by recording foods when they are consumed, the participant does not rely on memory to recall the information (15). Eating behaviors and patterns can also be addressed with this assessment tool. The limitations of this tool include a high respondent burden because of the need to keep the record with them at all times and record everything that is eaten, usually immediately after consumption. Additionally, the process of recording the items consumed can alter eating behaviors; respondents must be motivated and literate; and coding of the data is time-consuming (2). Collecting too few days of intake will not provide an accurate assessment of an individual's usual intake, and caution should be used when providing feedback to acknowledge the shortcomings of this assessment method.

24-Hour Recall

The 24-hour recall is a popular method to assess current dietary intake. In a structured interview, the respondent is asked to recall all foods and beverages consumed in the past 24 hours, including the amount consumed and details on the method of preparation. A single 24-hour recall provides an estimate of actual intake for a specific day but is not appropriate for estimating usual intake because of the daily variation in diet. To estimate usual intake, several 24-hour recalls would need to be collected, with the actual number depending on the nutrient of interest. However, in a research setting, a single 24-hour recall collected from groups of individuals can be used to adequately assess average intake of the groups.

The 24-hour recall is the dietary assessment method used by the U.S. Department of Agriculture (USDA) to assess the nutrient intakes of Americans in the current national nutrition survey known as *What We Eat in America* (17). To obtain the necessary level of detail on each recall, the USDA has developed a five-step multiple-pass method to administer the tool (4). The five steps include a quick list, a forgotten foods list, time and occasion, detail cycle, and the final review probe. The accuracy of the five-step method has been tested in normal, overweight, and obese women and was found to assess mean intake within 10% of actual intake that was measured by direct observation (4).

When used for counseling, the 24-hour recall is useful as a method to discuss general eating patterns, keeping in mind that a single day is not representative of overall diet. The 24-hour recall can be completed relatively quickly—in about 20 minutes. For some populations, this method may not be ideal because of poor memory or difficulty with estimating amounts. This method does not alter usual diet, although individuals may under- or overreport foods that are more "socially desirable" to appear healthier.

Food Frequency Questionnaire

The food frequency questionnaire (FFQ) is a dietary assessment tool used to assess usual intake by inquiring about frequency of past consumption of selected foods or food groups over a specific time (20). In research, this method is useful for assessing the relationship between diet and disease because it can be used to rank individuals by high and low intake. The FFQ may either be interviewer or self-administered; will not alter usual diet; and depending on the size of the questionnaire, takes between 20 and 30 minutes to complete.

The FFQ is composed of a food list, options for reporting the frequency of intake, and options for portion size. The food list used must be representative of the population being studied to ensure that the foods or food groups that are popular sources of nutrient intake are represented. This food list may be subdivided by food groups and typically contain 100 to 125 foods. The options used for collecting data about frequency of consumption include daily, weekly, monthly, and yearly; and the options depend on the purpose for assessing the diet.

An FFQ may or may not contain portion-size options. A nonquantitative FFQ only requires the individual to provide information about the frequency of consumption. For example, the individual would specify only if he or she ate or drank that item over a specified period (day, week, or month). A semiquantitative FFQ inquires about the frequency of consumption of a prespecified amount of food or beverage. Prespecified amounts, such as a slice of bread or glass of milk, are easier to report than items not typically consumed or easily quantifiable, such as chicken. A quantitative FFQ asks the individual to complete information on a portion size, but the portion-size options can range from small, medium, or large, to open-ended questions (20).

The FFQ relies on memory and may be challenging for participants to estimate the foods and beverages consumed over a prespecified length of time. The FFQ may require less administrative time than other methods because answers to the FFQ can be entered on scan sheets and the data entered directly into a database.

Diet History

The diet history is a combination of several diet assessment methods to provide a detailed assessment of health habits and usual eating patterns (1). The diet history was originally used in human growth and development studies to assess an individual's usual meal patterns, food preparation practices, and intake over a certain time, such as a month or year. This method, which is an interviewer-administered tool, includes a 24-hour recall and a food checklist for the past month. A 3-day food record may also be used as a cross-check of the data collected. Nutrition knowledge and training are generally necessary to probe for personal dietary habits and patterns, and a high level of respondent participation and cooperation is required. A diet history can provide an accurate assessment of usual diet (3) and does not alter usual diet. A limitation of this method includes interviews that can last 1 to 2 hours. Also, after data are collected, they must be coded and analyzed, processes that are labor intensive, difficult, and expensive.

Observation

Likely the best method to determine an individual's actual intake is to directly observe a patient during several days and record all foods and beverages consumed; however, this is not a realistic option in a free-living population. Using this method, a trained observer records all foods, beverages, and amounts consumed by an individual or group during mealtime. To accurately determine the amount consumed, the observer must know the exact amount the individual or group is served, which is why this method works well in controlled situations, such as metabolic units, institutionalized populations, and schools. The interviewer does not interact with the individuals consuming the food. This method is more often used to assess intake of a group because it is typically conducted during one period. The benefit of the observation method is the accuracy of the dietary intake data collected for the time assessed. The main limitations of this method are that it is very labor intensive and is not appropriate for assessing usual intake.

Summary of Dietary Assessment Tools

As illustrated by the descriptions, benefits, and limitations of each diet assessment tool, the choices for assessing diet are varied. Each dietary assessment tool has strengths and weaknesses, but the fitness professional will be more likely to use the 24-hour recall or diet record in counseling situations because of the ease of administration and the amount of data that can be collected quickly. Thus, the remaining sections in this chapter focus specifically on these two methods. It is important for fitness professionals to realize that the processes associated with assessing dietary intake are quite complicated and require a good bit of training and practice. This chapter provides an overview of the process, but readers are encouraged to work with dietitians or other nutrition specialists to hone their skills in this area.

OBTAINING THE DIETARY INTAKE

This section focuses on the steps that can be incorporated into dietary assessment to optimize the data quality obtained from 24-hour recalls and diet records. These steps include providing detailed, verbal and written, easy-to-understand instructions to the patient about recording intake and estimating portion size; probing either during the interview or after the completed recall has been received to elicit the necessary detail about intake and portion size; and scanning the completed assessment for missing values and outliers.

Completing the 24-Hour Recall and Diet Record

Usually, the 24-hour recall is completed by the interviewer and does not require instructions for the patient. The patient is asked to recall all foods and beverages consumed in the past 24 hours and to estimate the portion size of each item. The interviewer is responsible for recording the intake and probing for as much detail as possible. Table 14-1 contains a list of probing questions that will help with this task. It is important to ask open-ended questions, as well as portray a nonjudgmental expression when inquiring about an individual's intake.

When a patient is asked to keep a diet record for a predetermined number of days, detailed instructions are very useful because patients are typically sent home with a blank diary to complete. Box 14-1 provides instructions for recording food intake. The instructions should include general information about how to complete the record as well as the contact information of an individual able to assist with the process, if necessary. In addition, instructions for keeping the diet record should be reviewed with the patient to reinforce the importance of the exercise, answer questions, explain the level of detail needed for accurate assessment, and remind the patient not to omit foods or beverages or change intake.

TABLE 14-1. PROBES FOR IDENTIFYING DETAILS OF FOODS

TYPE OF INFORMATION	DID YOU SPECIFY?
Grains and Cereals	
Bread or tortilla	Brand, type (e.g., diet, regular, wheat, whole wheat, rye, flour vs corn)
Bakery items	Brand, type (bran, blueberry), how prepared (cake, raised), toppings
Cereal	Brand, type, anything added during preparation or consumption (sugar, fat)
Pasta, rice, and other grains	Brand; fat or salt added
Vegetables and Fruits	
Vegetables and fruit	Fresh, frozen, canned, dried; brand name; cooked or raw; juice: added sugar; salads: what was in salad; added fats, oils, or other toppings (e.g., croutons, sauces, bacon)
Dairy	
Milk	Brand, percent fat, anything added
Cheese	Brand, type (cheddar, American, cottage), version (lite, low fat, low sodium)
Yogurt	Brand, version, frozen or regular
Nondairy	Brand, powder or liquid
Other (ice cream, cream)	Brand, version, type, flavor
Meat, Poultry, and Fish	
Fresh cuts	Type of cut (e.g., T-bone, sirloin, thigh, breast, salmon, haddock)
	Fat trimmed or skin removed, before or after cooking
	Is reported weight for cooked or raw, with or without bone?
	Percent lean (hamburger)
	How prepared (baked, grilled, fried, barbecue)
	Fat, sauces and seasonings used during cooking
Cold cuts	Brand, version (e.g., lite hot dog, bun length, footlong), type (e.g., beef, turkey)
Canned tuna and salmon	Type (solid white, chunk light), packed in oil or water, reduced salt
Oils, Spreads, and Dressings	
Margarine	Brand, type (stick, tub, liquid), version (whipped, diet, lite)
Oils	Brand, type (corn, canola, olive)
Mayonnaise/salad dressings	Brand, type or flavor; version (low fat, nonfat, cholesterol free)
Other	
Mixed dishes	Is recipe included, brand, principal components
Pizza	Brand, thin or thick crust, toppings, diameter (e.g., 16 in, 20 in), how many pieces eaten
Soup	Brand or homemade, type or flavor, creamed, water or milk added
Other	Brand; include recipe, if possible; principal components; gravies and sauces
Beverages	Brand, sweetened or unsweetened, alcohol, diet or low cal, decaffeinated
Eggs	Whole, egg substitute, brand, how prepared
Crackers, snacks, chips	Brand, type, how prepared (e.g., microwave popcorn), size, handfuls, bowls (vitamins B_1 and B_2 food models, cups or ounces if they read it off the bag)
Pies, cakes	Brand, type, one or two crusts or layers, type of frosting

BOX 14-1   INSTRUCTIONS FOR RECORDING INTAKE

GENERAL INSTRUCTIONS FOR KEEPING A DIET RECORD

Write legibly.

Record for the specific number of days.

Record each meal, snack, and beverage *immediately* after you eat it. See instructions below.

Record each food on a separate line.

Leave one or two blank lines after each meal or snack.

If additional space is required for the same day, continue on an extra page.

INSTRUCTIONS FOR RECORDING OF FOODS

Write down every bit of food and beverage that goes into your mouth—even snacks—for the entire day!

Fully describe everything you eat and drink *in detail* (e.g., chicken thigh, skin not eaten; decaffeinated coffee; low-calorie French dressing; low-fat mayonnaise; whole milk).

Specify preparation methods (e.g., whether meat is breaded and fried, broiled, baked; vegetables cooked with fat).

List each separate ingredient for mixed dishes (sandwiches, casseroles, salads) on a separate line.

Record exact amounts of food and beverages. If possible, weigh and measure your foods. Example: ½ cup Cheerios and ½ cup 2% milk. Attach food labels or recipes, if possible.

Include anything that you add to your food at the table (e.g., baked potato with 1 tbs butter; coffee with 1 tsp sugar).

Try not to modify your eating habits.

Adapted with permission from the Cooper Institute, Dallas, Texas.

Recording Portion Size

The importance of estimating portion size should be emphasized to the patient. The expanding portion sizes of foods and beverages, coupled with the decrease in physical activity energy expenditure, are likely contributors to the current epidemic of overweight and obesity in the United States (22). Recent analyses from past national nutrition surveys indicate an increase in the portion size of several foods eaten inside and outside the home (12,14). Because weight reduction is a common reason for seeking dietary advice, inaccurate assessment of portion size may hide opportunities for improvement or modification of diet.

The estimation of portion size is one of the most challenging components of dietary assessment. Portion size can be determined by weighing food portions; visually estimating weights of foods; and making visual estimates of size through the use of household measures, food models, or photographs (21). The interviewer may suggest that the patient use common household items, such as scales, measuring cups, or a ruler, to assist with estimating portion size. Additionally, the patient may be asked to bring in recipes and food labels. Given that portion size is difficult to estimate and mistakes are often encountered during this step, a list of probes to assist with estimating portion size has been provided in Table 14-2. Specific attention should be given to the common mistake of confusing fluid and weight ounces when describing portion size.

ANALYZING THE DIETARY INTAKE

After dietary intake has been recorded and reviewed, the contents of the diet need to be analyzed. The goal of this step is to translate the food and beverage consumption data to nutrient intake or food group information, using nutrient composition or food group databases, respectively. Several resources are available to analyze dietary data, such as computerized database software, nutrient composition tables, and food manufacturer data.

Nutrient Composition Databases

Before the use of computerized databases, nutrition professionals looked up foods in published tables of nutrient composition, such as those found in Bowes and Church's Food Values of Portions Commonly Used (13). Each item

TABLE 14-2. PORTION SIZE PROBES

PORTION SIZES

How many?	Discrete numbers
Food model	Usual kitchen measures (e.g., cup, tablespoon, teaspoon, ounces)
	Ounces—fluid or weighed
	Reasonable
	Portion of model
Thickness of food or amount of ice in drink	Meat
	Cakes, brownies
	Unsliced bread
	Cubes or crushed
	A lot of ice, a little ice
	If the subject knows *exactly* how much he or she drank (e.g., one 12-oz can), you do not need to know if ice was used

was looked up individually, the nutrient content of the food was calculated and adjusted based on the reported portion size, and the nutrient values for each item were added to get an estimate of intake. This process is very time-consuming and tedious. The introduction of computerized nutrient databases has saved considerable time and effort. Several diet analysis software packages are available for purchase, and many may be downloaded free of charge from the Internet.

Additionally, in April 2003, the USDA made publicly available a user-friendly interface for downloading and using the Survey Nutrient Database, which is the most authoritative nutrient database available. The 2006 updated database includes more than 7,200 foods and 117 nutrients, as well as several options for coding portion size (18).

Government Guidelines

1.8.8-HFS: Knowledge of the USDA Food Pyramid and Dietary Guidelines for Americans

The Dietary Guidelines for Americans (16) have been the cornerstone of federal nutrition policy and nutrition education since 1980. The guidelines reflect a consensus of the most current science and medical knowledge available. To account for ongoing research efforts in nutrition and health, the guidelines are updated every 5 years. The next revision is due in 2010. The government convenes a panel of nutrition, medical, and epidemiologic experts to review the existing guidelines in light of new scientific data. The panel's recommendations are reviewed by government agencies and then provided to the public for comment. In addition, testing is done to determine consumer understanding of the guidelines before they are made final.

The current Dietary Guidelines include key recommendations from nine interrelated focus areas. The recommendations are based on the preponderance of scientific evidence for lowering risk of chronic disease and promoting health. It is important to remember that these are integrated messages that should be implemented as a whole. Taken together, they encourage most Americans to eat fewer calories, be more active, and make wiser food choices (Box 14-2).

Food Guide Pyramid

1.8.8-HFS: Knowledge of the USDA Food Pyramid and Dietary Guidelines for Americans

The Food Guide Pyramid was developed in 1992 as a graphic way to translate the Dietary Guidelines into practical recommendations for foods consumers need to eat daily to get the nutrients they need for good health. Given the significant advances in nutrition research over the past 12 years, the USDA updated the pyramid in 2005. The new pyramid, called MyPyramid (19), is personalized for an individual's age, height, weight, sex, and amount of regular activity. It provides detailed specific portion sizes

that a person needs to consume on a daily basis, divided into five food groups: grains, vegetables, fruits, milk, meat, and beans. MyPyramid also provides a meal-tracking system and physical activity recommendations.

Dietary Reference Intakes

Evaluating a patient's diet by analyzing the foods consumed is a perfectly adequate and efficient way to determine their dietary needs and is especially useful if you do not have more sophisticated tools, such as dietary analysis software, available to you. However, some patients may want information regarding specific nutrients. For example, a man with a family history of early heart attacks who is trying to lower his blood cholesterol level may want to evaluate his total fat and saturated fat intake. A postmenopausal woman may want to know how much calcium she is getting to determine if she should take a calcium supplement.

In an effort to make public health recommendations based on the latest research on nutrient needs, the federal government periodically commissions leading scientists in various areas of nutrient research to review the literature and establish estimates of nutrient intakes that can be used to assess and plan diets for generally healthy people. These are called the **Dietary Reference Intakes** (DRIs) (5–10). For macronutrients such as carbohydrate, fat, and protein, Acceptable Macronutrient Distribution Ranges (AMDRs) have recently been established (9).

The DRIs include three classifications that are of interest to fitness professionals. First, the Recommended Dietary Allowances (RDAs) and Adequate Intakes (AIs) can both be used as goals for patients. The RDAs are set to meet the nutrient needs of almost all individuals in a particular group (age, sex, pregnant, etc.). Second, when scientists establish an AI instead of an RDA for a nutrient, it is because they believe that the AI is adequate to meet the needs of all individuals in a group, but there are not sufficient data to establish an RDA for that particular nutrient. For some nutrients, there are enough data that support the setting of a Tolerable Upper Intake Level (UL). This level is the maximum daily intake that is likely to pose no risk or adverse effects. In most cases, the UL includes total daily intake from food, water, and supplements. Not all nutrients (e.g., thiamin, B_{12}, vitamin K) have a UL established for them, but that does not mean that it is safe to take them in amounts above the RDA or AI for these nutrients.

EVALUATING DIETARY INTAKE

After the results of a qualitative or quantitative analysis have been determined, the next step is to compare the results with dietary recommendations. Food and nutrient needs differ based on sex, age, physical activity level, life stage, and health status. Since the 1940s, the federal government has established guidelines for food and nutrient intake. Initially, the guidelines were designed to reduce the prevalence of nutrient deficiencies. As such, the dietary recommendations were used to establish policies for many

BOX 14-2   DIETARY GUIDELINES FOR AMERICANS

ADEQUATE NUTRIENTS WITHIN CALORIE NEEDS

Key Recommendations

- Consume a variety of nutrient-dense foods and beverages within and among the basic food groups while choosing foods that limit the intake of saturated and trans fats, cholesterol, added sugars, salt, and alcohol.
- Meet recommended intakes within energy needs by adopting a balanced eating pattern, such as the USDA Food Guide or the DASH Eating Plan.

WEIGHT MANAGEMENT

Key Recommendations

- To maintain body weight in a healthy range, balance calories from foods and beverages with calories expended.
- To prevent gradual weight gain over time, make small decreases in food and beverage calories and increase physical activity.

PHYSICAL ACTIVITY

Key Recommendations

- Engage in regular physical activity and reduce sedentary activities to promote health, psychological well-being, and a healthy body weight.
  - To reduce the risk of chronic disease in adulthood: Engage in at least 30 minutes of moderate-intensity physical activity, above usual activity, at work or home on most days of the week.
  - For most people, greater health benefits can be obtained by engaging in physical activity of more vigorous intensity or longer duration.
  - To help manage body weight and prevent gradual, unhealthy body weight gain in adulthood: Engage in approximately 60 minutes of moderate- to vigorous-intensity activity on most days of the week while not exceeding caloric intake requirements.
  - To sustain weight loss in adulthood: Participate in at least 60 to 90 minutes of daily moderate-intensity physical activity while not exceeding caloric intake requirements. Some people may need to consult with a healthcare provider before participating in this level of activity.
- Achieve physical fitness by including cardiovascular conditioning, stretching exercises for flexibility, and resistance exercises or calisthenics for muscle strength and endurance.

FOOD GROUPS TO ENCOURAGE

Key Recommendations

- Consume a sufficient amount of fruits and vegetables while staying within energy needs. Two cups of fruit and 2½ cups of vegetables per day are recommended for a reference 2,000-calorie intake, with higher or lower amounts depending on the calorie level.
- Choose a variety of fruits and vegetables each day. In particular, select from all five vegetable subgroups (dark green, orange, legumes, starchy vegetables, and other vegetables) several times a week.
- Consume 3 or more ounce-equivalents of whole-grain products per day, with the rest of the recommended grains coming from enriched or whole-grain products. In general, at least half the grains should come from whole grains.
- Consume 3 cups per day of fat-free or low-fat milk or equivalent milk products.
- Consume adequate protein. The daily recommended intake (DRI) for protein is $0.8 \text{ g} \cdot \text{kg}^{-1} \cdot \text{day}^{-1}$, however, with increased activity level, this intake may be increased to $1.5 \text{ g} \cdot \text{kg}^{-1} \cdot \text{day}^{-1}$ with the recommendation to not exceed $1.8 \text{ g} \cdot \text{kg}^{-1} \cdot \text{day}^{-1}$.

FATS

Key Recommendations

- Consume $<10\%$ of calories from saturated fatty acids and $<300 \text{ mg} \cdot \text{day}^{-1}$ of cholesterol, and keep trans fatty acid consumption as low as possible.
- Keep total fat intake between 20% and 35% of calories, with most fats coming from sources of polyunsaturated and monounsaturated fatty acids, such as fish, nuts, and vegetable oils.
- When selecting and preparing meat, poultry, dry beans, and milk or milk products, make choices that are lean, low-fat, or fat-free.
- Limit intake of fats and oils high in saturated and/or trans fatty acids, and choose products low in such fats and oils.

CARBOHYDRATES

Key Recommendations

- Choose fiber-rich fruits, vegetables, and whole grains often.
- Choose and prepare foods and beverages with little added sugars or caloric sweeteners, such as amounts suggested by the USDA Food Guide and the DASH Eating Plan.

BOX 14-2   DIETARY GUIDELINES FOR AMERICANS (Continued)

- Reduce the incidence of dental caries by practicing good oral hygiene and consuming sugar- and starch-containing foods and beverages less frequently.

SODIUM AND POTASSIUM

Key Recommendations

- Consume <2,300 mg (approximately 1 tsp of salt) of sodium per day.
- Choose and prepare foods with little salt. At the same time, consume potassium-rich foods, such as fruits and vegetables.

ALCOHOLIC BEVERAGES

Key Recommendations

- Those who choose to drink alcoholic beverages should do so sensibly and in moderation—defined as the consumption of up to one drink per day for women and up to two drinks per day for men.
- Alcoholic beverages should not be consumed by some individuals, including those who cannot restrict their alcohol intake, women of childbearing age who may become pregnant, pregnant and lactating women, children and adolescents, individuals

taking medications that can interact with alcohol, and those with specific medical conditions.
- Alcoholic beverages should be avoided by individuals engaging in activities that require attention, skill, or coordination, such as driving or operating machinery.

FOOD SAFETY

Key Recommendations

- To avoid microbial foodborne illness:
  - Clean hands, food contact surfaces, and fruits and vegetables. Meat and poultry should not be washed or rinsed.
  - Separate raw, cooked, and ready-to-eat foods while shopping, preparing, or storing foods.
  - Cook foods to a safe temperature to kill microorganisms.
  - Chill (refrigerate) perishable food promptly and defrost foods properly.
  - Avoid raw (unpasteurized) milk or any products made from unpasteurized milk, raw or partially cooked eggs or foods containing raw eggs, raw or undercooked meat and poultry, unpasteurized juices, and raw sprouts.

---

federal aid programs, such as the National School Lunch and the Women, Infants, and Children (WIC) programs. Dietary recommendations are still used for this purpose, but as the prevalence of chronic diseases, such as coronary heart disease, stroke, cancer, diabetes, and obesity, has grown in the past 50 years, the guidelines shifted to a dual focus of preventing deficiencies and promoting health.

In addition to providing the basis for many federal nutrition programs, current public health dietary recommendations are used as a basis for nutrition label information, military rations, the development of some food and nutritional products, and evaluation of the adequacy of intake for individuals and groups. The remainder of this section focuses on food and nutrient guidelines that fitness professionals would most likely use for evaluating dietary intake of individuals. Practical recommendations for using these guidelines are also provided. Diet can be evaluated at the food or nutrient level. For the former, you would use MyPyramid, whereas for the latter, you would use the DRIs. Regardless of the method you use, the steps are the same.

1. Convert foods and amounts eaten into food group servings or nutrients.
2. Determine the recommended intake of food groups or nutrients.

3. Compare the amount eaten with recommendations to determine dietary inadequacies.

Here again, be cautious because although these appear to be simple steps, the diet assessment process is not simplistic. It can be fraught with missing information, errors, and miscalculations, as described in earlier sections of this chapter. These errors can be compounded when dietary assessment is done by people with little or no training or experience. If fitness professionals feel uncomfortable with any part of this process, they should consult with or refer their patients to a registered dietitian. In addition, in many states, only registered dieticians or licensed nutritionists are legally able to analyze diets and counsel an individual regarding their diet. It is recommended that the exercise professional investigate the law in the state in which they are practicing to determine their scope of practice with respect to nutrition consulting.

Converting Foods and Amounts Eaten

Calculate nutrient intake by hand or by using computer software. The former requires you to list each food and the amount eaten. Then use a reference guide, such as Bowes and Church (13), to look up the amount of different nutrients in each food. Using computer software can be much faster and more accurate than the hand-tabulation

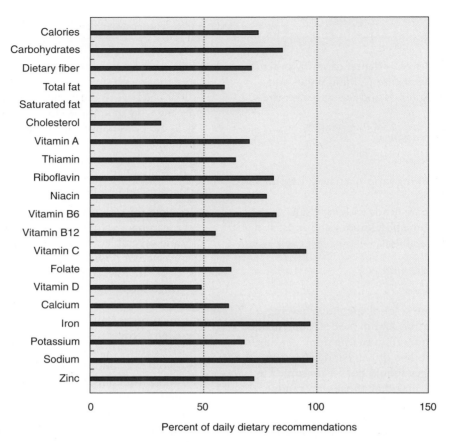

FIGURE 14-1. Sample nutrient analysis report.

method. Enter the foods and amount eaten into the dietary analysis software, and it calculates the quantity consumed for dozens of nutrients for each food. It then sums the quantity of each nutrient for all foods to generate a total daily intake for each nutrient. Many programs calculate an average nutrient intake amount for multiple days of food data as well.

Determine the Recommended Intake

In step one, determine nutrient intake either by hand calculation or by computer. Likewise, in step two, look up a patient's intake need for most nutrients in reference. Review the tables, and take note that nutrient needs sometimes differ from one age category to another or between sexes. Computerized dietary analysis software contains DRI information for each nutrient.

Compare the Amount Eaten with Recommendations

Determining nutrient adequacy simply means comparing actual intake with nutrient recommendations for a person based on his or her age and sex. Most nutrient analysis software programs have a database of the DRIs against which nutrient intake is compared. These applications often provide a tabular and graphic presentation of the adequacy of a patient's intake compared with the nutrient needs of some-

one of their sex and age. These are often given as percentages of recommended intake. For example, Figure 14-1 shows a graph that many applications may use.

This example shows that the patient did not meet her nutrient needs 100% exactly for a single nutrient. Does this mean she is nutritionally at risk? How should this be interpreted? There are several things to consider:

1. That dietary assessment information is an estimate: The report you generate from either a 24-hour recall or diet record is an estimate of nutrient intake. It is only as good as the completeness of the data provided to you, the quality of the analysis software you use to analyze the intake, and your data-entry accuracy.
2. Number of days recorded: One day's food record can have a high degree of variability compared with another day's. What you eat today may be very different from what you eat tomorrow or the next day, and what you eat in a single day is not likely to affect your health positively or negatively. It is most useful to smooth out the highs and lows in the daily variability of nutrient intake by averaging the nutrient values across several days.
3. Typical of usual intake: If the day (or days) the patient recorded were not very typical of his or her usual eating pattern, then the analysis may be skewed. For

example, a patient usually has a bowl of cereal and skim milk every morning, but on two of the days he recorded, he only ate a granola bar as he commuted to the courthouse for jury duty.

4. Accurate portion descriptions: Often people guess at the size of their portions or misinterpret information provided on their measuring tools.
5. Data entry errors: It is common to make a mistake in entering the many foods in a patient's dietary intake record. For example, misplacement of a decimal point can make 0.75 cup of Brussels sprouts 7.5 cups of sprouts! When the results seem skewed, review the data you entered to make sure you have selected the correct food option and entered the right portion amount.

If reviewing these issues does not at least somewhat account for any nutrient values below or above the recommended levels, it is rarely cause for alarm. Deficiency is not a concern until a patient is chronically below 66% of recommended intake. In general, if a patient is taking a multivitamin supplement, it is not usually included in the computer analysis, so it is likely the patient is getting an adequate intake. Excessive intake can occur when a patient chronically consumes levels above the UL from both diet and supplements.

In summary, this section has provided a step-by-step process for evaluating dietary intake. The fitness professional can use a food-focused evaluation process using MyPyramid or a nutrient-focused evaluation using the DRIs. The former is fairly simple and can be done without special software or references. The latter gives very specific information that may be important in some situations. Regardless of the method you use, you must translate the dietary evaluation into practical recommendations for changing food intake, and you must work with patients to help them set attainable, personal goals for dietary improvement.

PROVIDING USEFUL DIETARY FEEDBACK

> **1.9.1-HFS: List and apply behavioral strategies that apply to lifestyle modifications, such as exercise, diet, stress, and medication management.**

After the patient's diet is analyzed and evaluated, the next step is to educate them about the aspects of his or her diet that need to be changed to improve dietary intake. There are two components of giving feedback. The first is the content or the information given to the patient. The second component is the process or the way in which the information is provided.

Feedback Content

The task is to inform patients of the gaps that occur in their diets based on what they reported eating and what is recommended for them. These gaps can be characterized as underconsumption or overconsumption of foods

or nutrients. It is fairly easy to give feedback to close such gaps using specific foods and MyPyramid's food groups. Box 14-3 provides a list of practical recommendations for improving intake of foods in different food groups.

If the patient's diet has been evaluated using a nutrient analysis, it is necessary to convert nutrient needs to food-based recommendations. For example, if it has been determined that a patient is eating too much saturated fat, recommend that the patient reduce the intake of whole-milk dairy products, including cheese; choose small portions of meat; choose lean meats only; choose red meats less often; and limit butter and foods with hydrogenated fats. If a patient needs to increase her fiber intake, the fitness professional could advise that she eat more whole-grain products, fruits, vegetables, legumes, and nuts.

The Process of Giving Feedback

Identifying the gaps in what a patient eats and what is recommended for him is the first step in providing dietary guidance. Working with the patient to determine a plan for closing the gaps is the next step. This step requires an understanding about the behavior change process, and although this is covered elsewhere in this book, we have listed below several change strategies that fitness professionals can use to help patients succeed at improving their diets. It is important to note that the process is done collaboratively with patients. Simply telling patients what they need to change without providing assistance on how to do it on their own is not an effective way of giving feedback.

Educate on Dietary Gaps

This step provides the process in which the patient is informed of her dietary needs. It is important to share all needs while being mindful not to overwhelm the patient. Many patients are tempted to want to totally overhaul their eating habits based on the information provided. Point out early on in the feedback process that it is best that they choose one or two areas that they want to work on at first. After they have had success making those changes, they can refocus their efforts to address other areas.

Assess Readiness to Change

Patients may be more ready to change some aspects of their diet than others. For example, a patient may be more willing to incorporate more whole grains than increase dairy foods. It is important that it be determined which of the dietary improvement areas you have identified that the patient is most ready to change. This strategy has been discussed as it relates to physical activity readiness in Chapter 42 of this resource manual. It can easily be adapted to assessing readiness to change diet.

BOX 14-3   DIETARY FEEDBACK TIPS

BREAD, CEREAL, PASTA, AND RICE

Most people get adequate servings of the bread group. Because people often misjudge serving size (e.g., one bagel is equal to two to three servings), overconsumption is common.

Increase Servings

- Double up on servings of cereal, pasta, and rice.
- Enjoy low-fat breads as a snack. Choose whole-grain options whenever possible.

Decrease Servings

- Watch portion sizes. Measure cereal, rice, and pasta and weigh bread, muffins, and other bread foods to become familiar with the actual size of one serving.

Increase Whole Grains

- Start the day with a whole-grain breakfast cereal. Look for one that has at least 5 g of fiber per serving.
- Use 100% whole wheat bread.
- Make oatmeal a regular part of your diet.
- Double up on servings
- Try new whole grains such as bulgur (wheat berries), barley, amaranth, spelt, and quinoa in place of rice or pasta or as side dishes and salads.

VEGETABLES

Few people eat enough vegetables, and the vegetables they do eat are often limited to a few kinds, such as potatoes, corn, and iceberg lettuce.

Increase Servings

- Double and triple up on servings at meals.
- Order a side of vegetables when eating out.
- Enjoy large salads as a meal instead of a sandwich or burger. They can often count as two to four servings, depending on the size.
- Try vegetable juices as a refreshing alternative to soda.
- Eat vegetables and low-fat dips as healthy snack.
- Add extra veggies to soups, stews, and casseroles.

Other Suggestions

- Choose a variety of vegetables. Challenge your taste buds with sweet potatoes, rutabagas, Hubbard squash, kale, and other nutrient-packed veggies.
- Choose colorful vegetables such as carrots, melons, spinach, and tomatoes. Often, the more color, the more nutrients.
- Use canned or frozen vegetables to speed up the preparation process. Look for choices with no added sodium.

FRUITS

As with vegetables, fruits are underconsumed by most adults. They are packed with many nutrients.

Increase Servings

- Start your day with a glass of orange or grapefruit juice.
- Snack on fresh or dried fruits instead of chips or candy bars.
- Serve fruit as dessert and help yourself to seconds.

Other

- Like vegetables, choose a rainbow of colors.
- Pack frozen fruit in your lunch bag, and it will be thawed by the time the noon hour rolls around.

MEAT, POULTRY, FISH, EGGS, DRIED BEANS, AND MEAT ALTERNATIVES

Most people eat adequate amounts of meat and poultry, and some people eat these foods in excess.

Limit Meat Group Foods that are High in Total and Saturated Fat

- Choose lean cuts of meat. Cuts with the words "loin" or "round" in the name are usually good choices.
- Choose ground beef that is at least 90% lean.
- Trim visible fat from meat and poultry before cooking.
- Substitute two egg whites for one whole egg.
- Choose reduced-fat processed meats, cold cuts, and sausages. Check the Nutrition Facts label.

Choose Lean Meats and Meat Alternatives

- Go fishing for good nutrition by eating fish at least two servings a week. If you do not like to cook fish, make it your choice when eating out. Choose broiled or grilled fish, not battered and deep fried.
- Give soy and other plant-based meat alternates a try. Sausages, burgers, and chicken tenders are all available in veggie versions, and many grocery stores carry them. Look in the freezer section. Remember, do not expect them to taste just like meat, but enjoy them for their own delicious flavor.
- Eat several meatless meals each week. Look in cookbooks or online for vegetarian recipes.
- Get a leg up with legumes. Try different types of dried beans, peas, and lentils as meat substitutes in soups, salads, or casseroles.

MILK, YOGURT, AND CHEESE

Dairy foods are often overlooked by many adults who think only children need milk. Even people who are

BOX 14-3 DIETARY FEEDBACK TIPS (Continued)

lactose intolerant can (and should) enjoy dairy foods by using specially prepared dairy products.

Choose Low-fat and Nonfat Dairy Foods

- Use skim, 2%, or 1% milk or yogurt.
- Use reduced fat cheese or use less of regular cheese.
- Go easy on regular ice cream. Try low-fat or fat-free versions. Sorbet and sherbet are other low-fat choices.

Increase Dairy Foods

- Make hot cereals and condensed soups with skim milk instead of water.
- Enjoy fruit and low-fat yogurt smoothies for a quick, delicious meal or snack.
- Drink low-fat milk with meals instead of soda.

FATS, OILS, AND SWEETS

Foods in this category are high in calories, and many do not provide much in the way of nutrients; that, is they provide essentially empty calories. So, these foods should be used sparingly.

Limit Empty Calories

- Choose fruits and vegetables as snacks instead of candy.
- Cut amount of fat or oil called for in a recipe by one fourth or one third.
- Replace regular soda or sweetened soft drinks with diet versions or fruit juices or low-fat milk.

Other Ideas

- When choosing a fat for cooking, select vegetable oils, such as canola or olive oil, instead of using lard, butter, or shortening.
- Retrain your sweet tooth by gradually removing high-sugar foods from your diet.

Set Goals

People who are successful at changing habits challenge themselves by setting goals. However, it is not enough to simply state: "I want to eat better." Effective goals are those that are realistic (are within a patient's reach), specific (defined in behavioral terms), and measurable (will be able to know whether or not it was attained). Ask patients to state some short-term (1-day to 1-month) and long-term (more than 1-month) goals for the dietary improvement areas they are ready to change. Here is an example of a good goal: "On 5 of the next 7 days, I will eat at least five servings of fruits and vegetables." It is *realistic* because the patient was already eating three servings on most, but not all days. In addition, the patient recognizes that it is not likely that he is going to be able to get five servings every day, so he set the goal at five days. The goal is *specific* because it states what aspect of the diet (fruits and vegetables) he is going to change and to what extent. Finally, it is *measurable* because he defined a time frame (i.e., the next 7 days) and quantified the specific parameters of the goal.

Define an Action Plan

A goal is hollow unless it has an action plan to back it up. An action plan identifies the specific strategies the patient is going to use to attain his goal. Using the example goal given previously, the patient identified the following action plan: "Go to the store on my way home to buy orange juice, fresh strawberries, carrots, premixed salad, and frozen vegetables. Have orange juice for breakfast every morning. Take strawberries and carrots to work for snacks. Eat a big salad at lunch or dinner every weekday. Double up on servings of vegetables at dinner."

Identify a Self-monitoring Strategy

Daily logging helps patients identify whether they are on track toward their goals. Not only does self-monitoring help patients keep a record of what they are doing to attain their goals, it can also prompt patients to make better choices. Unlike keeping diet records for a dietary analysis, when patients are focusing on a specific goal, such as eating five or more servings of fruits and vegetables, they only need to focus on recording that specific behavior, simplifying the recording process a great deal.

Arrange Follow-up

Before the feedback session with your patient is ended, set a follow-up appointment. The follow-up can be done face to face, by telephone, or by electronic means, such as fax or email. The important thing is that patients know the availability of the fitness professional to discuss the success or difficulties they had with attaining their goals. This session is a good time to praise patients for their attainment of goals, problem solve difficulties, and set new goals. Many patients find the accountability of a follow-up contact to be very motivating. As stated earlier, this presentation is a rather simplistic overview of the process for helping patients take the information provided about their dietary needs and applying it to their particular lifestyle. The behavior change principles described in

Chapters 42 and 43 of this resource manual give a much more thorough review of the change process.

WHEN TO REFER PATIENTS

It is appropriate for fitness professionals to provide dietary guidance to patients who are generally healthy. Many of these patients are interested in improving their diets to lose weight, improve sports performance, or simply slow the development of age-related chronic diseases. There are, however, circumstances under which the fitness professional should refer patients to a registered or licensed dietitian. Patients who have special dietary needs, such as people with diabetes, renal problems, eating disorders, or other similar serious medical conditions, should be referred to a registered or licensed dietitian. To locate dietitians in your area to whom patients can be referred, check with your local hospital to find out if they provide outpatient services. Also, you can go to the American Dietetic Association's Web site at www.eatright.org. Look for the "Find a Nutrition Professional" section, and enter your patient's zip code.

SUMMARY

This chapter is intended to serve as a resource for fitness professionals interested in assessing diet by providing the descriptions of the diet assessment tools and their benefits and limitations. The steps to dietary assessment include identifying the purpose of diet assessment, selecting the appropriate diet assessment tool, obtaining the dietary intake from the individual, analyzing the data, evaluating the diet, and providing useful feedback. Assessing diet is a complex task and requires follow-through with each step to assist patients with reaching their goals.

REFERENCES

1. Burke B. Dietary history as a tool in research. *J Am Diet Assoc.* 1947;23:1041–1047.
2. Buzzard M. 24-hour dietary recall and food record methods. In Willett W, editor. *Nutritional Epidemiology.* 2nd ed. New York: Oxford University Press; 1998. p. 50–73.
3. Byers TE, Marshall JR, Anthony E, Fiedler R, Zielezny M. The reliability of dietary history from the distant past. *Am J Epidemiol.* 1987;125:999–1011.
4. Conway JM, Ingwersen LA, Vinyard BT, Moshfegh AJ. Effectiveness of the US Department of Agriculture 5-step multiple-pass method in assessing food intake in obese and non-obese women. *Am J Clin Nutr.* 2003;77:1171–1178.
5. Institute of Medicine. *Dietary Reference Intakes for Calcium, Phosphorous, Magnesium, Vitamin D and Fluoride.* Washington (DC): National Academies Press; 1997.
6. **Institute of Medicine.** *Dietary Reference Intakes for Thiamin, Riboflavin, Niacin, Vitamin B6, Folate, Vitamin B12, Pantothenic Acid, Biotin and Choline.* **Washington (DC): National Academies Press; 1998.**
7. Institute of Medicine. *Dietary Reference Intakes for Vitamin A, Vitamin K, Arsenic, Boron, Chromium, Copper, Iodine, Iron, Manganese, Molybdenum, Nickel, Silicon, Vanadium and Zinc.* Washington (DC): National Academies Press; 2001.
8. Institute of Medicine. *Dietary Reference Intakes for Vitamin C, Vitamin E, Selenium and Carotenoids.* Washington (DC): National Academies Press; 2000.
9. Institute of Medicine. *Dietary Reference Intakes for Energy, Carbohydrate, Fiber, Fat, Fatty Acids, Cholesterol, Protein and Amino Acids.* Food and Nutrition Board. Washington (DC): National Academies Press; 2005.
10. Institute of Medicine. *Dietary Reference Intakes for Water, Potassium, Sodium, Chloride, and Sulfate.* Food and Nutrition Board. Washington (DC): National Academies Press; 2004.
11. Lee RD, Nieman DC. *Nutritional Assessment.* 4th ed. New York: McGraw Hill; 2006. p. 1–12.
12. Nielson SJ, Popkin BM. Patterns and trends in food portion sizes, 1997–1998. *JAMA.* 2003;289:450–453.
13. Pennington JAT, Douglass JS. *Bowes and Church's Food Values of Portions Commonly Used.* 18th ed. Philadelphia: Lippincott Williams & Wilkins; 2004.
14. Smiciklas-Wright H, Mitchell D, Mickle SJ, Goldman JD, Cook A. Foods commonly eaten in the United States, 1989–1991 and 1994–1996: Are portion sizes changing? *J Am Diet Assoc.* 2003;103: 41–47.
15. Thompson FE, Byers T. Dietary assessment resource manual. *J Nutr.* 1994;124:2245s–2317s.
16. **U.S. Department of Agriculture and U.S. Department of Health and Human Services.** Dietary guidelines for Americans 2005. www.healthierus.gov/dietaryguidelines (accessed April 27, 2007).
17. U.S. Department of Agriculture, Agriculture Research Service Web site [Internet]. *What We Eat In America, NHANES 2003–2004: Documentation and Data Files.* 2006. www.ars.usda.gov/ba/bhnrc/fsrg(accessed April 19, 2007).
18. U.S. Department of Agriculture, Agricultural Research Service. USDA National Nutrient Database for Standard Reference, Release 19. Nutrient Data Laboratory Home Page; 2006. www.ars.usda.gov/ba/bhnrc/ndl (accessed April 27, 2007).
19. U.S. Department of Agriculture. MyPyramid Plan. www.mypyramid.gov (accessed May 5, 2007).
20. Willet W. Nature of variation in the diet. In: Nutritional Epidemiology. 2nd ed. New York: Oxford University Press; 1998. p. 33–49.
21. Young LR, Nestle M. Portion sizes in dietary assessment: issues and policy implications. *Nutr Rev.* 1995;53:149–159.
22. Young LR, Nestle M. The contribution of expanding portion sizes to the US obesity epidemic. *Am J Public Health.* 2002;92:246–249.

SELECTED REFERENCES FOR FURTHER READING

Charney P, Malone A. *ADA Pocket Guide to Nutrition Assessment.* Chicago: American Dietetic Association; 2004.
Pennington JA, Douglass JS. *Bowe and Church's Food Values of Portions Commonly Used.* Philadelphia: Lippincott Williams & Wilkins; 2004.

INTERNET RESOURCES

- American Dietetic Association: www.eatright.org
- Dietary Reference Intakes (DRI) and Recommended Dietary Allowances (RDA): www.nal.usda.gov/fnic/etext/000108.html
- MyPyramid Plan: www.mypyramid.gov
- Nutrition and Your Health: Dietary Guidelines for Americans 2005: www.healthierus.gov/dietaryguidelines

Psychosocial Status and Chronic Disease

Chronic diseases such as cardiovascular disease (CVD), cancer, chronic obstructive pulmonary disease (COPD), and diabetes account for more than 66% of deaths in the United States (30,114). Consequently, the alleviation of chronic disease is a priority of the Year 2010 Health Objectives for the nation (146). Chronic diseases typically progress through a series of stages characterized by increased morbidity and disability. Whereas the term *disease* is commonly used to describe pathologic or physiologic changes in the body, *illness* refers to the individual's ensuing adaptation to the disease.

Physical limitations and emotional issues surrounding chronic illness can have a devastating effect on the patient's quality of life. The influence of emotional distress on chronic illness is often underrecognized compared with other risk factors (106) despite a rapidly growing body of evidence showing a reciprocal relationship between psychosocial factors and chronic disease progression, in which emotional distress can be both a cause and consequence of chronic illness.

This chapter is directed to clinical exercise professionals who may have a limited background in psychology and the mental health aspects of disease prevention. It is intended to serve as a quick reference guide for those who need relevant information for professional and public education. The chapter does not provide a comprehensive review of the psychosocial literature associated with chronic illness. Instead, it focuses on the major chronic illnesses that account for much of the morbidity and mortality in the United States adult population, including CVD, stroke, heart failure, diabetes, chronic obstructive pulmonary disease (COPD), and asthma.

The chapter reviews epidemiologic and clinical research investigating the relationship between emotional distress and chronic disease. The evidence linking psychosocial factors to the onset and progression of chronic disease is examined. In addition to the three psychosocial domains identified in the Surgeon General's Report on Mental Health (147)—**life stress**, **depression**, and **anxiety**—consideration is given to the role of low **social**

> > > KEY TERMS

Anxiety: A perception of fear or apprehension that is accompanied by a state of heightened physiologic arousal that may include a surge in heart rate, sweating, and tensing of muscles.

Depression: The presence of a depressed mood or a markedly decreased interest in all activities, persisting for at least 2 weeks and accompanied by at least four of the following additional symptoms: changes in appetite, sleep disturbance, fatigue, psychomotor retardation or agitation, feelings of guilt or worthlessness, difficulty concentrating, and suicidal thoughts.

Hostility: An attitude of cynicism and mistrust that may provoke feelings of anger, irritation, and impatience.

Life stress: A combination of negative physiologic, cognitive, emotional, and behavioral responses that

occur in response to an individual's unique perception of life events.

Psychological traits: Persistent and stable enduring attributes or predispositions of an individual (e.g., type A pattern, which may be characterized by an overcommitment to work or completing tasks, competitiveness, an exaggerated need to achieve, free-floating hostility, and a propensity to become easily angered or annoyed).

Psychological states: Transient changes in mood that may reflect a person's circumstance at a particular point in time.

Social support: An affiliation with social networks that provide emotional support and assistance with aspects of daily living.

support and **psychological** **states** and **traits** (e.g., hostility).

The chapter also describes the impact of psychosocial and behavioral interventions on emotional distress. Particular attention is given to the role of cognitive behavioral therapy (CBT) because of its general application to numerous chronic conditions. CBT is a counseling method that is used by trained mental health specialists to change ineffective or unrealistic thought patterns and subsequently modify behavior. Consideration is also given to motivational interviewing, which has demonstrated success in the treatment of substance abuse (128) and has more recently been adapted to improve a wide range of problem behaviors in medical settings (24,42). Motivational interviewing is a patient-centered, directive method of communication that can be used by a wide variety of trained healthcare providers to enhance an individual's intrinsic motivation to change unhealthful behavior by exploring and resolving ambivalence (108). Finally, the chapter briefly reviews the direct role exercise may have in the reduction of emotional distress.

CHRONIC DISEASE AND ILLNESS

CARDIOVASCULAR DISEASE

1.9.7-CES: Identify the psychological issues associated with an acute cardiac event versus those associated with chronic cardiac conditions.

Approximately 15.8 million Americans have coronary heart disease (CHD); 5.6 million have cerebrovascular disease, and 5.2 million have heart failure (3). CVD is the most prevalent chronic illness in the United States (146). In reviewing the literature, it is clear that there is more research investigating the relationship between psychosocial factors and CVD than any other chronic illness. Therefore, a large portion of this chapter focuses on the CVD literature.

Evidence indicates there is a relationship between chronic life stress at work and the development of CVD. Stressful life events include the breakup of intimate personal relationships, death of a family member or friend, economic hardship, role conflict, work overload, racism and discrimination, poor physical health, accidental injuries, and intentional assaults of physical safety (66,87,93). Stressful life events may also reflect past events. Severe trauma in childhood, including sexual and physical abuse, may persist as stressors into adulthood or may make individuals more vulnerable to ongoing stress (22). Each individual exhibits a unique response to stressful life events that includes some combination of physiologic, cognitive, emotional, and behavioral characteristics that may be harmful to susceptible individuals.

In a meta-analysis of five different populations numbering more than 12,000 individuals and covering an 18- to 30-year period, work stress was associated with higher levels of cholesterol, systolic blood pressure (BP), and smoking behavior (123). Monotonous work, high-paced work, and job burnout have been correlated with an increased incidence of CHD (6). High-demand jobs with low-decision latitude have been associated with a fourfold increased risk of cardiovascular-related death (77). Work stress associated with high demand and low reward has also resulted in an increase in cardiac events (20,140) and the progression of carotid atherosclerosis (101). Researchers have identified that in a working population compared with a nonworking population, there is a 33% increase in relative risk of disease onset on Mondays (160). In a more recent study involving a sample of 170,000 men and women, death from CVD was 20% above the daily average on Mondays for those younger than age 50 years (45). In the 20-year follow-up of the Framingham Heart Study, the incidence of angina was two times greater among those who exhibited higher levels of worry, dissatisfaction with work, feeling undue time pressure, and competitive drive (43). Together, these studies indicate that there is strong association between this form of chronic stress and the development of CVD. Almost 4 decades ago, Holmes and Rahe (126) developed the Recent Life Change Questionnaire to assess the severity of typical stressful life events. Whereas the death of a spouse, divorce, and loss of a job were considered high stress, vacations and holidays were given a lower weighting. A retrospective recall identified that elevated scores on the survey were associated with higher rates of myocardial infarction (MI) or sudden cardiac death at 6-month follow-up (160).

Acute stress has been implicated in the triggering of cardiovascular events. Epidemiologic evidence has revealed that life-threatening situations such as earthquakes (78,95,143,145) and war (10,107) are associated with increased rates of MI and cardiac mortality. This observation does not appear to be limited to life-threatening situations. An increase in the rate of hospital admissions for MI and sudden cardiac death has been reported after important national soccer games (27,161). In an examination of the acute effect of anger as a trigger of MI, retrospective interviews of 1,623 post-MI patients identified a greater-than-twofold relative risk of MI after an episode of anger (109). Cross-sectional studies have yielded evidence that acute negative emotional states, such as anger, anxiety, and frustration (62), are associated with myocardial ischemia. In a retrospective analysis, the MILIS study (144) found that 49% of patients identified a possible exogenous trigger for their MI, including emotional upsets. It has been hypothesized that acute psychological triggers increase sympathetic nervous system activation, which then leads to increases in heart rate and BP, greater endothelial injury, and heightened hemostatic and platelet activation (151,153).

Depression takes a monumental toll on human suffering, lost productivity, and death. The 1-month community-based prevalence of major depression episodes is approximately 5% (13). However, the prevalence is three times higher among patients with CVD, and the point prevalence of major depression in the general population is 6.6% (26,79). When unrecognized, depression can result in excessive healthcare utilization.

Depression ranks among the top 10 causes of worldwide disability (112). Major depression is the most well-known mood disorder, but there are others, including bipolar disorder (one or more episodes of mania) and dysthymia (a chronic but less severe form of major depression) (147). Episodes of major depression are characterized by the presence of a depressed mood or a markedly decreased interest in all activities, persisting for at least 2 weeks and accompanied by at least four of the following additional symptoms: changes in appetite, sleep disturbance, fatigue, psychomotor retardation or agitation, feelings of guilt or worthlessness, problems concentrating, and suicidal thoughts. It is estimated that depression will rank as the second major cause of disability worldwide in the year 2020 (111).

The causes of depression are not fully known. It may be triggered by stressful life events, enduring stressful social conditions (e.g., poverty and discrimination), neurochemical imbalance in the brain, maladaptive cognitions, or a combination of these factors. Depression is twice as common in women as men.

Depression tends to be underdiagnosed and -treated in cardiac patients. Fewer than 25% of patients with major depression are recognized as being depressed by their cardiologists or general internists, and only about 50% of patients diagnosed as depressed receive treatment (103). The reasons for this finding are not clear, although it has been suggested that physicians may have difficulty differentiating between the symptoms of depression and those related to the disease (32). Depression can reduce the sensitivity of standard tests for CVD. In a study of nearly 1,400 patients undergoing standard single-photon emission computed tomography (SPECT) exercise testing, depressed patients had a higher rate of false-negative electrocardiogram (ECG) ischemia compared with nondepressed patients (91). Epidemiologic evidence demonstrates a significant prospective relationship between the occurrence of depression, or depressive symptoms, and the incidence of future cardiac events among healthy (5,9) and CVD populations (8,50,52) in many, but not all, studies (89,104). In a Finnish study of more than 95,000 individuals followed over 4 to 5 years, the highest risk of mortality occurred 1 month after bereavement, with more than a twofold risk for men and a threefold risk for women (75). Hopelessness, which is a component of depression, has shown a particularly strong link with sudden death and the development of CVD (5) and carotid atherosclerosis (45,46).

Anxiety disorders are the most prevalent mental disorders in adults (128), affecting twice as many women as men. These disorders include panic disorder, phobias, obsessive-compulsive disorder, posttraumatic stress disorder, and generalized anxiety disorder. Prevalence rates for all anxiety disorders in the general population are estimated to be 1% to 13% (4). Underlying this heterogeneous group of disorders is a state of heightened arousal or fear in relation to stressful events or feelings. The biological manifestations of anxiety, which are grounded in the "fight-or-flight" response, are unmistakable: they include surge in heart rate, sweating, and tensing of muscles. The Harvard Mastery of Stress Study, one of the longest prospective studies ever conducted in this field, revealed that severe anxiety and conflict with hostility were significant predictors of CVD and risk of overall future illness (134).

Social support has been widely recognized as an independent predictor of health and well-being in both general and clinical populations (74,149), especially among patients with cardiac disease. For example, low social support has been prospectively associated with poor clinical prognosis among patients with heart failure (110) and stable CVD (23,67,121,159). In addition, at least three relatively large-scale studies have found that low levels of support predicted an increased risk of mortality after an acute MI (11,60,155). In two large studies involving CVD patients, those at higher risk had significantly more socioeconomic difficulties while simultaneously lacking social support or social connections to deal with stress (74,159).

There are two broad categories of social support. Structural support refers to social networks and includes such indices as marital status, number of friends, and participation in church or civic organizations. Functional support refers to the perception of support and includes such elements as instrumental support (e.g., having someone who can assist in activities of daily living) and emotional support (e.g., having someone to talk to and whom you believe loves or cares for you [147]).

Studies on animals (73) and humans (7,14,35,71,86,120,132) have identified that psychological stress has an adverse impact on the cardiovascular system. The mechanism by which stress may influence atherogenesis involves a complex interaction of sympathetic arousal, hypothalamic stimulation, and adrenergic and neurohormonal responses that lead to increased BP, increased circulating catecholamine levels, and increased platelet activity (33,113,151). The resulting increased shearing forces of blood on the arterial wall lead to endothelial injury and arterial wall damage. Thus, chronic exposure to psychological stress promotes the development of atherosclerosis that may result in vasospasm (163), myocardial ischemia (18), coronary artery occlusion, MI, and increased incidence of ventricular arrhythmia, a known risk factor for sudden coronary death (34). These pathophysiologic mechanisms have been schematized by Rozanski et al. (133) in Figure 15-1.

Although conclusions regarding the mechanisms by which more chronic psychosocial factors contribute to cardiac events are not definitive, considerable evidence points to several mechanisms likely to be involved in the

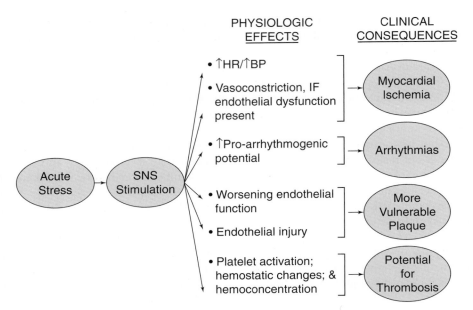

FIGURE 15-1. Pathophysiologic effects of acute psychosocial stress. Sympathetic nervous system (SNS) stimulation emanating from acute stress leads to a variety of effects, ranging from heart rate (HR) and blood pressure (BP) stimulation to direct effects on coronary vascular endothelium. Clinical consequences of these effects include myocardial ischemia, cardiac arrhythmias, and fostering of more vulnerable coronary plaques and hemostatic changes. These changes form a substrate for development of acute myocardial infarction and sudden cardiac death. (Adapted with permission from Rozanski A, Blumenthal JA, Kaplan J. Impact of psychological factors on the pathogenesis of cardiovascular disease and implications for therapy. *Circulation.* 1999;99:2192–2217.)

impact of depression on the prognosis of patients with established CVD. For example, it has been shown that depressed patients' exhibit increased sympathetic nervous system outflow and decreased parasympathetic function (153). This combination can lead to ventricular arrhythmias, platelet activation and aggregation, and increased myocardial oxygen consumption. It is plausible that these kinds of reactions could contribute to the pathophysiologic processes involved in the development of both CVD and MI. Increased activation of the pituitary adrenal axis in depressed patients has also been shown to produce high levels of cortisol (83), which can potentiate and prolong the effects of catecholamines (153).

Depression has been shown to be a predictor of poor adherence to a wide variety of medical treatment (26,40,109). A meta-analysis by Di Matteo et al. revealed that patients with chronic disease and depression were three times more likely to be nonadherent with medical treatment than nondepressed patients (38). In patients recovering from MI, there is evidence that depression is associated with poor adherence to cardiac rehabilitation and risk-factor modification (61). Consequently, depression may indirectly promote the progression of chronic illness by preventing adherence to other treatment regimens, such as healthy eating, physical activity and exercise, taking medications appropriately, abstaining from smoking, managing stress, and moderating alcohol consumption.

Psychosocial and Behavioral Interventions

Psychosocial and behavioral intervention trials in patients with CVD have reported mixed success. In a study of 107 cardiac patients with exercise-induced ischemia, a CBT-based approach to stress management was associated with improved psychosocial measures, a reduction in mental stress–induced ischemia (17), and fewer clinical events after a 5-year follow-up when compared with exercise therapy alone or usual care (15). In a review of other studies involving similar populations, CBT interventions have been reported to improve quality of life and reduce mortality in cardiac patients (100). However, in the Enhancing Recovery in Coronary Heart Disease (ENRICHD) Trial, a multicenter trial involving 2,481 post-MI patients with depression or low social support, CBT reduced depression levels but failed to yield a significant reduction in all-cause mortality and cardiac morbidity (162). Other trials (51,72) have also reported negative findings, and the failure of these brief interventions to alter psychosocial risk factors, such as anxiety and depression, may have been responsible for the lack of effect on "hard" clinical endpoints, such as mortality and morbidity.

The role of exercise as a stand-alone intervention in the prevention and management of CVD is well documented (148,156). However, it should be recognized that there is uncertainty about the extent to which clinical outcomes may have been directly or indirectly affected by improved psychosocial status as a result of exercise. Regardless, it is safe to conclude that exercise therapy added to a multi-intervention approach that includes behavioral cardiac risk modification, education, and counseling may enhance the improvements in CVD outcomes reported in exercise-only interventions (156). This finding is exemplified by the Lifestyle Heart Trial, which demonstrated that an intervention composed of exercise therapy, group support meetings, education and skills training in a low-fat diet, and daily stress management (i.e., yoga-derived stretching, breathing, meditation, imagery, and relaxation techniques) could assist a highly motivated group of cardiac patients to make comprehensive changes in lifestyle. Arteriographic data identified an average arterial stenosis regression from 40% to 37.8% in the intervention group compared with a progression from 42.7% to 46.1% in a usual care group at a 1-year follow-up (118). A 5-year follow-up showed continued progression in the control group and regression in the intensive lifestyle intervention group (119). Motivating CVD patients to adopt and maintain comprehensive changes in lifestyle is a challenge that faces healthcare professionals, and motivational interviewing is an innovative approach that has demonstrated efficacy in brief consultations. Scales et al. (139) found that compared with traditional cardiac rehabilitation, adding motivational interviewing coupled with brief skills-building sessions significantly lowers stress and enhances multiple health-related behaviors in CVD patients.

STROKE

Stroke and heart failure are especially important cardiovascular conditions that deserve attention because of the psychological sequelae associated with these chronic conditions and the need for more effective interventions. Stroke is the third leading cause of death in the United States and the leading cause of long-term disability (3). Each year, 700,000 people experience a new or recurrent stroke. The estimated direct and indirect cost of stroke for 2007 is approximately $62.7 billion (3).

The most common psychological reaction in individuals suffering a stroke is depression. The incidence of depression ranges from 25% to 79%, with most studies showing a rate of approximately 30% (81). The large variation in incidence is due to the timing of assessment relative to stroke onset and the instruments used to assess depression. A debate also exists as to whether depression following a stroke is organic or a result of the psychosocial adjustment required by the disease (81). Several factors may contribute to poststroke depression, including institutionalization, prestroke alcohol use, impairment of activities of daily living, and perception of social support. Poststroke depression has been found to be higher among older adults with similar chronic conditions causing similar physical disabilities (81). Finally, assessing depression in stroke patients is complicated by the fact that patients may exhibit lethargy, memory impairment, and difficulties because of dysphagia and/or other cognitive losses. Thus, family members and caregivers may need to be asked to help in the assessment process. Instruments such as the CES-D (125), used in epidemiologic studies of stroke, the Post-Stroke Depression Rating Scale (54), and the Structured Assessment of Depression in Brain Damaged Individuals (59) may help to define the nature and severity of poststroke depression.

Assessment and treatment is critical in this population as patients with poststroke depression utilize more healthcare resources. In a study of 2,405 veterans with poststroke depression, compared with 2,257 with other mental conditions, patients with poststroke depression had more inpatient hospitalization days and outpatient visits in the first 3 years following a stroke, even after adjustment for mental health clinic visits (57).

Psychological and Behavioral Interventions

Few intervention studies have shown success in decreasing depression in stroke patients. Psychological interventions have involved the use of healthcare disciplines, such as social workers and nurses, to provide counseling and support for patients following a stroke; CBT by therapists; and pharmacologic agents, such as the use of nortriptylline and selective serotonin reuptake inhibitors SSRIs (81,99,127). In a Cochrane review of interventions to treat depression after stroke involving nine trials and 780 subjects, Hackett and colleagues found no strong evidence of benefit of either pharmacotherapy or psychotherapy to enable complete remission of depression following stroke (64). However, patients did show improvement in scores on depression rating scales. In a merged analysis of three studies, Kimura et al., using the Hamilton interview, found that patients treated with nortriptylline compared with those in placebo groups showed significant reductions in depression scores as well as improvements in anxiety (80).

Because CBT by trained therapists has been shown to be an effective treatment in the general population and the elderly, it certainly deserves greater attention in depressed patients following a stroke. To date only a handful of studies with a small number of mildly to moderately depressed patients have been undertaken to determine the effects of CBT (162). Few studies have shown success, although investigators agree that further study is needed because of the success of using problem-solving, a component of CBT to improve family function poststroke. Problem-solving has also been shown to reduce depression in institutionalized older adults.

HEART FAILURE

Heart failure is a condition affecting more than 5 million patients in the United States alone and which is expected to increase substantially as the population ages (3). Over the past 10 years, heart failure has accounted for more than 1 million annual hospital admissions and an estimated $60 billion in annual healthcare expenditures (55). Like other chronic conditions, such as stroke, it is associated with disability and decline causing significant psychological distress (53).

Depression and anxiety and social isolation are common in patients with heart failure. In a meta-analysis of 36 studies, Rutledge et al. (135) found that depression was present in 21.5% of patients with heart failure, varying by the use of questionnaires versus diagnostic interviews (33.6% and 19.3%, respectively). Their results also indicate that depression is associated with a higher death rate (relative risk [RR] = 2.1, 95% confidence interval [CI] 1.7–2.6) and a trend toward increased healthcare use, hospitalization rates, and emergency room visits. Depression has been documented in both acute heart failure (70,145) and in those with chronic heart failure (150,157).

Although much less well studied, anxiety is also common in patients with heart failure. It is typically defined as a negative affective state with a component of fear because of an inability to predict, control, or obtain desired results in upcoming situations (71). Using the State-Trait Anxiety Scale to measure anxiety in 291 heart patients hospitalized as a result of cardiac events, Jiang et al. found that 29% had a state-A score ≥40, and 28% had a Trait-A score ≥40. These scores (≥40) have previously shown a threefold increased risk of cardiac events in post-MI patients. However, although relatively prevalent in this population with heart failure, and closely associated with depression, Jiang et al. did not find anxiety was highly correlated with mortality (70).

Konstam and colleagues (84) assessed both self-reported depression and anxiety in the Studies of Left Ventricular Dysfunction (SOLVD) trial as part of several psychological factors that might predict readmission and death. In this trial, neither depression nor anxiety were associated with worse outcomes (84). More recently, 153 patients in the Sudden Cardiac Death in Heart Failure Trial (SCD-Heft) participated in the Psychosocial Factors in Outcome Study (PFOS), which investigated the prevalence of depression and anxiety and the relationship of psychological factors to mortality in outpatients with heart failure. Although anxiety scores (≥40) measured by the State-Trait Anxiety Scale were high (45%), anxiety did not predict mortality (53). Thus, although these studies show a high prevalence of anxiety, it does not appear to reflect a worse heart failure outcome for patients with this condition.

A few studies have also shown a relationship between social support and heart failure and its relationship to mortality. For example, it has been shown that individuals who live alone with heart failure have a greater likelihood of developing depression within 1 year (65). After controlling for depression and heart failure severity, social isolation was also noted to increase mortality in outpatients with heart failure (110). Finally, after controlling for demographics, medical characteristics, and depression, emotional support—defined as the number of people available to talk over problems—was also an independent predictor of mortality in patients hospitalized with heart failure (88).

Psychosocial and Behavioral Interventions

Depression and anxiety in heart failure both appear to be associated with sympathetic activation and catecholamine release as well as abnormal platelet reactivity (69,135). Depression is associated with elevations of proinflammatory cytokines, including interleuken (IL-6), tumor necrosis factor alpha, and IL-1B. Exercise programs following heart failure appear to reduce IL-6 and tumor necrosis factor alpha levels in heart failure. Whether exercise and pharmacologic treatments for depression reduce symptoms and inflammation, showing a favorable outcome on morbidity and mortality in heart failure, has not been well studied. The Heart Failure ACTION study of close to 2,400 patients with heart failure involved in a randomized controlled trial of supervised and home exercise training may help to answer this important question (158). Results are expected in late 2008 and early 2009.

Although many more studies are needed with larger sample sizes to look at the effects of intervening in patients with heart failure with depression, anxiety, and social isolation to determine the effects on clinical outcomes, relief of symptoms may support patients with heart failure now. Thus, the use of CBT and exercise training may be appropriate interventions. SSRIs may also be used to treat depression and anxiety in this population (81,99).

DIABETES

Diabetes is a chronic disease caused by insulin deficiency, resistance to insulin action, or both. The estimated prevalence of physician-diagnosed diabetes was 15,200,000 in 2004. In addition, the prevalence of undiagnosed diabetes is 5 million (31). Diabetes is the leading cause of nontraumatic amputations ($\sim$157,000·year^{-1}), blindness among working-age adults ($\sim$20,000·year^{-1}), and end-stage kidney disease ($\sim$30,000·year^{-1}) (29). Stress, depression, and anxiety are more prevalent among patients with diabetes than the general population (122,130,142).

Evidence suggests that stress may precipitate the onset of diabetes or compromise glucose control after the disease is established (142). Glucose toxicity resulting from chronic, intermittent, stress-induced elevations in blood glucose further compromises pancreatic secretic ability (94), leading to the progression of the disease. However, evidence characterizing the effects of stress in type 1 diabetes is inconsistent. Human studies have shown that stress can stimulate hyperglycemia or hypoglycemia, or have no effect at all on glycemic status in established diabetes. More consistent evidence supports the role of stress in type 2 diabetes. Animal and human studies suggest that individuals with type 2 diabetes have altered adrenergic sensitivity in the pancreas, which could make them particularly sensitive to stressful life events. However, although substantial data link stress to the expression or control of type 2 diabetes (58), further evidence is needed. Moreover, few studies have followed patients long enough to determine the long-term consequences of stress in patients with diabetes.

Psychosocial and Behavioral Interventions

The few studies involving psychosocial and behavioral interventions in patients with diabetes have involved CBT, coping skills, empowerment, and diabetes management training. These approaches have been found to decrease diabetes-related anxiety and avoidance behaviors; enhance quality of life, coping ability, and emotional well-being; and, most importantly, improve self-care and glycemic control (58).

The Diabetes Prevention Program (DPP) Research Group (37) demonstrated the strong effect that physical activity and weight loss can exert in preventing the onset of diabetes in high-risk adults. Compared with usual care, there was a 58% reduction in the onset of diabetes over a period of approximately 3 years among individuals who were supported in their efforts to follow a healthful lifestyle. Although the intervention did not directly target stress management, these individuals received regular weekly support from a case manager and additional meetings with an exercise specialist, dietitian, and behavioral counselor. An intervention involving medication alone reduced the incidence of new cases by 31% (37). In another randomized controlled trial, the Finnish Diabetes Prevention Study (DPS) investigators used behavior modification techniques similar to the DPP that focused on intensively changing lifestyle. At the end of 4.5 years of follow-up, the DPS found that participants in the lifestyle intervention group who succeeded in increasing their physical activity were least likely to develop diabetes after controlling for changes in diet (90). Both the DPP and the DPS support the impact of lifestyle changes on preventing type 2 diabetes. Whether these types of interventions and other psychological/behavioral interventions can affect the status or complications in people with already established type 2 diabetes is largely unknown.

CHRONIC OBSTRUCTIVE PULMONARY DISEASE

Chronic obstructive pulmonary disease (COPD) is characterized by the presence of airflow obstruction resulting from chronic bronchitis and emphysema, two diseases that often coexist (146). It is the fourth leading cause of death in the United States, currently affecting 24 million individuals. Moreover, morbidity and mortality have not significantly declined in the past 20 years, and because of

an aging population with debilitating illness, COPD is expected to increase and become the third leading cause of death by 2020 (114). Chronic lower respiratory diseases rank as the fourth leading cause of death in the United States (82).

Common psychological reactions among patients with COPD include anger, frustration, guilt, dependency, and embarrassment (63,137). However, the most frequently observed psychological symptoms among patients with COPD are depression and anxiety. Studies have reported the prevalence of depression to be anywhere from 26% to 74% (2,68,137). One of the best studies of depression in COPD was a cross-sectional trial of 1,224 Veterans Administration patients with various chronic obstructive pulmonary diseases. Investigators used the Structured Clinical ID (SCID) interview and found that 39% were diagnosed with depression (116).

One of the main problems of measuring depression in patients with COPD is the overlap of symptoms of depression and COPD. Increased fatigue, sleep, and appetite problems and difficulties concentrating are associated with both depression and COPD, making the diagnosis difficult. Using instruments to address the overlap between depression and COPD may help to address this problem.

Depression can be aggravated in patients with COPD because of worsening dyspnea and fatigue, and perceived poor health, which in turn may decrease functional capacity and exercise tolerance. Therefore, it is important for clinicians to monitor quality of life over time to intervene appropriately. Depression has also been associated with a poorer survival and longer hospitalization stays. In a study of 376 consecutive COPD patients who were hospitalized and followed for 1 year, Ng and colleagues (115) found that the prevalence of depression on admission to hospital was 44.4%. Multivariate analysis revealed that depression was significantly associated with mortality (hazard rates, 1.93 CI 1.04–3.58), a longer index stay (mean 1.1 more days; $P = 0.02$) and total stay (mean 3.0 more days; $P = 0.047$), and worse physical and social functioning assessed by the St. George Respiratory Questionnaire (115).

Anxiety is another common psychological consequence of COPD. As many as 37% of patients with COPD may experience one or more panic attacks, which include bouts of intense anxiety, physiologic arousal, temporary cognitive impairment, and a desire to flee the situation (124). Dyspnea in conjunction with fear of suffocation and death is a source of significant anxiety in this population (137). The emotional arousal of anxiety increases ventilatory demands on the body, which may lead to hypoxia or hypercapnia. Increased physiologic arousal, in turn, exacerbates anxiety symptoms, which then produce greater insufficiency, resulting in a circular pattern that is difficult to break (147). The medical regimen of patients with COPD is often complex, with an average of six medications per patient (58). Consequently, nonadherence is high, with about 50% of the patients either over- or underutilizing their medications (39,69).

Psychosocial and Behavioral Interventions

For patients with COPD who are clinically depressed, pharmacologic treatments have been shown to decrease depression. Moreover, pulmonary rehabilitation programs have been shown to reduce both depression and anxiety and improve quality of life, even if patients did not show significant improvements in exercise performance (115). However, to date, no study has shown that psychotherapeutic interventions in depressed patients with COPD have been able to reduce mortality and hospitalizations.

Treatment studies involving patients with COPD have also shown that psychosocial intervention combined with exercise therapy improves mood, anxiety, and neurocognitive functioning (85). Psychological interventions on their own have been noted to reduce breathlessness and general disability and improve quality of life (129,131). In comparison, exercise-based interventions have tended to show additional benefits (44), with relief of dyspnea and improved functioning and control of the disease (12). However, these studies have been limited by small sample sizes, and as such, large-scale clinical trials are required before definitive conclusions can be drawn.

One of the largest studies of COPD undertaking pulmonary rehabilitation was performed with 590 patients who participated in 24 weeks of rehabilitation at the University of California, San Diego (152). These investigators found the 6-minute walk test, quality of life as measured by the Medical Outcomes Study SF-36, and the perception of dyspnea with activities of daily living all improved after 12 weeks of rehabilitation and were maintained at 24 weeks. The authors recommend that patients participate in supervised pulmonary rehabilitation for at least 24 weeks to gain and maintain optimal benefits (152).

ASTHMA

Asthma is a lung disease with recurrent exacerbations of airflow constriction, mucous secretion, and chronic inflammation of the airways, resulting in reduced airflow that causes symptoms of wheezing, coughing, chest tightness, and difficulty breathing. Data from the Behavioral Risk Factor Surveillance System (BRFSS) 2002 survey from the Centers for Disease Control indicated that 16 million U.S. adults had asthma, with the prevalence rates being higher among racial/ethnic minority populations (3.1% to 14.5%) compared with 7.6% among whites (28).

The emergency room has increasingly become a major source of asthma care, and the <1.9 million emergency room visits in 2002 represent a 30% increase in emergency room utilization over the past decade (102,105). Moreover, the annual direct and indirect costs have more than doubled, from $6.2 billion in 1990 to $12.7 billion in 1998 (154).

Research has demonstrated an association between emotional stress and various indices of impaired airway function, including increased breathlessness (dyspnea) and bronchoconstriction (1,119). As with patients with COPD, anxiety is common in patients with asthma, with panic disorder being particularly prevalent (96). Anxiety appears to be related to excessive use of bronchodilators, greater prescriptions for corticosteroid medication, more frequent hospital readmissions, and more lengthy hospitalizations, independent of pulmonary impairment (76). It has been well documented that individuals who have asthma also have a reduced quality of life, and quality of life tends to be lower in those with severe asthma (117). Ford et al., for example, showed that patients with asthma had a reduced quality of life compared with individuals who had never experienced asthma, and they experienced an average of 10 days of impaired physical or mental health, almost double that of those who had never had asthma (49).

Numerous studies report that the prevalence of depression in those with asthma ranges from 1% to 45% (117). The large variation in prevalence relates is the result of (a) symptoms of asthma that may be linked to depression that allow for misinterpretation, such as dyspnea, worsening at night, and morning symptoms; (b) use of corticosteroids, which has been hypothesized as a link between asthma and depression and which has been understudied; and (c) what is known as a feedback loop—depression, if diagnosed, leads to treatment nonadherence, nonadherence exacerbates asthma, and asthma exacerbations lead to increased depression, resulting in worsened outcomes (96). In addition, there has been a dearth of quality studies reviewing depression in those with asthma. Most studies are cross-sectional or retrospective in design, making it difficult to interpret the results.

Psychosocial and Behavioral Interventions

A limited number of psychological intervention studies have been done with patients with asthma. Therapies such as training in CBT, stress management, yoga, biofeedback, and symptom perception have been show to reduce measures of asthma morbidity and improve patient quality of life (97). In addition, because of its complex medication regimen, adherence has been one of the main foci of behavioral interventions (40,96). The primary intervention used is asthma education and management, which has been shown to improve measures such as frequency of asthma attacks and symptoms, medication adherence, and self-management skills (96). Although it is still unclear if exercise interventions in asthmatics improve pulmonary function and bronchial responsiveness, there is very good evidence that exercise training improves quality of life (138).

EXERCISE THERAPY TO REDUCE EMOTIONAL DISTRESS

The association between regular exercise and mood has been recognized since the late 1970s; however, the role of exercise as a clinical treatment for psychiatric disorders has only been explored recently (21). One of the original long-term prospective studies, the Alameda County Study (25), found that compared with individuals who were active at baseline, inactive participants were at a greater risk of high depression scores 9 years later. In addition, participants who increased their exercise levels across the first 9 years of the study were at no greater risk for depression after 18 years than those who exercised throughout the study. However, those who became inactive after the first 9 years were more likely to become depressed after 18 years relative to active participants. A meta-analysis of clinical trials (92) found that compared with no treatment, exercise reduced depression and was equally as effective as cognitive therapy. Also, evidence from cross-sectional and prospective studies suggests a dose–response effect of physical activity on depressive and anxiety disorders, although this relationship has not yet been found in clinical trials (41). Exercise has been shown to improve stress management ability, general feelings of well-being, self-esteem (48), and muscular tension (36). Clinically, exercise training potentially offers a vehicle for nonspecific psychological therapy. It also offers a specific psychological treatment that may be particularly effective for patients for whom more conventional psychological interventions are less acceptable (136).

A variety of mechanisms has been suggested for the therapeutic effects of exercise, including alterations in the central monoamine systems, improved regulation of the hypothalamic-pituitary-adrenal axis, and increased beta-endorphin levels. However, to date, there are no known studies that have directly assessed the mechanisms behind the exercise–mood relationship (21). Exercise training has also been shown to attenuate the cardiovascular response to emotional stressors (16,19,56,141). This response includes a decreased beta-adrenergic myocardial response to physical or behavioral challenges and an acute prophylactic effect in reducing BP response to psychological stressors (19,98). Additionally, there may be indirect effects of exercise on emotional distress. For example, the addition of diagnostic exercise testing can reassure anxious patients of safety and improve self-confidence (47). In summary, although good evidence suggests that increased physical activity and exercise training improve psychological distress, more high-quality studies are needed to identify if there is a dose–response relation-

ship and to identify the mechanisms by which exercise exerts its antidepressant and anxiolytic affects.

SUMMARY

Psychosocial factors, such as depression, anxiety, and low perceived social support, are common among patients living with chronic illness and appear to be both a cause and a consequence of several chronic medical conditions. However, future prospective studies that include valid measures to assess psychosocial factors and clinical outcomes associated with chronic illness are needed to further our understanding in this field of research.

Most people with psychosocial risk factors do not present themselves to mental health services for treatment. Therefore, systems need to be established to help non–mental health professionals, such as exercise specialists, to find ways to screen for emotional distress and recognize potential symptoms. Consideration should also be given to developing improved liaison relationships with psychological or behavioral specialists to facilitate more specialized interventions when appropriate. Individual or group CBT-based interventions have shown to be particularly effective in this regard. In addition, non–mental health specialists need to be encouraged and supported to develop skills that will enable them to better promote healthful behavior and emotional functioning in the overall treatment of individuals with chronic illness. For example, motivational interviewing, noted in Chapter 42, is one of several useful approaches that can be used by exercise professionals to meet this challenge.

REFERENCES

1. Affleck G, Apter A, Tennen H, et al. Mood states associated with transitory changes in asthma symptoms and peak expiratory flow. *Psychosom Med.* 2000;62:61–68.
2. Agle DP, Baum GL. Psychological aspects of chronic obstructive pulmonary disease. *Med Clin North Am.* 1977;61:749.
3. American Heart Association. *Heart Disease and Stroke Statistics–2007 Update.* Dallas (TX): American Heart Association; 2007.
4. American Psychiatric Association. *Diagnostic and Statistical Manual of Mental Disorders.* 4th ed. Washington (DC): American Psychiatric Association; 1994.
5. Anda R, Williamson D, Jones D, et al. Depressed affect, hopelessness, and risk of ischemic heart disease in a cohort of U.S. adults. *Epidemiology.* 1993;4:285–294.
6. Appels A, Schouten E. Burnout as a risk factor for coronary heart disease. *Behav Med.* 1991;17:53–59.
7. Bacon SL, Watkins LL, Babyak M, et al. The effects of daily stress on autonomic cardiac control in coronary artery disease patients. *Am J Cardiol.* 2004;93:1292–1294.
8. Barefoot JC, Helms MJ, Mark DB. Depression and long-term mortality risk in patients with coronary artery disease. *Am J Cardiol.* 1996;78:613–717.
9. Barefoot JC, Schroll M. Symptoms of depression, acute myocardial infarction, and total mortality in a community sample. *Circulation.* 1996;93:1976–1980.
10. Bergovec M, Mihatov S, Prpic H, et al. Acute myocardial infarction among civilians in the Zagreb city area. *Lancet.* 1992;339:303.

11. Berkman LF, Leo-Summers L, Horwitz RI. Emotional support and survival after myocardial infarction: a prospective, population-based study of the elderly. *Ann Intern Med.* 1992;117:1003–1009.

12. Berry MJ, Walschlager SA. Exercise training and chronic obstructive pulmonary disease: past and future research directions. *J Cardiopulm Rehabil.* 1998;18:181–191.

13. Blazer DG, Kessler RC, McGonagle KA, Swartz MS. The prevalence and distribution of major depression in a national community sample: the national co-morbidity survey. *Am J Psychiatry.* 1994;151:979–986.

14. Blazer DG. Social support and mortality in an elderly community program. *Am J Epidemiol.* 1984;115:684–694.

15. Blumenthal JA, Babyak M, Wei J, et al. Usefulness of psychosocial treatment of mental stress-induced myocardial ischemia in men. *Am J Cardiol.* 2002;89:164–168.

16. Blumenthal JA, Fredrikson M, Kuhn CM, et al. Aerobic exercise reduces levels of cardiovascular and sympathoadrenal responses to mental stress in subjects without prior evidence of myocardial ischemia. *Am J Cardiol.* 1990;65:93–98.

17. Blumenthal JA, Jiang W, Babyak MA, Krantz, et al. Stress management and exercise training in cardiac patients with myocardial ischemia: effects on prognosis and evaluation of mechanisms. *Arch Intern Med.* 1997;157:2213–2223.

18. Blumenthal JA, Jiang W, Waugh RA, et al. Mental stress-induced ischemia in the laboratory and ambulatory ischemia during daily life: association and hemodynamic features. *Circulation.* 1995;8: 2102–2108.

19. Boone JB, Probst MM, Rogers MW, Berger R. Post-exercise hypotension reduces cardiovascular responses to stress. *J Hypertens.* 1993;11:449–453.

20. Bosma H, Peter R, Siegrist J, Marmot M. Two alternative job stress models and the risk of coronary heart disease. *Am J Public Health.* 1998;88:68–74.

21. Brosse AL, Sheets ES, Lett HS, Blumenthal JA. Exercise and the treatment of clinical depression in adults: recent findings and future directions. *Sports Med.* 2002;12:741–760.

22. Browne A, Finkelhor D. Impact of child sexual abuse: a review of the research. *Psychol Bull.* 1986;99:66–77.

23. Brummett BH, Barefoot JC, Siegler IC, et al. Characteristics of socially isolated patients with coronary artery disease who are at elevated risk for mortality. *Psychosom Med.* 2001;63:267–272.

24. Burke BL, Arkowitz H, Dunn C. The effectiveness of motivational interviewing and its adaptations: what we know so far. In: Miller WR, Rollnick S, editors. *Motivational Interviewing: Preparing People to Change Addictive Behavior.* 2nd ed. New York: Guilford Press; 2002. p. 217–250.

25. Camacho TC, Roberts RE, Lazarus NB, et al. Physical activity and depression: evidence from the Alameda County study. *Am J Epidemiol.* 1991;134:220–231.

26. Carney RM, Freedland KE, Eisen SE, et al. Depression is associated with poor adherence to medical treatment regimen in elderly cardiac patients. *Health Psychol.* 1995;14:88–90.

27. Carroll D, Ebrahim S, Tiling K, et al. Admissions for myocardial infarction at World Cup football: database survey. *BMJ.* 2002;325: 21–28.

28. Centers for Disease Control and Prevention. Asthma prevalence and control characteristics by race/ethnicity—United States, 2002. *MMWR Morb Mortal Wkly Rep.* 2004;52:145°149.

29. Centers for Disease Control and Prevention. *Diabetes Surveillance.* Atlanta: U.S. Department of Health and Human Services, Centers for Disease Control and Prevention; 1997.

30. **Centers for Disease Control and Prevention. Mortality patterns: preliminary data; United States—1996. MMWR Morbid Mortal Wkly Rep. 1997;46:941–944.**

31. **Centers for Disease Control and Prevention. National Diabetes Fact Sheet: National Estimates and General Information on Diabetes in the United States. Atlanta: U.S. Department of Health**

and Human Services, Centers for Disease Control and Prevention; 1997.

32. Clarke DM. Psychological factors in illness and recovery. *N Z Med J.* 1998;111:410–412.

33. Coumel P, Leenhardt A. Mental activity, adrenergic modulation, and cardiac arrhythmias in patients with heart disease. *Circulation.* 1991;83:58–70.

34. Davis A, Natelson B. Brain-heart interactions: neurocardiology of arrhythmia and sudden death. *Tex Heart Inst J.* 1993;20:158–169.

35. Deanfield JE, Shea M, Kensett M, et al. Silent myocardial ischemia due to mental stress. *Lancet.* 1984;2:1001–1005.

36. DeVries H, Hams G. Electromyographic comparison of single dose of exercise and meprobamate as to effects on muscular relaxation. *Am J Phys Med.* 1972;51:130–141.

37. Diabetes Prevention Program Research Group. Reduction in the incidence of type 2 diabetes with lifestyle intervention or metformin. *N Engl J Med.* 2003;346:393–403.

38. Dimatteo MR, Lepper HS, Croghan TW. Depression as a risk factor for non-compliance with medical treatment: meta analysis of the effects of anxiety and depression on patient adherence. *Arch Intern Med.* 2000;160:2101–2107.

39. Dolce JJ, Crisp C, Manzella B, et al. Medication adherence patterns in chronic obstructive pulmonary disease. *Chest.* 1991;99:837.

40. Dunbar J. Predictors of patient adherence: patient characteristics. In: Shumaker SA, Schron EB, Ockene JK, editors. *The Handbook of Health Behavior Change.* New York: Springer Publishing; 1990. p. 348–360.

41. Dunn AL, Trivedi MH, O'Neal HA. Physical activity dose-response effects on outcome of depression and anxiety. *Med Sci Sports Exerc.* 2001;6(suppl.):S587–S597.

42. Dunn C, DeRoo L, Rivara, FP. The use of brief interventions adapted from motivational interviewing across behavioral domains: a systematic review. *Addiction.* 2001;96:1725–1742.

43. Eaker ED, Abbott RD, de Knell WB. Frequency of uncomplicated angina pectoris in type A compared with type B persons (the Framingham Study). *Am J Cardiol.* 1989;63:1042–1045.

44. Emery CF, Schein RL, Hauck ER, et al. Psychological and cognitive outcomes of a randomized trial of exercise among patients with chronic obstructive pulmonary disease. *Health Psychol.* 1998; 17:232–240.

45. Evans C, Chalmers J, Capewell S, et al. "I don't like Mondays"—day of the week of coronary heart disease death in Scotland: study of routine collected data. *BMJ.* 2000;320:218–219.

46. Everson SA, Kaplan GA, Goldberg DE. Hopelessness and 4-year progression of carotid atherosclerosis: the Kuopio ischemic heart disease risk factor study. *Arterioscler Thromb Vasc Biol.* 1997;17: 1490–1495.

47. Ewart CK, Taylor CB, Reese LB, DeBusk RF. Effects of early post-myocardial infarction exercise testing on self-perception and subsequent physical activity. *Am J Cardiol.* 1983;51:1076–1080.

48. Fillingim RB, Blumenthal JA. The use of aerobic exercise as a method of stress management. In: Lehrer PM, Woolfolk RL, editors. *Principles and Practice of Stress Management.* New York: Guilford Press; 1993. p. 443–4620.

49. Ford ES, Mannino DM, Homa DM, et al. Self-reported asthma and health-related quality of life: findings from the behavioral risk factor surveillance system. *Chest.* 2003;123:119–127.

50. Frasure-Smith N, Lesperance F, Junea M, et al. Gender, depression, and one-year prognosis after myocardial infarction. *Psychosom Med.* 1999;61:26–37.

51. Frasure-Smith N, Lesperance F, Prince RH, et al. Randomised trial of home-based psychosocial nursing intervention for patients recovering from myocardial infarction. *Lancet.* 1997;350: 473–479.

52. Frasure-Smith N, Lesperance F, Talajic M. Depression and 18-month prognosis after myocardial infarction. *Circulation.* 1995;91: 999–1005.

53. Friedmann E, Thomas SA, Liu F et al. Relationship of depression, anxiety, and social isolation to chronic heart failure outpatient mortality. *Am Heart J.* 2006;152:940.e1–940.e8.

54. Gainotti G, Azzoni A, Razzano C, et al. The post-stroke depression rating scale: a test specifically devised to investigate affective disorders of stroke patients. *J Clin Exp Neuropsychol.* 1997;19:340–356.

55. Galbreath AD, Krasuski RA, Smith B, et al. Long-term health care and cost outcomes of disease management in a large, randomized, community-based population with heart failure. *Circulation.* 2004;110:3518–3526.

56. Georgiades A, Sherwood A, Gullette ECD, et al. Effects of exercise and weight loss on mental stress-induced cardiovascular responses in individuals with high blood pressure. *Hypertension.* 2000;36:171–176.

57. Ghose SS, Williams LS, Swindle RW. Depression and other mental health diagnoses after stroke increase inpatient and outpatient medical utilization three years post-stroke. *Med Care.* 2005;43: 1259–1264.

58. Gonder-Frederick LA, Cox DJ, Ritterband LM. Diabetes and behavioral medicine: the second decade. *J Consult Clin Psychol.* 2002;70:611–625.

59. Gordon WA, Hibbard MR. Post-stroke depression: an examination of the literature. *Arch Phys Med Rehabil.* 1997;78: 658–663.

60. Gorkin L, Schron EB, Brooks MM, et al. Psychosocial predictors of mortality in the Cardiac Arrhythmia Suppression Trial-1 (CAST-1). *Am J Cardiol.* 1993;71:263–267.

61. Guiry E, Conroy, RM, Hickey N, Mulcahy R. Psychological response to an acute coronary event and its effect on subsequent rehabilitation and lifestyle change. *Clin Cardiol.* 1987;10:256–260.

62. Gullette EC, Blumenthal JA, Babyak M, et al. Effects of mental stress on myocardial ischemia during daily life. *JAMA.* 1997;277: 1521–1526.

63. Guyatt GH, Townsend M, Berman LB, Pugsley SO. Quality of life in patients with chronic airflow limitation. *Br J Dis Chest.* 1987;81:45.

64. Hackett ML, Anderson CS, House AO. Interventions for treating depression after stroke. *Cochrane Database Syst Rev.* 2004;(3): CD003437.

65. Havranek EP, Spertus JA, Masoudi FA, et al. Predictors of the onset of depressive symptoms in patients with heart failure. *J Am Coll Cardiol.* 2004;44:2333–2338.

66. Holmes T, Rahe R. The social readjustment rating scale. *J Psychosom Res.* 1967;11:213–218.

67. Horsten M, Mittleman MA, Wamala SP, et al. Depressive symptoms and lack of social integration in relation to prognosis of CHD in middle-aged women: the Stockholm Female Coronary Risk Study. *Eur Heart J.* 2000;21:1072–1080.

68. Isoaho R, Puolijoki H, Huhti E, et al. Chronic obstructive pulmonary disease and cognitive impairment in the elderly. *Int Psychogeriatr.* 1996;8:113.

69. James PNE, Anderson JB, Prior JG, et al. Patterns of drug taking in patients with chronic airflow obstruction. *Postgrad Med J.* 1985;61:7–10.

70. Jiang W, Alexander J, Christopher E, et al. Relationship of depression to increased risk of mortality and rehospitalization in patients with congestive heart failure. *Arch Intern Med.* 2001;161:1849–1856.

71. Jiang W, Babyak M, Krantz, DS, et al. Mental stress-induced myocardial ischemia and cardiac events. *JAMA.* 1996;25:1651–1656.

72. Jones DA, West RR. Psychological rehabilitation after myocardial infarction: multicentre randomized controlled trial. *BMJ.* 1996;313:1517–1521.

73. Kaplan JR, Manuck SB, Clarkson TB, et al. Social status, environment and atherosclerosis in cynomolgus monkeys. *Arteriosclerosis.* 1982;2:359–368.

74. Kaplan GA, Salonsen JT, Cohen RD, et al. Social connections and mortality from all causes and from cardiovascular disease: prospective evidence from eastern Finland. *Am J Epidemiol.* 1988;128:370–380.

75. Kaprio J, Koskenvuo M, Rita H. Mortality after bereavement: a prospective study of 95,647 persons. *Am J Publ Health.* 1987;77: 283–287.

76. Kaptein AA. Psychological correlates of length of hospitalization and rehospitalization in patients with acute, severe asthma. *Soc Sci Med.* 1982;16:725–729.

77. Karasek RA, Baker D, Marxer F, et al. Job decision latitude, job demands, and cardiovascular disease: a prospective study of Swedish men. *Am J Publ Health.* 1981;71:694–705.

78. Katsouyanni K, Kogevinas M, Trichopoulos D. Earthquake related stress and cardiac mortality. *Int J Epidemiol.* 1986;15:326–330.

79. Kessler RC, Berglund P, Demler O, et al. The epidemiology of major depressive disorder: results from the National Comorbidity Survey Replication (NCS-R). *JAMA.* 2003;289:3095–3105.

80. Kimura M, Tateno A, Robinson RG. Treatment of poststroke generalized anxiety disorder comorbid with poststroke depression: merged analysis of nortriptyline trials. *Am J Geriatr Psychiatry.* 2003;11:320–327.

81. Kneebone II, Dunmore E. Psychological management of post-stroke depression. *Br J Clin Psychol.* 2000;39:53–65.

82. Kochanek KD, Smith BL. Deaths: Preliminary Data for 2002. *Natl Vital Stat Rep.* 2004;52:13.

83. Koetnansky R. Catecholamines-corticosteroid interactions. In: Usdin E, Koetnansky R, Kopin IJ, editors. *Catecholamines and Stress.* Amsterdam: Elsevier/North Holland; 1980. p. 7.

84. Konstam V, Salem D, Puler H, et al. Baseline quality of life as a predictor of mortality and hospitalizations in 5,025 patients with congestive heart failure. *Am J Cardiol.* 1998;78:890–895.

85. Kozora E, Tran ZV, Make B. Neurobehavioral improvement after brief rehabilitation in patients with chronic obstructive pulmonary disease. *J Cardiopul Rehabil.* 2002;22:426–430.

86. Krantz DS, Helmers KF, Bairey NC, et al. Cardiovascular reactivity and mental stress-induced myocardial ischemia in patients with coronary artery disease. *Psychosom Med.* 1991;53:1–12.

87. Krieger N, Rowley DL, Herman AA, et al. Racism, sexism, and social class: implications for studies of health, disease, and well-being. *Am J Prev Med.* 1993;9 (suppl):82–122.

88. Krumholz HM, Butler J, Miller J, et al. Prognostic importance of emotional support for elderly patients hospitalized with heart failure. *Circulation.* 1998;97:958–964.

89. Lane D, Carroll D, Ring C, et al. In-hospital symptoms of depression do not predict mortality 3 years after myocardial infarction. *Int J Epidemiol.* 2002;31:1179–1182.

90. Laaksonen DE, Lindstrom J, Lakka TA, et al. Physical activity in the prevention of type 2 diabetes. *Diabetes.* 2005;54:158–165.

91. Lavoie KL, Fleet PP, Lesperance F, et al. Are exercise stress tests appropriate for assessing myocardial ischemia in patients with major depressive disorder? *Am Heart J.* 2004;148:621–627.

92. Lawlor DA, Hopker SW. The effectiveness of exercise as an intervention in the management of depression: systematic review and meta-regression analysis of randomised controlled trials. *BMJ.* 2001;322:763–767.

93. Lazarus RS, Folkman S. *Stress, Appraisal and Coping.* New York: Springer; 1984.

94. Leahy JL. Natural history of beta-cell dysfunction in NIDDM. *Diabetes Care.* 1990;13:992–1010.

95. Lear J, Kloner RA. The Northridge earthquake as a trigger for acute myocardial infarction. *Am J Cardiol.* 1996;77:1230–1232.

96. Lehrer P, Feldman J, Giardino N, et al. Psychological aspects of asthma. *J Consult Clin Psychol.* 2002;70:691–711.

97. Lehrer P, Smetankin A, Potapova T. Respiratory sinus arrhythmia biofeedback therapy for asthma: a report of 20 unmedicated pediatric cases using the Smetankin method. *Appl Psychophysiol Biofeedback.* 2000;25:193–200.

98. Light KC, Obrist PA, James SA, Strogatz DS. Cardiovascular responses to stress: II. Relationships to aerobic exercise patterns. *Psychophysiology.* 1987;24:79–85.

99. Lincoln NB, Flannaghan T, Phil M. Cognitive behavioral psychotherapy for depression following stroke: a randomized controlled trial. *Stroke.* 2003;34:111–115.

100. Linden W. Psychological treatments in cardiac rehabilitation: review of rationales and outcomes. *J Psychosom Res.* 2000;48:443–454.

101. Lynch JJ, Krause N, Kaplan GA, Salonen R, Salonen JT. Workplace demands, economic reward, and progression of carotid atherosclerosis. *Circulation.* 1997;96:302–307.

102. Mannino DM, Homa DM, Akinbami LJ, et al. Surveillance for asthma—United States, 1980–1999. *MMWR Surveill Summ.* 2002;51:1–3.

103. Mayou R, Foster A, Williamson B. Medical care after myocardial infarction. *J Psychosom Res.* 1979;23:23–26.

104. Mayou R, Gill D, Thompson DR, et al. Depression and anxiety as predictors of outcome after myocardial infarction. *Psychosom Med.* 2000;62:212–219.

105. McCaig LF, Burt CW. National Hospital Ambulatory Medical Care Survey: 2002 emergency department summary. *Adv Data.* 2004;340:1–34.

106. **McKenna MT, Taylor WR, Marks JS, Koplan JP. Current issues and challenges in chronic disease control. In: Brownson RC, Remington PL, Davis JR, editors. *Chronic Disease Epidemiology and Control.* Washington (DC): American Public Health Association; 1998. p. 1–26.**

107. Meisel SR, Kutz I, Dayan KI, et al. Effect of Iraq missile war on incidence of acute myocardial infarction and sudden death in Israeli civilians. *Lancet.* 1991;338:660–661.

108. Miller WR, Rollnick S. *Motivational Interviewing: Preparing People for Change.* 2nd ed. New York: Guilford Press; 2002.

109. Mittleman MA, MacLure M, Sherwood JB, et al. for the Determinants of Myocardial Infarction Onset Study Investigators. Triggering of acute myocardial infarction onset by episodes of anger. *Circulation.* 1995;92:1720–1725.

110. Murberg TA, Bru E. Social relationships and mortality in patients with congestive heart failure. *J Psychosom Res.* 2001;51:521–527.

111. Murray CJL, Lopez AD. Alternative projections of mortality and disability by cause 1990–2020: Global Burden of Disease Study. *Lancet.* 1997;349:1498–1504.

112. Murray CJL, Lopez AD. Evidence-based health policy: lessons from the Global Burden of Disease Study. *Science.* 1996;274:740–743.

113. Naesh O, Haedersdal C, Hindberg I, Trap-Jensen J. Platelet activation in mental stress. *Clinical Physiology.* 1993;13:299–307.

114. National Center for National Health Statistics. United States, 2002. *Natl Vital Stat Rep.* 2005;53(17):9.

115. Ng TP, Niti M, Tan WC, et al. Depressive symptoms and chronic obstructive pulmonary disease: effect on mortality, hospital readmission, symptom burden, functional status, and quality of life. *Arch Intern Med.* 2007;167:60–67.

116. Norwood R. Prevalence and impact of depression in chronic obstructive pulmonary disease patients. *Curr Opin Pulm Med.* 2006;12:113–117.

117. Opolski M, Wilson I. Asthma and depression: a pragmatic review of the literature and recommendations for future research. *Clin Pract Epidemiol Ment Health.* 2005;1:18.

118. Ornish D, Brown SE, Scherwitz LW, et al. Can lifestyle changes reverse coronary heart disease? The Lifestyle Heart Trial. *Lancet.* 1990;336:129–133.

119. Ornish D, Scherwitz LW, Billings JH, et al. Intensive lifestyle changes for reversal of coronary heart disease. *JAMA.* 1998;280:2001–2007.

120. Orth-Gomer K, Johnson JV. Social isolation and mortality: a six-year follow-up study of a random sample of the Swedish population. *J Chron Dis.* 1987;40:949–957.

121. Orth-Gomer K, Unden AL, Edwards ME. Social isolation and mortality in ischemic heart disease: a 10-year follow-up study of 150 middle-aged men. *Acta Medica Scandinavica.* 1988;224:205–215.

122. Peyrot M, Rubin RR. Levels and risks of depression and anxiety symptomatology among diabetic adults. *Diabetes Care.* 1997;20:585–590.

123. Pieper C, LaCroix A, Karasek R. The relationship of psychosocial dimensions on work with coronary heart disease. *Am J Epidemiol.* 1989;129:483–494.

124. Porzelius J, Vest M, Nochomovitz, M. Respiratory function, cognitions, and panic in chronic obstructive pulmonary patients. *Behav Res Ther.* 1992;30:75.

125. Radloff LS. The CES-D Scale: a self-report depressive scale for research in the general population. *Journal of Applied Psychological Measurement.* 1977;1:385–401.

126. Rahe RH, Romo M, Bennett L, Siltanen P. Recent life changes, myocardial infarction, and abrupt coronary death. *Arch Intern Med.* 1974;133:221–228.

127. Ramasubbu R. Relationship between depression and cerebrovascular disease: conceptual issues. *J Affect Disord.* 2000;57:1–11.

128. Regier DA, Farmer ME, Rae DS, et al. Comorbidity of mental disorders with alcohol and other drug abuse: results from the Epidemiologic Catchment Area (ECA) Study. *JAMA.* 1990;264:2511–2518.

129. Rietveld S, Everaerd W, Creer TL. Stress-induced asthma: a review of research and potential mechanisms. *Clin Exp Allergy.* 2000;30:1058–1066.

130. Robinson N, Fuller JH. Role of life events and difficulties in the onset of diabetes mellitus. *J Psychosom Res.* 1985;29:583–591.

131. Rose C, Wallace L, Dickson R, et al. The most effective psychologically-based treatments to reduce anxiety and panic in patients with chronic obstructive pulmonary disease (COPD): a systematic review. *Patient Education & Counseling.* 2002;47:311–318.

132. Rozanski A, Bairey N, Krantz, DS, et al. Mental stress and the induction of silent myocardial ischemia in patients with coronary artery disease. *N Engl J Med.* 1988;318:1005–1012.

133. Rozanski P, Blumenthal JA, Kaplan J. Impact of psychological factors on the pathogenesis of cardiovascular disease and implications for therapy. *Circulation.* 1999;99:2197–2217.

134. Russek LG, King SH, Russek SJ, Russek HI. The Harvard Mastery of Stress Study—35 year follow-up: prognostic significance of patterns of psychophysiological arousal and adaptation. *Psychiatr Med.* 1990;52:271–285.

135. Rutledge T, Reis VA, Linke SE, et al. Depression in heart failure: a meta-analytic review of prevalence, intervention effects, and associations with clinical outcomes. *J Am Coll Cardiol.* 2006;48:1527–1537.

136. Salmon P. Effects of physical exercise on anxiety, depression, and sensitivity to stress: a unifying theory. *Clin Psychol Rev.* 2001;21:33–61.

137. Sandhu HS. Psychosocial issues in chronic obstructive pulmonary disease. *Clin Chest Med.* 1986;7:629.

138. Satta A. Exercise training in asthma. *J Sports Med Phys Fitness.* 2000;40:277–283.

139. Scales R, Lueker RD, Atterbom HA, et al. Motivational interviewing and skills-based counseling to change multiple lifestyle behaviors [abstract]. *Ann Behav Med.* 1998;22D,20:68.

140. Siegrist J, Peter R, Junge A, et al. Low status control, high effort at work and ischemic heart disease: prospective evidence from blue-collar men. *Soc Sci Med.* 1990;331:1127–1134.

141. Sothman M, Hart B, Horn T. Plasma catecholamine response to acute psychological stress in humans: relation to aerobic fitness and exercise testing. *Med Sci Sports Exerc.* 1991;23:873–881.

142. Surwit RS, Schneider MS, Feinglos MN. Stress and diabetes mellitus. *Diabetes Care.* 1992;10:1413–1422.

143. Suzuki S, Sakamoto S, Miki S, Matsuo T. Hanshin-Awaji earthquake and acute myocardial infarction. *Lancet.* 1995;345:981.

144. Tofler GH, Stone PH, MacLure M, et al. Analysis of possible triggers of acute myocardial infarction (the MILIS Study). *Am J Cardiol.* 1990;66:22–27.

145. Trichopoulus D, Katsouyanni K, Zavitsanos X, et al. Psychological stress and fatal heart attack: the Athens 1981 earthquake natural experiment. *Lancet.* 1983;I:441–444.

146. U.S. Department of Health and Human Services Office of Public Health and Science. Healthy People 2010 Objectives: Draft for public comment. Washington (DC): U.S. Department of Health and Human Services Office of Public Health and Science; 1998.

147. U.S. Department of Health and Human Services. *Mental Health: A Report of the Surgeon General.* Rockville (MD): U.S. Department of Health and Human Services, Substance Abuse and Mental Health Services Administration, Center for Mental Health Services, National Institute for Mental Health, National Institute of Mental Health; 1999.

148. U.S. Department of Health and Human Services. *Physical Activity and Health: A Report of the Surgeon General.* Atlanta: Centers for Disease Control and Prevention, National Center for Chronic Disease Prevention and Health Promotion; 1996.

149. Uchino BN, Cacioppo JT, Kiecolt-Glaser JK. The relationship between social support and physiological processes: a review with emphasis on underlying mechanisms and implications for health. *Psychol Bull.* 1996;119:488–531.

150. Vaccarino V, Kasl SV, Abramson J, et al. Depressive symptoms and risk of functional decline and death in patients with heart failure. *J Am Coll Cardiol.* 2001;38:199–205.

151. Verrier RL, Dickerson LW. Autonomic nervous system and coronary blood flow changes related to emotional activation and sleep. *Circulation.* 1991;83(suppl 2):81–89.

152. Verrill D, Barton C, Beasley W, et al. The effects of short-term and long-term pulmonary rehabilitation on functional capacity, perceived dyspnea, and quality of life. *Chest.* 2005;128:673–683.

153. Vieth RC, Lewis N, Linares OA, et al. Sympathetic nervous system activity in major depression: basal and desipramine-induced alterations in plasma norepinephrine kinetics. *Arch Gen Psychiatry.* 1994;51:411–422.

154. Weiss KB, Sullivan SD. The health economics of asthma and rhinitis: I. Assessing the economic impact. *J Allergy Clin Immunol.* 2001;107:3–8.

155. Welin C, Lappas G, Wilhelmsen L. Independent importance of psychosocial factors for prognosis after myocardial infarction. *J Intern Med.* 2000;247:629–639.

156. **Wenger NK, Froehlicher ES, Smith LK, et al. *Cardiac Rehabilitation: Clinical Practice Guidelines.* Rockville (MD): Agency for Health Care Policy and Research and the National Heart, Lung and Blood Institute; 1995.**

157. Westlake C, Dracup K, Fonarow G, et al. Depression in patients with heart failure. *J Am Coll Cardiol.* 2004;44:2333–2338.

158. Whellan D, O'Connor C, Keteyian S, et al, on behalf of the HF-ACTION Investigators. Heart failure and a controlled trial investigating outcomes of exercise training (HF-ACTION): design and rationale. *Am Heart J.* 2007;153:201–211.

159. Williams RB, Barefoot JC, Califf RM, et al. Prognostic importance of social and economic resources among medically treated patients with angiographically documented coronary artery disease. *JAMA.* 1992;267:520–524.

160. Willich S, Hannelore L, Lewis M, et al. Weekly variation of acute myocardial infarction. *Circulation.* 1994;90:87–93.

161. Witte DR, Bots MI, Hoes AW, Grobbee DE. Cardiovascular mortality in Dutch men during the 1996 European football championship: longitudinal population study. *BMJ.* 2000;321:1332–1334.

162. Writing Committee for the ENRICHD Investigators. Effects of treating depression and low perceived social support on clinical events after myocardial infarction. *JAMA.* 2003;289:3106–3116.

163. Yeung AC, Vekshtein VI. Krantz DS, et al. The effect of atherosclerosis on the vasomotor response of the coronary arteries to mental stress. *N Engl J Med.* 1991;325:1551–1556.

SELECTED REFERENCES FOR FURTHER READING

Kneebone I, Dunmore E. Psychological management of post-stroke depression. *Br J Clin Psychol.* 2000;39:53–65.

Opolski M , Wilson M. Asthma and depression: a pragmatic review of the literature and recommendations for future research. *Clin Pract Epidemiol Ment Health.* 2005;1:1–7.

Rutledge T, Reis VA, Linke SE, et al. Depression in heart failure: a meta-analytic review of prevalence, intervention effects, and associations with clinical outcomes. *J Am Coll Cardiol.* 2006;48:1527–1537.

Smith TW, Kendall P, Keefe F, editors. Behavioral medicine and clinical health psychology. *J Consult Clin Psychol* [special issue] 2002;70:459–856.

INTERNET RESOURCES

- Cognitive behavior therapy: www.cognitive-behavior-therapy.org
- Mental health: A Report of the Surgeon General: www.surgeon-general.gov/library/mentalhealth/home.html
- Motivational interviewing: www.motivationalinterviewing.org

CHAPTER 16

Assessment of Psychosocial Status

This chapter focuses on assessment and treatment of common psychosocial and psychological correlates of cardiovascular disease (CVD), stroke, chronic obstructive pulmonary disease (COPD), and metabolic disease (obesity and diabetes), with an emphasis on stress, anxiety, and depression (SAD).

The development of behaviorally based management and prevention strategies for chronic disease is becoming an urgent priority, not only for healthcare providers, but as a matter of social and economic policy as well. The costs associated with healthcare are already staggering and will continue to increase in the coming years, fueled by our historic allegiance to end-state or tertiary models of medical care, an aging population, and spiraling costs of surgical, pharmacologic, and increasingly sophisticated technologic interventions. There is also an urgent need for prevention and long-term management strategies, especially for those diseases that are strongly correlated with lifestyle behavior patterns and that are the focus of this chapter: CVD, stroke, COPD, obesity, and

diabetes. Extensive research conducted in behavioral medicine and health psychology has documented the influence of psychological and social factors on illness, health, and well-being. The underlying model driving much of this research emphasizes the contributions of biological, psychological, and social influences on health and illness, and is referred to as the biopsychosocial model (83).

All healthcare professionals need to be familiar with ways in which biological, social, and psychological factors interact, producing illness, the cultural context of disease. The purpose of this chapter is to provide exercise professionals with an overview of clinical assessment and intervention strategies for three common forms of emotional distress as highlighted in the 1999 U.S. Surgeon General's Report on Mental Health: stress, anxiety, and depression, for which we use the acronym SAD. Significant distress may warrant a formal psychological clinical assessment, and it is useful to know some basic diagnostic nomenclature related to common psychological disorders,

Anxiety: Distressful emotional state marked by excessive anticipatory worry and tension.

Cognitive behavior therapy (CBT): A widely practiced, empirically validated method for treating common psychological disorders, including anxiety and depression. CBT focuses on helping patients become aware of how thoughts influence feelings and behavior, and how dysfunctional thoughts become linked to anxiety and depression. *Cognitive restructuring* is the general term used to describe CBT techniques designed to lessen the grip of maladaptive thought patterns on emotional states. CBT is strongly influenced both by behavior therapy and social cognitive theory.

Depression: A pervasive, enduring mood characterized by a low self-esteem, low energy, physical lethargy, and emotional distress. Isolated episodes

of a depressed mood are common; when frequent or prolonged, they may signify major depressive disorder, a DSM-IV/TR subcategory of the mood disorders.

Diagnostic and Statistical Manual of Mental Disorders, 4th Edition (DSM-IV): The current standard for psychiatric diagnosis, published by the American Psychiatric Association (APA) in 1994 and used by virtually all mental health professionals. A text revision (DSM-IV/TR) published in 2000 updated background information but did not alter diagnostic criteria (14,15).

Empirical: Founded on practical experience, rather than on reasoning alone, but not established scientifically.

Mood disorder: A diagnostic term in the DSM-IV/TR denoting a group of psychological disorders marked by disruption of normal mood (prevailing emotional tone) and affect (fluctuating emotional state). The most common mood disorders are major depressive disorder, bipolar disorder, dysthymic disorder, and cyclothymic disorder.

Perceived self-efficacy (PSE): The self-assessment of one's capabilities to perform or regulate behavior, based in Bandura's social cognitive theory. Perceived self-efficacy is the most influential psychological variable on a range of health and wellness behaviors.

Psychological disorder: A general term in the DSM-IV/TR used to denote a state of maladjustment marked by (a) subjective distress and/or (b)

functional impairment in activities of daily life. One or both of these criteria must be met, in addition to the criteria for specific disorders, in order for a person to be diagnosed with a psychological or mental disorder.

Social cognitive/social learning theory: Fundamental theories of behavior by Bandura that emphasize the role of social mediating factors on psychological development and learning.

Stress: The subjective experience of feeling overloaded or overwhelmed that results when personal resources (psychological or otherwise) are insufficient to meet existing challenges of daily life.

especially those involving anxiety and depression. It is also important to have a working knowledge of empirically validated interventions that have been developed to treat both clinically significant and subclinical manifestations of emotional distress.

This knowledge can be helpful in three ways. First, exercise professionals need to have a basic understanding of how anxiety, depression, and distress affect physical capabilities related to exercise testing and programming, both at a general level and in the context of specific disease. Knowing how to make appropriate adjustments or accommodations in designing exercise programs and determining how best to teach and motivate patients who are anxious, depressed, or highly stressed in terms of teaching and motivation strategies is important. Individualizing exercise protocols is significant. Second, and perhaps more significantly, exercise professionals need to be familiar with research documenting the positive effects of physical activity (Table 16-1) on stress, anxiety, and depression, and be able to apply this knowledge effectively with individual patients of increasingly diverse medical, social, and cultural backgrounds. In the case of patients diagnosed with anxiety or mood disorders, the latter being an umbrella term that encompasses depression, the exercise professional may be able to forge a collaboration with mental health professionals responsible for primary treatment of the disorder, in much the same way that productive working alliances are often formed with physicians treating patients for heart disease, hyper-

tension, or diabetes. This process can aid in the process of tailoring well-known general exercise guidelines (11,181) to the needs of specific individuals.

The importance of physical activity as a form of complementary health for both medically and psychologically based conditions cannot be overstated. With regard to the latter, both cost and social stigma inhibit many people from seeking treatment. For such individuals, being physically active can do much to reduce emotional distress in a cost-effective manner.

Finally, knowledge about psychological conditions and how emotional distress is affected by common diseases is essential information. This knowledge may help the exercise professional determine when consultation with mental health professionals may be warranted for patients whose medical management and exercise programming appear to be compromised. Working in a broad bio/psycho/social framework is believed to counteract the common tendency to become overly focused on the physical aspects of medical conditions.

The chapter begins by addressing common assessment procedures to clarify emotional distress patterns and determine whether formal clinical diagnoses are warranted. The next section focuses on a discussion of contemporary intervention models used to treat both clinical and subclinical manifestations of emotional distress. The final section of the chapter considers the implications of emotional distress in the context of four specific medical conditions: CVD, stroke, COPD, and the most common metabolic disorders, diabetes, obesity, and the metabolic syndrome.

TABLE 16-1. BENEFITS OF PHYSICAL ACTIVITY

Self-administration
Social acceptability
Decreased physical health risks
Ancillary strength and conditioning benefits
Convenience
Low cost
Minimal side effects

Adapted from Buckworth J, Dishman RK. *Exercise Psychology.* Champaign (IL): Human Kinetics; 2002. p. 13.

SURGEON-GENERAL'S MENTAL HEALTH REPORT: LIFE STRESS, ANXIETY, DEPRESSION

The 1999 Surgeon General's report provided a detailed overview of mental health issues in the U.S. just before the millennium (232). Based on a public health perspective, this report emphasized the need not only for epidemiologic monitoring and access to clinical mental health services, but health promotion and disease prevention initiatives as well. The report cited statistics underscoring the debilitating nature of mental disorders, which, at the time, ranked second only to CVD in terms of years lost to premature death and disability. The corresponding economic costs associated with mental illnesses are substantial and have been documented elsewhere (154). The report defined mental health as ". . . the successful performance of mental function, resulting in productive activities, fulfilling relationships with other people, and the ability to adapt to change and to cope with adversity" (232). It described a continuum linking mental health and mental illness, using language compatible with the DSM-IV/TR diagnostic system for diagnosing mental disorders, in addition to subclinical manifestations of distress not meeting formal diagnostic criteria. Finally, this report advocated a unified view of mind and body compatible with the biopsychosocial perspective described earlier (83) as a way of broadening the perspective on health and medical care and also reducing the social stigma attached to mental distress. This finding is the most significant aspect of the report because it clearly supports the use of empirically validated, psychosocial interventions in the context of treating known medical conditions. Both before and following publication of the Surgeon General's report, this integrative mind/body perspective has gradually been supplanting the historic, dichotomous view of mind and body as separate entities (120).

The Surgeon General's report was followed 2 years later by a report focusing on mental health needs in the context of cultural diversity (74). There are widely acknowledged disparities in healthcare services, delivery, and utilization, and this report, not as widely publicized as its predecessor, warrants careful attention as well in terms of the health and medical needs of patients from diversified cultural and racial backgrounds. Both reports have played an important role in stimulating thinking and research about how best to meet the psychological health needs of an increasingly diversified population.

THE BACKGROUND OF HEALTH PSYCHOLOGY AND BEHAVIORAL MEDICINE

Extensive research and clinical work in health psychology and behavioral medicine echo the sentiments of the Surgeon General's report. Three key principles in particular reflect an emerging consensus concerning the nature and maintenance of mental health: first, that mind and body interact reciprocally; second, that participatory healthcare is superseding medical disease management; and third, that the immune system serves as a critical point of integration between mind and body. The first principle concerns the reciprocal interaction between mental and physical health, a cornerstone not only of contemporary mental health practices (206), but also research on the relationship between personality (94) and exercise (170) and health. Of interest in this regard is a comment in the introduction to DSM-IV that the term *mental disorder* suggests an unfortunate distinction "that is a reductionistic anachronism of mind/body dualism" (14). It is also worth noting that the American College of Sports Medicine (ACSM) recently released a consensus statement aimed at physicians that advocated an integrative perspective on athletic training (114). This statement noted that physical injuries often have significant psychological sequelae and emphasized that psychological factors are related to injury vulnerability and rehabilitation outcomes.

Concerning participatory healthcare, infectious diseases no longer pose the greatest threats to health as they once did as the hallmark of late nineteenth and much of twentieth century medicine (94). Increasingly, lifestyle factors interacting with physical vulnerability result in chronic cardiovascular and metabolic diseases, which, along with cancer, are among the leading causes of mortality. As a result, lifestyle modifications and management of psychosocial factors are achieving parity with medical management of most chronic illnesses and offer enormous physical, psychological, and economic benefits to help prevent these conditions from developing in the first place. However, convincing people to take an active stance in regard to health maintenance and disease management/prevention has proven to be a significant challenge. One reason is that the concept of health itself has traditionally been defined as the absence of disease, a rather impoverished concept that does not offer any positive attributes to be cultivated in a proactive manner. Fortunately, contemporary formulations of health have expanded this early definition to include social and psychological factors that can be cultivated and contribute to an overall sense of well-being (200). A second factor acting against the proactive adoption of health behaviors concerns behavioral passivity, reflected, for example, in chronically low rates of regular physical activity (76) and more generally poor compliance with healthcare recommendations aimed at improving overall health (157,164).

There is substantial evidence that health promotion and a capacity for self-regulation are interrelated, much of it based on the research of psychologist Albert Bandura, a prominent figure in the area of social learning theory (32) and social cognitive theory (31). According to Bandura, self-regulation is a key factor not only in managing existing medical conditions but in disease prevention as well. Models of self-regulation entail three components: (a) monitoring health behavior; (b) goal setting; and (c) proactive enlistment of social and other resources to foster goal attainment (28). A discussion of the role of self-regulation and a related psychological characteristic, self-efficacy, will be presented later in the chapter. It is important to remember that intervention strategies based on social cognitive principles can be very effective in helping overcome behavioral passivity. Social cognitive theory underlies virtually all current intervention models in health psychology and behavioral medicine.

The third principle in contemporary health research concerns the critical role of research on ways the immune system influences mind/body interactions (65). Psychoneuroimmunology, the study of brain, immune system, and behavior interactions (151), emerged in research by Ader and Cohen (5) and documents ways in which the immune and nervous systems interact to affect emotions, behavior, and cognitive (thought) processes. Stress affects the immune system via the hypothalamic–pituitary–adrenal (HPA) axis (166,204) and accounts for the well-known observation that periods of high stress heighten susceptibility to illness. Social factors play a key role in mediating the effects of stress, either positively or negatively, as documented in extensive research by Cohen, Kiecolt-Glazer, and others (65,130). Other research in this area has documented the impact of immune system activity on mood states via production of cytokines as part of a restorative system that promotes an adaptive sort of depression associated with heart disease and athletic overtraining (150). Collectively, research in the area of psychoneuroimmunology has established a solid foundation for clinical healthcare practice that incorporates a range of psychosocial interventions, in addition to primary medical care.

The Surgeon General's 1999 report on mental health articulated a clear need for clinical services and resources to address a major health issue with psychological, social, and economic implications. Much still needs to be done to meet these needs. As noted in the Healthy People 2010 Midcourse Review (234), in the area of mental health and mental disorders, only 1 of 14 goals has been met or exceeded to date. In addition to traditional clinical services, more and better quality research (170) is needed to further document the impact of physical activity as an effective intervention for both clinically significant and subclinical conditions and ease the burden of delivering mental health services. Greater attention to disparities affecting access to health, wellness, and medical care is urgently needed, as is updated research pertaining to correlates of physical activity (229) to assist in the delivery of individually oriented, widely disseminated mental health resources. In the remainder of this chapter, the focus is on three key aspects of distress identified in the Surgeon General's report as affecting a significant percentage of the population, in terms of either diagnosable psychological disorders or subclinical patterns of distress: stress, and anxiety, and depression.

ASSESSMENT OF SOCIAL INFLUENCES ON EMOTIONAL DISTRESS

People experience significant fluctuations in both negative and positive emotions as a function of interpersonal influences. Extensive research has revealed that social influences can markedly affect psychological stress in either positive or negative ways. For example, researchers have demonstrated that the immune system interacts with the central nervous system, which is the conduit through which social and other environmental stimuli are processed (5,130,204). Social support can help strengthen immune system responses, reduce stress reactivity, and help mitigate the impact of CVD, acquired immunodeficiency syndrome (AIDS), COPD, cancer, and other challenging illnesses (5,65,130,204). Social support has been identified as a key variable affecting the onset, course, and outcome of heart disease (215), and it has been found to affect the immune system and metabolic conditions as well (231). Virtually all conceptual models of healthy psychological adjustment (for example, social cognitive theory) (27) and emotional adaptation (139), as well as systems of psychotherapy, incorporate social/interpersonal influences as an essential component.

The implications of the social/interpersonal influences for all healthcare providers are clear. First, it is important to be aware of, and sensitive to, the social context of healthcare services delivery. Interpersonal aspects of interactions between patients and professionals have a significant impact on the initiation, cultivation, and maintenance of healthcare practice. Second, social influences outside the immediate context of healthcare systems exert a powerful influence on health and psychological well-being. Finally, even though psychological, like medical, diagnoses are applied to the individual, they should be viewed in a broader context that includes interpersonal and social influences. In fact, as noted later in the discussion of clinical diagnosis, the DSM-IV diagnostic system includes a provision for rating the severity of psychosocial stressors that may affect the onset, course, and outcome of various disorders.

The field of psychological assessment has a long history that can be traced at least back to research on individual differences in mental abilities by Sir Francis Galton in England in the mid-nineteenth century. Subsequently, Freudian psychodynamic psychology stimulated interest in hypothetical unconscious forces believed to influence much of conscious behavior. This interest led to the development of projective tests that were believed capable of clarifying nonconscious drives and motives and found favor in early clinical assessments. Research on personality traits (relatively enduring predispositions) emerged in the mid-twentieth century, stimulated by the work of Allport (10), who analyzed and grouped thousands of terms in the English

TABLE 16-2. FIVE FACTOR MODEL OF PERSONALITY

Factor 1:	Neuroticism	Worry, anxiety prone
Factor 2:	Extraversion	Socially outgoing, gregarious
Factor 3:	Openness	Nondefensive, inquisitive
Factor 4:	Agreeableness	Socially oriented
Factor 5:	Conscientiousness	Dependable, reliable

From Costa PT, McCrae RR. Personality assessment in psychosomatic medicine. *Adv Psychosom Med.* 1987;17:71–82.

language into core dimensions or factors to describe individual differences. At present, the predominant model of personality structure with broadest clinical application is the five-factor model of McCrae et al., which is rooted in Allport's earlier work (67,158). The five-factor model (outlined in Table 16-2), utilizing the statistical technique of factor analysis, has identified dimensions that appear to reflect common, fundamental characteristics that are relatively enduring in nature. This model has been used extensively in personality research in various contexts, including health and physical activity (195).

In behavioral medicine, interest in personality traits and medical conditions was initially high (94). Perhaps best known in this regard is research on the type A personality pattern originally identified by Friedman and Rosenman (95) as predictive of heart disease risk. The original conception of the type A individual hypothesized that disease risk was due to a combination of impatience, low frustration tolerance, a fast-paced lifestyle, and poorly modulated anger. Subsequent research identified anger and hostility as key disease risk factors (33), a finding that has since been found to be of moderate predictive use in clinical applications. On the positive side, research by Antonovsky and others has focused on identifying personality traits associated with health, rather than illness. The salutogenic model of health was developed by Antonovsky (19); it focused on a trait termed *sense of coherence* (18) to explain the capacity of some individuals to remain physically and psychologically healthy despite exposure to chronically stressful circumstances.

Collectively, much of the research on personality and psychological trait factors, especially in the early years, focused on internal processes hypothesized to overt behavior. This research evolved independently of behavioral psychology, which emphasized the influence of external forces on behavior. This artificial dichotomy has gradually been bridged in contemporary psychology, beginning with Mischel's person by situation interactionist model of personality (167,168). Assessments conducted by clinical and health psychologists utilize a wide range of both trait and state measures, though the latter tend to predominate in healthcare settings where the emphasis is on relatively rapid assessment and circumscribed treatment of what is often transient psychological distress. Most clinics have neither time nor resources to conduct

extensive assessments required to diagnose disorders rooted in personality patterns, nor are they equipped to offer the sort of long-term treatment that these conditions tend to necessitate.

Depression, anxiety, and stress are examples of state-like measures that are the focus of considerable contemporary clinical interest. Recent epidemiologic data suggest that mood and anxiety disorders are highly prevalent, along with substance-use disorders (128), cutting across cultural and racial boundaries (207). It is important to have a practical understanding of each condition, as well as knowledge about how depression and anxiety are related to mental and medical disorders.

PSYCHOSOCIAL MODELS OF HEALTH BEHAVIOR

The gradual merging of research on personality traits and states that emphasized the influence of social and other environmental influences gradually led to the formulation of behaviorally based models that combined the influence of both groups of factors. A key figure in this evolution was Albert Bandura, a psychologist whose early work on observational learning (29) led to the subsequent formulation of social learning theory (32) and social cognitive theory (31), both of which emphasize the reciprocal interaction among cognitive processes, social influences, and behavioral inclinations. Bandura's research focused on how many behavioral responses are learned simply via observation and served as a critical bridge between early behavioral and current cognitive formulations of behavior acquisition and modifications that emphasize the influence of social mediators. Bandura is perhaps best known for the concept of **self-efficacy**, which refers to one's perception of having the necessary capabilities to learn and navigate the many challenges of daily life (30). Social cognitive theory is perhaps the most influential contemporary model of health behavior and self-efficacy the most widely researched and extensively validated variable in clinical health research.

There are other influential models of socially based health behavior as well, including the theory of reasoned action (84) and a closely related variant, the theory of planned behavior (7). The theory of reasoned action posited that the intention to perform a behavior is of primary importance in determining health behavior. The theory of planned behavior adds the dimension of perceived control as an additional influential factor. Subsequent research using both models has found them to be of varying utility in predicting patterns of health behavior adoption (42).

In addition, the transtheoretical model (TTM) is a highly influential model of health behavior (188). TTM is an overarching, integrative model of health behavior interventions that incorporates many different intervention techniques and conceptual approaches into a longitudinal approach that takes into account stages of readiness for change with respect to physical activity and other health behaviors. There are five stages: (a) precontemplation; (b) contemplation; (c) preparation; (d) action; and (e) maintenance. A key feature of this model is that it proposes a progressive shift from verbal (i.e., education, motivational) strategies to behaviorally based therapies (such as selective reinforcement), controlling environmental stimuli with each succeeding stage. Statewise progression is mediated by a cognitively based process, decisional balance, which evaluates positive and negative aspects of the associated changes. Progression from one stage to another is typically not linear, but rather marked by a series of advances and declines (189). Originally developed as model to guide therapy for eliminating negative health behaviors such as smoking, drug use, and risky sexual practices (190), the TTM has more recently been applied to cultivating positive behaviors as well, including exercise, where it appears to be moderately effective (222).

IMPLICATIONS FOR CLINICAL ASSESSMENT

Emotional distress can vary considerably in intensity and persistence. Emotional ups and downs are normal; what sets them apart from psychological disorders is the level of subjective distress that is the intensity, duration, and functional impairment they cause. Measures of psychological and emotional states can be rated on dimensional scales that assess intensity and pervasiveness. A variety of scales have been developed, primarily for use in clinical research, to assess depression, anxiety, stress, anger, and many other emotional characteristics linked to emotional distress. However, such scales do not provide a sufficient basis for clinical diagnosis, which involves a formal evaluative process conducted by mental health professionals. From a medical perspective, the purpose of diagnosis is to identify the underlying cause(s) of symptoms and specify treatment. Diagnosing psychological disorders serves a similar purpose, although it is seldom possible to isolate a specific cause because psychological disorders involve multiple contributory factors consistent with the biopsychosocial model. As a result, interventions frequently entail multiple components as well. For example, the diagnosis of depression, a mood disorder, might involve a coordinated treatment plan involving cognitive behavior therapy (CBT), anti-depressant medication, and exercise.

Whereas clinical research scales used to assess emotional states tend to be dimensional in nature, the DSM-IV is categorically based. It was developed by the American Psychiatric Association and is compatible with the International Classification of Diseases (ICD) system, published by the World Health Organization. The DSM-IV is strongly oriented toward an epidemiologic/disease model,

employing standardized, symptom-based diagnostic criteria for each psychological disorder. The DSM-IV comprises five axes or categories (Table 16-3). Axes 1 and 2 focus on psychological diagnoses, and axis 3 identifies any health-related problems or conditions. Axis 4 addresses psychosocial and environmental factors contributing to diagnosis. Axis 5 considers the clinician's diagnosis.

The DSM-IV is currently the most widely used clinical standard for diagnosing mental disorders, although it is not without critics (85). The diagnosis of mental disorders requires evidence of an established percentage of symptoms relative to the total, which constitutes a diagnostic threshold, below which the term *subclinical* is often used. In addition, to qualify as a mental disorder, symptoms need to be present for periods that vary with specific disorders. Clarifying periods help differentiate, for example, transient periods of depressed mood or anxiety that everyone experiences from more enduring periods of emotional distress that do not spontaneously resolve.

DSM-IV–based diagnoses typically draw on multiple types of information and may include data from clinical interviews, questionnaires to assess state and/or personality factors, case history material, collateral reports, and other sources. The use of multiple sources of information aids the process of cross-validating clinical impressions by

---

TABLE 16-3. DSM-IV AXES

Axis I	• Contains the majority of mental disorders, having a clear-cut onset and course (e.g. mood, substance abuse, anxiety disorders) • Multiple diagnoses are common, with high co-morbidity of mood and anxiety disorders (128)
Axis II	• Pervasive, long-standing conditions (e.g., personality disorders) • Personality disorders include acute maladaptive reactions and stable patterns of maladjustment that solidify with age (62) • Frequently co-occur with Axis I disorders (104)
Axis III	• Medical conditions contributing to onset, course, or outcome of a mental disorder • Based on International Classification of Disease (ICD) system
Axis IV	• Psychosocial and environmental factors contributing to diagnosis • Includes problems with social support, educational, occupation, or economic factors
Axis V	• Clinician's rating of overall adjustment • Used to help plan treatment and assess prognosis • Uses Global Assessment of Functioning (GAF) scale, a 100-point measure ranging from seriously impaired functioning (e.g., persistent risk of harming self or others; unable to care for self) to highly adaptive behavior

DSM-IV, *Diagnostic and Statistical Manual of Mental Disorders*, 4th ed.

From American Psychiatric Association. *Diagnostic and Statistical Manual of Mental Disorders*. 4th ed. Text Revision. Washington (DC): American Psychiatric Association; 2000.

avoiding excessive reliance on any single type of data. Thus, although questionnaires used to assess depression or anxiety may provide useful information, they are not sufficient to diagnose psychological disorders in either category. The DSM-IV system has other features that are important to understand. It is multiaxial in nature, employing five independent dimensions or axes (Table 16-3).

Exercise professionals are likely to work with individuals experiencing emotional distress, both at the level of subclinical intensity and psychological disorders based on DSM-IV criteria. An understanding of common forms of distress and related psychological disorders, especially anxiety and depression, and ways each of these affect behavior, cognitive processes, and emotional states is increasingly important owing to the widespread prevalence of these conditions. For years, anxiety and depression-related disorders, along with substance-use disorders, have been, and continue to be, the most prominent areas of clinical practice and research (37).

DEPRESSION

The key feature of depression is a negative emotional state marked by feelings of sadness and unhappiness, often accompanied by self-criticism and low self-esteem. Depressive-spectrum disorders, collectively referred to as mood disorders in DSM-IV, are among the most common mental disorders, affect approximately 10% of the population (128), and, along with bipolar disorder, a condition marked by mood swings ranging from depression to mania, extract a significant toll on work productivity (127) and social engagement (115). Depression is also linked to medical risk factors, including heart disease (16), and tends to have adverse effects on spouses and others who potentially could serve as sources of social support (221). People who are depressed typically experience a loss of physical and mental energy needed to handle everyday situations, and often present as lethargic or tired. A related term, *melancholia,* describes a pattern of such chronic and pervasive sadness that it appears to be almost "characterological" in nature. The concept of depression is intimately related to loss, bringing to mind states of grief or bereavement that would occur naturally in the context of, for example, the death of a loved one or the reaction to a catastrophic natural disaster, such as Hurricane Katrina. But such events are seldom at the root of sustained clinical depression, for which concepts such as loss or the perception of declining capabilities has more to do with negative self-appraisals, a pessimistic view of the world, and feelings of helplessness and hopelessness about the future. People who are depressed find that it blunts other emotional reactions, including bereavement (101). Psychiatrist Aaron Beck termed this observation the *cognitive triad of depression,* a central concept in cognitive therapy for depression and other emotional disorders first formulated in the 1960s. This

theory has undergone progressive evolution (39,40,61) to the point to which it is the most widely utilized, empirically validated clinical practice model. Persistence and severity of symptoms form the basis for diagnosing an actual disorder as opposed to a subclinical state. Depression is accompanied by significant health risks, including that of heart disease (16,56).

Other early and influential models of depression by Seligman and Lewinsohn emphasized, respectively, the importance of powerlessness, termed *learned helplessness,* and withdrawal from sources of behavioral reinforcement as important psychological contributors to depression (145,211,230). These models all converge in their emphasis on the importance of social factors with respect to onset, course, and amelioration of depressive symptoms. A review of the literature on social functioning in depression (115) described it as a prominent feature of depression and noted that neither pharmacologic nor psychological interventions effective in relieving cognitive and physical impairments necessarily restore social functioning to pre-depression levels.

Biological theories of depression have emphasized the role of neurotransmitter deficiencies, in particular biogenic amines, as a key contributory factor. Norepinephrine and serotonin are brain neurotransmitters that are the principle target of pharmacologic interventions to increase their activity level. Initially employing tricyclic antidepressants and later monoamine oxidase inhibitors (MAOIs), contemporary pharmacologic interventions for depression now favor selective serotonin uptake inhibitors (SSRIs) for routine cases (101). There is also evidence associating depression with dysregulation of the HPA axis, a key mediator of stress reactivity (166).

An important relative of depression in medical and athletic settings involves intense fatigue and mental exhaustion. Appels (21) devised a measure of vital exhaustion (the Maastricht Questionnaire) that was found to predict myocardial infarction in patients with heart disease (133). Similarly, athletic overtraining involves symptoms of depression, especially chronic fatigue, along with performance decrements and other impairments collectively labeled the *overtraining syndrome* (23,144), which involves dysregulation of the HPA stress reactivity system (160). An intriguing explanation for this syndrome has been offered by Nesse, who views depression as an adaptive response to overexertion that promotes energy conservation and restoration (173). Interesting support for this hypothesis comes from studies suggesting that production of cytokines in immunologic responses to inflammation signal a need for reallocating energy and reducing behavioral activation to fight infection, resulting in what is termed *sickness behavior* (69). Cytokine levels are elevated in clinical depression, and their production may be precipitated by stress (194), lending credibility to this energy conservation hypothesis concerning depressionlike behavior. The distinction between classic clinical depression and symptoms associated with CVD is currently the focus of significant research and analysis (70).

Depression is a **mood disorder**, of which the chief characteristic is relatively persistent alteration in mood or emotional tone. Table 16-4 depicts the three broad classes of mood disorders. To screen for depression, a two-item questionnaire has recently been proposed, inquiring whether within the preceding month patients have experienced either (a) "little interest or pleasure in doing things" or (b) "feeling down, depressed, or hopeless" (53). However, it should be noted that an actual diagnosis of depression can only be made by a healthcare professional, using the criteria set forth in the DSM-IV.

ANXIETY

The term *anxiety* is related to fear, in that both conditions generally involve heightened activation of the sympathetic nervous system (SNS). They differ in that anxiety is future oriented, whereas fear is a reaction to present threat or danger. Anxious people worry extensively about real or imagined future events over which they believe they have little control. Chronic anxiety is characterized by persisting apprehension that may or may not be attached to a specific source of concern. A focused object of concern is termed a *phobia*; anxiety that is not attached to a specific object or situation is described as *free floating* or *generalized anxiety*.

Anxiety is extremely common and is often referred to as the "common cold of psychopathology." Clinically, anxiety has high rates of comorbidity with other mental disorders, especially mood disorders. A large sample (43,93) survey conducted by the National Institute on Alcohol Abuse and Alcoholism (NIAAA) reported a 12-month prevalence of any form of anxiety disorder to be 11.1% (104). Efforts to control anxiety consume billions of dollars and double the cost for medical patients afflicted with anxiety (36). Anxiety symptoms are common secondary reactions to many medical disorders and appear to be predictive of coronary heart disease (CHD) risk independent of clinical depression (34), and even in healthy individuals, they are associated with inflammation and coagulation markers (186).

One reason for anxiety's prominence as a clinical disorder is that it is related to activation of the SNS. Normal SNS activation is adaptive and even protective, as when a reflexive fight-or-flight reaction is triggered in a risky or dangerous situation. Elevated heart rate, peripheral vasodilation, altered breathing, and diaphoresis are correlates of SNS activation (236). Activation of the SNS is normally balanced with that of the parasympathetic nervous system (PNS), which exerts a counterbalancing effect of energy restoration and recovery. A cardinal feature of most anxiety is unwarranted SNS activation in response to anticipated risk or danger, implying that it is (a) cognitively mediated and (b) future oriented. Either chronic or episodic SNS activation under circumstances that pose

TABLE 16-4. CLASSES OF MOOD DISORDERS

CLASS	DIAGNOSES INCLUDED
Depressive (or unipolar) disorders	**Major depressive disorder** • Most common mood disorder; at least one major episode • Two or more weeks of either diminished pleasure/interest in normal activities or depressed mood, and four of the following: weight change (<5% per month); altered sleep patterns; increased/decreased motor activity; fatigue; feeling worthless/guilty; poor concentration; persistent thoughts of death or suicide **Dysthymic disorder** • Chronically depressed for at least 2 years, and two of the following: altered appetite; minimal/excessive sleep; constant fatigue; poor self-esteem; hopelessness **Depressive disorder not otherwise specified (NOS)** • Atypical manifestations of depression • Often linked to other mental disorders
Bipolar disorders	**Bipolar I** • Episodes of mania (heightened energy and expansive mood) that alternate with depressive episodes • Previously known as manic-depressive illness **Bipolar II** • Periods of depression alternate with hypomanic episodes (less extreme elevations of mood and energy) **Cyclothymic disorder** • Chronic (at least 2 years) fluctuations in mood, alternating between hypomanic and depressive symptoms **Bipolar disorder NOS** • Atypical alternating mood patterns
Mood disorders that are due to a medical condition or substance abuse	• Mood disorders associated with **medical condition** (e.g., degenerative neurologic disorders, stroke, cancers) • Mood disorders associated with **substance use** (resulting from states of intoxication, withdrawal, or medication side effects) • Symptoms can be depressive or maniclike.

American Psychiatric Association. *Diagnostic and Statistical Manual of Mental Disorders*. 4th ed. Text Revision. Washington (DC): American Psychiatric Association; 2000.

no immediate danger can be highly debilitating and lead to additional anxiety, typically in the form of worry (47), as well as being associated with heightened hypertension risk related to both CHD and metabolic disorders (105).

The following are the primary subtypes of anxiety disorders in the DSM-IV: panic disorder with/without agoraphobia; phobias (agoraphobia; specific phobia; social phobia); obsessive-compulsive disorder; posttraumatic stress disorder; and generalized anxiety disorder (Table 16-5). As with mood disorders, there are additional subtypes related to medical conditions and substance-use disorders, and with atypical symptoms (i.e., not otherwise specified [NOS]).

As with mood disorders, anxiety disorders can be a result of certain medical conditions or psychoactive substances, including some medications. Panic attacks may be mistakenly perceived as heart attacks, owing to the prominence of tachycardia in conjunction with sudden SNS hyperactivation. For example, one study (242) found that roughly one third of emergency room visits for chest pain were linked to either panic disorder or depression. It is also the case that both anxiety and depression, either subclinical variants or full-blown DSM-IV disorders, can occur as secondary reactions to the stress associated with many medical disorders. As a result, it is important for exercise professionals to be sensitive to possible interactions between medical and psychological factors that contribute to the individual's overall level of adaptation. In addition, knowledge about side effects of pharmacotherapy for anxiety disorders is warranted (175), which is commonly employed either singly or in combination with psychotherapy (CBT). A brief screening measure for anxiety (53) poses three questions concerning symptoms within the preceding month: "being bothered by 'nerves,' or feeling anxious or on edge," "worrying about a lot of different things," and "having an anxiety attack (suddenly feeling fear or panic)."

STRESS

The term *stress* is interpreted in many different ways, but is rooted in engineering terminology, where it refers to deformation of an object (such as a steel beam) in response to an imposed load. This definition views stress as a stimulus. In health and medicine, the concept of stress is related to Bernard and Cannon's concept of internal responses that maintain physiologic balance despite environmental changes, which Cannon termed *homeostasis* and popularized in an early book (54). Lazarus et al. (143) define stress as the result of a cognitive appraisal process comparing situational demands with available coping resources; high stress occurs when perceived demands exceed resources. According to Lazarus (139, 141), stress is highly integrated with emotion, defined as "an organized, psychophysiologic reaction to ongoing relationships with the environment" (142). This conception is useful as everyday experience is marked by a range of emotional reactions to situations that pose challenges and evoke coping responses. Increasingly, research in this area is incorporating positive (e.g., hope, love) as well as negative (e.g., fear, anger, anxiety) emotions into the overall model (140).

Early interest in stress was stimulated by Selye, who formulated the general adaptation syndrome (GAS) based on early animal studies suggesting that a variety of physical stressors elicited a common, characteristic physiologic response pattern. There are three phases in the GAS: alarm, reaction, and exhaustion. The alarm phase entails physiologic arousal that increases metabolism and heightens vigilance, and is preparatory in nature. This

TABLE 16-5. SUBTYPES OF DSM-IV ANXIETY DISORDERS

Panic disorder with or without agoraphobia	*Panic attacks*: • Brief, unexpected, intense episodes of SNS activation peaking within a 10-minute period • Anxious apprehension about attacks or their reoccurrence *Agoraphobia*: • Situational avoidance (being in a crowd, being outdoors, etc.) perceived as risky and difficult to escape from • May be diagnostically linked to panic disorder, but can be diagnosed independently
Phobias	• Extreme anticipatory fear of specific objects or situations evoking anxiety symptoms comparable to panic attacks • Typically accompanied by recognition that fear is excessive or unwarranted • May become conditioned to virtually any object or situation
Obsessive-compulsive disorder	• Recurrent, uncontrolled obsessions (thoughts, impulses, images) and/or compulsions (repetitive behaviors) • Obsessions/compulsions generally acknowledged as unnecessary
Posttraumatic stress disorder	• Re-experiencing prior traumatic, catastrophic stressors 1 month or more after the event (termed *acute stress disorder* if reaction occurs within 1 month) • Avoidance of circumstances or cues related to trauma • Persisting, heightened SNS activation is common.
Generalized anxiety disorder	• Broadly based apprehension, unattached to specific object or situation • Heightened vigilance with moderately elevated SNS activation and chronic anticipatory worry

DSM-IV, *Diagnostic and Statistical Manual of Mental Disorders*, 4th ed; SNS, sympathetic nervous system.

phase is followed by sustained activation that underlies coping responses, followed by a phase of exhaustion and recovery. Chronic stress overloads the GAS, which functions best when only episodically activated. Selye distinguished between stress and eustress, the latter a positive stressor, as a way of emphasizing the possible adaptive, as well as maladaptive, aspects. Selye's research highlighted the importance of the HPA axis, which triggers secretion of cortisol from the adrenal cortex in response to prolonged stress. Research clearly demonstrates the key role of the HPA axis integrating the nervous, endocrine, and immune systems (166).

The HPA neuroendocrine axis and SNS make up two somewhat independent systems activated in response to stressful and/or anxiety-provoking circumstances. Functionally, it can be difficult to differentiate stress and anxiety, because both involve states of heightened physiologic arousal. One difference is cognitive: Anxiety is a response to anticipated risk or threat, whereas stress involves a state of physiologic adaptation to immediate concerns. Second, whereas anxiety is perceptible and unpleasant, signaled by SNS activation, stress reactions may involve less obvious patterns of arousal that evolve into chronically elevated activation in response to cortisol secretion. Third, stress has positive aspects in relation to, for example, exercise and performance contexts. Psychological and physiologic correlates of stress occur in a time-limited context that challenges coping resources and evokes adaptive emotional responses (140). Recently, the concepts of allostasis (stability in the context of change) and allostatic load (cumulative, pathologic stress adaptation) have been used to characterize neurologically based hormonal and cognitive changes reflecting adaptation to chronically variable environmental circumstances (159). Trait-based behavioral variations may predispose individuals to different stress-based diseases as a result of cumulative allostatic load (134).

Stress is associated with a range of health risk factors. Research in this area began with Holmes and Rahe's use of the Social Readjustment Rating Scale (SRRS) to predict illness onset (116), though this produced only modest correlations because of individual differences in response to specific stressful events. Stress is a common stimulus to overeating (106) and influences blood lipid levels via increased concentration of cortisol, catecholamines, and fatty acids (51). And as previously noted, various types of stressors can weaken immune system responses to viruses and other opportunistic pathogens (63,64). Psychosocial stressors have also been found to impede recovery from intensive training in athletes (184).

Stress and coping are inextricably linked, and many different strategies and programs have been developed outside the context of formal psychotherapy to help people manage stress. Lazarus characterized coping simply as how people manage stressful life events (141). In earlier writings (139,143), he used the terms *emotion focused* and *problem focused* to describe common ways of coping, the former involving cognitive interpretive strategies to reduce the emotional impact of stress, the latter taking direct action to deal with a stressor. Both are typically used at various times in the course of managing stressful events. Exercise (78) and meditation (125) are but two of many techniques found useful in helping to manage stress.

Despite its pervasive nature, stress does not have a corresponding discrete DSM-IV diagnosis. However, **posttraumatic stress disorder** and **acute stress disorder** are considered Axis I disorders involving reactions to specific catastrophic events well in excess of the severity needed to activate the HPA axis. In these disorders, symptoms may persist and often emerge well after the stressful event, whereas chronic stress reflects the cumulative impact of multiple day-to-day events that, either singly or collectively, overtax coping resources. One relevant DSM-IV diagnosis is psychological factors affecting physical condition, an Axis I disorder including what were previously referred to as psychosomatic disorders, reflecting the interplay between psychological and physical symptoms, and frequently attributed to stress (227). However, such interactions are based largely on correlational epidemiologic studies and await verification via more rigorous research methodology (129).

INTERVENTION MODELS AND STRATEGIES

The term *psychosocial intervention* is very broad and encompasses ways of helping people deal with emotional distress that include, but are not limited to, psychotherapy. Although pharmacotherapy is an obvious and well-proven means of providing relief for depression, anxiety, and other emotional disorders, there is increasing evidence that interpersonally based therapeutic interventions not only have strong empirical support (58), but also exert their effects at a neurobiological level (216).

Healthcare professionals are increasingly likely to encounter patients battling anxiety, depression, stress, and other challenging conditions in the context of treating primary diseases (136). Psychological problems cut across socioeconomic, cultural, and all other levels of society (110), and are of sufficient prevalence that there are not nearly enough psychotherapists to address these needs (188). Formal training in psychotherapy normally involves either medical or postgraduate education, the latter leading to either a master's or doctorate degree. The practice of psychotherapy is regulated in most cases by state boards that grant licenses or certificates to practice. There are, however, many ways in which healthcare professionals without such formal training can at least be sensitive to the psychosocial needs of their patients, know how to make appropriate referrals when warranted, and frequently intervene in effective ways to reduce patients' distress.

Psychotherapy incorporates aspects of interpersonal relationships common to other professional relationships, including those with healthcare providers, and several key factors have emerged that help account for its impact, including the therapeutic relationship; expectancy placebo factors; characteristics of the patient and extra therapeutic elements; and specific techniques (25). Self-disclosure is an important aspect of patient characteristics. Pennebaker, among others, has extensively documented the positive effects of both written and verbal narratives of stressful events on health and well-being, including immune system activity (182).

Although there are many forms of psychotherapy, virtually all employ (a) an emotionally charted relationship with a therapist, (b) a healing environment, (c) a conceptual rationale, and (d) procedures or techniques to provide relief (91). This section focuses on cognitive behavior therapy, the most widely practiced form of psychotherapy with well-validated applications for treating stress (161), depression (40), and anxiety (36).

Psychosocial interventions, including CBT, have solid empirical support (58) and broad application in health, medical, and psychiatric settings. Psychological interventions or CBT are also efficient and cost-effective means of treating emotional disorders (171), primarily in terms of reducing inpatient hospitalization time and work-related impairments for even serious psychological conditions (98). Psychosocial treatment for depression is a viable alternative to pharmacotherapy in primary care practice (208). In the area of behavioral medicine, Friedman et al. enumerated six routes through which psychosocial interventions could help contain costs, including (a) fostering active patient involvement in health and medical care; (b) reducing the negative and additive impact of stress on disease; (c) modifying overt behavior associated with destructive lifestyle patterns necessitating expensive end-stage medical care; (d) providing social support to buffer the impact of critical medical procedures, including cardiac surgery and cesarean sections; (e) identifying and treating psychological disorders underlying medical symptoms; and (f) reducing primary care usage by patients whose primary needs are emotional in nature, but expressed physically (somatization) (97).

COGNITIVE BEHAVIOR THERAPY

Cognitive behavior therapy is a problem-oriented, time-limited intervention model that views psychological distress as the result of negative thoughts based on either conscious or nonconscious unrealistic underlying assumptions about the world (cognitive schemas), such as "People should always treat me well" or "I should be perfect" (161) (Table 16-6). Clinically, its historical roots are in behaviorism, which emphasizes modifying overt

TABLE 16-6. KEY IMPLICATIONS OF COGNITIVE-BEHAVIOR THERAPY

- Form supportive, working relationship with patients.
- Treat patients as active collaborators in learning new skills.
- Promote self-efficacy by helping patients develop capabilities and self-confidence.
- Be aware of how thoughts, behavior, and emotions interact to affect motivation, learning, and retention.
- Listen to how patients talk about themselves for indications of positive or negative cognitions associated with distress (anxiety, depression, stress).
- Foster skills that have present-moment relevance.
- Provide encouragement and support in situations that evoke unwarranted anxiety and avoidant tendencies.
- Encourage patients to develop self-assessment and self-reinforcement capabilities as a means of promoting developmental autonomy.
- Use a "building block" approach to skill development: Break challenging tasks down into readily mastered components that build confidence and promote self-efficacy.
- Help patients enlist the social support in learning and maintaining new skills.

behaviors rather than thought patterns (92). CBT also incorporates social behavioral models, especially social learning and social cognitive theory (31,32), in terms of its emphasis on mediating factors such as self-efficacy to foster change in the face of depression, anxiety, or stress. CBT has widespread endorsement in behavioral medicine settings (82), perhaps because of its practical nature and amenability to empirical validation.

CBT combines cognitive restructuring with modifying underlying assumptions about the world reflected in conscious thought patterns and behaviorally based exposure. CBT encourages direct experience with the source of one's fear, or anxiety techniques to treat psychological problems (50). These components are often accompanied by training in relaxation techniques, such as progressive muscle relaxation and diaphragmatic breathing. Proponents of CBT have emphasized its specificity in treating anxiety, depression, and other disorders, akin to the medical model of diagnosis and treatment (37), but there is active debate as to whether such efficacy is due to specific or common factors characteristic of virtually all forms of psychotherapy (178,239). In fact, Barlow and others note that the concept of discrete DSM-IV diagnostic categories tends to accentuate differences that are difficult to empirically justify and, consequently, that developing specific treatment protocols for each disorder appears unwarranted (35). For example, the consistently high reported concordance between depression (mood) and anxiety disorders is consistent with this view (128). Barlow et al. have recently proposed a unified treatment model of CBT (35) with three factors: (a) modify antecedent cognitive appraisals that contribute to anticipatory emotional distress; (b) encourage acceptance, rather than avoidance or suppression, of unpleasant emotional states; (c) encourage behavioral activation in domains not limited by the disordered emotion. Practically, this entails helping people become aware of and limit negative anticipatory appraisals in circumstances otherwise likely to elicit stressful, depressive, or anxious reactions; encourage openness to emotional experiences, whether positive or negative; and facilitate active engagement in daily life. Of particular relevance for patients with the chronic illnesses described in this chapter, CBT has been validated for use with older patients, who are most vulnerable to these conditions (224).

Consistent with this unified treatment model, CBT is currently evolving in the direction of acceptance and mindfulness-based models of psychotherapy advocated by Hayes and others (108,109,209). These developments reflect the interesting influence of diverse influences, including cognitive theories of language and Buddhist meditation practices, united in the belief that detaching from and being less reactive to (hence accepting of) and aware (mindful) of thoughts and other elements of experience is therapeutically beneficial. Applications of this model in behavioral medicine, sports performance, and addiction treatment are now appearing in the literature (9,100,117,203). Of particular relevance are results of a recent study (79) reporting short-term autonomic and cardiovascular benefits from one component of a stress reduction protocol based on this model.

CBT interventions continue to be successfully utilized in medical and health applications, including managing stress associated with human immunodeficiency (HIV) diagnosis (17); preventing defibrillator shock (59); responding discriminatively to sudden chest pain (197); encouraging older adults to exercise (112); and reducing stress-related injury and illness among athletes (183). In general, CBT has attained parity with pharmacotherapy for treating depression and anxiety, and involving patients in the decision process is one way to enhance active engagement in treatment. CBT is a practical, problem-oriented form of psychotherapy. The basic principals can be readily applied in health and wellness, as well as in clinical settings.

EXERCISE AND PSYCHOSOCIAL FACTORS

Exercise professionals are in an especially advantageous position to help patients deal with symptoms of anxiety, depression, and stress because exercise and physical activity have well-documented positive effects on these conditions. However, the effects of stress, anxiety, and depression on exercise motivation need to be taken into account to increase the likelihood of exercise initiation and maintenance. There are numerous cognitive and behavioral determinants of physical activity (52,214), and it is important to have a working knowledge of how these can affect day-to-day behavior. Stress-prone individuals are vulnerable to fatigue and unfavorable appraisals of their capacity to cope with the inevitable challenges in becoming and staying physically active. Anxiety triggers apprehension and worry about future outcomes, even in the context of potentially enjoyable activities, whereas depression saps both psychological and physical energy, triggering pessimistic cognitive appraisals and crippling self-doubts. All three undermine self-efficacy in different ways.

However, there is growing evidence that physical activity and exercise can help reduce distress associated with symptoms of stress (198), anxiety (147), and depression (177), and exercise guidelines for work with clinical populations have been published (165). Early research shows that exercise alleviates negative emotional states employed with nonclinical samples, i.e. physically fit individuals, athletes, state-based measures of emotionality, and, frequently, relatively high-intensity exercise. Comparatively few studies were conducted using clinical populations. Furthermore, the absence of conceptual models linking emotions to physical activity and lack of integration with extant psychiatric diagnostic nomenclature limited clinical applications of the early research literature. Finally, stress, anxiety, and depression are associated with advanced age, which imposes its own constraints on physical activity.

Despite these caveats, there is increasing evidence from recent longitudinal epidemiologic and clinical studies attesting to the positive effects of physical activity based on clinical samples to reinforce the conclusions of earlier studies (38,107). In addition, contemporary conceptually driven models integrating physical activity, neurobiological structures, cognitive functions, and emotional reactivity have stimulated research on the impact of even low-intensity or dose activity on emotional states (81). The emergence of the interdisciplinary field of "exercise" psychology, with a corresponding emphasis on health optimization in clinical settings that has occurred in recent years, has developmental roots in exercise physiology, behavioral medicine, and health psychology. However, the impact of physical activity across the full spectrum of both anxiety and mood clinical disorders has not been systematically evaluated, being limited largely to panic disorder (176) and moderate intensity depression (177).

Exercise professionals need to integrate knowledge of exercise prescription techniques with sensitivity to psychosocial factors when designing programs for patients expressing symptoms of stress, anxiety, and/or depression. The importance of gauging the impact of exercise—itself a stressor—on overall cumulative stress level (i.e., the allostatic load) cannot be overstated. The common channel factor here is the HPA axis, which, as noted earlier, is designed to modulate the impact of short-term, rather than chronic, stress. Although it has been hypothesized that exercise-based stress may reduce the impact of stress in other modalities (the cross-stressor adaptation hypothesis), supportive evidence is equivocal (78,219), although research is ongoing (220). Although this hypothesis has some validity with respect to people who are physically fit, adjusting exercise prescriptions in response to varying self-reported stress is recommended (2), especially to avoid overtaxing unfit patients or those with chronic medical conditions whose immune system may be compromised either by the disease or as a result of treatment side effects.

It may seem paradoxical that physical activity appears to reduce symptoms of both anxiety and depression, the latter involving heightened SNS arousal, the former a reduction in overall activation. Psychological benefits accrue from both aerobic and nonaerobic forms of exercise, eliminating physiologic conditioning per se as the principal explanatory factor (187). In part, this finding can be explained by nonspecific aspects of any psychological intervention described earlier (25), including expectancy factors and a positive therapeutic relationship. Physical activity may be beneficial in other ways as a temporary distraction (26,192) and as a way to enhance self-efficacy (30), the perception of fitness (187), and perhaps even alterations in trait factors as well (72), independent of measurable changes in fitness. Physiologically, regular physical activity helps modulate SNS and HPA activation, a contributing factor to both anxiety- and depression-spectrum disorders. Furthermore, as noted earlier, the high comorbidity of depression and anxiety disorders suggests at least a partial underlying etiologic commonality. It has been suggested that a unifying factor concerning the benefits of physical activity may in fact lead to an overarching increase in stress resilience, mediated by both cognitive and physiologic mechanisms (202). Finally, neurocognitive changes associated with exercise suggest a generalized positive impact on central nervous system (CNS) functioning that may indeed have implications for emotional, cognitive, and behavioral well-being (225).

A particular challenge facing exercise professionals is how to help emotionally distressed patients work with the low level of physical conditioning common in anxiety and depression (155,191). Exacerbating this problem is the inevitable experience of most individuals initiating exercise programs; that the experience is not particularly pleasant and that perceptible benefits take time to accrue. Self-consciousness and skill deficits are also potential issues to be faced. Anxious individuals—those with panic disorder in particular—may be conditioned to experience physiologic arousal as both unpleasant and, because of prior elicitation during panic attacks, embarrassing or even dangerous. Anticipating the worst, they may worry about the possibility of injury or other negative outcomes. And those who experience chronic SNS activation may find even modest exercise-induced stimulation excessive rather than invigorating. Depressed individuals pose unique challenges as well (210), in terms of low

TABLE 16-7. GUIDELINES FOR THE TREATMENT OF EMOTIONAL DISTRESS

- Know symptoms of common psychological disorders and medications used to treat them.
- Listen attentively to patients without minimizing their concerns; know how and where to refer patients for professional help if needed.
- Conduct thorough assessment of physical capabilities and motivational factors. Anxiety is linked to worry and fear, depression to self-criticism, both of which can decrease motivation.
- Encourage enjoyable, nonthreatening, easily accessible exercise; link it to being active outside scheduled sessions.
- Eliminate obstacles, establish reasonable goals, and help patients integrate physical activity into daily life.
- Incorporate patients in planning and assessing of exercise programs to enhance active collaboration and counteract passivity associated with anxious worry and depressive pessimism.
- Adopt a nonjudgmental, problem-solving stance when difficulties with compliance arise. Emphasize immediate benefits rather than long-term outcomes; minimize significance of lapses.
- Watch for resistance to change that can sabotage progress; address it directly and collaboratively. Reinforce positive behaviors unrelated to depression or anxiety to sidestep negative effects on motivation.

From O'Neal HA, Dunn AL, Martinsen EW. Depression and exercise. *Int J Sport Psychol.* 2000;31:110–135.

motivation, chronic inactivity, and a pessimistic view of the world. In working with depressed or anxious patients, the recommendations listed in Table 16-7, although developed primarily for depressed individuals, are useful in either case. Especially important in this work is anticipating and making allowances for cognitively based motivational barriers to progress when initiating exercise programs (24). The following guidelines adapted from O'Neal et al. (177), although developed for depression, are very useful for other types of emotional distress as well.

Finally, emerging clinical practice and research on mindfulness emphasizes the value of keeping one's attention focused in the present moment. Being mindful can help anxious or depressed patients avoid being distracted by past or future concerns and help cultivate an appreciation for present-moment experience. Currently, applications of mindfulness in exercise tend to emphasize non-Western practices such as Yoga and Tai 'Chi (138), but in fact, a much broader framework exists in Western psychology underlying its incorporation into many other aspects of daily life (203).

CLINICAL APPLICATIONS

CARDIOVASCULAR DISEASE

Psychosocial interventions for CVD patients have involved both preventive and postmyocardial infarct applications. Beginning with early efforts to identify psychological precursors of cardiac events (33,95,96), accumulating data has shown that psychosocial factors, stress, and emotional reactivity in particular are significant predictors of CVD risk. Moreover, emotional distress and anxiety are associated with heightened risk of sudden cardiac death (126). A related factor, heightened cardiovascular reactivity, may be a risk factor as well, although supportive evidence has been considered equivocal (135). Recently, however, convincing evidence links depression, dysfunctional autonomic nervous system activity with both mortality and morbidity associated with CVD (56). These relationships may be mediated in part by immune system dysregulation, marked by cytokine production, which has deleterious cardiac effects and produces depression symptoms (180).

More recent research continues to validate this relationship, particularly with respect to anxiety and depression. Rozankis et al. (199) cited evidence linking CVD risk to the following five domains: (a) depression, (b) anxiety, (c) personality traits, (d) social isolation, and (e) chronic stress. All of these factors appear to contribute to endothelial damage as a function of stress and, in addition for some individuals, SNS hyperactivation. A recent analysis of data from the Normative Aging Study, a longitudinal study of aging in men, revealed a dose-response relationship between negative emotionality and CVD incidence (228). A more recent study derived from this database revealed that anxiety and a factor characterized as "general emotional distress" was a significant predictor of CVD risk. Similar results were also recently reported from a moderately sized sample of men and women in the Pittsburgh Healthy Heart Project, where it was reported that somatic symptoms of depression in particular compared with measures of anxiety and hostility are linked to early-stage CVD (226).

Overall, studies of patients with CVD support the value of psychosocial, lifestyle, and related complementary interventions. An early meta-analysis based on 23 randomized control studies (146) concluded that adding a psychosocial intervention component to standard cardiac care not only reduced psychological distress, but mortality and morbidity as well. Several specific outcome studies are especially notable. The Stanford Coronary Risk Intervention Project (SCRIP) employed a multicomponent treatment package to reduce multiple CVD risk factors via lifestyle modification involving diet, exercise, and medication. Over a 4-year period, there was a significant decline in coronary artery stenosis, documented by angiography.

Ornish and colleagues (179) reported that radical lifestyle alterations over a 5-year period in patients with known CVD showed an angiographically documented slight reduction in coronary artery stenosis compared with a significant increase in patients receiving usual medical care. Intervention components consisted of a low-fat vegetarian diet, aerobic exercise, smoking cessation, and stress-reduction training in the context of a supportive social milieu. Coronary perfusion abnormalities

also decreased as a result of the intervention (103). The Ornish program has subsequently been employed in multiple clinical settings, and a recent composite analysis based on data from eight independent medical centers reported positive changes in both physiologic (lipids, body fat, blood pressure) and psychosocial (quality of life, stress, depression, hostility) measures (8).

Multicomponent interventions such as these are clearly effective in reducing CVD risk, but make it difficult to specify the nature of the treatment effects. Nonetheless, they underscore the importance of lifestyle factors in risk management, an obvious point of emphasis in any exercise program for medical patients. It is also important to emphasize that CVD is frequently accompanied by emotional reactivity (stress, anxiety, depression) reflecting either the primary (stress-based) impact of the disease itself or a secondary reaction, and that this emotional reactivity should be addressed either in terms of the general guidelines previously enumerated or via referral to an appropriate mental health specialist. Although exercise may be an effective antidote for depression, dealing with cognitively based motivational factors requires interpersonal skill, sensitivity, and patience. Exercise professionals working with CVD (and other controlled chronic illnesses) would do well to augment their training in developing aerobic, strength, and flexibility programs with relaxation and other stress management skills. Of clinical significance is evidence that depressive symptoms may reflect "vital exhaustion," an inflammation-based precursor of myocardial infarction (MI) in some patients (21,22).

Similar issues arise with post-MI or ischemic CVD patients, exacerbated by the psychological trauma of an acute, life-threatening event. Depression in particular, as well as anxiety and other manifestations of emotional stress, are both common and persistent in the aftermath of MI, and depression in particular is predictive of subsequent 18-month cardiac mortality (93). Depressed patients are also less likely to follow through on recommendations to reduce risk of subsequent MIs (243).

However, despite widespread prevalence, there is presently no consensus concerning the relationship between CVD-based depression syndrome and standard psychiatric diagnosis with respect to underlying cause(s) or optimal treatment (119). Nonetheless, the frequency with which this condition is encountered makes clinical management a high priority (233). The AACVPR recently issued a position statement advocating early screening and treatment of post-MI depression (113) in the context of cardiac rehabilitation. Both antidepressants (SSRIs) and CBT, either singly or in combination, were identified as effective treatment options.

The effects of psychosocial interventions have been studied following both MI and ischemia (43,45). Ischemic heart disease is of particular interest because of its close association with stress and further complications, including MI. In a landmark study, the effects of aerobic exercise and a stress management program (SMP) on postischemic patients were compared with usual medical care over a 5-year period in older male and female CVD patients (43). The SMP was based on cognitive/social learning principles (similar to CBT) and also included training in progressive muscle relaxation (PMR) and electromyography (EMG) biofeedback. Participants in the SMP experienced fewer subsequent cardiac events and also incurred lower medical costs. This study was subsequently replicated using a stronger research design (45), at which time both SMP and exercise were found to reduce depression, distress, and cardiovascular abnormalities in comparison with usual medical care. Components of the SMP that could be adapted for use with exercise patients include (a) education concerning stress and cardiac function, (b) training in learning to recognize the impact of negative thoughts and acquire relaxation skills, and (c) establishing a supportive social network.

Similar results for post-MI patients were reported by the same research group in a large-scale, multicenter, randomized control trial to evaluate the impact of exercise and CBT on post-MI depression, mortality, and subsequent adverse events in older men and women. The Enhancing Recovery in Coronary Heart Disease (EN-RICHD) study found that aerobic exercise in particular was helpful in reducing mortality and subsequent infarction in MI patients with either depression or low social support (44). In contrast, neither medication nor CBT for depression affected mortality more than usual care, but patients who were unresponsive to either intervention had elevated risk of late mortality (55). In a separate analysis, CBT was found to have a modest positive impact on quality of life (71).

Neither CBT nor other psychosocial interventions are really intended to directly affect biological markers of health or disease, and it is no surprise when such negative findings are reported, as was recently the case (60). Rather, such practices are more likely to affect psychologic mediators, such as self-efficacy and self-regulatory skills, which in turn affect motivation and treatment adherence (217). The impact of such interventions can be further amplified if implemented not only by patients, but by family members as well, who are also otherwise vulnerable to emotional distress and ineffective coping strategies (221).

STROKE

CVD, including stroke, ranks second worldwide in all-cause mortality (48). Stroke has devastating consequences, and prevention is not only desirable, but feasible in the majority of cases. Pharmacologic treatments for precursors of stroke, including hypertension, clot formation, and elevated lipids, are routinely recom-

mended (48), but diet, exercise, stress management, and other lifestyle modifications contribute significant protective effects as well. Management of emotional problems is also important, because both anxiety and depression contribute to risk of hypertension, a precursor of stroke (124).

In addition to physical and cognitive impairments, stroke impairs psychological functioning. Depression is a common sequel, and it appears appropriate to consider psychosocial interventions in the aftermath (174). Poststroke depression is related to both cerebral localization and secondary emotional reactions. In addition, management must take into account degree of cognitive and motor impairment present; obviously, presence of aphasia and other communicative impediments would interfere with psychotherapy. However, for patients without disabling language impairments, cognitively oriented interventions are recommended (132). A recent review and formulation of a biosocial approach to poststroke depression (156) recommended increasing emphasis on cognitive and behavioral management strategies in addition to pharmacotherapy. The behaviorally oriented model of depression by Lewinsohn et al. (145) is potentially applicable because of its emphasis on formulating pleasant experiences and positively reinforcing social interactions. An added advantage of such an approach is that it can incorporate caregivers and others in the patient's network as therapeutic resources. Reducing risk of subsequent stroke is another important intervention target, as suggested by results of a health promotion program for African-American stroke survivors, in which a 12-week intervention showed significant, positive changes in lipid levels, fitness, strength, and social isolation (196). Clearly, however, prevention of stroke is preferable to postincident intervention, and exercise specialists are a key resource in encouraging those at risk to develop healthy lifestyle patterns to reduce contributory risk factors.

CHRONIC OBSTRUCTIVE PULMONARY DISEASE

Chronic obstructive pulmonary disease, defined as "non-reversible pulmonary function impairment," is the fourth leading cause of death in the United States (153). Like CVD and stroke, it extracts a substantial personal, social, and economic toll, owing to the debilitating symptoms, functional impairment, and need for long-term care. The clinical course of COPD is a spiraling cycle that begins with dyspnea and progresses through reduced physical activity, deconditioning, and ultimately to a state of disability (20). Guidelines for clinical care (1) have traditionally emphasized smoking cessation, pharmacologic management, and pulmonary rehabilitation. Training to minimize dyspnea and promote physical activity are important treatment components and appear to be effective if consistently utilized (201). However, the cost of such interventions can be substantial to begin with and escalate over time (185), and may not address psychological factors (depression and anxiety) that can limit treatment adherence and exacerbate symptomatology.

Psychosocial interventions designed to foster active self-management and to limit the adverse impact of depression and anxiety are a relatively recent addition to clinical practice that appear to be effective if consistently utilized (201). Incorporating psychosocial interventions into routine COPD rehabilitation is of relatively recent origin, despite the fact that both depression and anxiety are common comorbid factors that markedly attenuate quality of life (68) and may interfere not only with rehabilitation, but also with effective self-regulation of lifestyle behaviors. For example, smoking is strongly linked to COPD; the 2002 National Health Interview Surveys reported that 36.2% of adults with COPD were smokers. In addition, it is astonishing that only half reported trying to stop smoking, and of these, only 14.6% succeeded in eliminating this life-threatening habit (205). Significantly, this same survey reported that fewer than 25% of current smokers or recent quitters reported receiving cessation advice from healthcare professionals, but even advice and social support may not be enough to help patients change their behavior (241). Ironically, smoking is negatively associated with long-term treatment participation, according to interviews conducted with long-term (11-year) survivors involved in the Lung Health Study (218).

Dyspnea, a key symptom, creates acute distress symptoms of anxiety and even panic. Not surprisingly, anxiety disorder in patients with COPD reportedly occurs at two to three times the rate of the general population and significantly more frequently than in most other medical conditions (49). This finding may in part account for high rates of emergency room visits and utilization of other forms of healthcare resources, which to some extent can be contained by applying a model of chronic illness management used successfully with other diseases that encourages informed decision making, self-management, and use of authoritative information (4).

Both CBT and SSRI antidepressants have been effectively used to treat psychosocial distress in COPD, although medications sometimes used to treat depression and anxiety, including tricyclic antidepressants and benzodiazepines, are not recommended (53). CBT helps reduce the impact of negative, sometimes catastrophic thinking by teaching patients to monitor (i.e., notice) rather than become preoccupied with mental rumination. It is also paired with some form of relaxation training to help counteract accompanying SNS activation. These techniques are helpful with older adults (224) and especially applicable with COPD patients. In one study, a two-hour, group-based CBT session teaching cognitive and relaxation strategies with follow-up home practice

for 6 weeks reduced anxiety and depression symptoms significantly more than an education-only control condition (137). A promising intervention currently under way utilizes a group-based CBT intervention to foster increased compliance with physical activity recommendations in COPD patients, using a model successful with other chronic medical conditions (90).

METABOLIC DISEASE

Diabetes

Physical activity and metabolism are interdependent, and physical inactivity is associated with physiologic changes that alter energy balance, increase insulin resistance, promote muscle atrophy, and consequently further reduce exercise capacity (41). In diabetes, metabolic processes are disrupted either because of inadequate pancreatic insulin secretion (type 1) or resistance to cellular insulin absorption (type 2); gestational diabetes is another form associated with pregnancy. The long-term consequences of uncontrolled diabetes are profound, resulting in chronic disability and global systemic failure. Among its effects are vision loss (as a result of retinopathy), kidney failure, peripheral neuropathy, and CNS dysfunction affecting multiple organs and functions (12). Type 1 diabetes can be managed with supplementary insulin, but the process of monitoring and stabilizing insulin levels requires constant attention and care. Type 2 diabetes is strongly influenced by diet and physical activity and thus potentially at least can be controlled by lifestyle adjustments. However, both type 1 diabetes and obesity are reaching epidemic proportions in Westernized countries, affecting not only adults but increasingly children as well. The problem of insulin resistance is of relatively recent origin and has profound implications for health on a global scale (240) because it is linked to a lethal syndrome of risk factors, including obesity, elevated low-density lipoprotein (LDL) cholesterol, low high-density lipoprotein (HDL) cholesterol, hyperglycemia, hypertension associated with type 2 diabetes, and CVD (162).

The American Diabetes Association (ADA) recognizes physical activity as a potential therapeutic agent for both type 1 and type 2 diabetes, provided it is preceded by a thorough medical assessment to evaluate cardiovascular, retinal, and CNS status. Prescriptive guidelines have been published by ADA and recently summarized (13). Physical activity is especially helpful in regulating insulin activity in overweight individuals, and there appears to be a dose-response effect related more to exercise volume than intensity (118).

The potential of physical activity for insulin regulation warrants consideration of psychosocial factors related to motivation, self-efficacy, and self-regulation. Both cognitive and behavioral strategies appear to be helpful in this regard for type 2 diabetes (131). Depression is a key factor, affecting more than 25% of type 1 and 2 diabetic patients and having a negative impact on insulin, medication, and dietary management (148), all of which in turn affect physical activity level, and the relationship is reciprocal. The presence of depression in diabetes is associated with functional disability—the capacity or lack thereof to carry out daily activities (80). A recent review of psychological complications linked to diabetes (6) concluded that although several moderator variables (including age, sex, and social support) influence the nature and severity of such impairments, educating patients and physicians about their manifestations and effects is critically important. Treatment options include CBT, family/social, and problem-oriented interventions. Several studies employing CBT-based interventions support this recommendation.

The effects of a group-based diabetic education program plus CBT (compared with education alone) on DSM-based major depression in type 2 diabetic patients was evaluated in one study (149). More than three fourths of those in the CBT group showed a significant decline on depression inventory scores, versus approximately one fourth of those in the education-only condition. Significantly, glycemic levels (glycosylated hemoglobin, Hba1c) improved as well, suggesting improved self-management.

More recently, short-term, group-based CBT was effective in improving self-efficacy and mood in adult type I diabetic patients with poor glycemic control, nearly half of whom likely experienced clinically significant depression (235). However, the treatment effect of CBT did not differ from that of an education-based control group, nor was there is a significant improvement in glycemic control. Self-care behavior was the target of a short-term, CBT-based intervention in adult diabetic patients, who attended six sessions focusing on obstacles to self-care, cognitive factors, and ways to promote self-regulation. At the program's conclusion, participants showed an improvement in goal setting, and those who engaged in self-monitoring (using activity records) achieved the greatest behavioral changes.

Obesity

Like diabetes, obesity is a health problem of epidemic proportions. It is associated with risk of metabolic and other disorders, and rates of both obesity and diabetes are increasing in virtually all segments of the population (169). Currently, more than half the U.S. population is classified as overweight (body mass index [BMI] ≥25) or obese (BMI >30). To counteract excess weight, the ACSM advocates combining increased energy expenditure with reduced intake to effect controlled, gradual loss (122), and there is ample evidence that physical activity lowers insulin resistance, a stimulus to weight gain (73). Empirically validated procedures to control obesity include surgery, pharmacotherapy, and behavioral strate-

gies (66). However, losing weight and, more importantly, keeping it off, is not easy. For this reason, behavioral and cognitive-behavioral interventions have been developed to enhance motivation and persistence. Early behavioral models focused on environmental cues, such as stimuli to eating, and advocated controlling exposure, whereas subsequent interventions adopted a broader focus, incorporating emotional and cognitive factors (88). These elements are integrated into CBT via strategies that include (a) self-monitoring dysfunctional thoughts, (b) controlling access to eating cues (stimulus control), (c) cognitive restructuring related to maladaptive beliefs about weight and how to control it, (d) effective stress management, and (e) social support (89).

Structured interventions based on CBT have tended to emphasize in particular the common problem of regaining weight previously lost. Long-term weight maintenance may entail a combination of ongoing weight monitoring, cognitive strategies to help avoid negative thinking that can cause relapses, and behavioral programming to control energy expenditure and intake (66). Despite such efforts, long-term compliance tends to be low (163), but it can be improved when CBT is embedded in an interdisciplinary treatment framework, including nutritional counseling and exercise, as reported in one study that involved an initial 6-week hospitalization stay (102). Following up behavioral intervention with a program of monitored physical activity has also been shown to be effective in long-term weight loss (237), further underscoring the importance of physical activity in managing obesity, especially at relatively high volumes (123). However, physical activity alone does not appear to ensure weight loss maintenance, as reported by a recent study comparing the effects of a CBT-based intervention with a behaviorally oriented program emphasizing physical activity, which found that the cognitively based intervention results in significantly greater weight loss and maintenance (223).

Collectively, these studies suggest that cognitive-based strategies are helpful in controlling obesity, especially in the context of an integrative management program that includes, but is not limited to, physical activity. Both psychological (213) and activity-based (212) interventions are empirically validated weight management strategies, the effects of which appear to be most likely sustained when they are combined. A recent review of both short- and long-term results of behavioral/cognitive-behavioral interventions advocated an approach that is (a) goal oriented; (b) process oriented; and (c) strives for small, incremental changes (238). The emphasis on "process" factors is especially relevant for clinical exercise specialists working with obese patients. It advocates helping patients specify what it is they want to modify and how to bring this about based on an analysis of behavior chains that can lead to episodes of overeating or other behaviors incompatible with goals (e.g., lose weight, alter body composition). Consistent with previous recommendations, the basic intervention model teaches self-monitoring, stimulus control, and cognitive restructuring in the context of programs designed to provide structure and social support.

Metabolic Syndrome

Much of what has been said about diabetes and obesity can be applied to the metabolic syndrome (MS), a related and potentially lethal mix of central obesity plus two of several additional symptoms (elevated triglycerides, low HDL, high blood pressure, and elevated fasting glucose level), according to the International Diabetes Federation (IDF) consensus statement (121). A similar definition, focusing on cholesterol management, was previously formulated by the National Cholesterol Education Program Adult Treatment Panel III (172) and is widely cited. A recent epidemiologic study (3) reported that IDF-based prevalence rates may be even higher than the figure of nearly 25% reported using ATP III criteria (86). It is especially alarming not only that the MS is increasing rapidly in adults, but that childhood obesity, now at an epidemic level, is an early risk factor (46). Prevalence rates are also high in African-American women (62).

Psychosocial interventions for the MS have focused on behavioral, cognitive, and emotional aspects. It has recently been hypothesized that SNS overactivation may be a significant contributor (152), and consequently, management techniques to reduce SNS activation are likely to prove helpful. According to these authors, both diet and physical activity can have this effect, but in addition, CBT-based interventions should be considered as well. Significantly, depression has recently been shown to be an MS risk factor (111), independent of variations in clinical definitions (193).

Because of the multifaceted nature of MS, it is important to integrate intervention strategies (57). As with the other metabolic disorders discussed in this section, weight management is of critical importance and can best be achieved via CBT-based strategies for increasing energy output via physical activity and reducing weight via controlling eating patterns. Concurrent management of emotional disorders, especially depression, via CBT and/or pharmacotherapy should be considered a primary factor for immediate attention, as should treatment of hypertension, which places patients at risk for further cardiovascular complications, including stroke and diabetes (99).

The MS calls for radical lifestyle changes that can be a daunting challenge for healthcare professionals and patients alike. Weight management and increasing physical activity are of fundamental importance, but it is important to have an overall plan that addresses the many complications that accompany this disorder. An extremely useful overview of lifestyle interventions has recently been proposed (87) that is relevant not only for MS specifically, but also for the spectrum of metabolic conditions discussed in this chapter. The key components of this intervention model are as follows:

A. Preliminary assessment of obesity level, eating and exercise patterns, emotional status, and degree of motivation.
B. Lifestyle interventions, incorporating (a) setting reasonable goals for weight loss, (b) raising self-awareness as a means of enhancing self-regulation, (c) developing a problem-solving attitude toward common compliance problems, (d) stress management skills, (e) cognitive restructuring, (f) relapse prevention strategies, (g) social support, (h) behavioral contracting to increase health-oriented behaviors, and (i) pharmacotherapy as needed.

SUMMARY

Psychosocial interventions can have a significant impact on increasing healthy behaviors and eliminating those that are harmful. All of the diseases discussed in this chapter—CVD, stroke, COPD, diabetes, obesity, and the metabolic syndrome—are largely preventable via healthy lifestyle patterns. Unfortunately, we are currently facing the prospect of increases in most of these conditions because of an aging population, lack of prevention-oriented initiatives at a sociocultural level, and an overall largely sedentary population (77). Moreover, there has been insufficient progress on amelioration of psychological conditions, including the SAD trio (stress, anxiety, depression) discussed here, despite the attention called to these conditions by the U.S. Surgeon General years ago in the context of an integrated view of mental and physical health. And the recent Healthy People 2010 Midcourse Review (234) revealed that of 14 objectives related to promoting mental health and treating mental illness, only three had moved toward or met the targeted goal.

There are, however, some promising developments, including formation of the New Freedom Commission on Mental Health, designed to address three problems with the current system: (a) the stigma associated with mental illness, (b) disparities in mental health care, and (c) a fragmented delivery system (75). There is also a clear trend toward greater integration of psychosocial interventions with traditional medical treatment of chronic disease, consistent with Engle's biopsychosocial model (83). Clinical exercise professionals can play an important role in this more integrative management of chronic illnesses by developing a sensitivity to psychologically based impediments to physical activity, knowing when to refer patients for mental health services, and incorporating basic elements of the cognitive-behavioral perspective described here into their day-to-day work as a way of encouraging self-efficacy and self-regulatory capacities.

REFERENCES

1. ACCP/AACVPR Pulmonary Rehabilitation Guidelines Panel. Pulmonary rehabilitation: Joint ACCP/AACVPR evidence-based guidelines. *Chest.* 1997;112:1363–1396.

2. Adams KJ, Salmon P. Acute adjustments for stress. *Strength and Conditioning Journal.* 2002;24(1):63–64.

3. Adams RJ, Appleton S, Wilson DH, et al. Population comparison of two clinical approaches to the metabolic syndrome. *Diabetes Care.* 2005;28(11):2777–2779.

4. Adams SG, Smith PK, Allan PF, Anzueto A, Pugh JA, Cornell JE. Systematic review of the chronic care model in chronic obstructive pulmonary disease prevention and management. *Arch Int Med.* 2007;167:551–561.

5. Ader R, Cohen N. Behaviorally conditioned immunosuppression. *Psychosom Med.* 1975;37(4):333–340.

6. Adili F, Larijani B, Haghighatpanah M. Diabetic patients: psychological aspects. *Ann N Y Acad Sci.* 2006;1084:329–349.

7. Ajzen I. *Attitudes, Personality, and Behavior.* Chicago: Dorsey Press; 1988.

8. Aldana SG, Greenlaw R, Thomas D, et al. The influence of an intense cardiovascular disease risk factor modification program. *Prev Cardiol.* 2004;7(1):19–25.

9. Allen NB, Blaskhi G, Gullone E. Mindfulness-based psychotherapies: a review of conceptual foundations, empirical evidence and practical considerations. *A N Z J Psychiatry.* 2006;40: 285–294.

10. Allport G. *Personality: A Psychological Interpretation.* New York: Holt; 1937.

11. American College of Sports Medicine. *ACSM's Guidelines for Exercise Testing and Prescription.* 8th ed. Philadelphia: Lippincott Williams and Wilkins; 2009.

12. American Diabetes Association. Diagnosis and classification of diabetes mellitus. *Diabetes Care.* 2007;30(S1):S42–S47.

13. American Diabetes Association. Physical activity/exercise and diabetes. *Diabetes Care.* 2004;27(S1):S58–S62.

14. American Psychiatric Association. *Diagnostic and Statistical Manual of Mental Disorders.* 4th ed. Washington (DC): American Psychiatric Association; 1994.

15. American Psychiatric Association. *Diagnostic and Statistical Manual of Mental Disorders.* 4th ed. Text Revision. Washington (DC): American Psychiatric Association; 2000.

16. Anda R, Williamson D, Jones D, et al. Depressed affect, hopelessness, and the risk of ischemic heart disease in a cohort of U.S. adults. *Epidemiology.* 1993;4:285–294.

17. Antoni MH, Baggert L, Ironson G, et al. Cognitive behavioral stress management intervention buffers distress responses and immunological changes following notification of HIV-1 seropositivity. *J Consult Clin Psych.* 1991;59:906–915.

18. Antonovsky A. The structure and properties of the sense of coherence scale. *Soc Sci Med.* 1993;36:725–733.

19. Antonovsky A. *Unraveling the Mystery of Health: How People Manage Stress and Stay Well.* San Francisco: Jossey-Bass; 1987.

20. Anzueto A. Clinical course of chronic obstructive pulmonary disease: review of therapeutic interventions. *Am J Med.* 2006;119 (10A):S46–S53.

21. Appels A. Psychological prodromata of myocardial infarction and sudden death. *Psychoth Psychosom.* 1980;34(2–3):187–195.

22. Appels A, Bar FW, Bar J, Bruggeman C, de Baets M. Inflammation, depressive symptomatology, and coronary artery disease. *Psychosom Med.* 2000;62(5):601–605.

23. Armstrong LE, VanHeest JL. The unknown mechanism of the overtraining syndrome. *Sports Med.* 2002;32(3):185–209.

24. Artal M, Sherman C. Exercise against depression. The Physician and Sportsmedicine [Internet]. 1998;26(10). Available from: <www.physsportsmed.com/issues/1998/10Oct/artal.htm>. Accessed May 4, 2001.

25. Asay TP, Lambert MJ. The empirical case for the common factors in therapy: quantitative findings. In: Hubble M, Duncan BL, Miller SD, editors. *The Heart and Soul of Change: What Works in Therapy.* Washington (DC): American Psychological Association; 1999. p. 23–55.

26. Bahrke MS, Morgan WP. Anxiety reduction following exercise and meditation. *Cog Ther Res.* 1978;2(4):323–333.

27. Bandura A. Health promotion by social cognitive means. *Health Educ Behav.* 2004;31(2):143–164.

28. Bandura A. The primacy of self-regulation in health promotion. *Appl Psych: An Int Review.* 2005;54(2):245–254.

29. Bandura A. *Principles of Behavior Modification.* New York: Rinehart & Winston; 1969.

30. Bandura A. *Self-Efficacy: The Exercise of Control.* New York: Freeman; 1997.

31. Bandura A. *Social Foundations of Thought and Action: A Social Cognitive Theory.* Englewood Cliffs (NJ): Prentice-Hall; 1986.

32. Bandura A. *Social Learning Theory.* Englewood Cliffs (NJ): Prentice-Hall; 1977.

33. Barefoot JC, Dahlstrom WG, Williams RB. Hostility, CHD incidence, and total mortality: a 25-year follow-up study of 255 physicians. *Psychosom Med.* 1983;45(1):59–63.

34. Barger SD, Sydeman SJ. Does generalized anxiety disorder predict coronary heart disease risk factors independent of major depressive disorder? *J Affect Disord.* 2005;88(1):87–91.

35. Barlow D, Allen LB, Choate ML. Toward a unified treatment for emotional disorders. *Behav Ther.* 2004;3 (2):205–230.

36. Barlow DH. *Anxiety and Its Disorders: The Nature and Treatment of Anxiety and Panic.* 2nd ed. New York: Guilford; 2002.

37. Barlow DH, editor. *Clinical Handbook of Psychological Disorders.* 3rd ed. New York: Guilford; 2001.

38. Bartholomew JB, Morrison D, Ciccolo JT. Effects of acute exercise on mood and well-being in patients with major depressive disorder. *Med Sci Sports Exerc.* 2005;37(12):2032–2037.

39. Beck AT. *Depression: Clinical, Experimental, and Theoretical Aspects.* New York: Harper and Row; 1967.

40. Beck AT, Rush AJ, Shaw BF, Emery G. *Cognitive Therapy of Depression.* New York: Guilford; 1979.

41. Biolo G, Ciocchi B, Piccoli A, et al. Metabolic consequences of physical inactivity. *J Renal Nutr.* 2005;15(1):49–53.

42. Blue CL. The predictive capacity of the theory of reasoned action and the theory of planned behavior in exercise research: an integrated literature review. *Res Nurs Health.* 1995;18(2): 105–121.

43. Blumenthal JA, Babyak M, Wei J, et al. Usefulness of psychosocial treatment of mental stress-induced myocardial ischemia in men. *Am J Cardiol.* 2002;89:164–168.

44. Blumenthal JA, Babyak MA, Carney RM, et al. Exercise, depression, and mortality after myocardial infarction in the ENRICHD trial. *Med Sci Sports Exerc.* 2004;36(5):746–755.

45. Blumenthal JA, Sherwood A, Babyak MA, et al. Effects of exercise and stress management training on markers of cardiovascular risk in patients with ischemic heart disease. *JAMA.* 2005;293: 1626–1634.

46. Boney CM, Verma A, Tucker R, Vohr BR. Metabolic syndrome in childhood: association with birth weight, maternal obesity, and gestational diabetes mellitus. *Pediatrics* 2005;115(3):e290–e296.

47. Borkovec TD, Inz J. The nature of worry in generalized anxiety disorder: a predominance of thought activity. *Behav Res Ther.* 1990;28(2):153–158.

48. Brass LM. Strategies for primary and secondary stroke prevention. *Clin Cardiol.* 2006;29(10S):II21–II7.

49. Brenes GA. Anxiety and chronic obstructive pulmonary disease: prevalence, impact, and treatment. *Psychosom Med.* 2003;65:963–970.

50. Brewin CR. Theoretical foundations of cognitive-behavioral therapy for anxiety and depression. *Ann Review Psychol.* 1996;47: 33–57.

51. Brindley DN, McCann BS, Niaura R, Stoney CM, Suarez EC. Stress and lipoprotein metabolism: modulators and mechanisms. *Metabolism*. 1993;42(9, S1):3–15.

52. Buckworth J, Dishman RK. *Exercise Psychology*. Champaign (IL): Human Kinetics; 2002.

53. Burgess A, Kunik ME, Stanley MA. Chronic obstructive pulmonary disease: assessing and treating psychological issues in patients with COPD. *Geriatrics*. 2005;60(12):18–21.

54. Cannon WB. *The Wisdom of the Body*. New York: Norton; 1939.

55. Carney RM, Blumenthal JA, Freedland KE, et al. Depression and late mortality after myocardial infarction in the Enhancing Recovery in Coronary Heart Disease (ENRICHD) study. *Psychosom Med*. 2004;66:466–474.

56. Carney RM, Freedland KE, Veith RC. Depression, the autonomic nervous system, and coronary heart disease. *Psychosom Med*. 2005;67(S1):S29–S33.

57. Cassells HB, Haffner SM. The metabolic syndrome: risk factors and management. *J Cardiovasc Nurs*. 2006;21(4):306–313.

58. Chambliss DL, Baker MJ, Baucom DH, et al. Update on empirically validated therapies, II. *Clin Psychol*. 1998;51(1):3–16.

59. Chevalier P, Cottraux C, Mollard E, et al. Prevention of implantable defibrillator shocks by cognitive behavioral therapy: a pilot trial. *Am Heart J*. 2006;151:191.e1–.e6.

60. Claesson M, Birgander LS, Jansson JH, et al. Cognitive-behavioural stress management does not improve biological cardiovascular risk indicators in women with ischaemic heart disease: a randomized-controlled trial. *J Int Med*. 2006;260:320–331.

61. Clark DA, Beck AT. *Scientific Foundations of Cognitive Theory and Therapy of Depression*. New York: Wiley; 1999.

62. Clark LA. Assessment and diagnosis of personality disorder: perennial issues and an emerging reconceptualization. *Ann Rev Psychol*. 2007;58:227–257.

63. Cohen S. The Pittsburgh common cold studies: psychosocial predictors of susceptibility to respiratory infectious illness. *Int J Behav Med*. 2005;12(3):123–131.

64. Cohen S, Frank E, Doyle WJ, Skoner DP, Rabin BS, Gwaltney JM. Types of stressors that increase susceptibility to the common cold in healthy adults. *Health Psychol*. 1998;17(3):214–223.

65. Cohen S, Herbert TB. Health psychology: psychological factors and physical disease from the perspective of human psychoneuroimmunology. *Ann Rev Psychol*. 1996;47:113–142.

66. Cooper Z, Fairburn CG. A new cognitive behavioral approach to the treatment of obesity. *Behav Res Ther*. 2001;39:499–511.

67. Costa PT, McCrae RR. Personality assessment in psychosomatic medicine. *Adv Psychosom Med*. 1987;17:71–82.

68. Cully JA, Graham DP, Stanley MA, et al. Quality of life in patients with chronic obstructive pulmonary disease and comorbid anxiety or depression. *Psychosomatics*. 2006;47:312–319.

69. Dantzer R, Kelley KW. Twenty years of research on cytokine-induced sickness behavior. *Brain Behav Immun*. 2007;21(2):153–160.

70. Davidson KW, Rieckmann N, Rapp MA. Definitions and distinctions among depressive syndromes and symptoms: implications for a better understanding of the depression-cardiovascular disease association. *Psychosom Med*. 2005;67(S1):S6–S9.

71. de Leon M, Czajkowski SM, Freedland KE, et al. The effect of a psychosocial intervention and quality of life after acute myocardial infarction: the Enhancing Recovery in Coronary Heart Disease (ENRICHD) clinical trial. *J Cardiopulm Rehabil*. 2006;26(1):9–13.

72. de Morr MHM, Beem AL, Stubbe JH, Boomsa DI, de Gues EJC. Regular exercise, anxiety, depression and personality: a population-based study. *Prev Med*. 2006;42(4):273–279.

73. DeFronzo RA, Sherman RS, Kraemer N. Effect of physical training on insulin action in obesity. *Diabetes*. 1987;36(12):1379–1385.

74. **U.S. Department of Health and Human Services.** *Mental Health: Culture, Race, and Ethnicity—A Supplement to Mental Health: A Report of the Surgeon General*. **Rockville (MD): US Department of Health and Human Services, Substance Abuse and Mental Health Services Administration, Center for Mental Health Services, National Institute for Mental Health; 2001.**

75. U.S. Department of Health and Human Services. New Freedom Commission on Mental Health. *Achieving the Promise: Transforming Mental Health Care in America. Final Report*. [Internet]. 2003. Available from: www.mentalhealthcommission.gov/reports/FinalReport/. DHHS Pub. No. SMA-03-3832. Accessed April 30, 2007.

76. Dishman R. Exercise adherence. In: Singer R, Murphey M, Tennant LK, editors. *Handbook of Research on Sport Psychology*. New York: Macmillan; 1993. p. 779–798.

77. Dishman RK, Buckworth J. Increasing physical activity: a quantitative synthesis. *Med Sci Sports Exerc*. 1996;28(6):706–719.

78. Dishman RK, Jackson EM. Exercise, fitness, and stress. *Int J Sports Psychol*. 2000;31(2):175–203.

79. Ditto B, Echlache M, Golman N. Short-term autonomic and cardiovascular effects of mindfulness body scan meditation. *Ann Behav Med*. 2006;32(3):227–234.

80. Egede LE. Diabetes, major depression, and functional disability among U.S. adults. *Diabetes Care*. 2004;27(2):421–428.

81. Ekkekakis P, Acevedo EO. Affect responses to acute exercise: toward a psychobiological dose-response model. In: Acevedo E, Ekkekakis P, editors. *Psychobiology of Physical Activity*. Champaign (IL): Human Kinetics; 2006. p. 91–109.

82. Emmelkamp PM, van Oppen P. Cognitive interventions in behavioral medicine. *Psychother Psychosom*. 1993;59(3–4):116–130.

83. Engle GL. The need for a new medical model: a challenge for biomedicine. *Science*. 1977;196(4286):129–136.

84. Fishbein M. A theory of reasoned action: some applications and implications. *Nebr Symp Motiv*. 1980;27:65–116.

85. Follete WC. Introduction to the special section on the development of theoretically coherent alternatives to the DSM system. *J Consult Clin Psychol*. 1996;64(6):1117–1119.

86. Ford ES, Giles WH, Dietz WH. Prevalence of the metabolic syndrome among US adults. *JAMA*. 2002;287(3):356–359.

87. Foreyt JP. Need for lifestyle intervention: how to begin. *Am J Cardiol*. 2005;96(Suppl):11E–14E.

88. Foreyt JP, Goodrick KK. Evidence for success of behavior modification in weight loss and control. *Ann Int Med*. 1993;119(7 part 2):698–701.

89. Foreyt JP, Poston, WS. What is the role of cognitive-behavior therapy in patient management? *Obesity Res*. 1998;6(SI):18S–22S.

90. Foy CG, Wickley KL, Adair N, et al. The reconditioning exercise and chronic obstructive pulmonary disease trial II (REACT II): rationale and study design for a clinical trial of physical activity among individuals with chronic obstructive pulmonary disease. *Contemp Clin Trials*. 2006;27:135–146.

91. Frank JD, Frank JB. *Persuasion and Healing: A Comparative Study of Psychotherapy*. Baltimore: Johns Hopkins University Press; 1991.

92. Franks CM. *Behavior Therapy: Appraisal and Status*. New York: McGraw-Hill; 1969.

93. Frasure-Smith N, Lesperance F, Talajic M. Depression and 18-month prognosis after myocardial infarction. *Circulation*. 1995;91:999–1005.

94. Friedman HS. Personality and disease: overview, review, and preview. In: Friedman H, editor. *Personality and Disease*. New York: Wiley; 1990. p. 3–13.

95. Friedman M, Rosenman RH. Association of specific overt behavior pattern with blood and cardiovascular findings. *JAMA*. 1959;169(12):1286–1296.

96. Friedman M, Rosenman RH. *Type A Behavior and Your Heart*. New York: Knopf; 1974.

97. Friedman R, Sobel D, Myers P, Caudill M, Benson H. Behavioral medicine, clinical health psychology, and cost offset. *Health Psychol*. 1995;14(6):509–518.

98. Gabbard GO, Lazar SG, Hornberger J, Spiegel D. The economic impact of psychotherapy: a review. *Am J Psych*. 1997;154(2):147–155.

99. Ganne S, Arora S, Karam J, McFarlane SI. Therapeutic interventions for hypertension in metabolic syndrome: a comprehensive approach. *Exp Rev Cardiovasc Ther.* 2007;5(2):201–11.

100. Gardner FL, Moore ZE. A mindfulness-acceptance-commitment-based approach to athletic performance enhancement: theoretical considerations. *Behav Ther.* 2004;35:707–723.

101. Gelenberg AJ, Hopkins HS. Assessing and treating depression in primary care medicine. *Am J Med.* 2007;120:105–108.

102. Golay A, Buclin S, Ybarra J, et al. New interdisciplinary cognitive-behavioral-nutritional approach to obesity treatment: a 5-year follow-up study. *Eat Weight Disord.* 2004;9(1):29–34.

103. Gould KL, Ornish D, Scherwitz L, et al. Changes in myocardial perfusion abnormalities by positron emission tomography after long-term, intense risk factor modification. *JAMA.* 1995;274(11):894–901.

104. Grant BF, Hasin DS, Stinson, et al. Co-occurrence of 12-month mood and anxiety disorders and personality disorders in the US: Results from the national epidemiology survey on alcohol and related conditions. *J Psychiatr Res.* 2005;39:1–9.

105. Grassi G. Sympathetic overdrive and cardiovascular risk in the metabolic syndrome. *Hypertens Res.* 2006;29:839–847.

106. Greeno CG, Wing RR. Stress-induced eating. *Psychol Bull.* 1994;115(3):444–464.

107. Harris AHS, Cronkite R, Moos R. Physical activity, exercise coping, and depression in a 10-year cohort study of depressed patients. *J Affecte Disord.* 2006;93:79–85.

108. Hayes S. Acceptance and commitment therapy, relational frame theory, and the third wave of behavioral and cognitive therapies. *Behav Ther.* 2004;35(4):639–665.

109. Hayes SC, Linehan VM, Linehan MM. *Mindfulness and Acceptance: Expanding the Cognitive-Behavioral Tradition.* New York: Guilford; 2004.

110. Hays PA. *Addressing Cultural Complexities in Practice: A Framework for Clinicians and Counselors.* Washington (DC): American Psychological Association; 2001.

111. Heiskanen TH, Niskanen LK, Hintikka JJ, et al. Metabolic syndrome and depression: a cross-section analysis. *J Clin Psych.* 2006;67(9):1422–1427.

112. Herning MM, Cook JH, Schneider JK. Cognitive behavioral therapy to promote exercise behavior in older adults: implications for physical therapists. *Journal of Geriatric Physical Therapy.* 2005;28(2):34–38.

113. Herridge ML, Stimler CE, Southard DR, et al. Depression screening in cardiac rehabilitation: AACVPR task force report. *J Cardiopulm Rehabil.* 2005;25:11–13.

114. Herring SA, Boyajian-O'Neill LA, Coppel DB, et al. Psychological issues related to injury in athletes and the team physician: a consensus statement *Med Sci Sport Exerc.* 2006; 38:2030–2034.

115. Hirschfeld RM, Montgomery SA, Keller MB, et al. Social functioning in depression: a review. *Clin Psych.* 2000;61(4):268–275.

116. Holmes TH, Rahe, RH. The social readjustment rating scale. *J Psychosom Res.* 1967;11(2):213–218.

117. Hoppes K. The application of mindfulness-based cognitive interventions in the treatment of co-occurring addictive and mood disorders. *CNS Spectrums.* 2006;11(11):829–851.

118. Houmard JA, Tanner JJ, Slentz CA, et al. Effect of the volume and intensity of exercise training on insulin sensitivity. *J Appl Physiol.* 2004;96:101–106.

119. Huffman JC, Smith FA, Quinn DK, Fricchione GL. Post-MI psychiatric syndromes: six unanswered questions. *Harvard Rev Psychiatry.* 2006;14(6):305–318.

120. Institute of Medicine. *Health and Behavior: The Interplay of Biological, Behavioral, and Societal Influences.* Washington (DC): National Academy Press; 2001.

121. International Diabetes Foundation. The IDF consensus worldwide definition of the metabolic syndrome. [Internet]. 2006. Available from: www.idf.org/webdata/docs/MetS_def_update2006.pdf. Accessed April 21, 2007.

122. Jakicic JM, Clark K, Coleman E, et al. American College of Sports Medicine position stand. Appropriate intervention strategies for weight loss and prevention of weight regain for adults. *Med Sci Sports Exerc.* 2001;33(12):2145–2156.

123. Jakicic JM, Otto AD. Treatment and prevention of obesity: What is the role of exercise? *Nutr Rev.* 2006;64(2 part 2):S57–S61.

124. Jonas BS, Franks P, Ingram DD. Are symptoms of anxiety and depression risk factors for hypertension? Longitudinal evidence from the National Health and Nutrition Examination Survey I Epidemiological Follow-Up Study. *Arch Fam Med.* 1997;6(1):43–49.

125. Kabat-Zinn J. *Full Catastrophe Living: Using the Wisdom of Your Body and Mind to Face Stress, Pain, and Illness.* New York: Delta; 1990.

126. Kawachi I, Sparrow D, Vokonas PS, Weiss ST. Symptoms of anxiety and risk of coronary heart disease: the normative aging study. *Circulation.* 2007;90:2225–2229.

127. Kessler RC, Akiskal HS, Amers M, et al. Prevalence and effects of mood disorders on work performance in a nationally representative sample of U.S. workers. *Am J Psychiatry.* 2006;163:1561–1568.

128. Kessler RC, Chiu WT, Demler O, Walters EE. Prevalence, severity, and comorbidity of 12-month DSM-IV disorders in the National Comorbidity Survey Replication. *Arch Gen Psychiatry.* 2005;62:617–627.

129. Ketterer MW, Mahr G, Goldberg AD. Psychological factors affecting a medical condition: ischemic coronary heart disease. *J Psychosom Res.* 2000;48:357–367.

130. Kiekolt-Glaser JK, Newton T. Marriage and health: his and hers. *Psychol Bull.* 2001;127(4):472–503.

131. Kirk AF, Mutrie N, MacIntyre PD, Fisher MB. Promoting and maintaining physical activity in people with type 2 diabetes. *Am J Prev Med.* 2004;27(4):289–296.

132. Kneebone II, Dunmore E. Psychological management of post-stroke depression. *Br J Clin Psychol.* 2000;39(1):53–65.

133. Kop WJ, Appels AP, Mendes de Leon CF, et al. Vital exhaustion predicts new cardiac events after successful coronary angioplasty. *Psychosom Med.* 1994;56:281–287.

134. Korte SM, Koolhaas JM, Wingfield JC, McEwen BS. The Darwinian concept of stress: benefits of allostasis and costs of allostatic load and the trade-offs in health and disease. *Neurosci Biobehav Rev.* 2005;29:3–38.

135. Krantz DS, Manuck SB. Acute psychophysiologic reactivity and risk of cardiovascular disease: a review and methodologic critique. *Psychol Bull.* 1984;96(3):43–464.

136. Krishnan KR. Treatment of depression in the medically ill. *J Clin Psychopharmacol.* 2005;25(S1):S14–S18.

137. Kunik ME, Braun U, Stanley MA, et al. One session cognitive behavioural therapy for elderly patients with chronic obstructive pulmonary disease. *Psychol Med.* 2001;31(4):717–723.

138. La Forge R. Aligning mind and body: exploring the disciplines of mindful exercise. *ACSM's Health and Fitness Journal.* 2005;9(5):7–13.

139. Lazarus RS. *Emotion and Adaptation.* New York: Oxford University Press; 1991.

140. Lazarus RS. How emotions influence performance in competitive sports. *Sport Psychol.* 2000(b);14(3):229–252.

141. Lazarus RS. *Stress and Emotion: A New Synthesis.* New York: Springer; 1999.

142. Lazarus RS. Toward better research on stress and coping. *Am Psychol.* 2000(a);55(6):665–673.

143. Lazarus RS, Folkman S. *Stress, Appraisal, and Coping.* New York: Springer; 1984.

144. Lehman M, Foster C, Keul J. Overtraining in endurance athletes: a brief review. *Med Sci Sports Exerc.* 1993;25(7):854–862.

145. Lewinsohn PM, Weinstein MS, Shaw DA. Depression: a clinical-research approach. In: Rubin R, Franks CM, editors. *Advances in Behavior Therapy.* New York: Academic Press; 1969. p. 231–240.

146. Linden W, Stossel C, Maurice J. Psychosocial interventions for patients with coronary artery disease: a meta-analysis. *Arch Int Med.* 1996;156 (7):745–752.

147. Long BC, van Staval R. Effects of exercise training on anxiety: a meta-analysis. *J Appl Sport Psychol.* 1995;7(2):167–189.

148. Lustman PJ, Clouse RE. Depression in diabetic patients: the relationship between mood and glycemic control. *J Diabetes Complications.* 2005;19:113–122.

149. Lustman PJ, Griffith LS, Freedland KE, et al. Cognitive behavior therapy for depression in type 2 diabetes mellitus: a randomized, controlled trial. *Ann Int Med.* 1998;129(8):613–621.

150. Maier SF, Watkins LR. Cytokines for psychologists: implications of bidirectional immune-to-brain communication for understanding behavior, mood, and cognition. *Psychol Rev.* 1998;105(1):83–107.

151. Maier SF, Watkins LR, Fleshner M. Psychoneuroimmunology: the interface between behavior, brain, and immunity. *Am Psychol.* 1994;49(12):1004–1017.

152. Mancia G, Bousquet P, Elghozi JL, et al. The sympathetic nervous system and the metabolic syndrome. *J Hypertens.* 2007;25: 909–920.

153. Mannino DM, Homa DM, Akinbami LJ, Ford ES, Redd SC. Chronic obstructive pulmonary disease surveillance—United States, 1971–2000. Surveillance Summaries [Internet]. 2000; 51(SS06). Available from: www.cdc.gov/mmwr/preview/ mmwrhtml/ss5106a1. htm. Accessed May 25, 2007.

154. Marcotte DE, Wilcox-Gök V. Estimating earnings losses due to mental illness: a quantile regression approach. *J Ment Health Policy Econ.* 2003;6:123–134.

155. Martinsen E. Exercise and depression. *Int J Sport Exerc Psychol.* 2005;3(4):469–483.

156. Mast BT, Vedrody S. Poststroke depression: a biopsychosocial approach. *Curr Psychiatry Rep.* 2006;8(1):25–33.

157. **Mazzeo RS, Cavanagh P, Evans WJ, et al. American College of Sports Medicine Position Stand: Exercise and physical activity for older adults. *Med Sci Sports Exerc.* 1998;30(6):992–1008.**

158. McCrae RR, Allik J, editors. *The Five-Factor Model of Personality Across Cultures.* New York: Kluwer Academic/Plenum; 2002.

159. McEwen B. Protective and damaging effects of stress mediators: central role of the brain. *Dialogues in Clinical Neuroscience.* 2006;8(4):367–381.

160. Meeusen R. Physical activity and neurotransmitter release. In: Acevedo E, Ekkekakis P, editors. Psychobiology of Physical Activity. Champaign (IL): Human Kinetics; 2006. p. 129–143.

161. Meichanbaum D. *Cognitive Behavior Modification: An Integrative Approach.* New York: Plenum; 1977.

162. Meigs JB. Epidemiology of the insulin resistance syndrome. *Curr Diab Rep.* 2003;3(1):73–79.

163. Melchionda N, Besteghi L, Di Domizio S, et al. Cognitive behavior therapy for obesity: one-year follow-up in a clinical setting. *Eat Weight Disord.* 2003;8(3):188–193.

164. Melzer K, Kayser B, Pichard C. Physical activity: the health benefits outweigh the risks. *Curr Opin Clin Nutr Metab Care.* 2004;7: 641–647.

165. Meyer T, Broocks A. Therapeutic impact of exercise on psychiatric diseases: guidelines for exercise testing and prescription. *Sports Med.* 2000;30(4):269–279.

166. Miller GE, Chen E, Zhou ES. If it goes up, must it come down? Chronic stress and the hypothalamic-pituitary-adrenocortical axis in humans. *Psychol Bull.* 2007;133(1):25–45.

167. Mischel W. *Personality and Assessment.* New York: Wiley; 1968.

168. Mischel W, Shoda Y. A cognitive-affective system theory of personality: reconceptualizing situations, dispositions, dynamics, and invariance in personality structure. *Psychol Rev.* 1995;102(2): 246–268.

169. Mokdad AH, Ford ES, Bowman BA, et al. Prevalence of obesity, diabetes, and obesity-related health risk factors, 2001. *JAMA.* 2003;289(1):76–79.

170. Morgan WP. Methodological considerations. In: Morgan W, editor. *Physical Activity and Mental Health.* Washington (DC): Taylor and Francis; 1997. p. 3–32.

171. Mumford E, Schlesinger HJ, Glass GV, Patrick C, Cuerdon T. A new look at evidence about reduced cost of medical utilization following mental health treatment. *J Psychother Pract Res.* 1998;7:65–86.

172. **NCEP Adult Treatment Panel III. Executive summary of the third report of the National Cholesterol Education Program (NCEP) expert panel on detection, evaluation, and treatment of high blood cholesterol in adults (Adult Treatment Panel III). *JAMA.* 2001;285(19):2486–2497.**

173. Nesse R. Is depression an adaptation? *Arch Gen Psychiatry.* 2000;57(1):14–20.

174. Nicholl CR, Lincoln NB, Muncaster K, Thomas S. Cognitions and post-stroke depression. *Br J Clin Psychol.* 2002;41:221–231.

175. Nutt DJ, Ballenger JC, Sheehan D, Wittchen HU. Generalized anxiety disorder: comorbidity, comparative biology, and treatment. *Int J Neuropsychopharmacol.* 2002;5(4):315–325.

176. O'Connor PJ, Raglin JS, Martinsen EW. Physical activity, anxiety and anxiety disorders. *Int J Sport Psychol.* 2000;31:136–155.

177. O'Neal HA, Dunn AL, Martinsen EW. Depression and exercise. *Int J Sport Psychol.* 2000;31:110–135.

178. Ogden J. Some problems with social cognitive models: a pragmatic and conceptual analysis. *Health Psychol.* 2003;22(4):424–428.

179. Ornish D, Scherwitz LW, Billings JH, et al. Intensive lifestyle changes for reversal of coronary heart disease. *JAMA.* 1998;280(23):2001–2007.

180. Pasic J, Levy WC, Sullivan MD. Cytokines in depression and heart failure. *Psychosom Med.* 2003;65:181–193.

181. **Pate RR, Pratt M, SN Blair, et al. Physical activity and public health: a recommendation from the Centers for Disease Control and Prevention and the American College of Sports Medicine. *JAMA.* 1995;273(5):402–407.**

182. **Pennebaker JW, editor. *Emotion, Disclosure, and Health.* Washington (DC): American Psychological Association; 1995.**

183. Perna FM, Antoni MH, Baum A, et al. Cognitive behavioral stress management effects on injury and illness among competitive athletes: a randomized clinical trial. *Ann Behav Med.* 2003;25(1): 66–73.

184. Perna FM, McDowell SL. Role of psychological stress in cortisol recovery from exhaustive exercise among elite athletes. *Int J Behav Med.* 1995;2(1):13–26.

185. Pierson DJ. Clinical practice guidelines for chronic obstructive pulmonary disease: a review and comparison of current resources. *Respir Care.* 2006;51(3):277–288.

186. Pitsavos C, Panagiotakos DB, Papageorgiou C, et al. Anxiety in relation to inflammation and coagulation markers, among healthy adults: the ATTICA study. *Atherosclerosis.* 2006;185:320–326.

187. Plante TG. Could the perception of fitness account for many of the mental and physical health benefits of exercise? *Adv Mind Body Med.* 1999;15:291–301.

188. Prochaska JO. How do people change, and how can we change to help many more people? In: Hubble M, Duncan BL, Miller SD, editors. *The Heart and Soul of Change: What Works in Therapy.* Washington (DC): American Psychological Association; 1999. p. 227–255.

189. Prochaska JO, DiClemente CC. Transtheoretical therapy: toward a more integrative model of change. *Psychotherapy: Theory, Research and Practice.* 1982;19:276–288.

190. Prochaska JO, Johnson S, Lee P. The transtheoretical model of behavior change. In: Shumaker S, Schron EB, Ockene JK, McBee WL, editors. *The Handbook of Health Behavior Change.* 2nd ed. New York: Springer; 1998. p. 59–84.

191. Raglin JS. Anxiolytic effects of physical activity. In: Morgan W, editor. *Physical Activity and Mental Health.* Washington (DC): Taylor and Francis; 1997. p. 107–126.

192. Raglin JS, Morgan WP. Influence of vigorous exercise on mood state. *Behav Therapist.* 1985;8(9):179–183.

193. Raikkonen K, Matthews KA, Kuller LH. Depressive symptoms and stressful life events predict metabolic syndrome among middle-aged women. *Diabetes Care.* 2007;30:872–877.

194. Raison CL, Capuron L, Miller AH. Cytokines sing the blues: inflammation and the pathogenesis of depression. *Trends Immunol.* 2006;27(1):23–31.

195. Rhodes RE, Smith, NE. Personality correlates of physical activity: a review and meta-analysis. *Br J Sports Med.* 2006;40(12): 958–965.

196. Rimmer JH, Braunschweig C, Silverman K, et al. Effects of a short-term health promotion intervention for a predominantly African-American group of stroke survivors. *Am J Prev Med.* 2000;18(4): 332–338.

197. Robertson N. Unexplained chest pain: a review of psychological conceptualizations and treatment efficacy. *Psychol Health Med.* 2006;11(2):255–263.

198. Rostad FG, Long BC. Exercise as a coping strategy for stress: a review. *Int J Sport Psychol.* 1996;27(2):197–222.

199. Rozanski A, Blumenthal JA, Kaplan J. Impact of psychological factors on the pathogenesis of cardiovascular disease and implications for therapy. *Circulation.* 1999;99:2192–2217.

200. Ryff CD, Singer B. The contours of positive human health. *Psychological Inquiry.* 1998;9(1):1–28.

201. Salman GF, Mosier MC, Beasley BW, Calkins DR. Rehabilitation for patients with chronic obstructive pulmonary disease: meta-analysis of randomized controlled trials. *J Gen Int Med.* 2003;18(3):213–221.

202. Salmon P. Effects of physical exercise on anxiety, depression, and sensitivity to stress: a unifying theory. *Clin Psychol Rev.* 2001;21 (1):33–61.

203. Salmon P, Sephton S, Weissbecker I, Hoover K, Ulmer C, Studts JL. Mindfulness meditation in clinical practice. *Cogn Behav Pract.* 2004;11:434–446.

204. Sapolsky RM. *Why Zebras Don't Get Ulcers.* 3rd ed. New York: Henry Holt; 2004.

205. Schiller JS, Ni H. Cigarette smoking and smoking cessation among persons with chronic obstructive pulmonary disease. *AM J Health Promot.* 2006;20(5):319–323.

206. Schneiderman N, Siegel SD. Mental and physical health influence each other. In: Lilienfeld S, O'Donohue WT, editors. *The Great Ideas of Clinical Science: 17 Principles That Every Mental Health Professional Should Understand.* New York: Routledge/Taylor and Francis; 2007. p. 329–346.

207. Schraufnagel TJ, Wagner AW, Miranda J, Roy-Byrne PP. Treating minority patients with depression and anxiety: What does the evidence tell us? *Gen Hosp Psychiatry.* 2006;28(1):27–36.

208. Schulberg HS, Katon W, Simon GE, Rush AJ. Treating major depression in primary care practice: an update of the Agency for Health Care Policy and Research Practice guidelines. *Arch Gen Psychiatry.* 1998;55(12):1121–1127.

209. Segal Z, Williams JM, Teasdale JD. *Mindfulness-Based Cognitive Therapy for Depression: A New Approach to Preventing Relapse.* New York: Guilford; 2002.

210. Seime RJ, Vickers KS. The challenges of treating depression with exercise: from evidence to practice. *Clin Psychol Sci Prac.* 2006;13: 194–197.

211. Seligman MEP. *Helplessness: On Depression, Development, and Death.* 2nd ed. New York: W.H. Freeman; 1991.

212. Shaw K, Gennat H, O'Rourke P, Del Mar C. Exercise for overweight or obesity. Cochrane Database of Systematic Reviews [Internet]. 2006;18(4). Available from: \www.thecochranelibrary.com. 10.1002/ 14651858.CD003817.pub3. Accessed May 27, 2007.

213. Shaw K, O'Rourke P, Del Mar C, Kenardy J. Psychological interventions for overweight or obesity. Cochrane Database of Systematic Reviews [Internet]. 2005;18(2). Available from: www.thecochrane library. com. 10.1002/14651858.CD003818.pub2. Accessed May 27, 2007.

214. Sherwood NE, Jeffrey RW. The behavioral determinants of exercise: implications for physical activity interventions. *Annu Rev Nutr.* 2000;20:21–44.

215. Shumaker SA, Czajkowski SM, editors. *Social Support and Cardiovascular Disease.* New York: Plenum; 1994.

216. Siegel DJ. An interpersonal neurobiology approach to psychotherapy. *Psychiatric Annals.* 2006;36(4):248–256.

217. Sniehotta FF, Scholz U, Schwarzer R, et al. Long-term effects of two psychological interventions on physical exercise and self-regulation following coronary rehabilitation. *Int J Behav Med.* 2005; 12(4):244–255.

218. Snow WM, Connett JE, Sharma S, Murray RP. Predictors of attendance and dropout at the Lung Health Study 11-year follow-up. *Contemp Clin Trials.* 2007;28:25–32.

219. Sothman M, Buckworth J, Claytor RP, Cox RH, White-Welkley JE, Dishman RK. Exercise training and the cross-stress adaptation hypothesis. *Exerc Sport Sci Rev.* 1996;24:267–287.

220. Sothmann MS. The cross-stressor adaptation hypothesis and exercise training. In: Acevedo E, Ekkekakis P, editors. *Psychobiology of Physical Activity.* Champaign (IL): Human Kinetics; 2006. p. 149–160.

221. Spangenberg JJ, Theron JC. Stress and coping strategies in spouses of depressed patients. *J Psychol.* 1999;133(3):253–262.

222. Spencer L, Adams TB, Malone S, Roy L, Yost E. Applying the transtheoretical model to exercise: a systematic and comprehensive review of the literature. *Health Promot Pract.* 2006;7(4):428–443.

223. Stahre L, Tarnell B, Hakanson CE, Hallstrom T. A randomized controlled trial of two weight-reducing short-term group treatment programs for obesity with an 18-month follow-up. *Int J Behav Med.* 2007;14 (1):48–55.

224. Stanley MA, Beck JG, Novy DM, et al. Cognitive-behavioral treatment of late-life generalized anxiety disorder. *J Consult Clin Psychol.* 2003;71(2):309–319.

225. Stein DJ, Collins M, Daniels W, Noakes TD, Zigmond M. Mind and muscle: the cognitive-affective neuroscience of exercise. *CNS Spectrums.* 2007;12(1):19–22.

226. Stewart JC, Janicki DL, Muldoon MF, Sutton-Tyrrell K, Kamarck TW. Negative emotions and 3-year progression of subclinical atherosclerosis. *Arch Gen Psychiatry.* 2007;64(2):225–233.

227. Stoudemire A, Hales RE. Psychological and behavioral factors affecting medical conditions and DSM-IV: an overview. *Psychosomatics.* 1991;32(1):5–13.

228. Todaro JF, Shen B, Niaura R, Spiro A, Ward K. Effect of negative emotions on frequency of coronary heart disease (the Normative Aging Study). *Am J Cardiol.* 2003;92:901–902.

229. Trost SG, Owen N, Bauman AE, Sallis JF, Brown W. Correlates of adults' participation in physical activity: review and update. *Med Sci Sports Exerc.* 2002;34(12):1996–2001.

230. Turner RW, Ward MF, Turner DJ. Behavioral treatment for depression: an evaluation of therapeutic components. *J Clin Psychol.* 1979;35(1):166–175.

231. Uchino BN, Cacioppo JT, Keicolt-Glaser JK. The relationship between social support and physiological processes: a review with emphasis on underlying mechanisms and implications for health. *Psychol Bull.* 1996;119(3):488–531.

232. **U.S. Department of Health and Human Services. *Mental Health: A Report of the Surgeon General.* Rockville (MD): Department of Health and Human Services, Substance Abuse and Mental Health Services Administration, Center for Mental Health Services, National Institute for Mental Health; 1999.**

233. **U.S .Department of Health and Human Services. *Post-Myocardial Infarction Depression.* Rockville (MD): Agency for Healthcare Research and Quality; 2005.**

234. **U.S. Department of Health and Human Services, Office of the Secretary. *Healthy People 2010 Midcourse Review.* Washington (DC): Department of Health and Human Services, Office of Public Health and Science; 2006.**

235. van der Ven NC, Hogenelst MH, Tromp-Wever AM, et al. Short-term effects of cognitive behavioral group training (CBGT) in

adult type 1 diabetes patients in prolonged poor glycaemic control: a randomized controlled trial. *Diabet Med.* 2005;22: 1619–1623.

236. Vander A, Sherman J, Luciano D. *Human Physiology: The Mechanism of Body Function.* 8th ed. New York: McGraw-Hill; 2001.

237. Villanova N, Pasqui F, Burzacchini S, et al. A physical activity program to reinforce weight maintenance following a behavior program in overweight/obese subjects. *Int J Obes.* 2006;30:697–703.

238. Wadden TA, Crerand CE, Brock J. Behavioral treatment of obesity. *Psychiatr Clin North Am.* 2005;28:151–170.

239. Wampold BE. *The Great Psychotherapy Debate: Models, Methods, and Findings.* Mahweh (NJ): Lawrence Erlbaum; 2001.

240. Wilcox G. Insulin and insulin resistance. *Clin Biochem Rev.* 2005;26:19–39.

241. Wilson JS, Fitzsimons D, Bradbury I, Elborn JS. Does additional support by nurses enhance the effect of a brief smoking cessation intervention in people with moderate to severe chronic obstructive pulmonary disease? A randomized controlled trial. *Int J Nurs Stud.* 2007;45(4):508–517.

242. Yinclinc KW, Wulsin LR, Arnold LM, Rouan GW. Estimated prevalences of panic disorder and depression among consecutive patients in an emergency department with acute chest pain. *Gen Int Med.* 1993;8(5):231–235.

243. Ziegelstein RC, Fauerbach JA, Stevens SS, Romanelli J, Richter DP, Bush DE. Patients with depression are less likely to follow recommendations to reduce cardiac risk during recovery from a myocardial infarction. *Arch Int Med.* 2000;160(12):1818–1823.

SELECTED REFERENCES FOR FURTHER READING

Christensen AJ, Martin R, Smyth J, editors. *Encyclopedia of Health Psychology.* Philadelphia: Springer; 2004.

Sarafino EP. *Health Psychology: Biopsychosocial Interactions.* 6th ed. New York: John Wiley & Son; 2008.

INTERNET RESOURCES

- American Psychological Association (APA): www.apa.org
- National Alliance of Mental Illness (NAMI): www.nami.org
- National Institutes of Mental Health (NIMH): www.nimh.gov
- National Library of Medicine (NLM): www.nlm.nih.gov/medlineplus/mentalhealth.html

CHAPTER 17

Body Composition Status and Assessment

> **1.3-HFS: Knowledge of and ability to discuss the physiologic basis of the major components of physical fitness: flexibility, cardiovascular fitness, muscular strength, muscular endurance, and body composition.**

Body composition is a term that describes the relative proportions of fat, bone, and muscle mass in the human body. Measurement of body composition has become standard practice for exercise professionals (44). Valuable information regarding percent body fat, fat distribution, and lean tissue mass may be gained through body composition assessment. Such information may be pertinent to athletic performance and for reducing risk factors associated with musculoskeletal injury and disease. This chapter discusses body composition assessment and compares commonly employed methods for making these measurements.

RATIONALE FOR BODY COMPOSITION ASSESSMENT

The assessment of body composition has many benefits in children, adolescents and teenagers, adults, and elderly populations. Estimation of body fat percentage provides critical information concerning health and fitness. An excess amount of body fat, or **obesity** (especially in the abdominal area), is linked to several diseases including type 2 diabetes mellitus, hypertension, hyperlipidemia, cardiovascular disease (CVD), and certain types

> > > KEY TERMS

Anthropometry: Measurement of the human body. Such measurements include height, weight, circumferences, girths, and skinfolds.

Bland-Altman analysis: A statistical procedure used to compare a test criterion with a standard criterion.

Body fat percentage: The magnitude of fat tissue within the human the body. Percent body fat can only be estimated, as no direct measurement methods are available for living organisms.

Component-based methods: A system of detailed taxonomies that separates the body into different components (e.g., fat tissue, lean tissue, bone density, body water).

Obesity: A major public health concern affecting more than 90 million Americans in which an excess of nonessential body fat is observed.

Overfat: Expression of a percent body fat in excess of the desired range.

Overweight: A weight in excess of a recommended range or standard. One example was the 1983 Metropolitan Life Insurance Table, which established an optimal weight range for men and women with small, medium, and large frames. It is important to note that overweight does not necessarily reflect obesity. Thus, *overweight* is a term more suited for sedentary populations and not athletes or individuals who exercise regularly.

Property-based methods: Measurement of specific properties, such as body volume, decay properties of specific isotopes, or electrical resistance.

Standard error of the estimate: A statistic used to express the amount of variability (error) from predictions. The prediction error of a test score can be expressed as the standard error of the estimate (SEE). Similar to the standard deviation, the SEE is generally expressed as a $\pm$ around the mean score. Using the bell-shaped curve for normal distribution, ± 1 SEE unit refers to 68% of the population—that is, 68% of the population will be within the score $\pm$ the SEE. For example, a predicted percent body fat of $20 \pm 3.5\%$ means that 68% of the population studied will have a percent body fat between 16.5% and 23.5%.

of cancer (17), thereby leading to increased morbidity and mortality. The mortality rate increases by 50% to 100% when the body mass index (BMI) is equal to or greater than 30 kg·m^{-2}. Indeed, central or visceral obesity appears to serve as platform for a cascade of events that can result in a variety of clinical health problems. In addition to the greater risk of serious illness, obesity poses other mechanical limitations that limit performance of activities of daily living. For example, obesity has been linked to disc degeneration and low back pain (59), increased risk of joint injury and osteoarthritis (89), and reduced cognitive performance (37). Because of the current epidemic of obesity in the United States, detection of obesity is of primary importance for health and exercise science professionals.

Body composition measurement is also useful for those individuals with a low **body fat percentage**. During times of malnutrition (i.e., eating disorders) and in some weight-controlled sports, body fat levels and water content can fall to dangerously low levels. Sports such as gymnastics, wrestling, and bodybuilding require athletes to compete at either low weight or body fat. For wrestling, the American College of Sports Medicine (ACSM) has documented via a position stand the "weight cutting" procedures commonly used by wrestlers and the low percent body fat recorded in some wrestlers in season (3). Procedures such as excessive exercise; fasting; food restriction; and various dehydration techniques, such as rubber suits, steam rooms, and pharmaceutical use elicit rapid weight loss, much of which comes in the form of water weight, which poses inherent health risks. Regular body composition assessment can be used as a monitoring tool to benefit these individuals. With some methodologies, not only can percent body fat be estimated, but total body water can be estimated as well. In fact, the National Collegiate Athletic Association (NCAA) has recommended assessing body composition preseason in wrestling to establish a minimum body weight for each wrestler [fat-free mass (FFM) + 5% body fat] (16).

Measurement of muscle mass and bone mineral density (BMD) have several important ramifications. In the clinical setting, assessment of muscle mass and BMD can be used to assess the effects of aging and disease. Sarcopenia is the degenerative loss of skeletal muscle mass and strength as a result of aging and reduced physical activity. A progressive reduction in BMD—i.e., osteopenia and osteoporosis—may occur with aging and physical inactivity. Sarcopenia and a loss of muscle mass reduces ability to perform activities of daily living; alters metabolism, muscle, and bone function; and increases the risk of musculoskeletal injury (19,57). Thus, body composition assessment in the clinical setting can be used to monitor the progression of disease or muscle/bone enhancement as a result of therapeutic or pharmaceutical intervention. Body composition assessment is particularly important in populations with pulmonary disease, as prolonged use of steroid therapies adversely affects BMD, often resulting in increased risk of falls, broken bones, or compression fractures of the spine. In apparently healthy or athletic populations, body composition assessment can be used to quantify changes in muscle mass and BMD as a result of physical training (11). These measurements may be used for individualization of exercise prescriptions and for evaluation of the efficacy of the training program.

LEVELS OF BODY COMPOSITION

Body composition may be described at five levels: atomic, molecular, cellular, tissue, and whole body (65,73). Basic elements are found at the atomic level. Out of all the elements found in nature, about 50 are found in the human body. Of these, oxygen, carbon, hydrogen, and nitrogen account for >95% of body mass, and other key elements, such as sodium, potassium, phosphorous, calcium, chloride, magnesium, and sulfur, raise the total to nearly 99.5% of body mass (65). At the molecular level, the major components are water, lipids, protein, minerals, and carbohydrates. At the cellular level, the critical components are the cell mass (e.g., muscle, nerve, connective tissue, and adipocytes), extracellular fluid, and extracellular solids. At the tissue level, body composition analyses focus on skeletal muscle, bone, blood, visceral organs, and adipose tissue. Adipose tissue includes adipocytes with collagenous fibers, fibroblasts, capillaries, and extracellular fluid. Lastly, the whole body level entails body mass, size, stature, volume, density, and proportions. Most of the body composition assessments discussed in this chapter entail measurements at the whole body level.

BODY COMPOSITION MODELS

Body composition methods can be categorized as being direct, indirect, or doubly indirect (88). A direct method (i.e., chemical analysis of the whole body or cadaver) is not suitable in the living human body. Thus, indirect or doubly indirect methods are preferred. Indirect methods (e.g., hydrostatic weighing) were derived from the direct method, and doubly indirect methods (e.g., skinfolds) were generally derived from an indirect method. Therefore, doubly indirect methods are generally prone to greater measurement error in comparison to the direct (chemical analysis) method. Table 17-1 categorizes many popular body composition assessment methods into indirect or doubly indirect.

Indirect methods are based on either property or component (42) approaches. **Property-based methods** involve the measurement of specific properties, such as body volume, decay properties of specific isotopes, or electrical resistance, e.g., estimation of total body water (TBW) from tritium dilution. The development of in vivo neutron activation analysis, for example, has made possible

TABLE 17-1. CATEGORIZATION OF COMMON BODY COMPOSITION ASSESSMENT TECHNIQUES

ASSESSMENT TECHNIQUE	METHOD	COMPONENT MODEL
Skinfolds	Doubly indirect	Largely 2C (some multiple C equations)
Bioelectrical impedance	Doubly indirect	3C
Near-infrared interactance	Doubly indirect	2C
Hydrodensitometry	Indirect	2C
CT and MRI scans	Indirect	Multiple C
Plethysmography: air displacement	Indirect	2C
Dual-energy x-ray absorptiometry (DXA)	Indirect	3C

CT, computed tomography; MRI, magnetic resonance imaging.

Method: direct, indirect, or doubly indirect (see text for complete explanation). Component model: 2C (two compartment), 3C (three compartment), multiple C (more than 2C) (see text for complete explanation).

nondestructive chemical analysis by measuring the radiation given off during the decay of excited atoms (23). **Component-based methods** depend on well-established models, usually ratios of measurable quantities to components that are assumed to be constant, both within and between individuals. The measured quantity is first assessed using a property-based method, and the component is estimated by application of the model. Thus, FFM can be estimated from TBW by use of tritium dilution, and subsequently, fat mass can be calculated.

Two types of mathematical approaches are used to estimate body composition with property- and component-based methods. The model approach, which depends on the ratio between a particular constituent and the component of interest, was illustrated earlier. In the second approach, regression analysis is used with experimental data to derive an equation that relates a measured property or component to an unknown (estimated) component. Equations for estimating percent body fat from skinfold thickness or bioelectrical impedance are developed in this manner—e.g., doubly indirect. Direct methods represent the most fundamental approach to assessment, property-based methods are one step removed, and component-based methods are two steps removed. Assessment methods are structured so that measurement errors are propagated from level to level.

Different models have been proposed for characterizing human body composition by compartments with the sum totaling the individual's body weight or mass. The two-compartment (2C) model partitions body mass into fat mass and FFM (12,78) and has the widest application to body composition analysis. It is limited by the assumptions that water and mineral contents of the body remain constant throughout life and between all individuals, and that the density of FFM is constant among all individuals. The assumption related to FFM composition is known to be violated by age, sex, and ethnicity differences.

Multicompartment models have been developed because of violation of the inherent assumptions of the 2C model. These models divide the body into more than two compartments and require fewer assumptions about the composition of the FFM. Thus, multicompartment models may provide more accurate results. However, their applica-

tion requires additional measurements (e.g., TBW, bone mineral content); therefore, the theoretic reduction in total error may be offset by an increased technical error in measuring multiple components. Multicompartment models include the three-compartment (3C) and four-compartment (4C) models. The 3C model includes fat mass, but also partitions FFM into TBW and dry FFM. The 4C model partitions body mass into fat mass, FFM, TBW, BMD, and the residual dry FFM. In addition, 4C models (7,41) often serve as the criterion model for body composition measurement in validation studies. The choice of an appropriate model depends on the component of FFM that is expected to vary the most from population norms. When equipment is limited and 3C and 4C models are not feasible, population-specific equations (that use a 2C model) that are adjusted for differences in FFM can be used to improve accuracy (see GETP8 Table 4-4). Population-specific equations appropriate for children and older adults, various racial or ethnic groups, athletic groups, and some clinical populations should result in more accurate estimates than generalized equations. (44,61)

METHODOLOGIES IN BODY COMPOSITION ASSESSMENT

> **1.3.7-HFS:** Knowledge of the advantages/disadvantages and limitations of the various body composition techniques including but not limited to air displacement plethysmography (BOD POD), dual energy x-ray absorptiometry (DEXA), hydrostatic weighing, skinfolds, and bioelectrical impedance.

As discussed earlier, there are no direct in vivo methods available to measure different body composition compartments. Rather, most body composition measurements involve indirect assessment, or estimation. Comparative studies between different methods are numerous, as each method has advantages and disadvantages. Critical to these comparisons is the establishment of a criterion or standard method. Evaluation of each technique for accuracy, validity, and reliability is critical for assessment. The decision on which method to use depends on several factors, including the needs of the individual, purpose of the evaluation, cost of the measurements or equipment needed, availability of each assessment tool, training of the technician, and the weighed advantages/disadvantages of each. In this chapter, each body composition assessment tool listed below is discussed. These basic and advanced measures include:

- Height
- Body weight and mass
- BMI
- Waist and hip circumferences
- Hydrodensitometry (underwater weighing)
- Skinfold assessments
- Bioelectrical impedance
- Near-infrared interactance
- Air displacement plethysmography
- Computed tomography scans
- Magnetic resonance imaging scans
- Ultrasound
- Isotopic dilution
- Dual-energy x-ray absorptiometry (DXA)

HEIGHT, BODY WEIGHT, AND BODY MASS INDEX

> **1.3.9-HFS: Skill in measuring skinfold sites, skeletal diameters, and girth measurements used for estimating body composition.**

Measurements of height and body weight are simple to perform and rapid to complete. Height should be assessed with a stadiometer (a vertical ruler mounted on a wall with a wide horizontal headboard). Although many commercial scales have an attached vertical ruler, these devices are less reliable and not recommended. Standards for height measurements include the following: (a) subject removes shoes; (b) subject stands straight up with heels together; (c) subject takes a deep breath and holds it; and (d) subject stands with head level, looking straight ahead. The height of the subject is then recorded in inches or centimeters (1 in = 2.54 cm). Failure to follow these standards reduces reliability and accuracy.

Body weight and body mass is best measured on a calibrated physician's scale with a beam and moveable weights. If other types of commercial scales are used, it is recommended they be calibrated using standardized

weights or compared with measured weight from the beam-type scale. Clothing is the major measurement issue for body weight assessment. The type and amount of clothing must be standardized (Box 17-1). Ideally, measurements should be completed with minimal clothing. However, this recommendation may not be feasible in many instances, so a facility should adopt the most reasonable clothing policy for their population. Individuals should remove their shoes and any excess layers of clothing (e.g., coats), empty their pockets, and remove jewelry and cell phones. A reasonable standard in many fitness environments is shorts and a T-shirt. Body weight can change at various times of day because of meal/beverage consumption, urination, defecation, and potential dehydration/water loss. Thus, a standard time (e.g., early in the morning) relative to exercise and nutritional intake will increase the consistency of measurements. Body weight is recorded in either pounds or kilograms (1 kg = 2.2 lbs).

BMI is used to assess an individual's mass relative to height [BMI $(kg \cdot m^{-2})$ = body mass (kg)/height (m^2)]. BMI has been used to determine risk of developing type 2 diabetes, hypertension, and CVD according to standards developed by the Expert Panel on the Identification, Evaluation, and Treatment of Overweight and Obesity in Adults (68). According to current BMI $(kg \cdot m^{-2})$ standards: (a) individuals with a BMI <18.5 are classified as underweight; (b) a BMI of 18.5 to 24.9 is normal; (c) a BMI of 25 to 29.9 indicates overweight; (d) a BMI of 30 to 39.9 is obese; and (e) a BMI >40 indicates morbid obesity. Thus, a BMI range of 30 to 40 indicates a moderate risk for disease development, whereas a BMI >40 indicates a high risk of developing metabolic disease. Criticisms of the use of BMI are that it is a relatively poor predictor of **body fat percentage** and may result in inaccurate classifications (normal, overweight, obese) for some individuals, particularly those who are muscular or athletic or who play collegiate or professional sports. The standard error of the estimate (SEE) for predicting percent body fat from BMI is ±5%, thereby demonstrating the criticism of BMI to be valid. The error is particularly high when BMI equations are used to predict percent body fat in athletic populations, e.g., body builders (85). BMI does not differentiate fat mass from FFM. Hence, BMI may be more acceptable in clinical or sedentary populations.

BOX 17-1	**STANDARDS FOR BASIC BODY COMPOSITION MEASUREMENTS**

MEASUREMENT	INSTRUMENT	STANDARDIZATION
Waist circumference	Tension-controlled tape	See GETP8 Box 4-1
Weight	Balance beam scale	Nude or hospital gown
		or
		Facility-developed standard
Height	Stadiometer	No shoes, heels together, after a deep inhalation, head level

The accuracy of BMI is highly questionable in athletes and individuals who exercise regularly. In a recent study examining body composition in National Football League (NFL) football players, every player (including kickers and punters) was classified as overweight, obese, and very obese using BMI as a standard, despite having body fat percentages of 6.3% to 18.5% (with offensive linemen at 25.1%) (55). Thus, BMI is not a particularly useful body composition analysis tool in resistance-trained populations. Misclassification of body weight is not prevalent in nonathletic adult populations who are weight stable or who have gained weight in their adult years. Thus, BMI should provide a reasonably accurate classification in these individuals.

WAIST-TO-HIP RATIO

> **1.3.12-HFS: Ability to locate common sites for measurement of skinfold thickness and circumferences (for determination of body composition and waist-to-hip ratio).**

The waist-to-hip ratio (WHR) is a ratio measurement of the circumferences of the waist to that of the hip. It is an indicator of body fat distribution. Body fat distribution has been recognized as a predictor of risk factors for disease. A high WHR ratio may indicate visceral obesity. Visceral obesity increases the risk for hypertension, type 2 diabetes, hyperlipidemia, metabolic syndrome, and CVD. Standardization of circumference measurement technique for the WHR is critical for accuracy and reliability. The waist circumference is measured around the smallest area of the waist, typically approximately 1 inch (2.54 cm) above the umbilicus or navel. The hip circumference is taken around the largest area of the buttocks. Multiple measurements should be taken until each is within ¼ inch of each other. Typically, men between the ages of 20 and 70 with a WHR ranging from 0.89 to 0.99 (and greater) are at high risk for disease. Women of similar ages with a WHR of 0.78 to 0.84 and higher are also at greater risk of metabolic disease (43). Younger adults are at a very high risk when WHR values are greater than 0.95 and 0.86 for men and women, respectively. These values rise to 1.03 and 0.90, respectively, for ages 60 to 69.

HYDRODENSITOMETRY (UNDERWATER OR HYDROSTATIC WEIGHING)

Underwater or hydrostatic weighing (also known as hydrodensitometry) has traditionally been considered the criterion method for body composition analysis even though it is considered an indirect method. Hydrostatic weighing (HW) is based on Archimedes' principle for determining body density. Archimedes' principle states that a body immersed in water is subjected to a buoyant force that results in a loss of weight equal to the weight of the displaced water. Subtracting the body weight measured in the water during submersion from the body weight measured on land provides the weight of the displaced water. Body fat contributes to buoyancy because the assumed density of fat (0.9007 $g \cdot cm^{-3}$) is less than water (1 $g \cdot cm^{-3}$), whereas FFM (≥ 1.100 $g \cdot cm^{-3}$) exceeds the density of water. Density is inversely related to body fat. Thus, HW is based on the equation: body density = mass $\cdot$ volume^{-1}. A volumetric analysis of the body is possible with HW, as body volume can be determined via hydrodensitometry or air displacement plethysmography. Body density is then converted to percent body fat using a two-compartment (2C: fat and FFM) model equation, such as the Siri (78) or Brozek (12) body density equations. As a criterion measure, other popular methods of body composition analyses (e.g., skinfolds, bioelectrical impedance) are usually validated against HW. Thus, HW can be very accurate when methods are followed correctly.

Several variables must be known to use HW. These include:

1. Residual volume—the amount of air remaining in the lungs following full expiration. Residual volume can be measured or predicted using a combination of age, sex, and height. A substantial amount of air left in the lungs increases buoyancy, which may be mistaken as additional body fat.
2. Density of the water—this varies with water temperature, as buoyancy decreases with warmer temperatures.
3. The amount of trapped gas in the gastrointestinal system—typically a predicted constant of 100 mL is used.
4. Dry body weight.
5. Body (wet) weight fully submerged in water.

Body density may then be calculated and converted to percent body fat using a 2C model prediction equation.

When performing HW, the subjects should wear a tight-fitting bathing suit that traps little air, remove all jewelry, and have urinated/defecated before assessment. In addition, the subject should be 2 to 12 hours postabsorptive and avoid foods that may have increased gas in the gastrointestinal tract. Menstruation may pose a problem for women because of associated water gain, thus, women should try to avoid being tested within 7 days of menstruation. The equipment used for HW may vary. The tank can be made of stainless steel, fiberglass, ceramic tile, Plexiglas®, or other material and should be at least 4 × 4 × 5 feet (36). A chair or seat suspended from a scale (many times a cadaver or vegetable scale is used) or force transducer is needed to allow subjects to be weighed while completely submerged underwater. The subject is weighed on land to determine dry weight, and the mass is converted to grams. The temperature of the water should be between 33° and 36° C, and the density can be determined based on temperature. Subjects subsequently enter the tank, remove potential trapped air from the skin, hair, suit, etc., and attain a seated position. Once seated and chair height adjusted, the subject fully expires as much air as possible before leaning forward to be weighed. The subject should be weighed five to ten times while submerged underwater for 5 to 10 seconds. Movement in the chair should be minimized to reduce scale fluctuations. Typically, the highest of the weights or the average of the three highest weights are used for analysis. It is important to factor in the weight of the chair in addition to any weight belts used to encourage complete submersion when determining underwater weight. Residual lung volume can be measured directly (which increases accuracy) in some systems or estimated based on height and age:

- Men: RV (L) = [0.019 × ht (cm)] + [0.0155 × age (yrs)] − 2.24

$$(10)$$

- Women: RV (L) = [0.032 × ht (cm)] + [0.009 × age (yrs)] − 3.90

$$(70)$$

Body density (BD) may then be calculated using the following equation:

- BD = Mass in air/[([Mass in air − Mass in water]/Water density) − (RV + 100)]
  Masses are in grams
  RV = mL

Body fat can then be calculated using either the Siri (75) or Brozek (12) equations:

- Siri: % Fat = $\dfrac{457}{BD}$ − 414.2

- Brozek: % Fat = $\dfrac{495}{BD}$ − 450

The test–retest reliability of HW has been shown to be high in most cases (R = 0.95) (61), although in certain groups of the population (e.g., African Americans, youths, elderly individuals), the error magnitude may be higher because certain density assumptions are known to be invalid in these populations. High correlation coefficients and similar percent body fat estimates have been shown between HW and a 4C model in athletes (85). Although the density of lean tissue is assumed to be 1.100 $g \cdot cm^{-3}$ for all, this value differs in African Americans (>1.11 g/cm^3) and youths (< 1.09 $g \cdot cm^{-3}$), which is suspected to be the major factor with the higher error magnitude (64). In addition, the density of FFM varies between individuals, resulting in a body fat SEE of about ±2.7%, even when the technique is performed flawlessly (61). Major practical limitations to HW include space and plumbing requirements, the cost and specialized use of the equipment needed, the time involved in each measurement, the need for an accurate residual volume measurement, and the inherent fear and discomfort many individuals have being fully submerged in water. Because of these limitations, HW is not used in many fitness or medical centers.

SKINFOLD MEASUREMENT

> **1.3.12-HFS: Ability to locate common sites for measurement of skinfold thickness and circumferences (for determination of body composition and waist-to-hip ratio).**

One of the more popular and practical methods used in the determination of percent fat is the skinfold thickness measurement. Skinfold measurement predicts percent body fat reasonably well if performed properly by a trained technician using a high-quality skinfold caliper (i.e., a Lange or Harpenden caliper that provides a constant pressure of ~10 $g \cdot mm^{-2}$). However, skinfold analysis provides only an estimate of body density and percent body fat and is based largely on the 2C model (there are a few multicompartment models that use skinfold analysis). Skinfold analysis is based on the principle that the amount of subcutaneous fat (fat immediately below the skin) is directly proportional to the total amount of body fat. The proportion of subcutaneous to total fat varies with sex, age, race or ethnicity, and other factors. Numerous regression equations using a combination of multiple skinfold sites have been developed to predict body density and fat from skinfold measurements. These multiple regression equations are either general or population-specific for sex, age, race or ethnicity, and activity or sport status.

The number of sites needs to be predetermined based on the regression equation or methods used (i.e., 3-, 4-, or 7-site). A fold of skin is firmly grasped between the thumb and index finger of the left hand (about 8 cm apart on a line perpendicular to the long axis of the site) and lifted away from the body while the subject is relaxed. A slight muscular contraction of the subject or finger roll of the fold itself ensures that subcutaneous tissue (skin, fat) is measured and not skeletal muscle. For obese individuals, a large grasping area (i.e., >8 cm) may be needed. While the caliper is facing up, the jaws of the caliper are then placed over the skinfold 1 cm below the fingers of the tester. The grip of the caliper is released, and the skinfold measurement is subsequently taken within 2 to 3 seconds. All measurements are taken on the right side of the body in duplicate or triplicate for consistency between measurements to the nearest 0.5 mm. If there is more than a 3-mm difference between readings, then a fourth measurement may be needed. It is important to rotate through the measurement sites as opposed to taking two or three measurements sequentially from the same site (see Fig. 17-1 for a description of selected skinfold sites). Each site is averaged and summed to estimate percent body fat via a regression equation or prediction table. The specific skinfold equation used must match the anatomic measurement description specific to the equation, as there are reported differences in skinfold anatomic site descriptions and measurement techniques. Therefore, major limitations to the skinfold procedure are the amount of technician training in equation selection, accuracy of skinfold site measurement, selection of appropriate calipers, and measurement technique. It has been suggested that a tester measure approximately 50 to 100 individuals to attain a high level of competency (36). Common sites assessed are:

- Abdominal: Vertical fold; 2 cm to the right side of the umbilicus

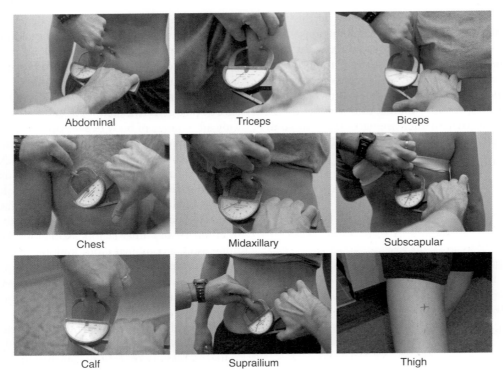

Abdominal	Triceps	Biceps
Chest	Midaxillary	Subscapular
Calf	Suprailium	Thigh

FIGURE 17-1. Skinfold measures.

- Triceps: Vertical fold; on the posterior midline of the upper arm, halfway between the acromion and olecranon processes, with the arm held freely to the side of the body
- Biceps: Vertical fold; on the anterior aspect of the arm over the belly of the biceps muscle, 1 cm above the level used to mark the triceps site
- Chest/pectoral: Diagonal fold; one half the distance between the anterior axillary line and the nipple (men), or one third the distance between the anterior axillary line and the nipple (women)
- Medial calf: Vertical fold; at the maximum circumference of the calf on the midline of its medial border
- Midaxillary: Vertical fold; on the midaxillary line at the level of the xiphoid process of the sternum (an alternate method is a horizontal fold taken at the level of the xiphoid/sternal border in the midaxillary line)
- Subscapular: Diagonal fold (at a 45-degree angle), 1 to 2 cm below the inferior angle of the scapula
- Suprailiac: Diagonal fold; in line with the natural angle of the iliac crest taken in the anterior axillary line immediately superior to the iliac crest
- Thigh: Vertical fold; on the anterior midline of the thigh, midway between the proximal border of the patella and the inguinal crease (hip)

Reliability and accuracy of skinfold measurement are specific to the skinfold regression equation used. Variability in percent body fat prediction from skinfold analysis is approximately ±3.5% (SEE), assuming that appropriate techniques and equations have been used (61). In those with abdominal subcutaneous fat that is not easily grasped because of marked abdominal obesity, skinfold assessment may not be accurate, and other body composition assessment techniques may be required for accurate body composition assessment.

BIOELECTRICAL IMPEDANCE

Bioelectrical impedance analysis (BIA) is a noninvasive and easy-to-administer body composition assessment tool. A variety of different BIA analyzers are commercially available that range in utility and price. The premise underlying this procedure is that fat-free tissue in the body is proportional to the electrical conductivity of the body (6). A small electrical current is sent through the body (from ankle to wrist), and the impedance to that current is measured. The theory underlying BIA is that lean tissue (i.e., mostly water and electrolytes) is a good electrical conductor (low impedance), whereas fat is a poor electrical conductor and acts as impedance to electrical current. BIA estimates TBW and uses equations for percent body fat (based on a 3C model) based on assumptions about hydration levels and the exact water content of various tissues (43). A single frequency (50 kHz) low-level current (500 mA) is used to measure whole-body impedance using four electrodes placed on the legs and arms. Unlike lower-frequency current (<50 kHz), which flows through the extracellular fluid, higher frequencies penetrate the cell membranes and flow through both the intracellular and extracellular fluid. Thus, total body impedance at the constant frequency of 50 kHz primarily reflects the volumes of water (intracellular and extracellular fluid) and muscle compartments constituting the FFM. Most studies examining BIA have used the equation: $V = pL^2 \cdot R^{-1}$, where V is the volume of the conductor (i.e., TBW), p is the specific resistance of the tissue, L is the length of the conductor, and R is the observed resistance (36).

The methods used in BIA testing are relatively simple. The subject lies supine on a nonconductive surface with arm and legs at the side, not in contact with the rest of the body. The right hand and foot are prepared with an alcohol pad, then allowed to dry. Source electrodes are placed on the distal metacarpal of the right index finger and the distal metatarsal of the right big toe, and the reference (detecting) electrodes are placed on the right wrist (bisecting the ulnar and radial styloid processes) and the right ankle (midpoint on the line bisecting the medial and lateral malleoli). The voltage drop between reference electrodes is the impedance. Newer BIA equipment is simpler to use and requires the subject to either stand on the machine (i.e., electronic digital platform scale with built-in stainless steel footpad electrodes) with both feet or hold the BIA analyzer in both hands. Accuracy among different BIA models varies greatly.

Most BIA machines use different equations that account for the differences in water content and body density between different sexes, ages, and races or ethnicities, as well as by physical activity status. The BIA technology has been shown to be reliable for single measurements and measurements taken up to 5 days (36). It is important when performing a BIA assessment that the subject has not eaten or consumed a beverage within 4 hours of the test, has not exercised within 12 hours of the test, has not consumed alcohol or diuretics before testing, has completely voided the bladder within 30 minutes of the test, and has had minimal consumption of diuretic agents, such as chocolate or caffeine. In addition, glycogen stores can affect impedance and can be a factor during times of weight loss. If possible, BIA measurements should not be taken before menstruation to avoid the possible effects of water retention in women. BIA manufacturers also recommend avoiding this method of body composition assessment with pregnant women and those with implanted electrical devices, such as a pacemaker. The reported SEE for BIA is between ±2.7 and 6.3%, which is greater than that reported for skinfold analysis (36). Although high correlations between BIA and other criterion methods have been established, percent body fat from BIA appears to be consistently overestimated for lean individuals and underestimated for obese persons. In athletes, BIA has been shown to significantly underestimate percent body fat when compared with HW (18). Compared with DXA, BIA has been shown to underestimate percent body fat and overestimate lean tissue mass (9). However, BIA has been shown to detect similar changes in percent body fat during weight loss comparable with the magnitude of change determined via DXA (32).

Subject factors, technical skill, the prediction equation used, and the instruments used all affect the accuracy of BIA. To reduce measurement error, analyzers should be calibrated before measurement, and the same instrument (or at least brand when applicable) should be used when following changes in body composition within an individual. Hydration, temperature, and exercise status must be controlled to stabilize resistance measurements. Technician error is minor if standard procedures for subject and electrode positioning are followed. Finally, error can be reduced by selecting appropriate prediction equations according to age, sex, ethnicity, and level of physical activity, and by using an equation developed on a BIA unit similar to the one being used for testing.

Recent studies indicate that it may be possible to estimate extracellular and intracellular water compartments along with TBW (6,63) with newer multiple-frequency BIA. As a result, this methodology may be less affected by hydration status and may be a better estimate of FFM. Multiple-frequency BIA may also enhance the clinical application of BIA to assess changes and shifts between intracellular and extracellular fluid compartments associated with certain diseases, as well as accurate hydration status.

NEAR-INFRARED INTERACTANCE

Near-infrared interactance (NIR) is based on principles of light absorption and reflection using near-infrared spectroscopy to provide information about the chemical composition of the body. A light wand device is positioned perpendicularly on a body part (typically on the anterior midline of the biceps brachii, midway between the antecubital fossa and the acromion process), and infrared light is emitted at specific wavelengths (i.e., 940 and 950 nm). The absorption of the infrared beam is subsequently measured via a silicon-based detector, which is expressed as two optical densities. Prediction equations estimate percent body fat via optical density, sex, height, and body weight. Some research indicates that NIR is valid and reliable for body composition assessment in female athletes (31). However, the SEE associated with NIR has been shown to be higher than other assessment tools, i.e., skinfolds and BIA (10,31). NIR has also been shown to overpredict percent body fat in obese women (72) and has shown constant error values ranging from 6.5% to 14.7% in overpredicting percent body fat in young wrestlers (48). Even when NIR equations are adjusted for constant error values, the error rate in youth wrestlers is still approximately 2% to 3% (47), suggesting unacceptable prediction errors for these populations. In addition, NIR has been shown be least effective for monitoring body composition changes following resistance and aerobic training (11). Some commercial versions of NIR (e.g.,

Futrex-5000, -5500, -6000, -6100) are portable and require minimal technician training, making them attractive to the health and fitness industry. However, a major limitation is the relatively small sampling area on the body for NIR absorption. The SEE reported for NIR varies more than ±5.0 percent body fat (24). Thus, because of the inaccuracies cited above and the high SEE reported in most NIR studies, this body composition assessment technique is not recommended for routine use in apparently healthy, athletic, or clinical populations.

AIR DISPLACEMENT PLETHYSMOGRAPHY

Body volume can be measured by air displacement rather than water displacement. Air displacement plethysmography (ADP) is suggested as an alternative body composition assessment technique to HW for individuals who may experience difficulty with HW. This technique offers several advantages over other reference methods, including safety. ADP is usually a quick and comfortable assessment, is noninvasive, and accommodates children, adults, obese, elderly, and disabled individuals (28). However, a major disadvantage for ADP is initial cost of purchasing the ADP unit. The only commercial system (BOD POD®, Life Measurement Instruments, Concord, CA) available at the time of this writing uses a dual-chamber (e.g., 450 L for the subject test chamber, 300 L for the reference chamber) plethysmograph that measures body volume via changes in air pressure, i.e., using Boyle's law ($P1 \cdot P2^{-1} = V2 \cdot V1^{-1}$), within a closed two-compartment chamber. A plethysmograph is an instrument for measuring volume or changes in volume. The plethysmograph also includes an electronic weighing scale, computer, and software system. The volume of air displaced is equal to body volume and is calculated indirectly by subtracting the volume of air remaining in the chamber when subject is inside from the volume of air in the chamber when it is empty. A diaphragm (which separates the two internal chambers) oscillates back and forth to create volume changes that produce pressure changes in the two chambers. The subject needs to wear a bathing suit (or minimal clothing, such as Lycra® biking shorts) and a swim cap and then sits quietly during testing while a minimum of two measurements (within 150 mL of each other) are taken. Subsequently, thoracic gas volume is measured during normal breathing (i.e., via the "panting" method, for which the subject breathes normally into a tube connected within the chamber, followed by three small puffs after the airway tube becomes momentarily occluded at the midpoint of exhalation). Corrected body volume (raw body volume – thoracic gas volume) is then calculated (36). Sources of error include (a) interlaboratory variation, (b) variations in testing conditions, (c) performing testing while not in a fasting state, (d) air that is not accounted for in the lungs or that is trapped within clothing and bodily hair, and (e) body moisture

and/or increased body temperature (28,29). Percent body fat may also be underestimated by nearly 3% if a swimming cap is not worn and the subject has hair covering a large portion of his face (45).

After body density has been determined, percent body fat can be calculated. Most prediction equations used to convert body density to percent body fat using ADP are similar to HW, although body density measured via ADP does result in consistently higher values compared with HW (36). Reliability of ADP in adults has been shown to be good (within-subject coefficients of variation (CVs) = 1.7% to 4.3%) (5,15,28). In addition, ADP has shown to be valid in comparison to HW and DXA. In comparison with HW, ADP has been shown to range by −4.0% to 1.9% and SEE of 1.8% to 2.3% in adults and −2.9% to 2.6% and SEE of 3.3% in children (28). In comparison to DXA, ADP has been shown to range by −3.0% to 2.2% and SEE of 2.4% to 3.7% in adults and −3.9% to −0.1% and SEE of 3.4% to 4.1% in children (4,28). In comparison to 4C models, ADP has been shown to underestimate percent body fat by nearly 2% in women (30). Recently, it has been shown that ADP is valid in comparison to HW in subjects classified as overweight (BMI = 27.1 $kg \cdot m^{-2}$), obese (BMI = 34.0 $kg \cdot m^{-2}$), and severely obese (BMI = 47.2 $kg \cdot m^{-2}$) (34). Compared with HW and DXA, ADP has been shown to produce similar measurements (percent body fat = 0.5%, SEE = 2.9%) in collegiate female athletes (5) and collegiate wrestlers (18), overestimate percent body fat in collegiate female athletes (86), and underestimate percent body fat by about 2% in collegiate football players (15). Last, ADP has been shown to be an effective body composition assessment technique for monitoring changes during weight loss. In comparison with DXA, ADP assessment of percent body fat during weight loss programs of 8 weeks to 16 months has been shown to be similar in absolute changes, although ADP underestimated percent body fat by 2% to 4% (66,91) and overestimated percent body fat by about 5% (32) in the pre- and postexperimental periods. Thus, ADP is effective for measuring changes over time provided standardized techniques are used.

COMPUTED TOMOGRAPHY SCANS AND MAGNETIC RESONANCE IMAGING

Cross-sectional imaging of the whole body is an available technique for body composition analysis. All major organs and tissues can be viewed with computed tomography (CT) and magnetic resonance imaging (MRI). These imaging techniques can produce scans that can noninvasively quantify the volume of certain body tissues, such as regional fat distribution. A total body composition analysis is possible with sequential "slicing" through the body and assumptions for tissue densities. These scans use a multicompartment model for body composition. For CT scans, the x-ray passes through the subject and creates cross-sectional slices approximately 10 mm thick. The image represents a 2-D map of pixels corresponding to a 3-D section of volume elements (voxels). Each pixel has a numeric value called the *attenuation coefficient* that helps differentiate tissues based on the density and electrons per unit mass (36), and an image is created via a process known as *windowing*. The ratios of electrons to mass for carbon, nitrogen, and oxygen are 0.5, whereas hydrogen is 1.0, thus making it easier to separate adipose tissue from other tissues. For MRI scans, the image is created by interaction of hydrogen atoms via the magnet creating a magnetic field. With the hydrogen protons aligned within the field, a pulsed radio frequency is applied, causing the hydrogen protons to absorb energy, and subsequently, an image is generated. The image is made up of T1 (time required for protons to return to original position, longitudinal relaxation) and T2 (images generated that provide information on tissue differences, transverse relaxation) information. Mostly, tissue area within the CT scan or MRI is calculated by segmentation techniques. Fat and lean tissue can be quantified by selecting regions of interest on the scan. The area of each region is determined by multiplying the number of pixels by their known area. Both MRI and CT scans have been validated compared with cadavers for determining interstitial and subcutaneous adipose tissue (67). These scans may provide an additional benefit in that a relative analysis of muscle and bone density can be performed. Both MRI and CT scans provide valuable information regarding intra-abdominal fat and could be useful in clinical settings and research. The use of radiation in CT scans may limit its usefulness for children and some adults. Scanning is typically associated with a high cost (especially MRI), making it impractical.

ULTRASOUND

The use of ultrasound for body composition assessment has been in existence for many years. Ultrasound provides sonic energy at frequencies well above the audible range in humans (i.e., 20 Hz–20 kHz) (36). The sonic energy (pulse or vibration) is propagated through the tissues at a specific velocity. For example, skeletal muscle has a density of 1.07 $g \cdot cc^{-1}$ and a velocity of 1,570 $m \cdot s^{-1}$, whereas fat has a density of 0.90 $g \cdot cc^{-1}$ and a velocity of 1,440 $m \cdot s^{-1}$ (36). Subsequently, the pattern depends on its wavelength (frequency) and the density of the tissues. Part of the energy is reflected while the rest is refracted where the tissue density dictates the magnitude of reflection. Pulsed ultrasound imaging technology measures the reflection. In A-mode ultrasound, a pulse is sent from the probe through the subject and back (similar to an echo), and the depth (time of echo) is visually shown on an oscilloscope. B-mode ultrasound collects similar information, but adds the positioning of the echo in a two-dimensional plane, as well as the memory to recall previous echoes. The probe (transducer) is coupled to an echo camera that converts the impulses into a recognizable image. B-mode ultrasonography is the most practical for body composition assessment.

The reliability and validity of B-mode ultrasound body fat measurements have been established. Reliability coefficients of $R > 0.90$ for various regions measured have been reported (8,36). Research has validated ultrasound compared with other techniques (40,52). Compared to skinfolds for measuring subcutaneous fat, ultrasound has shown high correlation coefficients (40,52) and may be more accurate for actual subcutanenous fat thickness (90). In fact, B-mode ultrasound has been shown to be superior to skinfolds for measuring subcutaneous fat in obese adults and children (56,77) and reliable and valid for measuring visceral fat (1,80). Total percent body fat can be predicted via regression equations (using various sites of subcutaneous fat measurements) that estimate body density similar to skinfold analyses (25). Critical to reliable ultrasonic measurement is standardization of technique. The technician needs to be able to standardize the exact site locations of measurement and apply uniform and constant pressure on the probe throughout, as an imbalance can alter adipose tissue distribution significantly (36).

ISOTOPIC DILUTION

Isotopic dilution enables measurement of TBW and estimation of FFM and percent body fat. TBW is calculated from the compartment volume, which is the ratio of the dose of a tracer to its concentration in the bodily compartment after equilibration is achieved within the body (36). Common tracers used in isotopic dilution are D_2O, ^{18}O, and tritiated water (^3H_2O). Following a baseline fluid sample (e.g., blood, urine, saliva), a tracer dose of labeled water is given, a second fluid sample (administered about 2–4 hours after equilibration) is collected, and then these are analyzed via mass spectroscopy or gas chromatography (36). TBW may be calculated by dilution space (L)/1.041 (83). Because the mean hydration fraction of FFM is about 73.2%, FFM = TBW (kg)/0.732 (83), and fat mass may be calculated by subtracting FFM from total body mass.

Test-retest reliability of isotopic dilution is very good. However, isotopic dilution does have a few limitations. Technical errors can occur with the methodology. Hydrogen tracers (2%–4%) may exchange with nonaqueous hydrogen, thereby altering fat mass by up to 1.4 kg and percent body fat by approximately 2% (36). Correction factors (0.5%–4%) may be needed to account for errors in the calculation of isotopic dilution space. In addition, isotopic dilution is costly, which may further limit its use.

DUAL-ENERGY X-RAY ABSORPTIOMETRY

Dual-energy x-ray absorptiometry is based on a 3C model of total body mineral stores, FFM, and fat mass. The principle of absorptiometry is based on exponential attenuation of x-rays at two energies as they pass through the body.

DXA machines are commonly used in hospitals and research facilities and have largely replaced dual-photon absorptiometry (which uses a radionuclide, such as gadolinium, to generate gamma rays) in many settings (51). X-rays are generated at two energies (either alternating voltages or constant potentials) via a low-current x-ray tube located underneath the DXA machine. A detector positioned overhead on the scanning arm and interface with a computer is also needed for scanning an image. Following system calibration and removal of metallic objects from the subject, the subject is instructed to lie motionless and is secured with VELCRO® straps on the lower leg and feet on a scanning bed. The individual is then scanned rectilinearly from head to toe for a duration of 5 to 25 minutes, depending on the type of scan. Newer DXA units have greatly reduced total scan time, making it more practical and easy to administer. The x-rays are delivered at 2 photon energies (between 38 and 140 keV, depending on the manufacturer), and the differential attenuation is used to estimate bone mineral content and soft tissue composition (i.e., a 2C model). Soft tissue measurements can only be made in regions where no bone is present. The ratio of soft tissue attenuation of the low- and high-energy beams is measured as follows: soft tissue attenuation (low and high energy) = proportion of fat (fat attenuation) + proportion of lean tissue (attenuation of lean tissue) (51). Thus, a 3C model is seen as soft tissue mass is divided into FFM and fat mass. Lohman (61) reported a precision for the DXA technique of about 1% with a SEE of about 1.8% body fat. A DXA scan generates pertinent information regarding the masses (g) of fat, lean tissue, and bone mineral content and density $(g \cdot cm^{-2})$ for the total body and for specific regions, e.g., the head, trunk, and limbs (Fig. 17-2).

DXA has many advantages for measurement of body composition. It is easy to administer, and subjects have a higher comfort level compared with other techniques, such

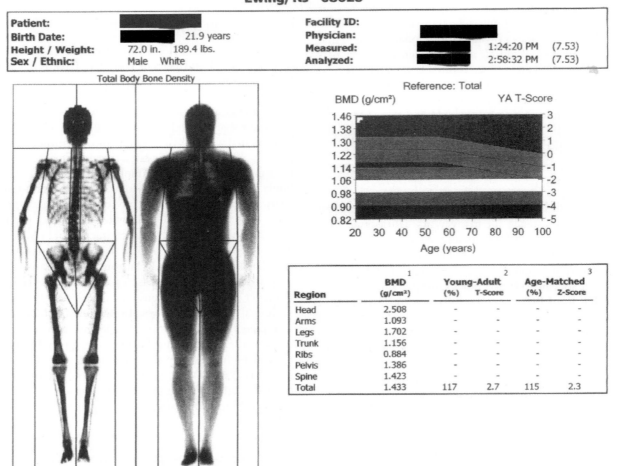

FIGURE 17-2. Sample DXA scan report.

ANCILLARY RESULTS [Total Body]

Region	BMD (g/cm²)	Young-Adult[1] (%)	T-Score	Age-Matched[2] (%)	Z-Score[3]	BMC (g)	Area (cm²)
Head	2.508	-	-	-	-	595	237
Arms	1.093	-	-	-	-	544	497
Legs	1.702	-	-	-	-	1,515	890
Trunk	1.156	-	-	-	-	1,357	1,174
Ribs	0.884	-	-	-	-	491	555
Pelvis	1.386	-	-	-	-	539	389
Spine	1.423	-	-	-	-	328	230
Total	1.433	117	2.7	115	2.3	4,011	2,799

BODY COMPOSITION

Region	Tissue (%Fat)	Region (%Fat)	Tissue (g)	Fat (g)	Lean (g)	BMC (g)	Total Mass (kg)
Left Arm	9.1	8.6	5,162	467	4,695	266	-
Left Leg	19.2	18.2	14,288	2,737	11,551	735	-
Left Trunk	18.5	17.8	19,948	3,685	16,263	699	-
Left Total	17.0	16.2	42,201	7,164	35,037	2,013	-
Right Arm	9.1	8.6	5,415	490	4,925	278	-
Right Leg	19.2	18.2	14,929	2,861	12,068	780	-
Right Trunk	18.5	17.8	18,381	3,394	14,987	658	-
Right Total	17.0	16.2	41,054	6,973	34,081	1,998	-
Arms	9.1	8.6	10,577	958	9,619	544	-
Legs	19.2	18.2	29,216	5,598	23,619	1,515	-
Trunk	18.5	17.8	38,330	7,079	23,619	1,357	-
Total	17.0	16.2	83,255	14,137	69,118	4,011	87.3

FIGURE 17-2. Continued.

as HW. Analytically, DXA software provides a great deal of information for the user. Regional body composition measurements are particularly attractive for clinical and research utilities. For example, BMD assessments of the lumbar spine, proximal femur, and forearm are useful in the diagnosis of osteoporosis (2). In fact, DXA has been shown to be a very reliable analytic tool for body composition measurements in clinical populations, including those with gastrointestinal, renal, endocrinologic, pulmonary, hepatic, bone, neuromuscular, and metabolic/nutritional disorders (2). Regional measurement of FFM is very attractive for examining the effects of various exercise programs, such as resistance training on muscular hypertrophy (87). DXA uses low-level radiation and is safe, fast, and accurate. A whole-body measurement is <5 μSv, which is close to background radiation levels (6–20 μSv) (26,51) and less than CT scans (58), chest x-ray (12–50 μSv), and lumbar spine x-ray (700–820 μSv) (2,25).

There are some limitations associated with DXA measurements. An individual's size is of some concern. A very tall person or individual of large weight (e.g., >300 lbs) may extend beyond the measurable range on the scanner table or have to maintain a "cramped" position, which can distort regional measurements. The DXA machines (e.g., General Electric Lunar, Hologic, and Norland) are also large and expensive, although the machines are becoming more accessible in number. Because of the expense of the DXA equipment, these machines are typically found in a clinical or research setting. DXA assumes the same amount of fat lies over bone as over neighboring bone-free tissue, which could potentially reduce accuracy in the limb and trunk regions (33). An increase in tissue anterior-posterior thickness in obese individuals could also reduce accuracy via attenuation of the dual energy rays (33). DXA assumes a constant hydration state (73.2%) and electrolyte content in lean tissue; thus, a change in hydration status could have a small effect of soft tissue attenuation (33,51). Last, user error can occur when delineating regional measurements, thereby demonstrating the importance of a single user for sequential testing.

There is concern over the lack of standardization between DXA equipment manufacturers. Differences exist in hardware, calibration methodology, and software that elicit different body composition results between machines

(2,33,54,82). The imaging geometry—e.g., the older-style pencil versus the newer fan beam—may be a source of variation. A pencil beam is coupled to a single detector and scans the whole body in a raster, whereas a fan beam is coupled to a multidetector (because z/x-rays overlap) linear array that distributes the x-rays across a wider area for a whole body scan (2). Fan-beam systems also have a higher x-ray flux and better image quality (2). Different manufacturers have different arrangements for x-ray distribution, number, and alignment of detectors (61). Genton et al. (33) reported that fat mass varied between DXA devices of different manufacturers and with different software used by the same manufacturer by 0.4 to 4.4 kg (0.5%–6.9%). In addition, body fat measurements have been shown to vary by about 1.7% when repeated measurements are taken on different DXA machines from the same manufacturer (81). CVs between DXA devices have been reported to be <5.2% (20,38), although the CV may be <1% when the same machine is used (69). Thus, for high reliability of measurements, it is strongly recommended that DXA scans be performed on the same machine for repeated intrasubject measurements.

DXA has been shown to correlate highly with HW and other multicompartment models (i.e., 4C) in athletes and in young, middle-aged, or elderly men and women. However, **Bland-Altman** analyses have shown that DXA typically registered higher body fat percentages (i.e., 1%–2%) for total body measurements (53,69,85). This procedure is commonly used to assess how well some "experimental" result compares with that of a result from a more sophisticated or criterion method. DXA has also been shown to overestimate percent body fat in young (±4.5%) and elderly (±2.2%) women, but to underestimate percent body fat in young (±0.9%) and elderly men (±1.7%) (14). DXA correlates strongly, but also underestimates, total fat mass by approximately 0.7 kg (76). In one investigation, when lard was added to either the trunk or thigh regions, DXA was able to quantify the additional mass as 96% fat (53), but was only able to identify approximately 62% of lard in the trunk as fat and >80% in the legs in another study (76). Regional body composition assessment has produced varying results, although DXA is valid for measuring abdominal adiposity (35). In some studies, DXA has been shown to underestimate central body fat (35,36) and to overestimate fat mass in the thigh and calf areas compared with CT scans (76). It is important to note that DXA alone cannot distinguish intra-abdominal from subcutaneous fat (51). Although the results of most validation studies show DXA to be an accurate tool for body composition assessment, limitations render it from becoming a gold standard at the current time. Lastly, DXA has been shown to be a reliable tool for monitoring body composition changes over time (91) and has been shown to be more sensitive for assessing small changes in body composition in postmenopausal women than HW and other multicompartment methods (49). Box 17-2 summarizes the pros and cons of body composition techniques.

BODY COMPOSITION ASSESSMENT IN CHILDREN AND ADOLESCENTS

It has been shown that >15% of children aged 6 to 19 years in the United States are overweight (71), and more than 2 million children are considered extremely obese (50). The prevalence of the metabolic syndrome in children is roughly 4%, with estimates reaching as high as 50% in obese youth populations (39). With the rise in childhood obesity in the United States, body composition measurement in children and adolescents has become a very important assessment tool. However, these populations can be difficult to assess because of the effects of growth/maturation on FFM, fat mass, and hydration state. Several studies have examined skinfolds, BMI, ADP, BIA, HW, and DXA assessments in children and adolescents. In comparison to 4C models, DXA and ADP have correlated very highly (27,79), but DXA has been shown to underestimate percent body fat in lean subjects and overestimate fat in heavier subjects (27,79). Overall, percent body fat obtained with DXA has been approximately 1% to 1.7% higher than in 4C models (27,79). Skinfolds are commonly used and have been shown to correlate highly with DXA (13). However, selection of the appropriate equation is critical, as more than 15 researchers have developed specific equations for children and adolescents, but few have correlated well to DXA (75). Several studies have shown ADP and skinfolds to provide accurate assessments of body composition in children compared with DXA (21,22), with absolute percent body fat values higher in DXA (60). However, BIA has been shown to underestimate percent body fat considerably (21) (sometimes, by as much as 12.8%) to overestimate FFM (46), and to overestimate changes in percent body fat over time (22). In obese children, ADP has been shown to correlate highly with DXA, with absolute percent body fat values being higher in DXA by about 3% to 5% (74). HW has been shown to produce similar percent body fat values compared with DXA (60) but to underestimate percent body fat (27) in children. HW has been considered unsuitable in children because of the difficulty in following the procedures of being submerged underwater and exhaling completely (21,27,79).

BODY FAT PREDICTION EQUATION SELECTION

Since the early 1950s, more than 100 regression equations have been developed to predict body density and percent body fat. Prediction equations may be either general or population specific. Population-specific equations may underestimate or overestimate body composition if they are applied to individuals from other populations. In contrast, generalized equations can replace several equations as they can be applied to diverse populations. Generalized

BOX 17-2   SUMMARY OF BODY COMPOSITION TECHNIQUES

TECHNIQUE	PROS OR ADVANTAGES	CONS OR DISADVANTAGES

SKINFOLD ANALYSIS

- Highly regarded technique yet prone to many sources of error
- Technician training and anatomic site selection important
- Equation(s) selected should be specific to population tested
- Many skinfold formulas exist from one to ten sites
- Standard error of the estimate (SEE) is approximately ±3.5% (differs with each equation)

BIOELECTRICAL IMPEDENCE

- Less technician training required compared with skinfold measurement
- Numerous pretest control conditions need to be followed by the patient (anything that affects hydration status)
- SEE is approximately ±3.5% to 5% (differs with each equation)

HYDRODENSITOMETRY

- Procedure is time consuming
- Equipment is fairly expensive and requires adequate space, plumbing, and high maintenance
- Criterion-reference (or gold) standard
- Some patients may not be able to perform the procedure (complete water submersion at full exhalation)
- Requires measurement of residual lung volume (additional equipment needed)
- SEE is approximately ±2.5%

NEAR-INFRARED INTERACTANCE

- Limited research on this procedure compared with other techniques

- Very little technician training needed
- SEE is approximately ±5% (differs with each equation)

CLINICAL ASSESSMENT PROCEDURES: COMPUTED TOMOGRAPHY SCANS AND MAGNETIC RESONANCE IMAGING SCANS

- Procedures are time-consuming
- Equipment is very expensive and is accessible only in clinical facilities
- Has numerous clinical applications
- SEE is not yet fully developed (more research data are needed)

PLETHYSMOGRAPHY: AIR DISPLACEMENT

- Equipment is expensive and is generally accessible only in research facilities
- No physical performance requirements for patient (advantage compared with hydrodensitometry)
- Does require special clothing (tight-fitting Lycra-type material)
- SEE is approximately ±2.2% to 3.7% (more research data are needed)

DUAL-ENERGY X-RAY ABORPTIOMETRY

- Equipment is expensive and is generally accessible only in clinical or research facilities
- Has more clinical utility than just percent body fat (also bone density)
- Can provide regional measurements on the body
- SEE is approximately ±1.8 % (more research data are needed)

---

equations are developed from heterogeneous samples and account for differences in age, sex, ethnicity, and other characteristics by including these variables as predictors in the equation.

To develop prediction equations, it is necessary to select a large representative sample of a specific population. The predictor variables (e.g., height and weight, sex, age, race or ethnicity, skinfolds, or bioelectrical impedance) and the criterion estimates of body composition are measured in the same subjects, and the equation is then developed using appropriate statistical methods. The usefulness of the equation depends on the strength of association between the variables and the accuracy with which the dependent variable is estimated. Useful equations give estimates of percent fat or FFM that are reasonably well correlated ($r > 0.80$) with the criterion measure. Moreover, the means and standard deviations of the estimated and criterion scores should be nearly equal, and the SEE for predicting the criterion from the estimated values is between $\pm 2.5\%$ to 3.5% for percent body fat (84). To select the most appropriate equation, the following questions should be considered (84):

1. To whom is the specific percent body fat equation applicable? Age, ethnicity, sex, physical activity level, and estimated amount of body fat all influence which equation should be used.

2. Was an appropriate compartment model used to develop the equation? Errors from the compartment model contribute to the equation's total error. For example, multicompartment models require fewer assumptions and give more accurate reference measurements than methods based on the 2C model. Equations derived from 3C and 4C models should be used in populations for whom the assumptions underlying the 2C model are not valid.

3. Was a representative sample of the population studied? Large, randomly selected samples are needed to ensure that the data are representative of the population. If random sampling is not possible and convenience samples are used, the prediction equation may be acceptable as long as a sufficient number of subjects are studied. Large sample sizes yield stable and valid equations.

4. How were the predictor variables measured? When any equation is applied, it is important that the predictor variables be measured in the same way as the original investigators to minimize prediction errors.

5. Was the equation cross-validated in another sample of the population? Investigator/laboratory differences can reduce equation accuracy. Thus, the equation should be tested (i.e., cross-validated) in other samples of the same population.

6. Does the equation give accurate estimates of percent body fat? In validation studies, when estimating body fat, the multiple correlations between variables should be $R^2 > 0.80$, and SEEs should range from 2.5% to 3.5%.

INTERPRETATION OF BODY FAT PERCENTAGE ESTIMATES

Interpretation of body fat percent estimates is complicated by three factors: (a) there are no universal standards for percent body fat that have been established and accepted; (b) all methods of measurement are indirect, so error needs to be considered; and (3) there is no universally accepted criterion measurement method.

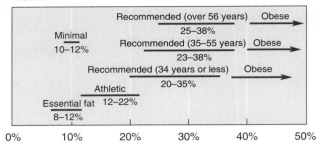

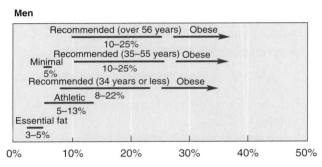

FIGURE 17-3. Percent body fat standards for men and women.

BODY FAT PERCENTAGE STANDARDS

Although national standards have been developed and accepted for BMI and waist circumference (GETP8 Tables 4.2 and 4.3; Fig. 17-3), none exist for estimates of body fat percent. Thus, practitioners must choose from many classifications proposed by textbook authors, researchers, and programs (62). Standards may be based on health or physical performance, but only sex is considered a differentiating factor in percent body fat classifications. However, it is well known that body fat increases with age from the late teens/early 20s up to the sixth decade of life. The magnitude of increase in body fat with age is associated with lifestyle factors that affect energy intake and expenditure.

Since 1981, subsequent releases of the *ACSM Guidelines for Exercise Testing and Prescription* have included the normative-based standards developed by the Cooper Institute in Dallas, Texas. These norms were revised in 1994 and were developed using skinfold measurements to estimate body fat percent in a population of predominately white and college-educated men and women (GETP8 Tables 4-5 and 4-6). These norms provide percentiles that differ by sex and age (ranging from 20 to 60+ years). The average (fiftieth percentile) for young (20–29 years) men and women is 15.9% and 22.1%, respectively. The average increases to 23.5% and 30.9% for elderly (60+ years) men and women, respectively (62). The difference from the tenth to nineteenth percentile is approximately 16% points in men and 17% points in women within each age grouping.

MEASUREMENT ERROR CONSIDERATIONS

Body fat percent data should be presented and interpreted with the SEE term for the methods used (e.g., 22% ± 3.5%). Minimally, ±1 SEE unit should be used; however, if the 95% confidence interval (CI) limits are desired, then ±2 SEE units are required. A major concern in interpreting body fat percent values is the relatively large SEE of the measurements. This concern is shown by viewing the SEE of ±3.5% for skinfold equations. For example, a 45-year-old woman who had skinfolds taken and a percent body fat of 28.5% (thirty-eighth percentile) could be as low as 21.5% (eightieth percentile) or as high as 35.5% (<tenth percentile) when considering the 95% CI (±2 SEE). Because of the lack of accepted national standards and the large SEE, interpretation of percent body fat estimates need to be interpreted with caution and shared with patients only after careful explanation of the meaning of the values. The most appropriate use of these estimates may be for serial measurements over time or to evaluate responses to diet or physical activity where the same measurement procedure (i.e., instrument and technician) is used.

SUMMARY

Excess body fat is detrimental to overall health and physical performance. Measurement and quantification of body fat is of great importance for allied health professionals, fitness practitioners, and athletic personnel. In most nonathletic adults, a reasonable assessment of excess weight (fat) status can be determined from simple measurements of height, weight, or body mass and waist circumference. These measurements are easy to obtain, do not require extensive training to perform, and do not require expensive equipment. Advanced body composition estimates can be made when specific information is needed, equipment is available, and trained technicians perform the assessments. It is important for users of these advanced body fat estimation methods to understand the error associated with these measurements, to use the SEE in reporting body composition results, and to strictly adhere to the procedures outlined in this chapter when assessing body composition.

REFERENCES

1. Abe T, Kawakami Y, Sugita M, Yoshikawa K, Fukunaga T. Use of B-mode ultrasound for visceral fat mass evaluation: comparisons with magnetic resonance imaging. *Appl Human Sci.* 1995;14:133–139.
2. Albanese CV, Diessel E, Genant HK. Clinical applications of body composition measurements using DXA. *J Clin Densitom.* 2003; 6:75–85.
3. **American College of Sports Medicine. Position stand: Weight loss in wrestlers.** *Med Sci Sports Exerc.* **1996;28:ix–xii.**
4. Ball SD, Altena TS. Comparison of the Bod Pod and dual energy x-ray absorptiometry in men. *Physiol Meas.* 2004;25:671–678.
5. Ballard TP, Fafara L, Vukovich MD. Comparison of Bod Pod® and DXA in female collegiate athletes. *Med Sci Sports Exerc.* 2004;36: 731–735.

6. Baumgartner RN. Electrical impedance and total body electrical conductivity. In... Roche AF, Heymsfield SB, Lohman TG, editors. *Human Body Composition.* Champaign (IL): Human Kinetics; 1996. p. 79–107.
7. Baumgartner RN, Heymsfield SB, Lichtman S, Wang J, Pierson RN. Body composition in elderly people: effect of criterion estimates on predictive equations. *Am J Clin Nutr.* 1991;53:1345–1353.
8. Bellisari A, Roche AF, Siervogel RM. Reliability of B-mode ultrasonic measurements of subcutaneous adipose tissue and intraabdominal depth: comparisons with skinfold thicknesses. *Int J Obes Relat Metab Disord.* 1993;17:475–480.
9. Bolanowksi M, Nilsson BE. Assessment of human body composition using dual-energy x-ray absorptiometry and bioelectrical impedance analysis. *Med Sci Monit.* 2001;7:1029–1033.
10. Boren HG, Kory RC, Snyder JC. The Veteran's Administration Army Coorperative Study of Pulmonary Function. II. The lung volume and its subdivisions in normal men. *Am J Med.* 1966;41:96–114.
11. Broeder CE, Burrhus KA, Svanevik LS, Volpe J, Wilmore JH. Assessing body composition before and after resistance or endurance training. *Med Sci Sports Exerc.* 1997;29:705–712.
12. Brozek J, Grande F, Anderson J, et al. Densitometric analysis of body composition: revision of some quantitative assumptions. *Am N Y Acad Sci.* 1963;110:113–140.
13. Buison AM, Ittenbach RF, Stallings VA, Zemel BS. Methodological agreement between two-compartment body-composition methods in children. *Am J Hum Biol.* 2006;18:470–480.
14. Clasey JL, Kanaley JA, Wideman L, et al. Validity of methods of body composition assessment in young and older men and women. *J Appl Physiol.* 1999;86:1728–1738.
15. Collins MA, Millard-Stafford ML, Sparling PB, et al. Evaluation of the BOD POD® for assessing body fat in collegiate football players. *Med Sci Sports Exerc.* 1999;31:1350–1356.
16. Committee refines wrestling safety rules. *The NSCA News* 1998; 35:1.
17. Despres JP, Lemieux I. Abdominal obesity and metabolic syndrome. *Nature.* 2006;444:881–887.
18. Dixon CB, Deitrick RW, Pierce JR, Cutrufello PT, Drapeau LL. Evaluation of the BOD POD and leg-to-leg bioelectrical impedance analysis for estimating percent body fat in National Collegiate Athletic Association Division III collegiate wrestlers. *J Strength Cond Res.* 2005;19:85–91.
19. Dutta C. Significance of sarcopenia in the elderly. *J Nutr.* 1997;127 (suppl.):992S–993S.
20. Economos CD, Nelson ME, Fiatarone MA, et al. A multi-center comparison of dual energy x-ray absorptiometers: in vivo and in vitro soft tissue measurement. *Eur J Clin Nutr.* 1997;51:312–317.
21. Eisenmann JC, Heelan KA, Welk GJ. Assessing body composition among 3- to 8-year old children: anthropometry, BIA, and DXA. *Obes Res.* 2004;12:1633–1640.
22. Elberg J, McDuffie JR, Sebring NG, et al. Comparison of methods to assess change in children's body composition. *Am J Clin Nutr.* 2004;80:64–69.
23. Ellis KJ. Whole-body counting and neutron activation analysis. In: Roche AF, Heymsfield SB, Lohman TG, editors. *Human Body Composition.* Champaign (IL): Human Kinetics; 1996. p. 45–61.
24. Erickson JM, Stout JR, Eveertourch TK, et al. Validity of self-assessment techniques for estimating percent body fat in men and women. *J Strength Cond Res.* 1998;12:243–247.
25. Fanelli MT, Kuczmarski RJ. Ultrasound as an approach to assessing body composition. *Am J Clin Nutr.* 1984;39:703–709.
26. Fewtrell MS. Bone densitometry in children assessed by dual x ray absorptiometry: uses and pitfalls. *Arch Dis Child.* 2003;88:795–798.
27. Fields DA, Goran MI. Body composition techniques and the four-compartment model in children. *J Appl Physiol.* 2000;89:613–620.
28. Fields DA, Goran MI, McCory MA. Body composition assessments via air displacement plethysmography in adults and children: a review. *Am J Clin Nutr.* 2002;75:453–467.

29. Fields DA, Higgins PB, Hunter GR. Assessment of body composition by air-displacement plethysmography: influence of body temperature and moisture. *Dynamic Medicine.* 2004;3:3.

30. Fields DA, Wilson D, Gladden LB, et al. Comparison of the BOD POD with the four-compartment model in adult females. *Med Sci Sports Exerc.* 2001;33:1605–1610.

31. Fornetti WC, Pivarnik JM, Foley JM, Fiechtner JJ. Reliability and validity of body composition measures in female athletes. *J Appl Physiol.* 1999;87:1114–1122.

32. Frisard MI, Greenway FL, Delany JP. Comparison of methods to assess body composition changes during a period of weight loss. *Obes Res.* 2005;13:845–854.

33. Genton L, Hans D, Kyle UG, Pichard C. Dual-energy x-ray absorptiometry and body composition: differences between devices and comparison with reference methods. *Nutrition.* 2002;18:66–70.

34. Ginde SR, Geliebter A, Rubiano F, et al. Air displacement plethysmography: validation in overweight and obese subjects. *Obes Res.* 2005;13:1232–1237.

35. Glickman SG, Marn CS, Supiano MA, Dengel DR. Validity and reliability of dual-energy x-ray absorptiometry for the assessment of abdominal obesity. *J Appl Physiol.* 2004;97:509–514.

36. Graves JE, Kanaley JA, Garzarella L, Pollock ML. Anthropometry and body composition assessment. In: Maud PJ, Foster C, editors. *Physiological Assessment of Human Fitness.* 2nd ed. Champaign (IL): Human Kinetics; 2006. p. 185–225.

37. Gunstad J, Paul RH, Cohen RA, Tate DF, Spitznagel MB, Gordon E. Elevated body mass index is associated with executive dysfunction in otherwise healthy adults. *Compr Psychiatry.* 2007;48(1):57–61.

38. Guo Y, Franks PW, Brookshire T, Tataranni PA. The intra- and inter-instrument reliability of DXA based on ex vivo soft tissue measurements. *Obes Res.* 2004;12:1925–1929.

39. Harrell JS, Jessup A, Greene N. Changing our future: obesity and the metabolic syndrome in children and adolescents. *J Cardiovasc Nurs.* 2006;21:322–330.

40. Haymes EM, Lundegren HM, Loomis JL, Buskirk ER. Validity of the ultrasonic technique as a method of measuring subcutaneous adipose tissue. *Ann Hum Biol.* 1976;3:245–251.

41. Heymsfield SB, Lichtman S, Baumgartner RN, et al. Body composition of humans: comparison of two improved four-compartment models that differ in expense, technical complexity, and radiation exposure. *Am J Clin Nutr.* 1990;52:52–58.

42. Heymsfield SB, Wang ZM, Withers RT. Multicomponent molecular level models of body composition. In: Roche AF, Heymsfield SB, Lohman TG, editors. *Human Body Composition.* Champaign (IL): Human Kinetics; 1996. p. 129–147.

43. Heyward VH, Stolarczyk LM. *Applied Body Composition Assessment.* Champaign (IL): Human Kinetics; 1996. p 82.

44. Heyward VH, Wagner DR. *Applied Body Composition Assessment.* Champaign (IL): Human Kinetics; 2004.

45. Higgins PB, Fields DA, Hunter GR, Gower BA. Effect of scalp and facial hair on air displacement plethysmography estimates of percentage of body fat. *Obes Res.* 2001;9:326–330.

46. Hosking J, Metcalf BS, Jeffery AN, Voss LD, Wilkin TJ. Validation of foot-to-foot bioelectrical impedance analysis with dual-energy x-ray absorptiometry in the assessment of body composition in young children: the early bird cohort. *Br J Nutr.* 2006;96:1163–1168.

47. Housh TJ, Johnson GO, Housh DJ, et al. Accuracy of near-infrared interactance instruments and population-specific equations for estimating body composition in young wrestlers. *J Strength Cond Res.* 2004;18:556–560.

48. Housh TJ, Stout JR, Johnson GO, Housh DJ, Eckerson JM. Validity of near-infrared interactance instruments for estimating percent body fat in youth wrestlers. *Pediatr Exerc Sci.* 1996;8:69–76.

49. Houtkooper LB, Going SB, Sproul J, Blew RM, Lohman TG. Comparison of methods for assessing body-composition changes over 1 y in postmenopausal women. *Am J Clin Nutr.* 2000;72:401–406.

50. Inge TH, Xanthakos SA, Zeller MH. Bariatric surgery for pediatric extreme obesity: now or later? *Int J Obes.* 2007;31:1–14.

51. Jebb SA. Measurement of soft tissue composition by dual energy x-ray absorptiometry. *Br J Nutr.* 1997;77:151–163.

52. Jones PR, Davies PS, Norgan NG. Ultrasonic measurements of subcutaneous adipose tissue thickness in man. *Am J Phys Anthropol.* 1986;71:359–363.

53. Kohrt WM. Preliminary evidence that DEXA provides an accurate assessment of body composition. *J Appl Physiol.* 1998;84:372–377.

54. Koo WWK, Hammami M, Shypailo RJ, Ellis KJ. Bone and body composition measurements of small subjects: discrepancies from software for fan-beam dual energy x-ray absorptiometry. *J Am Coll Nutr.* 2004;23(6):647–650.

55. Kraemer WJ, Torine JC, Silvestre R, et al. Body size and composition of National Football League players. *J Strength Cond Res.* 2005;19:485–489.

56. Kuczmarski RJ, Fanelli MT, Koch GG. Ultrasonic assessment of body composition in obese adults: overcoming the limitations of the skinfold caliper. *Am J Clin Nutr.* 1987;45:717–724.

57. Lane JM, Serota AC, Raphael B. Osteoporosis: differences and similarities in male and female patients. *Orthop Clin North Am.* 2006;37:601–609.

58. Laskey MA, Phil D. Dual-energy x-ray absorptiometry and body composition. *Nutrition.* 1996;12:45–51.

59. Liuke M, Solovieva S, Lamminen A, et al. Disc degeneration of the lumbar spine in relation to overweight. *Int J Obes.* 2005;29:903–908.

60. Lockner DW, Heyward VH, Baumgartner RN, Jenkins KA. Comparison of air-displacement plethysmography, hydrodensitometry, and dual x-ray absorptiometry for assessing body composition of children 10 to 18 years of age. *Ann N Y Acad Sci.* 2000;904:72–78.

61. Lohman TG. *Advances in Body Composition Assessment.* Champaign (IL): Human Kinetics; 1992.

62. Lohman TG, Houtkooper LB, Going SB. Body composition assessment: body fat standards and methods in the field of exercise and sports medicine. *ACSM Health & Fitness Journal.* 1997;1:30–35.

63. Lukaski HC, Siders WA. Validity and accuracy of regional bioelectrical impedance devices to determine whole-body fatness. *Nutrition.* 2003;19(10):851–857.

64. Malina RM. Regional body composition: age, sex, and ethnic variation. In: Roche AF, Heymsfield SB, Lohman TG, editors. *Human Body Composition.* Champaign (IL): Human Kinetics; 1996. p. 217–255.

65. Malina RM. Body composition in athletes: assessment and estimated fatness. *Clin Sports Med.* 2007;26:37–68.

66. Minderico CS, Silva AM, Teixeira PJ, et al. Validity of air-displacement plethysmography in the assessment of body composition changes in a 16-month weight loss program. *Nutr Metab.* 2006;3:32.

67. Mitsiopoulos N, Baumgartner RN, Heymsfield SB, et al. Cadaver validation of skeletal muscle measurement by magnetic resonance imaging and computerized tomography. *J Appl Physiol.* 1998;85:115–122.

68. **National Heart, Lung, and Blood Institute. *Clinical Guidelines on the Identification, Evaluation, and Treatment of Overweight and Obesity in Adults: The Evidence Report.* Bethesda (MD): National Institutes of Health, National Heart, Lung, and Blood Institute. U.S. Department of Health and Human Services, Public Health Service; 1998.**

69. Norcross J, Van Loan MD. Validation of fan beam dual energy x ray absorptiometry for body composition assessment in adults aged 18–45 years. *Br J Sports Med.* 2004;38:472–476.

70. O'Brien RJ, Drizd TA. Roentgenographic determination of total lung capacity: normal values from a national population survey. *Am Rev Respir Dis.* 1983;128:949–952.

71. Ogden CL, Flegal KM, Carroll MD, Johnson CL. Prevalence and trends in overweight among US children and adolescents, 1999–2000. *JAMA.* 2002;288:1728–1732.

72. Panotopoulos G, Ruiz JC, Guy-Grand B, Basedevant A. Dual x-ray absorptiometry, bioelectrical impedance, and near infrared interactance in obese women. *Med Sci Sports Exerc.* 2001;33:665–670.

73. Pietrobelli A, Wang Z, Heymsfield SB. Techniques used in measuring human body composition. *Curr Opin Clin Nutr Metab Care.* 1998;1:439–448.

74. Radley D, Gately PJ, Cooke CB, et al. Percentage fat in overweight and obese children: comparison of DXA and air displacement plethysmography. *Obes Res.* 2005;13:75–85.

75. Rodriguez G, Moreno LA, Blay MJ, et al. Body fat measurement in adolescents: comparison of skinfold thickness equations with dual-energy x-ray absorptiometry. *Eur J Clin Nutr.* 2005;59:1158–1166.

76. Salamone LM, Fuerst T, Visser M, et al. Measurement of fat mass using DEXA: a validation study in elderly adults. *J Appl Physiol.* 2000;89:345–352.

77. Semiz S, Ozgoren E, Sabir N. Comparison of ultrasonographic and anthropometric methods to assess body fat in childhood obesity. *Int J Obes.* 2007;31:53–58.

78. Siri WE. The gross composition of the body. *Adv Biol Med Physiol.* 1956;4:239–280.

79. Sopher AB, Thornton JC, Wang J, et al. Measurement of percentage of body fat in 411 children and adolescents: a comparison of dual-energy x-ray absorptiometry with a four-compartment model. *Pediatrics.* 2004;113:1285–1290.

80. Stolk RP, Wink O, Zelissen PMJ, et al. Validity and reproducibility of ultrasonography for the measurement of intra-abdominal adipose tissue. *Int J Obes.* 2001;25:1346–1351.

81. Tataranni PA, Pettitt DJ, Ravussin E. Dual energy x-ray absorptiometry: inter-machine variability. *Int J Obes Relat Metab Disord.* 1996;20:1048–1050.

82. Tothill P, Avenell A, Reid DM. Precision and accuracy of measurements of whole-body bone mineral: comparisons between Hologic, Lunar and Norland dual-energy x-ray absorptiometers. *Br J Radiol.* 1994;67:1210–1217.

83. Tylavsky FA, Lohman TG, Dockrell M, et al. Comparison of the effectiveness of 2 dual-energy X-ray absorptiometers with that of total body water and computed tomography in assessing changes in body composition during weight change. *Am J Clin Nutr.* 2003;77:356–363.

84. **U.S. Department of Health and Human Services.** *Basic Data on Anthropometric Measurements and Angular Measurements of the Hip and Knee Joints for Selected Age Groups 1–74 Years of Age (1971–1975). Atlanta, GA. DHHS Publication No. (PHS) 81–1669, Series II, No. 219, 2003.*

85. Van Marken Lichtenbelt WD, Hartgens F, Vollaard NBJ, Ebbing S, Kuipers H. Body composition changes in bodybuilders: a method comparison. *Med Sci Sports Exerc.* 2004;36:490–497.

86. Vescovi JD, Hildebrandt L, Miller W, Hammer R, Spiller A. Evaluation of the BOD POD for estimating percent fat in female college athletes. *J Strength Cond Res.* 2002;16:599–605.

87. Volek JS, Ratamess NA, Rubin MR, et al. The effects of creatine supplementation on muscular performance and body composition responses to short-term resistance training overreaching. *Eur J Appl Physiol.* 2004;91:628–637.

88. Wang ZM, Heshka S, Pierson RN, et al. Systematic organization of body composition methodology: an overview with emphasis on component-based methods. *Am J Clin Nutr.* 1995;61:457–465.

89. Wearing SC, Hennig EM, Byrne NM, Steele JR, Hills AP. Musculoskeletal disorders associated with obesity: a biomechanical perspective. *Obes Rev.* 2006;7:239–250.

90. Weits T, van der Beek EJ, Wedel M. Comparison of ultrasound and skinfold caliper measurement of subcutaneous fat tissue. *Int J Obes.* 1986;10:161–168.

91. Weyers AM, Mazzetti SA, Love DM, et al. Comparison of methods for assessing body composition changes during weight loss. *Med Sci Sports Exerc.* 2002;34:497–502.

SELECTED REFERENCES FOR FURTHER READING

American College of Sports Medicine. *ACSM's Guidelines for Exercise Testing and Prescription.* 8th ed. Philadelphia: Lippincott, Williams, and Wilkins; 2008.

American College of Sports Medicine. *ACSM's Health-Related Physical Fitness Assessment Manual.* 2nd ed. Philadelphia: Lippincott, Williams, and Wilkins; 2007.

Heymsfield SB, Lohman T, Wang Z, Going SB. *Human Body Composition.* 2nd ed. Champaign (IL): Human Kinetics; 2006.

Heyward VH, Wagner DR. *Applied Body Composition Assessment.* 2nd ed. Champaign (IL): Human Kinetics; 2004.

Hoffman J. *Norms for Fitness, Performance, and Health.* Champaign (IL): Human Kinetics; 2006.

Lohman TG, Roche AF, Martorell R, editors. *Anthropometric Standardization Reference Manual.* Champaign (IL): Human Kinetics; 1988.

Maud PJ, Foster C. *Physiological Assessment of Human Fitness.* 2nd ed. Champaign (IL): Human Kinetics; 2006.

National Heart, Lung, and Blood Institute. *Clinical Guidelines on the Identification, Evaluation, and Treatment of Overweight and Obesity in Adults: The Evidence Report.* Bethesda (MD): National Institutes of Health, National Heart, Lung, and Blood Institute, U.S. Department of Health and Human Services, Public Health Service; 1998.

INTERNET RESOURCES

- Body Fat Lab: www.shapeup.org/bodylab/default.php
- Body Composition Tests: www.americanheart.org/presenter.jhtml?identifier=4489
- National Center for Health Statistics. National Health and Nutrition Examination Survey. www.cdc.gov/nchs/nhanes.htm
- National Heart Lung and Blood Institute: Clinical Guidelines on the Identification, Evaluation, and Treatment of Overweight and Obesity in Adults: www.nhlbi.nih.gov/guidelines/obesity/ob_home.htm
- National Institutes of Health: Calculate your body mass index: www.nhlbisupport.com/bmi
- Overweight Children: www.americanheart.org/presenter.jhtml?identifier=4670

SECTION

II

Exercise Testing

ADAM DeJONG, MA, FACSM, *Section Editor*

> **1.3.7-CES: Conduct pre-exercise test procedures.**

> **1.3.16-CES: Evaluate medical history and physical examination findings as they relate to health appraisal and exercise testing.**

> **1.3.2-HFS: Knowledge of the value of the health/medical history.**

> **1.3.3-HFS: Knowledge of the value of a medical clearance before exercise participation.**

> **1.3.13-HFS: Ability to obtain a health history and risk appraisal that includes past and current medical history, family history of cardiac disease, orthopedic limitations, prescribed medications, activity patterns, nutritional habits, stress and anxiety levels, and smoking and alcohol use.**

Exercise is a safe activity for most individuals. However, risks such as sudden cardiac death and myocardial infarction are associated with beginning an exercise program or performing an exercise test (26). The benefits and risk associated with physical activity and exercise testing are discussed in Chapter 1 of Guidelines of Exercise Testing and Prescription, 8th edition (GETP8). The preparticipation health screen reduces the risk of an untoward event associated with starting an exercise program or performing an exercise test by identifying known diseases and risk factors for coronary artery disease. Furthermore, identification of additional factors that require special consideration when developing an appropriate exercise prescription and exercise program can optimize adherence, minimize risk, and maximize benefits. The purposes of the preparticipation health screen include the following:

- Identification of individuals with medical contraindications for exclusion from exercise programs until those conditions have been abated or controlled
- Recognition of persons with clinically significant disease who should participate in a medically supervised exercise program
- Detection of individuals at increased risk for disease because of age, symptoms, and/or risk factors who should undergo a medical evaluation and exercise testing before initiating an exercise program or increasing the frequency, intensity, or duration of their current program
- Recognition of special needs of individuals that may affect exercise testing and programming

This chapter will focus on preparticipation health screening for (a) individuals beginning an exercise program, (b) athletes participating in sports, and (c) individuals before an exercise test. In addition to preparticipation health screening, aspects of the pretest evaluation will be discussed.

PREPARTICIPATION SCREENING BEFORE BEGINNING AN EXERCISE PROGRAM

> **1.3.16-CES: Evaluate medical history and physical examination findings as they relate to health appraisal and exercise testing.**

> **1.3.2-HFS: Knowledge of the value of the health/medical history.**

> > > **KEY TERMS**

Aneroid: Without fluid; denoting a form of barometer without mercury, in which the varying air pressure is indicated by a pointer governed by the movement of the elastic wall of an evacuated chamber. Also used to denote a mercury-free pressure gauge used with some sphygmomanometers.

Coarctation: Pertaining to a constriction, stricture, or stenosis.

Peripheral: Situated nearer the periphery of an organ or part of the body in relation to a specific reference point; opposite of *central*.

> **1.3.3-HFS: Knowledge of the value of a medical clearance before exercise participation.**

> **1.3.4-HFS: Knowledge of and the ability to perform risk stratification and its implications toward medical clearance before administration of an exercise test or participation in an exercise program.**

> **1.3.13-HFS: Ability to obtain a health history and risk appraisal that includes past and current medical history, family history of cardiac disease, orthopedic limitations, prescribed medications, activity patterns, nutritional habits, stress and anxiety levels, and smoking and alcohol use.**

Preparticipation health screenings can be either self-administered or performed by an appropriately trained healthcare professional (see Appendix D, GETP8). A self-administered questionnaire such as the American Heart Association (AHA)/American College of Sports Medicine (ACSM) Health/Fitness Facility Preparticipation Screening Questionnaire (2) or Physical Activity Readiness Questionnaire (PAR-Q) (7) are considered the minimally accepted screening tools that alert the health fitness professional to recommend medical clearance before beginning an exercise program. The AHA/ACSM Health/Fitness Facility Preparticipation Screening Questionnaire and PAR-Q screening tools are explained in detail and sample forms provided in Chapter 2 of the GETP8. Individuals classified as "low risk" may safely pursue physical activity (see Risk Stratification in Chapter 2 of GETP8).

PREPARTICIPATION SCREENING FOR COMPETITIVE ATHLETES

> **1.3.16-CES: Evaluate medical history and physical examination findings as they relate to health appraisal and exercise testing.**

> **1.3.2-HFS: Knowledge of the value of the health/medical history.**

> **1.3.3-HFS: Knowledge of the value of a medical clearance before exercise participation.**

> **1.3.4-HFS: Knowledge of and the ability to perform risk stratification and its implications toward medical clearance before administration of an exercise test or participation in an exercise program.**

> **1.3.13-HFS: Ability to obtain a health history and risk appraisal that includes past and current medical history, family history of cardiac disease, orthopedic limitations, prescribed medications, activity patterns, nutritional habits, stress and anxiety levels, and smoking and alcohol use.**

Sudden death in young competitive athletes has sparked interest in prevention of these untimely deaths.

The American Heart Association released recommended guidelines for preparticipation screenings for cardiovascular abnormalities in competitive athletes in 2007. These recommendations were published in the journal *Circulation* and are available online at http://circ.ahajournals. org/cgi/reprint/115/12/1643 (16). Currently, high schools and colleges do not have mandated standards for screening athletes. Generally, athletes are cleared to participate in sports by a physician or other trained healthcare provider. However, past medical history (PMH) and physical examination (PE) alone are not sufficiently sensitive in detecting cardiovascular abnormalities that are linked to sudden death in youth athletes. The AHA recommends a 12-element Preparticipation Cardiovascular Screening of Competitive Athletes, which is presented in Table 18-1. Should an athlete have any one or more of the 12 items, a referral for a cardiovascular evaluation is recommended (16).

PREPARTICIPATION SCREENING BEFORE EXERCISE TESTING/PRESCRIPTION

> **1.3.2-HFS: Knowledge of the value of the health/medical history.**

> **1.3.3-HFS: Knowledge of the value of a medical clearance before exercise participation.**

> **1.3.4-HFS: Knowledge of and the ability to perform risk stratification and its implications toward medical clearance before administration of an exercise test or participation in an exercise program.**

> **1.3.13-HFS: Ability to obtain a health history and risk appraisal that includes past and current medical history, family history of cardiac disease, orthopedic limitations, prescribed medications, activity patterns, nutritional habits, stress and anxiety levels, and smoking and alcohol use.**

A more detailed and structured preparticipation assessment should be performed on individuals who are considered moderate to high risk. The preparticipation screen before exercise testing focuses on a comprehensive assessment that guides the health fitness professional in making decisions regarding the patient's optimal care (6).

IMPORTANCE OF PRE-EXERCISE TESTING EVALUATION

A comprehensive preparticipation assessment should include a PMH, PE, laboratory testing, and electrocardiograph (ECG) monitoring (3,22). The focus of the examination is on detection of risk factors that can be directly modified (22). According to the American Thoracic Society and American College of Chest Physicians

TABLE 18-1. THE 12-ELEMENT AMERICAN HEART ASSOCIATION RECOMMENDATIONS FOR PREPARTICIPATION CARDIOVASCULAR SCREENING OF COMPETITIVE ATHLETES

Medical history[a]

Personal history

1. Exertional chest pain/discomfort
2. Unexplained syncope/near-syncope[b]
3. Excessive exertional and unexplained dyspnea/fatigue, associated with exercise
4. Prior recognition of a heart murmur
5. Elevated systemic blood pressure

Family history

6. Premature death (sudden and unexpected, or otherwise) before age 50 years as a result of heart disease in ≥1 relative
7. Disability from heart disease in a close relative <50 years of age
8. Specific knowledge of certain cardiac conditions in family members: hypertrophic or dilated cardiomyopathy, long-QT syndrome or other ion channelopathies, Marfan syndrome, or clinically important arrhythmias

Physical Examination

9. Heart murmur[c]
10. Femoral pulses to exclude aortic coarctation
11. Physical stigmata of Marfan syndrome
12. Brachial artery blood pressure (sitting positions)[d]

[a]Parental verification is recommended for high school and middle school athletes.

[b]Judged not to be neurocardiogenic (vasovagal); of particular concern when related to exertion.

[c]Auscultation should be performed in both supine and standing positions (or with Valsalva maneuver), specifically to identify murmurs of dynamic left ventricular outflow tract obstruction.

[d]Preferably taken in both arms.

Source: Reprinted with permission from Maron BJ, Thompson PD, Ackerman MG, et al. (16). Recommendations and considerations related to preparticipation screening for cardiovascular abnormalities in competitive athletes: 2007 update: a scientific statement from the American Heart Association Council on Nutrition, Physical Activity, and Metabolism: endorsed by the American College of Cardiology Foundation. *Circulation.* 2007;115(12):1643–1655.

(3), a comprehensive preparticipation assessment allows the clinician to:

- Determine reasons for clinical exercise testing
- Form a clinical diagnosis
- Determine medications that may alter heart rate and blood pressure (BP) responses with exercise
- Identify risk factors for cardiovascular, pulmonary, musculoskeletal, and metabolic disorders

Accurate, yet simple methods of risk assessment are important for patient care (6). Evidence suggests that an aggressive risk factor management program clearly improves patient survival, reduces recurrent events and the need for interventional procedures, and improves the quality of life for individuals with atherosclerosis. However, reports indicate a large proportion of individuals in whom therapies are indicated are *not* receiving those therapies in actual clinical practice (25). Therefore, a link is missing between the knowledge of risk factor management and the actual practice of risk factor management. The AHA and American College of Cardiology (ACC) continue to urge all healthcare settings to have a specific plan to identify persons with known risk factors, provide healthcare providers with useful reminder clues based on the guidelines, and continuously assess the outcomes achieved in providing all appropriate therapies to all of the patients who can benefit from them (25). Furthermore, the health fitness professional should focus on identifying patients at an earlier stage of their disease and encourage participation in a comprehensive cardiovascular risk reduction program so that individuals may realize the benefits that primary prevention can provide (22).

Many times, the health fitness professional is the first to identify individuals in need of risk factor reduction.

The health fitness professional should create an environment supportive of risk factor change, including long-term reinforcement of adherence to lifestyle and drug interventions. Because risk factors have heredity and environmental factors, not only should risk factor reduction be implemented for the patient, but a family-centered approach to primary prevention is recommended. The family-centered approach would include avoidance of tobacco (including secondhand smoke), healthy dietary patterns, weight control, and regular, appropriate exercise (22).

PAST MEDICAL HISTORY

> **1.3.13-HFS: Ability to obtain a health history and risk appraisal that includes past and current medical history, family history of cardiac disease, orthopedic limitations, prescribed medications, activity patterns, nutritional habits, stress and anxiety levels, and smoking and alcohol use.**

The PMH of the patient initiates the preparticipation process (3,22). The PMH may include the following information:

- Demographic information (patient's name, address, admission date, date of birth, etc.)
- Medical diagnosis, and past and present conditions or diseases
- Recent or past surgeries
- Current medications (antiplatelet agents/anticoagulants, angiotensin-converting enzyme [ACE] inhibitors, β-blockers, etc.) (27)

- Medical test results (laboratory such as Hb$_{A1c}$, radiologic test, etc.)
- Functional status/activity level
- Social history (cultural/religious beliefs that could affect care, available social support)
- Employment status (full time or part time, retired or student, workplace demands)
- General health status (rating of the patient's health during the past year)
- Social/health habits (past and current alcohol, tobacco, and exercise habits) (3,15,27)
- Family health history (heart disease, diabetes, arthritis, osteoporosis, and other conditions)
- Patient goals (15)

Components of the medical history are further explained in Box 3.1 of GETP8. All information obtained in the PMH is used to provide quality care in determination of functional goals/outcomes for the patient.

PHYSICAL EXAMINATION

After obtaining the PMH, each patient is risk stratified to determine necessary components of the physical examination (3,22). Components of the pre-exercise test physical examination are located in Box 3.2 of GETP8.

Heart Rate Examination

> **1.3.3-CES: Describe anatomic landmarks as they relate to exercise testing and programming (e.g., electrode placement, BP).**

> **1.3.4-CES: Locate and palpate anatomic landmarks of radial, brachial, carotid, femoral, popliteal, and tibialis arteries.**

> **1.3.8-HFS: Skill in accurately measuring heart rate, BP, and obtaining rating of perceived exertion (RPE) at rest and during exercise according to established guidelines.**

Exercise professionals can obtain an index of resting heart rate by measuring **peripheral** pulses. The two most commonly used anatomic palpation sites are the carotid and radial artery. The radial pulse (wrist pulse) is felt by palpating the radial artery and is pictured in Figure 18-1. The radial artery is a smaller, terminal branch of the brachial artery located on the lateral side (thumb side) of the wrist (19).

The carotid pulse (neck pulse) is felt by palpating the common carotid artery in the side of the neck and is illustrated in Figure 18-2. The common carotid artery lies in the groove between the trachea and the infrahyoid muscles and is easily palpated just deep to the anterior border of the sternocleidomastoid muscle (19).

Other anatomic landmarks for palpation of heart rate include the brachial, femoral, popliteal, tibialis posterior, and dorsalis pedis artery, which are illustrated in

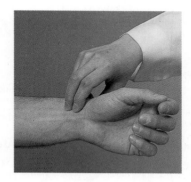

FIGURE 18-1. Palpation site for radial pulse. (From Bickley LS, Szilagyi P. Bates' *Guide to Physical Examination and History Taking.* 8th ed. Philadelphia: Lippincott Williams & Wilkins; 2003.)

Figure 18-3. The procedure for taking a pulse for determination of heart rate is as follows:

1. Locate an anatomic palpation site.
2. Place the index and third finger over the palpation site (avoid using the thumb).
3. Gently press down with the two fingers over the palpation site.
4. Count the number of pulsations for a specific time period (e.g., 10, 15, 20, or 30 seconds).
5. Begin counting the first pulsation as 0 when timing is initiated simultaneously or, if a lag time occurs after the start time and the first pulsation, begin with the number 1 for determining number of pulsations.
6. Determine heart rate based upon the number of pulsations in a given time period.
   10 seconds = multiply number of pulsations by 6
   15 seconds = multiply number of pulsations by 4
   20 seconds = multiply number of pulsations by 3
   30 seconds = multiply number of pulsations by 2

Accuracy of heart rate increases with longer palpation times. For instance, taking heart rate for 30 seconds is more accurate than taking it for 10 seconds. However, heart rate will decrease significantly once exercise has

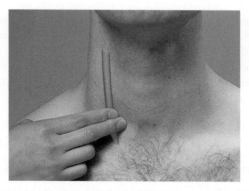

FIGURE 18-2. Palpation site for carotid pulse. (From Bickley LS, Szilagyi P. Bates' *Guide to Physical Examination and History Taking.* 8th ed. Philadelphia: Lippincott Williams & Wilkins; 2003.)

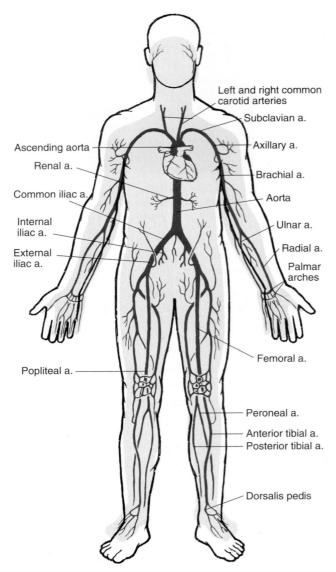

Left and right common carotid arteries
Subclavian a.
Ascending aorta
Axillary a.
Renal a.
Brachial a.
Common iliac a.
Aorta
Internal iliac a.
Ulnar a.
External iliac a.
Radial a.
Palmar arches
Femoral a.
Popliteal a.
Peroneal a.
Anterior tibial a.
Posterior tibial a.
Dorsalis pedis

FIGURE 18-3. Palpation sites for pulse in the human body. (From *Stedman's Medical Dictionary.* 27th ed. Baltimore: Lippincott Williams & Wilkins; 2000.)

stopped. Thus, estimation of exercise heart rate is normally taken in the initial 15 seconds after ceasing exercise.

During an exercise test, palpation of pulse may become difficult because of the patient's movement. Other options for monitoring an exercise heart rate are ECG monitoring, heart rate monitors, and stethoscope auscultation at the point of maximal intensity.

Blood Pressure Examination

> **1.1.3-CES: Identify the cardiorespiratory responses associated with postural changes.**

> **1.3.17-CES: Accurately record and interpret right and left arm pre-exercise BPs in the supine and upright positions.**

> **1.3.8-HFS: Skill in accurately measuring heart rate, BP, and obtaining RPE at rest and during exercise according to established guidelines.**

> **1.3.11-HFS: Ability to locate the brachial artery and correctly place the cuff and stethoscope in position for BP measurement.**

> **1.3.15-HFS: Ability to explain the purpose and procedures and perform the monitoring (heart rate, RPE, and BP) of patients before, during, and after cardiorespiratory fitness testing.**

The accuracy of BP measurements is critical in the clinical setting (17). The gold standard for determining arterial BP is direct intra-arterial measurement with a catheter. However, this method is inappropriate for the asymptomatic individual or for public health screening. The indirect method is the most commonly used method of measurement (23). Mercury and aneroid sphygmomanometers are the most popular devices for measuring BP (4), and all devices should be calibrated before their use to increase accuracy. The American Association for the Advancement of Medical Instrumentation (www.aami.org) publishes protocols for establishing accuracy of sphygmomanometers. Note that mercury devices are being phased out due to environmental concerns. Additionally, O'Brien et al. (21) validated several BP devices for clinical use in hospitals, home-use devices, and ambulatory devices.

Blood pressure measurements are obtained when an artery is occluded by an inflatable cuff, and BP is determined either oscillometrically or by auscultation of Korotkoff sounds (4). The most common method used for BP determination is auscultation of the brachial artery (28), as shown in Figure 18-4. Other auscultation sites include the ankle or thigh, which may be necessary for individuals with peripheral arterial disease in determining ankle brachial index or in individuals that are morbidly obese (11). Proper procedures for a resting BP assessment are presented in Box 3-4 of GETP8. Improper assessment procedures lead to inaccurate measurements, which may lead to an underestimation or overestimation of the individ-

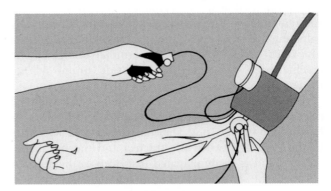

FIGURE 18-4. Blood pressure assessment in upper arm. (From Weber J, Kelley J. *Health Assessment in Nursing.* 2nd ed. Philadelphia: Lippincott Williams & Wilkins; 2003.)

TABLE 18-2. ACCEPTABLE BLADDER DIMENSIONS (in cm) FOR ARMS OF DIFFERENT SIZES[a]

CUFF	BLADDER WIDTH (cm)	BLADDER LENGTH (cm)	ARM CIRCUMFERENCE RANGE AT MIDPOINT (cm)
Newborn	3	6	≤6
Infant	5	15	6–15[b]
Child	8	21	6–15[b]
Small adult	10	24	22–26
Adult	13	30	27–34
Large adult	16	38	35–44
Adult thigh	20	42	45–52

[a]There is some overlapping of the recommended range for arm circumferences to limit the number of cuffs; it is recommended that the larger cuff be used when available.

[b]To approximate the bladder width:arm circumference ratio of 0.40 more closely in infants and children, additional cuffs are available.

ual's true BP. Common BP procedure mistakes include using an inappropriately sized cuff, failing to allow adequate rest before the measurement, deflating the cuff too fast, not measuring in both arms, and failing to palpate maximal systolic pressure before auscultation (18).

Considerable BP variability can occur with respiration, emotion, exercise, meals, tobacco, alcohol, temperature, bladder distension, and pain. Furthermore, BP can be influenced by age, race, and circadian rhythm variation. Ideally, the patient should be relaxed in a quiet room at a comfortable temperature with a short rest period before BP measurement (4). The examination should include an appropriate measurement of BP, with verification in the contralateral arm (28). Blood pressure measurements should be modified in persons with mastectomy (11), lymphedema (1,11), or arteriovenous fistulas (8,11) so that measurements are taken on the unaffected arm (1). Blood pressure measurements may be taken in the lower extremity (e.g., thigh or calf muscle) if a patient is suspected of having **coarctation** of the aorta or other type of obstructive aortic disease (11).

When choosing a BP cuff, it is essential that the cuff and bladder fit appropriately. A bladder that is too small will lead to an overestimation of BP, whereas a bladder that is too large will lead to an underestimation of BP. Recommended bladder dimensions are presented in Table 18-2 (4).

The posture of the subject should be noted before exercise testing. Generally, BP increases from the lying to the sitting or standing position. However, BP measurements are unlikely to be different if the arm is supported at heart level. Antihypertensive drugs can lead to postural hypotension; thus, BP should be measured both lying and standing (4).

Supporting the arm during BP assessment is necessary to prevent possible increases (up to 10%) in diastolic blood pressure (DBP) associated with an isometric muscle action of the unsupported arm. Furthermore, placing the arm in a dependent position below the level of the heart leads to an overestimation of systolic blood pressure (SBP) and DBP, whereas raising the arm leads to an underestimation of SBP and DBP. Many BP devices are inaccurate if the wrist is not held at the heart level during measurement (4).

During BP assessment, the BP cuff is inflated above the individual's SBP, which leads to complete artery occlusion and an elimination of audible sounds. Once the cuff pressure decreases to the individual's SBP, turbulent blood flow in the artery causes audible sounds (Korotkof sounds). The SBP is determined when the first of two or more Korotkof sounds are heard (phase 1). Turbulent blood flow continues until the cuff pressure reaches the individual's DBP; at that time, smooth blood flow occurs, and the Korotkof sounds disappear. The DBP is determined just before the disappearance of Korotkof sounds (phase 5) (28). A description of auscultatory sounds are presented in Table 18-3 (5,9). In addition to listening to Korotkoff sounds, palpation is useful in patients in whom auscultatory endpoints are difficult to judge (e.g., during exercise, pregnant, etc.). With this technique, the brachial artery is palpated during BP assessment. The cuff is inflated to approximately 30 mm Hg above the point at which the pulse disappears. The cuff is then slowly

TABLE 18-3. KOROTKOFF SOUNDS (5,9)

Phase 1 (SBP)	First, initial sound of faint, repetitive, and clear tapping sounds. The phase 1 sounds approximate the SBP—the maximum pressure that occurs near the end of systole of the left ventricle.
Phase 2	A soft tapping or murmur sound that has a swishing quality. Phase 2 sounds begin 10–15 mm Hg after the onset of sound or below the phase 1 sound.
Phase 3	Return of loud, tapping sounds, which are crisper and louder than phase 1 or 2 sounds.
Phase 4 (true DBP)	Sounds become muffled and are less distinct and less audible. Sounds may be described as soft or blowing
Phase 5 (clinical DBP)	Complete disappearance of sound that usually occurs 8–10 mm Hg from phase 4.

SBP, systolic blood pressure; DBP, diastolic blood pressure.

deflated, and the observer determines the SBP at which the pulse reappears. Palpation is important because phase I sounds sometimes disappear as pressure is reduced and then reappear at a lower level, leading to SBP being underestimated unless already determined by palpation (5).

Ambulatory BP monitoring is useful for evaluation of "white-coat" hypertension. Ambulatory BP is taken every 15 to 30 minutes during the day to determine BP in a 24-hour period. Generally, ambulatory BP values will be lower than clinic readings (28). According to the Seventh Report of the Joint National Committee on Prevention, Detection, Evaluation, and Treatment of High Blood Pressure (JNC7) (28), all individuals with documented hypertension should have a PE that includes the following:

- Examination of optic fundi
- Calculation of body mass index
- Auscultation for carotid, abdominal, and femoral bruits
- Palpation of the thyroid gland
- Examination of the heart and lungs
- Examination of the abdomen for enlarged kidneys, masses, and abnormal aortic pulsation
- Palpation of the lower extremities for edema and pulses
- A neurologic assessment

Laboratory Tests

Additional laboratory tests may be necessary based on information obtained from the PMH. Cholesterol testing is outlined by the National Cholesterol Education Program (NCEP) and classifications are presented in Table 3.2 of the GETP8. Further blood profile analysis may provide useful information regarding the individual's overall health status. Table 3.3 of the GETP8 provides normal ranges for selected blood chemistries.

RISK STRATIFICATION

> **1.3.6-CES: Identify individuals for whom physician supervision is recommended during maximal and submaximal exercise testing.**

> **1.10.6-CES: Risk stratify individuals with cardiovascular, pulmonary, and metabolic diseases, using appropriate risk stratification methods and understanding the prognostic indicators for high-risk individuals.**

> **1.3.3-HFS: Knowledge of the value of a medical clearance before exercise participation.**

> **1.3.4-HFS: Knowledge of and the ability to perform risk stratification and its implications toward medical clearance before administration of an exercise test or participation in an exercise program.**

> **1.3.23-HFS: Ability to identify individuals for whom physician supervision is recommended during maximal and submaximal exercise testing.**

> **2.2.1-HFS: Knowledge of cardiovascular risk factors or conditions that may require consultation with medical personnel before testing or training, including inappropriate changes of resting or exercise heart rate and BP; new onset discomfort in chest, neck, shoulder, or arm; changes in the pattern of discomfort during rest or exercise; fainting or dizzy spells; and claudication.**

> **3.2.1-HFS: Knowledge of pulmonary risk factors or conditions that may require consultation with medical personnel before testing or training, including asthma, exercise-induced asthma/bronchospasm, extreme breathlessness at rest or during exercise, bronchitis, and emphysema.**

> **4.2.1-HFS: Knowledge of metabolic risk factors or conditions that may require consultation with medical personnel before testing or training, including obesity, metabolic syndrome, thyroid disease, kidney disease, diabetes or glucose intolerance, and hypoglycemia.**

> **5.2.1-HFS: Knowledge of musculoskeletal risk factors or conditions that may require consultation with medical personnel before testing or training, including acute or chronic back pain, osteoarthritis, rheumatoid arthritis, osteoporosis, inflammation/pain, and low back pain.**

The exercise test is considered a diagnostic tool rather than a therapy tool and thus does not have a direct effect on patient outcomes. The risk of exercise testing in appropriately selected candidates is extremely low. The main argument for not performing an exercise test in many clinical situations is that the test would not be cost-effective in that given situation (12).

Risk stratification is important for identifying individuals for whom physician supervision is recommended during maximal and submaximal exercise. A detailed risk stratification process can be found in Chapter 2 and Chapter 3 of the GETP8. Individuals unable to exercise because of physical limitations, such as arthritis, severe peripheral vascular disease, severe chronic obstructive pulmonary disease, or general debility, should undergo pharmacologic stress testing in combination with an imaging modality (12).

Pulmonary risk factors that may require consultation with medical personnel before exercise testing include asthma, exercise-induced asthma/bronchospasm, extreme dyspnea at rest or during exercise, bronchitis, or emphysema. Individuals with pulmonary risk factors should have spirometry (see Table 3.4 of GETP8) and maximal voluntary ventilation (MVV) measured. Furthermore, if hypoxemia is suspected, pre-exercise arterial blood gases should be obtained (3).

Metabolic risk factors that may require consultation with medical personnel before exercise testing include metabolic syndrome, obesity, thyroid disease, kidney disease, diabetes, glucose intolerance, and/or hypoglycemia. Before exercise testing, laboratory tests should be obtained to ensure that the individual's blood chemistry profiles are within normal limits.

Musculoskeletal risk factors that may require consultation with medical personnel before exercise testing include acute/chronic back pain, osteoarthritis, rheumatoid arthritis, osteoporosis, and/or joint inflammation/pain. Modifications to the exercise test may be necessary to avoid exacerbating musculoskeletal problems.

PATIENT PREPARATION

BEFORE TESTING

> **1.3.9-CES: Instruct the test participant in the use of the RPE scale and other appropriate subjective rating scales, such as the dyspnea, pain, claudication, and angina scales.**

> **1.3.18-CES: Describe and analyze the importance of the absolute and relative contraindications and test termination indicators of an exercise test.**

> **1.4.14-CES: Obtain and interpret a pre-exercise standard and modified (Mason-Likar) 12-lead ECG on a participant in the supine and upright position.**

> **1.4.15-CES: Ability to minimize ECG artifact.**

> **1.7.11-CES: Describe relative and absolute contraindications to exercise training.**

> **1.3.5-HFS: Knowledge of relative and absolute contraindications to exercise testing or participation.**

> **1.3.6-HFS: Knowledge of the limitations of informed consent and medical clearance before exercise testing.**

> **1.3.8-HFS: Skill in accurately measuring heart rate, BP, and obtaining RPE at rest and during exercise according to established guidelines.**

> **1.3.13-HFS: Ability to obtain a health history and risk appraisal that includes past and current medical history, family history of cardiac disease, orthopedic limitations, prescribed medications, activity patterns, nutritional habits, stress and anxiety levels, and smoking and alcohol use.**

> **1.3.14-HFS: Ability to obtain informed consent.**

> **1.3.15-HFS: Ability to explain the purpose and procedures and perform the monitoring (heart rate, RPE, and BP) of patients before, during, and after cardiorespiratory fitness testing.**

> **1.3.16-HFS: Ability to instruct participants in the use of equipment and test procedures.**

> **1.3.17-HFS: Ability to explain purpose of testing, determine an appropriate submaximal or maximal protocol, and perform an assessment of cardiovascular fitness on the treadmill or the cycle ergometer.**

Each patient should be carefully prepared before all exercise testing. Ideally, a detailed set of instructions should be provided to the patient when the testing appointment is made. Verbal and written instructions are recommended to reduce test anxiety and to standardize the response to testing. Instructions before testing should include avoiding eating and smoking for a minimum of 3 hours before testing and 8 hours before nuclear imaging study. Individuals should wear comfortable footwear and loose-fitting clothing. Each individual should be instructed on whether medications should be tapered, discontinued, or continued for the test based on physician orders. Individuals should avoid unusual physical efforts for at least 12 hours before testing (10,24).

A history and physical examination that focuses on risk factors should be conducted before the exercise test to determine any signs and symptoms of cardiovascular risk factors, pulmonary risk factors, metabolic syndrome risk factors, musculoskeletal risk factors, and neurologic restrictions (24). Furthermore, contraindications to testing should be determined before exercise testing (10). Contraindications to exercise testing are located in GETP8, Chapter 3 (Box 3.5). In addition, determining the individual's current physical activity level can aid in the selection of an appropriate testing protocol. Informed consent (see GETP8, Chapter 3 Figure 3.1) should be signed and included in the exercise test record. The informed consent must accurately describe all procedures and potential risks/benefits associated with these procedures. Specific instructions should be given on how to perform the exercise test, purpose of the test, and a brief demonstration of the test procedure (e.g., walking on treadmill, riding bicycle). Furthermore, any questions that the patient has should be addressed (10,24).

Individuals undergoing an exercise stress test with ECG should follow skin preparation guidelines to ensure adequate monitoring during the test. Improper skin preparation can lead to ECG artifact. Electrode resistance should be reduced to ≤5000Ω by removing the superficial layer of skin. The area where electrodes will be applied should be shaved and cleaned with an alcohol-saturated gauze pad to remove oil from the skin. Once the skin has dried, the electrode-placement areas should be rubbed with fine sandpaper or a commercially prepared abrasive to remove the superficial layer of skin (10,24).

A standing ECG and BP is recorded to determine vasoregulatory abnormalities and positional changes. Once a standing ECG and BP are obtained, the individual should be instructed, using verbal and written explanations, on all scales that will be used. The subjective rating of intensity of exertion is obtained with the Borg scale of perceived exertion (see Chapter 4 of GETP8 Table 4.7) (10). Depending on the individual's PMH and current signs/symptoms, other scales such as dyspnea, pain, claudication, and angina scales (see Chapter 5 of GETP8 Figure 5.4) may be necessary.

PROTOCOL SELECTION

> **1.3.5-CES: Select an appropriate test protocol according to the age, functional capacity, physical ability, and health status of the individual.**

> **1.3.19-CES: Select and perform appropriate procedures and protocols for the exercise test, including modes of exercise, starting levels, increments of work, ramping versus incremental protocols, length of stages, and frequency of data collection.**

Protocol selection is an important consideration that should be based on the individual's PMH, preparticipation screening, and physical examination. The healthcare provider must determine which device (treadmill, cycle ergometer, etc.) is necessary and then determine an appropriate protocol (12). Protocols for clinical exercise testing include a low-load initial warm-up, a progressive uninterrupted exercise with increasing loads and an adequate time interval in each level, and a recovery period (10). The exercise protocols can be submaximal or symptom limited. Submaximal protocols have a predetermined endpoint, often defined as a peak heart rate of 120 beats per minute or 70% of the predicted maximum heart rate or a peak metabolic equivalent (MET) level of 5 (12,13). Symptom-limited tests continue until the individual presents with signs or symptoms that require termination of exercise testing (12,14). The treadmill, cycle ergometer, and arm ergometer are used for dynamic exercise testing. Treadmills are the most common modality for exercise testing in the United States. One major limitation of using a cycle ergometer for exercise testing is that quadriceps muscle fatigue often occurs before the subject reaches maximum oxygen uptake (12).

The most commonly used protocols following an acute myocardial infarction include the modified Bruce, the modified Naughton, and the standard Bruce (12,13). Much of the published data regarding stress testing, however, are based on the Bruce protocol. Protocols with the largest increments in work rate, like the Bruce protocol, demonstrate decreased ratios of oxygen uptake to work rate (10,20). An optimum protocol selection will include testing that lasts 6 to 12 minutes and can be adjusted to the subject's capabilities (10).

Ramping treadmill or cycle ergometer protocols offer the advantage of steady gradual increases in work rate and enhanced estimation of functional capacity (12,20). These protocols start at relatively low treadmill speeds, and the speed is gradually increased until the individual is at a comfortable walking pace. The incline or grade is progressively increased at fixed intervals (e.g., 60 seconds), start-

ing at 0% grade. The increase in grade is determined based on the person's estimated functional capacity so that the test will be completed in 6 to 12 minutes. Steady states are not reached in ramp protocols. Underestimation or overestimation of functional capacity will result if the test is prematurely terminated or if the test becomes too long (10). Ramp protocols have not been widely studied in patients early after myocardial infarction (12). Exercise capacity should be reported in estimated METs of exercise. Furthermore, the nature of protocol and minutes of exercise should be recorded (12).

The 6-minute walk test is a functional test that can be used to evaluate exercise capacity in individuals with marked left ventricular dysfunction or peripheral arterial disease. This protocol uses a submaximal level of stress, and ECG monitoring is normally not done, thus limiting its diagnostic accuracy (10).

Protocols for arm ergometry testing require that the subject is seated upright with the fulcrum of the handle adjusted at shoulder height. The arm should be slightly bent at the elbow during the farthest extension movements. Cycling speed of 60 to 75 revolutions $\cdot$ minute^{-1} must be maintained, with a work rate increase of 10 W per 2-minute stage (10,24).

Cycle Ergometer

Cycle ergometers must have handlebars and an adjustable seat (24). Advantages of a cycle ergometer include decreased energy cost and noise production as compared with the treadmill. Furthermore, during cycle ergometer testing, the upper-body motion is reduced, making it easier to obtain BP measurements and to record the ECG. A major disadvantage to cycle ergometer testing is the discomfort and fatigue of the quadriceps muscle. Because of leg fatigue, the subject may stop the exercise test before reaching a true VO$_2$ max (10). Cycle ergometry is an alternative for individuals with orthopedic, peripheral vascular, or neurologic limitations that restrict weight-bearing exercise. Work intensity is adjusted by changes in resistance and/or cycling pedal rate. Work rate is typically calculated in watts or kilopond-meters per min (kpm $\cdot$ min^{-1}).

Stationary bicycles used for exercise testing are either mechanically braked or electronically braked. Mechanically braked ergometers require that a specified cycling rate be maintained to keep a constant work rate (e.g., Monarch). Electronically braked ergometers automatically adjust internal resistance to maintain specified work rates according to the cycling rate. Either type of stationary bicycle is used for exercise testing as long as the ergometer has the capability to adjust the work rate in specific increments either automatically or manually (24).

Treadmill

Treadmills used for exercise testing should have front and/or side rails. Subjects should be encouraged to minimize handrail holding during testing, using only their fingers to maintain balance once they are accustomed to walking on the treadmill (10). A treadmill should be electrically driven and accommodate up to at least 157.5 kg (350 lb) (24). The treadmill should be able to change speed and grades (10). Treadmill speed should range between 26.8 m·min^{-1} (1 mph) and at least, 214.4 m·min^{-1} (8 mph). The elevation or grade should be electronically controlled and be able to move from no elevation to 20% elevation. All facilities should make sure that treadmills meet electrical safety standards according to the model of treadmill used. The treadmill platform should be at a minimum of 127 cm (50 in) in length and 40.64 cm (16 in) in width. Models with side platforms are recommended to allow the patient to adapt to the moving belt before stepping onto the belt. All treadmills must have a visible emergency stop button that is accessible to staff and to the patient. Many models also have a clip on emergency stop apparatus so that if the patient moves too far away, the magnet will pull away from the treadmill and stop the treadmill (e.g., if the patient is falling) (24).

Arm Ergometer

Arm exercise testing is an alternative for exercise testing of individuals with lower-extremity impairments. Arm ergometers are either mechanically braked or electronically braked similar to the cycle ergometers (24). Protocols may begin in the range of 20 to 25 W and increase by 10 to 20 W per stage, which typically lasts 2 minutes (10). Blood pressure should be evaluated regularly. At lower resistance levels, this may be done by removing one hand for BP evaluation while continuing to crank with the other hand. However, at higher resistances, this becomes difficult, and often an intermittent protocol is implemented, with approximately 1 minute rest between stages to take BP.

CALIBRATION OF TESTING EQUIPMENT

 1.3.11-CES: Describe the importance of accurate and calibrated testing equipment (e.g., treadmill, ergometers, electrocardiograph, gas analysis systems, and sphygmomanometers) and ability to recognize and remediate equipment that is no longer properly calibrated.

1.3.10-HFS: Knowledge of calibration of a cycle ergometer and a motor-driven treadmill.

Each facility should record dates that equipment calibrations are performed as part of the facility's quality assurance procedures. At a minimum, equipment should be calibrated on a monthly basis and more frequently if many tests are performed. The product's operation manual, provided by the manufacturer, will provide specific directions on calibration and preventive maintenance. The user must assure that all measurements are accurate and maintain a calibration logbook so that long-term trends can be monitored (3). General calibration procedures are provided in

the next section of this chapter for the treadmill, bicycle ergometery, arm ergometer, and indirect calonmetry systems.

Treadmill

Both speed and grade/incline must be calibrated on the treadmill. To calibrate speed, the treadmill belt length must be measured. Normally, the manufacturer will supply the belt length, but if this information is not available, the belt can be measured with a measuring tape. A reference mark is made on the belt, the treadmill is turned on at a specified speed (e.g., 2 miles·hour^{-1} or 53.6 m·min^{-1}), and treadmill belt revolutions are counted for 1 minute. The following equation is used to calculate the actual treadmill speed:

$$\frac{\text{Belt length (inches)} \times \text{number of revolutions per minute}}{1,056}$$

The constant of 1,056 represents the conversion of inches per minute to miles per hour.

The actual treadmill speed is compared with the speed indicator on the treadmill. Both of these values should be in agreement, and if these values are different, the treadmill will need to be calibrated according to the manufacturer recommendations. These calibration procedures should be repeated for several different speeds that are commonly used in exercise testing protocols (e.g., 1.7 miles·hour^{-1} or 45.56 m·min^{-1}). Initially, all speed calibrations should be calibrated without a subject on the treadmill. After the initial calibration, a moderately heavy subject (75 to 100 kg) should walk on the treadmill to ensure accurate calibration with someone walking on the treadmill (24).

Treadmill grade/incline calibration is performed by measuring a fixed distance on the floor and determining the difference in height of the treadmill over the fixed distance. To begin, the treadmill elevation is set to 0%, and a carpenter's level is placed on the treadmill to determine the actual elevation. If the elevation does not read 0% when it is level, adjust the grade/incline until it reads 0%. Next, mark two points on the treadmill 50 cm (20 in) apart along the length of the treadmill. Elevate the treadmill to 20% grade, and measure the distance of each point to the distance of the floor. The following equation is used to determine grade:

$$\frac{\text{Distance 1} - \text{Distance 2}}{\text{Fixed distance}}$$

If the actual result is not 20%, the elevation meter should be adjusted. A check of 5%, 10%, and 15% grade is recommended (24). Most of todays equipment contain an electronic calibration procedure. Often speed or grade adjustments require biomedical engineering assistance.

Ergometers

Ergometers are either mechanically braked or electronically braked. Each type of ergometer requires different calibration techniques. Mechanically braked ergometers depend on resistance and cycling rate in revolutions·minute^{-1}.

Therefore, the belt tension must be adjusted appropriately, and the flywheel should be cleaned to ensure smooth operation. Electronically braked ergometers normally require special instruments to calibrate, thus calibration procedures are normally provided by the manufacturer or by the institutional biomedical engineering department (24).

During calibration of the mechanically braked ergometer, the belt is removed from the flywheel. The pendulum weight is set at 0, and a known weight (e.g., 3 kg, 5 kg) is attached to the belt. A reading of the weight on the ergometer should correspond to the known weight added to the belt. If the scale shows an incorrect reading, the adjusting screw on the ergometer should be turned until the scale reads the appropriate weight (24).

If an ergometer has a lateral friction device, the ergometer is placed on two chairs so that the brake scale plate is vertical. The brake regulator is released, and a known metric weight is hung on the brake arm using a wire S-hook. The fastening screw of the shock absorber is loosened, and the scale should correspond to the exact amount of the weight attached to the brake arm. The pointer should always be read from directly above. If the scale is inaccurate, the regulating nut should be turned. When the pointer indicates the same figure as the weight attached, the ergometer is correctly calibrated (24).

Electrocardiograph

Electrocardiograph machines should be calibrated before exercise testing. Each machine will have a 1-mV button to press. Once the button is pressed, the stylus should deflect 10 small boxes or 2 large boxes on the electrocardiogram paper. If the stylus does not deflect 10 small boxes, follow the calibration procedures supplied by the manufacturer to correct discrepancies.

Gas Exchange Analysis

The analysis of respiratory gases was once limited to specialized laboratories, but is now increasingly available in both clinical and health fitness settings. Today there are several manufacturers of integrated gas analysis systems (aka, metabolic cart) that allow cardiorespiratory exercise testing to be administered by persons of various academic backgrounds. Although these systems can produce valid and reliable data, this is dependent on the proper maintenance, calibration and testing procedures. It is important that staff is properly trained, preferably by the manufacturer (24). Although it varies by manufacturer and model, systems usually must be calibrated prior to testing. Typically this calibration involves the measurement of flow, the analysis of oxygen and carbon dioxide, and the timing (i.e., phase delay) of the two.

Recognizing the potential for data validity problems with cardiorespiratory exercise testing, the American Thoracic Society with the American College of Chest Physicians (3) suggest that laboratories regularly perform quality assurance testing by having a ". . .a healthy member of the laboratory staff perform a constant work rate test at several workloads at regular intervals. . ." This would serve as a reason check of the system and the staff's procedures. Unfortunately, little quality assurance outcome data is available at this time for comparison. In addition to this physiologic testing, mechanical devices (e.g., dry gas validators) are also available that are not limited by the biologic variation that is inherent in a healthy volunteer. The number of laboratories that institute such procedures is unknown.

In addition to the above, staff should know the typical physiologic response (rest through maximum) of the patients being tested. This knowledge can be useful to "reason check" the system during a test. If non-physiologic data is observed at rest or during exercise, sources of error can be considered (e.g., air leak around the mask) and corrected, or a test can be restarted or rescheduled if necessary.

Sphygmomanometer

The **aneroid** sphygmomanometer can be calibrated using the standard mercury sphygmomanometer. The needle on the aneroid sphygmomanometer should read zero when no air pressure is inside the cuff. Figure 18-5 is a

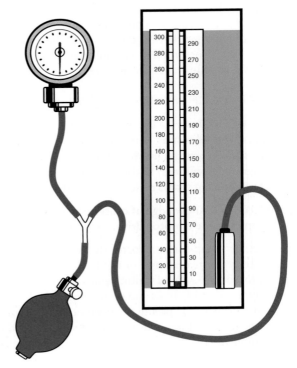

FIGURE 18-5. Blood pressure calibration setup. (From *ACSM's Health Related Physical Fitness Assessment Manual.* 2nd ed.)

drawing of the calibration setup. Steps for calibration include (9):

1. Wrap the aneroid sphygmomanometer cuff around a large can or bottle (similar in circumference to the upper arm). Be sure that the aneroid gauge is readable.
2. Connect the tube from the aneroid sphygmomanometer cuff that would go from the hand bulb to one end of the Y connector. *Note:* Some stethoscopes may have a Y connector on them, so you could use that connector.
3. Connect the other end of the Y connector to the tube that would go from the hand bulb to the mercury sphygmomanometer.
4. Connect the third end of the Y connector to a hand bulb (an extra piece of tubing may be necessary to do this).
5. Pump the hand bulb so that a reading is obtained on the aneroid gauge (e.g., 60 mm Hg).
6. Observe and record the level of the mercury in the mercury sphygmomanometer.
7. Deflate the bladder and repeat the same procedure several more times choosing different pressures (e.g., 80, 120 mm Hg).

A mathematic correction formula can be determined based on the differences between the aneroid and mercury sphygmomanometers. For instance, if the aneroid and mercury sphygmomanometer are always off so that the mercury level always reads 4 mm more than the aneroid gauge, then add 4 mm Hg to every pressure recorded with that aneroid sphygmomanometer (9).

SUMMARY

Preparticipation screenings help identify risk factors for individuals beginning an exercise program, competing in athletics, or completing an exercise test. Risk factor identification is based on the individual's PMH and PE. The preparticipation screening assists the healthcare professional in determining which protocol and modality to use for the individual's exercise test. Furthermore, the healthcare professional should understand proper calibration and use of all equipment commonly used for exercise testing.

REFERENCES

1. American Cancer Society Web site [Internet]. Oklahoma City (OK): American Cancer Society. Available from: www.cancer.org/docroot/CRI/content/CRI_2_6X_Lymphedema_5.asp?sitearea=. Accessed April 2, 2007.
2. **American College of Sports Medicine Position Stand and American Heart Association. Recommendations for cardiovascular screening, staffing, and emergency policies at health/fitness facilities.** *Med. Sc. Sports Exerc.* 1998;30(6):1009–1018.
3. American Thoracic Society, American College of Chest Physicians. ATS/ACCP statement on cardiopulmonary exercise testing. *Am. J Respir Crit Care Med.* 2003;167(2):211–277.
4. Beevers G, Lip GY, O'Brien E. ABC of hypertension: Blood pressure measurement. Part I—sphygmomanometry: factors common to all techniques. *BMJ.* 2001;322(7292):981–985.
5. Beevers G, Lip GY, O'Brien E. ABC of hypertension: Blood pressure measurement. Part II—conventional sphygmomanometry: technique of auscultatory blood pressure measurement. *BMJ.* 2001;322(7293):1043–1047.
6. **Braunwald E, Antman EM, Beasley JW, et al. ACC/AHA 2002 guideline update for the management of patients with unstable angina and non-ST-segment elevation myocardial infarction: summary article: a report of the American College of Cardiology/American Heart Association task force on practice guidelines (committee on the management of patients with unstable angina).** *Circulation.* 2002;106(14):1893.
7. Canadian Society for Exercise Physiology Web site [Internet]. Gloucester (ON): Canadian Society for Exercise Physiology. Available from: www.csep.ca/communities/c574/files/hidden/pdfs/par-q.pdf. Accessed May 21, 2007.
8. Cygnes Business Media Web site [Internet]. Mission Hills (CA): EMS Magazine. Available from: http://www.emsresponder.com/publication/article.jsp?pubId=1&id=1799. Accessed April 12, 2007.
9. Dwyer GB, Davis SE. Resting and exercise blood pressure and heart rate. In: *ACSM's Health-Related Physical Fitness Assessment Manual.* Baltimore (MD): Lippincott Williams & Wilkins; 2008. p. 30.
10. **Fletcher GF, Balady GJ, Amsterdam EA, et al. Exercise standards for testing and training: a statement for healthcare professionals from the American Heart Association.** *Circulation.* 2001;104(14):1694.
11. Gardner AW. Exercise training for patients with peripheral artery disease. *Phys Sportsmed.* [Internet]. 2001;29(7). Available from: http://www.physsportsmed.com/issues/2001/08_01/gardner.htm. Accessed April 25, 2007.
12. **Gibbons RJ, Balady GJ, Bricker JT, et al. ACC/AHA 2002 guideline update for exercise testing: summary article. A report of the American College of Cardiology/American Heart Association task force on practice guidelines (committee to update the 1997 exercise testing guidelines).** *J Am Coll Cardiol.* 2002;40.
13. Hamm LF, Crow RS, Stull GA, et al. Safety and characteristics of exercise testing early after acute myocardial infarction. *Am J Cardiol.* 1989;63(17):1193–1197.
14. Jain A, Myers GH, Sapin PM, et al. Comparison of symptom-limited and low level exercise tolerance tests early after myocardial infarction. *J Am Coll Cardiol.* 1993;22(7):1816–1820.
15. Kettenbach G. *Writing Soap Notes.* 3rd ed. Philadelphia (PA): FA Davis Company; 2004. 208 p.
16. **Maron BJ, Thompson PD, Ackerman MJ, et al. Recommendations and considerations related to preparticipation screening for cardiovascular abnormalities in competitive athletes: 2007 update: a scientific statement from the American Heart Association Council on Nutrition, Physical Activity, and Metabolism: endorsed by the American College of Cardiology Foundation.** *Circulation.* 2007; 115(12):1643–1655.
17. McAlister FA, Straus SE. Evidence based treatment of hypertension. Measurement of blood pressure: an evidence based review. *BMJ.* 2001;322(7291):908–911.
18. McKay DW, Campbell NR, Parab LS, et al. Clinical assessment of blood pressure. *J Hum Hypertens.* 1990;4(6):639–645.
19. Moore KL, Agur AM. Neck. In: Taylor C, editor. *Essential Clinical Anatomy.* Baltimore (MD): Lippincott Williams & Wilkins; 2007. p. 599.
20. Myers J, Buchanan N, Walsh D, et al. Comparison of the ramp versus standard exercise protocols. *J Am Coll Cardiol.* 1991;17(6):1334–1342.
21. O'Brien E, Waeber B, Parati G, et al. Blood pressure measuring devices: recommendations of the European Society of Hypertension. *BMJ.* 2001;322(7285):531–536.
22. **Pearson T, Blair S, Daniels S, et al. AHA guidelines for primary prevention of cardiovascular disease and stroke: 2002 update: Consensus panel guide to comprehensive risk reduction for adult patients without coronary or other atherosclerotic vascular diseases.** *Circulation.* 2002;106(3):388.

23. Perloff D, Grim C, Flack J, et al. Human blood pressure determination by sphygmomanometry. *Circulation.* 1993;88(5):2460–2470.

24. **Pina IL, Balady GJ, Hanson P, et al. Guidelines for clinical exercise testing laboratories: a statement for healthcare professionals from the Committee on Exercise and Cardiac Rehabilitation, American Heart Association.** *Circulation.* **1995;91(3):912–921.**

25. Smith S, Blair S, Bonow R, et al. AHA/ACC Guidelines for preventing heart attack and death in patients with atherosclerotic cardiovascular disease: 2001 update: a statement for healthcare professional from the American Heart Association and the American College of Cardiology. *Circulation.* 2001;104(13):1577.

26. Thompson PD. Cardiovascular risks of exercise: avoiding sudden death and myocardial infarction. Phys. Sportsmed. [Internet]. 2001;29(4). Available from: http://www.physsportsmed.com/issues/2001/04_01/thompson.htm. Accessed May 15, 2007.

27. **U.S. Department of Health and Human Services.** *Clinical Guidelines on the Identification, Evaluation, and Treatment of Overweight and Obesity in Adults: The Evidence Report.* **Bethesda (MD): National Heart, Lung, and Blood Institute; 1998. 262 p.**

28. **U.S. Department of Health and Human Services.** *The Seventh Report of the Joint National Committee on Prevention, Detection, Evaluation, and Treatment of High Blood Pressure (JNC7)—Complete Report.* **Bethesda (MD): National Heart, Lung, and Blood Institute; 2004. 86 p.**

SELECTED REFERENCES FOR FURTHER READING

Chung EK, Tighe D. *A Pocket Guide to Stress Testing.* Oxford (England): Blackwell Science; 1997.

Ellestad MH. *Stress Testing: Principles and Practice.* 5th ed. New York: Oxford University Press, Inc.; 2003.

INTERNET RESOURCES

- American Heart Association: www.americanheart.org/presenter.jhtml? identifier=3004540
- American Thoracic Society: www.thoracic.org/sections/publications/statements/pages/pfet/cardioexercise.html

Cardiorespiratory and Health-Related Physical Fitness Assessments

CARDIORESPIRATORY AND HEALTH-RELATED PHYSICAL FITNESS ASSESSMENT

> **1.3.1-HFS: Knowledge of and ability to discuss the physiologic basis of the major components of physical fitness: flexibility, cardiovascular fitness, muscular strength, muscular endurance, and body composition.**

> **1.3.20-HFS: Ability to analyze and interpret information obtained from the cardiorespiratory fitness test and the muscular strength and endurance, flexibility, and body composition assessments for apparently healthy individuals and those with controlled chronic disease.**

The potential to assess levels of physical fitness begins with understanding what comprises physical fitness. In the American College of Sports Medicine (ACSM)'s *Health-Related Physical Fitness Assessment Manual, Sec-* *ond Edition*, physical fitness is described as a "dynamic construct in that it is continually growing in importance to everyday life and health," and the author proposes that physical fitness, as a construct, can essentially be defined by its five health-related components (1). These components are cardiorespiratory fitness, muscular strength, muscular endurance, flexibility, and body composition (1).

Each component of physical fitness has a strong relationship with good health, is characterized by an ability to perform daily activities with vigor, and demonstrates the traits and capacities associated with a reduction in risk for developing diseases associated with physical inactivity (37). Individually and collectively, the health-related components of physical fitness relate closely with disease prevention and health promotion, and can each be modified with regular physical activity and exercise to positively affect disease risk (50).

The health benefits associated with regular physical activity and exercise (Box 19-1) are apparent. Recently

---

> > > KEY TERMS

Blood pressure: The force of blood against the walls of the arteries and veins created by the heart as it pumps blood to the body.

Body composition: The relative proportion of fat to fat-free tissue in the body.

Cardiac output (CO): The product of heart rate times stroke volume; the volume of blood pumped by the heart in 1 minute.

Cardiorespiratory (CR) endurance: The ability to perform large muscle, dynamic, moderate-to-high intensity exercise for prolonged periods.

Flexibility: The maximum range of motion around a joint.

Heart rate (HR): The number of times the heart contracts, usually expressed in beats per minute.

Maximal oxygen consumption: The maximal rate of oxygen that can be used for production of adenosine triphosphate (ATP) during exercise.

Muscle endurance: The ability of a muscle group to perform repeated contractions over a period of time sufficient to cause muscular fatigue or to maintain a specific percentage of maximum voluntary contraction for a prolonged period of time.

Muscle strength: The maximal force (expressed in newtons, kilograms, or pounds) that can be generated by a specific muscle or muscle group.

Risk stratification: Modeling that attempts to classify individuals (based on health conditions) into low, moderate, and high risk for untoward events during exercise.

Stroke volume (SV): The volume of blood ejected per heart beat.

BOX 19-1 BENEFITS OF REGULAR PHYSICAL ACTIVITY AND/OR EXERCISE*

Improvement in Cardiovascular and Respiratory Function
- Increased maximal oxygen uptake due to both central and peripheral adaptations
- Lower minute ventilation at a given submaximal intensity
- Lower myocardial oxygen cost for a given absolute submaximal intensity
- Lower heart rate and blood pressure at a given submaximal intensity
- Increased capillary density in skeletal muscle
- Increased exercise threshold for the accumulation of lactate in the blood
- Increased exercise threshold for the onset of disease signs or symptoms (e.g., angina pectoris, ischemic ST-segment depression, claudication)

Reduction in Coronary Artery Disease Risk Factors
- Reduced resting systolic/diastolic pressures
- Increased serum high-density lipoprotein cholesterol and decreased serum triglycerides
- Reduced total body fat, reduced intra-abdominal fat
- Reduced insulin needs, improved glucose tolerance

Decreased Mortality and Morbidity
Primary prevention (i.e., interventions to prevent an acute cardiac event)
- Activity and/or fitness levels are associated with lower death rates from coronary artery disease
- Higher activity and/or fitness levels are associated with lower incidence rates for combined cardiovascular diseases, coronary artery disease, cancer of the colon, and type 2 diabetes
- Secondary prevention (i.e., interventions after a cardiac event [to prevent another])
- Based on meta-analyses (pooled data across studies), cardiovascular and all-cause mortality are reduced in post-myocardial infarction patients who participate in cardiac rehabilitation exercise training, especially as a component of multifactorial risk factor reduction
- Randomized controlled trials of cardiac rehabilitation exercise training involving postmyocardial infarction patients do not support a reduction in the rate of nonfatal reinfarction

Other Postulated Benefits
- Decreased anxiety and depression
- Enhanced feelings of well-being
- Enhanced performance of work, recreational, and sport activities

*Adapted from United States Department of Health and Human Services: Physical activity and health: a report of the Surgeon General Atlanta, GA: US Department of Health and Human Services, Centers for Disease Control and Prevention, National Center for Chronic Disease Prevention and Health Promotion, 1996; Pollock ML, Gaesser GA, Butcher JD. The recommended quantity and quality of exercise for developing and maintaining cardiorespiratory and muscular fitness, and flexibility in healthy adults. Med Sci Sports Exerc 1998;30:975–991; Frankline BA, Roitman JL. Cardiorespiratory adaptations to exercise. In: Roitman JL, ed. ACSM's Resource Manual for Guidelines for Exercise Testing and Prescription. Baltimore: Williams & Wilkins, 1998:156–163; Wenger NK, Froelicher ES, Smith LK, et al. Cardiac rehabilitation. Clinical practice guidelines No. 17. Rockville, MD: US Department of Health and Human Services, Public Health Service, Agency for Health Care Policy and Research and the National Heart, Lung and Blood Institute, AHCPR Publication No. 96–0672, October 1995; and Whaley MH, Kaminsky LA. Epidemiology of physical activity, physical fitness and selected chronic diseases. In: Roitman JL, ed. ACSM's Resource Manual for Guidelines for Exercise Testing and Prescription. Baltimore: Williams & Wilkins, 1998:13–26.

more emphasis, however, has been placed on the measurement of health-related physical fitness rather than on skill-related physical fitness (agility, balance, coordination, speed, power, reaction time) (9). As the definition offered by the U.S. Centers for Disease Control and Prevention states, "the five health-related components of physical fitness are more important to public health than are the components related to athletic ability" (50). Thus, physical fitness assessment and programming on both the primary and secondary intervention levels provide a foundation to improve health, and should, therefore, focus on the components of health-related physical fitness.

The purpose of this chapter is to provide a detailed desciption of how to assess each component of health-related physical fitness in presumably healthy adults. Figure 19-1 provides a summary of tests that may be used to measure each individual component of health-related physical fitness.

REASONS FOR THE ASSESSMENT OF HEALTH-RELATED FITNESS

To determine the effectiveness of a preventive or rehabilitative fitness program, it is essential that a baseline evaluation is completed and that periodic follow-up measurement of the health-related components of physical fitness are evaluated. Additional reasons for measurement of health-related fitness include the following (1):

- To educate participants about their current level of health-related physical fitness
- To use data from fitness assessments to individualize exercise programs
- To evaluate an exercise program's effectiveness
- To inspire individuals to take action to improve their health-related physical fitness
- To improve a participant's risk stratification status

Cardiorespiratory Fitness:	Body Composition:	Muscular Strength:
• Field Tests: i.e., Step Tests, 1.5 Mile Walk/Run, One Mile Walk Test • Submaximal Tests: i.e., YMCA Submaximal Cycle Test & Astrand-Ryhming Cycle Test • Maximal Tests: Graded Exercise Test	• Height/Weight & Body Mass Index • Circumferences & Waist-to-Hip Ratio • Skinfolds • Bioelectrical Impedance • Underwater Weighing Flexibility: • Sit and Reach Test • Modified Sit and Reach Test	• Hand Grip Test • One RM (repetition maximum) Muscular Endurance: • Sit-ups • Curl-ups • Pushups • YMCA Bench Press Test

FIGURE 19-1. Summary of Tests for Measuring Each Component of Health-Related Physical Fitness (From: American College of Sports Medicine. Health-Related Physical Fitness Assessment Manual. 2nd edition. Philadelphia: 2008. Lippincott Williams & Wilkins.)

BASIC PRINCIPLES AND GUIDELINES SURROUNDING HEALTH-RELATED FITNESS TESTING

The ideal approach to identifying an individual's physical fitness is to assess each component of health-related physical fitness separately, then compare the individual's assessment data with normative data for each component. The information obtained from fitness testing, in combination with the individual's health and medical information, can then be used by the health and fitness professional to identify and assist in achieving specific fitness goals. While several tests are available for each fitness component, consideration of a multitude of issues needs to occur prior to determining the appropriate task. These include (6):

- Ease of test administration (How easy is it for the patient to perform the test? Can the test administrator and the patient interract during the test?)
- Ease of normative data comparison (How applicable and well-developed are the normative standards for any given mode of testing?)
- Economic issues, such as the cost of the test, equipment, and personnel
- Validity and reliability of test results
- Patient needs, preferences, current fitness level, and risk stratification

The ideal health-related physical fitness test is reliable, valid, objective, relatively inexpensive, and easy to administer. It should provide information on an individual's current state of fitness and should be able to reflect any change related to participation in physical activity or exercise. Additionally, the information obtained from the fitness test should be comparable to a previously completed fitness evaluation or available normative data.

PREACTIVITY SCREENING

Preactivity screening gathers pertinent demographic, medical, and personal information which is then used to reduce the occurrence of unwanted and potentially dangerous events during a fitness assessment or exercise session.

The primary reasons for conducting preactivity screening include (1):

- Identification of medical contraindications (reasons not to test) to performing specific health-related fitness assessments
- Identification of those patients who should receive a medical evaluation before participating in specific health-related fitness assessments
- Identification of those patients who should be medically supervised during health-related fitness assessments
- Identification of any other health/medical concern or condition that may alter testing format (i.e., diabetes mellitus, orthopedic injuries, readiness for exercise, etc.)

PRETEST INSTRUCTIONS

 1.3.8-CES: Describe basic equipment and facility requirements for exercise testing.

Pretest instructions are to be provided and adhered to before arrival at the testing facility. Care should be taken to ensure patient safety and comfort before administering a fitness test. At a minimum, it is recommended that individuals complete a questionnaire, such as the Physical Activity Readiness Questionnaire (PAR-Q; see *GETP8*, Chapter 2). A listing of preliminary instructions can be found in the *GETP8* Chapter 3 under Participant Instructions. These instructions, however, should be modified to meet needs and circumstances of the testing situation. Guidelines for preactivity screening are listed in Box 19-2.

TEST ENVIRONMENT

To minimize test anxiety, it is recommended that the test environment is controlled, including room temper-

---

BOX 19-2   GUIDELINES FOR PREACTIVITY SCREENING

- Consult a physician before participating in health-related physical fitness assessment or any exercise program:
  - If you are a man 45 or older, or a woman 55 or older
  - If you are planning to perform vigorous physical activity
  - If you are new to exercise and/or not accustomed to exercise
  - If you are in doubt about your health status
- Conduct a medical history/health habits questionnaire including but not limited to:
  - Family history
  - History of various diseases and illnesses, including cardiovascular disease
  - Surgical history

- Past and present health behaviors/habits (such as a history of cigarette smoking and physical inactivity)
- Current use of various drugs and/or medications
- Specific history of any signs or symptoms suggesting cardiovascular disease or any other chronic disease
- Physical Activity Readiness Questionnaire (PAR-Q; a minimal standard for entry into a moderate-intensity exercise program that was developed as a simpler alternative to the health habits questionnaire and designed to prevent patients from participating in physical activities that may be too strenuous for them; see the ACSM/AHA form in GETP8 Figure 2.2)
- Medical/health examination

From: American College of Sports Medicine. Health-Related Physical Fitness Assessment Manual. 2nd edition. Philadelphia: 2008. Lippincott Williams & Wilkins.

---

ature and ventilation. The test procedures should be well explained, and the test environment should be quiet and private. The room should be equipped with a comfortable seat and/or examination table to be used for resting blood pressure (BP), heart rate (HR), and/or electrocardiographic (ECG) recordings. The professional conducting the test should be relaxed and confident. Testing procedures should not be rushed, and all procedures must be clearly explained before initiating the process. The participant should confirm understanding of the testing procedures, and informed consent should be obtained before continuing with the procedures. General pretest instructions are provided in Box 19-3. Box 19-4 provides recommendations for maintaining a conducive testing environment, and Box 19-5 lists pretest organization and order of testing procedures.

TEST ORDER

To prepare for testing, the following should be completed before the participant arrives at the test site:

- Assure that all forms, score sheets, tables, graphs, and other testing documents are organized and available for the test's administration.
- Equipment should have been calibrated within the past month to ensure accuracy (e.g., metronome, cycle ergometer, treadmill, sphygmomanometer, skinfold calipers).
- Testing equipment should be organized in a sequence that prevents stressing the same muscle group repeatedly.
- Have appropriate informed consent form available.

- Ensure that the appropriate room temperature (68°F–72°F [20°C–22°C]) and humidity (<60%) are maintained.

During the administration of multiple tests, the sequence can be very important. Testing order should include resting measurements of HR, BP, height, weight, and body composition, followed by tests of cardiorespiratory endurance, muscular fitness, and flexibility. When multiple fitness components are assessed in a single session, the order of the testing is extremely important. For example,

---

BOX 19-3   GENERAL PRETEST INSTRUCTIONS TO THE PARTICIPANT

1. Wear loose-fitting, comfortable clothes that will easily allow for participation in an exercise test.
2. Avoid food, alcohol, and caffeine for at least 3 hours before the fitness assessment.
3. Drink plenty of fluids in the 24 hours preceding the assessment.
4. Avoid stenuous exercise on the day of the test.
5. Sleep for at least 6 to 8 hours the night before the test.
6. All pretest instructions should be provided to the participant ahead of time and adhered to by the participant before his/her arrival at the testing facility.

From: American College of Sports Medicine. Health-Related Physical Fitness Assessment Manual. 2nd edition. Philadelphia: 2008. Lippincott Williams & Wilkins.

BOX 19-4	RECOMMENDATIONS FOR MAINTAINING AN ENVIRONMENT CONDUCIVE TO EFFECTIVE, LOW-ANXIETY, HEALTH-RELATED FITNESS TESTING

1. Maintain room temperature of 68°F to 72°F (20°C–22°C) and humidity of <60%.
2. Room should be private, quiet, and well ventilated.
3. Test subject should be made comfortable during resting measures and all nonstrenuous assessment procedures.
4. Test administrator should be relaxed and confident.

From: American College of Sports Medicine. Health-Related Physical Fitness Assessment Manual. 2nd edition. Philadelphia: 2008. Lippincott Williams & Wilkins.

testing cardiorespiratory endurance after assessing muscular fitness (which elevates HR) can produce inaccurate results. Likewise, perspiration may make skinfold assessment more difficult.

To preserve the validity and reliability of fitness assessment results, professionals are encouraged to pay close attention to the details throughout the entire assessment to minimize variance in test results. These recommendations, and those identified previously in this chapter, can save the test administrator time and allow for a more relaxed environment for the test participant.

BOX 19-5	THE PRETEST ORGANIZATION AND ORDER OF TESTING PROCEDURES

- Assure all forms, score sheets, tables, graphs, and other testing documents are organized and available for the test's administration.
- Calibrate all equipment a minimum of once each month to ensure accuracy (e.g., metronome, cycle ergometer, treadmill, sphygmomanometer, skinfold calipers).
- The test session should be reasonably paced and not rushed for time.
- The participant should receive a clear explanation of all procedures associated with the assessment process (informed consent).
- Resting measures (including heart rate, blood pressure, body composition assessment) should be performed first, followed by cardiorespiratory fitness assessment, then tests of muscular fitness and flexibility.
- Organize equipment so that tests can follow in sequence without stressing the same muscle group repeatedly.
- Provide informed consent form (see GETP8 Figure 3.1).

From: American College of Sports Medicine. Health-Related Physical Fitness Assessment Manual. 2nd edition. Philadelphia: 2008. Lippincott Williams & Wilkins.

RISK STRATIFICATION

> **1.3.4-HFS: Knowledge of and the ability to perform risk stratification and its implications toward medical clearance before administration of an exercise test or participation in an exercise program.**

> **2.2.1-HFS: Knowledge of cardiovascular risk factors or conditions that may require consultation with medical personnel before testing or training, including inappropriate changes of resting or exercise HR or exercise HR and BP; new onset discomfort in chest, neck, shoulder, or arm; changes in the pattern of discomfort during rest or exercise; fainting or dizzy spells; and claudication.**

> **2.2.4-HFS: Knowledge of the effects of the above diseases and conditions on the cardiorespiratory responses at rest and during exercise.**

> **3.21-HFS: Knowledge of pulmonary risk factors or conditions that may require consultation with medical personnel before testing or training, including asthma, exercise-induced asthma/bronchospasm, extreme breathlessness (at rest or during exercise), bronchitis, and emphysema.**

> **4.2.1-HFS: Knowledge of metabolic risk factors or conditions that may require consultation with medical personnel before testing or training, including obesity, metabolic syndrome, thyroid disease, kidney disease, diabetes or glucose intolerance, and hypoglycemia.**

> **5.2.1-HFS: Knowledge of musculoskeletal risk factors or conditions that may require consultation with medical personnel before testing or training, including acute or chronic back pain, osteoarthritis, rheumatoid arthritis, osteoporosis, inflammation/pain, and low back pain.**

> **1.3.6-CES: Identify individuals for whom physician supervision is recommended during maximal and submaximal exercise testing.**

The ACSM has a specific set of guidelines for preactivity screening termed *risk stratification* (see Chapters 2 and 3 in GETP8). There are three risk stratification categories (low, moderate, and high risk) (Box 19-6). Risk stratification is used to help determine an appropriate course of

BOX 19-6	INITIAL ACSM RISK STRATIFICATION

Low Risk
Younger individuals[*] who are asymptomatic and meet no more than one risk factor threshold from Box 19-7

Moderate Risk
Older individuals (men ≥45 years of age; woman ≥55 years of age) or those who meet the threshold for two or more risk factors from Box 19-7

High Risk
Individuals with one or more signs/symptoms listed in Box 19-8 or known cardiovascular,[†] pulmonary,[‡] or metabolic[§] disease

---

[*]Men < 45 years of age; women < 55 years of age.

[†]Cardiac, peripheral vascular, or cerebrovascular disease.

[‡]Chronic obstructive pulmonary disease, asthma, interstitial lung disease, or cystic fibrosis.

[§]Diabetes mellitus (types 1 and 2), thyroid disorders, renal or liver disease.

action for an individual by identifying the need for a medical examination before proceeding with a health-related physical fitness test.

Risk stratification and medical clearance prior to exercise testing, should also coincide with the gathering of information to identify signs and symptoms or known history of cardiovascular, pulmonary, and/or metabolic disease in their test participants. ACSM, in collaboration with other national organizations, provides test administrators with guidelines for recognizing and understanding the impact on exercise testing of these signs and symptoms (5,13). Boxes 19-7, 19-8, and 19-9 provide guidelines for risk stratification and assist in identifying individuals who may be candidates for physician supervision during an exercise test.

RESTING MEASURES: MEASUREMENT OF RESTING HEART RATE, BLOOD PRESSURE, AND BODY COMPOSITION

> **1.3.8-HFS: Skill in accurately measuring HR, BP, and obtaining rating of perceived exertion (RPE) at rest and during exercise according to established guidelines.**

> **1.3.15-HFS: Ability to explain the purpose and procedures and perform the monitoring (HR, RPE, and BP) of patients before, during, and after cardiorespiratory fitness testing.**

RESTING HEART RATE, STROKE VOLUME, AND CARDIAC OUTPUT

> **1.1.12-HFS: Ability to describe normal cardiorespiratory responses to static and dynamic exercise in terms of HR, stroke volume, cardiac output, BP, and oxygen consumption.**

> **1.1.13-HFS: Knowledge of the HR, stroke volume, cardiac output, BP, and oxygen consuption responses to exercise.**

Heart rate (HR) is the number of times the heart contracts, usually expressed in beats per minute. Stroke volume (SV) is the volume of blood ejected from the heart per beat. Cardiac output is the product of HR times SV, or the volume of blood pumped by the heart in 1 minute. Improvements in cardiorespiratory fitness resulting from chronic exercise training improves the heart's efficiency by increasing the SV. Improvements in fitness that increase the SV result in a lower resting and exercise HR, which can be used as an indicator of cardiorespiratory fitness.

Heart rate can be measured using manual palpation, via a HR monitor (25); auscultation with a stethoscope, or use of an electrocardiogram. For greater accuracy it is recommended that resting HR be measured by palpation at the radial artery for a full 60-second count prior to health-related fitness testing. More detailed information regarding HR measurement can be found in Chapter 18 of this manual.

RESTING BLOOD PRESSURE

> **1.1.27-HFS: Knowledge of BP responses associated with acute exercise, including changes in body position.**

> **1.3.17-CES: Accurately record and interpret right and left arm pre-exercise BPs in the supine and upright positions.**

Blood pressure is defined as the force of blood, in millimeters of mercury (mm Hg), against the walls of the arteries and veins created by the heart as it pumps blood through the body. Blood pressure is created and altered by changes in the diameter of the more elastic blood vessels as they constrict and relax in response to various stimuli (such as blood volume, stress, and blood flow changes related to the support of bodily functions like digestion and exercise). Atherosclerosis, caused by *plaque* buildup, can also cause changes in BP by narrowing the diameter of the blood vessels. The process for accurately detecting resting BP can be found in Chapter 18 of this resource manual and in Chapter 3 of GETP8.

Blood pressure assessment during exercise is more challenging than taking a BP measurement at rest. Although the technique used for measuring BP during

BOX 19-7	**CORONARY ARTERY DISEASE RISK FACTOR THRESHOLDS FOR USE WITH ACSM RISK STRATIFICATION**

POSITIVE RISK FACTORS	**DEFINING CRITERIA**
1. Family history	Myocardial infarction, coronary revascularization, or sudden death before 55 years of age in father or other male first-degree relative, or before 65 years of age in mother or other female first-degree relative.
2. Cigarette smoking	Current cigarette smoker or those who quit within the previous 6 months
3. Hypertension	Systolic blood pressure $\geq$ 140 mmHg or diastolic $\geq$90 mmHg, confirmed by measurements on at least two separate occasions, or antihypertensive medication
4. Dyslipidemia	Low-density lipoprotein (LDL) cholesterol >130 mg$\cdot$dL^{-1} (3.4 mmol$\cdot$L^{-1}) or high-density lipoprotein (HDL) cholesterol <40 mg$\cdot$dL^{-1} (1.03 mmol$\cdot$L^{-1}), or on lipid-lowering medication. If total serum cholesterol is all that is available use >200 mg$\cdot$dL^{-1} (5-2mmol$\cdot$L^{-1}) rather than LDL >130 mg$\cdot$dL^{-1}
5. Impaired fasting glucose	Fasting blood glucose $\geq$ 100mg$\cdot$dL^{-1} (5.6 mmol$\cdot$L^{-1}) confirmed by measurements on at least two separate occasions
6. Obesity	Body mass index >30 kg$\cdot$m^{-2} or Waist girth >102 cm for men and >88 cm for women or Waist/hip ratio: $\geq$0.95 for men and $\geq$0.86 for women
7. Sedentaty lifestyle	Persons not participating in a regular exercise program or not meeting the minmal physical activity recommendations from the U. S. Surgeon General's Report.

Negative Risk Factors	**Defining Criteria**
1. High serum HDL cholesterol	>60 mg$\cdot$dL^{-1} (1.6mmol$\cdot$L^{-1})

Hypertension threshold based on National High Blood Pressure Education Program. The Seventh Report of the Joint National Committee on Prevention, Detection, Evaluation, and Treatment of High Blood Pressure (JNG7) 2003-03-5233.

Lipid thresholds based on National Cholesterol Education Program. Third Report of the National Cholesterol Education Program (NCEP) Expert Panel on Detection, Evaluation, and Treatment of High Blood Cholesterol in Adults (Adult Treatment Panel III). NIH Publication No. 02–5215, 2002.

Impaired Fg threshold based on Expert Committee on the Diagnosis and Classification of Diabetes Mellitus. Follow-up report on the diagnosis of diabetes mellitus. Diabetes Care 2003;26:3160–3167

Obesity thresholds based on Expert Panel on Detection, Evaluation, and Treatment of Overweight and Obesity in Adults. National Institutes of Health. Clinical guidelines on the identification, evaluation, and treatment of overweight and obesity in adults—the evidence report. Arch Int Med 1998:158:1855–1867.

Sedentary lifestyle thresholds based on United States Department of Health and Human Services. Physical activity and health: a report of the Surgeon General. 1996.

†Professional opinions vary regarding the most appropriate markers and thresholds for obesity and therefore, allied health professionals should use clinical judgment when evaluating this risk factor.

‡Accumulating 30 minutes or more of moderate physical activity on most days of the week.

§Notes: It is common to sum risk factors in making clinical judgments If HDL is high, subtract one risk factor from the sun of positive risk factors, because high HDL decreases CAD risk.

BOX 19-8	**MAJOR SIGNS OR SYMPTOMS SUGGESTIVE OF CARDIOVASCULAR AND PULMONARY DISEASE***

- Pain, discomfort (or other anginal equivalents) in the chest, neck, jaw, arms, or other areas that may be due to ischemia
- Shortness of breath at rest or with mild exertion
- Dizziness or syncope
- Orthopnea or paroxysmal nocturnal dyspnea
- Ankle edema
- Palpitations or tachycardia
- Intermittent claudication
- Known heart murmur
- Unusual fatigue or shortness of breath with usual activities

*These symptoms must be interpreted in the clinical context in which they appear because they are not all specific for cardiovascular, pulmonary, or metabolic disease.

	LOW RISK	MODERATE RISK	HIGH RISK
BOX 19-9 — ACSM RECOMMENDATIONS FOR (A) CURRENT MEDICAL EXAMINATION* AND EXERCISE TESTING BEFORE PARTICIPATION AND (B) PHYSICIAN SUPERVISION OF EXERCISE TESTS			
A.			
Moderate exercise[†]	Not necessary[‡]	Not necessary	Recommended
Vigorous exercise[§]	Not necessary	Recommended	Recommended
B.			
Submaximal test	Not necessary	Not necessary	Recommended
Maximal test	Not necessary	Recommended[||]	Recommended

* Within the past year.

[†]Moderate exercise is defined as activities that are approximately 3 to 6 METs or the equivalent of brisk walking at 3 to 4 mph for most healthy adults (13). Nevertheless, a pace of 3 to 4 mph might be considered to be "hard" to "very hard" by some sedentary, older persons. Moderate exercise may alternatively be defined as an intensity well within the individual's capacity, one that can be comfortably sustained for a prolonged period of time (~45 min), which has a gradual initiation and progression, and is generally noncompetitive. If an individual's exercise capacity is known, relative moderate exercise may be defined by the range 40 to 60% maximal oxygen uptake.

[‡]The designation of "Not necessary" reflects the notion that a medical examination, exercise test, and physician supervision of exercise testing would not be essential in the preparticipation screening; however, they should not be viewed as inappropriate.

[§]Vigorous exercise is defined as activities of 16 METs. Vigorous exercise may alternatively be defined as exercise intense enough to represent a substantial cardiorespiratory challenge. If an individual's exercise capacity is known, vigorous exercise may be defined as an intensity of 60% maximal oxygen uptake.

[||]When physician supervision of exercise testing is "Recommended," the physician should be in close proximity and readily available should there be an emergent need.

exercise is not unlike that used for resting measurement, significant practice is required to master this skill.

Exercise BP is an important physiologic indicator of an individual's work intensity during exercise and is often used as a criterion for test termination (43). Additionally, systolic BP also serves as an indicator of left ventricular function during exercise and should rise with exercise intensity. Diastolic blood pressure, however, typically remains constant during exericse or may decrease slightly.

DETERMINATION OF BODY COMPOSITION

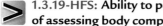 **1.3.9-HFS: Skill in measuring skinfold sites, skeletal diameters, and girth measurements used for estimating body composition.**

1.3.12-HFS: Ability to locate common sites for measurement of skinfold thicknesses and circumferences (for determination of body composition and waist-to-hip ratio).

1.3.19-HFS: Ability to perform various techniques of assessing body composition.

Body composition is the relative proportion of fat to fat-free tissue in the body. It is an important measure as excess body fat, particularly when located centrally around the abdomen, is associated with increased disease risk (31). Currently, it is estimated that approximately two thirds of American adults are now classified as overweight (body mass index [BMI] ≥ 25 kg·M^{-2}), and approximately 32% are classified as obese (BMI ≥ 30 kg·M^{-2})

(33). In addition, the more than twofold increase in adult obesity between 1980 and 2004 coincides with 13% increase in the prevalence of overweight children between 1970 and 2004 (33,34,49). Unfortunately, this trend shows no signs of slowing in the near future (33,34).

Estimation of body composition can be accomplished using both laboratory and field techniques that vary in terms of complexity, cost, and accuracy. Although various assessment techniques are briefly reviewed in this section, the detail associated with obtaining measurements and calculating estimates of body fat for all of these techniques is beyond the scope of this chapter. More detailed descriptions of each technique are available in Chapter 17 of this resource manual and elsewhere (21,40).

The assessment of body composition can be helpful in establishing optimal weight for health and physical performance (40). Currently, hydrostatic or underwater weighing (UWW) is considered the most accurate measure and is considered the gold standard of body composition analysis. However, UWW requires expensive equipment and a certain amount of inconvenience to the subject. Thus, to alleviate the cost and inconvenience associated with UWW, measurements of height, weight, circumferences, and skinfolds are more frequently used to estimate body composition. Although skinfold measurement is more difficult than other anthropometric procedures, as a technique, it provides a better estimate of body fatness than those based solely on height, weight, and circumferences (29). Table 19-1 provides a summary of ratings for the validity and objectivity among various body composition methods. Regardless of the technique used to assess body composition, the technician must be

TABLE 19-1. RATINGS OF THE VALIDITY AND OBJECTIVITY OF BODY COMPOSITION METHODS

METHOD	PRECISION	OBJECTIVITY	ACCURACY	VALID EQUATIONS	OVERALL
Body mass index	1	1	4, 5	4,5	4
Near infrared interactance	1	1, 2	4	4	3.5
Skinfolds	2	2, 3	2, 3	2,3	2.5
Bioelectric impedance	2	2	2, 3	2, 3	2.5
Circumferences	2	2	2, 3	2,4	3.0

1, excellent; 2, very good; 3, good; 4, fair; 5, unacceptable.

Precision is reliability within investigators; objectivity is reliability between investigators; accuracy refers to comparison with a criterion method; valid equations are cross-validated.

From: American College of Sports Medicine. Health-Related Physical Fitness Assessment Manual. 2nd edition. Philadelphia: 2008. Lippincott Williams & Wilkins.

adequately trained and routinely practiced in the techniques to obtain accurate results.

ANTHROPOMETRIC METHODS

Anthropometry is the measurement of the human body and indicates measurements of height, weight, circumferences/girths, and skinfold measurement. The correct measurement of height is accomplished with the shoes off and the subject standing upright and looking straight ahead while taking in and holding a deep breath. The subject's height can be recorded in centimeters (cm) or inches (in) and can be used in various normative equations.

The measurement of weight should occur without shoes and excess clothing. The subject's weight can be recorded in pounds (lbs) or kilograms (kg) and compared with the recommendations of the National Institutes for Health (Table 19-2). These recommendations should be used with caution, however, as they do not take into consideration excess lean body weight.

Body Mass Index

Body mass index is used to assess weight relative to height ($kg \cdot m^{-2}$). The Expert Panel on the Identification, Evaluation, and Treatment of Overweight and Obesity in Adults (13) identifies those with a BMI of 25.0 to 29.9 $kg \cdot m^{-2}$ as overweight and those having a ≥ 30.0 $kg \cdot m^{-2}$ as obese. BMI >30 $kg \cdot m^{-2}$ is associated with an increased risk of hypertension, total cholesterol/high-density lipoprotein (HDL) cholesterol ratio, coronary artery disease, and mortality. However, similar to height/weight charts, BMI fails to distinguish between body fat, muscle mass, or bone (39). The use of specific BMI values to predict percentage body fat and health risk can be found in Table 4-2 of the GETP8 (16).

Circumferences

Circumferences, or girths, are used to estimate body composition and provide specific reference to the distribution of fat in the body. The pattern of body fat distribution is recognized as an important predictor of the health risks associated with obesity (51). Increased fat distribution on the trunk (android obesity) is positively correlated with an increased risk of hypertension, metabolic syndrome, type 2 diabetes, dyslipidemia, coronary artery disease, and premature death when compared with individuals whose fat is distributed in the hip and thigh region (gynoid obesity) (13).

Using circumference measures as a means for estimating body composition has the advantage of being easy to learn, quick to complete, and inexpensive. Various translational equations are available for men and women to convert girth measurements to body fat estimations across a range of ages (47,48). Accuracy of circumference measures vary, but can range within 2.5% to 4% of the body composition if precise circumference measures

TABLE 19-2. SUGGESTED BODY WEIGHTS FOR ADULTS

HEIGHT[1]	WEIGHT IN POUNDS[2]	
	19 TO 34 YEARS	35 + YEARS
5'0"	97–128	108–138
5'1"	101–132	111–143
5'2"	104–137	115–148
5'3"	107–141	119–152
5'4"	111–146	122–157
5'5"	114–150	126–162
5'6"	118–155	130–167
5'7"	121–160	134–172
5'8"	125–164	138–178
5'9"	129–169	142–183
5'10"	132–174	146–188
5'11"	136–179	151–194
6'0"	140–184	155–199
6'1"	144–189	159–205
6'2"	148–195	164–210
6'3"	152–200	168–216
6'4"	156–205	173–222
6' 5"	160–211	177–228
6'6"	164–216	182–234

[1]Without shoes.

[2]Without clothes.

(From *Understanding Adult Obesity*, National Institute of Diabetes and Digestive and Kidney Diseases. National Institutes of Health, U S. Department of Health and Human Services)

are obtained and the subject's characteristics match those of the original validation population. An improvement in measurement accuracy can occur when duplicate measurements are obtained at each site using a cloth tape measure with a spring-loaded handle (e.g., Gulick tape measure). In addition, measurements should be obtained in a rotational order instead of consecutively.

Waist circumference can be used as an indicator of disease risk, as abdominal obesity has been identified as a predictor of disease. Although all fitness assessments should include a minimum of waist circumference or BMI, it is preferable that both be performed when evaluating for risk stratification. The classification of disease risk based on both BMI and waist circumference is shown in Table 4-1 of the GETP8 (13). Additionally, risk stratification is now available for adults based on waist circumference measures (see Table 4-3 of the GETP8)(7). This assessment can be used alone or in conjunction with BMI to estimate chronic disease risk. A description of circumference sites and procedures for measurement is provided in Chapter 17 of this manual.

Waist-to-Hip Ratio

A simple method for estimating body fat distribution is the waist-to-hip ratio (WHR). The WHR is the circumference of the waist divided by the circumference of the hips (8). Disease risk increases with increased WHR, and standards for risk vary with age and sex. For example, disease risk is considered *very high* for young men when WHR exceeds 0.95 and for young women when WHR exceeds 0.86. In addition, for those age 60 to 69 years, the WHR values are <1.03 for men and <0.90 for women, respectively, for the same risk classification (13,21).

Skinfold Measurement

> **1.3.7-HFS: Knowledge of the advantages/disadvantages and limitations of the various body composition techniques, including but not limited to air displacement plethysmography (BOD POD®), dual energy x-ray absorptiometry (DEXA), hydrostatic weighing, skinfolds, and bioelectrical impedance.**

Although skinfold measurement is more difficult than other anthropometric procedures, it provides a better estimate of body fitness than those measures based solely on height, weight, and circumference (29). Skinfold measurements correlates well ($r = 0.70–0.90$) with underwater weighing in the determination of body composition (41). As it is assumed that the amount of subcutaneous fat is proportional to the total amount of body fat, then approximately one third of the total body fat is located beneath the skin. This proportion of subcutaneous-to-total fat, however, varies with sex, age, and

ethnicity (40), and regression equations must be used to accurately convert a sum of skinfolds to percent body fat. A standardized description of skinfold sites and procedures is presented in Chapter 17 of this book.

The accuracy of predicting percent fat from skinfolds approximates 3.5% (21). This accuracy, however, can vary because of many factors, including poor technique and/or inexperienced evaluator, an extremely obese or lean subject, and an improperly calibrated caliper (20).

The use of skinfold measurements to predict percent body fat and body density depends on regression equations and various equations that have been developed to assist the professional. Box 19-10 lists generalized equations that allow calculation of body composition from skinfolds (20,24), whereas population-specific equations are provided by Heyward and Stolarczyk in Table 4-4 of the GETP8 (21).

More detailed information concerning the standardization of skinfold measurements, as well as formulas for assessing body composition using skinfold calibration, is available in Chapter 17 of this manual.

Bioelectrical Impedance Analysis

> **1.3.7-HFS: Knowledge of the advantages/disadvantages and limitations of the various body composition techniques including but not limited to air displacement plethysmography (BOD POD®), dual energy x-ray absorptiometry (DEXA), hydrostatic weighing, skinfolds, and bioelectrical impedance.**

Bioelectrical impedance analysis (BIA) provides a noninvasive and easy-to-administer mechanism for assessing body composition that uses a small electrical current that is passed through the body. The resistance to this current is measured by the BIA analyzer and is used to estimate the percent body fat.

BIA can be assessed using a handheld device or by stepping on a specialized scale that has BIA capabilities. The basic premise behind the procedure is that the volume of fat-free tissue in the body will be proportional to the electrical conductivity of the body, as lean tissue contains mostly water (>90%) and electrolytes and is a good electrical conductor. Therefore, the faster the current is conducted (and the less resistance it encounters), the greater the amount of lean tissue present.

BIA can be used to estimate percent body fat; however, assumptions must be made regarding the hydration status of the subject. Therefore, the following conditions must be controlled to ensure that accurate measurements are obtained (1):

- The subject should not eat or drink within 4 hours of the test, should not consume alcohol within 48 hours of the test, and should not exercise within 12 hours of the test.

BOX 19-10 GENERALIZED SKINFOLD EQUATIONS

MEN

- **Seven-Site Formula** (chest, midaxillary, triceps, subscapular, abdomen, suprailiac, thigh)
  Body density = 1.112 − 0.00043499 (sum of seven skinfolds)
  + 0.00000055 (sum of seven skinfolds)^2
  − 0.00028826 (age) *[SEE 0.008 or ~3.5% fat]*
- **Three-Site Formula** (chest, abdomen, thigh)
  Body density = 1.10938 − 0.0008267 (sum of three skinfolds)
  + 0.0000016 (sum of three skinfolds)^2
  − 0.0002574 (age) *[SEE 0.008 or ~3.4% fat]*
- **Three-Site Formula** (chest, triceps, subscapular)
  Body density = 1.1125025 − 0.0013125 (sum of three skinfolds)
  + 0.0000055 (sum of three skinfolds)^2
  − 0.000244 (age) *[SEE 0.008 or ~3.6% fat]*

WOMEN

- **Seven-Site Formula** (chest, midaxillary, triceps, subscapular, abdomen, suprailiac, thigh)
  Body density = 1.097 − 0.00046971 (sum of seven skinfolds)
  + 0.00000056 (sum of seven skinfolds)^2
  − 0.00012828 (age) *[SEE 0.008 or ~3.8% fat]*
- **Three-Site Formula** (triceps, suprailiac, thigh)
  Body density = 1.099421 − 0.0009929 (sum of three skinfolds)
  + 0.0000023 (sum of three skinfolds)^2
  − 0.0001392 (age) *[SEE 0.009 or ~3.9% fat]*
- **Three-Site Formula** (triceps, suprailiac, abdominal)
  Body density = 1.089733 − 0.0009245 (sum of three skinfolds)
  + 0.0000025 (sum of three skinfolds)^2
  − 0.0000979 (age) *[SEE 0.009 or ~3.9% fat]*

Adapted from Jackson AS, Pollock ML. Practical assessment of body composition. *Phys Sport Med.* 1985;13:76–90. Pollock ML, Schmidt DH, Jackson AS. Measurement of cardiorespiratory fitness and body composition in the clinical setting. *Comp Ther.* 1980;6:12–17.

- The subject should completely void his/her bladder by urinating within 30 minutes of the test.
- The subject should not take any nonprescribed diuretics within 7 days of the test (caution: those on prescribed diuretics for hypertension or other health problems should **not** discontinue these medications) and should discontinue use of substances that can result in a diuretic response (such as caffeine, chocolate, etc.).

As long as stringent protocols are followed and valid equations are used, the accuracy of BIA testing is similar to that of skinfolds (19). Procedures for using BIA to assess body composition are explained in detail in Chapter 17 in this manual.

DENSITOMETRY

Whole body density, which uses the ratio of body mass to body volume, can also be utilized to estimate body composition. This technique is generally considered the crite-rion standard for determining body composition and is divided into two components: fat mass and fat-free mass. Although the benefit of this mechanism is its high degree of accuracy, it is limited in its ability to accurately determine body density via body volume. Although body mass can easily be measured by using body weight, body volume must be obtained using various other techniques, including hydrodensiometry or plethysmography.

Hydrodensiometry (Underwater Weighing)

Underwater weighing (UWW) is known as the gold standard or criterion method for body composition analysis, and all other methods of body composition analysis (e.g. skinfolds, BIA, etc.) are based on values obtained via this mechanism. UWW uses Archimedes' principle, which states that the density of the body is equal to the mass of the body divided by its volume. As bone and muscle tissue are denser than water and fat tissue is less dense, the loss of weight in water allows body volume to be calculated.

Thus, a person with a higher fat-free mass for the same total body mass weighs more in water and has a higher body density and lower percentage of body fat (41).

Although hydrostatic weighing is a standard method for measuring body volume and, therefore, body composition, it requires special equipment, the accurate measurement of residual volume, and significant cooperation by the subject (17). Thus, the following variables must be known to ensure accuracy (1):

1. Residual volume: The amount of air remaining in the lungs after full expiration; excess air adds to buoyancy and could falsely be measured as additional body fat.
2. Water density: Water density varies with its temperature, and buoyancy decreases with warmer temperatures.
3. Trapped gas in the subject's gastrointestinal system: As this is difficult to measure and could subsequently cause added buoyancy, a constant of 100 mL is used for all trapped gas in the gastrointestinal system.
4. Body weight: Body weight in the air (dry) and fully submerged in the water (wet).

Recommended procedures for UWW, as well as formulas for the conversion of body density to body composition, are provided in Chapter 17 of this manual.

Plethysmography

Recent advances now allow for body volume to be measured by air rather than water displacement. This can be accomplished by using a dual-chambered plethysmograph that measures body volume by changes in pressure in a closed chamber (12). The advantage of plethysmography is that it reduces anxiety as compared with UWW, which has allowed it to become an increasingly accepted method for determining body composition (12,17,29). A more detailed explanation of this technique can be found in Chapter 17 of this resource manual.

OTHER TECHNIQUES FOR BODY COMPOSITION ASSESSMENT

Dual energy x-ray absorptiometry (DEXA) and total body electrical conductivity (TOBEC) are reliable and accurate measures of body composition. These measures, however, are rarely used in general health fitness testing because of the cost and the need for highly trained personnel (42). Detailed explanations of these techniques are found in Chapter 17 of this manual.

BODY COMPOSITION NORMS

There are no universally accepted norms for body composition; however, Tables 4-5 and 4-6 of the GETP8 provide selective normative values of percent body fat for men and women, respectively. A consensus opinion for an exact percentage body fat value associated with optimal health has yet to be defined; however, a range 10% to 22% for men and 20% to 32% for women is considered satisfactory for normal health (28).

CARDIORESPIRATORY FITNESS

Cardiorespiratory fitness (CRF) is determined by one's ability to perform dynamic exercise at moderate to high intensities, utilizing large muscle groups, for prolonged periods. The ability to perform such exercise depends on the functional ability of the respiratory, cardiovascular, and skeletal muscle systems.

CRF is well established as a health-related index of fitness, as (a) a low level of CRF is associated with a markedly increased cardiovascular and all-cause mortality, (b) increasing CRF results in a reduction in all-cause mortality, and (c) high levels of CRF are related to increased levels of habitual physical activity, which in turn is correlated with significant health benefits (6,7,42). The assessment of CRF is fundamentally important as part of a primary or secondary prevention program.

REASONS FOR MEASURING CARDIORESPIRATORY FITNESS

> **1.3.17-HFS: Ability to explain purpose of testing, determine an appropriate submaximal or maximal protocol, and perform an assessment of cardiovascular fitness on the treadmill or cycle ergometer.**

Identification of CRF can assist the professional by providing valuable information that can be used to determine the intensity, duration, and mode of exercise recommended as part of an exercise program. Additionally, the measurement of CRF following the initiation of an exercise training program can serve as motivation to the patient as reason for continuing with a regular exercise program and may encourage the addition of other modes of exercise to improve overall fitness. Lastly, the assessment of CRF can assist in identifying, diagnosing, and prognosing health/medical situations.

HOW CARDIORESPIRATORY FITNESS IS MEASURED AND EXPRESSED: MAXIMAL OXYGEN UPTAKE

> **1.3.5-CES: Select an appropriate test protocol according to the age, functional capacity, physical ability, and health status of the individual.**

Maximal oxygen uptake ($\dot{V}O_{2max}$) is widely considered the best measure of CRF. Maximal oxygen uptake can be defined as the product of the maximal cardiac output ($L \cdot min^{-1}$) and arterio-venous oxygen difference ($mL \cdot O_2$ per L blood). Variations resulting from sex, age, and fitness level are noted in $\dot{V}O_{2max}$ and result primarily from differences in maximal cardiac output. Thus, the functional capacity of the heart is the primary predictor of $\dot{V}O_{2max}$.

$\dot{V}O_{2max}$ is measured using open-circuit spirometry that requires the subject to breathe through a low-resistance mouthpiece with his/her nose occluded while pulmonary ventilation and expired fractions of oxygen (O_2) and carbon dioxide (CO_2) are measured or calculated. Today, the measurement of $\dot{V}O_{2max}$ is less labor intensive in that data printouts and detailed graphics are provided on a breath-by-breath basis (11). However, this test remains highly specialized, and the administration of the test and interpretation of results should be reserved for trained professional with a thorough understanding of exercise science. Additionally, because of the costs associated with the equipment, space, and personnel needed to complete this testing, $\dot{V}O_{2max}$ testing is generally reserved for research or clinical laboratory settings.

$\dot{V}O_{2max}$ can be estimated using a variety of submaximal and maximal exercise tests. Although not as accurate as directly measuring $\dot{V}O_{2max}$, these tests provide validated estimates by examining (a) the physiologic response to submaximal exercise (e.g., HR at a specified power output) as compared with correlations with directly measured $\dot{V}O_{2max}$, or (b) one's test performance measures (e.g., distance completed within a specified amount of time) as compared with correlations with directly measured $\dot{V}O_{2max}$.

Because of the numerous options for assessing CRF, the choice of which test to use is important. Some factors to consider when choosing test type are (1):

- Length of the test
- Willingness of the participant
- Cost of the test to administer
- What the personnel need is (i.e., qualifications)
- What equipment and facilities are needed for the test
- Whether physician supervision is needed
- Whether there are any safety concerns
- Needs to be met to preserve accuracy of the data being collected

CONTRAINDICATIONS TO EXERCISE TESTING

Before initiating an exercise test, the risk for performing the test must be weighed against the potential benefits. Box 19-11 outlines both relative and absolute contraindications to exercise testing. Performing the pre-exercise test evaluation and the careful review of prior medical history, as described in the *GETP8* and in related chapters of this manual, assists in identifying potential contraindications to exercise testing and increases the safety of the exercise test.

Individuals identified as having absolute contraindications should not be tested until such conditions are stabilized or adequately treated. Those with relative contraindications may be tested only after careful evaluation to determine if the benefits obtained from test completion outweigh the risk involved. However, certain clinical situations may preclude the use of contraindications to determine testing risk—such as soon after acute myocardial infarction, revascularization procedure, or bypass surgery—or to determine the need for, or benefit of, drug therapy.

MAXIMAL VERSUS SUBMAXIMAL EXERCISE TESTING

> **1.3.12-CES: Obtain and recognize normal and abnormal physiologic and subjective responses (e.g. symptoms, ECG, BP, HR, RPE and other scales, oxygen saturation, and oxygen consumption) at appropriate intervals during the test.**

> **1.7.9-CES: Identify patients who require a symptom-limited exercise test before exercise training.**

> **1.3.23-HFS: Ability to identify individuals for whom physician supervision is recommended during maximal and submaximal exercise testing.**

> **1.3.22-HFS: Ability to modify protocols and procedures for cardiorespiratory fitness tests in children, adolescents, and older adults.**

> **4.2.1-HFS: Knowledge of metabolic risk factors or conditions that may require consultation with medical personnel before testing or training, including obesity, metabolic syndrome, thyroid disease, kidney disease, diabetes or glucose intolerance, and hypoglycemia.**

The use of maximal or submaximal exercise testing depends on the information desired, the personnel available to perform the test, and the equipment available for testing purposes. Maximal exercise testing offers increased sensitivity in the diagnosis of coronary artery disease in asymptomatic individuals and provides a better estimate of $\dot{V}O_{2max}$ (see Chapter 5 of the GETP8). The disadvantage, however, of using maximal exercise testing to determine $\dot{V}O_{2max}$ is that patients are required to exercise to the point of volitional fatigue, thus potentially requiring medical supervision (see Chapter 2 of the GETP8) and the availability of emergency equipment.

Submaximal exercise can provide reasonable estimates of $\dot{V}O_{2max}$ by considering test duration at a given workload on an ergometer and using the established prediction equations found in Chapter 7 of ACSM's GETP8. Additionally, submaximal exercise testing estimates $\dot{V}O_{2max}$ through the determination of the HR response to one or more submaximal work rates. Lastly, the use of submaximal BP, workload, RPE, and other subjective indices (pain/discomfort) can provide valuable information regarding one's functional response to exercise.

BOX 19-11   CONTRAINDICATIONS TO EXERCISE TESTING

ABSOLUTE

- A recent significant change in the resting ECG suggesting significant ischemia, recent myocardial infarction (within 2 days), or other acute cardiac event
- Unstable angina
- Uncontrolled cardiac dysrhythmias causing symptoms or hemodynamic compromise
- Symptomatic severe aortic stenosis
- Uncontrolled symptomatic heart failure
- Acute pulmonary embolus or pulmonary infarction
- Acute myocarditis or pericarditis
- Suspected or known dissecting aneurysm
- Acute systemic infection, accompanied by fever, body aches, or swollen lymph glands

RELATIVE[a]

- Left main coronary stenosis
- Moderate stenotic valvular heart disease
- Electrolyte abnormalities (e.g., hypokalemia, hypomagnesemia)
- Severe arterial hypertension (i.e., systolic BP of (200 mm Hg and/or a diastolic BP of (110 mm Hg) at rest
- Tachydysrhythmia or bradydysrhythmia
- Hypertrophic cardiomyopathy and other forms of outflow tract obstruction
- Neuromuscular, musculoskeletal, or rheumatoid disorders that are exacerbated by exercise
- High-degree atrioventricular block
- Ventricular aneurysm
- Uncontrolled metabolic disease (e.g., diabetes, thyrotoxicosis, or myxedema)
- Chronic infectious disease (e.g., mononucleosis, hepatitis, AIDS)
- Mental or physical impairment leading to inability to exercise adequately

[a]Relative contraindications can be superseded if benefits outweigh risks of exercise. In some instances, these individuals can be exercised with caution and/or using low-level end points, especially if they are asymptomatic at rest.

Modified from Gibbons RJ, Balady GJ, Bricker J, et al. ACC/AHA 2002 guideline update for exercise testing: a report of the American College of Cardiology/American Heart Association Task Force on Practice Guidelines (Committee on Exercise Testing) [Internet]. 2002. [cited 2007 June 15]. Available from: www.acc.org/clinical/guidelines/exercise/dirIndex.htm

The following are assumed to have been met when estimating $\dot{V}O_{2max}$ from the submaximal HR response:

- A steady-state HR is achieved and is consistent for each work rate
- HR and work rate exists as a linear relationship
- The $\dot{V}O_{2max}$ is indicated by the maximal workload
- There is a uniform maximal HR for a given image
- Mechanical efficiency is the same for everyone
- The subject is not on medications that alter HR

Submaximal exercise test are typically performed on low- to moderate-risk individuals, based on ACSM guidelines for risk stratification. General Procedures for Submaximal Testing of Cardiorespiratory Fitness, which provides professionals with a quick-reference guide to test administration, can be found in Box 19-12.

PRETEST INSTRUCTIONS FOR CARDIORESPIRATORY FITNESS ASSESSMENT

To standardize the testing conditions, increase the predictive accuracy for identifying CRF, and ensure the safety of the patient, the following general instructions should be provided (1):

- Abstain from eating at least 4 hours before testing (though patients who experience hypoglycemia may

be advised to have a light, healthy snack of protein and carbohydrate combination 2 to 3 hours before the test, and all patients should be encouraged to eat something light and well balanced in the 12 hours preceding the 4-hour pretest fast).
- Abstain from strenuous exercise for at least 24 hours before the test.
- Abstain from consuming caffeine-containing products for a minimum of 12 to 24 hours before the test.
- Abstain from using products containing nicotine for at least 3 hours and from consuming alcohol for at least 24 hours before the test.
- Consult the test administrator and/or physician for advice on the use of medications before testing (medications affecting resting or exercise HR, such as β-blockers, may affect test accuracy).

TEST MODE FOR MEASURING CARDIORESPIRATORY FITNESS: PROCEDURES AND PROTOCOLS FOR STEP TESTS, FIELD TESTS, SUBMAXIMAL EXERCISE TESTS, AND MAXIMAL EXERCISE TESTS

 1.3.16-HFS: Ability to instruct participants in the use of equipment and test procedures.

BOX 19-12 GENERAL PROCEDURES FOR SUBMAXIMAL TESTING OF CARDIORESPIRATORY FITNESS

1. Obtain resting heart rate and BP immediately before exercise in the exercise posture.
2. The client should be familiarized with the ergometer. If using a cycle ergometer, properly position the client on the ergometer (i.e., upright posture, five-degree bend in the knee at maximal leg extension, hands in proper position on handlebars).
3. The exercise test should begin with a two- to three-minute warm-up to acquaint the client with the cycle ergometer and prepare him or her for the exercise intensity in the first stage of the test.
4. A specific protocol should consist of 2- or 3-minute stages with appropriate increments in work rate.
5. Heart rate should be monitored at least two times during each stage, near the end of the second and third minutes of each stage. If heart rate >110 beats·min^{-1}, steady-state heart rate (i.e., two heart rates within 5 beats·min^{-1}) should be reached before the workload is increased.
6. Blood pressure should be monitored in the last minute of each stage and repeated (verified) in the event of a hypotensive or hypertensive response.
7. Perceived exertion and additional rating scales should be monitored near the end of the last

minute of each stage using either the 6–20 or 0–10 scale (Table 4-8 of GETP8).
8. Client appearance and symptoms should be monitored and recorded regularly.
9. The test should be terminated when the subject reaches 70% heart rate reserve (85% of age-predicted maximal heart rate), fails to conform to the exercise test protocol, experiences adverse signs or symptoms, requests to stop, or experiences an emergency situation.
10. An appropriate cool-down/recovery period should be initiated consisting of either:
    a. Continued exercise at a work rate equivalent to that of the first stage of the exercise test protocol or lower; or
    b. A passive cool-down if the subject experiences signs of discomfort or an emergency situation occurs
11. All physiologic observations (e.g., heart rate, BP, signs and symptoms) should be continued for at least 5 minutes of recovery unless abnormal responses occur, which would warrant a longer posttest surveillance period. Continue low-level exercise until heart rate and BP stabilize, but not necessarily until they reach pre-exercise levels.

From: American College of Sports Medicine. Health-Related Physical Fitness Assessment Manual. 2nd edition. Philadelphia: 2008. Lippincott Williams & Wilkins.

> **1.3.17-HFS: Ability to explain purpose of testing, determine an appropriate submaximal or maximal protocol, and perform an assessment of cardiovascular fitness on the treadmill or the cycle ergometer.**

Step Tests

Step tests have been used for fitness testing for more than 50 years. Step tests are practical for exercise testing in that they can be used in a field or laboratory setting, can be submaximal or maximal in nature, require little or no testing equipment, are easily transportable, requires little practice, are usually of short duration, and are an advantageous mode to utilize with most populations (30). Unlike traditional fitness testing, evaluation of CRF from step tests is usually done via the evaluation of recovery HR. The Queens College (or McArdle) Step Test is described in detail in Box 19-13. Other common step protocols are also available (i.e., Forestry Test and Harvard Step Test) and differ from the Queens College step test in either step height and/or test time (1). Also, the Canadian Home Fitness test has demonstrated that testing for CRF can be performed on a large scale and at a low cost (3,4,44).

Field Tests for the Prediction of Cardiorespiratory Fitness

> **1.3.34-CES: Ability to perform a 6-minute walk test and appropriately utilize the results to assess prognosis, fitness, and/or improvement.**

Field tests are often used to measure CRF in large groups of apparently healthy subjects (30). Field tests offer many benefits over other forms of laboratory testing in that they are easy to administer, are inexpensive, and can be performed wherever a measured distance is available.

Several disadvantages are associated with using field tests for the prediction of CRF, including the inability to control the setting and the potential for the tests to become maximal or near maximal tests. In addition, field tests are unmonitored and can be highly affected by an individual's motivation or pacing ability. Thus, for these reasons, field tests are not recommended for individuals at moderate to high risk of cardiovascular or musculoskeletal complications.

Field tests can utilize various modes of exercise, including walking, running, a walk-run, cycling, and swimming.

BOX 19-13   QUEENS COLLEGE STEP TEST

The Queens College Step Test is also known as the McArdle Step Test.

1. The step test requires that the individual step up and down on a standardized step height of 16.25 in (41.25 cm) for 3 minutes. (Many gymnasium bleachers have a riser height of 16.25 in.)

2. The men step at a rate (cadence) of 24 per minute, whereas the women step at a rate of 22 per minute. This cadence should be closely monitored and set with the use of an electronic metronome. A 24 per minute cadence means that the complete cycle of step up with one leg, step up with the other, step down with the first leg, and finally step down with the last leg is performed 24 times in a minute (up one leg, up the other leg, down the first leg, down the other leg). Commonly we set the metronome at a cadence of four times the step rate, in this case 96 beats per minute for men, to coordinate each leg's movement with a beat of the metronome. The women's step rate would be 88 beats per minute. Although it may be possible to test more than one patient at a time, depending on equipment, it would be difficult to test men and women together.

3. After the 3 minutes are up, the patient stops and palpates the pulse or has the pulse taken (at the radial site, preferably) while standing within the first 5 seconds. A 15-second pulse count is then taken. Multiply this pulse count by 4 to determine heart rate (HR) in beats per minute (bpm). The recovery HR should occur between 5 and 20 seconds of immediate recovery from the end of the step test.

The subject's $\dot{V}O_{2max}$ in $mL \cdot kg^{-1} \cdot min^{-1}$ is determined from the recovery HR by the following formulas:

For men:

$$VO_{2max} (mL \cdot kg^{-1} \cdot min^{-1}) = 111.33 - (0.42 \cdot HR)$$

For women:

$$VO_{2max} (mL \cdot kg^{-1} \cdot min^{-1}) = 65.81 - (0.1847 \cdot HR)$$
$$HR = \text{recovery HR (bpm)}$$

For example:

If a man finished the test with a recovery HR of 144 bpm (36 beats in 15 seconds), then:

$$VO_{2max} (mL \cdot kg^{-1} \cdot min^{-1}) = 111.33 - (0.42 \cdot 144)$$
$$= 50.85 \ mL \cdot kg^{-1} \cdot min^{-1}$$

From: American College of Sports Medicine. Health-Related Physical Fitness Assessment Manual. 2nd edition. Philadelphia: 2008. Lippincott Williams & Wilkins.

The most common field tests used for the prediction of CRF, however, are those requiring a timed completion of a set distance (i.e., 1.5-mile run) or a maximal distance measurement (i.e., 12-minute run). Box 19-14 provides procedures for the 1.5-mile run and the 12-minute walk/run test, and Box 19-15 gives the Rockport 1-mile walk test procedures.

SUBMAXIMAL EXERCISE TESTS FOR THE PREDICTION OF CARDIORESPIRATORY FITNESS

Submaximal exercise testing can be a valid and reliable method for predicting CRF when done in a laboratory setting. These exercise tests usually involve use of a step test, treadmill, or cycle ergometer. The cycle ergometer is the most preferred mode for laboratory testing because of its ability to reproduce work output. For more information about work output and choice of testing mode, consult ACSM's *Health-Related Physical Fitness Assessment Manual, Second Edition* (1). Box 19-16 provides general procedures for submaximal exercise testing using a cycle ergometer.

To achieve valid results during submaximal exercise testing, it is essential that an accurate measurement of HR

is achieved. Typically, HR is obtained by palpation; however, the accuracy of this method varies with the experience and technique of the fitness professional. Alterations to palpation which may increase accuracy of HR measurement include the use of an ECG, HR monitor, or a stethescope.

Additionally, submaximal HR response can be altered by several environmental (i.e., heat and humidity), dietary (i.e., caffeine, time since last meal), and behavioral (i.e., anxiety, smoking, previous activity) factors (see pretest instructions earlier in this chapter) that must be controlled for, as previously discussed.

Assumptions of Submaximal Prediction of Cardiorespiratory Fitness

The following list of assumptions is specific to submaximal testing (1).

- A linear (straight line) relationship exists between VO_2 and HR within the range of 110 to 150 bpm. It is at this point that SV has reached a plateau (approximately 40%–50% of max), and the HR and oxygen consumption track linearly.

BOX 19-14 1.5-MILE RUN AND 12-MINUTE WALK/RUN TEST PROCEDURES

1.5-MILE RUN TEST

This test is contraindicated for unconditioned beginners, individuals with symptoms of heart disease, and those with known heart disease or risk factors for heart disease. Your patient should be able to jog for 15 minutes continuously to complete this test and obtain a reasonable prediction of their aerobic capacity.

1. Ensure that the area for performing the test measures out to be 1.5 miles in distance. A standard quarter-mile track would be ideal (6 laps = 1.5 miles).
2. Inform the patient of the purposes of the test and the need to pace over the 1.5-mile distance. Effective pacing and the subject's motivation are key variables in the outcome of the test.
3. Have the patient start the test; start a stopwatch to coincide with the start. Give your patient feedback on time to help them with pacing.
4. Record the total time to complete the test and use the formula below to predict cardiorespiratory fitness in $mL \cdot kg^{-1} \cdot min^{-1}$

For men and women:

$$VO_{2max} (mL \cdot kg^{-1} \cdot min^{-1}) = 3.5 + 483/Time$$

Time = time to complete 1.5 miles in nearest hundredth of a minute

For example:

If time to complete 1.5 miles was 11:12 (11 minutes and 12 seconds), then the time used in the formula would be 11.2 (12/60=0.2).

$$VO_{2max} (mL \cdot kg^{-1} \cdot min^{-1}) = 3.5 + 483/11.2$$
$$= 46.6 \ mL \cdot kg^{-1} \cdot min^{-1}$$

12-MINUTE WALK/RUN TEST PROCEDURES

A popular variation of the 1.5-mile run test is the 12-minute walk/run test popularized by Dr. Ken Cooper of the Aerobics Institute in Dallas, Texas. This test requires the patient to cover the maximum distance in 12 minutes by either walking, running, or using a combination of walking and running. The distance covered in 12 minutes needs to be measured and expressed in meters.

The prediction of aerobic capacity from the 12-minute walk/run test is:

$$VO_{2max} (mL \cdot kg^{-1} \cdot min^{-1}) = (distance \ in \ meters - 504.9)/44.73$$

From: American College of Sports Medicine. Health-Related Physical Fitness Assessment Manual. 2nd edition. Philadelphia: 2008. Lippincott Williams & Wilkins.

BOX 19-15 ROCKPORT 1-MILE WALK TEST PROCEDURE

This test may be useful for those who are unable to run because of a low fitness level and/or injury. The patient should be able to walk briskly (get their exercise heart rate [HR] above 120 bpm) for 1 mile to complete this test.

1. The 1-mile walk test requires that the subject walk 1 mile as fast as possible around a measured course. The patient must not break into a run! Walking can be defined as having contact with the ground at all times (running involves an airborne phase). The time to walk this 1 mile is measured and recorded.
2. Immediately at the end of the 1-mile walk, the patient counts the recovery HR or pulse for 15 seconds and multiplies by 4 to determine a 1-minute recovery HR (bpm). In another version of the test, HR is measured in the final minute of the 1-mile walk (during the last quarter mile).

The formula for VO_{2max}, $mL \cdot kg^{-1} \cdot min^{-1}$ is sex specific (i.e., the constant of 6.315 is added to the formula for men only).

$$VO_{2max} (mL \cdot kg^{-1} \cdot min^{-1}) = 132.853 - (0.1692 \cdot WT)$$
$$- (0.3877 \cdot AGE) + (6.315, for \ men) - (3.2649 \cdot TIME)$$
$$- (0.1565 \cdot HR)$$

WT = weight in kilograms

AGE = in years

TIME = time for 1 mile in nearest hundredth of a minute (e.g., 15:42 = 15.7

HR = recovery HR in bpm

This formula was derived on apparently healthy individuals ranging in age from 30 to 69 years of age.

For example:

32-year-old male; 68 kg (150 lbs)

1 mile = 10:35 (10.58); HR = 136

$$VO_{2max} (mL \cdot kg^{-1} \cdot min^{-1}) = 132.853 - (0.1692 \cdot 68)$$
$$- (0.3877 \cdot 32) + (6.315) - (3.2649 \cdot 10.58) - (0.1565 \cdot 136)$$
$$= 59.4 \ mL \cdot kg^{-1} \cdot min^{-1}$$

From: American College of Sports Medicine. Health-Related Physical Fitness Assessment Manual. 2nd edition. Philadelphia: 2008. Lippincott Williams & Wilkins.

BOX 19-16	GENERAL PROCEDURES FOR LABORATORY SUBMAXIMAL EXERCISE TEST FOR CARDIORESPIRATORY FITNESS USING A CYCLE ERGOMETER

1. The exercise test should begin with a 2- to 3-min warm-up to acquaint the client with the cycle ergometer and prepare him or her for the exercise intensity in the first stage of the test.
2. The specific protocol consists of 3-min stages with appropriate increments in work rate.
3. The client should be properly positioned on the cycle ergometer (i.e., upright posture, 5° bend in the knee at maximal leg extension, hands in proper position on handlebars).
4. Heart rate should be monitored at least two times during each stage, near the end of the second and third minutes of each stage. If heart rate > 110 beats·min^{-1}, steady state heart rate (i.e., two heart rates within 6 beats·min^{-1}) should be reached before the work rate is increased.
5. Blood pressure should be monitored in the later portion of each stage and re-peated (verified) in the event of a hypotensive or hypertensive response.
6. Perceived exertion should be monitored near the end of each stage using either the 6–20 or the 0–10 scale.
7. Client appearance and symptoms should be monitored regularly.
8. The test should be terminated when the subject reaches 85% of age-predicted maximal heart rate (70% of heart rate reserve), fails to conform to the exercise test protocol, experiences adverse signs or symptoms, requests to stop, or experiences an emergency situation.
9. An appropriate cool-down/recovery period should be initiated consisting of either:
   a. continued pedaling at a work rate equivalent to that of the first stage of the exercise test protocol or lower; or,
   b. a passive cool-down if the subject experiences signs of discomfort or an emergency situation occurs.
10. All physiologic observations (e.g., heart rate, blood pressure, signs and symptoms) should be continued for at least 4-min of recovery unless abnormal responses occur, which would warrant a longer posttest surveillance period.

From: American College of Sports Medicine. Health-Related Physical Fitness Assessment Manual. 2nd edition. Philadelphia: 2008. Lippincott Williams & Wilkins.

- Maximum HR (HR$_{max}$), which must be predicted for submaximal ergometer testing, can be estimated or predicted as a function of age (HR$_{max}$ = 220 – age).

  Unfortunately, a large variation exists in the age-prediction of HR$_{max}$, and this assumption may provide for the greatest source of error in the submaximal prediction of CRF (3).
- Steady state heart rate (HR$_{ss}$) can be achieved in 3 to 4 minutes at a constant, submaximal work output. HR$_{ss}$ is ensured by consecutive HR measurements being within six beats of each other. Thus, the achievement of HR$_{ss}$ during the protocol is essential for valid results.
- A cadence of 50 revolutions per minute (rpm) is typically considered comfortable and mechanically efficient in most individuals. It is assumed that each subject expends the same amount of energy and has the same absolute oxygen requirements at the same work output on the cycle. Maintaining a constant pedal rate on a mechanically braked ergometer is essential to ensure a constant power output.
- The HR at two separate work outputs can be plotted as the HR – VO$_2$ relationship and extrapolated to the estimated HR$_{max}$. The YMCA submaximal cycle ergometer protocol and the Bruce Submaximal treadmill protocol are both multistage tests that utilize a minimum of two stages to predict CRF. The Åstrand protocol prediction is based on the HR$_{ss}$ at a single work stage.

Sources of Error in Submaximal Prediction

A submaximal exercise test requires predetermined test endpoints for satisfactory completion of the test. General indications for stopping an exercise test in low-risk adults can be found in Box 19-17. In addition to terminating the test because of completion of the protocol, the health/fitness professional should consider test termination if the patient's HR exceeds 85% of his/her age-predicted HR$_{max}$, as this exposes the subject to near maximal exertion and increases the risk of cardiovascular or orthopedic complications.

Submaximal Protocols for Predicting Cardiorespiratory Fitness

As discussed previously in this chapter, various modes of exercise can be utilized in the completion of submaximal

BOX 19-17 GENERAL INDICATIONS FOR STOPPING AN EXERCISE TEST IN LOW-RISK ADULTS[A] (ABSOLUTE AND RELATIVE)

ABSOLUTE INDICATIONS

- Drop in systolic blood pressure of >10 mm Hg from baseline[a] blood pressure despite an increase in workload when accompanied by other evidence of ischemia
- Moderately severe angina (defined as 3 on standard scale)
- Increasing nervous system symptoms (e.g., ataxia, dizziness, or near syncope)
- Signs of poor perfusion (cyanosis or pallor)
- Technical difficulties monitoring the ECG or systolic blood pressure
- Subject's desire to stop
- Sustained ventricular tachycardia
- ST elevation (+1.0 mm) in leads without diagnostic Q-waves (other than V_1 or aVR)

RELATIVE INDICATIONS

- Drop in systolic blood pressure of >10 mm Hg from baseline[a] blood pressure despite an increase in workload in the absence of other evidence of ischemia
- ST or QRS changes such as excessive ST depression (≥ 2 mm horizontal or downsloping ST-segment depression) or marked axis shift
- Arrhythmias other than sustained ventricular tachycardia, including multifocal PVCs, triplets of PVCs, supraventricular tachycardia, heart block, or bradyarrhythmias
- Fatigue, shortness of breath, wheezing, leg cramps, or claudication
- Development of bundle-branch block or intraventricular conduction delay that cannot be distinguished from ventricular tachycardia
- Increasing chest pain
- Hypertensive response (systolic blood pressure of >250 mm Hg and/or a diastolic blood pressure of >115 mm Hg).

ECG, electrocardiogram; PVC, premature ventricular contraction.

[a]Baseline refers to a measurement obtained immediately before the test and in the same posture as the test is being performed.

Reprinted with permission from Gibbons RJ, Balady GJ, Bricker JT, et al. Pretest Likelihood of atherosclerotic cardiovascular disease (CVD). ACC/AHA 2002 Guideline Update for Exercise Testing; a report of the American College of Cardiology/American Heart Association Task Force on Practice Guidelines; Committee on Exercise Testing, 2002. *Circulation.* 2002;106(14):1883–92.

exercise tests. Most common modes of exercise for laboratory-based exercise testing includes the motor-driven treadmill and the mechanically braked cycle ergometer. Although both provide adequate mechanisms for completion of submaximal testing, each has inherent advantages and disadvantages that must be considered. Common protocols utilized in predicting CRF using submaximal exercise testing can be found in Boxes 19-18 through 19-21, Table 19-3 and Figure 19-2.

MAXIMAL EXERCISE TESTING

Maximal exercise testing is the most challenging of all physical fitness assessment tests for both the patient and the test technician. Also called a graded exercise test (GXT) or stress test, these tests use incremental changes in workload until peak exertion/exhaustion is achieved. Although many exercise professionals may not be involved in maximal exercise testing, they should be aware of the purposes, procedures, protocols, and contraindications to this type of exercise test.

More information on maximal exercise testing can be found in Chapters 21 and 22 of this resource manual.

Purposes of Maximal Exercise Testing

The maximal GXT has four primary purposes:

1. Screening for the presence of disease
2. Diagnosis of a disease when symptoms are present
3. Prognosis of the patient relative to their coronary artery disease and/or other disease history
4. Guiding the management of an individual, including for use as an exercise prescription

Procedures for Maximal Exercise Testing

Decisions concerning the use of a maximal GXT include the identification of who should have the test, whether a physical examination should be performed before the test, whether a physician should be present for the test, and what personnel will be needed to conduct the test.

BOX 19-18	SUBMAXIMAL CYCLE ERGOMETER TEST PROCEDURES: MULTISTAGE PROTOCOL

In summary, the patient performs a multistage protocol based on the response to the first stage. The total test may last from 6 to 12 minutes.

1. Explain the test to your patient. Be sure you have adequately screened your patient via a Health History Questionnaire and/or a PAR-Q and performed ACSM risk stratification. *Note:* Physician supervision is not necessary with submaximal testing in low- and moderate-risk adults. More information on this can be found in ACSM's GETP8.

2. In addition, you should have already ensured that your patient has followed some basic pretest instructions for this submaximal test: wearing comfortable clothing; having plenty of fluids beforehand; avoiding alcohol, tobacco, and caffeine within 3 hours of the test; avoiding strenuous exercise on the day of the test; and having adequate sleep the night before the test.

3. Explain informed consent. The safety of this test is reported as >300,000 tests performed without a major complication. It is very important the patient understands that he or she is free to stop the test at any time, but he or she is also responsible for informing you of any and all symptoms that might develop.

4. You should also discuss with your patient the concept of your general preparedness to handle any emergencies. The details of general preparedness include the testing environment and emergency plan/procedures. Also, an explanation of the rating of perceived exertion (RPE) scale is warranted at this time (Table 4-7 of GETP8). An example of some verbal directions you could read to your patient before asking him or her to use the RPE scale to give a general rating is: "Rate your feelings that are caused by exercise using this scale. The feelings should be general, about your whole body. We will ask you to select one number that most accurately corre-

sponds to your perception of your total body feeling. You can use the verbal qualifiers to help you select your RPE number. There is no right or wrong answer. Use any number that you think is appropriate."

5. Take the baseline or resting measures of heart rate and blood pressure with your patient seated. If necessary, these seated measurements can be performed on the cycle ergometer.

6. Adjust seat height. The knee should be flexed at approximately 5 to 10 degrees in the pedal-down position with the toes on the pedals. Another way to check seat height is to have your patient place the heels on the pedals; with the heels on the pedals, the leg should be straight in the pedal-down position. Also, you can align the seat height with you patient's greater trochanter, or hip, with your patient standing next to the cycle. Most important is for your patient to be comfortable with the seat height. Have your patient turn the pedals to test for the seat height appropriateness. While pedaling, your patient should be comfortable, and there should be no rocking of the hips (you can check on hip rocking by viewing your patient from behind). Also, be sure your patient maintains an upright posture (by adjusting the handlebars, if necessary) and does not grip the handlebars too tight.

7. START THE TEST. Have your patient freewheel, without any resistance (0 kg), at the pedaling cadence of 50 rpm. A brief period of approximately 2 to 3 minutes should suffice for this freewheeling period. Remember, some subjects may have a difficult time with freewheeling. Maintaining 50 rpm throughout the test is essential. The rpm may vary between about 48 and 52 rpm; any more variance than this may invalidate the test.

8. Set the first work output according to YMCA protocol. The first work output, for everyone, is 150 $kp \cdot m \cdot min^{-1}$ (50 rpm $\cdot$ 0.5 kp). The YMCA protocol is found in Boxes 19-19 and 19-20.

From: American College of Sports Medicine. Health-Related Physical Fitness Assessment Manual. 2nd edition. Philadelphia: 2008. Lippincott Williams & Wilkins.

Who Should Have a Maximal Graded Exercise Test?

 1.7.9-CES: Identify patients who require a symptom-limited exercise test before exercise training.

ACSM's GETP8 addresses the appropriate candidates for a maximal GXT by applying the concept of risk

stratification (discussed earlier in this chapter and in Chapter 18 of this manual). According to these guidelines, patients younger than age 45 (men) or 55 (women) are not recommended to have a maximal exercise test before starting an exercise program. It is recommended, however, that patients who are at a

BOX 19-19 YMCA SUBMAXIMAL CYCLE ERGOMETER PROTOCOL

1. Start the clock/timer. It may be best to think of timing each stage (e.g., 3 minutes) rather than the entire test time. Therefore, you may wish to reset the time at the end of each stage. In reality, timing of this test is the most difficult part for individuals to learn. Suggested timing sequence for each stage of the test are included below.

2. Measure the heart rate (HR) after 2 minutes into the first work rate or stage. Count HR for at least 10 to 15 seconds. Some suggest a 30-second count for more accuracy, but it may be impractical to spend a full 30 seconds of each minute counting the HR. The use of an HR monitor may be helpful; however, it should only be used as a teaching aid to check your results by palpation. Record the HR on the test form.

3. Measure and record the blood pressure (BP) one time during each stage; usually after having completed the 2-minute HR of that stage. ACSM's GETP8 for test termination and BP is applicable.
   - BP >250/115 mm Hg
   - Significant drop (>10 mm Hg) in systolic blood pressure or a failure to rise with an increase in exercise intensity

4. Ask your patient for the RPE for that stage. Choose either the 6–20 scale or the 0–11 scale. These scales were discussed earlier. Be sure to monitor your patient for general appearance and any symptoms that may develop.

5. Take another HR after the BP and RPE measurements, around 3 minutes into the stage. Record the HR on the appropriate testing data form.

   Compare minute 2 HR to minute 3 HR during each stage:
   A. If there is a difference of within 5 bpm, consider that work rate or stage finished. Steady state conditions apply.
   B. If there is a difference of >5 bpm, continue on for another minute (i.e., minute 4 of that stage) and check HR again. Do not change to the next stage until you have a steady-state heart rate HR_{SS} (difference within 5 bpm). If you fail to have your

patient achieve an HR_{SS} for a stage, then you may have to discontinue the test and plan to test again on another day. It has been noted that up to 10% of individuals who are tested with this protocol are unable to obtain HR_{SS} in a stage.

In summary:
HR_{SS} (within 5 bpm): Go to step 7
No HR_{SS} (>5 bpm) achieved: Continue stage until HR_{SS}

6. Regularly check the work output of the cycle ergometer using the pendulum resistance scale on the side of the ergometer and the rpm of your patient. For the resistance, do not use the scale on the top front panel of the cycle ergometer for measurement. Adjust the work output if necessary. Regularly check your patient's rpm and correct if necessary.

7. After completing the first stage of 150 $kp \cdot m \cdot min^{-1}$ compare your patient's HR_{SS} to the protocol sheet. Adjust resistance appropriately for the second stage based on HR response to first stage. This is a multistage test; the patient will perform at least two stages.
   - You need to obtain HR_{SS} from a stage (within 6 bpm).
   - The test requires completion of at least two separate stages with HR_{SS} at each stage.
   - Consider for the test results the third minute HR as the HR_{SS}, if it is a steady state (for plotting or calculations) for that stage.
   - These two stages must have HRs between 110 bpm and 85% of age-predicted maximum heart rate (APMHR) to be used in the plotting and calculation of VO_{2max}.

8. Allow your patient to cool down after the last stage of the protocol is complete. Have your patient continue to pedal at 50 rpm, and adjust the resistance down to 0.5 to 1 kp for 3 minutes of cool-down or recovery. Take your patient's HR and BP at the end of the 3-minute active recovery period. Next, allow him or her to sit quietly in a chair for 2 to 3 minutes to continue the recovery process. Be sure to check the HR and BP before allowing them to leave the lab. It is hoped that the HR and BP will approach the resting measures.

From: American College of Sports Medicine. Health-Related Physical Fitness Assessment Manual. 2nd edition. Philadelphia: 2008. Lippincott Williams & Wilkins.

BOX 19-20	SUGGESTED STAGE PROCEDURES FOR YMCA SUBMAXIMAL CYCLE ERGOMETER TEST

0:00–0:45	Monitor your client's work output (cadence and resistance)
0:45–1:00	Pulse count for 15 seconds (for practice)
1:00–1:45	Monitor your client's work output (cadence and resistance)
1:45–2:00	Pulse count for 15 seconds (2 min HR)
2:00–2:30	Stage BP check
2:30–2:45	Stage RPE check
2:45–3:00	Pulse count for 15 seconds (3 min HR)

From: American College of Sports Medicine. Health-Related Physical Fitness Assessment Manual. 2nd edition. Philadelphia: 2008. Lippincott Williams & Wilkins.

BOX 19-21	ASTRAND SUBMAXIMAL CYCLE ERGOMETER TEST PROCEDURES

In summary, the patient performs a 6-minute submaximal exercise session on the cycle ergometer. Thus, this is typically a single-stage test. The heart rate (HR) response to this session will determine the maximal aerobic capacity by plotting the HR response to this one stage on a nomogram.

The calibration of the cycle ergometer is the same as in the YMCA protocol:

1. Explain the test to your patient: same as in the YMCA protocol.
2. Explain informed consent: same as in the YMCA protocol.
3. You should also discuss with your patient the concept of your general preparedness to handle any emergencies: same as in the YMCA protocol.
4. Take the baseline or resting measures of HR and blood pressure (BP) with your patient seated: same as in the YMCA protocol.
5. Adjust seat height: same as in the YMCA protocol.
6. START THE TEST. Have your patient freewheel, without any resistance (0 kg), at the pedaling cadence of 50 rpm. Maintaining 50 rpm throughout the test is essential.
7. Set the first stage's work output according to protocol table 19-3.
8. Start the clock/timer.
9. Measure the HR after each minute starting at minute 2. Count the HR for 10 to 15 seconds. You may wish to use a heart rate monitor, only as a teaching tool. Record the HR on the test form.
10. Measure and record the blood pressure after the 3-minute HR; ACSM guidelines for test termination and BP are applicable.
11. The fifth and sixth minute HR will be used in the test determination of VO_{2max} as long as there is not more than a 6-beat difference between the two HRs.

The following applies for steady-state heart rate (HR_{SS}):

If there is a difference of ≤6 bpm, then consider the test finished.

If there is a difference of >6 bpm, then continue for another minute and check HR again.

12. Regularly check the work output of the cycle ergometer using the pendulum resistance scale on the side of the ergometer and the rpm of subject. For the resistance, do not use the scale on the top front panel for measurement. Adjust the work output if necessary.
13. Regularly check your patient's rpm and correct if necessary.

The Astrand protocol requires the following for test completion:

You need to obtain HR_{SS} from the test with the fifth and sixth minute HR (within 6 bpm).

For the best (most accurate) prediction of V_{O2max}, the HR should be between 125 and 170 bpm.

If the HR response to the initial work rate is not above 125 bpm after 6 minutes, then the test is continued for another 6-minute interval by increasing the work rate by 300 $kp \cdot m \cdot min^{-1}$ (0.5kp).

The HR at the fifth and sixth minutes, if acceptable to the criteria above, is averaged for the nomogram method.

14. Allow your patient to cool down after the protocol is complete. Have your patient continue to pedal at 50 rpm, and adjust the resistance down to 0.5 to 1 kp for 3 minutes of cool-down or recovery. Take your patient's HR and BP at the end of the 3-minute active recovery period. Next, allow your patient to sit quietly in a chair for 2 to 3 minutes to continue the recovery process. Be sure to check your patient's HR and BP before allowing your patient to leave the lab. It is hoped that the HR and BP will approach the resting measures.

From: American College of Sports Medicine. Health-Related Physical Fitness Assessment Manual. 2nd edition. Philadelphia: 2008. Lippincott Williams & Wilkins.

TABLE 19-3. ÅSTRAND CYCLE SUBMAXIMAL CYCLE ERGOMETER TEST INITIAL WORKLOADS

This protocol table is designed as a guide. The protocol is designed to elicit an HR of between 125–170 bpm by 6 minutes. You can adjust the work output as necessary during the test (usually after the first 6 minutes) to achieve an HR in or near this range-in your subject.

INDIVIDUAL	WORK OUTPUT ($kp \cdot m \cdot min^{-1}$)
Men	
Unconditioned	300–600
Conditioned	600–900
Women	
Unconditioned	300–450
Conditioned	450–600
Poorly Conditioned or Older Individuals	300

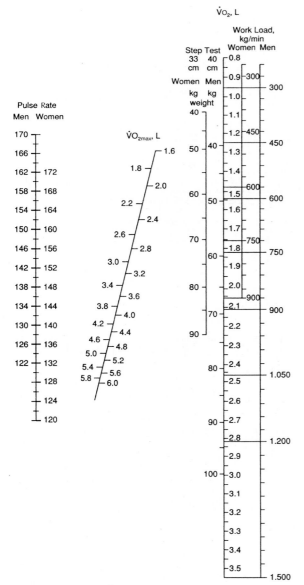

FIGURE 19-2. Modified Åstrand-Ryhming nomogram (from ACSM's Health-Related Physical Fitness Assessment Manual 2e) and reference (4).

moderate or high risk for disease have a maximal GXT with a medical examination before starting a vigorous exercise program.

Personnel Needs for Conducting the Maximal Graded Exercise Test

> **1.3.23-CES: Ability to identify individuals for whom physician supervision is recommended during maximal and submaximal exercise testing.**

Research indicates that allied health personnel (i.e., exercise physiologists or nurses) who have been adequately trained can safely perform maximal exercise testing (15). These personnel should be healthcare professionals who are certified at the basic life support (advanced life support preferred) level and have a professional certification (ACSM Clinical Exercise Specialist or Registered Clinical Exercise Physiologist). Personnel should be skilled at monitoring HR, BP, and signs and symptoms suggesting the presence of disease or exercise intolerance. In addition, personnel should understand ECG interpretation and be able to recognize myocardial ischemia and rhythm disturbances (15).

The *GETP8* also recommends that those patients who are low risk and younger than age 45 (men) or 55 (women) may have a maximal GXT without physician supervision. Patients at moderate or high risk are recommended to have a physician within close proximity to the testing area who will be readily available in the event of an emergency situation that might occur during the maximal GXT.

Qualified personnel, independent of job title, should be aware of, and adhere to, the recommendations found in the *ACSM GETP8* regarding test contraindications, test termination criteria, and emergency procedures.

Protocols for Maximal Exercise Testing

> **1.3.12-CES: Obtain and recognize normal and abnormal physiologic and subjective responses (e.g. symptoms; ECG, BP, HR, RPE, and other scales; oxygen saturation; and oxygen consumption) at appropriate intervals during the test.**

Traditionally, the treadmill has been the most utilized mode for testing in the United States. Treadmill walking involves the use of a large muscle mass, enabling the subject to generally achieve a greater physiologic maximum. Utilization of a cycle ergometer, which is much more quadriceps specific, generally results in a reduced $\dot{V}O_{2max}$. However, other modes of testing and protocols are available and appropriate for special populations. A visual summary of common protocols used for maximal exercise testing can be found in Figure 19-3.

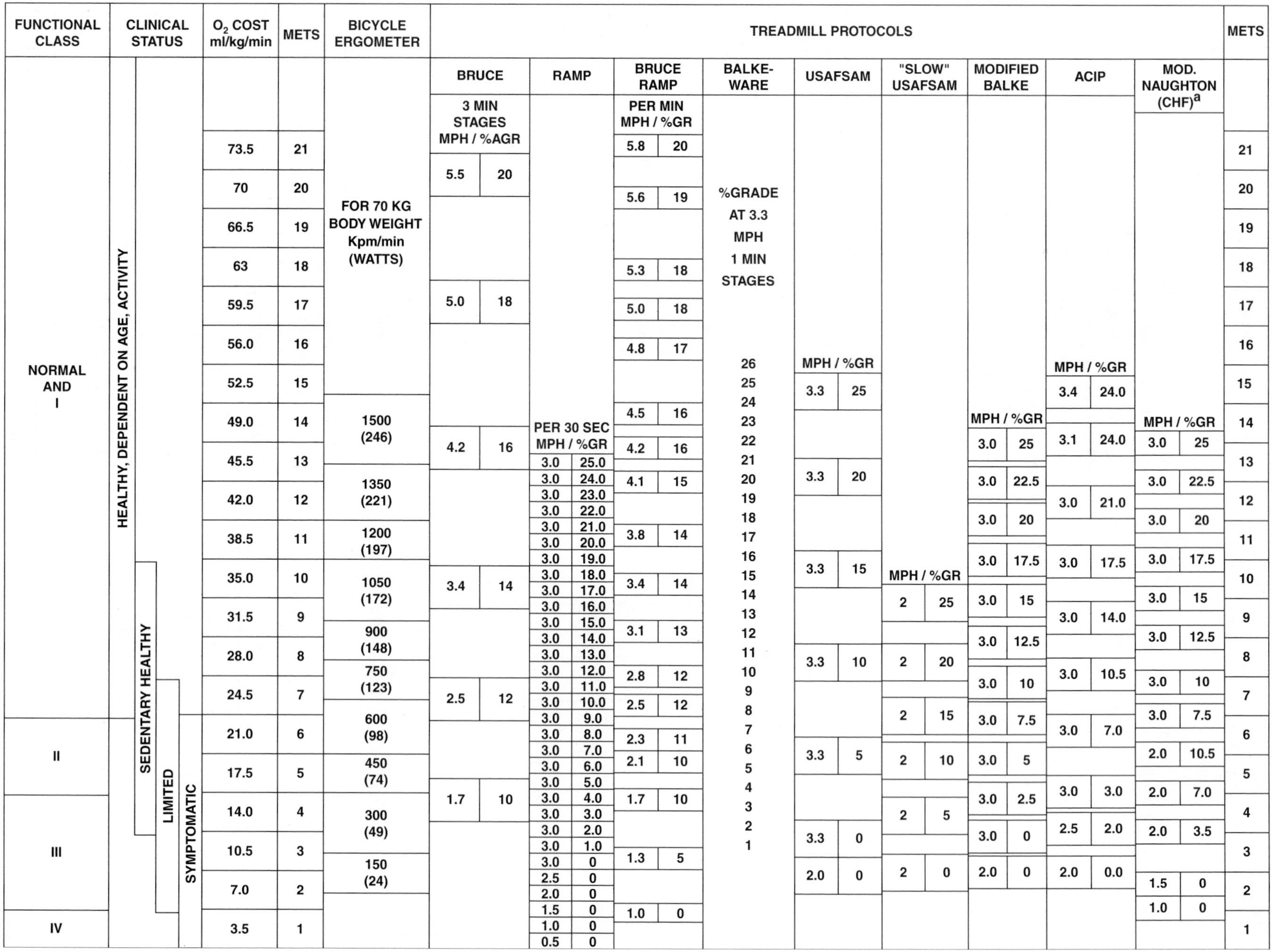

FIGURE 19-3. Visual Summary of Protocols for Maximal Exercise Testing (from ASCM's GETP8.)

[a] There are multiple variations of the modified Naughton protocol.

FUNCTIONAL CLASS	CLINICAL STATUS	O₂ COST ml/kg/min	METS	BICYCLE ERGOMETER (FOR 70 KG BODY WEIGHT Kpm/min (WATTS))	BRUCE (3 MIN STAGES MPH / %AGR)	RAMP (PER 30 SEC MPH / %GR)	BRUCE RAMP (PER MIN MPH / %GR)	BALKE-WARE (%GRADE AT 3.3 MPH 1 MIN STAGES)	USAFSAM (MPH / %GR)	"SLOW" USAFSAM (MPH / %GR)	MODIFIED BALKE (MPH / %GR)	ACIP (MPH / %GR)	MOD. NAUGHTON (CHF)[a] (MPH / %GR)	METS
NORMAL AND I	HEALTHY, DEPENDENT ON AGE, ACTIVITY	O_2 cost												METS
		73.5	21											21
		70	20		5.5 / 20		5.8 / 20							20
		66.5	19				5.6 / 19							19
		63	18				5.3 / 18							18
		59.5	17		5.0 / 18		5.0 / 18							17
		56.0	16				4.8 / 17		3.3 / 25					16
		52.5	15				4.5 / 16			2 / 25		3.4 / 24.0		15
		49.0	14	1500 (246)	4.2 / 16	3.0 / 25.0	4.2 / 16		3.3 / 20		3.0 / 25	3.1 / 24.0	3.0 / 25	14
		45.5	13	1350 (221)		3.0 / 23.0	4.1 / 15				3.0 / 22.5		3.0 / 22.5	13
		42.0	12	1200 (197)		3.0 / 21.0	3.8 / 14		3.3 / 15	2 / 20	3.0 / 20	3.0 / 21.0	3.0 / 20	12
		38.5	11	1050 (172)	3.4 / 14	3.0 / 19.0	3.4 / 14				3.0 / 17.5	3.0 / 17.5	3.0 / 17.5	11
		35.0	10	900 (148)		3.0 / 17.0	3.1 / 13		3.3 / 10	2 / 15	3.0 / 15	3.0 / 14.0	3.0 / 15	10
		31.5	9	750 (123)		3.0 / 15.0	2.8 / 12				3.0 / 12.5		3.0 / 12.5	9
SEDENTARY HEALTHY		28.0	8	600 (98)		3.0 / 13.0	2.5 / 12		3.3 / 5	2 / 10	3.0 / 10	3.0 / 10.5	3.0 / 10	8
		24.5	7	450 (74)	2.5 / 12	3.0 / 11.0	2.3 / 11				3.0 / 7.5	3.0 / 7.0	3.0 / 7.5	7
		21.0	6	300 (49)		3.0 / 9.0	2.1 / 10		3.3 / 0	2 / 5	3.0 / 5		2.0 / 10.5	6
II	LIMITED	17.5	5	150 (24)	1.7 / 10	3.0 / 7.0	1.7 / 10				3.0 / 2.5	3.0 / 3.0	2.0 / 7.0	5
III		14.0	4			3.0 / 5.0			2.0 / 0	2 / 0	3.0 / 0	2.5 / 2.0	2.0 / 3.5	4
	SYMPTOMATIC	10.5	3			3.0 / 3.0	1.3 / 5				2.0 / 0	2.0 / 0.0	1.5 / 0	3
		7.0	2			3.0 / 1.0 / 3.0 / 0	1.0 / 0						1.0 / 0	2
IV		3.5	1			2.5 / 0 / 2.0 / 0 / 1.5 / 0 / 1.0 / 0 / 0.5 / 0								1

TREADMILL PROTOCOLS

(BALKE-WARE: %GRADE at 3.3 MPH, 1 MIN STAGES: 26, 25, 24, 23, 22, 21, 20, 19, 18, 17, 16, 15, 14, 13, 12, 11, 10, 9, 8, 7, 6, 5, 4, 3, 2, 1)

Measurements Taken during Exercise Testing

Common variables measured during maximal exercise testing include HR, BP, RPE, ECG, and subjective measurements of signs or symptoms related to coronary ischemia. In addition, direct measurements of ventilatory responses and expired gases can also be observed during maximal exercise testing. Typically, BP and HR are measured at rest, during each exercise stage, and during recovery. In addition, ECG measurements are observed during these same intervals.

During exercise, exercise-induced measurements, including RPE, gas exchange, and signs or symptoms related to cardiovascular or pulmonary disorders should be observed. These measures should be obtained routinely throughout the examination and throughout recovery. Box 19-22 provides the recommended sequence for measurement of HR, BP, RPE, and ECG during exercise testing.

Test Termination Criteria

> **1.3.21-HFS: Ability to identify appropriate criteria for terminating a fitness evaluation and demonstrate proper procedures to be followed after discontinuing such a test.**

Graded exercise testing, whether maximal or submaximal, is considered safe when subjects are appropriately screened and testing guidelines are followed. Occasionally, the test may have to be terminated before the subject achieves $\dot{V}O_{2max}$ because of volitional fatigue or a predetermined endpoint (i.e., 50% to 70% heart rate reserve or 70% to 85% age-predicted maximal HR). Box 19-23 provides indications for terminating exercise testing during maximal GXT. In addition, there may be instances when an exercise test should be stopped for other reasons. Some of these were outlined previously in Box 19-17, as *General Indications for Stopping an Exercise Test in Low-Risk Adults.*

CRITERION-REFERENCED STANDARDS VERSUS NORMATIVE DATA

Upon completion of an exercise test, the results should be interpreted by comparing the test results with established standards or norms. Traditionally, two sets of standards are utilized for comparisons: criterion-referenced standards and normative standards. Criterion-referenced standards are those that are considered desirable to achieve based on external criteria and may use adjectives such as "excellent" or "poor" in the data interpretation tables. Criterion-referenced standards exist mostly in cardiorespiratory fitness evaluations and in body fat analyses. These standards, however, are open to subjective interpretation, and disagreement is still present among "experts" as to what these results truly mean when used for interpretation.

Normative standards (norms) are based on previous performances by a similar group of individuals. Norms compare how the patient performed versus other like individuals, and the data are presented using percentile values to assist in identifying level of CRF.

Evaluative decisions about a patient's health-related physical fitness can be based on either criterion-referenced standards or normative standards. Traditionally, in the fitness assessment arena, a greater amount of focus in placed on normative standards as opposed to criterion-referenced standards.

INTERPRETATION OF RESULTS

When utilizing submaximal exercise testing to establish one's fitness status, the accuracy of the comparison with published norms depends on the similarities of the groups being compared and the testing methodology used. Although maximal exercise testing reduces some of the error involved in determining CRF, the utilization of submaximal exercise testing introduces assumptions that can be easily met (e.g., steady-state HR can be verified) and others (e.g., estimated maximal HR) that introduce errors into the prediction of $\dot{V}O_{2max}$. However, as a straightforward assessment of results, it can be assumed that a reduction in HR response during serial, submaximal exercise testing over a period of weeks or months in response to a fixed work rate indicates an improved CRF. Therefore, despite the differences in test accuracy and various errors introduced with each methodology, virtually all evaluations can establish a baseline and be used to track progress relative to improvement in fitness.

MUSCULAR FITNESS ASSESSMENT

> **1.3.18-HFS: Ability to describe the purpose of testing, determine appropriate protocols, and perform assessments of muscular strength, muscular endurance, and flexibility.**

Muscular fitness integrates muscular strength, muscular endurance, and flexibility, and is an integral portion of total health-related fitness (2,35). Testing for these components of fitness should be accomplished following a CRF assessment to allow the muscles to warm up and to reduce the risk for muscle injury during testing. The development and maintenance of muscular fitness contributes to health by increasing fat-free mass and resting metabolic rate, maintaining bone mass, stimulating modest improvements in cardiovascular fitness, and improving the ability to perform activities of daily living (ADL). Additional information on muscle fitness, including more in-depth information on muscle fitness assessment techniques, can be found in Chapter 20 of this manual.

BOX 19-22 SEQUENCE OF MEASURES FOR HR, BP, RPE, AND ELECTROCARDIOGRAM (ECG) DURING EXERCISE TESTING

Pre-Test

1. 12-lead ECG in supine and exercise postures
2. Blood pressure measurements in the supine position and exercise posture

Exercise*

1. 12-lead ECG recorded during last 15 seconds of every stage and at peak exercise (3-lead ECG observed/recorded every minute on monitor)
2. Blood pressure measurements should be obtained during the last minute of each stage[†]
3. Rating scales: RPE at the end of each stage, other scales if applicable

Post-Test

1. 12-lead ECG immediately after exercise, then every 1 to 2 minutes for at least 5 minutes to allow any exercise-induced changes to return to baseline
2. Blood pressure measurements should be obtained immediately after exercise, then every 1 to 2 minutes until stabilized near baseline level.
3. Symptomatic ratings should be obtained using appropriate scales as long as symptoms persist after exercise

*In addition, these referenced variables should be assessed and recorded whenever adverse symptoms or abnormal ECG changes occur.

[†]*Note:* An unchanged or decreasing systolic blood pressure with increasing workloads should be retaken (i.e., verified immediately)

From: American College of Sports Medicine. Health-Related Physical Fitness Assessment Manual. 2nd edition. Philadelphia: 2008. Lippincott Williams & Wilkins.

MUSCULAR STRENGTH

Muscular strength is defined as the maximal force (expressed in newtons, kilograms, or pounds) that can be generated by a specific muscle or muscle group (37). It is specific to the muscle group being tested, the type of contraction (static or dynamic, concentric or eccentric), the speed of the contraction, and the joint angle being tested (1). Because of the specificity of strength measurement, there is no single test for total body muscle strength.

BOX 19-23 INDICATIONS FOR TERMINATING EXERCISE TESTING*

Absolute

- Drop in systolic blood pressure of 210 mmHg from baseline blood pressure despite an increase in workload, when accompanied by other evidence of ischemia
- Moderate to severe angina
- Increasing nervous system symptoms (e.g., ataxia, dizziness, or near syncope)
- Signs of poor perfusion (cyanosis or pallor)
- Technical difficulties monitoring the ECG or systolic blood pressure
- Subject's desire to stop
- Sustained ventricular tachycardia
- ST elevation ($\geq$1.0 mm) in leads without diagnostic Q-waves (other than V_1 or aVR)

Relative

- Drop in systolic blood pressure of $\geq$10 mmHg from baseline blood pressure despite an increase in workload, in the absence of other evidence of ischemia
- ST or QRS changes such as excessive ST depression ($>$2 mm horizontal or downsloping ST-segment depression) or marked axis shift
- Arrhythmias other than sustained ventricular tachycardia, including multifocal PVCs, triplets of PVCs, supraventricular tachycardia, heart block, or brady-arrhythmias
- Fatigue, shortness of breath, wheezing, leg cramps, or claudication
- Development of bundle-branch block or intraventricular conduction delay that cannot be distinguished from ventricular tachycardia
- Increasing chest pain
- Hypertensive response[†]

*Reprinted. with permission from Gibbons RA, Balady GJ, Beasely JW, et al. ACC/AHA guidelines for exercise testing. *J Am Coll Cardiol.* 1997:30 260–315.

[†]Systolic blood pressure of more than 250 mmHg and/or a diastolic blood pressure of more than 115 mmHg.

The measurement of muscle force production is used for assessing muscular strength, identifying weaknesses in muscle groups, monitoring progress in the rehabilitation of muscles, and measuring the effectiveness of training (1).

Strength can be assessed either statically (no overt muscular movement or limb movement) or dynamically (movement of an external load or body part, in which the muscle changes length). A variety of devices are available to measure static strength, including cable tensiometers and handgrip dynamometers. These measures, however, cannot be generalized for total body strength, as they are specific to both the muscle group and joint angle tested (10). In addition, the measure of the peak force development during these tests is referred to as the maximum voluntary contraction (MVC).

Common techniques/protocols for measuring muscular strength include the 1-repetition maximum (RM) bench press test, the 1RM leg press test, and isokinetic testing. The 1-repetition maximum (1RM) test identifies the greatest resistance that can be moved through the full range of motion in a controlled manner and has traditionally been used as the standard measure of dynamic strength. Recently, multiple RM tests have been used, such as 4- or 8RM, as a measure of muscular strength to allow the participant to integrate evaluation into their training program (36). Difficulty remains in trying to estimate a 1RM value from multiple RM tests; however, this is generally not necessary. For instance, the number of lifts one can perform at a fixed percent of 1RM for different muscle groups (e.g., leg press versus bench press) varies tremendously, thus rendering an estimate of 1RM impractical (22,23). Still, the use of the 1RM remains a popular measure (27). Traditional measures of upper-body strength utilize 1RM values for the bench press or military press, whereas 1RM indices of lower-body strength include leg press or leg extension. Norms—which are based on resistance lifted divided by body mass—for the bench press and leg press are provided in Tables 19-4 and 19-5, respectively. Box 19-24 provides the basic steps in 1RM (or any multiple RM) testing following familiarization/practice sessions (27).

Isokinetic testing differs from dynamic muscle testing in that it involves the assessment of constant-speed muscular contraction against accommodating resistance. The speed of movement is controlled and the amount of resistance is proportional to the amount of force produced throughout the full range of motion. Commercial devices are available that will measure the peak force and torque at various joints (knee, hip, shoulder, elbow), yet these pieces of equipment are limited by their cost (18).

MUSCULAR ENDURANCE

Muscular endurance is the ability of a muscle group to repeatedly perform muscular contractions over a period

TABLE 19-4. NORMS FOR UPPER BODY STRENGTH[*,†]

	AGE				
PERCENTILE	20–29	30–39	40–49	50–59	60+
Men					
90	1.48	1.24	1.10	.97	.89
80	1.32	1.12	1.00	.90	.82
70	1.22	1.04	.93	.84	.77
60	1.14	.98	.88	.79	.72
50	1.06	.93	.84	.75	.68
40	.99	.88	.80	.71	.66
30	.93	.83	.76	.68	.63
20	.88	.78	.72	.63	.57
10	.80	.71	.65	.57	.53
Women					
90	.90	.76	.71	.61	.64
80	.80	.70	.62	.55	.54
70	.74	.63	.57	.52	.51
60	.70	.60	.54	.48	.47
50	.65	.57	.52	.46	.45
40	.59	.53	.50	.44	.43
30	.56	.51	.47	.42	.40
20	.51	.47	.43	.39	.38
10	.48	.42	.38	.37	.33

[*]One repetition maximum bench press, with bench press weight ratio = weight pushed/body weight ratio.

[†]Data provided by the Institute for Aerobics Research, Dallas. TX (1994). Adapted from *ACSM's Guidelines for Exercise Testing and Prescription*. 8th ed, 2009. Study population for the data set was predominantly white and college educated. A Universal dynamic variable resistance (DVR) machine was used to measure the I-RM. The following may be used as descriptors for the percentile rankings: well above average (90), above average (70), average (50); below average (30), and well below average (10).

TABLE 19-5. NORMS FOR LEG STRENGTH[*,†]

	AGE				
PERCENTILE	20–29	30–39	40–49	50–59	60+
Men					
90	2.27	2.07	1.92	1.80	1.73
80	2.13	1.93	1.82	1.71	1.62
70	2.05	1.85	1.74	1.64	1.56
60	1.97	1.77	1.68	1.58	1.49
50	1.91	1.71	1.62	1.52	1.43
40	1.83	1.65	1.57	1.46	1.38
30	1.74	1.59	1.51	1.39	1.30
20	1.63	1.52	1.44	1.32	1.25
10	1.51	1.43	1.35	1.22	1.16
Women					
90	1.82	1.61	1.48	1.37	1.32
80	1.68	1.47	1.37	1.25	1.18
70	1.58	1.39	1.29	1.17	1.13
60	1.50	1.33	1.23	1.10	1.04
50	1.44	1.27	1.18	1.05	.99
40	1.37	1.21	1.13	.99	.93
30	1.27	1.15	1.08	.95	.88
20	1.22	1.09	1.02	.88	.85
10	1.14	1.00	.94	.78	.72

*One repetition maximum leg press with leg press weight ratio = weight pushed body weight.

†Data provided by the Institute for Aerobics Research, Dallas, TX (1994). Adapted from *ACSM's Guidelines for Exercise Testing and Prescription*, 8th ed, 2009 Study population for the data set was predominantly white and college educated. A Universal dynamic variable resistance (DVR) machine was used to measure the I-RM. The following may be used as descriptors for the percentile rankings: well above average (90), above average (70), average (50); below average (30), and well below average (10).

that is sufficient to cause muscular fatigue, or the ability to maintain a percentage of MVC for an extended period. Common assessments for muscular endurance include the YMCA Bench Press Test, push-up test, and the partial curl-up (crunch) test. Procedures for the push-up and curl-up (crunch) tests are offered in Box 19-25. Norms and position for partial curl-up are offered in Table 19-6 and Figure 19-4, respectively. Norms for push-ups are listed in Table 19-7. Procedures for assessing muscle endurance via the YMCA Bench Press are provided in Box 19-26. Norms for the YMCA Bench Press Test are presented in Table 19-8.

BOX 19-24   1RM BENCH PRESS TEST PROCEDURES

1. The subject should warm up by completing several submaximal repetitions (at 40%–60% of perceived maximum).
2. Select an initial weight that is within the subject's perceived capacity (~50%–70% of capacity).
3. With the subject keeping his/her back on the bench, both feet on the floor, and hands shoulder width apart with palms up on the bar, determine the 1RM (or any multiple RM) within four trials with rest periods of 3 to 5 minutes between trials (a spotter should be present for all lifts and assists the subject with liftoff.) The subject starts the lift with the bar in the up position with arms fully extended, then lowers the bar to the chest and pushes it back up until the arms are locked. Be sure to encourage regular breathing and avoid breath holding during exertion.

4. Following a 1-minute rest with light stretching, the subject does three to five repetitions at 60% to 80% of perceived maximum.
5. Further lifts should include the addition of a small amount of weight, and a 1RM lift is attempted. This continues until the subject cannot lift the desired weight. The goal is to find the 1RM in three to five maximal efforts. The greatest amount of weight lifted is considered the 1RM.
6. For the determination of the amount of weight lifted compared with the individual's body weight (for norms comparison purposes), divide the maximum weight lifted in pounds by the subject's weight in pounds.

Note: The above procedure can also be used for the 1RM leg press.

Special Considerations

> **1.7.8-CES: Demonstrate exercise equipment adaptations necessary for different age groups, physical abilities, and other potential contributing factors.**

Older Adults

Utilizing muscular strength and muscular endurance assessments, in combination with other aspects of health-related physical fitness, for older adults can aid in the detection of deteriorating health while yielding important information that can be used to design an individualized exercise program to improve strength and functional independence. The Senior Fitness Test (SFT) was developed in response to a need for specialized tools that improved the overall assessment capabilities for older persons to assess the key physiologic parameters (e.g., strength, endurance, agility, and balance) needed to perform activities that become increasingly difficult as one ages (39). The SFT meets scientific standards for reliability and validity, is an easy to administer field test, and has normative data for older men and women (44). Two specific tests included in the SFT, the 30-second chair stand and the single arm curl, can be used to safely

and effectively assess muscular strength and muscular endurance in a majority of older adults.

Coronary Heart Disease Patients

Moderate-intensity resistance training, when performed 2 to 3 days per week, has been shown to be safe and effective for improving muscular fitness, preventing and managing certain chronic medical conditions, modifying coronary risk factors, and enhancing psychosocial well-being in those with and without cardiovascular disease. Consequently, influential health organizations, including the American Heart Association and ACSM, support the inclusion of resistance training exercises as a beneficial adjunct to endurance exercises for individuals with cardiovascular disease (36).

Those cardiac patients deemed low-risk (e.g., persons without resting or exercise-induced evidence of myocardial ischemia, severe left ventricular dysfunction, or complex ventricular dysrhythmias, and with normal or near-normal CRF) can perform moderate to high intensity (e.g., 40%–80% 1RM) resistance testing and training safely. Additionally, research does not support the occurrence of an abnormal cardiovascular "pressor response" in cardiac patients or those with controlled hypertension, indicating strength testing and training

---

BOX 19-25 PUSH-UP AND CURL-UP (CRUNCH) TEST PROCEDURES FOR MEASUREMENT OF MUSCULAR ENDURANCE*

Push-up

1. The push-up test is administered with male subjects starting in the standard "down" position (hands pointing forward and under the shoulder, back straight, head up, using the toes as the pivotal point) and female subjects in the modified "knee push-up" position (legs together, lower leg in contact with mat with ankles plantar-flexed, back straight, hands shoulder width apart, head up, using the knees as the pivotal point).
2. The subject must raise the body by straightening the elbows and return to the "down" position, until the chin touches the mat. The stomach should not touch the mat.
3. For both men and women, the subject's back must be straight at all times and the subject must push up to a straight arm position.
4. The maximal number of push-ups performed consecutively without rest is counted as the score.

5. The test is stopped when the client strains forcibly or is unable to maintain the appropriate technique within two repetitions.

Curl-Up (Crunch)

1. Individual assumes a supine position on a mat with the knees at 90 degrees. The arms are at the side, palms facing down with the middle fingers touching a piece of masking tape. A second piece of masking tape is placed 10 cm apart. Shoes remain on during the test.
2. A metronome is set to 50 beats·min^{-1} and the individual does slow, controlled curl-ups to lift the shoulder blades off the mat (trunk makes a 30-degree angle with the mat) in time with the metronome at a rate of 25 per minute. The test is done for 1 minute. The low back should be flattened before curling up.
3. Individual performs as many curl-ups as possible without pausing, to a maximum of 25.[‡]

*Canadian Society for Exercise Physiology. The Canadian Physical Activity, Fitness & Lifestyle Approach: CSEP-Health & Fitness Program's Health Related Appraisal & Counselling Strategy, 3rd ed. Canadian Society for Exercise Physiology, 2003.

[†]Alternatives include: 1) having the hands held across the chest, with the head activating a counter when the trunk reaches a 30-degree position and placing the hands on the thighs and curling up until the hands reach the knee caps. Elevation of the trunk 30 degrees is the important aspect of the movement.

[‡]An alternative includes doing as many curl-ups as possible in 1 minute.

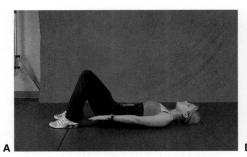 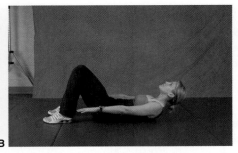

FIGURE 19-4. Position for Curl-Up and Partial Curl-Up (from ACSM's Health-Related Physical Fitness Assessment Manual 2e).

TABLE 19-6. FITNESS CATEGORIES BY AGE GROUPS AND GENDER FOR PARTIAL CURL-UP*

	AGE									
CATEGORY	20–29		30–39		40–49		50–59		60–69	
GENDER	M	F	M	F	M	F	M	F	M	F
Excellent	25	25	25	25	25	25	25	25	25	25
Very good	24	24	24	24	24	24	24	24	24	24
	21	18	18	19	18	19	17	19	16	17
Good	20	17	17	18	17	18	16	18	15	16
	16	14	15	10	13	11	11	10	11	8
Fair	15	13	14	9	12	10	10	9	10	7
	11	5	11	6	6	4	8	6	6	3
Needs improvement	10	4	10	5	5	3	7	5	5	2

*The Canadian Physical Activity, Fitness & Lifestyle Approach: CSEP-Health & Fitness Program's Health-Related Appraisal and Counseling Strategy. 3rd ed. Reprinted with permission from the Canadian Society for Exercise Physiology, 2003

should be safe to include in comprehensive evaluation and training programs. However, data on the safety of muscular fitness testing in moderate- to high-risk cardiac patients, especially those with poor left ventricular function, are limited and require additional investigation (36).

Current guidelines suggest that the following contraindications be recognized when considering muscular strength and endurance testing: unstable angina, uncontrolled hypertension (systolic BP ≥160 mm Hg and/or diastolic BP ≥100 mm Hg), uncontrolled dysrhythmias, poorly managed or untreated heart failure, severe stenotic or

TABLE 19-7. FITNESS CATEGORIES BY AGE GROUPS AND GENDER FOR PUSH-UPS*

	AGE									
CATEGORY	20–29		30–39		40–49		50–59		60–69	
GENDER	M	F	M	F	M	F	M	F	M	F
Excellent	36	30	30	27	25	24	21	21	18	17
Very good	35	29	29	26	24	23	20	20	17	16
	29	21	22	20	17	15	13	11	11	12
Good	28	20	21	19	16	14	12	10	10	11
	22	15	17	13	13	11	10	7	8	5
Fair	21	14	16	12	12	10	9	6	7	4
	17	10	12	8	10	5	7	2	5	2
Needs improvement	16	9	11	7	9	4	6	1	4	1

*The Canadian Physical Activity, Fitness & Lifestyle Approach: CSEP-Health & Fitness Program's Health-Related Appraisal and Counseling Strategy 3rd ed. Reprinted with permission from the Canadian Society for Exercise Physiology, 2003

BOX 19-26 YMCA BENCH PRESS TEST

1. Use a 35-pound barbell setup for women or an 80-pound barbell setup for men.
2. Set the metronome to 60 beats per minute; the subject's lifting cadence will be 30 lifts or reps per minute.
3. Have the subject lie back down on the bench with both feet on the floor.
4. A spotter should hand the barbell to the subject and be available throughout the test to grasp the barbell when necessary
5. The subject will start with the weight in the down position (weight resting on chest) and with elbows flexed. Hands should grip the bar at shoulder width with palms up.
6. The subject will press the weight and lower the weight at the cadence of 30 repetitions per minute. Each repetition must consist of full movement of the barbell from elbows flexed with the barbell resting on the chest to arms fully extended. The cadence of 30 repetitions per minute must be maintained.
7. The subject completes the test for the maximum number of repetitions before fatigue or breaking of the lifting cadence. Compare the subject's maximum number of reps with the norms.

From: American College of Sports Medicine. Health-Related Physical Fitness Assessment Manual. 2nd edition. Philadelphia: 2008. Lippincott Williams & Wilkins.

regurgitant valvular disease, and hypertrophic cardiomyopathy (36). In addition, it is suggested that those with cardiac disease should also have well-preserved left ventricular function and CRF (>5 or 6 metabolic equivalents) without anginal symptoms or ischemic ST-segment changes to participate in traditional resistance training programs (14,36). Significant care should be taken during preparticipation screening, and proper supervision should be provided in an effort to reduce the risk of a serious cardiac event during muscular strength and endurance testing.

Children and Adolescents

As with other fitness parameters, muscular fitness is recognized as an important component of health-related fitness in children and adolescents. Enhancing muscular strength and muscular endurance in youth provides significant benefits, including the development of proper posture, reducing injury risk, enhancing body composition, and improving motor performance skills. Muscular strength and muscular endurance are typically assessed with push-up and abdominal curl-up tests and standardized testing procedures with

TABLE 19-8. ENDURANCE BENCH-PRESS TEST—TOTAL LIFTS

AGE (yrs)	18–25		26–35		36–45	
GENDER	M	F	M	F	M	F
Excellent	44–64	42–66	41–61	40–62	36–55	33–57
Good	34–41	30–38	30–37	29–34	26–32	26–30
Above average	29–33	25–28	26–29	24–28	22–25	21–24
Average	24–28	20–22	21–24	18–22	18–21	16–20
Below average	20–22	16–18	17–20	14–17	14–17	12–14
Poor	13–17	9–13	12–16	9–13	9–12	6–10
Very poor	0–10	0–6	0–9	0–6	0–6	0–4

AGE (yrs)	46–55		56–65		>65	
GENDER	M	F	M	F	M	F
Excellent	28–47	29–50	24–41	24–42	20–36	18–30
Good	21–25	20–24	17–21	17–21	12–16	12–16
Above Average	16–20	14–18	12–14	12–14	10	8–10
Average	12–14	10–13	9–11	8–10	7–8	5–7
Below average	9–11	7–9	5–8	5–6	4–6	3–4
Poor	5–8	2–6	2–4	2–4	2–3	0–2
Very Poor	0–2	0–1	0–1	0–1	0–1	0

Note: Women use a 35-pound bar; men, 80 pounds Maximum repetitions in time to metronome at 30 lifts per minute.

Source: Adapted from YMCA. *Y'S Way to Fitness,* 4th ed., 1998. Reprinted with permission from the YMCA of the USA.

normative comparison data are currently available to use with children and adolescents.

Strength and weakness can be assessed in children using various muscular fitness measures. Data derived from these tests can be used to develop an individualized fitness program, and to motivate participants to continue with and progress in their current exercise program. To enhance safety and to ensure adequate completion of each exercise, fitness professionals should demonstrate the proper skill techniques and ensure proper technique is being followed.

FLEXIBILITY

Flexibility is defined as the functional ability of a joint to move through its full range of motion (ROM). *Functional ability* refers to movement through the ROM without incurring pain or a limit to performance. Flexibility is joint specific, because it depends on the muscle and joint that is being evaluated. It also depends on the distensibility of the joint capsule, adequate warm-up,

muscle viscosity, and the compliance of ligaments and tendons.

Assessment of flexibility is important as there is an associated decrease in performance of activities of daily living with inadequate flexibility. While no single test can truly characterize one's flexibility, the sit-and-reach test is the most widely used test for flexibility assessment. The sit-and-reach test is a reflection of hamstring, hip, and lower-back flexibility, which is important to the prevention of chronic lower back pain and the promotion of a healthy lifestyle (26,31).

Trunk flexion test procedures (for the sit-and-reach test) are provided in Box 19-27. Procedures for the YMCA Sit-and-Reach Test are also provided (Box 19-28). Fitness categories by age groups and sex for trunk forward flexion using a sit-and-reach box are provided in Table 19-9. Percentiles by age group and sex for the YMCA Sit-and-Reach Test (inches) are presented in Table 19-10.

Overall ROM at any joint can be measured. In addition, postural analysis and body alignment are also im-

---

BOX 19-27   TRUNK FLEXION (SIT-AND-REACH) TEST PROCEDURES*

Pretest: Participant should perform a short warm-up prior to this test and include some stretches (e.g., modified hurdler's stretch). It is also recommended that the participant refrain from fast, jerky movements, which may increase the possibility of an injury. The participant's shoes should be removed.

1. For the Canadian trunk forward flexion test, the client sits without shoes and the soles of the feet flat against the flexometer (sit-and-reach box) at the 26-cm mark. Inner edges of the soles are placed within 2 cm of the measuring scale. For the YMCA sit and reach test, a yardstick is placed on the floor and tape is placed across it at a right angle to the 15-inch mark. The participant sits with the yardstick between the legs, with legs extended at right angles to the taped line on the floor. Heels of the feet should touch the edge of the taped line and be about 10 to 12 inches apart. (Note the zero point at the foot/box interface and use the appropriate norms.)
2. The participant should slowly reach forward with both hands as far as possible, holding this position

approximately 2 seconds. Be sure that the participant keeps the hands parallel and does not lead with one hand. Fingertips can be overlapped and should be in contact with the measuring portion or yard-stick of the sit-and-reach box.

3. The score is the most distant point (in centimeters or inches) reached with the fingertips. The best of two trials should be recorded. To assist with the best attempt, the participant should exhale and drop the head between the arms when reaching. Testers should ensure that the knees of the participant stay extended: however, the participant's knees should not be pressed down. The participant should breathe normally during the test and should not hold his or her breath at any time. Norms for the Canadian test are presented in Table 19-9. Note that these norms use a sit-and-reach box in which the "zero" point is set at the 26-cm mark. If you are using a box in which the zero point is set at 23 cm (e.g., Fitnessgram), subtract 3 cm from each value in this table. The norms for the YMCA test are presented in Table 19-10.

*Diagrams of these procedures are available from Golding LA, Myers CR, Sinning WE. YMCA Fitness Testing and Assessment Manual, 4th ed. YMCA of the USA, 101 N. Wacker Drive, Chicago, IL 60606. Canadian Society for Exercise Physiology. The Canadian Physical Activity, Fitness & Lifestyle Approach: CSEP-Health & Fitness Program's Health-Related Appraisal & Counseling Strategy. 3rd ed. Canadian Society for Exercise Physiology, 2003.

From: American College of Sports Medicine. Health-Related Physical Fitness Assessment Manual. 2nd edition. Philadelphia: 2008. Lippincott Williams & Wilkins.

BOX 19-28 YMCA SIT-AND-REACH TEST PROCEDURES

1. Before administering the sit-and-reach test, offer the individual the opportunity to do some stretching exercises and light to moderate aerobic exercise (5–10 minutes) to warm up the muscles. Inquire whether the subject has any back problems before administering the protocol. If the subject has a back problem or a history of back problems.
2. Make sure they have an adequate aerobic and muscular warm-up.
3. Have them take a few practice tries before the actual measure and inquire if it bothers the back, or skip the test.

4. A yardstick is placed on the floor and tape is placed across it at a right angle to the 15-inch mark.
5. The subject sits with the yardstick between the legs and the legs extended at right angles to the taped line on the floor. Heels of the feet should touch the edge of the taped line and be about 10 to 12 inches apart.
6. Table 19-9 contains the YMCA Sit-and-Reach Test norm data.

portant to assess. ACSM's *Health-Related Physical Fitness Assessment Manual* (1) provides thorough step-by-step instructions for measuring these, which are, unfortunately, outside of the scope of this chapter.

SUMMARY

The assessment of an individual's health-related physical fitness can provide valuable information to help develop a safe, effective, and individualized exercise program. The development of an exercise program requires careful consideration to the medical/health history, preactivity screening (including risk stratification), and the individual responses to the selected tests of health-related physical fitness. The following is a summary of chapter points:

- The first step in any assessment of health-related physical fitness is to perform a preactivity screening, including a medical/health history, risk stratification, and (possibly) a physical examination.
- Test procedures should be selected according to the population being tested, facilities and equipment available, and the qualifications of those performing the tests.
- There are various techniques available to assess body composition, including height/weight charts, BMI, anthropometric measurements, and percent body fat prediction.
- Cardiorespiratory fitness can be assessed using several techniques that can be classified as either laboratory or field tests for the estimation and/or measurement of $\dot{V}O_{2max}$.
- Several submaximal cycle and treadmill protocols exist that can be used to estimate cardiorespiratory fitness.

TABLE 19-9. FITNESS CATEGORIES BY AGE GROUPS AND GENDER FOR TRUNK FORWARD FLEXION USING A SIT-AND-REACH BOX (cm)[*,†]

	AGE									
PERCENTILE	20–29		30–39		40–49		50–59		60–69	
GENDER	M	F	M	F	M	F	M	F	M	F
Excellent	40	41	38	41	35	38	35	39	33	35
Very good	39	40	37	40	34	37	34	38	32	34
	34	37	33	36	29	34	28	33	25	31
Good	33	36	32	35	28	33	27	32	24	30
	30	33	28	32	24	30	24	30	20	27
Fair	29	32	27	31	23	29	23	29	19	26
	25	28	23	27	18	25	16	25	15	23
Needs improvement	24	27	22	26	17	24	15	24	14	22

*The Canadian Physical Activity, Fitness & Lifestyle Approach: CSEP-Health & Fitness Program's Health-Related Appraisal & Counseling Strategy. 3rd ed. Reprinted with permission from the Canadian Society for Exercise Physiology, 2003.

†Note: These norms are based on a sit-and-reach box in which the "zero" point is set at 26 cm. When using a box in which the zero point is set at 23 cm, subtract 3 cm from each value in this table.

TABLE 19-10. PERCENTILES BY AGE GROUPS AND GENDER FOR YMCA SIT-AND-REACH TEST (Inches)*

	AGE											
PERCENTILE	18–25		26–35		36–45		46–55		56–65		>65	
GENDER	M	F	M	F	M	F	M	F	M	F	M	F
90	22	24	21	23	21	22	19	21	17	20	17	20
80	20	22	19	21	19	21	17	20	15	19	15	18
70	19	21	17	20	17	19	15	18	13	17	13	17
60	18	20	17	20	16	18	14	17	13	16	12	17
50	17	19	15	19	15	17	13	16	11	15	10	15
40	15	18	14	17	13	16	11	14	9	14	9	14
30	14	17	13	16	13	15	10	14	9	13	8	13
20	13	16	11	15	11	14	9	12	7	11	7	11
10	11	14	9	13	–	12	6	10	5	9	4	9

* Based on data from YMCA of the USA (reference 18). The following may be used as descriptors for the percentile rankings: well above average (90), above average (70), average (50), below average (30), and well below average (10)

- Maximal exercise testing using various treadmill or cycle ergometer protocols exist for determining cardiorespiratory fitness.
- The assessment of muscular strength, muscular endurance, and flexibility is often grouped together and can occur using several different testing measures.

REFERENCES

1. American College of Sports Medicine. *Health-Related Physical Fitness Assessment Manual.* 2nd ed. Baltimore: Lippincott Williams & Wilkins; 2008.
2. **American College of Sports Medicine. Position Stand: The recommended quantity and quality of exercise for developing and maintaining cardiorespiratory and muscular fitness, and flexibility in healthy adults.** *Med Sci Sports Exerc.* 1998;30:975–991.
3. Astrand P-O. Aerobic work capacity in men and women with special reference to age. *Acta Physiol Scand.* 1960;49(suppl):45–60.
4. Astrand P-O, Ryhming I. A nomogram for calculation of aerobic capacity (physical fitness) from pulse rate during submaximal work. *J Appl Physiol.* 1954;7:218–221.
5. **Balady GJ, Chaitman B, Driscoll D, et al. American College of Sports Medicine and American Heart Association Joint Position Statement: Recommendations for cardiovascular screening staffing, and emergency procedures at health/fitness facilities.** *Med Sci Sports Exerc.* 1998;30:1009–1018.
6. Blair SN, Kohl HW 3rd, Barlow LE, et al. Changes in physical fitness and all-cause mortality: a prospective study of healthy and unhealthy men. *JAMA.* 1995;273:1093–1098.
7. Blair SN, Kohl HW 3rd, Paffenbarger RS Jr, et al. Physical fitness and all-cause mortality: a prospective study of healthy men and women. *JAMA.* 1989;262:2395–2401.
8. Bray GA. Don't throw the baby out with the bath water. *Am J Clin Nutr.* 2004;79:347–349.
9. Caspersen CJ, Powell KE, Christenson GM. Physical activity, exercise, and physical fitness: definitions and distinctions for health-related research. *Public Health Rep.* 1985;100:126–131.
10. Clarkson H. *Musculoskeletal Assessment, Joint Range of Motion and Manual Muscle Strength.* Baltimore: Lippincott Williams & Wilkins; 1999.
11. Davis JA. Direct determination of aerobic power. In: Maud PJ, Foster C, editors. *Physiological Assessment of Human Fitness.* Champaign (IL): Human Kinetics; 1995. p. 9–17.
12. Dempster P, Aitkens S. A new air displacement method for the determination of human body composition. *Med Sci Sports Exerc.* 1995;27:1692–1697.
13. Folsom AR, Kaye SA, Sellers TA, et al. Body fat distribution and 5-year risk of death in older women. *JAMA.* 1993;269:483–487.
14. Franklin BA, Gordon NF. *Contemporary Diagnosis and Management in Cardiovascular Exercise.* Newtown (PA): Handbooks in Healthcare; 2005.
15. Franklin BA, Gordon S, Timmis GC, et al. Is direct physician supervision of exercise stress testing routinely necessary? *Chest.* 1997;111:262–265.
16. Gallagher D, Heymsfield SB, Heo M, et al. Healthy percentage body fat ranges: an approach for developing guidelines based on body mass index. *Am J Clin Nutr.* 2000;72:694–701.
17. Going BS. Densitometry. In: Roche AF, Heymsfield SB, Lohman TG, editors. *Human Body Composition.* Champaign (IL): Human Kinetics; 1996. p. 3–23.
18. Graves JE, Pollock ML, Bryant CX. Assessment of muscular strength and endurance. In: Roitman JL, editor. *ACSM's Resource Manual for Guidelines for Exercise Testing and Prescription.* 4th ed. Baltimore: Lippincott Williams & Wilkins; 2001. p. 376–380.
19. Hendel HW, Gotfredsen A, Hojgaard L, et al. Change in fat-free mass assessed by bioelectrical impedance, total body potassium and dual energy x-ray absorptiometry during prolonged weight loss. *Scand J Clin Lab Invest.* 1996;56:671–679.
20. Heyward VH. Practical body composition assessment for children, adults, and older adults. *Int J Sport Nutr.* 1998;8:285–307.
21. Heyward VH, Stolarczyk LM, editors. *Applied Body Composition Assessment.* Champaign (IL): Human Kinetics; 1996. p. 12.
22. Hoeger WW, Barette SL, Hale DR. Relationship between repetition and selected percentages of one repetition maximum. *J Appl Sport Sci Res.* 1987;1:11–13.
23. Hoeger WW, Hopkins DR, Bareete SL. Relationship between repetitions and selected percentages of one repetition maximum: a comparison between untrained and trained males and females. *J Appl Sport Sci Res.* 1990;4:47–54.
24. Jackson AS, Pollock ML. Practical assessment of body composition. *Phys Sport Med.* 1985;13(3):76–90.
25. Leger L, Thivierge M. Heart rate monitors: validity, stability and functionality. *Phys Sport Med.* 1988;16:143–151.
26. Liemohn WP, Sharpe GL, Wasserman JF. Lumbosacral movement in the sit-and-reach and in Cailliet's protective-hamstring stretch. *Spine.* 1994;19:2127–2130.
27. Logan P, Fornasiero D, Abernathy P, et al. Protocols for the assessment of isoinertial strength. In: Fore CJ, editor. *Physiological Tests for Elite Athletes.* Champaign (IL): Human Kinetics; 2000. p. 200–221.
28. Lohman TG. Body composition methodology in sports medicine. *Phys Sports Med.* 1982;10:47–58.

29. Lohman TG, Houtkooper L, Going SB. Body fat measurement goes high-tech. *ACSM's Health & Fitness Journal* 1997;1(1):30–35.

30. McConnell TR. Cardiorespiratory assessment of apparently healthy populations. In: Roitman JL, editor. *ACSM Resource Manual for Guidelines for Exercise Testing and Prescription.* 4th ed. Baltimore: Williams & Wilkins; 2001. p. 361–375.

31. Minkler S, Patterson P. The validity of the modified sit-and-reach test in college-age students. *Res Q Exerc Sport.* 1994;65: 189–192.

32. National Institutes of Health. Health implications of obesity. *Ann Intern Med.* 1985;163:1073–1077.

33. Ogden CL, Carroll MD, Curtin LR, et al. Prevalence of overweight and obesity in the United States, 1999–2004. *JAMA* 2006;295: 1549–1555.

34. Ogden CL, Flegal KM, Carroll MD, et al. Prevalence and trends in overweight among US children and adolescents, 1999–2000. *JAMA.* 2002;288:1728–1732.

35. Palmer ML, Epler ME, editors. *Fundamentals of Musculoskeletal Assessment Techniques.* 2nd ed. Philadelphia: Lippincott-Raven; 1998.

36. **Expert Panel on the Identification, Evaluation, and Treatment of Overweight and Obesity in Adults. Executive summary of the clinical guidelines on the identification, evaluation, and treatment of overweight and obesity in adults.** *Arch Intern Med.* **1998;158: 1855–1867.**

37. **U.S. Department of Health and Human Services.** *Physical Activity and Health: A Report of the Surgeon General.* **Atlanta (GA): U.S. Department of Health and Human Services, Centers for Disease Control and Prevention, National Center for Chronic Disease Prevention and Health Promotion; 1996.**

38. **Pollock ML, Franklin BA, Balady GJ, et al. Resistance exercise in individuals with and without cardiovascular disease: benefits, rationale, safety, and prescription: an advisory from the American Heart Association.** *Circulation.* **2000;101:828–833. p. 15.**

39. President's Council on Physical Fitness. Definitions: health, fitness, and physical activity. PCPFS *Research Digest.* 2000. www.fitness. gov/digestg_mar2000.htm. Last accessed on 11/11/08.

40. Rikli R, Jones CJ. *Senior Fitness Test Manual.* Champaign (IL): Human Kinetics; 2001. p. 1–14.

41. Rimm EB, Stampfer MJ, Giovannucci E, et al. Body size and fat distribution as predictors of coronary heart disease among middle-aged and older US men. *Am J Epidemiol.* 1995;141:1117–1127.

42. Roche AF. Anthropometry and ultrasound. In: Roche AF, Heymsfield SB, Lohman TG, editors. *Human Body Composition.* Champaign (IL): Human Kinetics; 1996. p. 167–189.

43. Roche AF, Heymsfield SB, Lohman TG, editors. *Human Body Composition.* Champaign (IL): Human Kinetics, 1996; p. 19.

44. Sesso HD, Paffenbarger RS Jr, Lee IM. Physical activity and coronary heart disease in men: The Harvard Alumni Health Study. *Circulation.* 2000;102:975–980.

45. Shephard RJ, Thomas S, Weller I. The Canadian Home Fitness Test: 1991 update. *Sports Med.* 1991;11:358–366.

46. **Seventh Report of the Joint Committee on Prevention, Detection, Evaluation, and Treatment of High Blood Pressure (JNCVIII).** *JAMA.* **2003;289:2560–2572.**

47. **Third Report of the National Cholesterol Education Program (NCEP). Expert Panel on Detection, Evaluation, and Treatment of High Blood Cholesterol in Adults. National Institutes of Health National Heart, Lung, and Blood Institute. NIH Publication No. 02-8215, September, 2002.**

48. Tran ZV, Weltman A. Generalized equation for predicting body density of women from girth measurements. *Med Sci Sports Exerc.* 1989;21:101–104.

49. Tran ZV, Weltman A. Predicting body composition of men from girth measurements. *Hum Biol.* 1988;60:167–175.

50. Troiano RP, Flegal KM. Overweight children and adolescents: description, epidemiology, and demographics. *Pediatrics.* 1998;101: 497–504.

51. Van Itallie TB, editor. Topography of body fat: relationship to risk of cardiovascular and other diseases. In: Lohman TG, Roche AF, Martorell R, editors. *Anthropometric Standardization Reference Manual.* Champaign (IL): Human Kinetics; 1988. p. 16.

SELECTED REFERENCES FOR FURTHER READING

Gleim GW, McHugh MP. Flexibility and its effects on sports injury and performance. *Sports Med.* 1997;24:289–299.

Heyward VH, Wagner DR. *Applied Body Composition Assessment.* 2nd ed. Champaign (IL): Human Kinetics; 2004.

Thacker SB, Gilchrist J, Stroup D, et al. The impact of stretching on sports injury risk: a systemic review of the literature. *Med Sci Sports Exerc.* 2004;36:371–378.

Yasmura S, Wang J, Peirson RN, editors. In vivo body composition studies. *Ann N Y Acad Sci.* 2000;904:1–631.

INTERNET RESOURCES

American College of Sports Medicine (ACSM): www.acsm.org
American Council on Exercise (ACE): www.acefitness.org
National Heartt, Lung, Blood Institute of the National Institutes of Health (NHLBI): www.nhlbi.nih.gov/guidelines/cholesterol/
National Strength and Conditioning Association (NSCA): www.nsca-lift.org

Skeletal muscle has several functions, including force generation, movement stimulation, joint stability, and caloric expenditure. Relative and absolute muscular assessment has relevance in athletics, general fitness, and clinical settings. Strength, endurance, power generation, physical work capacity, and flexibility are measurable components of muscular health and fitness. Endurance is examined both for duration of sustained (*isometric/static*) muscle contraction, as well as repetitive skeletal motion (*dynamic*), and refers to a muscle's ability to resist or delay the onset of fatigue. Each of these measures is both clinically and practically relevant and may be utilized to assess functional capacity and performance (34). Flexibility or *range of motion* (ROM) is another muscular fitness parameter for both performance enhancement and rehabilitation, and is commonly evaluated and employed when prescribing an exercise regimen. This chapter reviews characteristics of strength generation, assessment techniques for muscular strength and flexibility, and practical applications of each.

PRINCIPLES OF MUSCULAR FUNCTION

MUSCLE FIBER RECRUITMENT

 1.1.19-HFS: Knowledge of the structure and function of the skeletal muscle fiber.

 1.1.20-HFS: Knowledge of the characteristics of fast- and slow-twitch muscle fibers.

Athletes, exercise professionals, and coaches consistently seek strength, endurance, and functional improvements by striving for a competitive edge to maximize performance. Physical therapists, athletic trainers, and other exercise professionals employ similar techniques and principles for rehabilitation and performance enhancement. Assessment and training techniques are vital to this process, and several parameters should be considered. *Specificity* refers to the type of training necessary to maximize performance of a given sport or activity, including muscle fiber recruitment and isolation; accordingly, it is a primary consideration when designing an exercise program. Other considerations include baseline health status and muscular fitness, program progression, training modalities and techniques, joint flexibility, and ROM. Specificity involves identifying realistic training goals and limitations and choosing baseline assessments that may be augmented or enhanced by an appropriate exercise prescription. Knowledge of exercise modalities required to meet specific goals will assist the exercise professional in developing the program. For example, if a patient is interested in an endurance activity, such as cross-country skiing, training should focus on aerobic metabolism and recruitment of appropriate muscle fiber types (Table 20-1). Although training will include both aerobic and anaerobic activities, the program should be designed specifically for muscular and cardiovascular demands of cross-country skiing. In such situations, cross-training, high-repetition sets, and other endurance training techniques should be considered before high-resistance, low-repetition exercises primarily used for power training.

Type I muscle fibers are primarily used during sustained endurance activities. Muscle fibers classified as type II are generally recruited for higher-intensity, power-oriented resistance exercises and shorter bouts of work. Table 20-1 details the characteristics of varied muscle fiber types; however, the relative exercise intensity and duration will largely determine the predominant type(s) and recruitment of motor units (19). Muscular fitness assessments attempt to examine a person's ability to recruit a predominant fiber type and test either for endurance, power, maximal force production, or combinations thereof. Techniques of assessment are parameter specific. Many parameters, including safety, should be considered before testing. For example, muscular endurance may be evaluated with decreased risk of injury as less acute strain is placed on joints and bones susceptible to injury. Maximal muscle force is accurately predicted and represented by use of *one repetition maximum* (1RM) for a given exercise. On the other hand, endurance protocols may be safer and also represent an accurate predictor of maximal force production (34).

TABLE 20-1. CHARACTERISTICS OF MUSCLE FIBER TYPES

FIBER TYPE	TYPE I FIBERS	TYPE IIA FIBERS	TYPE II FIBERS	TYPE IIB FIBERS
Contraction time	Slow	Moderately fast	Fast	Very fast
Size of motor neuron	Small	Medium	Large	Very large
Resistance to fatigue	High	Fairly high	Intermediate	Low
Activity used for	Aerobic	Long-term anaerobic	Short-term anaerobic	Short-term anaerobic
Maximum duration of use	Hours	<30 minutes	<5 minutes	<1 minute
Force production	Low	Medium	High	Very high
Mitochondrial density	High	High	Medium	Low
Capillary density	High	Intermediate	Low	Low
Oxidative capacity	High	High	Intermediate	Low
Glycolytic capacity	Low	High	High	High
Major storage fuel	Triglycerides	Creatine phosphate, glycogen	Creatine phosphate, glycogen	Creatine phosphate, glycogen

MUSCULAR FORCE DEVELOPMENT

 1.1.22-HFS: Knowledge of twitch, summation, and tetanus with respect to muscle contraction.

Muscular contractions are stimulated by the central nervous system in response to release of acetylcholine at the neuromuscular junction. Cellular voltage changes (action potentials) generated by neurologic stimulation release calcium ions (Ca^{2+}) into the interstitial space. A chemical reaction occurs with intracellular adenosine triphosphate (ATP) produced by metabolizing creatine phosphate and glycogen. A positive voltage change stimulates cross-bridge formation and a power stroke between actin and myosin filaments, thereby shortening the sarcomere. This process is repeated in a progressive manner for individual muscle fibers. Additional fiber recruitment leads to more cross-bridge formations and greater relative force production, ultimately achieving the maximum voluntary contraction (MVC). The number of fibers recruited is related to the strength and frequency of neurologic stimulus (19) from a motor neuron, termed *motor unit recruitment*. Although mitochondrial activity plays a significant role in longer duration fiber recruitment, during resistance exercises energy is supplied predominantly from phosphagen pools and glycolysis within the sarcoplasm. Motor unit recruitment depends on the amount of force and/or power required for the given movement and the level of motor control. Movement requiring a considerable power output will recruit more muscle fibers simultaneously; however, fine motor control will be sacrificed, and vice versa.

MECHANICS OF FORCE DEVELOPMENT

1.1.3-HFS: Knowledge of the following action terms: inferior, superior, medial, lateral, supination, pronation, flexion, extension, adduction, abduction, hyperextension, rotation, circumduction, agonist, antagonist, and stabilizer.

1.1.4-HFS: Knowledge of the plane in which each movement action occurs and the responsible muscles.

1.1.5-HFS: Knowledge of the interrelationships among center of gravity, base of support, balance, stability, posture, and proper spinal alignment.

Human movement is based on a system involving three classes of levers. Figure 20-1 illustrates classifications of levers with corresponding anatomic examples. As shown, each system combines three separate components: force application (muscular insertion), fulcrum or center of rotation (joint center), and resistance application (center of gravity), all applied along a lever arm (bone). Anatomic levers are primarily third-class levers, as the muscle insertion is commonly distal to the joint center and proximal to the resistance application. The perpendicular distance measured between the joint center and muscle insertion, termed the *force arm*, provides the lever with mechanical torque required for movement. The distance measured from the joint center and the point of resistance application (often identified as the center of mass for the limb and any external resistance[s]) is termed the *resistance arm*. Thus, using a shovel during digging represents a third-class lever. The hand supporting the top of the shovel signifies the fulcrum, the hand placed on the shovel's shaft is the force application point, and load combined with the mass of the shovel below the axis of rotation provides the resistance. To lift a heavier load, the force application should be as close to the resistance as possible; however, if the hands are too close together, the mass would be very difficult to lift. The latter position (hands close together) with a relatively short force arm and long resistance arm represents the system most common in the human body. Force arms in our systems are significantly shorter than natural resistance arms (consider the distance from the elbow joint to the biceps brachii insertion versus the joint to the hand holding a dumbbell or other resistance), which does not allow for a significant *mechanical advantage*. Because most human levers are third class, they offer the advantage of greater ROM and movement velocity at the expense of maximal force production. Figure 20-2 represents the various forces acting on the elbow during flexion. Contraction of elbow flexors (force M) produces torque, causing movement

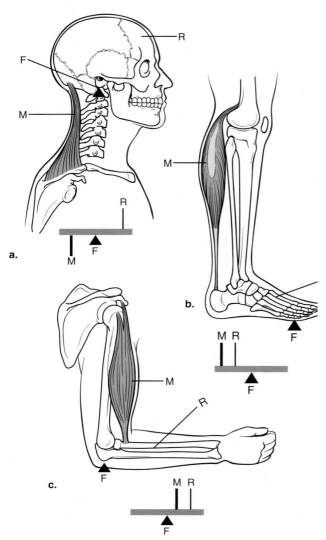

FIGURE 20-1. Classes of Anatomical Levers. Class 1 (a), class 2 (b), and class 3 (c). F, fulcrum (joint center); M, force generation (muscle); R, resistance (center of gravity, external load). Anatomic examples are illustrated. Recall most human examples are class 3. From Kreighbaum E, Barthals K. *Biomechanics: A Qualitative Approach for Studying Human Movement.* New York: Allyn and Bacon; 1996.

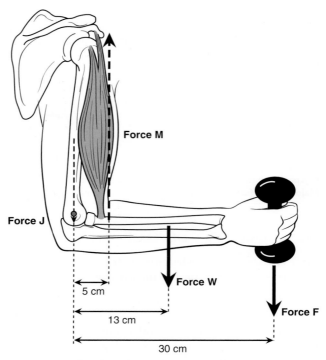

FIGURE 20-2. Mechanical representation of force and torque development in the elbow, where force M is muscular force generation in response to force W and force F. Distances indicated represent moments created by the bony lever of the forearm at various points relative to the joint fulcrum. Force J represents joint reaction force produced during muscular contraction.

against opposing resistance(s). Measures indicated are force and resistance movement arms; however, note that measures will vary depending on body size and stature.

The point of attachment of a tendon to bone is its *insertion*. At any given point in the joint's ROM, the tendon and bone create an angle of insertion, or *angle of muscle pull*. Muscle force can be separated into two components; *turning* (rotary) and *stabilizing*. Acting concurrently, muscle contractions create a torque (which moves the lever about the fulcrum) and a joint stabilizing effect. The turning force acts perpendicular to the lever (bone), and the stabilizing force acts parallel and toward the joint center. Relative to joint ROM, the angle of muscle pull increases or decreases. As the muscle angle of pull increases, approaching 90 degrees, muscle force becomes

increasingly more rotary. Therefore, muscles with relatively small angles of pull provide strong stabilizing components to the affected joint. Likewise, muscles involved with large joint ROM will have progressively larger angles of pull. When the angle of muscle pull reaches exactly 90 degrees, muscle force produced is entirely rotary and no longer has a stabilizing effect on the joint. This implies maximal turning force production of the muscle at exactly 90 degrees. In a few cases, the angle of pull exceeds 90 degrees, with full joint ROM creating a dislocating force. The parallel component of the muscle force is now oriented away from the joint's center; however, the muscle will not be able to create significant force to cause an actual dislocating effect. When a muscle's angle of muscle pull reaches 45 degrees, the turning and stabilizing components are equal. Consequently, muscles display characteristics relative to their potential angles of muscle pull. Small degrees of muscle pull contribute primarily to stabilization, and those that approach or exceed 90 degrees of pull can be considered primary movers for a ROM. For example, the coracobrachialis muscle has small relative changes of angle during shoulder flexion and is primarily considered a stabilizer as opposed to the biceps brachii, in which the angle of muscle pull ranges from approximately 10 degrees at full extension to beyond 90 degrees at full elbow flexion. Thus, muscle angle of pull is different than joint angle and degrees of ROM. Figure 20-3

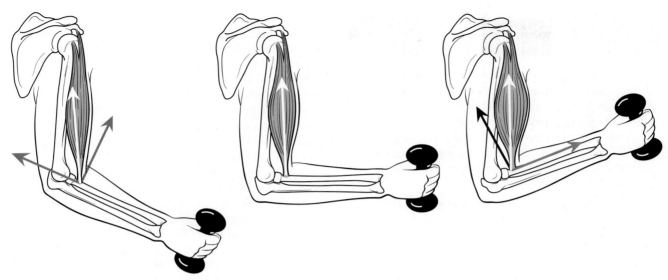

FIGURE 20-3. Force component vectors representing rotary force (red), stabilizing force (gray), dislocating force (black), and muscle force orientation (white). Note as muscle insertion angle changes from A (45 degrees) to B (90 degrees) to C (>90 degrees), force vectors shift properties from stabilizing/rotary, purely rotary, and dislocating/rotary, respectively.

illustrates force component vectors at varying degrees of joint movement.

SKELETAL MUSCLE RESPONSE TO RESISTANCE EXERCISE

MUSCLE FIBER ADAPTATION

> **1.1.23-HFS: Knowledge of the principles involved in promoting gains in muscular strength and endurance.**

> **1.1.36-HFS: Knowledge of the following terms: progressive resistance, isotonic/isometric, concentric, eccentric, atrophy, hyperplasia, hypertrophy, sets, repetitions, plyometrics, Valsalva maneuver.**

The acute and chronic responses to resistance exercise and *resistance training* (RT) have been previously reported (3,46,57). *Resistance exercise* refers to a single bout of variable resistance exercise, whereas RT describes a long-term program of progression and overload leading to some or all of the benefits detailed in Table 20-2 (46,57). Controversy exists about whether measurable strength gains associated with RT are the result of *hyperplasia* or *hypertrophy*. Generally, strength gains after RT are attributable to increased fiber size (12,35) rather than additional fiber production. Unfortunately, cross-sections of muscle fibers large enough to analyze are difficult to obtain in human subjects for ethical and practical reasons. The relative contributions from neurologic adaptations and muscular hypertrophy to strength enhancements are largely determined by age, training status, and genetic predisposition. Training stimuli will dictate the physiologic

TABLE 20-2. COMPARISON OF THE EFFECTS OF AEROBIC AND RESISTANCE TRAINING ON SELECTED PHYSIOLOGIC VARIABLES

PHYSIOLOGIC VARIABLE	AEROBIC EXERCISE	RESISTANCE EXERCISE
Bone mineral density	↑↑	↑↑
Body composition		
% fat	↓↓	↓
Lean body mass	↔	↑↑
Muscular strength	↔	↑↑↑
Glucose metabolism		
Insulin response	↓↓	↓↓
Basal insulin levels	↓	↓
Insulin sensitivity	↑↑	↑↑
Serum lipids		
High-density lipoprotein	↑↔	↑↔
Low-density lipoprotein	↓↔	↓↔
Resting heart rate	↓↓	↔
Stroke volume, rest and maximal	↑↑	↔
Cardiovascular dynamics		
Resting systolic blood pressure	↓↔	↔
Resting diastolic blood pressure	↓↔	↓↔
Submaximal exercise RPP	↓↓↓	↓↓
Maximal oxygen uptake	↑↑↑	↑↔
Overall endurance time	↑↑↑	↑↑
Basal metabolism	↑	↑↑
Health-related quality of life	↑↔	↑↔

RPP, rate pressure product.

↑ indicates values increase; ↓, values decrease; ↔, values remain unchanged; ↑ or ↓, small effect; ↑↑ or ↓↓, medium effect; ↑↑↑ or ↓↓↓, large effect.

From Williams M, Haskell W, Ades P, et al. Resistance exercise in individuals with and without cardiovascular disease: 2007 update: a scientific statement from the American Heart Association Council on Nutrition, Physical Activity, and Metabolism. *Circulation*. 2007;116:572–584.

BOX 20-1	MUSCLE FIBER MEASURE-MENT TECHNIQUES

Histologic cross-sectioning methods extract muscle fiber, commonly from the belly of the muscle, and fibers are counted utilizing ATPase staining. ATPase staining allows for relatively accurate counting of total fiber number and percentage of each fiber type. Limitations to this technique make it difficult to know whether accurate counts are indeed obtained.

Nitric acid digestion is a more definitive method of isolating and counting muscle fibers accurately. Direct counts using this technique may result in an underestimation of total fiber number.

responses underlying muscular improvements. Prolonged endurance training may stimulate metabolic and muscle morphology changes, including mitochondria biogenesis, type II to type I fiber-type transformation, and adjusted substrate metabolism (12). Likewise, heavy resistance exercise will augment contractile proteins that are responsible for hypertrophy and increased MVC (12). Some highly advanced training techniques may lead to hyperplasia of skeletal muscle tissue (5). Hyperplasia has been reported as a result of both exercise and stretch overload of skeletal muscle using nitric acid digestion and cross-section techniques (5) (Box 20-1). However, it remains unclear whether this methodology and these findings, derived primarily from animal models, can be extrapolated to human physiology.

Loss of skeletal muscle (*atrophy*) is a natural physiologic response to disuse as a result of injury, immobilization, sedentary lifestyle, and/or certain disease processes. Atrophy causes reduced muscle protein synthesis (56), usually first in type II fibers, and muscle protein degradation primarily in type I fibers. Force generation capacity diminishes as muscle atrophy occurs, contributing to generalized weakness. Atrophy occurs as a result of a change in balance between protein synthesis and degradation, during which there is a down-regulation of the former and enhancement of the latter. *Sarcopenia* is associated with "body wasting" and is common in elderly persons and patients suffering from chronic diseases or medical conditions, congestive heart failure, chronic obstructive pulmonary disease, and liver failure (15). Resistance training programs have obvious benefits for reversing atrophy, as well as sarcopenia, associated with varied clinical pathologies (47). Selective fiber-type atrophy associated with congestive heart failure, for example, has been shown to be reversible with participation in a RT program (46).

Initial strength gains when beginning an RT program may be attributable to neurologic adaptations in the skeletal muscle motor units (22). Synchronization of motor units leading to more succinct recruitment of muscle fibers is believed to initiate considerable gains in strength and coordination, particularly early in training. Increases in microvascularization and capillary density serve to enhance oxygen delivery to skeletal muscle, thereby improving energy production and muscular endurance (35,55). Some research has demonstrated no change in capillary density per muscle fiber with high-intensity and eccentric RT (25). Others have reported little or no change or enhancements in muscle capillary density, depending on the training protocol used (35). Collectively, these data support the principle of training specificity and suggest that type I fibers demonstrate that vascular adaptations improve aerobic endurance.

Architectural changes in skeletal muscle after both concentric and eccentric RT affect torque production capabilities and fiber length and may contribute to improvements in MVC (9). Other adaptations associated with strength improvements include more actin/myosin cross-bridge formations (22,25). Microscopic increases are not only observed in actin and myosin proteins, but also in connective tissue proteins like titin and nebulin, increases in the muscle cross-sectional area, and increased myofibril density. Functional adaptations to training are determined by the volume (*sets* × *reps* × *weight*), intensity, and frequency of exercise (12). It has been shown that muscle fiber number increases during fetal growth and that postnatal improvements in strength are due to hypertrophy (36). Some evidence suggests that both hypertrophy and hyperplasia are responsible for strength gains early in life. For example, using nitric acid digestion measurement techniques (Box 20-1), both exercise and stretch overload have been shown to result in significant increases in muscle fiber number, signifying hyperplasia (35).

Progressive overload is essential for promoting increases in muscular fitness. Plateaus often occur in novice exercisers, as not enough emphasis is placed on progression early in training. Modest increments in exercise regimens will promote rapid improvements in muscular strength and endurance. Promoting adaptation without causing overuse injury is a key component to planning and executing training programs. Wolff's law illustrates progressive adaptation and remodeling of bony tissue and may be extrapolated to connective and muscle tissue. This law demonstrates adaptation both to underutilization (atrophy) and to overutilization (injury). Progressive tissue adaptation is maximized within the "physiologic training zone," during which training intensity can be enhanced without causing tissue damage (Fig. 20-4). Periodization training programs may be used to avoid plateaus and ensure adequate progression. For example, a training program may incorporate seasonal cycles or advancing monthly intensity and modality changes.

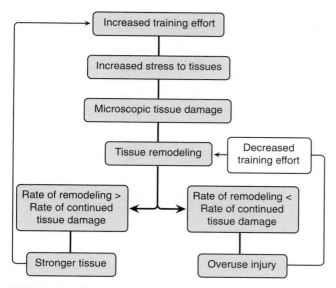

FIGURE 20-4. Tissue adaptation to training stimulus. Appropriate stress on muscle or connective tissue results in remodeling and stronger tissue. Overuse injury occurs when tissue continues to be trained and damaged without adequate remodeling time.

SPECIAL POPULATION AND SAFETY CONSIDERATIONS

> **1.1.11-CES: Knowledge of acute and chronic adaptations to exercise for those with cardiovascular, pulmonary, and metabolic demands.**

> **1.3.30-CES: Discuss the appropriate use of static and dynamic resistance exercise for individuals with cardiovascular, pulmonary, and metabolic disease.**

> **1.7.20-CES: Describe the importance of, and appropriate methods for, resistance training in older adults.**

> **1.1.36-HFS: Knowledge of the following terms: progressive resistance, isotonic/isometric, concentric, eccentric, atrophy, hyperplasia, hypertrophy, sets, repetitions, plyometrics, Valsalva maneuver.**

Resistance training has been shown to elicit overall muscular strength and endurance improvements with an adequate dosage. Blood pressure, heart rate response, *rate pressure product* (RPP), body composition, and biochemical markers, such as lactic acid accumulation (23), nitric oxide (21), and creatine kinase (21) may be monitored selectively during RT and muscle testing. Ongoing research in special populations is consistently demonstrating the safety of RT using higher exercise intensities. Higher-intensity training (>80% 1RM) regimens have been examined in healthy elderly men (22), women (53), patients with heart disease (2,7,8,36,53,57) and cancer (51), and other clinical populations that may benefit from increases in muscular fitness. Collectively, these findings demonstrate cardioprotective benefits of high-intensity resistance training in varied populations. Tradi-

tionally, resistance training, specifically with higher intensities, has been contraindicated in coronary patients because of concerns regarding the potential for cardiovascular events. Extensive research has now shown RT to be safe and effective in achieving improvements in muscular strength in selected low-to-moderate-risk cardiac and other chronically ill patients (45). In fact, cardiac demands during RT may be less than that of prescribed aerobic exercise training in these individuals, if it is executed following established guidelines (14,51). This area of investigation warrants future study, because RT at both high and low intensities may benefit certain patient subsets (e.g., stable coronary artery disease, congestive heart failure, peripheral vascular disease).

Breath holding during exercise or daily lifting activities may allow for an increase in force generation; however, it is not recommended and may compromise safety. This technique, which is referred to as the *Valsalva maneuver*, may elicit a dramatic and potentially dangerous rise and fall in systolic blood pressure, resulting in dizziness, cardiac dysrhythmias, and related syncope. Cardiac and chronically debilitated patients have been cautioned against performing this maneuver and are instructed in proper lifting and breathing patterns (18). Exhalation during the concentric phase of lifting and inhalation during eccentric contraction is the recommended breathing pattern for individuals with and without heart disease.

MUSCULAR FITNESS ASSESSMENT

> **1.1.23-HFS: Knowledge of the principles involved in promoting gains in muscular strength and endurance.**

Muscular assessment is important for defining a baseline fitness level and gauging subsequent improvements. Muscular fitness testing can be done at all levels, from novice to advanced athletes; however, protocols and techniques should be adjusted to accommodate specific levels of fitness and strength. The evaluation must consider varied parameters to ensure that valuable and reliable measurements are obtained.

Muscular strength is defined as peak *force* (Newton) or *torque* (Newton-meters) developed during MVC under standardized or unique conditions (49). Strength and power are assessed for four main purposes: to quantify relative significance of strength and power for athletic events and other activities, to identify deficiencies in muscular function so that serial improvements might be monitored (strength diagnosis), to evaluate the potential of individuals for particular athletic pursuits, and to assess the effects of training and rehabilitation programs (1).

Coaches, clinical exercise specialists, health fitness specialists, therapists, athletic trainers, atheletic team scouts, and lay persons have differing interests in musculoskeletal strength assessments. Muscular strength is frequently difficult to assess because of the level of specificity and reproducibility of the parameter being measured. Accuracy of measurements is paramount to maintain the integrity of the sport and chronicle performance statistics. The crucial determinants of musculoskeletal testing include *reliability*, *reproducibility*, and *accuracy* of measurements.

In addition to athletes, the general public may derive considerable benefits from an accurate musculoskeletal fitness assessment. Many health and fitness clubs offer initial fitness assessments to determine baseline measures and to assist in goal setting for their patients. This session will often include both a cardiorespiratory fitness assessment and musculoskeletal strength and flexibility analysis. Allied health and medical professionals may utilize muscular strength, endurance, and ROM assessments before and after a course of rehabilitation to determine the effectiveness of treatments and modalities. Accuracy and standardization of measurements is crucial to deriving optimal clinical outcomes, reimbursement, and patient satisfaction.

TECHNIQUES AND LIMITATIONS

> **1.1.24-HFS: Knowledge of muscle fatigue as it relates to mode, intensity, duration, and the accumulative effects of exercise.**

> **1.3.18-HFS: Ability to describe the purpose of testing, determine appropriate protocols, and perform assessments of muscular strength, muscular endurance, and flexibility.**

> **1.3.20-HFS: Ability to analyze and interpret information obtained from the cardiorespiratory fitness test and the muscular strength and endurance, flexibility, and body composition assessments for apparently healthy individuals and those with controlled chronic disease.**

Maximal *dynamic* strength has been reported in the scientific literature and may be assessed by varied protocols and techniques; however, the 1RM test remains the gold standard when evaluating MVC. *Isotonic* contraction suggests a constant resistance throughout a given ROM, which, in the human body, is difficult to maintain. As previously discussed, insertion angles determine whether a muscle is primarily a stabilizer or agonist; however, the angle of insertion changes throughout a joint's ROM, thereby altering the rotary force potential. Although the term *isotonic* is used to describe resistance throughout ROM, muscle force generation is a function of insertion angle, velocity of movement, and required acceleration or deceleration for the movement. According to the length-tension relationship of muscle force development, tension increases at longer resting lengths and decreases as the muscle shortens.

One repetition maximum is defined as the highest progressive load that can be lifted through full ROM one time (16). Once one full repetition is completed, the subject is to attempt another without rest; however, if the second repeti-

TABLE 20-3. NORMATIVE BENCH PRESS DATA BASED ON 1RM TESTS[a]

BENCH PRESS NORMS FOR MEN

Percentile	AGE				
	20–29	30–39	40–49	50–59	60+
90	1.49	1.24	1.10	0.97	0.89
80	1.39	1.12	1.00	0.90	0.82
70	1.29	1.04	0.93	0.84	0.77
60	1.20	0.98	0.88	0.79	0.72
50	1.10	0.93	0.84	0.75	0.68
40	1.00	0.88	0.80	0.71	0.66
30	0.90	0.83	0.76	0.68	0.63
20	0.81	0.78	0.72	0.63	0.57
10	0.71	0.71	0.65	0.57	0.53

BENCH PRESS NORMS FOR WOMEN

Percentile	AGE				
	20–29	30–39	40–49	50–59	60+
90	0.75	0.76	0.71	0.61	0.64
80	0.70	0.70	0.62	0.55	0.54
70	0.65	0.63	0.57	0.52	0.51
60	0.60	0.60	0.54	0.48	0.47
50	0.56	0.57	0.52	0.46	0.45
40	0.51	0.53	0.50	0.44	0.43
30	0.47	0.51	0.47	0.42	0.40
20	0.42	0.47	0.43	0.39	0.38
10	0.37	0.42	0.38	0.37	0.33

[a]Values are relative to body weight (1RM/body weight).

Adapted from the University of Texas and the Cooper Institute, Dallas, Texas.

tion is not completed maintaining correct form and posture, the 1RM has been achieved. Reproducibility of the test may vary slightly depending on the technician and the equipment employed, which should be standardized for retesting. Commonly, the 1RM is accepted throughout the industry as a muscle-group–specific measure of strength (16,20). For example, Table 20-3 shows normative and predictive data of 1RM for the bench press. A similar table and another for leg strength can be found in the GETP8 (Tables 4-9 and 4-10).

The 1RM technique has been used safely to assess strength in many populations, including healthy adults (43), athletes (13), elderly persons, and those with chronic disease (2,7,21,23,36,53). Orthopedic limitations should always be considered and testing avoided or terminated if the loaded movement causes pain or exacerbates an existing medical condition. Accordingly, 1RM evaluation may be contraindicated for a patient with rheumatoid arthritis who is experiencing shoulder (glenohumeral joint) pain. Although the 1RM assessment remains the most accurate and effective measure of strength, prediction equations (Box 20-2) using lighter loads and more repetitions (i.e., a

BOX 20-2 REPETITION MAXIMUM PREDICTION EQUATION (11)

$$1RM = wt.\ lifted\ /\ \{1 + (0.033(n)\};$$
where n = repetitions to failure

3RM, 5RM, or 10RM) are available (11). As more repetitions are incorporated into the assessment, however, the muscle will become increasingly reliant on endurance fibers and less on true force generation. One repetition maximum testing can be performed for muscle isolation exercises (leg extension for quadriceps strength) or for multijointed and complex exercises (bench press for pectorals, triceps brachii, and anterior shoulders). More dynamic movements, such as standing squats, may also be tested for strength; however, higher-repetition tests are recommended to lower the risk of injury because of excessive joint and connective tissue loading. Table 20-4 provides % 1RM information to help guide higher-repetition tests. Box 20-3 describes the 1RM protocol for testing.

Equipment considerations during 1RM testing are important. For example, a 1RM exercise performed for upper-body strength is the bench press. Consider the bar thickness (Olympic vs. 2-inch vs. 3-inch bar) for this test as it has a significant effect on measured values in resistance-trained individuals. Similarly, bent-over row and dead-lift strength testing demonstrate significant decreases in 1RM values for the 2-inch and 3-inch bars, respectively, as compared with an Olympic bar. Moreover, these measures correlate significantly with isometric grip strength (48). These data suggest that selecting ergonomically appropriate

equipment will minimize extraneous muscle fatigue and difficulty maintaining posture and body mechanics.

Dynamometry is a testing modality currently used to assess force-generation capability and performance associated with activities during which the load or movement velocity remains constant. Various forms of dynamometry are useful for evaluating *isotonic*, *isokinetic*, and *isometric* contractions.

Power is defined as the rate at which mechanical work is performed under a defined set of conditions. This parameter is of particular interest to many athletes and professional trainers and should be evaluated within the context of a given event (1). Although strength and power are closely related and are often considered in tandem, for optimal measures they should be evaluated independently. Dynamometric evaluation of strength and power is possible, although methodologically challenging. Athletic skills and events often involve considerable variability, making the biomechanics difficult to isolate and evaluate independently and in real time. Technology, such as digital movement analysis, has advanced dramatically and has allowed for these data to be routinely applied to training programs. Identifying the load for peak power output is often the variable to be quantified. However, assessment of maximal or near maximal power output is possible through incremental loading of working muscle (24). This recent finding diminishes the importance of identifying one load for maximal power output in athletes. Although significant progress has been made, current understanding of power and force capacity related to human biomechanics is incomplete; therefore, our ability to apply assessment methodologies to actual events is limited.

Isometric dynamometry measures MVC achieved at specific joint angles against a fixed object. Muscle tension is quantified by a device connected to a strain gauge, cable tensiometer, force platform, or force transducer. This information is subsequently conveyed to the patient or trainer and provides a useful index of strength at a given joint angle (58). Isometric MVC varies, as both joint angles and muscle angles of pull change; therefore, one must conduct serial muscle strength assessments at exactly the same joint angles. Test-retest reliability of isometric dynamometry depends on the consistency of the joint angle, among other parameters (29) (Box 20-4). During isometric training, muscular strength benefits may be realized at the joint angle maintained during contraction, with a potential carryover effect extending to ±15 degrees from the training position. Isometric exercises may also be effective when training individuals for whom movement elicits pain, such as those with rheumatoid arthritis or orthopedic injuries. Initiating muscle contraction at a fixed angle may not provoke the magnitude of pain that occurs with dynamic exercise.

The *rate of force development* (RFD) is often used to assess athletic power; it represents the muscular force produced immediately upon contraction and is commonly measured using isometric dynamometry. Despite the lack of dynamic measures involved with this assessment, RFD

BOX 20-3 REPETITION MAXIMUM TESTING PROCEDURE

1. Complete a light warm-up with muscle groups to be tested
2. 1-minute rest period
3. Estimate and complete movement with a workload that will allow three to five repetitions to fatigue
4. 2-minute rest period
5. Estimate near maximum workload and complete set to fatigue
6. 2-minute rest period
7. Increase load progressively for one to three additional sets until maximum load completed for 1RM is achieved
8. If single repetition is failed, reduce load by 2.5% to 5% for upper-body or 5% to 10% for lower-body exercises
9. Reattempt 1RM

Set is completed either when two to three repetitions are completed successfully or form is compromised during subsequent repetitions; 1RM must be completed, maintaining proper biomechanical form for the exercise. Retesting should be completed using identical procedures to ensure reliability of measures.

BOX 20-4	CONSIDERATIONS FOR TEST–RETEST RELIABILITY AND CONSISTENCY (20)

SUBJECT-RELATED FACTORS

- Age
- Sex
- Weight
- Athletic conditioning
- Orthopedic disability
- Side dominance

TESTING-RELATED FACTORS

- Warm-up procedures
- Starting position and posture
- Joint stabilization
- Alignment of anatomic and dynamometer axis of rotation
- Lever arm length and position
- Muscle preloading and/or stretch reflex

DURING MOVEMENT

- Velocity of contraction
- Rest intervals
- Patient feedback
- Joint angle and ROM tested
- Mode of contraction (isometric, isokinetic, isodynamic)

POSTTESTING

- Type of data analyzed
- Data analysis

has reliably predicted athletic performance requiring sudden bursts of muscular strength (28,37). A high jumper, for example, requires a sudden burst of strength from leg extensor muscles to clear the height of the bar. Immediate force development is crucial to overcome gravitational forces adequately to complete the jump successfully. Although the propelling movements may be difficult to assess, RFD provides a useful measure when evaluating a high jumper's potential performance.

When assessing the utility of isometric dynamometry, consider the subject's posture, body mechanics, and how difficult the position might be to reproduce. Careful attention must be paid to such details to extrapolate these data to potential performance indicators. Isometric tests should mimic specific tasks as closely as possible. Accordingly, testing angles should approximate to those at which peak force generation is required for a given movement or activity. Some authorities suggest testing should be done only at the angle of insertion capable of greatest force generation (for example, 90 degrees for the biceps brachii in elbow flexion), which would improve retest reliability (1).

Isoinertial dynamometry refers to continuous resistance to movement and accurately describes external loading through a ROM as in weight lifting or training. Although RT is often characterized as isotonic, isoinertial reflects the change in load as joint angle varies, thereby increasing or decreasing the mechanical leverage of the joint. Isotonic is used for constant and equal loading throughout a ROM or action. A maximum isoinertial force is a measure of a person's 1RM as previously described, and because of its dynamic nature, it has greater usefulness and practical application than isometric measures. Measurements of isoinertial force capability are performed using weighted systems (e.g., weighted squat jump), machines with loading throughout the ROM, or hydraulic loading devices.

One repetition maximum testing offers excellent test-retest reliability for field studies and can be employed to assess maximal isoinertial force. However, regression equations that have been developed to predict may often overestimate actual measured values. Overestimation of a person's strength may be potentially hazardous at high loads as orthopedic injuries and cardiovascular events are more likely to occur. Trainer intuition and progressive overloading should be used to evaluate strength for given exercises, thereby reducing the potential for musculoskeletal injury and related complications.

Isokinetic dynamometry measures torque and power through the ROM when the joint angular velocity remains constant. Analysis of agonist/antagonist torque, analysis of power-velocity and torque-velocity curves, and comparisons between limbs are representative applications of such devices. Researchers commonly use isokinetic dynamometry with excellent reliability and consistency, as numerous extraneous variables can be accounted for and eliminated. It might be difficult to extrapolate measurements into practical applications because isolation of individual movements is rarely seen in sports or activities of daily living. Isokinetic evaluations have been used extensively in endurance studies, physical rehabilitation, and biomechanical analysis, and to further clarify the intricacies of movement with good *internal validity*. The last suggests that there is a causal relationship between a treatment or stimulus and an outcome from which a therapist might draw conclusions.

In addition to dynamometry, tensiometers are instruments commonly used for measuring isometric strength. Tensiometers include a steel cable, a testing table, wall hooks, and a goniometer. A strap is attached to the moving limb while the cable is fixed to an immovable object, placing the joint at the desired angle for measurement based on the goniometer reading (see flexibility assessment section for discussion of goniometers). The patient is asked to exert as much force as possible against the strap (maximal contraction) and hold for a minimum of 5 seconds. The tensiometer measures the maximum force exerted in pounds. Muscular strength at several joint angles can be measured during a testing session. Three trials should be completed, with the highest measure recorded as strength at a given joint angle.

TESTING SAFETY AND EQUIPMENT CONSIDERATIONS

A gradual and progressive, pretest warm up is recommended prior to resistance training and testing. The warm-up serves to increase blood flow to primary muscles and connective tissues and may reduce the risk of injury during testing; moreover, it should be part of a well-designed RT program. During the maximal lift, proper posture and mechanics must be maintained to maximize contractile force capabilities of agonist muscle(s). It is recommended that the eccentric phase of a lift be completed with half the velocity of the concentric phase. *Concentric* lifting time of 3 to 5 seconds is appropriate to achieve MVC for the lift and ensures volitional fatigue in muscle fibers; however, exercise intensity and overload is greater during the *eccentric* phase of movement. Initial weight can be accurately estimated based on previous training loads, self-reported lifting capability, or a practice set performed before the testing (17). Rest between successive attempts should be no less than 3 minutes to ensure full recovery of muscle fibers until a second repetition cannot be completed.

In addition to muscular strength assessment, 1RM may also be used to estimate training levels for a given exercise. Once 1RM is determined, considerable information can be extracted. As previously discussed, to stimulate appropriate muscle protein synthesis for hypertrophy, higher weights (60%–80% 1RM) may be used during a particular exercise (12). For endurance improvements, a lighter load (up to 50% of 1RM) is used for the same exercise, using more repetitions (12). These 1RM percentages will vary with patients with a chronic disease (e.g. heart disease) age and ASM versus leg exercise. Knowledge of a person's 1RM is crucial when attempting to maximize eccentric contraction using muscular overload during a particular exercise. Accordingly, loading with 110% to 130% of 1RM, eccentric contractions are maximized until muscle fiber failure occurs. Heavy eccentric training, however, should only be done with appropriate supervision.

Retesting provides measurable outcomes of the training program and should be done with consistency. To ensure the retest is valid, careful consideration to reproducing the baseline methodology should be used. If testing was initially done on resistance training equipment, the same equipment should be used for retesting. More complex movements, however, may be more difficult to recreate.

For example, the environment during a vertical jump test should be carefully recorded initially and reconstructed using the same equipment, flooring, and footwear. Measured strength gains after a given training program provide useful feedback and motivation to the patient and are valid if testing was done appropriately before, at given intervals, and after the physical conditioning regimen. Although regression equations may be used to predict 1RM, some professionals have used isometric grip strength to predict overall muscle strength; however, this methodology has limitations for predicting 1RM (49,50).

Although 1RM is an excellent measure of force generation and power capabilities, functional performance is often of greater interest in athletics and during activities of daily living. Strength is often a poor predictor of skill and performance during a given task (34). There appears to be no relationship between the relative improvement in 1RM and functional performance in skilled athletes (40). Optimal performance in dynamic skills requires unique physical attributes; moreover, improvements in performance are not always paralleled by increases in muscular strength (40). Relative muscle endurance was found to accurately predict 1RM bench press in college students after a RT program (34), suggesting that this methodology may provide reliable estimations of strength.

Although many athletic RT regimens emphasize strength and power improvements, training effectiveness should be evaluated beyond the MVC and include functional performance tests, such as the athlete's vertical jump or sprint times (42). Testing protocols specifically designed for a given sport or event are more accurate for evaluating performance of the skills involved, rather than for making predictions based on other parameters. For example, standard anthropometric, strength, and power assessments were shown to be inadequate predictors of sprint performance (32). Similarly, isometric testing of muscle activation and force development at various joint angles proved to be a poor predictor of dynamic performance (41), further demonstrating the need to measure performance variables beyond the MVC.

RELIABILITY OF ASSESSMENT

> **1.1.24-HFS: Knowledge of muscle fatigue as it relates to mode, intensity, duration, and the accumulative effects of exercise.**

> **1.3.20-HFS: Ability to analyze and interpret information obtained from the cardiorespiratory fitness test and the muscular strength and endurance, flexibility, and body composition assessments for apparently healthy individuals and those with controlled chronic diseases.**

The test-retest reliability of isokinetic, isometric, and isoinertial dynamometry is normally high; however, one should consider all variables before reporting and applying data from any assessment. Factors influencing reliability during testing include the individual's athletic ability, instructions provided, recent bouts of exertion to fatigue, selected testing angles, postures, and, most importantly, a standardized testing environment. Although many of these variables are often controlled and/or explained with ease, one must consider them before investing time and effort into the procedures. Consistency in performing assessment tests is paramount to translating findings into practice (29). Potentially confounding variables during comparison include athletic history, subject age and anthropometrics, rest between tests, points of resistance application, joint axis alignment, specific equipment utilized during assessment, and whether positive/negative feedback was given to participants. Biomechanical torque production will vary based on joint angle measurements and the position in which neutral or zero angles are determined. During a knee extension, for example, minimal consistency is noted throughout the literature, allowing for variability in the reports of torque production (29). Consistency in the velocity of muscular contraction during a given range of motion is also crucial for retesting, as the force-velocity curve demonstrates (discussed elsewhere). Such an oversight will lead to inconclusive data. Box 20-4 summarizes some considerations during testing and retesting of muscular strength and performance.

In practice, strength is often assessed by a therapist or athletic trainer using *manual muscle testing*. Relative unilateral strength is commonly used to establish a baseline or monitor progress during rehabilitation. The patient is asked to move through either a full ROM or to their pain threshold. At the end of the ROM, the therapist or trainer provides immovable stationary resistance on the movement and requests an isometric contraction from the patient. Force production is scored numerically by the therapist on a subjective scale ranging from 0 to 5. Zero represents no perceivable contraction, whereas 5 demonstrates complete ROM without difficulty resisting. A subjective assessment such as this, although common, may be confounded by the examiner's ability to produce more force than the test subject through a given ROM (39). If, for example, more torque force is produced by the patient than the therapist, weakness becomes difficult or impossible to detect. This scenario may be significantly limiting with a lower-extremity test (e.g., knee extension) and an examiner with insufficient leverage, either from lower relative muscular strength or ineffective mechanical positioning (39). Although the reliability of manual muscle testing may be low, this methodology has proven to be useful for subjective assessment and field testing of varied movements and muscle groups.

As is the case with most objective measures, such as muscular strength and flexibility, assessments must be both *valid* and *reliable*. A reliable test will essentially replicate the same results under the same conditions, whereas a valid one will measure what it is intended to be measured. Careful attention must be paid to ensure testing validity, thereby reporting accurate and applicable physiologic responses. Conversely, an invalid test might still be repeatable, and therefore will still be reliable.

CLINICAL RELEVANCE AND APPLICATION

> **1.3.20-HFS: Ability to analyze and interpret information obtained from the cardiorespiratory fitness test and the muscular strength and endurance, flexibility, and body composition assessments for apparently healthy individuals and those with controlled chronic diseases.**

Strength and movement efficiency are measured using dynamometry and other methods that may be useful when attempting to predict a person's health and/or performance of activities of daily living or athletic skills. Testing should be specific to the movement or physical challenge (i.e., athletics, rehabilitation); however, the prognostic value of performance testing decreases with more complex sports or activities. For example, if an athlete is tested for power generated during a vertical jump, it will not necessarily translate into his or her timing or speed during a 100-m sprint (41). If testing is performance specific and sport oriented, it may be possible to reliably predict athletic performance in a competitive environment.

Test-specific training is accepted for performance outcome measures where necessary or applicable (i.e., lower-extremity power training for vertical jump test performance during basketball tryouts). However, changes to an athlete's training program should not be based on modulations in actual performance, rather on performance measures. Isokinetic and isometric test results are widely considered poor predictors of training-induced performance improvements (38,41,58). Trainers should perform an activity needs assessment and closely match testing protocols with desired performance outcomes whenever possible.

As is the case with many testing protocols and procedures, normative or average data are desired for comparison. Reliable data are often unavailable for accurate comparisons because of significant variability in testing procedures, equipment used, and individual parameters that are inadequately controlled for across study groups (i.e., prior training, medical history, orthopedic limitations, etc.). There are, however, normative values for widely used and reproducible movements, such as the vertical jump, grip strength, curl-ups, and leg power production (watts), that can be used for comparison with other individuals of similar age and body weight (44). Table 20-3 provides an example of bench press normative data.

Analysis or results from such testing can be useful for goal setting, training program design, and individual motivation for initiating or modifying a training program. When adequate normative values for muscle strength are not available, relative comparisons may become necessary. Comparative pre- and posttraining assessments are common among teams and small groups for movements or skills that do not have normative data available. Although not advised for widespread recommendation, such techniques may be used for motivation or to evaluate a given group of athletes or individuals. For example, bench press data may not be specific to football offensive linemen; however, upper-body strength was identified as a measurement of interest by this cohort. Relative to those on the team, testing and retesting provides baseline, averages, and improvements. The latter is especially important for gauging the effectiveness of varied training regimens or protocols. Similarly, power skating is paramount to success as a hockey player; however, data may not be available for a specific level of player for speed between blue lines on a hockey rink. Simple field testing of explosive power translating to speed over this distance can easily demonstrate associated improvements after a specific training program.

BODY STATURE AND TESTING

> **1.1.34-HFS: Knowledge of the effect of the aging process on the musculoskeletal and cardiovascular structure and function at rest, during exercise, and during recovery.**

It has been theorized that increasing body mass will translate into increased force production capabilities. As a trained person's body mass increases, muscle cross-section also increases, thereby providing additional force generation capabilities or strength (27). Conversely, individuals with longer limbs should be able to generate higher angular velocities that would affect their torque generation capabilities. If individuals are considered geometrically similar and moment arms change proportionally to a segment's length (Fig. 20-2), torque potential should be consistent across all body types. Consequently, differences in force production capability are proportional to anatomic cross-section of skeletal muscle, not mechanical leverage, and have been normalized for body size mathematically.

As previously discussed, anatomic force arms are measured from the joint center (fulcrum) and the point of muscular insertion. This distance is genetically determined, and a small difference in force arm size can have major effects both on muscle recruitment and torque-generating capabilities. Anatomic force arm length varies considerably between individuals and may be related to body stature. However, this theory and its application are limited by a lack of consideration or correction for body composition, specifically lean body mass as well as subject age. Because aging is associated with atrophy and sarcopenia, significant changes in torque-generation capability may be largely age related. Normalization techniques are available and applicable for increased reliability of outcomes for muscle strength testing; however, body size remains an independent variable to consider relative to functional performance (27).

As training programs progress from beginner to advanced levels, careful consideration must be paid to assessment techniques and how these influence exercise prescription. Whether working with an Olympic power lifter or a weekend warrior, the exercise professional must be aware of the patient's current physical capabilities to establish training goals and objectives. For muscle strength testing to be worthwhile, as many variables as possible should be considered. Increasingly, performance testing will become more sophisticated and computer based; however, patient safety remains the most important focus and concern.

TECHNOLOGIC INSTRUMENTATION

Development of computerized equipment and instruments has accelerated dramatically over the past two decades. From video imaging to digital re-creation of the most complex athletic skills and movements, technology provides opportunity for creative exercise design, including training specificity. Dynamic force output is commonly measured using computer-aided isokinetic dynamometers. Resistance is modulated to match the force generated by the muscle and torque output, respectively.

Electromyography (EMG) is the study of motor unit activity in skeletal muscle. During movement, the EMG graphically records electrical activity stimulated by individual motor units. Isolating individual muscles involved in a given movement is achieved by proper placement of electrodes. From complex athletic movements to pathologic muscular conditions, EMG testing can provide valuable adjunctive analyses to a testing laboratory. A thorough and working knowledge of neuromuscular anatomy is critical for effective EMG testing. Development of treatment strategies and training programs can be greatly enhanced using EMG equipment, when available.

Computer-generated animations allow therapists and trainers to design physical conditioning programs specifically for complex, dynamic, and high-velocity movements. Segmentation of movements (i.e., pitcher's arm during throwing motion) now permits a complete and thorough analysis, potentially identifying areas of improvement or potential injury. In highly skilled athletes, a competitive edge is crucial. Digital analysis of the sport's movement patterns may provide this opportunity for sport-specific training.

Beyond movement analysis, technology is providing opportunities to study effects of training interventions on biological and physiologic markers. Skeletal muscle proteins, tissue adaptations, and early-response genes are being isolated and studied, which may lead to innovative training techniques and new concepts for musculoskeletal fitness (12). Knowledge of mechanisms and exercise-induced adaptation pathways in skeletal muscle is important for our understanding of disease processes, attenuation of the aging process, and peak performance in athletics (12).

As noted above, specificity of training remains an important thread in assessment techniques. Technologic advances may be paralleled by higher levels of performance. Training regimens and exercise program design must be modified according to new information and advancing technology to meet this objective. Similarly, in clinical settings, patients may be provided with enhanced specificity in their rehabilitation and regimens that potentially offer accelerated recoveries.

FLEXIBILITY AND RANGE OF MOTION

ASSESSMENT

> **1.1.3-HFS: Knowledge of the following muscle action terms: inferior, superior, medial, lateral, supination, pronation, flexion, extension, adduction, abduction, hyperextension, rotation, circumduction, agonist, antagonist, and stabilizer.**

Every joint in the body has an acceptable ROM, which is dependent on a variety of factors, including genetics, orthopedic health, surgeries to the articulating bones or joints, muscular tension, and strength. The joint's ability to pass through a given ROM without significant impingement or restriction is its *flexibility*. Measurement and assessment of flexibility and ROM is particularly useful in athletic training, rehabilitation, and conditioning settings; however, the findings can be misleading if performed without standard procedures, calibration, and instruments. Table 20-5 shows estimates of normal ROM in male subjects. A variety of measuring procedures exists that may lead modest variability of measurements.

The most common instrument used for measuring joint ROM is the two-arm *goniometer* (Fig. 20-5). This device is portable, relatively easy to use, and inexpensive; moreover, the measurements obtained are highly reproducible. The transparent plastic device includes two arms with a protractor for measuring degrees of joint displacement. One arm remains fixed to the proximal articulating segment, and the other adjusts through the ROM with the distal segment, measuring the resulting degree of move-

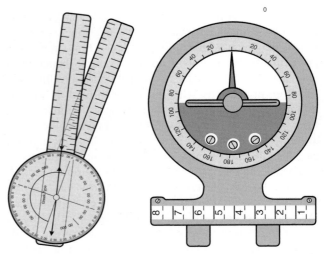

FIGURE 20-5. Devices used for measuring joint range of motion. *Left:* standard goniometer. *Right:* mechanical inclinometer.

ment. The center of the protractor remains fixed at the joints' axis of rotation. Limitations of the conventional goniometer include difficulty stabilizing moving segments and visually determining a vertical axis; however, impressive validity and reliability has been demonstrated if proper procedures are followed (33). Goniometers of various size and shapes have been developed to minimize limitations of the traditional design and allow for accurate measurement with small and larger joints (33).

Spinal and other complex movements, including supination, pronation, ankle inversion, and eversion, are difficult if not impossible to assess with a traditional goniometer. Such data are more accurately measured using an *inclinometer* (Fig. 20-5). Inclinometers use a universal center of gravity to establish a starting point that remains constant from test to test. The pendulum-weighted inclinometer indicates degrees of motion using a weighted needle and protractor. Difficulties positioning and securing the device has led to its modification and alteration. This makes both electronic and mechanical inclinometers adaptable and reliable in a variety of situations and environments (33).

A recommendation from the American Medical Association (4) suggests that ROM should be measured using three consecutive trials and averaged as the true value. If the average ROM is 50 degrees, three of the measurements must fall within ±5 degrees of the mean. If the average is <50 degrees, three measurements must fall within 10 degrees of average. Such measures may be taken up to six times, until they meet the criteria; otherwise, they are considered invalid (33).

Range of motion of the spine and other joints can be accurately evaluated using video motion analysis. Originally used in gait analysis by kinesiology laboratories, the technology has been adapted for measurement of ROM in given joints. Both postural angles and dynamic movement capabilities may be measured using these techniques. Dynamic

TABLE 20-4. LOAD-REPETITION RELATIONSHIPS FOR RESISTANCE TRAINING

% 1RM	REPETITIONS POSSIBLE, n
60	17
70	12
80	8
90	5
100	1

1RM, one repetitive maximum.

From Williams M, Haskell W, Ades P, et al. Resistance exercise in individuals with and without cardiovascular disease: 2007 update: a scientific statement from the American Heart Association Council on Nutrition, Physical Activity, and Metabolism. *Circulation.* 2007;116:572–584.

rather than static studies more accurately measure naturally occurring movements. *Digitation* utilizes reflective markers placed on the skin as reference points. Range of motion is measured based on angular changes during movement. Validity and reliability of testing and retesting measurements can vary with reference reflector placement (33).

FACTORS INFLUENCING RELIABILITY AND VALIDITY

 1.1.7-HFS: Knowledge of the stretch reflex and how it relates to flexibility.

 1.3.18-HFS: Ability to describe the purpose of testing, determine appropriate protocols, and perform assessments of muscular strength, muscular endurance, and flexibility.

As with strength testing, consistency and accuracy during flexibility assessment are critical. Several factors that may compromise accuracy include anatomic landmark identification, positioning and stabilization of the body, application and stabilization of the measurement device, consistency in technique and protocol, appropriate recording of measures, and recognition of limiting factors or situations during recording. In order for a specific joint ROM to be compared with available norms, standardized landmarks for each measurement should be identified and used whenever possible. Several commonly measured joints have standard landmarks identified and should be used consistently when measuring ROM, including the knee, elbow, hip, and ankle. Inaccurate identification of bony or surface landmarks is a common source of error during assessment; therefore, knowledge of surface anatomy is required before accurate measurements can be recorded. Several authors have reported ROM measures and techniques that vary considerably from those of the American Medical Association (4) standards discussed in this chapter. Table 20-5 provides ROM norms expressed as degrees according to the American Academy of Orthopedic Surgeons (10).

When using a goniometer, the proximal segment of the joint should be stabilized, and the distal segment remains freely moveable. Body position should be conducive to the movement being measured and comfortable for the subject. Joints can be measured in varied positions; however, reliability depends on reproducibility of the position. The patient should be able to maintain the given position without extraneous movement during the measurement. Careful consideration of the movement requirements and complexity should be made before selecting the appropriate assessment tool.

In addition to stabilizing body segments, the measurement device must also be properly positioned to ensure data accuracy. The technician should be familiar with the device being used, as well as the methodology and biomechanics. Inappropriate placement and use of the

TABLE 20-5. AVERAGE RANGE OF MOTION ESTIMATES FROM THE AMERICAN ACADEMY OF ORTHOPEDIC SURGEONS

JOINT	MOVEMENT	AVERAGE ROM (IN DEGREES)
Shoulder		
	Horizontal flexion	135
	Horizontal	—
	Neural abduction	170
	Flexion	158
	Extension	53
	Internal rotation	70
	External rotation	90
Elbow		
	Flexion	146
	Extension	0
Forearm		
	Pronation	71
	Supination	84
Wrist		
	Flexion	73
	Extension	71
	Radial deviation	19
	Ulnar deviation	33
Hip		
	Flexion	113
	Extension	28
	Abduction	48
	Adduction	31
	Internal rotation	45
	External rotation	45
Knee		
	Flexion	134
	Extension	0
Ankle		
	Plantar flexion	48
	Dorsi flexion	18
Foot		
	Inversion	33
	Eversion	18

ROM, range of motion.

From Boone D, Azen S. Normal range of motion of joints in male subjects. *J Bone Joint Surg.* 1979;61-A(5):756–759.

device represents a major source of error in many studies examining ROM (33). On the other hand, limitations based on equipment design are inevitable. As a result of its size and shape, for example, the inclinometer is often more difficult to stabilize than a traditional goniometer, causing it to move or wobble during measurements. Mounting devices for inclinometers have been developed that may reduce the associated measurement error. In addition to device size and shape, stabilizing tools against limbs and joints with pathology and pain (such as in rheumatoid arthritis or scleroderma) may pose a challenge for assessors. Repeated adjustment of device position may be required in such cases.

Range of motion measurements are most accurately made using a universal starting point with the body in the *anatomic position*. Anatomic position is defined by a person standing upright, feet facing forward, arms resting at their sides with palms facing forward (anterior). Standard points of reference are important for consistency in reporting data and for retesting purposes. For example, Table 20-5 lists elbow extension as a movement with 0 degrees of ROM. In the anatomic position, the elbow is fully extended and is a natural starting point for measurement. However, what is considered anatomic "zero" may be different in this scenario if the patient has a shorter-than-normal olecranon process, allowing the elbow to extend beyond standard anatomic position. Detailed recording and reproducible methodology are important in this case to allow for accurate retesting.

Basic understanding of anatomy and the movement being measured is helpful during testing. The ROM being tested often involves complex movements or postures, and reproduction through several trials may be required for accurate measurement. Therefore, adequate instruction and practice by the patient may be warranted. This will not only increase the reproducibility and reliability of the measurements, it will also provide a warm-up for the joint(s) being measured. Some questions remain regarding the optimal number of repetitions required for accurate measurement; however, most authorities favor multiple repetitions and either a "best number" or average value recorded as the ROM (33,44). Using different devices for retesting is not advised, as reliability is compromised. Likewise, measurements such as ROM and flexibility should be re-evaluated by the same technician whenever possible. Moreover, accuracy of retesting is improved if initial procedures are well documented and the methodology and equipment are replicated in several studies.

SIT-AND-REACH EVALUATION

 1.3.18-HFS: Ability to describe the purpose of testing, determine appropriate protocols, and perform assessments of muscular strength, muscular endurance, and flexibility.

Hamstring and lower back flexibility are often measured using a *sit-and-reach test*. Done either with a sit-and-reach box or with a properly placed tape measure, this test is valid and reliable for evaluating general flexibility. The box has a fixed ruler that will measure the farthest point the patient reaches during three trials, which should be considered their numeric score for subsequent comparison. The patient is instructed to sit comfortably, legs extended, with their feet positioned against the measuring box and toes pointed upward. He/she bends forward from the waist, reaching forward with their fingertips as far as possible, holding the position for 2 seconds without bouncing, with farthest distance reached on the box or measuring tape being recorded. The methodology should incorporate a preliminary warm-up before any flexibility assessment, including the sit and reach.

STRETCHING

 1.1.7-HFS: Knowledge of the stretch reflex and how it relates to flexibility.

Along with RT and cardiovascular exercise, flexibility training is part of a complete training program. Athletes, healthy and aging adults, and those with chronic disease affecting muscular performance may benefit from participation in a flexibility program (30,47). The primary goal of stretching is to alter tendon inflexibility, which contributes to a reduced joint ROM; specifically, elasticity is improved acutely and chronically through stretching. This results in both a transient increase in musculotendon unit length resulting from actin-myosin complex relaxation (52) and chronic alteration of the extracellular matrix (54). Stretching should be incorporated into warm-up and cool-down phases of exercise (47).

Stretching programs will vary depending on specific goals: whether for improved athletic performance, injury rehabilitation, or general fitness. The volume of stretching required for a positive effect may vary. Three primary forms of stretching are presented: static, *proprioceptive neuromuscular facilitation* (PNF), and dynamic stretching. *Static*, as the term implies, is done with no movement either passively or actively. The muscle is moved into position and held for several seconds (15–60 seconds is recommended by the American College of Sports Medicine [47]), not beyond mild discomfort. The stretch may be repeated; however, research has not shown a great deal of benefit with repeating beyond four cycles (54). PNF, also termed *tense/relax*, combines isometric contraction with passive static stretching in series for a specific muscle. Isometric contraction for 6 seconds is followed with 10 to 30 seconds of passive stretching and repeated. *Dynamic* stretching involves movement of the targeted joint. Different from *ballistic*, dynamic stretching incorporates muscle tension development and is performed actively. This technique has been described as a sport- or function-specific warm-up (26). Ballistic stretching involves bouncing, or rapid movements, in an attempt to hold the motion at peak tension. For example, for the sit-and-reach test, correct form is a slow reach to maximal tension, a brief hold of the position, and a return to resting. This would be a static, active stretch. Trying to maximize the test by bouncing forward and pushing the limit would be considered ballistic.

Muscle groups isolated during exercise and/or muscles crossing major moving joints should be stretched two to three times each week or more. Although stretching may be done any time of the day for beneficial results, a warm-up or exercise stimulus should precede it. It has been thought that stretching before an athletic event would help with force production, performance, and delay soreness associated with training. However, recent research suggests that acute bouts of stretching might have detrimental effects on performance parameters, such as jumping ability (6), balance (31), reaction time, and torque-generation capabilities

(31). Consensus remains, however, that stretching is an important component of exercise and should be incorporated into musculoskeletal analysis, fitness, and training.

REFERENCES

1. Abernethy P, Wilson G, Logan P. Strength and power assessment: issues, controversies, and challenges. *Sports Med.* 1996;19(6): 401–417.
2. Adams KJ, Barnard KL, Swank AM, Mann E, Kushnick MR, Denny DM. Combined high-intensity strength and aerobic training in diverse phase II cardiac rehabilitation patients. *J Cardiopulm Rehabil.* 1999;19(4):209–215.
3. **American College of Sports Medicine. Position Stand on progression models in resistance training for healthy adults.** *Med Sci Sports Exerc.* 2002;34(2):364–380.
4. American Medical Association. *Guides to the Evaluation of Permanent Impairment.* 4th ed. Chicago: American Medical Association; 1993.
5. Antonio J, Gonyea WJ. Skeletal muscle hyperplasia. *Med Sci Sports Exerc.* 1993;25(12):1333–1345.
6. Behm DG, Kibele A. Effects of differing intensities of static stretching on jump performance. *Eur J Appl Physiol.* 2007;101(5): 587–594.
7. Beniamini Y, Rubenstein JJ, Faigenbaum AD, Lichtenstien AH, Crim MC. High-intensity strength training of patients enrolled in an outpatient cardiac rehabilitation program. *J Cardiopulm Rehabil.* 1999;19(1):8–17.
8. Beniamini Y, Rubenstein JJ, Zaichkowsky LD, Crim MC. Effects of high-intensity strength training on quality of life parameters in cardiac rehabilitation patients. *Am J Cardiol.* 1997;80(7):841–846.
9. Blazevich AJ, Cannavan D, Coleman DR, Horne S. Influence of concentric and eccentric resistance training on architectural adaptation in human quadriceps muscles. *J Appl Physiol.* 2007;103(5): 1565–1575.
10. Boone D, Azen S. Normal range of motion of joints in male subjects. *J Bone Joint Surg.* 1979;61-A(5):756–759.
11. Brzycki M. Strength testing: predicting a one-rep max from a reps-to-fatigue. *Journal of Physical Education, Recreation and Dance.* 1993;64(1):88–90.
12. Coffey VG, Hawley JA. The molecular bases of training adaptation. *Sports Med.* 2007;37(9):737–763.
13. Cronin JB, Jones JV, Hagstrom JT. Kinematics and kinetics of the seated row and implications for conditioning. *J Strength Cond Res.* 2007;21(4):1265–1270.
14. DeGroot DW, Quinn TJ, Kertzer R, Vroman NB, Olney WB. Circuit weight training in cardiac patients: determining optimal workloads and safety for energy expenditure. *J Cardiopulm Rehabil.* 1998; 18(2):145–152.
15. Estrada M, Kleppinger A, Judge JO, Walsh SJ, Kuchel GA. Functional impact of relative versus absolute sarcopenia in healthy older women. *J Am Geriatr Soc.* 2007;55(11):1712–1719.
16. Fernandez, R. One repetition maximum clarified. *J Orthop Sports Phys Ther.* 2001;31:264.
17. Fleck SJ, Kraemer WJ. *Designing Resistance Training Programs.* Champaign (IL): Human Kinetics; 1987.
18. Franklin BA, Bonzheim K, Gordon S, Timmis GC. Snow shoveling: a trigger for acute myocardial infarction and sudden coronary death. *Am J Cardiol.* 1996;77:855–858.
19. Fuglevand AJ, Segal SS. Simulation of motor unit recruitment and microvascular unit perfusion: spatial considerations. *J Appl Physiol.* 1997;83(4):1223–1234.
20. Grimsby O. More on 1RM testing. *J Orthpo Sports Phys Ther.* 2001;31:264–265.
21. Guzel NA, Hazar S, Erbas D. Effects of different resistance exercise protocols on nitric oxide, lipid peroxidization and creatine kinase activity in sedentary males. *J Sports Sci Med.* 2007;6:417–422.
22. Hagerman FC, Walsh WJ, Staron RS, et al. Effects of high-intensity resistance training on untrained older men. I. Strength, cardiovascular, and metabolic responses. *J Gerontol.* 2000;55A(7):B336–B346.
23. Hale T. History of developments in sport and exercise physiology: A.V. Hill, maximal oxygen uptake and oxygen debt. *J Sports Sci.* 2008;26(4):365–400.
24. Harris NK, Cronin JB, Hopkins WG. Power outputs of a machine squat-jump across a spectrum of loads. *J Strength Cond Res.* 2007; 21(4):1260–1264.
25. Hather BM, Tesch PA, Buchanan P, Dudley GA. Influence of eccentric actions on skeletal muscle adaptations to resistance training. *Acta Physiol Scand.* 1991;143:177–185.
26. Holcomb WR. Stretching and warm up. In: Baechle TR, Earle RW, editors. *Essentials of Strength Training and Conditioning.* 2nd ed. Champaign (IL): Human Kinetics; 2000. p. 321–342.
27. Jaric S. Muscle strength testing: use of normalization for body size. *Sports Med.* 2002;32(10):615–631.
28. Jaric S, Ristanovc D, Corcos M. The relationship between muscle kinetic parameters and kinetic variables in a complex movement. *Eur J Appl Physiol.* 1989;59:770–776.
29. Keating J, Matyas T. The influence of subject and test design on dynamometric measurements of extremity muscles. *Phys Ther.* 1996;76(8):866–889.
30. Kokkonen J, Nelson AG, Eldredge C, Winchester JB. Chronic static stretching improves exercise performance. *Med Sci Sports Exerc.* 2007;39(10):1825–1831.
31. Kreighbaum E, Barthels K. *Biomechanics: A Qualitative Approach for Studying Human Movement.* New York: Allyn and Bacon; 1996.
32. Kukolj M, Ropret R, Ugarokovic D, Jaric S. Anthropometric, strength, and power predictors of sprinting performance. *J Sports Med Phys Fitness.* 1999;39:120–122.
33. Lea R, Gerhardt J. Current concepts review: range of motion measurements. *J Bone Joint Surg.* 1995;77(5):784–798.
34. Mayhew JL, Ball TE, Arnold MD, Bowen JC. Relative muscular endurance performance as a predictor of bench press strength in college men and women. *J Appl Sports Sci Res.* 1992;6(4):200–206.
35. McCall GE, Byrnes WC, Dickinson A, Pattany PM, Fleck SJ. Muscle fiber hypertrophy, hyperplasia, and capillary density in college men after resistance training. *J Appl Physiol.* 1996;81(5):2004–2012.
36. McCartney N, McKelvie RS, Haslam DR, Jones NL. Usefulness of weightlifting training in improving strength and maximal power output in coronary artery disease. *Am J Cardiol.* 1991;67(11): 939–945.
37. Mero A, Luhtanen P, Viitasalo T. Relationship between maximal running velocity, muscle fibre, characteristics, force production, and force relaxation of sprinters. *Scand J Sports Sci.* 1981;3: 16–22.
38. Mirkov D, Nedeljkovic A, Milanovic S, Jaric S. Muscle strength testing: evaluation of tests of explosive force production. *Eur J Appl Physiol.* 2004;91:147–154.
39. Mulroy S, Lassen K, Chambers S, Perry J. The ability of male and female clinicians to effectively test knee extension strength using manual muscle testing. *J Orthop Sports Phys Ther.* 1997;26(4): 192–199.
40. Murphy AJ, Wilson GJ. Poor correlations between isometric tests and dynamic performance: relationship to muscle activation. *Eur J Appl Physiol.* 1996;73:353–357.
41. Murphy AJ, Wilson GJ. The ability of tests of muscular function to reflect training-induced changes in performance. *J Sports Sci.* 1997; 15:191–200.
42. Murphy A, Wilson G. The assessment of human dynamic muscular function: a comparison of isoinertial and isokinetic tests. *J Sports Med Phys Fitness.* 1996;36(3):169–177.
43. Okamoto T, Masuhara M, Ikuata K. Combined aerobic and resistance training and vascular function: effect of aerobic exercise before and after resistance training. *J Appl Physiol.* 2007;103(5): 1655–1661.
44. Payne N, Gledhill N, Katzmarzyk P, Jamnik P, Keir P. Canadian muskuloskeletal fitness norms. *Can J Appl Physiol.* 2000;25(6): 430–442.

45. Pierson LM, Herbert WG, Norton HJ, et al. Effects of combined aerobic and resistance training versus aerobic training alone in cardiac rehabilitation. *Eur J Cardiovasc Prev Rehabil.* 2001;21(2):101–110.

46. Pollock M, Franklin B, Balady G, et al. Resistance exercise in individuals with and without cardiovascular disease: benefits, rationale, safety, and prescription. An advisory from the Committee on Exercise, Rehabilitation, and Prevention, Council on Clinical Cardiology, American Heart Association. *Circulation.* 2000;101:828–833.

47. Pollock MJ, Gaesser GA, Butcher JD, Despres JP, Dishman RK, Franklin BA, Garber CE. ACSM Position Stand: The recommended quantity and quality of exercise for developing and maintaining cardiorespiratory and muscular fitness, and flexibility in healthy adults. *Med Sci Sports Exerc.* 1998;30(6):975–991.

48. Ratamess N, Faigenbaum A, Mangine G, Hoffman J, Kang J. Acute muscular strength assessment using free weight bars of different thickness. *J Strength Cond Res.* 2007;21(1):240–244.

49. Sale DG. *Testing Strength and Power: Physiological Testing of the High-Performance Athlete.* Champaign (IL): Human Kinetics; 1991. p. 21–103.

50. Sale DG, Martin JE, Moroz DE. Hypertrophy without increased isometric strength after weight training. *Eur J Appl Physiol.* 1992;64: 51–55.

51. Schneider CM, Hsieh CC, Sprod LK, Carter SD, Hayward R. Cancer treatment-induced alterations in muscular fitness and quality of life: the role of exercise training. *Ann Oncol.* 2007;18(12): 1957–1962.

52. Smith A. The warm up procedure: to stretch or not to stretch. *J Orthop Sports Phys Ther.* 1994;19:12–17.

53. Taaffe DR, Pruitt L, Pyka G, Guido D, Marcus R. Comparative effects of high- and low-intensity resistance training on thigh muscle strength, fiber area, and tissue composition in elderly women. *Clin Physiol.* 1996;16(4):381–392.

54. Taylor DC, Dalton JD, Seaber AV, Garrett WE. Viscoelastic properties of muscle-tendon units: the biomechanical effects of stretching. *Am J Sports Med.* 1990;18:300–309.

55. Tesch PA, Thorsson A, Colliander EB. Effects of eccentric and concentric resistance training on skeletal muscle substrates, enzyme activities and capillary supply. *J Appl Physiol.* 1984;56:35–38.

56. Vescovo G, Ravara B, Dalla Libera L. Skeletal muscle myofibrillar protein oxidation and exercise capacity in heart failure. *Basic Res Cardiol.* 2008;103(3):285–290.

57. **Williams M, Haskell W, Ades P, et al. Resistance exercise in individuals with and without cardiovascular disease: 2007 update: a scientific statement from the American Heart Association Council on Nutrition, Physical Activity, and Metabolism. *Circulation.* 2007;116:572–584.**

58. Wilson GJ, Murphy AJ. The use of isometric tests of muscular function in athletic assessment. *Sports Med.* 1996;22(1):19–37.

SELECTED REFERENCES FOR FURTHER READING

Abernethy PJ, Jurimae J, Logan PA, et al. Acute and chronic response of skeletal muscle to resistance exercise. *Sports Med.* 1994;17:22–38.

Gleim GW, McHugh MP. Flexibility and its effects on sports injury and performance. *Sports Med.* 1997;24:289–299.

Kraemer WJ, Ratamess NA. Fundamentals of resistance training: progression and exercise prescription. *Med Sci Sports Exerc.* 2004;36: 674–688.

Stone MH, Fleck SJ, Triplett NT, Kraemer WJ. Health- and performance-related potential of resistance training. *Sports Med.* 1991;11: 210–231.

Thacker SB, Gilchrist J, Stroup D, et al. The impact of stretching on sports injury risk: a systematic review of the literature. *Med Sci Sports Exerc.* 2004;36:371–378.

Winett RA, Carpinelli RN. Potential health-related benefits of resistance training. *Prev Med.* 2001;33:503–513.

INTERNET RESOURCES

- American College of Sports Medicine (ACSM): www.acsm.org
- American Council on Exercise (ACE): www.acefitness.org
- International Fitness Association: www.ifafitness.com/stretch/index.html
- National Strength and Conditioning Association (NSCA): www.nsca-lift.org

Clinical Exercise Testing Procedures

> **1.3.24-CES: Understand and apply pretest likelihood of coronary artery disease (CAD), the positive and negative predictive values of various types of stress tests (e.g., electrocardiogram [ECG] only, stress echo, radionuclide), and the potential of false-positive/negative and true-positive/negative results.**

> **1.4.18-CES: Identify the causes of false-positive and false-negative exercise ECG responses and methods for optimizing sensitivity and specificity.**

Exercise testing is an extension of the history and physical examination and has been of recognized clinical value for

> > > KEY TERMS

Akinesis: Absence of movement, such as that observed in areas of the myocardium that have been infarcted.

Augmentation: Enhancement of movement.

Bruits: A harsh or musical intermittent auscultatory sound on physical examination of the heart or blood vessels that are near the surface of the body.

Clubbing: A condition affecting the fingers and toes in which proliferation of distant soft tissues, especially the nail beds, results in thickening and widening of the extremities of the digits. The nail beds are abnormally curved and are excessively compressible. The skin over them is red and shiny.

Chronotropic: Affecting the heart rate.

Cyanosis: A dark bluish or purplish discoloration of the skin and mucous membranes caused by deficient oxygenation of the blood.

Diagnosis: The determination of the presence of a disease.

Differential diagnosis: The determination of which of two or more diseases with similar symptoms is the one from which the patient is suffering. In clinical practice, the physician examines the patient and develops a "shopping list" of potential problems. Diagnostic tests are then used to rule out items on the list. If an item cannot be ruled out, then it is likely to be included in the diagnosis.

Dyskinesis: Abnormal movement, such as of a myocardial wall.

Edema: An accumulation of an excessive amount of watery fluid in intra- or extra-cellular tissues.

False-negative: An initial negative diagnostic assessment that is ultimately untrue.

False-positive: An initial positive diagnostic assessment that is ultimately untrue.

Ischemic: Inadequate circulation of blood to a tissue.

Hypokinesis: Diminished or slow movement.

Predictive value: Calculated as a number of true-positive tests divided by the number of true-positive plus the number of false-positive tests. This provides the percentage of tests that effectively identify disease in a population with the disease.

Pretest likelihood: The probability that an individual has a given disease based on history and physical findings before performing a diagnostic test.

Prevalence: The percentage of individuals in a population with a particular disease at any point in time.

Prognosis: The probable outcome of a disease.

Hemodynamic: Affecting heart rate and blood pressure.

Sensitivity: The percentage of individuals with a disease who have a positive diagnostic test.

Specificity: The percentage of healthy individuals who have a negative diagnostic test.

True-negative: A diagnostic finding that is apparently negative (e.g., normal) and ultimately is true.

True-positive: A diagnostic finding that is apparently positive (e.g., abnormal) and ultimately is true.

at least 50 years. Traditionally, exercise testing has been a preliminary step in the diagnosis of coronary artery disease (CAD), the primary diagnostic criteria being ST-segment changes on the electrocardiogram (ECG) and their correlation with symptoms (e.g., angina pectoris, shortness of breath) that are consistent with a diagnosis of exertional myocardial ischemia. Exercise tests have established value in the evaluation of patients with an intermediate likelihood of CAD and are of lesser value in patients with either very low or very high pretest likelihood of CAD. In view of the limited sensitivity and specificity of ST-segment changes during exercise testing and the likelihood that the reported sensitivity and specificity (60%–70%) of exercise testing is influenced by workup bias, the true sensitivity and specificity of exercise testing may be as low as 40% to 50% (27). With this in mind, the value of exercise testing in asymptomatic patients for the detection of occult CAD remains controversial. Although screening tests are probably of value, the risk of false-positive results is not trivial and needs to be considered carefully. Beyond this, the limitation of coronary angiography as the gold standard, particularly with reference to detecting unstable plaques, suggests that the traditional view of exercise testing must be reconsidered. Within the past several years, the application of exercise testing has been broadened in response to a better understanding of the considerable prognostic information to be derived from the exercise test (7,8, 19,28,29,34,39,44,47), particularly the use of exercise test scores combining exercise capacity, ECG abnormalities, hemodynamic abnormalities, and symptoms (3,34).

WHY DO AN EXERCISE TEST?

There are several reasons, or **indications**, for conducting a clinical exercise test (see GETP8 Chapter 5). These indications are enumerated in Box 21-1. Essentially, there are three reasons for performing an exercise test: (a) for diagnostic purposes, (b) for functional evaluation, and (c) to determine prognosis or risk (e.g., surgical risk). Before assuming the risk of conducting an exercise test, one must always be certain that the indications for the test are sufficient to justify the risk of exercise testing. An understanding of the indications for the test will dictate how the relative criteria for terminating the test are judged and how the test results are evaluated. For example, the attitude taken when conducting a test on an otherwise healthy individual at risk for occult cardiovascular disease (CVD) will be somewhat different than in a patient with a clinical presentation suggestive of stable angina pectoris. Likewise, the interpretative approach will be quite different when one is trying to make a new diagnosis of exertional myocardial ischemia versus trying to define **prognosis** in a patient with known CAD.

PRELIMINARY DECISIONS

> **1.3.2-CES: Knowledge of exercise testing procedures for various clinical populations, including those individuals with cardiovascular, pulmonary, and metabolic diseases in terms of exercise modality, protocol, physiologic measurements, and expected outcomes.**

| **BOX 21-1** | **CLINICALLY ACCEPTED REASONS FOR PERFORMING AN EXERCISE TEST, INCLUDING THE LEVEL OF EVIDENCE SUPPORTING THE INDICATION[a]** |

Extension of the history and physical (allowing the physician to examine the patient during symptoms) (I)

Evaluate exertional discomfort (I)

    Chest discomfort

    Dyspnea

    Leg discomfort

    Palpitations

    Cerebral symptoms

Evaluate the presence of occult coronary artery disease (Ia, IIb)

    Risk stratification in patients with known cardiovascular disease (I)

Follow-up of therapy (IIa)

Exercise prescription (IIb)

Class I: Conditions for which there is evidence and/or general agreement that a given procedure or treatment is useful and effective.

Class II: Conditions for which there is conflicting evidence and/or a divergence of opinion about the usefulness/efficacy of a procedure or treatment.

    IIa: Weight of evidence/opinion is in favor of usefulness/efficacy.

    IIb: Usefulness/efficacy is less well established by evidence/opinion.

Class III: Conditions for which there is evidence and/or general agreement that the procedure/treatment is not useful/effective and in some cases may be harmful.

[a]Adapted from Gibbons RJ, Balady GJ, Bricker Jt, et al. ACC/AHA 2002 Guideline update for exercise testing: a report of the American College of Cardiology/American Heart Association Task Force on Practice Guidelines (Committee on Exercise Testing). 2002. American College of Cardiology Web site. Available at: www.acc.org/clinical/guidelines/exercise/dirindex.htm.

> **1.3.5-CES: Select an appropriate test protocol according to the age, functional capacity, physical ability, and health status of the individual.**

> **1.3.16-CES: Evaluate medical history and physical examination findings as they relate to health appraisal and exercise testing.**

> **1.3.5-HFS: Knowledge of relative and absolute contraindications to exercise testing or participation.**

Before conducting an exercise test, several things must be considered that will affect the information to be derived from the test. These include the indications and contraindications to exercise testing, the mode of exercise, the endpoint of the exercise test, the protocol, safety considerations, and medication decisions.

In the most general sense, the overriding concept is that exercise testing is an extension of the history and physical examination designed to allow the physician to evaluate the patient in circumstances that will provoke the signs or symptoms of exertional myocardial ischemia or other manifestations of CVD or pulmonary disease. There are both absolute and relative contraindications to exercise testing, which are presented in GETP8 Box 3-5. For the most part, contraindications are based on decisions designed to avoid unstable **ischemic**, **rhythm**, or **hemodynamic** conditions or other situations in which the risk associated with exercise testing is likely to exceed the information to be gained from the exercise test. The number of conditions considered to be absolute contraindications has decreased over the past 50 years. At the same time, the general practice of exercise testing has become safer (16). Given that there is a certain risk of complications during exercise testing (16), subjects should provide informed consent before undergoing testing (see GETP8, Fig. 3-1). As a general principle, the person actually conducting the test should review the informed consent with the patient immediately before the test, even if the patient has already signed the form. It is particularly important to tell the patient what they are likely to feel during the test (e.g., "I'm going to try to make you have that chest discomfort you were telling your doctor about. If you don't get the pain, I'm still going to make your legs get very tired and make you get sweaty and out of breath."). At this time, it is worth reviewing the history, current medications, and indications for the test with the patient, along with current or recent changes in symptoms, to ensure that the goals of the test are well understood by both the patient and laboratory personnel. Lastly, the resting ECG should be examined before beginning the test, first to identify contraindications for testing and second to make sure that the resting ECG is sufficiently normal to allow for interpretation of changes that might occur during the exercise test. In the case of more than minimal abnormalities of the resting ECG, consider-

ation should be given to adjunctive procedures, if the test is designed to make a new diagnosis. Radionuclide myocardial perfusion imaging and either radionuclide or echocardiographic measurements of left ventricular function are the most commonly used adjunctive procedures. (see Chapter 22). Imaging tests are not necessary for tests with the goal of determing functional capacity.

Exercise mode may play a role in the results of the exercise test. In the United States, treadmill walking is the most preferred mode during an exercise test, whereas in Europe, a cycle is most likely preferred. For those less trained on a cycle, the typical peak work capacity and VO_2 will be reduced by about 10%. This may influence both functional and prognostic assessments that rely on establishing precise peak exercise work rates. Certainly, other modes of exercise testing are appropriate for those with lower-limb limitations (e.g., arm ergometry) or those who are overweight (e.g., seated stepping).

PERSONNEL

Before about 1980, a **graded exercise test (GXT)** in a clinical setting was primarily (90%) supervised by a cardiologist. Since that time, GXTs have been performed by many healthcare professionals, including clinical **exercise physiologists** and clinical exercise specialists. The American Heart Association guidelines for exercise testing laboratories state that the paramedical personnel listed previously, when appropriately trained and possessing specific performance skills (e.g., American College of Sports Medicine certification), can safely supervise clinical GXTs (49).

For graded exercise testing of patients with high-risk medical conditions, such as heart failure or high-grade dysrhythmias, direct physician supervision is suggested. Otherwise, having a supervising physician in the immediate area and readily available to respond to emergencies and questionable interpretations is acceptable. When comparing physician with nonphysician supervision of exercise testing, four studies reported that the average morbidity and mortality rates during a GXT with physician supervision (>85% of the tests directly supervised by a physician) were 3.6 and 0.44 per 10,000 tests, respectively (4,53–55). In three studies involving nonphysician supervision, average morbidity and mortality rates of 2.4 and 0.77 per 10,000 tests were observed, respectively (18,26,30). These data suggest that no differences exist in morbidity and mortality rates related to graded exercise testing between direct physician and paramedical staff supervision. In addition, when a symptom-limited GXT is performed on a high-risk population (**left ventricular dysfunction** with **ejection fraction** <35%), nonphysician supervision has been observed to be safe when a physician is immediately available (55). Additional personnel should include a trained technician with skills in informed consent, medical history, ECG preparation and equipment function, blood pressure, and patient interaction. If utilized, this staff person should also have the ability to maintain and operate gas exchange analysis equipment (2).

PROTOCOL

 1.3.19-CES: Select and perform appropriate procedures and protocols for the exercise test, including modes of exercise, starting levels, increments of work, ramping versus incremental protocols, length of stages, and frequency of data collection.

The exercise protocol represents a convenient way to conduct the exercise examination for both the patient and the professional supervising the test. There are several general principles that can be applied to the selection of the exercise protocol. The initial level of exertion should be clearly submaximal, the increments between stages should be comparatively small and of consistent size, the protocol should allow easy estimation of the exercise capacity, and the test should be time efficient for both patient and health professional. The Bruce treadmill protocol is the most widely used exercise protocol in the United States (6,45). From the standpoint of physician familiarity, availability of equations to predict functional capacity (14,36,42), and efficiency of health professional and patient time, the Bruce treadmill protocol is very good. However, this protocol is ideal only for younger individuals with a fairly normal exercise capacity and a good ability to communicate with the professional conducting the test. For older and more debilitated patients, the high starting aerobic requirements (~5 metabolic equivalents [METs]) and the large increases between stages make the Bruce protocol less than optimal and encourages extensive handrail support, which compromises accurate evaluation of exercise capacity (23,36). In response to these limitations, modifications of the Bruce protocol and many other treadmill and cycle protocols have been developed. Most recently, patient-specific ramping protocols have gained popularity (12,23,25,42,48) (see GETP8 Figure 5-3 for many popular protocols).

MONITORING AND TERMINATION

 1.4.6-CES: Define the ECG criteria for initiating and/or terminating exercise testing or training.

Heart rate, blood pressure, and perceived exertion using the Borg rating of perceived exertion scale should be monitored and recorded throughout the test (20). Heart rate should be observed to increase with increasing workloads and not be used as a criterion to stop a symptom-limited test. Blood pressure and perceived exertion should be assessed in the final 30 to 60 seconds of a stage and again at peak exercise and into recovery of at least 6 to 8 minutes. During each stage of the exercise test, the ECG should be monitored for ST-segment abnormalities and other electrocardiographic manifestations of myocardial ischemia, and for arrhythmias. Standard chest pain evaluation—and, if indicated, evaluation for dyspnea and

claudication pain—should also be assessed at the end of each stage and more often if these symptoms are present.

Termination criteria for exercise testing are well established (see GETP8 Box 5-2). In general, the test should be continued until the clinical question that prompted the exercise test to be ordered has been answered. Arbitrary termination based on a predetermined workload or percent of the age-predicted heart rate (HR) is difficult to justify. Such practices tend to heavily stress the most debilitated patients and suboptimally challenge healthy well-conditioned patients. Particularly considering the power of exercise capacity as a prognostic marker (44), failure to take the patient to either a fatigue or symptom/sign limitation (i.e., symptom-limited test) results in a failure to acquire information that is very important. However, after clearly abnormal findings have been documented, there is little justification for continuation of the test. Some clinicians view the achievement of 85% of the age-predicted maximal HR as adequate stress for revealing exertional ischemia. This practice is based on older observations that 50% of ischemic abnormalities were observed by the time 85% of age-predicted maximal HR was achieved. The sensitivity of exercise testing is increased in tests in which more than 85% of the age-predicted HR is achieved. Thus, it makes more sense to argue that achievement of a particular percent of maximal HR is primarily a "security blanket" in an otherwise normal test. In the context of interpreting a clinically indicated test with no abnormal findings, clinicians are compelled to ask themselves if they have really ruled out exertional ischemia, or if something may have been missed. Given that severe exercise in a previously sedentary person is a well-established trigger of acute myocardial infarction (38,57), and the likelihood that patients receiving reassurance after a normal exercise test result might be willing to engage in severe exercise, the risk of missing an abnormal finding by inadequately stressing the patient is clinically relevant. Accordingly, it seems reasonable to argue that the best place to provoke abnormal findings is in the exercise laboratory, where complications can be more readily identified and addressed appropriately.

POSTEXERCISE

 1.3.20-CES: Describe and conduct immediate postexercise procedures and various approaches to cool-down and recognize normal and abnormal responses.

 1.4.10-CES: Describe the diagnostic and prognostic significance of ischemic ECG responses and arrhythmias at rest, during exercise, or recovery.

A decision needs to be made concerning procedures immediately following the exercise test. Older studies suggest that the sensitivity of ST-segment changes can be maximized by placing the patient in a sitting or supine position immediately following exercise (5,21,27). However, more recent data focusing on the prognostic value of exercise testing have demonstrated the important data derived from the pattern of HR and blood pressure (BP) recovery during the postexercise period (3,7,8,28,29,37,39). These data suggest that the gain in ECG sensitivity from passive postexercise recovery is less than the information that can be gained by choosing to continue light exercise during the recovery period. Thus, it is probably best to perform a short period of low-intensity exercise during the postexercise period to document the recovery pattern of HR and BP. Further, because profound hypotension during recovery, resulting from a large drop in venous return, can itself cause significant exertional ischemia by decreasing perfusion pressure into the myocardium, performing gentle exercise may support venous return and thus hemodynamic stability. The moments immediately after the exercise test are also uniquely "teachable moments" during which the clinician conducting the exercise test can communicate with the patient (e.g., the value of habitual exercise, weight loss, stopping smoking, or the safety of resuming activities that the patient might fear).

SAFETY

Exercise testing is generally quite safe. The classical data of Rochemis and Blackburn (53) suggested that the risk of serious complications was on the order of 6/10,000 tests. More recent data suggest that the risk of serious complications is <2/10,000 tests (45). Most of these tests were in patients without established heart disease. Proper attention to contraindications for exercise testing, careful monitoring during the test, and recognizing criteria for terminating the exercise test all contribute to improved safety.

In tests that are performed for diagnostic purposes, medications that might mask ischemic or hemodynamic abnormalities may be withdrawn long enough before the test to allow the test to be diagnostically adequate, although many centers encourage patients to continue to take all medications on the day of testing (20). In the case in which the exercise test is being performed to evaluate the effectiveness of therapy, medications should be continued because the clinical question to be answered is how effectively the treatment protocol is working (20).

INTERPRETATIVE STRATEGY

> **1.2.11-CES: Describe the cardiorespiratory and metabolic responses in myocardial dysfunction** and ischemia at rest and during exercise.

> **1.3.21-CES: Record, organize, perform, and interpret necessary calculations of test data.**

> **1.3.24-CES: Understand and apply pretest likelihood of CAD, the positive and negative predictive** values of various types of stress tests (e.g., ECG only,

stress echo, radionuclide), and the potential of false-positive/negative and true-positive/negative results.

> **1.3.29-CES: Identify the variables measured during cardiopulmonary exercise testing (e.g., heart rate, blood pressure, rate of perceived exertion, ventilation, oxygen consumption, ventilatory threshold, pulmonary circulation) and their potential relationship to cardiovascular, pulmonary, and metabolic disease.**

> **1.4.10-CES: Describe the diagnostic and prognostic significance of ischemic ECG responses and arrhythmias at rest, during exercise, or recovery.**

> **1.4.16-CES: Describe the diagnostic and prognostic implications of the exercise test ECG and hemodynamic responses.**

> **1.3.20-HFS: Ability to analyze and interpret information obtained from the cardiorespiratory fitness test and the muscular strength and endurance, flexibility, and body composition assessments for apparently healthy individuals and those with controlled chronic disease.**

Interpreting exercise test results should be accomplished within the clinical context of the reasons for ordering the exercise test. At least five factors must be considered during the interpretation of the exercise test—including clinical responses, ECG responses, exercise capacity, hemodynamic responses, and the integrated response—as reflected by exercise test scores.

The *clinical response* to the exercise test must be evaluated in terms of the clinical context of the test. The clinical context is well reflected by the pretest likelihood of ischemic CAD that was the indication for the exercise test (see GETP8 Table 5-1). This concept is well expressed in terms of Bayes theorem of conditional probability. Bayes theorem states that the probability of having disease is determined by the disease probability before the test and by the probability a true result will be provided by the test. For CAD, well-accepted quantitative guidelines have been established.

Symptoms observed during the exercise test must be interpreted in terms of their correspondence to the patients' presenting symptoms. In the case of chest discomfort that is potentially angina pectoris, the timing and character of the chest discomfort must be carefully considered. It is also important to recognize that in older patients, dyspnea is often an angina equivalent. Ideally, the appearance of symptoms will be correlated with either ECG or hemodynamic abnormalities. However, these can be masked by baseline ECG abnormalities, arrhythmias, pacemaker activity, or medications. There is a tendency for fewer symptoms to be observed during exercise testing than during spontaneous activity, perhaps because of the influence of warm-up during exercise testing (35).

Changes in the *ST segments* of the ECG are the traditional interpretative sign related to the presence of exertional ischemia (see Chapter 27). ST segment depression that is >1 mm magnitude and is horizontal or downsloping in nature and persists for 80 msec after the J point is considered the minimal diagnostic threshold to support a diagnosis of exertional myocardial ischemia. In the case of ST-segment depression (or elevation), there is usually a lead with the greatest degree of ST change, surrounded by leads with progressively less ST change. Although it is common to refer to ST-segment changes relative to an area of the heart that might be ischemic or even to a particular coronary artery that might have an obstructive lesion, ischemic abnormalities map onto the surface of the chest fairly poorly. Using the traditional criteria of a 70% narrowing of at least one epicardial artery, the sensitivity and specificity of ECG exercise testing is on the order of 70% and 80%, respectively. However, there is likely a significant workup bias, and the true sensitivity may be as low as 40% (28). Beyond this, high-grade angiographic lesions are probably not an ideal criterion against which to evaluate exertional ischemia or diagnose atherosclerotic CAD. ST-segment changes that occur early during an exercise test, are evident in multiple leads, or persist into recovery predict either severe single-vessel CAD or multivessel disease.

Dysrhythmias, especially ventricular dysrhythmias, are particularly disturbing during exercise testing because they are widely thought to portend a catastrophic hemodynamic collapse (see Chapter 27). In general, dysrhythmias that increase in frequency or complexity with progressive exercise, are associated with ischemia, or are associated with hemodynamic instability are thought to be more malignant than isolated dysrhythmias. Recent evidence indicating that high-grade dysrhythmias occurring during exercise or in recovery are associated with a poor long-term prognosis have served to reinforce the traditional concern about the ominous nature of dysrhythmias (19).

Exercise capacity has always been viewed as an important aspect of exercise testing. A high maximal oxygen uptake ($\dot{V}O_{2max}$) can be inferred to predict a relatively high cardiac output and therefore the absence of serious limitations of left ventricular function. Within the past decade, several studies have been published demonstrating the profound importance of exercise capacity relative to the prognosis of patients with CVD (33,44). Either absolute or age/sex normalized exercise capacity is highly related to survival. A significant issue relative to exercise capacity is the imprecision of estimating exercise capacity from exercise performance. The error in estimating exercise capacity from various published prediction equations is about ±1 MET (1,12,14,23,25,42). This is comparatively unimportant (<10% error) in young, healthy individuals with 13- to 15-MET exercise capacities, but is much more significant (15%–25% error) in individuals with reduced exercise capacities typical of those observed in patients with CVD (4–8 METs). In view of the prognostic importance of exercise capacity, the frequent custom of stopping the

exercise test early because the subject has reached an arbitrary HR (or percent of an assumed maximal HR) is difficult to justify. Conversely, but more importantly, the spurious elevation of the estimated functional capacity resulting from the practice of allowing patients to use handrail support inaccurately implies a more favorable prognosis than is justified. Although some of the equations for predicting functional capacity from exercise performance account for handrail support, their relative prediction error is larger than when the patient is not allowed to use handrail support (36). In the case when equations that assume no handrail support are used, or when the supposed steady-state MET requirement for the terminal stage is used to predict functional capacity, the prediction errors may be quite large.

Exercise capacity is best understood in terms of the age- and sex-predicted norms. Historically, this has been difficult because age and sex average values derived from a sedentary population, in a species that is clearly not designed to be sedentary, are hardly appropriate as a basis for interpretation. Morris et al. (40) have presented data based on physically active individuals, which probably should be the interpretative norm. Although these data are for men, other data can be used to estimate appropriate age-related values for women (see GETP8, Table 4-8). In the pioneering approach advocated by Bruce, exercise capacity was reported in terms of functional aerobic impairment (6). However, because physically fit patients have a negative functional aerobic impairment, because negative numbers are intuitively difficult to understand, and because the original concept was anchored in the relative disability approach to heart disease that arose following World War II (but is no longer relevant), the concept of functional aerobic impairment has become less popular. Accordingly, simple percentages of the age- and sex-predicted norm are now most widely reported.

> ### 1.3.23-CES: Describe normal and abnormal chronotropic and inotropic responses to exercise testing and training.

Hemodynamic responses have historically been used to identify high-risk situations during exercise testing. Abnormalities in either the pattern or magnitude of the systolic BP response have long been recognized for their prognostic significance. A decrease in systolic BP—especially to below the pre-exercise level, particularly when linked with ECG abnormalities or symptoms—during the course of an exercise test is widely taken as a marker of a decreasing cardiac output and has represented an unequivocal criterion to terminate an exercise test.

A relatively recent development in our understanding of exercise testing is in the data regarding the prognostic significance of hemodynamic responses during and immediately after exercise testing (2,5,6,23,24,31,41). Lauer (28) has presented evidence that patients who cannot achieve an adequate HR response to exercise (**chronotropic incompetence**) have an unfavorable prognosis beyond that accounted for by symptoms or ECG changes. The most widely accepted cutpoint is a failure to achieve 80% of the predicted HR reserve in patients with no pharmacologic reason to have a limitation in the HR response. The prognostic value of a poor HR response is as great as an exercise-induced myocardial perfusion deficit. An abnormal chronotropic response apparently provides information that is independent of myocardial perfusion because the combination of perfusion deficit and an abnormal chronotropic index suggests a worse prognosis than either abnormality alone (28). In a similar fashion, the failure of the HR to recover promptly after exercise provides independent information related to prognosis (28). Logistic regression analysis suggests that a failure to decrease HR by 12 bpm during the first minute of recovery is strongly associated with death during the follow-up period (28). The unfavorable prognosis conveyed by the failure of HR to recover is apparently related to the inability to reassert vagal control over HR, which is independently known to predispose to arrhythmic heart conditions (28).

EXERCISE TEST SCORES

Within the past decade, the use of exercise test scores that combine both favorable and unfavorable information derived during the exercise test into a single prognostically useful term has gained popularity (32,34). Although the concept of exercise test scores has been around for a generation, the most widely accepted and used is the Duke score (34). (*Note:* The Duke score should be used only in patients referred for testing to evaluate chest pain and who do not have known cosonary disease.) The Duke nomogram (see GETP8 Fig. 6-2) balances a favorable result (exercise capacity) against two unfavorable results (the magnitude of ST-segment depression and the presence and severity of angina pectoris). The calculated score has been shown to be related to 5-year survival rate and allows the categorization of patients into low-, moderate-, and high-risk subgroups. This categorization may guide the physician caring for the patient toward conservative or aggressive therapies, depending on classification. The Duke score can also be used in combination with other simple hemodynamic findings, such as an abnormal pattern of recovery of HR or the combination of an abnormal chronotropic index and an abnormal HR recovery (28). Each of these abnormalities of exercise testing contributes independent prognostic information. Although there is a general belief that physicians informally integrate much of this information without the specific calculation of a specific exercise test score, recent data suggest that estimates of the presence of CAD provided by scores are superior to physician estimates and analysis of ST-segment changes alone (32).

HEART RATE PERFORMANCE CURVE

Although not as well tested relative to prognostic risk, there is independent information to be gained from the pattern of increase in HR during exercise. In the majority of healthy individuals, the rate of increase in HR is negatively accelerated at exercise intensities above the second ventilatory threshold (50). In about 5% of healthy individuals and a high percentage of individuals with CVD, the HR performance curve is positively accelerated (50). Independent data suggest that this change in the rate of increase in HR is a method of supporting cardiac output in individuals who have large decreases in stroke volume at high exercise intensities (17). These data are supported by findings in athletes that the negative HR deflection is evident only in cases in which the SV has begun to decline (31). Because the hallmark response during exertional ischemia is a decrease in stroke volume (SV) (secondary to the well-known decrease in left ventricular [LV] ejection fraction [13] during ischemia), it is unclear why the HR performance curve is positively, rather than negatively, accelerated. From a commonsense standpoint, it can be argued that the positive acceleration of the HR performance curve either limits the expansion of the LV end-diastolic volume (which often increases inappropriately in patients with exertional ischemia) or simply is an attempt to defend cardiac output in the face of a falling SV (17).

BLOOD PRESSURE RESPONSE

> **1.3.12-CES: Obtain and recognize normal and abnormal physiologic and subjective responses** (e.g., symptoms, ECG, blood pressure, heart rate, rate of perceived exertion and other scales, oxygen saturation, and oxygen consumption) at appropriate intervals during the test.

Systolic BP normally increases in a negatively accelerated manner during incremental exercise. The magnitude of increase approximates 10 mm Hg per MET, with a minimal increase of 10 mm Hg from rest to maximal exercise being considered normal (see GETP8 Box 6-1). An absolute peak systolic pressure of >250 mm Hg or a relative increase of >140 mm Hg above resting levels is considered a hypertensive response and is predictive of future resting hypertension (1). In patients with limitations of cardiac output, there is either an inappropriately slow increase in BP or a decrease in systolic BP midway through the exercise test. A decrease of systolic BP to below the resting value or by >10 mm Hg after a preliminary increase, particularly in the presence of other indices of ischemia, is grossly abnormal (see GETP8 Box 6-1). Diastolic BP is difficult to measure with accuracy during exercise testing. An increase by >10 mm Hg is generally considered to be an abnormal finding and may be consistent with exertional ischemia, as is an increase to >115 mm Hg (1).

During the postexercise period, systolic BP normally decreases promptly (3,37). Several recent investigators have demonstrated that a delay in the recovery of systolic BP is highly related both to ischemic abnormalities and to a poor prognosis (3,37). As a general principle, the 3-minute postexercise systolic BP should be <90% of the systolic BP at peak exercise. If peak exercise BP cannot be measured accurately, the 3-minute postexercise systolic BP should be less than the systolic BP measured 1 minute after exercise. Although not yet as well documented, abnormalities of the systolic BP recovery ratio may be more prognostically discriminative than abnormalities of the HR recovery pattern.

RESPIRATORY GAS EXCHANGE

 1.1.8-CES: Describe the methodology for measuring peak oxygen consumption ($\dot{V}O_{2peak}$).

Although the majority of exercise testing is performed without direct measurements of respiratory gas exchange, such measurements have been shown to be clinically useful. A major advantage of measuring gas exchange is the more accurate measurement of functional capacity. A complete review of this topic can be found in the American Thoracic Society/American College of Chest Physicians statement on cardiopulmonary gas exchange methods (2). Also see Arena et al. in selected references for further reading. When exercise capacity is directly measured, values for $\dot{V}O_{2max}$ collected over periods of <30 seconds may significantly overestimate exercise capacity. In addition to a more accurate measurement of exercise capacity, gas exchange exercise testing may be particularly useful in defining prognosis (and thus helping to define the timing of transplantation) in patients with heart failure (33,41,43,51) and may help to guide the differential diagnosis in patients with possible cardiovascular or respiratory disease (10,56). Gas exchange measurements also allow the determination of ventilatory threshold, which is a marker of sustainable exercise capacity (11) and a critical factor in terms of defining appropriate exercise training intensity. Gas exchange measurements are also of particular value in the diagnosis of multiorgan system disease. For example, patients who smoke and who are being evaluated for potential CAD are just as likely to have a pulmonary disease as to have heart disease. A test that evaluates only the cardiovascular aspects of their disease is unlikely to lead to successful treatment outcomes.

RADIONUCLIDE IMAGING

 1.3.1-CES: Describe common procedures and apply knowledge of results from radionuclide imaging (e.g., thallium, technetium, sestamibi, tetrafosmin, single-photon-emission computed tomography [SPECT]), stress echocardiography, and pharmacologic testing (e.g., dobutamine, adenosine, persantine).

In patients in whom the resting ECG is abnormal, exercise testing may be coupled with various techniques designed to either augment the information provided by the ECG or to replace the ECG when resting abnormalities make evaluation of changes during exercise impossible. Various radioisotopes can be used effectively either to evaluate the presence of perfusion, which is the index event in exertional ischemia, and the beginning of the "ischemic cascade" (22,24,46), or of abnormalities of ventricular function that often occur with myocardial infarction or exertional ischemia (9,13,15,52). However, even in the presence of a nondiagnostic ECG, all other aspects of the exercise test should remain the same, including HR and BP monitoring during and after exercise, symptom evaluation, rhythm monitoring, and exercise capacity. It is fair to say that one of the important mistakes of the 1980–2000 period in exercise testing was that the value of simple exercise test parameters was ignored in the enthusiasm for optimizing cardiac imaging.

Myocardial perfusion imaging can be performed with a variety of agents and imaging approaches, although the two most common isotopes are [201]Thallium or [199m]Technetium Sestamibi (Cardiolyte). Delivery of the isotope is proportional to coronary flow, and these agents exchange across cell membranes of metabolically active tissue either actively (Thallium) or passively (Sestamibi). In the case of myocardial infarction, the necrotic tissue does not result in uptake of the isotope, and thus a permanent (**nonreversible, or fixed, perfusion deficit**) reduction of tracer activity is observed on the image. In the case of exertional ischemia, the tissue uptake in the ischemic region is reduced during exercise by virtue of the relative reduction of blood flow (and thus isotope) to the ischemic tissue during exercise. This abnormality is reversed when the myocardial perfusion is evaluated at rest. Thus, a **reversible perfusion deficit** is diagnostic of exertional ischemia. [201]Thallium is the traditionally used isotope and has the advantage of redistributing itself during the recovery period after exercise, meaning that only one isotope injection is required. However, [201]Thallium emits a low energy photon and thus, even when combined with SPECT imaging, is often less than ideal. [199m]Technetium Sestamibi is a much better isotope in that it emits a higher-energy photon, which makes for improved imaging and is the preferred isotope. However, because it does not automatically redistribute within the myocardium, two injections (rest and exercise) are required to determine whether an exercise-related perfusion deficit is reversible or fixed. The advantage of [199m]Technetium Sestamibi is that it may be used to measure ventricular function and myocardial perfusion at the same time.

Ventricular function can be evaluated with radioisotopes, often using [199m]Technetium. This isotope can be used to tag red cells and then imaged over a somewhat prolonged period of time (60–120 seconds) using an ECG **gated blood pool** approach to make movies of brightest spot in the chest—the heart—as it changes its volume throughout the cardiac cycle. From this movie image, the contraction pattern of different walls of the heart can be evaluated. Because ischemic muscle, or scar tissue, does not contract well, the regional wall motion will deteriorate through the course of an exercise test as exertional ischemia emerges. Additionally, the global function of the left ventricle can be evaluated using the left ventricular ejection fraction (LVEF). Decreases in the LVEF are routine findings in the presence of myocardial ischemia (9,13,15,52). Using an alternative technique, the passage of a bolus of isotope can be followed on its **first pass** through the central circulation. Although technically more difficult than the gated blood pool technique, by concentrating the isotope, it is possible to achieve very-high-quality images.

In patients incapable of exercising, it is also possible to perform either myocardial perfusion or ventricular function studies with pharmacologic stress, but these techniques are beyond the scope of this chapter. Further information is provided in Chapter 22.

ECHOCARDIOGRAPHIC IMAGING

Just as adjunctive studies can be performed using radioisotopes to visualize myocardial perfusion and ventricular function, it is possible to use ultrasound to image the heart in relation to exercise (or pharmacologic) stress. Although not suitable for evaluating myocardial perfusion, it is relatively simple to make an echocardiographic examination of the heart before and after a conventional exercise test. Echocardiographic examination allows evaluation of wall motion, wall thickening, and valve function. Although it is theoretically possible to perform an echocardiographic examination during the course of upright cycle ergometer exercise, it is technically challenging. Typical practice is to have the patient lie down immediately following completion of the exercise test in the left lateral decubitus position. This allows optimization of the echocardiographic window to the heart. Regional wall motion of various segments of the left ventricle is assessed. Deterioration in regional wall motion with exercise is a sign of myocardial ischemia. LVEF before and after exercise is also measured. Normally, postexercise imaging in the upright position gives a spuriously high LVEF and normalization of wall motion abnormalities (9). However, the volume loading associated with assuming a supine position allows for adequate resolution of left ventricular dysfunction associated with exercise. Imaging techniques, such as radionuclide perfusion and echocardiography allow localization of myocardial ischemia. Further information is provided in Chapter 22.

SUMMARY

Recent evidence suggests that there is much more information in the simple incremental exercise test that formerly believed. However, these data are more important in terms of defining prognosis than in making a specific diagnosis of obstructive CAD. Changes in the ST segments of the ECG are not the only feature of this contemporary approach to evaluating exercise test results. An extremely important feature is the functional exercise capacity, as this serves as a surrogate of cardiac output, which is likely to be depressed in almost any pathologic state. The prognostic impression gained from the exercise capacity is typically balanced by either ECG or symptomatic evidence of exertional myocardial ischemia. This relationship is well expressed in exercise test scores, such as the Duke score. Lastly, hemodynamic responses have been shown to be very powerful prognostic markers. It is reasonable to suggest that if all of the components of the standard exercise test are put together that exercise testing may provide as significant information as myocardial perfusion scans or ventricular function measurements, which are the sine qua non of noninvasive diagnostics for more than two decades.

REFERENCES

1. American College of Sports Medicine: Position stand: exercise and hypertension. *Med Sci Sports Exerc.* 2004;36:533–553.
2. American Thoracic Society/American College of Chest Physicians: ATS/ACCP Statement on Cardiopulmonary Exercise Testing. *Am J Respir Crit Care Med.* 2003;167:211–277.
3. Amon KW, Richards KL, Crawford MH. Usefulness of the postexercise response of systolic blood pressure in the diagnosis of coronary artery disease. *Circulation.* 1984;70:951–956.
4. Atterhog JH, Jonsson B, Samuelsson R. Exercise testing: a prospective study of complication rates. *Am Heart J.* 1979;98:572–579.
5. Bigi R, Cortigiani L, Gregori D, et al. Exercise versus recovery electrocardiography in predicting mortality in patients with uncomplicated myocardial infarction. *Eur Heart J.* 2004;25:558–564.
6. Bruce RA, Hosmer F, Kusumi K. Maximal oxygen intake and nomographic assessment of functional aerobic impairment in cardiovascular disease. *Am Heart J.* 1973;85:546–562.
7. Cole CR, Blackstone EH, Pashkow FJ. Heart rate recovery immediately after exercise as a predictor of mortality. *N Engl J Med.* 1999;341:1351–1357.
8. Cole CR, Foody JM, Blackstone EH, Lauer MS. Heart rate recovery after submaximal exercise testing as a predictor of mortality in a cardiovascularly healthy cohort. *Ann Intern Med.* 2000;132:552–555.
9. Dymond DS, Foster C, Grenier RP, et al. Peak exercise and immediate post exercise imaging for the detection of left ventricular functional abnormalities in coronary artery disease. *Am J Cardiol.* 1984; 53:1532–1537.
10. Eschenbacher WL, Mannina A. An algorithm for the interpretation of cardiopulmonary exercise tests. *Chest.* 1990;97:263–267.
11. Foster C, Cotter H. Blood lactate, respiratory and heart rate markers of the capacity for sustained exercise. In: Maud PJ, Foster C, editors. *Physiological Assessment of Human Fitness.* 2nd ed, Champaign (IL): Human Kinetics; 2005. p. 63–76.
12. Foster C, Crowe AJ, Daines E, et al. Predicting functional capacity during treadmill testing independent of exercise protocol. *Med Sci Sports Exerc.* 1996;28:752–756.
13. Foster C, Georgakopoulous N, Meyer K. Physiological and pathological aspects of exercise left ventricular function. *Med Sci Sports Exerc.* 1998;30:S379–S386.
14. Foster C, Jackson AS, Pollock ML, et al. Generalized equations for prediction of functional capacity from treadmill performance. *Am Heart J.* 1984;107:1229–1237.

15. Foster C, Pollock ML, Anholm JD, et al. Work capacity and left ventricular function during rehabilitation after myocardial revascularization surgery. *Circulation*. 1984;69:748–755.

16. Foster C, Porcari JP. The risks of exercise training. *J Cardiopulm Rehabil*. 2001;21:347–352.

17. Foster C, Spatz P, Georgakopoulos N. Left ventricular function in relation to the heart rate performance curve. *Clin Exerc Physiol*. 1999;1:29–32.

18. Franklin BA, Dressendorfer R, Bonzbeim K, et al. Safety of exercise testing by non-physician health care providers: eighteen year experience [abstract]. *Circulation*. 1995;92(Suppl I):1–37.

19. Frolkis JP, Pothier CE, Blackstone EH, Lauer MS. Frequent ventricular ectopy after exercise as a predictor of death. *N Engl J Med*. 2003;348:781–790.

20. **Gibbons RJ, Balady GJ, Bricker JT, et al. ACC/AHA 2002 guideline update for exercise testing: a report of the American College of Cardiology/American Heart Association Task Force on Practice Guidelines (Committee on Exercise Testing). 2002. American College of Cardiology Web site. Available at: www.acc.org/clinical/guidelines/exercise/dirIndex.htm.**

21. Gutman RA, Alexander ER, Li YB, et al. Delay of ST depression after maximal exercise by walking for 2 minutes. *Circulation*. 1970; 42:229–235.

22. Hammond HK, Kelly TL, Froelicher VF. Noninvasive testing in the evaluation of myocardial ischemia: agreement among tests. *J Am Coll Cardiol*. 1985;5:59–69.

23. Haskell WL, Savin W, Oldridge N, DeBusk R. Factors influencing estimated oxygen uptake during exercise testing soon after myocardial infarction. *Am J Cardiol*. 1982;50:299–304.

24. Heller GV, Ahmed I, Tilkemeier PL, et al. Influence of exercise intensity on the presence, distribution and size of thallium-201 defects. *Am Heart J*. 1992;123:909–916.

25. Kaminsky LA, Whaley MH. Evaluation of a new standardized ramp protocol: the BSU/Bruce Ramp protocol. *J Cardiopulm Rehabil*. 1998;18:438–444.

26. Knight JA, Laubach CA, Butcher RJ, et al. Supervision of clinical exercise testing by exercise physiologist. *Am J Cardiol*. 1995;75: 390–391.

27. Lachterman B, Lehmann KG, Abrahamson D, Forelicher VF. Recovery only ST-segment depression and the predictive accuracy of the exercise test. *Ann Intern Med*. 1990;112:11–16.

28. Lauer MS. Exercise electrocardiogram testing and prognosis: novel markers and predictive instruments. In: Balady GJ, editor. *Cardiol Clin*. 2001;19:401–414.

29. Lauer MS, Francis GS, Okin PM. Impaired chronotropic response during exercise stress testing as a predictor of mortality. *JAMA*. 1999;281:524–529.

30. Lem V, Krivokapich J, Child JS. A nurse-supervised exercise stress testing laboratory. *Heart Lung*. 1985;14:280–284.

31. Lepretree P-M, Foster C, Koralsztein J-P, Billat VL. Heart rate deflection point as a strategy to defend stroke volume during incremental exercise. *J Appl Physiol*. 2005;98:1660–1665.

32. Lipinski M, Froelicher V, Atwood E, et al. Comparison of treadmill scores with physician estimates of diagnosis and prognosis in patients with coronary artery disease. *Am Heart J*. 2002;143: 650–658.

33. Mancini DM, Eisen H, Kussmaul W, et al. Value of peak exercise oxygen consumption for optimal timing of cardiac transplantation in ambulatory patients with heart failure. *Circulation*. 1991;83: 778–786.

34. Mark DB, Shaw L, Harrell FE, et al. Prognostic value of a treadmill exercise score in outpatients with suspected coronary artery disease. *N Engl J Med*. 1991;325:849, 853.

35. Maybaum S, Ilan M, Mogilevsky J, Tzivoni D. Improvement in ischemic parameters during repeated exercise testing: a possible model for myocardial preconditioning. *Am J Cardiol*. 1996;78: 1087–1091.

36. McConnell TR, Foster C, Conlin NC, Thompson NN. Prediction of functional capacity during treadmill testing: effect of handrail support. *J Cardiopulm Rehabil*. 1991;11:255–260.

37. McHam SA, Marwick TH, Pashkow FJ, Lauer MS. Delayed systolic blood pressure recovery after graded exercise: an independent correlate of angiographic coronary disease. *J Am Coll Cardiol*. 1999;34: 754–759.

38. Mittleman MA, Maclure M, Tofler GH. Triggering of acute myocardial infarction by heavy physical exertion: protection against triggering by regular exertion. *N Engl J Med*. 1993;329:1677–1683.

39. Morshedi-Meibodi A, Larson MG, Levy D, et al. Heart rate recovery after treadmill exercise testing and risk of cardiovascular disease events (the Framingham Heart Study). *Am J Cardiol*. 2002;90:848–852.

40. Morris CK, Myers J, Froelicher VF, et al. Nomogram based on metabolic equivalents and age for assessing aerobic exercise capacity in men. *J Am Coll Cardiol*. 1993;22:175–182.

41. Myers J. Effect of exercise training on abnormal ventilatory responses to exercise in patients with chronic heart failure. *Congest Heart Fail*. 2000; 6:243–249.

42. Myers J, Bellin D. Ramp exercise protocols for clinical and cardiopulmonary exercise testing. *Sports Med*. 2000;30:23–29.

43. Myers J, Madhavan R. Exercise testing with gas exchange analysis. In: Balady GJ, editor. *Cardiol Clin*. 2001;19:433–446.

44. Myers J, Prakash M, Froelicher V, et al. Exercise capacity and mortality among men referred for exercise testing. *N Engl J Med*. 2002;346:793–801.

45. Myers JN, Voodi L, Froelicher VF. A survey of exercise testing: methods, utilization, interpretation, and safety in the VAHCS. *Med Sci Sports Exerc*. 2000;32:S143.

46. Nesto RW, Kowalchuk GJ. The ischemic cascade: temporal sequence of hemodynamic, electrocardiographic and symptomatic expressions of ischemia. *Am J Cardiol*. 1987;59:23C–30C.

47. Nissines SI, Makikallio TH, Seppanen T, et al. Heart rate recovery after exercise as a predictor of mortality among survivors of acute myocardial infarction. *Am J Cardiol*. 2003;91:711–714.

48. Peterson MJ, Pieper CF, Morey MC. Accuracy of VO_2max prediction equations in older adults. *Med Sci Sports Exerc*. 2003;35:145–149.

49. **Pina IL, Balady GJ, Hanson P, et al. Guidelines for clinical exercise testing laboratories: a statement for healthcare professionals from the committee on exercise and cardiac rehabilitation, American Heart Association. *Circulation*. 1995;91(3):912–921.**

50. Pokan R, Hofmann P, von Duvillard SP. The heart rate performance curve and left ventricular function during exercise in patients after myocardial infarction. *Med Sci Sports Exerc*. 1998;30:1475–1480.

51. Ramos-Barbon D, Fitchett D, Gibbons WJ, et al. Maximal exercise testing for the selection of heart transplantation candidates: limitation of peak oxygen consumption. *Chest*. 1999;115:410–417.

52. Rerych SK, Scholz PM, Newman GE, et al. Cardiac function at rest and during exercise in normals and in patients with coronary heart disease. *Ann Surg*. 1978;187:449-463.

53. Rochemis P, Blackburn H. Exercise tests: a survey of procedures, safety and litigation experience in approximately 170,000 tests. *JAMA*. 1971;217:1061–1066.

54. **Rodgers GP, Ayanian JZ, Balady G, et al. American College of Cardiology/American Heart Association clinical competence statement on stress testing. A report of the American College of Cardiology/American Heart Association/American College of Physicians–American Society of Internal Medicine Task Force on Clinical Competence. *Circulation*. 2000;102:1726–1738.**

55. Squires RW, Allison TG, Johnson BD, Gau GT. Non-physician supervision of cardiopulmonary exercise testing in chronic heart failure: safety and results of a preliminary investigation. *J Cardiopulm Rehabil*. 1999;19:249–253.

56. Wasserman K. Diagnosing cardiovascular and lung pathophysiology from exercise gas exchange. *Chest*. 1997;112:1091–1101.

57. Willich SN, Lewis M, Lowell H. Physical exertion as a trigger of acute myocardial infarction. *N Engl J Med*. 1993;329:1684–1690.

SELECTED REFERENCES FOR FURTHER READING

Arena R, Myers J, Williams MA, et al. Assessment of functional capacity in clinical and research settings: A Scientific Statement from the AHA Committed on Exercise, Rehabilitation, and Prevention of the Council on Clinical Cardiology and the Council on Cardiovascular Nursing. *Circulation* 2007;116:329–343.

Froelicher VF, Myers J. *Exercise and the Heart.* 5th ed. Philadelphia: Saunders; 2006.

Froelicher VF, Myers JN. *Manual of Exercise Testing.* Amsterdam: Mosby Elsevier; 2006.

Wassermann K, Hansen JE, Sue DY, Stringer WW, Whip BJ. *Principles of Exercise Testing and Interpretation.* 4th ed. Baltimore: Lippincott, Williams & Wilkins; 2004.

INTERNET RESOURCES

- American College of Cardiology/American Heart Association Clinical Competence Statement on Stress Testing, 2000: http://circ.ahajournals.org/cgi/content/full/102/14/1726
- American College of Cardiology/American Heart Assocation 2002 Guideline Update for Exercise Testing: www.americanheart.org/presenter.jhtml?identifier=3005237
- American Heart Association. Scientific Statement: Exercise standards for testing and training. 2001: http://circ.ahajournals.org/cgi/content/full/104/14/1694

Diagnostic Procedures for Cardiovascular Disease

> **1.3.2-HFS: Knowledge of the value of the health/medical history.**

> **1.3.4-HFS: Knowledge of and the ability to perform risk stratification and its implications toward medical clearance before administration of an exercise test or participation in an exercise program.**

The diagnosis of cardiovascular disease is made using a medical history, physical examination, and a variety of noninvasive and invasive tests. These tests are ordered by physicians (typically internists and cardiologists) and should follow the recommendations made by the American College of Cardiology (ACC) and the American Heart Association (AHA) Task Forces (10,11).

Current guidelines grade both the strength of the evidence and the degree to which an action should or should not be undertaken. The ACC/AHA Task Force applies a grade of A, B, or C based on data derived from multiple randomized clinical trials or meta-analyses (level A); data derived from a single randomized trial or nonrandomized studies (level B); and information derived only from consensus opinion of experts, case studies, or standard of care (level C). From this evidence, three levels or classes of recommendations for performing a certain diagnostic test or treatment are made. Class I indicates conditions for which there is evidence and/or general agreement that a given procedure or treatment is beneficial, useful, and effective, and in general suggests an action *should be done*; class II

> > > KEY TERMS

Akinesis: Absence of contraction of a myocardial segment.

Augmentation: Enhancement of contraction of a myocardial segment.

Bruits: A harsh or musical intermittent auscultatory sound, especially an abnormal one.

Differential diagnosis: The determination of which of two or more diseases with similar symptoms is the one from which the patient is suffering, by a systematic comparison and contrasting of the clinical findings.

Dyskinesis: Absence of contraction and movement of a myocardial segment outward with systole.

Edema: An accumulation of an excessive amount of watery fluid in cells or intercellular tissues.

False-negative: An initial negative diagnostic assessment that is ultimately untrue.

False-positive: An initial positive diagnostic assessment that is ultimately untrue.

Gold standard: The diagnostic test that serves as the comparison for all other tests evaluating the same condition, disease, or physiologic response.

Hypokinesis: Diminished or reduced contraction of a myocardial segment.

Predictive value: The probability of disease being present/absent in the setting of a positive/negative test.

Pretest likelihood: The probability that an individual has a given disease, based on physical and history findings before the performance of a diagnostic test.

Prevalence: The number of cases of a disease existing in a given population at a specific period of time (*period prevalence*) or at a particular moment in time (*point prevalence*).

Sensitivity: The proportion of affected individuals who give a positive test result for the disease that the test is intended to reveal.

Specificity: The proportion of individuals with negative test results for the disease that the test is intended to reveal.

True-negative: Denoting an initial negative diagnostic assessment that is ultimately true.

True-positive: Denoting an initial positive diagnostic assessment that is ultimately true.

indicates conditions for which there is conflicting evidence and/or a divergence of opinion about the usefulness/efficacy of a procedure or treatment (subdivided into class IIa, for which the weight of evidence/opinion is in favor of usefulness/efficacy, interpreted as "probably should do it," and class IIb, for which the usefulness/efficacy is less well established by evidence/opinion, interpreted as "can consider doing it"); and class III indicates conditions for which there is evidence and/or general agreement that aprocedure/treatment is not useful/effective and in some cases may be harmful, and in general suggests that the action *should not* be done. An example of a guideline statement is the ACC/AHA 2005 guideline update for the management of patients with heart failure with the following, which is listed as a class IIa recommendation: "Maximal exercise testing with measurement of respiratory gas exchange is reasonable to identify high-risk patients presenting with HF [heart failure] who are candidates for cardiac transplantation or other advanced treatments. (Level of Evidence: B)" (10).

Clinical exercise professionals should be familiar with both the general decision-making process of cardiovascular diagnosis and the specific diagnostic procedures used to make the diagnosis. Often in the cardiac rehabilitation setting, for instance, patients ask about diagnostic procedures and why a diagnostic assessment was or was not performed. Even though clinical exercise professionals would not be expected to provide a definitive answer to these types of questions, they can provide some insight during a teaching moment with the patient, provided they have the requested knowledge. Specific questions concerning diagnosis, prognosis, and management should be referred to the patient's physician.

Additionally, there is an increasing role for the clinical exercise professional in the administration and preliminary interpretation of some cardiac diagnostic procedures. Often, noninvasive cardiology laboratories and other settings in which cardiac stress imaging is performed use these individuals to perform technical duties and supervise exercise testing or cardiac physiologic response to pharmacologic agents (adenosine, dipyridamole, or dobutamine).

This chapter focuses on common forms of cardiovascular testing that are relevant to the clinical exercise specialist. It is important to keep in mind that testing serves many important clinical functions, including screening for disease, making a diagnosis when symptoms are present, indicating prognosis when disease status is known, and, finally, guiding the management of the patient.

HISTORY AND PHYSICAL EXAMINATION

 1.3.2-HFS: Knowledge of the value of the health/medical history.

1.3.33-CES: Recognition of the value of heart and lung sounds in the assessment of patients with cardiovascular and/or pulmonary disease.

BOX 22-1	**EIGHT SYMPTOMS OF HEART DISEASE**

1. Chest discomfort
2. Dyspnea (shortness of breath with exertion)
3. Orthopnea (shortness of breath with lying down)
4. Paroxysmal nocturnal dyspnea (waking at night short of breath)
5. Peripheral edema
6. Cardiac palpitations
7. Syncope (fainting)
8. Cough

The cornerstone of the evaluation and clinical workup of the patient with suspected heart disease is the history and physical examination. This is the basis of any subsequent cardiovascular testing that may be performed. The history and physical examination may be performed by a physician, midlevel provider (physician assistant, nurse practitioner), or other qualified personnel (e.g., clinical exercise physiologist) who is working with a patient during the clinical encounter.

When evaluating a patient for the first time, it is always best to perform a complete history and physical and obtain as many of the previous medical records as possible. Creation of a problem list and list of current medications and allergies to medications is essential. It is only with a complete knowledge of all of the patient's health and medical information that an accurate diagnosis and effective treatment plan can be designed. The eight symptoms most common to patients with heart disease are listed in Box 22-1.

Each patient should be questioned regarding the presence of these symptoms at each visit. For each symptom, additional information needs to be obtained, such as how long ago it began, the duration of the symptom with each occurrence, any precipitating event, and how the patient relieves the discomfort. The most common symptom in those with cardiac disease is chest discomfort. With chest discomfort, the key components to assess include (a) location and type of sensation; (b) if it occurs with myocardial stress, such as exertion or mental stress; and (c) if it is relieved by using nitroglycerin or rest and relaxation. If a patient has only one of these components, then it is considered "nonangina" pain; if he or she has two components, then it is "atypical" angina; and if the patient has all three components, then it is considered "typical" angina (11). It should be noted that women can have more atypical chest pain that is determined to be ischemic in nature than men. It should also be noted that patients with diabetes more commonly have atypical features or no symptoms at all of ischemia despite the presence of significant coronary disease.

Angina typically presents as a dull pressure or burning type (also, gripping, heavy, suffocating, tightness, burning, or aching are used to describe the sensation) discomfort in the chest, jaw, shoulder, back, or arm. It usually occurs with physical exertion or emotional stress and is relieved with rest or nitroglycerine use. It is incorrect to ask about chest pain. Most patients do not experience pain in their chest as a symptom of heart disease. Rather, they may describe the discomfort as "bothersome" rather than painful. By asking about chest pain, many patients with heart disease may be missed. Discomfort that persists for hours or days, is localized to a small area defined by a fingertip, or is sharp in nature is less likely to be angina. The other symptoms listed in Box 22-1 may occur in association with angina or with other types of cardiac disease (e.g., valvular, nonischemic heart failure, arrhythmias).

The history intake should also include an evaluation of the risk factors associated with cardiac disease (listed in order of frequency): obesity (body mass index >30 $kg \cdot m^{-2}$), sedentary lifestyle, hypertension (17), metabolic syndrome, diabetes, dyslipidemia (14), smoking, and a family history of heart disease in a parent or sibling before age 55 years for men and 65 years for women (GETP8 Box 3.1). Any previous history of cardiovascular disease should also be noted (myocardial infarction, prior revascularization, stroke, or known peripheral arterial disease). All patients identified with risk factors, whether cardiovascular disease reported by the patient or not, should be counseled about the risk factors, educated about how lifestyle plays a central role in risk factor and disease development, and treated accordingly. The clinician may also consider ordering laboratory tests for fasting blood lipids (total cholesterol, high- and low-density lipoproteins [HDL-C and LDL-C], and triglycerides), hemoglobin (anemia evaluation), and fasting blood glucose (diabetes evaluation) (see GETP8, Box 3.3). In some instances, blood lipids and glucose may be assessed at the time of the clinic visit using point-of-care testing procedures.

The physical examination should include blood pressure; pulse; respiratory rate; and body weight, including the body mass index. The person who places the patient in the exam room typically determines the vital signs. The general physical examination performed by the clinician is best approached by inspection, palpation, auscultation, and percussion.

Inspection includes assessment of the patient's general condition, such as the appearance of distress; the color and texture of the skin; the presence of cyanosis or **edema** of the extremities; the presence of skin lesions or jugular venous distention. Palpation involves feeling the major arteries—including the abdominal aorta, femoral, pedal, radial, and carotid arteries—to determine the presence and magnitude of the pulse, and in the case of the abdominal aorta, to estimate its size. The apex of the left ventricle (LV) can be palpated to determine if cardiac enlargement is present. Peripheral edema is assessed by palpation, first to determine its presence and second to grade its severity. Percussion of vital organs is performed next but is of little value in the assessment for cardiac disease. The final step of the physical examination is auscultation. Each of the major arteries should be evaluated for **bruits**. The lungs are auscultated for signs of pneumonia, emphysema, or heart failure, and the heart is auscultated for regularity of rhythm, murmurs, and extra sounds.

For patients with symptoms that are potentially related to myocardial ischemia, a resting electrocardiogram (ECG) should be performed. It is useful as a baseline for future reference and as a screen for previous or current cardiac problems, including infarction, arrhythmia, and left ventricular hypertrophy (LVH). It is also an important aid for determining the type of diagnostic test to next perform. For instance, any pre-existing abnormality may suggest the need to add an imaging study to a graded exercise test to evaluate the patient with ischemic symptoms.

DETERMINING THE GOALS OF CARDIOVASCULAR TESTING

SCREENING FOR CORONARY ARTERY DISEASE

> **1.3.4-HFS: Knowledge of and the ability to perform risk stratification and its implications toward medical clearance before administration of an exercise test or participation in an exercise program.**

The clinician should estimate the coronary heart disease risk (myocardial infarction or death) using the Framingham or other scoring scheme based on age, sex, total cholesterol or LDL-C, HDL-C, blood pressure, diabetes, and smoking (Fig. 22-1) (25). In general, when the coronary heart disease risk exceeds 20% over 10 years (or 2% per year), then a patient is considered at high risk, and position papers support the action of using exercise stress testing as a screening test for significant coronary artery disease (CAD) (21).

EVALUATION OF CHEST DISCOMFORT

There is a broad differential diagnosis for chest discomfort (Box 22-3). The Diamond and Forrester model uses age,

BOX 22-2	FOUR MAJOR APPLICATIONS OF CARDIOVASCULAR TESTING
	Screening
	Diagnosis
	Prognosis
	Management

Estimate of 10-Year Risk for Men
(Framingham Point Scores)

A

Age, y	Points
20–34	−9
35–39	−4
40–44	0
45–49	3
50–54	6
55–59	8
60–64	10
65–69	11
70–74	12
75–79	13

B

Total Cholesterol, mg · dL⁻¹	Age 20–39	Age 40–49	Age 50–59	Age 60–69	Age (y) 70–79
< 160	0	0	0	0	0
160–199	4	3	2	1	0
200–239	7	5	3	1	0
240–279	9	6	4	2	1
≥ 280	11	8	5	3	1

C

	Age 20–39	Age 40–49	Age 50–59	Age 60–69	Age (y) 70–79
Nonsmoker	0	0	0	0	0
Smoker	8	5	3	1	1

D

HDL, mg · dL⁻¹	Points
≥ 60	−1
50–59	0
40–49	1
< 40	2

E

Systolic BP, mmHg	If Untreated	If Treated
< 120	0	0
120–129	0	1
130–139	1	2
140–159	1	2
≥ 160	2	3

F

Point Total	10-Year Risk, %
< 0	< 1
0	1
1	1
2	1
3	1
4	1
5	2
6	2
7	3
8	4
9	5
10	6
11	8
12	10
13	12
14	16
15	20
17	25
≥ 17	≥30

Estimate of 10-Year Risk for Women
(Framingham Point Scores)

A

Age, y	Points
20–34	−7
35–39	−3
40–44	0
45–49	3
50–54	6
55–59	8
60–64	10
65–69	12
70–74	14
75–79	16

B

Total Cholesterol, mg · dL⁻¹	Age 20–39	Age 40–49	Age 50–59	Age 60–69	Age (y) 70–79
< 160	0	0	0	0	0
160–199	4	3	2	1	1
200–239	8	6	4	2	1
240–279	11	8	5	3	2
≥ 280	13	10	7	4	2

C

	Age 20–39	Age 40–49	Age 50–59	Age 60–69	Age (y) 70–79
Nonsmoker	0	0	0	0	0
Smoker	9	7	4	2	1

D

HDL, mg · dL⁻¹	Points
≥ 60	−1
50–59	0
40–49	1
< 40	2

E

Systolic BP, mmHg	If Untreated	If Treated
< 120	0	0
120–129	1	3
130–139	2	4
140–159	3	5
≥ 160	4	6

F

Point Total	10-Year Risk, %
< 9	< 1
9	1
10	1
11	1
12	1
13	2
14	2
15	3
16	4
17	5
18	6
19	8
20	11
21	14
22	17
23	22
25	27
≥ 25	≥30

FIGURE 22-1. Estimation of coronary heart disease risk (nonfatal myocardial infarction or death) using the Framingham equation. HDL, high-density lipoprotein; BP, blood pressure. Add points accordingly for A–E and determine 10-year risk % in F.

BOX 22-3	DIFFERENTIAL DIAGNOSIS OF CHEST DISCOMFORT

CARDIAC

- Angina
- Acute coronary syndrome
- Mitral valve prolapse
- Pericarditis
- Aortic stenosis
- Aortic dissection

GASTROINTESTINAL

- Peptic ulcer disease
- Esophageal spasm or reflux disease
- Cholecystitis or cholelithiasis

PULMONARY

- Pneumonia
- Pleurisy
- Pulmonary embolism

MUSCULOSKELETAL

- Costochondritis

TRAUMA

- Cervical and thoracic spine disorders

sex, and discomfort type (see previous discussion of typical, atypical, and noncardiac chest discomfort in this chapter) to determine the probability of CAD (8). Their scheme stratifies the patient's risk into a low-, intermediate-, or high-risk group, which is used to determine the next step in the evaluation process (GETP8 Table 5.1). In general, those in whom a low probability of CAD is suspected based on the history and physical examination should be considered for treatment of cardiac disease risk factors and assessed for a noncardiac cause of their symptoms (e.g., referrals for gastrointestinal testing, pulmonary function testing, musculoskeletal assessment). However, patients with risk stratified into the intermediate- or high-risk groups should be assessed using diagnostic tests for cardiac disease. Intermediate-risk patients, who are appropriate candidates for a graded exercise test, should undergo an ECG or an ECG plus imaging (radionuclide or echocardiography) stress test. Pharmacologic stress assessment is considered when a patient cannot perform exercise on a treadmill. Patients who are in the high-risk group may begin with an exercise test or directly undergo cardiac catheterization, depending on their individual clinical situation. Cardiac catheterization is also appropriate for those who are initially categorized as intermediate risk and move into the high-risk group after stress testing. As a general rule of thumb, when a patient has a pretest probability

of >80% for significant coronary disease, it is more clinically cost-effective to move directly to coronary angiography as the initial step (24).

DETERMINING PROGNOSIS

Conventional exercise stress testing gives considerable prognostic information concerning cardiovascular and all-cause mortality. As covered elsewhere in this text (Chapter 21), there is a strong relationship between work capacity (as expressed in metabolic equivalents [METs]) and survival. The Duke Treadmill Score is an example of how METs, as well as other information, can be integrated to predict risk of future events (18). One important variable to report is the heart rate recovery. A heart rate recovery of <12 beats/minute has been related to cardiovascular deconditioning and predicts an overall higher mortality in many studies that is independent from other information on the stress test (1). Importantly, directly measured peak oxygen consumption expressed in $mL \cdot kg^{-1} \cdot min^{-1}$ is considered the best single predictor of survival among all of the diagnostic tests available in medicine today (10). Use of peak oxygen consumption has specific applications in determining prognosis in systolic heart failure and consideration of patients who may require heart transplant (peak oxygen consumption $<10–14$ $mL \cdot kg^{-1} \cdot min^{-1}$) (16). In addition, peak oxygen consumption has been recently shown to be predictive of complications in obese patients undergoing elective noncardiac surgery (19).

GUIDING MANAGEMENT

> **1.6.2-CES: Describe indications and limitations for medical management and interventional techniques in different subsets of individuals with CAD and peripheral artery disease.**

The most common application of stress testing in terms of management is the determination of ischemic threshold. In a patient with established CAD, irrespective of whether angioplasty or bypass surgery has been performed, there is atherosclerosis throughout the coronary tree, and the exercise capacity and the level of activity on which symptoms and/or signs of ischemia develop is critical. It is important to keep in mind that ischemia can manifest itself according to symptoms (chest discomfort, dyspnea), ST-segment elevation or depression, and, in some instances, by ventricular arrhythmias (7). The clinician's counseling concerning job functions, leisure activity, exercise, and prescription of medications is very much dependent on the results of stress testing in the presence of known CAD. It is important for the clinical exercise physiologist to convey the important information discussed above to give the clinician the clearest picture possible with respect to the patient's ischemic heart disease and response to exercise stress.

DECISION STATISTICS OF DIAGNOSTIC TESTS

The ability of a diagnostic test to accurately identify individuals with heart disease is dependent on the sensitivity and specificity of the test, as well as the prevalence of the disease in the population being tested. Bayes theorem clarifies the importance that these variables play in the selection of the appropriate test in the workup of patients for heart disease. Depending on the specific test and patient and on the pretest likelihood (low, intermediate, or high) of the patient's having heart disease, physicians have a variety of clinical tests at their disposal that can be performed. The following paragraphs define the terms used in the process of determining and understanding about the accuracy of these diagnostic tests.

A positive test result is considered one in which the clinical judgment is that the patient evaluated has an abnormality that was identified by the test. Likewise, a negative test result is one that did not find an abnormality—or in others words, the finding was normal. It must be understood that any clinical test, even if considered the **gold standard**, will not always correctly identify whether a person has or does not have an abnormality. When the test result is considered positive and the patient is later found to not have the abnormality, the test result is then considered a **false-positive** result. On the other hand, if a test result is determined to be negative and later the patient is found to have the abnormality or disease, the initial test is considered a **false-negative** result. And likewise, tests that accurately assess a patient as positive or negative for an abnormality or disease are considered **true-positive** and **true-negative** results, respectively.

Based on this knowledge, the **sensitivity** and **specificity** of a type of clinical test can be determined (see GETP8 Box 6.2 to determine how to calculate sensitivity and specificity). Sensitivity refers to how often the test uncovers an abnormality or disease in a population with the abnormality or disease. Specificity is the percentage of tests that are negative or normal in a population without the abnormality or disease. For any type of clinical test, the success of a test to uncover an abnormality, if it is present, is only as good as the technical performance of the test, the appropriateness of the test for the person being evaluated, and the interpretation or clinical judgment of the clinician who evaluates the test results. It is important to remember that sensitivity and specificity are terms applied to the performance of a diagnostic test in a population.

The **predictive value** of a clinical test provides us with insight into the ability of a test to accurately determine the presence or absence of an abnormality or disease in a single person. The predictive value relies on the test sensitivity and specificity and the **prevalence** of disease in the population being tested. Thus, the **positive predictive value** is the probability of disease being present in a person with a positive test. Conversely, the **negative predictive value** is the probability of disease being absent in a person with a negative test. As such, it is important that the proper population, techniques, and interpretation be applied to any clinical test to enhance the predictive value. It is this criterion on which studies in the literature are evaluated and recommendations made for diagnostic testing. Table 22-1 provides an overview of the sensitivity, specificity, and predictive values of various cardiac tests that are presented in the next several sections.

There are two statistical methods used to evaluate the overall value of a diagnostic test. The **diagnostic accuracy** is the ability of the test to make the correct determination—that is, be positive when disease is present and be negative when disease is absent—and holds the test at a single cutpoint. In a 2×2 table, diagnostic accuracy is the correct two cells divided by all four cells. The other statistical method used to evaluate diagnostic tests is the **receiver operating characteristic curve** (ROC curve). This is a plot of sensitivity (true positives) on the x axis and 1-specificity (false negatives) on the y axis. The ROC curve is important because it gives information about the test performance through a range of values and allows one to determine the optimal cutpoint for a positive test. In general, an ROC curve with 50% of the area under the curve is considered useless (no different than tossing a coin), 70% is considered moderately useful, and >80% considered extremely useful.

TABLE 22-1. COMPARISON OF TESTS FOR SENSITIVITY, SPECIFICITY, AND PREDICTIVE ACCURACY

GROUPING	STUDIES, n	TOTAL PATIENTS, n	SENSITIVITY, %	SPECIFICITY, %	PREDICTIVE ACCURACY, %
Standard exercise test	147	24,047	68	77	73
Thallium scintigraphy	59	6,038	85	85	85
SPECT	30	5,272	88	72	80
Adenosine SPECT	14	2,137	89	80	85
Exercise echocardiography	58	5,000	84	75	80
Dobutamine echocardiography	5	<1,000	88	84	86
Dobutamine scintigraphy	20	1,014	88	74	81
Coronary calcium score	16	3,683	60	70	65

SPECT, single-photon emission computed tomography.

Adapted from www.cardiology.palo-alto.med.va.gov/slides/ExerciseTest.ppt.

HOW TO DECIDE WHICH DIAGNOSTIC TEST TO SELECT

As mentioned in the previous section, it is important to select the appropriate test for the patient and the indication (screening, diagnosis, prognosis, or management).

The decision tree in Figure 22-2 was developed by the ACC and the AHA (12). It can be used to illustrate to clinical exercise personnel how decisions are made during the diagnosis of CAD. The next several sections review the common diagnostic methods for CAD. These techniques are from the ACC/AHA guidelines for stable angina (11).

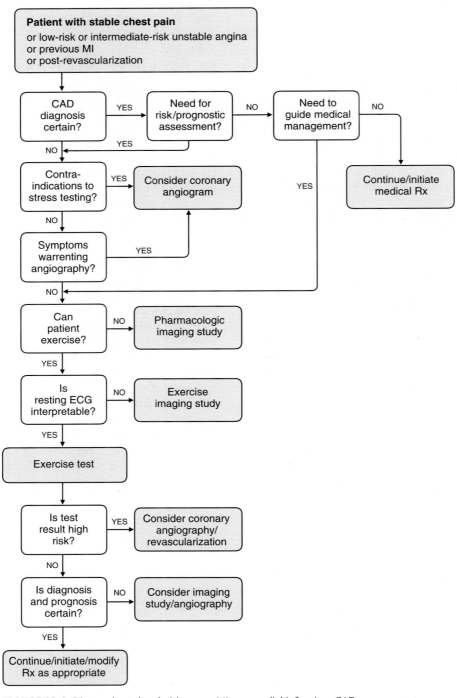

FIGURE 22-2. Diagnostic testing decision tree. MI, myocardial infarction; CAD, coronary artery disease; ECG, electrocardiography.

GRADED EXERCISE TESTING WITH ELECTROCARDIOGRAPHY

In-depth information regarding the performance and interpretation of graded exercise tests can be found in Chapter 21 and in GETP8 Chapters 5 and 6. This section discusses only the decision-making process with respect to the entire process of patient evaluation for ischemia. The decision to perform a graded exercise test should be made based on several criteria, including the pretest likelihood that the patient has CAD (see GETP8 Table 5.1), whether the patient can adequately exercise to symptom-limited maximum, and whether the ECG will be interpretable at peak exercise for possible ischemia.

Patients with repolarization abnormalities (left bundle branch block [LBBB], LVH, using digoxin, are not appropriate candidates for graded exercise testing without imaging when the indication is screening or diagnosis of CAD. However, those with right bundle branch block or <1 mm ST-segment depression (not including V1–3) can be tested. Box 22-4 lists the types of patients who are appropriate and inappropriate candidates for diagnostic testing using graded exercise testing without imaging. Those in the inappropriate category should be considered for stress testing with imaging, for angiography if considered at an intermediate or high risk, or for noncardiac testing or risk factor treatment if considered low risk. Depending on the interpretation of the graded exercise test (see Chapter 21 and GETP8 Chapter 6), a recommendation for no further testing (negative test result) or for further testing (equivocal or positive test result) is made. When the indications are prognosis and management, information other than the ECG findings becomes more valuable, and often testing without adjunctive imaging is performed.

There is a clinical workup "gap" between what is recommended by the ACC/AHA Guidelines for Exercise Testing and what is commonly practiced by the medical community when faced with making a decision about a patient requiring assessment for heart disease (12). The guidelines recommend that patients with chest discomfort, a normal resting ECG, and the ability to ambulate be scheduled for an exercise test with ECG monitoring alone. In clinical practice, many physicians faced with this scenario begin with an imaging test. Instead, an exercise test with imaging is recommended by the guidelines as an initial diagnostic test for patients with an abnormal resting ECG, those who are unable to walk, and those with a history of coronary bypass surgery. Although this strategy provides a slight improvement in predictive accuracy over the stress ECG combined with the Duke Treadmill Score (18) (see GETP8 Figure 6.2), it does so at a significantly increased cost. Many believe the one exception to this rule is women. Women commonly have exercise-induced ECG changes without ischemia resulting in lower sensitivity and specificity, thus, in women with chest discomfort, some sort of adjunctive imaging is commonly performed (20).

IMAGING METHODS

> **1.3.1-CES: Describe common procedures and apply knowledge of results from radionuclide imaging (e.g., thallium, technetium, sestamibi, tetrafosmin, single-photon emission computed tomography [SPECT]), stress echocardiography, and pharmacologic testing (e.g., dobutamine, adenosine, persantine)**

BOX 22-4   CANDIDATES FOR EXERCISE ELECTROCARDIOGRAPHIC ASSESSMENT (REGULAR STRESS TESTING WITHOUT IMAGING)

APPROPRIATE CANDIDATES/APPLICATIONS

Able to exercise to achieve adequate myocardial stress (i.e., >85% of predicted peak heart rate or double product > ~ 24,000

If repolarization abnormality is either right bundle branch block or (<1 mm ST-segment depression not caused by digoxin use

Screening for significant coronary artery disease (CAD) when the 10-year Framingham risk is >20%

Diagnosis of chest discomfort in intermediate-risk patients based on age, sex, and symptoms

Prognosis of patients with established CAD, heart failure, and for entry into cardiac rehabilitation

Guiding medical and revascularization therapy in patients with established CAD

INAPPROPRIATE CANDIDATES

Women with baseline ST/T wave abnormalities

Low or high risk of ischemic heart disease, including asymptomatic patients with possible ischemia during ambulatory electrocardiographic monitoring or those with acute coronary syndromes

Pre-existing repolarization abnormalities (left bundle branch block, left ventricular hypertrophy with strain, digoxin, ventricular pacing, nonspecific ST-segment depression >1 mm)

Pre-excitation syndrome (Wolff-Parkinson-White)

Patients unable to exercise to an adequate myocardial stress level (i.e., <85% of predicted peak heart rate or double product < ~24,000) because of arthritis, pulmonary disease, or peripheral vascular disease

Imaging techniques for the diagnosis of CAD provide slightly higher sensitivity and specificity than exercise testing with ECG analysis. Candidates for imaging studies, versus stress ECG, are those with an uninterpretable ECG and those unable to exercise to a level high enough to produce an adequate myocardial stress. In general, imaging studies allow for the patient to be further risk stratified to either a low- or high-risk group. If the test is equivocal, then either a different imaging test or coronary angiography may be suggested as a next step in the diagnostic process. These imaging techniques are categorized as echocardiography or myocardial perfusion imaging and are reviewed in the next several sections (also see GETP8 Chapter 5).

ECHOCARDIOGRAPHY

> **1.3.1-CES: Describe common procedures and apply knowledge of results from radionuclide imaging (e.g., thallium, technetium, sestamibi, tetrafosmin, single-photon emission computed tomography [SPECT]), stress echocardiography, and pharmacologic testing (e.g., dobutamine, adenosine, persantine).**

Over the past 25 years, echocardiography has become the second most frequently ordered test in the evaluation of cardiac patients after the resting ECG. With its high resolution, echocardiography provides a very accurate anatomic view of the heart. Doppler allows the evaluation of the physiology (e.g., blood flow) of the heart. The two procedures are almost always used in combination and provide an assessment of pathophysiology of cardiac disease processes. The principle of cardiac ultrasound is that high-frequency sound waves bouncing off cardiac structures and returning to the transducer provide information regarding that structure. The time it takes for the sound wave to return to the transducer is twice the time (which can be converted to distance) that it takes to travel from the transducer to the structure, such as a wall of the LV or a valve. By analyzing all of the returning sound waves with computers, it is possible to identify multiple structures and their relationships to each other. This allows the measurement of chamber size and wall motion, as well as identifying valvular structures and pericardial effusions.

Cardiac Doppler assessment uses the principle of Doppler shift to evaluate intracardiac blood flow. The frequency of the returning sound wave varies depending on whether the object is moving toward or away from the transducer. For example, whereas objects moving toward the transducer reflect a sound wave with a higher frequency than the emitted sound wave, objects traveling away from the transducer have a lower frequency. Therefore, blood flow toward the transducer can be distinguished from blood flow away from the transducer. Using Doppler, blood velocity and volumetric flow can be measured to determine intracardiac gradients, valve areas, valvular regurgitation, and intracardiac pressures.

Exercise echocardiography combines surface echocardiography and graded exercise testing (3,22). The echocardiographic images are obtained at rest and within 1 to 2 minutes after exercise. These images are then viewed using a side-by-side digital display format that allows the visualization of cardiac function both at rest and during exercise. Exercise echocardiography allows assessment of wall motion abnormalities, ejection fraction, and systolic and diastolic function. The normal response to exercise is for the LV to decrease in size, the ejection fraction to increase, and **augmentation** of LV wall motion to occur. Patients with ischemia have normal wall motion at rest and during exercise develop **hypokinesis** or **akinesis** of the LV wall(s) being supplied by an artery with 70% or more stenosis. Patients with a previous myocardial infarction (MI) have akinesis, or possibly **dyskinesis**, of the infarcted wall at rest as well as with exercise. Dilatation of the LV with exercise is a sign of triple-vessel disease.

It is always best to use exercise to deliver the increased myocardial oxygen demand because this best replicates the physiologic processes leading to ischemia. However, some patients may not be able to perform exercise. Intravenous dobutamine, a beta-adrenergic–stimulating agent, offers a pharmacologic alternative for patients who are unable to exercise. Infusion of an incremental dose of dobutamine evokes a positive inotropic and chronotropic response. Unlike dipyridamole and adenosine, dobutamine closely parallels the exercise response by creating an oxygen supply and demand imbalance. In cases in which a patient who is scheduled for a "nonexercise" stress test is actually able to perform an adequate amount of exercise, an alternate plan using graded exercise testing should be discussed. Dobutamine echocardiography has a special value in the detection of myocardial viability. In a hypokinetic segment at rest that is viable but served by a critically diseased vessel, low-dose dobutamine will induce hyperkinesis, and this will degrade to hypo- and then akinesis at higher levels. This so-called triple-phase response has a high predictive value for myocardial viability and response to revascularization.

When to Use Echocardiography

Echocardiography is useful at *rest* in patients who present with symptoms suggestive of valvular disorders, pericardial disease, or LV dysfunction. *Exercise* echocardiography is useful for those with suspected ischemic heart disease and improves the predictive accuracy of the graded exercise test from about 75% to 80%–85%. This improved predictive accuracy remains even after excluding normal submaximal stress tests and nondiagnostic exercise ECGs (10). An increased test predictive accuracy, compared with exercise ECG assessment alone, has also been observed in a population with a high prevalence of symptomatic CAD (3). Specificity is also enhanced by exercise echocardiography (3).

BOX 22-5 | **CANDIDATES FOR REST AND EXERCISE ECHOCARDIOGRAPHY ASSESSMENT WITH ECHOCARDIOGRAPHY (STRESS-ECHO)**

APPROPRIATE CANDIDATES

Rest

Suspected valvular disease

Suspected ventricular dysfunction

Patients with systolic murmur suggestive of aortic stenosis

Exercise

Women with baseline ST/T-wave abnormalities

Intermediate pretest probability of coronary artery disease and uninterpretable rest electrocardiogram (high- and low-risk patients may also be considered but may be more appropriate for myocardial perfusion imaging studies)

Previous revascularization (percutaneous coronary intervention or coronary artery bypass surgery) and questions concerning segmental myocardial viability

INAPPROPRIATE CANDIDATES

Rest

Patients with multiple myocardial infarctions

Those with complex wall motion abnormalities

Those with a poor imaging window (e.g., obese patients and patients with chronic obstructive pulmonary disease)

Exercise

Those who cannot adequately ambulate (may be more suitable to perform a pharmacologic test)

Box 22-5 identifies candidates for resting and/or exercise echocardiographic testing and those for whom testing would be inappropriate. In addition, stress echocardiography is useful in patients with a high likelihood of false-positive test results, such as women, and in patients with concurrent valvular or primary myocardial disease. Stress echocardiography is less useful in patients with multiple MIs, complex wall motion abnormalities, or a poor imaging window (e.g., obese individuals or those with chronic obstructive pulmonary disease).

MYOCARDIAL PERFUSION IMAGING

> **1.3.1-CES: Describe common procedures and apply knowledge of results from radionuclide imaging (e.g., thallium, technetium, sestamibi, tetrafosmin, single-photon emission computed tomography [SPECT]), stress echocardiography, and pharmacologic testing (e.g., dobutamine, adenosine, persantine).**

Radionuclide imaging, in combination with exercise or pharmacologic stress, is a commonly applied means for diagnosing CAD (2). Use of radionuclide imaging is indicated in follow-up of patients with abnormal ECG test findings and in the diagnostic evaluation of women, patients taking digitalis, and those with an abnormal resting ECG (i.e., LBBB, LVH, Wolff-Parkinson-White syndrome, intraventricular conduction defects, and resting ST-T wave abnormalities). It is also useful for the assessment of myocardial perfusion in patients with angiographically documented CAD and to study myocardial viability.

Thallium 201 (^{201}Th) and technetium 99m (^{99m}TC) injected at peak exercise and at rest are proportionally distributed within the myocardium in relation to regional myocardial blood flow and muscle viability. Newer $_{99m}$TC-based radiopharmaceutical flow tracers, such as sestamibi, provide diagnostic benefits over $_{201}$Th on the basis of their physical and biological attributes. $_{99m}$TC sestamibi has a higher energy output and a shorter half-life than $_{201}$Th. This allows administration of a larger dose, providing superior images. Also, the traditional stress–rest $_{201}$Th scan can be replaced with a protocol in which the rest images are acquired before stress, reducing the time required for the study and allowing acquisition of ECG-gated functional images.

In a normal myocardium, rest and stress images show accumulation of the isotope throughout the LV, reflecting integrity of regional blood supply. In areas of decreased perfusion, there is delayed uptake and slower washout. The presence of a perfusion defect on the stress images not present on the rest images suggests ischemia. Areas of scar from previous infarction characteristically show no uptake, either at rest or with stress. In addition to uniformity of isotopic uptake, ventricular size, wall motion, ejection fraction, and wall thickness can be assessed.

The diagnostic accuracy of $_{201}$Th and $_{99m}$TC are similar (6). Recent advances in radionuclide imaging, such as quantification of radionuclide data, tomographic imaging, and SPECT have enhanced the sensitivity and specificity beyond that provided by planar imaging. A review of studies using SPECT analysis indicated an overall sensitivity of 89% and a specificity of 70% (2).

As stated previously, it is always best to use exercise to deliver the myocardial stress in patients. However, some patients may not be able to exercise. In these cases, pharmacologic techniques, including the use of dipyridamole or adenosine, which are coronary artery selective vasodilators, can be used. With exercise, the myocardial oxygen demand is increased, and after it exceeds the ability of oxygen delivery by the blood, ischemia can be detected, if present. Use of the coronary artery vasodilators results in a mismatch of blood flow increase between the normal and diseased coronary arteries that can be detected on the perfusion imaging studies. Alternatively, as with echocardiography, dobutamine can be used with nuclear perfusion imaging. It is important for the clinical personnel to realize that when monitoring the ECG during pharmacologic stress testing, ischemic ST-segment changes are much less common than in conventional exercise stress testing. However, when ischemic ST-changes do occur, they have a very high (>90%) positive predictive value for significant CAD and should always be flagged (6).

When to Use Myocardial Perfusion Imaging

Myocardial perfusion imaging is most useful in patients who are intermediate- (or high-) risk patients for CAD, have abnormal ECG findings (LBBB, paced rhythm), have a history of bypass surgery, or have poor echocardiographic images (Box 22-6). Additionally, those who cannot exercise are candidates for pharmacologic imaging studies using dipyridamole, adenosine, or dobutamine. However, adenosine and dipyridamole cannot be used in patients with reactive airway disease because severe bronchospasm may occur. In addition, dobutamine in certain cases cannot be used because of the risks of serious arrhythmias.

POSITRON EMISSION TOMOGRAPHY

Positron emission tomography (PET) scanning is one of the most accurate methods for noninvasively identifying and assessing the severity of CAD. There are two specific clinical applications for PET scanning in patients with suspected CAD. The first is the noninvasive detection of coronary artery stenosis. This is performed using a PET perfusion agent at rest and during pharmacologic vasodilatation similar to that done for pharmacologic nuclear scintigraphy(5). Radionuclide tracers used to diagnose coronary artery stenosis are nitrogen-13, ammonia, and rubidium-82. Reviews of PET indicate higher sensitivity and specificity (~93%) than with SPECT. In institutions with both SPECT and PET scanning, PET scanning is typically reserved for patients with equivocal SPECT scans. Recent data suggest PET scanning generates superior imaging in the obese compared with nuclear scintigraphy because of the higher energy of the radiotracers used and less attenuation of the nuclear image data with PET acquisition. The second and more frequent clinical application of PET is the assessment of myocardial viability in patients with CAD and LV impairment, which is useful in determining if revascularization would be beneficial. Hibernating myocardium can be differentiated from scar using fluorine-18 fluorodeoxyglucose. In a summary of three studies that included 313 patients, if PET scanning demonstrated myocardial viability, mortality was reduced from 41% in a medically treated population to 8% in the surgically revascularized group (23).

CARDIAC MAGNETIC RESONANCE IMAGING

> **1.3.32-CES: Recognize the emergence of new imaging techniques for the assessment of heart disease (e.g., computed tomography [CT] angiography).**

Magnetic resonance imaging (MRI) provides an anatomic view of the heart by measuring the emitted electromagnetic waves from resonating nuclei and locating these nuclei in space. Because of a natural high contrast that exists between blood and cardiac tissue, no contrast agent is needed to identify the blood pool. In cardiology, MRI is used primarily to evaluate the patient for structural heart disease. The most frequent uses are to (a) assess the extent of damage to the LV as a complication of ischemic

---

BOX 22-6   CANDIDATES FOR NUCLEAR MYOCARDIAL PERFUSION IMAGING (STRESS-NUCLEAR)

APPROPRIATE CANDIDATES

Women with baseline ST/T-wave abnormalities

Those who have an uninterpretable resting electrocardiogram (i.e., left bundle branch block, left ventricular hypertrophy, digoxin, >1 mm ST-segment depression)

Use in conjunction with pharmacologic modes if patient cannot exercise

Those unable to achieve a high heart rate or systolic blood pressure

Intermediate- and high-risk symptomatic patients

INAPPROPRIATE CANDIDATES

Those who have contraindications to testing

In those patients with a history of bronchospasm, use of adenosine or dipyridamole is contraindicated

In those patients with a history or high risk of serious arrhythmias, use of dobutamine is contraindicated

BOX 22-7	CANDIDATES FOR CORONARY COMPUTED TOMOGRAPHIC ANGIOGRAPHY

APPROPRIATE CANDIDATES	INAPPROPRIATE CANDIDATES
Suspected coronary artery disease (CAD) based on history and physical (chest discomfort)	Asymptomatic patients
Intermediate pretest probability of CAD	Significant chronic kidney disease or allergic reaction to iodinated contrast
Uninterpretable baseline electrocardiogram, inability to exercise	Hyperparathyroidism or known disorders of calcium/phosphate metabolism
Uninterpretable/equivocal completed stress test with or without imaging	Medically unstable patients (noncardiac medical problems)

heart disease; (b) assess the type of cardiomyopathy and quantify physiologic parameters, such as wall stress and LV volume; (c) visualize the pericardium and assess its thickness in pericardial disease; (d) evaluate intracardiac and pericardial neoplastic disease; (e) provide information regarding morphology, size of shunts, and valvular function in congenital heart disease; and (f) evaluate the thoracic aorta for dissection, false lumens, periaortic disease, and abnormalities of the thoracic aortic arch (15).

Cardiac MRI can be used as the imaging method for pharmacologic stress with adenosine, dipyridamole, or dobutamine. Like echocardiography, wall motion can be evaluated. In addition, the degree of perfusion and late enhancement of the myocardium can be seen, giving the clinician an idea of how much ventricular damage is present.

CORONARY COMPUTED TOMOGRAPHY ANGIOGRAPHY

 1.3.31-CES: Understand the basic principle and methods of coronary calcium scoring using computed tomography (CT) methods.

1.3.32-CES: Recognize the emergence of new imaging techniques for the assessment of heart disease (e.g., CT angiography).

Computed tomography has been used for decades to image motionless solid organs, such as the brain, abdominal organs, etc. However, CT of the heart has only recently been mastered, using technology that acquires images very rapidly and timed (gated) to the cardiac cycle. This technology is called multidetector-row cardiac CT angiography (CTA). This form of imaging supplanted earlier forms of electron-beam computed tomography (EBCT), which could only evaluate the coronaries for the presence of calcium. Modern CTA gives a full evaluation of the degree of coronary calcium and generates a calcium score. Anatomic studies indicate that all human atheroma become calcified, beginning at the necrotic core of the lesion. Thus, the presence of coronary calcification represents the presence of atherosclerosis. The U.S. Centers for Medicare and Medicaid Services

(CMS) approved reimbursement for CTA in 2006, however, reimbursement from other carriers is still regionally determined. CTA generates images of the coronary arteries that are comparable to conventional angiography. A recent randomized trial by Goldstein et al. demonstrated that CTA was superior to conventional chest pain and stress test evaluations done in the emergency department in patients with acute chest discomfort (13). Given the much lower cost of CTA compared with forms of stress imaging, we can expect a growing number of patients to be referred for this form of testing. The ACC/AHA currently list suspected CAD as a class IIa, level of evidence B, indication for CTA (15). The circumstances that are considered appropriate for use of CTA include intermediate pretest probability of CAD, uninterpretable baseline ECG, inability to exercise, or uninterpretable/equivocal completed stress test with or without imaging (Box 22-7). Already clinicians are witnessing the integration of information from multiple imaging modalities. A common scenario is the discovery of moderate CAD by CTA. The next question is whether the lesion is hemodynamically significant, calling for a form of stress imaging. The most sophisticated approach thus far is CTA-PET, in which patients in the same scanner undergo anatomic CTA with pharmacologic stress imaging using PET (9). Computer algorithms then attempt to match up coronary anatomy with perfusion territories seen on PET.

CORONARY ANGIOGRAPHY

1.4.1-CES: Summarize the purpose of coronary angiography.

Coronary angiography using the cardiac catheterization technique is considered the gold standard for assessing the presence of CAD (11,12). Given the time, expense, and invasive nature of the test, it is often considered as a last-resort for diagnostic testing on the large menu of tests currently available.

The technique requires the placement of a catheter through an incision in the common femoral artery (done in >95% of cases), radial artery, or brachial artery. The catheter is then guided through the femoral or brachial artery to the location of the coronary arteries. Iodinated contrast media is injected during radiographic fluoroscopy, which allows for its visualization while flowing through the coronary tree. An area of narrowing can then be identified, located with respect to the coronary artery anatomy, and quantified for the amount of stenosis within a given artery. Angiography cannot determine if a coronary artery lesion is flow limiting and causing ischemia during stress, and, therefore, most patients undergoing this test are previously symptomatic. However, the assumption that an identified lesion is causing ischemia can be made. Generally, coronary artery stenosis of 70% or more is required to cause ischemia. Those lesions between 50% and 70% of lumen diameter are considered borderline significant and are only considered clinically important if they corresponded to abnormalities seen on the stress imaging test or the patient is experiencing typical angina. Lesions ≤50% of lumen diameter are not generally thought to cause ischemia.

When to Use Angiography

> **1.6.1-CES: Describe percutaneous coronary interventions (PCI) and peripheral interventions as an alternative to medical management or bypass surgery.**

Referral for angiography is appropriate when noninvasive assessment cannot be made because of contraindications, test inadequacy, or in symptomatic patients who are considered to be at high risk for CAD either before or after noninvasive testing. Additionally, patients who have an equivocal noninvasive test, and thus an uncertain diagnosis, are also potential candidates for referral for coronary angiography. Most commonly, coronary angiography is appropriate for patients with acute symptoms (acute coronary syndromes) in the hospital and for those outpatients with positive noninvasive studies discussed above. Box 22-8 presents appropriate and inappropriate patients for angiography referral. A trend is to combine the diagnostic and therapeutic parts of the procedure with the aim in most patients to perform angiography and move into a coronary angioplasty with stenting during the same procedural setting.

INTRAVASCULAR ULTRASOUND

In addition to the standard cardiac catheterization assessments commonly performed, many laboratories also offer intracoronary diagnostic procedures to evaluate the severity of coronary artery stenosis. Atherosclerotic plaque development in the wall of the coronary artery results in a remodeling process of the entire blood vessel, which helps to maintain the lumen diameter. Traditional coronary angiography allows only for the visualization of the lumen of the coronary artery and thus may underestimate the size of a plaque in a remodeled artery. Also, coronary

---

BOX 22-8   CARDIAC CATHETERIZATION AND CORONARY ANGIOGRAPHY

APPROPRIATE CANDIDATES

Positive stress testing with or without imaging

Very high pretest probability of coronary artery disease (CAD) based on clinical evaluation

Known CAD in the setting of acute coronary syndrome

INAPPROPRIATE CANDIDATES

Asymptomatic patients

Patients who are deemed not candidates for revascularization

Significant chronic kidney disease or allergic reaction to iodinated contrast (relative contraindications)

---

angiographic evaluation of coronary artery stenosis frequently identifies a lesion that appears "borderline significant" (i.e., stenoses of 50%–70%). Further evaluation of these lesions using intravascular ultrasound (IVUS), intravascular Doppler (coronary flow velocity), and fractional flow reserve helps to determine which of these stenoses requires revascularization with either percutaneous coronary intervention (PCI) or coronary bypass surgery.

During diagnostic evaluation, IVUS provides the visualization of the lumen and wall of the vessel and provides the size of the plaque. During interventional angiography, IVUS can be used after angioplasty to evaluate vessel patency and to look for complications such as coronary artery dissection. Additionally, IVUS is used in coronary stenting to provide information about the deployment of the stent. The most common use of IVUS at this time is to assess the severity and significance of left main coronary lesions, which are found incidentally. These lesions may not have been suggested by noninvasive imaging but, when present, can lead to higher rates of sudden death.

Intravascular Doppler techniques provide information about the amount of obstruction to blood flow from an individual plaque within a coronary artery. By measuring the velocity of blood flow at the level of the lesion and determining the vessel's cross-sectional area, an estimate of coronary blood flow distal to the coronary stenosis can be made. Adenosine, a vasodilator that is infused into the coronary artery, is used to assess coronary artery vasodilatation. Normal coronary arteries increase blood flow by 250% or more in response to the adenosine challenge. Increases of <250% suggest that the distal vasculature is maximally dilated and that the coronary stenosis is limiting vasodilatation and thus negatively affecting blood flow.

Fractional flow reserve is a measure of the pressure across a section of a coronary artery. It is performed using small guide wires capable of measuring pressure. A decrease in pressure across a coronary artery stenosis indicates a reduction in blood flow. Fractional flow reserve of <0.75 suggests the lesion is significantly affecting blood flow and likely resulting in ischemia.

These adjunctive techniques are time consuming and require the coronary arteries to be instrumented with wires and equipment, which runs the risk of inducing coronary ischemia or infarction. Thus, they are infrequently done and are reserved for the most difficult cases in the catheterization laboratory (4).

SUMMARY

Diagnostic testing in cardiovascular disease is done for screening, diagnosing, assessing prognosis, and guiding therapy. Exercise capacity is the most important prognostic variable for cardiac and all-cause mortality. Graded exercise testing, with or without imaging (echocardiography or radionuclide methods), CTA, and coronary angiography are the primary methods to detect CAD. Cardiac MRI has emerged as the test of choice for structural and congenital heart disease, particularly when it involves the great vessels and aorta. In the future, screening CTA to identify preclinical disease or the status of existing disease composition and structure may become mainstream and is likely to change the practice of preventive cardiology. The concept of reduction in cardiac risk to treatment of known and proven CAD by CTA is likely to gain popularity among clinicians and patients alike.

REFERENCES

1. Aktas MK, Ozduran V, Pothier CE, Lang R, Lauer MS. Global risk scores and exercise testing for predicting all-cause mortality in a preventive medicine program. *JAMA*. 2004;22;292(12):1462–1468.
2. American Society of Nuclear Cardiology. Imaging guidelines for nuclear cardiology procedures. American Society of Nuclear Cardiology. Myocardial perfusion stress protocols. *J Nucl Cardiol*. 1996;3(3):G11–15.
3. Armstrong WF, Pellikka PA, Ryan T, Crouse L, Zoghbi WA. Stress echocardiography: recommendations for performance and interpretation of stress echocardiography. Stress Echocardiography Task Force of the Nomenclature and Standards Committee of the American Society of Echocardiography. *J Am Soc Echocardiogr*. 1998; 11(1):97–104.
4. Bashore TM, Bates ER, Kern MJ, et al. American College of Cardiology/American Heart Association. American College of Cardiology/Society for Cardiac Angiography and Interventions clinical expert consensus document on cardiac catheterization laboratory standards: summary of a report of the American College of Cardiology Task Force on Clinical Expert Consensus Documents. *Catheter Cardiovasc Interv*. 2001;53(2):281–286.
5. Bateman TM. Cardiac positron emission tomography and the role of adenosine pharmacologic stress. *Am J Cardiol*. 2004;94(2A): 19D–24D; discussion 24D–25D.
6. Cortigiani L, Lombardi M, Michelassi C, Paolini EA, Nannini E. Significance of myocardial ischemic electrocardiographic changes during dipyridamole stress echocardiography. *Am J Cardiol*. 1998;82(9):1008–1012.
7. Davies RF, Goldberg AD, Forman S, et al. Asymptomatic Cardiac Ischemia Pilot (ACIP) study two-year follow-up: outcomes of patients randomized to initial strategies of medical therapy versus revascularization. *Circulation*. 1997;95(8):2037–2043.
8. Diamond GA, Forrester JS. Analysis of probability as an aid in the clinical diagnosis of coronary-artery disease. *N Engl J Med*. 1979; 300:1350–1358.
9. Di Carli MF, Dorbala S, Hachamovitch R. Integrated cardiac PET-CT for the diagnosis and management of CAD. *J Nucl Cardiol*. 2006;13(2):139–144.
10. Franklin BA. Survival of the fittest: evidence for high-risk and cardioprotective fitness levels. *Curr Sports Med Rep*. 2002;1(5): 257–259.
11. Gibbons RJ, Abrams J, Chatterjee K, et al. ACC/AHA 2002 guideline update for the management of patients with chronic stable angina: a report of the American College of Cardiology/American Heart Association Task Force on Practice Guidelines (Committee to Update the 1999 Guidelines for the Management of Patients with Chronic Stable Angina); 2002. Available at: www.acc.org/ clinical/ guidelines/stable/stable.pdf.
12. Gibbons RJ, Balady GJ, Bricker JT, et al. ACC/AHA 2002 guideline update for exercise testing: a report of the American College of Cardiology/American Heart Association Task Force on Practice Guidelines (Committee on Exercise Testing); 2002. Available at: www.acc.org/clinical/guidelines/exercise/dirindex.htm.
13. Goldstein JA, Gallagher MJ, O'Neill WW, Ross MA, O'Neil BJ, Raff GL. A randomized controlled trial of multi-slice coronary computed tomography for evaluation of acute chest pain. *J Am Coll Cardiol*. 2007;49(8):863–871.
14. Grundy SM, Cleeman JI, Merz CN, et al. National Heart, Lung, and Blood Institute, American College of Cardiology Foundation, American Heart Association: Implications of recent clinical trials for the National Cholesterol Education Program Adult Treatment Panel III guidelines. *Circulation*. 2004;110(2):227–239.
15. Hendel RC, Patel MR, Kramer CM, et al. American College of Cardiology Foundation Quality Strategic Directions Committee Appropriateness Criteria Working Group, American College of Radiology, Society of Cardiovascular Computed Tomography, Society for Cardiovascular Magnetic Resonance, American Society of Nuclear Cardiology, North American Society for Cardiac Imaging; Society for Cardiovascular Angiography and Interventions, Society of Interventional Radiology. ACCF/ACR/SCCT/SCMR/ ASNC/NASCI/SCAI/ SIR 2006 appropriateness criteria for cardiac computed tomography and cardiac magnetic resonance imaging: a report of the American College of Cardiology Foundation Quality Strategic Directions Committee Appropriateness Criteria Working Group, American College of Radiology, Society of Cardiovascular Computed Tomography, Society for Cardiovascular Magnetic Resonance, American Society of Nuclear Cardiology, North American Society for Cardiac Imaging, Society for Cardiovascular Angiography and Interventions, and Society of Interventional Radiology. *J Am Coll Cardiol*. 2006;48(7):1475–1497.
16. Hunt SA, Abraham WT, Chin MH, et al. American College of Cardiology, American Heart Association Task Force on Practice Guidelines, American College of Chest Physicians, International Society for Heart and Lung Transplantation, Heart Rhythm Society. ACC/AHA 2005 guideline update for the diagnosis and management of chronic heart failure in the adult: a report of the American College of Cardiology/American Heart Association Task Force on Practice Guidelines (Writing Committee to Update the 2001 Guidelines for the Evaluation and Management of Heart Failure): developed in collaboration with the American College of Chest Physicians and the International Society for Heart and Lung Transplantation; endorsed by the Heart Rhythm Society. *Circulation*. 2005;112(12):e154–235.

17. Joint National Committee on Prevention, Detection, Evaluation, and Treatment of High Blood Pressure. The seventh report of the Joint National Committee on Prevention, Detection, Evaluation, and Treatment of High Blood Pressure. *JAMA*. 2003;209:2560–2572.

18. Mark DB, Shaw L, Harrell FE, et al. Prognostic value of a treadmill exercise score in outpatients with suspected coronary artery disease. *N Engl J Med*. 1991;325:849–853.

19. McCullough PA, Gallagher MJ, deJong AT, et al. Cardiorespiratory fitness and short-term complications after bariatric surgery. *Chest*. 2006;130(2):517–525.

20. Mieres JH, Shaw LJ, Arai A, et al. Cardiac Imaging Committee, Council on Clinical Cardiology, and the Cardiovascular Imaging and Intervention Committee, Council on Cardiovascular Radiology and Intervention, American Heart Association. Role of noninvasive testing in the clinical evaluation of women with suspected coronary artery disease: consensus statement from the Cardiac Imaging Committee, Council on Clinical Cardiology, and the Cardiovascular Imaging and Intervention Committee, Council on Cardiovascular Radiology and Intervention, American Heart Association. *Circulation*. 2005;111(5):682–696.

21. Pearson TA, Blair SN, Daniels SR, et. al. AHA guidelines for primary prevention of cardiovascular disease and stroke: 2002 Update: Consensus Panel Guide to Comprehensive Risk Reduction for Adult Patients Without Coronary or Other Atherosclerotic Vascular Diseases. American Heart Association Science Advisory and Coordinating Committee. *Circulation*. 2002;106(3): 388–391.

22. Quinones MA, Douglas PS, Foster E, et al. American College of Cardiology, American Heart Association, American College of Physicians, American Society of Internal Medicine Task Force on Clinical Competence. American College of Cardiology/American Heart Association clinical competence statement on echocardiography: a report of the American College of Cardiology/American Heart Association/American College of Physicians—American Society of Internal Medicine Task Force on Clinical Competence. *Circulation*. 2003;107(7):1068–1089.

23. Schelbert HR. 18F-deoxyglucose and the assessment of myocardial viability. *Semin Nucl Med*. 2002;32(1):60–69.

24. Sox HC, Hickam DH, Marton KI, et al. Using the patient's history to estimate the probability of coronary artery disease: a comparison of primary care and referral practices [published erratum appears in *Am J Med*. 1990;89:550]. *Am J Med*. 1990;89:7–14.

25. Wilson PWF, D'Agostino RB, Levy D, Belanger AM, Silbershatz H, Kannel WB. Prediction of coronary heart disease using risk factor categories. *Circulation*. 1998;97:1837–1847.

SELECTED REFERENCES FOR FURTHER READING

Cheitlin MD, Armstrong WF, Aurigemma GP, et al. ACC/AHA/ASE 2003 guideline update for the clinical application of echocardiography: a report of the American College of Cardiology/American Heart Association Task Force on Practice Guidelines (ACC/AHA/ASE Committee to Update the 1997 Guidelines for the Clinical Application of Echocardiography); 2003. Available at: www.acc.org/clinical/guidelines/echo/index.pdf.

Ehrman JK, Gordon PM, Visich PS, Keteyian SJ. *Clinical Exercise Physiology*. 2nd ed.; Champaign (IL): Human Kinetics; 2008.

Klocke FJ, Baird MG, Bateman TM, et al. ACC/AHA/ASNC guidelines for the clinical use of cardiac radionuclide imaging: a report of the American College of Cardiology/American Heart Association Task Force on Practice Guidelines (ACC/AHA/ASNC Committee to Revise the 1995 Guidelines for the Clinical Use of Radionuclide Imaging); 2003. Available at: www.acc.org/clinical/guidelines/radio/rni_fulltext.pdf.

INTERNET RESOURCES

- American College of Cardiology: www.acc.org
- American Heart Association: Scientific statements and practice guidelines topic list: www.americanheart.org/presenter.jhtml?identifier=2158
- International Atherosclerosis Society: www.athero.org

Diagnostic Procedures in Patients with Pulmonary Diseases

Lung disease can generally be classified into one of three categories: obstructive, restrictive, or vascular disease. Patients with lung disease often develop shortness of breath precipitated by exercise or strenuous conditions as the first symptom regardless of the type of disease process that is present. Although this presenting symptom is the same, the pathophysiology associated with the development of such symptomatology is varied depending on the underlying disease process. This chapter addresses the pathophysiology and associated limitations of each of these disease processes, and the clinical assessment of patients with lung disease.

NORMAL VENTILATORY MECHANICS

> **3.2.1-HFS: Knowledge of pulmonary risk factors or conditions that may require consultation with medical personnel before testing or training, including asthma, exercise-induced asthma/bronchospasm, extreme breathlessness at rest or during exercise, bronchitis, and emphysema.**

During normal inspiration, the diaphragm contracts and moves downward, and the rib cage moves upward and outward. A negative pressure within the thorax develops and causes air to move into the lungs from the mouth. During normal expiration, the diaphragm relaxes and moves upward, and the rib cage moves inward, allowing air to move from the lungs to the mouth. Expiration is assisted by the elastic recoil of the lung parenchyma.

The larger airways remain open during inspiration and expiration because they are supported by cartilage in their walls. As the size of the airway decreases, the amount of cartilage present in the airway wall is reduced. The smallest airways have no cartilage and are tethered open by the surrounding meshwork of the lung, which includes the alveoli. During inspiration, these smaller airways are pulled open by the development of negative intrathoracic pressure resulting in traction of the airways. During expiration, these airways may collapse because of the positive intrathoracic pressure causing a reduction in the lung volume and traction over the smaller airways (Fig. 23-1).

> > > KEY TERMS

Asthma: A continuum of disease processes characterized by inflammation of the airway wall.

Chronic bronchitis: A clinical diagnosis for patients who have chronic cough and sputum production.

Chronic obstructive pulmonary disease (COPD): A group of lung diseases (e.g., emphysema, chronic bronchitis, asthma) that result in airflow obstruction.

Dyspnea: The perception of shortness of breath.

Emphysema: A pathologic or anatomic description marked by abnormal permanent enlargement of the respiratory bronchioles and alveoli accompanied by destruction of the lung parenchyma.

Hypercapnia: Excess carbon dioxide in the blood.

Hypoxemia: Deficient oxygenation of the blood.

Pulmonary hypertension: An elevation in the blood pressure within the arteries of the lung.

Restrictive lung disease: A group of diseases characterized by the inability to normally inflate the lungs.

Timed walk test: One of a variety of tests (e.g., 6-minute walk test, shuttle walk test, endurance shuttle walk test) used to assess functional status. The distance walked over a certain period of time is measured during these tests.

Vascular lung disease: A group of diseases that affect the vascular supply (pulmonary arteries, capillaries, and veins) of the lung.

Polycythemia: Excess red blood cells often secondary to hypoxemia.

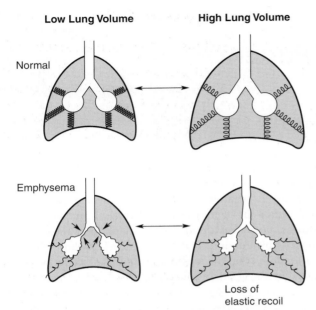

FIGURE 23-1. Small airways are tethered open by radial traction of lung tissue. Airway caliber depends on recoil of the lung, which is greater at high lung volume; hence, airway caliber is also greater at a high lung volume. In diseases in which elastic recoil is lost, small airways are prone to dynamic collapse when pressure outside the airway becomes more positive, as during forced expiration.

OBSTRUCTIVE AIRWAY DISEASES

> **1.1.30-HFS: Knowledge of how each of the following differs from the normal condition: dyspnea, hypoxia, and hyperventilation.**

> **1.1.14-CES: Identify normal and abnormal respiratory responses during rest and exercise as assessed during a pulmonary function test (i.e., forced vital capacity [FVC], maximum voluntary ventilation [MVV], forced expiratory volume in 1 second [FEV1.0], flow volume loop).**

> **1.2.15-CES: Recognize the pathologic process that various risk factors contribute for the development of cardiac, pulmonary, and metabolic diseases (e.g., smoking, hypertension, abnormal blood lipid values, obesity, inactivity, sex, genetics, diabetes).**

> **1.3.3-CES: Describe anatomic landmarks as they relate to exercise testing and programming (e.g., electrode placement, blood pressure).**

CHRONIC OBSTRUCTIVE PULMONARY DISEASE

Chronic obstructive pulmonary disease (COPD) is a common disorder characterized by progressive expiratory airflow obstruction. Symptoms develop insidiously over many years and include **dyspnea** at rest and with exertion, cough, and sputum production. The obstructive airway diseases include emphysema, chronic bronchitis, and asthma. Although these are often considered to be distinct entities, their physiologic and clinical features often overlap in individual patients.

Chronic obstructive pulmonary disease is characterized by nonuniform narrowing of airways secondary to inflammation. The airway narrowing increases resistance to airflow and results in uneven distribution of ventilation and expiratory flow limitation (Fig. 23-2). Loss of elastic recoil of the lung occurs, causing the small airways to close at an abnormally high lung volume, resulting in an increase in residual volume (RV) at the end of a forced expiration (also known as air trapping). Air trapping causes an increase in the total lung capacity and causes the diaphragm to flatten, ultimately causing a mechanical disadvantage for contraction (Fig. 23-3). All of these mechanisms lead to an increase in the work of breathing, which results in dyspnea for the patient.

Emphysema

> **1.1.14-CES: Identify normal and abnormal respiratory responses during rest and exercise as assessed during a pulmonary function test (i.e., FVC, MVV, FEV$_{1.0}$, flow volume loop).**

> **1.2.15-CES: Recognize the pathologic process that various risk factors contribute for the development of cardiac, pulmonary, and metabolic diseases (e.g., smoking, hypertension, abnormal blood lipid values, obesity, inactivity, sex, genetics, diabetes).**

> **1.3.33-CES: Recognition of the value of heart and lung sounds in the assessment of patients with cardiovascular and/or pulmonary disease.**

Emphysema is a type of COPD in which destruction of lung parenchyma and smaller airways occurs. A variety of mechanisms are responsible for this lung tissue destruction: protease–antiprotease imbalance, chronic inflammation, and pulmonary vascular wall thickening and smooth muscle proliferation (21,26,57). The inflammation is a result of exposure to cigarette smoke (37,52) and is mediated by a variety of inflammatory cell types (macrophages, lymphocytes, and neutrophils). For example, cigarette smoke stimulates alveolar macrophages to release tumor necrosis factor (TNF)-alpha, which leads nuclear factor-KappaB (NKF-B) protein production and subsequently interleukin-8 (IL-8), which then activates neutrophils. IL-8 activates the gene for MMP9, which is an enzyme that destroys elastin. Transforming growth factor (TGF)-beta is also released and causes fibrosis of the small airways. Other mechanisms (e.g., reduced histone deacetylation) are being uncovered that contribute to this inflammatory response (6,42,48).

As a result of these pathologic processes, the lung loses its elasticity and its elastic recoil pressure. Small airways lose traction with the surrounding alveolar walls

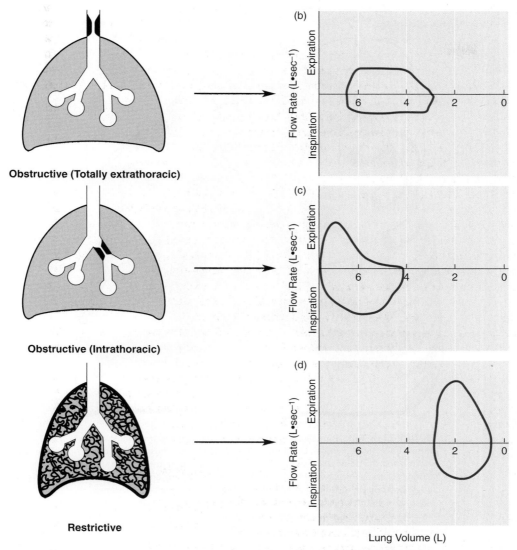

FIGURE 23-2. Maximal flow–volume curves in a normal subject, a patient with obstructive airways disease, and a patient with restrictive lung disease.

and become easily collapsible during expiration. Distribution of ventilation is nonuniform, and alterations in perfusion occur. Ventilation occurs in areas in which the capillary bed has been destroyed and an increase in dead space ventilation occurs.

In an attempt to overcome this elevation in dead space ventilation and alteration of the normal ventilation–perfusion balance, a patient with emphysema must maintain a high minute-ventilation (by initially increasing the breath to breath tidal volume [V_T] and, once this is maximized, by then increasing the respiratory rate). With all of these physiologic changes, an increase in the work of breathing occurs. A larger-than-normal supply of oxygen is needed by the respiratory muscles to maintain a stable ventilatory process. Oxygen supply is then diverted from the gut toward the respiratory muscles. An increase in overall metabolism occurs, resulting in malnutrition.

Functional skeletal muscle (in terms of strength and endurance) is lost, and severe muscular deconditioning occurs.

Patients with emphysema alter their pattern of breathing in an attempt to reduce the work of breathing. Air trapping can be decreased by breathing through pursed lips. This causes external resistance to flow and maintains a more positive intra-airway pressure during exhalation, minimizing compression of the small airways.

Patients with pure emphysema are often known as "pink puffers." They report significant dyspnea, are barrel-chested because of the marked lung hyperinflation, and have little cough or sputum production. They are typically thin with general muscle wasting. With mild to moderate emphysema, the arterial oxygen and carbon dioxide tensions are relatively normal. As the disease progresses, arterial oxygen tension may decrease (first during

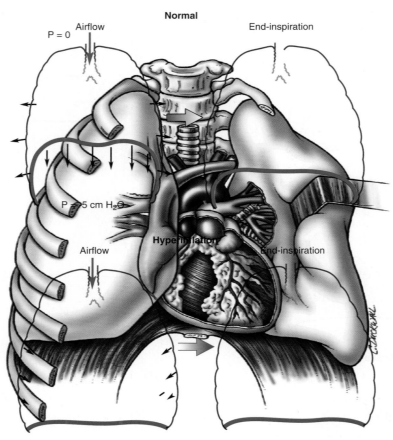

FIGURE 23-3. Top: Normally, the diaphragm is dome shaped, with most of the muscle fibers nearly vertical. Diaphragm contraction causes muscle fibers to shorten and the dome to descend, simultaneously expanding the rib cage. These actions generate a negative pressure inside the thorax causing airflow into the lungs. **Bottom:** In the lung that is hyperinflated (as in a patient with chronic obstructive pulmonary disease), the diaphragm loses its dome shape. With contraction, the diaphragm cannot descend normally, which can create a paradoxical inward movement of the lower rib cage.

exercise and then while at rest). Progressive elevation in pulmonary artery pressure may eventually develop and be followed by right heart failure (Fig. 23-4) (28). The diagnosis of emphysema is based on the patient's history and abnormal pulmonary function tests showing a reduced FEV_1/FVC ratio, elevated total lung capacity (TLC), and a reduced diffusing capacity for carbon monoxide.

Chronic Bronchitis

Chronic bronchitis is another type of COPD and is characterized by chronic cough and mucous production. Unlike emphysema, which primarily involves abnormalities within the lung parenchyma and smaller airways, chronic bronchitis primarily involves the large airways. The intrathoracic pressure generated by muscular effort and lung elastic recoil is normal in patients with chronic bronchitis. Airway wall injury occurs because of the effects of infiltration of inflammatory cells and mucous gland enlargement. As the body attempts to repair the inflamed areas, structural remodeling occurs, with an increase in the deposition of collagen in the airway walls

(52). Such bronchial and peribronchiolar inflammation results in further airway narrowing, ultimately resulting in an increase in airway resistance (34,35). Those areas of the lung that have an elevation in airway resistance receive little ventilation. The blood flow to these areas remains unchanged or decreased, causing underventilation and overperfusion. This ventilation–perfusion imbalance leads to arterial **hypoxemia**, which, in turn, may lead to increased pulmonary vascular resistance and pulmonary arterial hypertension. Eventually, right ventricular failure (cor pulmonale) may develop (Fig. 23-5). Hypoxemia stimulates the production of erythropoietin, resulting in excess blood volume (also known as secondary polycythemia). Polycythemia may lead to a high blood viscosity, increasing flow resistance in blood vessels and further compromising blood flow.

A typical patient with severe chronic bronchitis is known as a "blue bloater" because he/she exhibits a stocky habitus with central and peripheral cyanosis. Reduced airflow rate is associated with only mildly increased lung volumes and a relatively normal rate of oxygen transfer across

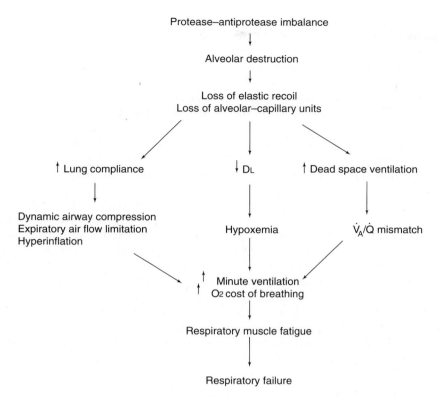

FIGURE 23-4. Progression of emphysema. $\dot{V}_A/\dot{Q}$ ventilation-perfusion ratio. DL, lung diffusion capacity.

the alveolar–capillary membrane (normal diffusing capacity for carbon monoxide). Secondary derangements in ventilatory control may develop, resulting in an elevation in the arterial carbon dioxide tension. Patients with chronic bronchitis tend to maintain low minute ventilation, which may further decrease during sleep and may result in nocturnal hypoxemia. The diagnosis of chronic bronchitis is based on the patient's history and abnormal pulmonary function tests (showing a reduced FEV_1/FVC ratio without a response to bronchodilators, mildly increased TLC, and a normal diffusing capacity).

Chronic cough and sputum production

↓

Expiratory airflow limitation
progressive dyspnea on exertion

↓

Progressive $\dot{V}_A/\dot{Q}$ mismatch
↓Arterial pO_2
↑Arterial pCO_2

↓

Pulmonary hypertension
Right heart strain
Polycythemia

↓

Right heart failure

FIGURE 23-5. Progression of chronic bronchitis.

Asthma

Asthma is yet another type of COPD characterized by increased airway reactivity resulting in widespread reversible narrowing of the airways. Its episodic nature and reversibility are important features separating it from the two other major types of obstructive airways disease (i.e., emphysema and chronic bronchitis). The airway reactivity is often in response to one of a variety of stimuli. Although a precipitating factor often cannot be accurately identified in most instances, it is possible to identify a specific agent (e.g., pollens, dust mites, chemical, animal dander, drugs, exposure to cold, and exercise). In such instances, appropriate avoidance of the precipitating agent is recommended.

Like the other obstructive lung diseases, the pathophysiology of asthma is related to an underlying inflammatory response. Asthma is often initiated by an antigen presented to the airway. An antibody to that antigen is produced, ultimately resulting in the release of various chemical mediators from mast cells and eosinophils. This response promotes ongoing inflammation of the airway walls and airway smooth muscle (4,25). The airway lumen becomes structurally changed and becomes occluded by a combination of mucus and denuded epithelium. Abnormal collagen deposition in the airways and subepithelial fibrosis subsequently develops and results in persistent airway narrowing (50).

The clinical symptoms of a patient with asthma are similar to those of the other obstructive lung diseases.

Shortness of breath and wheezing are commonly present. The diagnosis is made by using a combination of the patient's history, clinical examination, and pulmonary function tests. Reduced maximal expiratory flow rates, increased expiratory airway resistance, and elevated RV and TLC, which are corrected with the administration of a bronchodilator, are hallmarks of this disease. Bronchial hyperresponsiveness to methacholine (a medication that causes airway irritation) may be seen in those patients who have asthma and have normal pulmonary function tests. In some patients, asthma is only present during or after exercise and can be diagnosed based on the clinical history and measurement of pulmonary function tests following an exercise challenge (31).

Some patients with asthma may develop an acute worsening of symptoms. During this acute exacerbation, the lung units distal to the areas of airway narrowing are underventilated, resulting in ventilation perfusion imbalance. Initially, hyperventilation occurs, and the arterial oxygen tension remains normal and the arterial carbon dioxide tension decreases. As the exacerbation worsens, the distribution of ventilation and perfusion becomes more imbalanced, resulting in a decrease in the arterial oxygen tension and an increase in the arterial carbon dioxide tension. This can ultimately lead to respiratory failure.

CLINICAL FEATURES AND LABORATORY ASSESSMENT OF PATIENTS WITH CHRONIC OBSTRUCTIVE PULMONARY DISEASE

Most patients with COPD are current or former smokers. The development of symptoms may lag up to 20 years after the initiation of cigarette smoking. Many factors appear to play a role in the development of COPD. The amount and duration of cigarette use, a family history of lung disease (e.g., alpha-1 antitrypsin deficiency), childhood illnesses such as asthma and allergies, and a complete work history are important to know in an attempt to help determine the underlying basis for the COPD. Interestingly, sex also appears to play an important role in the development of lung disease, with women being more prone to developing lung disease at an earlier age than men (13,21).

Early in the course of the disease, there are no physical examination abnormalities. As the disease progresses, wheezing may be noted only on a forced expiration maneuver, and hyperinflation of the lung and chest wall occurs. A decrease in breath sounds with a decrease in movement of the diaphragm and a decrease in heart sounds become noticeable. A prolongation of the time for a forced expiration (>3 seconds) is seen. With ongoing progression, the patient may use techniques that are more effective to reduce the work of breathing, such as leaning forward with the arms outstretched and weight supported by the palms or breathing using pursed lips. If cor pulmonale develops, neck vein distention, enlarged liver, and peripheral edema may be seen.

Routine laboratory testing supplements the patient's history and physical examination. A chest radiograph is essential to confirm the presence of COPD (e.g., through the presence of lung hyperinflation, increase in the retrosternal airspace, flattening of the diaphragm, and enlargement of the pulmonary artery) and also to determine whether there may be another cause for dyspnea (e.g., pleural effusion, lung cancer, congestive heart failure).

An electrocardiogram (ECG) is helpful to determine whether cardiac disease may be present. Measurement of oxyhemoglobin saturation by cutaneous pulse oximetry or arterial blood gas analysis will help determine the presence of hypoxemia. With the latter, arterial carbon dioxide tension can also be determined. Measurement of hemoglobin will help to determine the duration of hypoxemia, particularly in the instance in which the hematocrit is $>50 \text{ g} \cdot \text{dL}^{-1}$, suggesting hypoxemia of long-standing duration. Computed tomography (CT) scanning of the chest will help to assess the lung parenchyma and to evaluate for other intrathoracic pathology (e.g., masses, pleural disease).

Measurement of pulmonary function tests should be performed on all patients suspected of having lung disease. In addition, pulmonary function testing in the form of simple spirometry should be performed for all smokers older than age 45 years and for any smoker who has respiratory symptoms (e.g., cough, sputum production, dyspnea), regardless of age (19,43,44). The pulmonary function testing should include measurement of TLC, RV, vital capacity (VC), inspiratory capacity (IC), forced expiratory volume in 1 second (FEV_1) and in 6 seconds (FEV_6), forced vital capacity (FVC), peak expiratory flow rate (PEFR), and diffusing capacity for carbon monoxide (Dl_{CO}). Although some of the measures (e.g., TLC, VC, RV, Dl_{CO}) require the use of sophisticated equipment, many (e.g., FEV_1, FEV_6, FVC) can be performed using very simple equipment. Pulmonary function testing will often help in the determination of the type of lung disease process that is present (Table 23-1).

TABLE 23-1. PULMONARY FUNCTION TESTING: INTERPRETATION FOR VARIOUS DISEASE STATES

	OBSTRUCTIVE	RESTRICTIVE	VASCULAR
FEV_1 (L)	↓	↓	↔
FVC (L)	↓	↓	↔
FEV_1/FVC (FEV_1/FEV_6)	↓	↔ or ↓	↔
TLC (L)	↑	↓	↔
VC (L)	↓	↓	↔
FRC (L)	↑	↓	↔
RV (L)	↑	↓	↔
Dl_{CO}	↔ or ↓	↔ or ↓	↓

↔, no change; ↑, increased; ↓, decreased. ↔ or ↑, no change early in disease process, increase late in disease; ↔ or ↓, no change early in disease process, decrease late in disease; Dl_{CO}, diffusing capacity for carbon monoxide; FEV_1, forced expiratory volume in one second; FRC, functional residual capacity; FVC, forced vital capacity; RV, residual volume; TLC, total lung capacity; VC, vital capacity.

BOX 23-1   ABNORMALITIES NOTED DURING EXERCISE IN PATIENTS WITH CHRONIC OBSTRUCTIVE PULMONARY DISEASE

Dyspnea

Leg discomfort

Reduced maximal oxygen consumption

Reduced work rate

High dead space ventilation (V_D/V_T)

Decreased V_T response with increased respiratory rate

Reduced inspiratory capacity with exercise (i.e., dynamic hyperinflation)

Variable arterial oxyhemoglobin desaturation

VD, dead space; VT, tidal volume.

Pulmonary function testing is helpful not only with the diagnosis of the disease but also with determination of the severity of the disease process. The FEV_1 is the best correlate with morbidity and mortality in these patients, and several proposals for staging have been developed using the FEV_1. The American Thoracic Society suggests staging based on the severity of airflow obstruction: stage I is an FEV_1 of >50% predicted, stage II is an FEV_1 of 35% to 49% predicted, and stage III is an FEV_1 of <35% predicted (3). In general, patients with stage I disease have little impairment in their quality of life. Patients with stage II disease have significant impairments in their quality of life, and patients with stage III disease are significantly impaired, often requiring many hospitalizations for severe exacerbations.

More recently, another staging system has been proposed by the Global Initiative for Lung Disease (GOLD Guidelines) panel and is characterized based on not only the spirometry but also on the patient's symptoms (41). Stage I (mild COPD) is characterized by a patient who has mild airflow limitation (FEV_1/FVC <70% but FEV_1 >80% predicted) and usually, but not always, has symptoms. Stage II (moderate COPD) is characterized by a patient who has worsening airflow limitation (FEV_1 between 30% and 80% predicted) and who has progression of symptoms to include dyspnea with exertion. Stage III (severe COPD) is characterized by a patient who has severe airflow limitation (FEV_1 <30% predicted) and the presence of respiratory failure or clinical signs of right heart failure. The latter staging system is the becoming the more widely accepted severity staging system for patients with COPD.

EXERCISE LIMITATIONS IN CHRONIC OBSTRUCTIVE PULMONARY DISEASE

> **1.1.14-CES: Identify normal and abnormal respiratory responses during rest and exercise as assessed during a pulmonary function test (i.e., FVC, MVV, $FEV_{1.0}$, flow volume loop).**

Exercise intolerance (either through the development of shortness of breath or easy fatigability) is invariably present in a patient with COPD. As the disease progresses, dyspnea and fatigability at even minimal levels of exercise can occur. A variety of factors are involved in exercise intolerance for patients with COPD: ventilatory abnormalities (impaired respiratory system mechanics and ventilatory muscle dysfunction), metabolic and gas exchange abnormalities, peripheral muscle dysfunction, and cardiovascular abnormalities (Box 23-1).

Ventilatory abnormalities are the primary cause for exercise limitation in patients with COPD. Airflow limitation, prominent on maximal expiratory efforts, occurs secondary to loss of elastic recoil of the lung parenchyma, airway inflammation, and airway collapse. As exercise effort increases (e.g., during exercise), expiratory flow increases to a point beyond which further effort does not produce any further increase in expiratory flow (Fig. 23-6) and results in exercise limitation. In patients with normal ventilatory mechanics, only a small fraction of the expiratory flow is used during tidal breathing, and airflow limitation is never reached, either at exercise or during rest. In patients with COPD, the anatomic and physiologic processes causing expiratory flow limitation (noted as scalloping of the expiratory portion of the flow volume curve) may be so severe in some that even during tidal breathing, expiratory limitation is reached. Patients

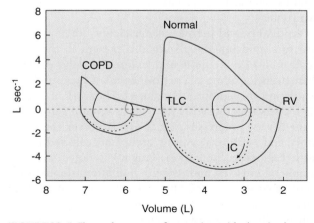

FIGURE 23-6. Flow volume curve for a patient with chronic obstructive pulmonary disease (COPD) (rest and exercise). IC, inspiratory capacity; RV, residual volume; TLC, total lung capacity.

with expiratory airflow limitation cannot reach the increased demands placed on the ventilatory system during exercise by increasing their expiratory flow as would occur in normal individuals.

As expiratory flow limitation occurs, the lung cannot fully empty during resting breathing. This is particularly worsened during exercise. As a result of this expiratory flow limitation, end-expiratory lung volume remains elevated, and *dynamic hyperinflation* of the respiratory system occurs. Dynamic hyperinflation results in a decrease in the inspiratory capacity and places severe mechanical constraints on V_T expansion during exercise despite an increase in the respiratory drive (16,39). The reduction in resting inspiratory capacity and resting expiratory flow limitation results in poorer exercise performance (10,38).

Dynamic hyperinflation also causes increased elastic loading of the inspiratory muscles. Alterations of the normal length–tension relationship of the inspiratory muscles (e.g., the diaphragm, sternomastoids, and scalenes) compromise the ability of these muscle groups to function efficiently. As exercise increases, progressive limitation of the normal increase in V_T despite maximal inspiratory efforts occurs because of this dynamic hyperinflation. In fact, dyspnea is likely more related to the effects of dynamic hyperinflation than it is to airflow obstruction. An increase in muscle oxygen utilization and muscle work occur in response to these pathophysiologic processes.

Gas exchange abnormalities (e.g., hypoxemia and hypercapnia) are commonly seen in patients with COPD. Airflow limitation results in an uneven distribution of ventilation with blood perfusion. Destruction of the lung parenchyma (e.g., as might occur in patients with emphysema), alveolar hypoventilation (e.g., as might occur in patients with chronic bronchitis), and an elevation in the resting physiologic dead space that does not decrease with exercise also may play a role in the gas exchange abnormalities. As patients exercise, the gas exchange abnormalities become more prominent, resulting in worsening hypoxemia.

Ventilatory and peripheral muscle dysfunction (both structural and functional) are also present in these patients (11,14). Strength and endurance (the primary characteristics of muscle performance) of the muscles of ventilation are significantly reduced. The work of breathing increases significantly for a given level of ventilation as the disease progresses (Fig. 23-7). However, the ventilatory and peripheral muscle groups are affected differently. Endurance limitation (fatigue) is noted with the peripheral muscles, and strength limitation is noted with the ventilatory muscles. Muscle biopsy of the peripheral muscles of a patient with COPD show a consistent reduction in type I (slow-twitch, low-tension, fatigue-resistant) fibers and an increase in type II (fast-twitch, high-tension) fibers. At a microscopic level, these mus-

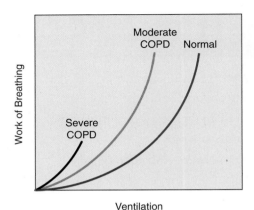

FIGURE 23-7. Work of the respiratory muscles increases as ventilation increases. As chronic obstructive pulmonary disease (COPD) progresses, the work of breathing is higher than normal at any given level of ventilation. In addition, the maximum work that can be generated by the respiratory muscles is diminished as the disease progresses.

cles show increased oxidative stress, increased apoptosis, and inflammatory changes. The systemic inflammatory state that is present in patients with COPD is only now being more fully understood as a causative mechanism for the local and systemic complications associated with the disease (7,45,54,61).

The skeletal muscle dysfunction results from a variety of pathophysiologic mechanisms. Hypoxia and oxidative stress (caused by reactive oxygen species, oxygen free radicals), disuse atrophy (deconditioning), malnutrition, skeletal muscle myopathy, and weight loss with altered substrate (e.g., amino acid, anabolic steroids, leptin) metabolism have all been shown to be associated with muscle dysfunction in patients with COPD. Current evidence also suggests an alteration of the oxidative capacity (reduction in citrate synthase and hydroxyacyl-CoA dehydrogenase activities and increase in glycolytic activities) of both the peripheral skeletal muscles and the ventilatory muscles, along with a reduction in the capillary density in patients with COPD (29).

RESTRICTIVE LUNG DISEASE

Restrictive lung diseases reduce lung volume through their involvement of the lung parenchyma or thoracic cage. There are more than 200 disorders that can affect the pleural space (e.g., hemothorax, pleural effusion), alveoli (e.g., pulmonary alveolar proteinosis, pneumonia), interstitial space (e.g., interstitial lung disease), neuromuscular system (e.g., myasthenia gravis, spinal cord injury), and thoracic cage (e.g., kyphoscoliosis, ankylosing spondylitis) and can result in a restrictive lung process. A patient with restrictive lung disease develops dyspnea (often first noted during exertion) that is related to the reduction in lung volume caused by the underlying disease process.

CLINICAL EVALUATION AND LABORATORY ASSESSMENT OF PATIENTS WITH RESTRICTIVE LUNG DISEASE

The initial evaluation of the patient should include a complete history and physical examination. The patient often seeks medical attention because of progressive shortness of breath (particularly with exertion) or a nonproductive cough. The history is helpful to elicit clues to the diagnosis, particularly when interstitial lung disease is being considered as a potential cause (Box 23-2). Attention should be paid to the patient's occupational history, environmental exposure history, medication history, family history, and smoking history.

The shortness of breath develops insidiously because a patient will often decrease his/her level of activity to compensate for the impairment. As the shortness of breath progresses and interferes with the patient's activities of daily living, medical attention is then sought. The duration of shortness of breath is helpful in the evaluation process. A short, rapid onset of symptoms is suggestive of hypersensitivity pneumonitis, eosinophilic pneumonia, or alveolar hemorrhage syndromes. A more prolonged course, with the development of symptoms over years or longer, is more characteristic of the interstitial lung diseases (particularly idiopathic pulmonary fibrosis).

The physical examination may be helpful but often not until the patient has developed significant symptoms. A thorough examination of the patient, with particular attention to the chest and neuromuscular systems, is important. A decrease in excursion of the chest with an increase in respiratory rate at rest is often present. A decrease in breath sounds over one side of the chest is seen in patients with pleural disease; an anatomic deformity of the chest and thoracic cage is seen in patients with kyphoscoliosis; and fine-end inspiratory rales (Velcro crackles) are seen in patients with interstitial fibrosis. Weakness of the extremities is present in patients with neuromuscular disease (e.g., myasthenia gravis). Arthritis can be associated with collagen vascular diseases or sarcoid. Integration of the history and physical findings should then prompt further diagnostic testing.

A chest radiograph should initially be performed. This helps to assess the lung volume, structure of the chest wall and thorax, and presence or absence of pleural, interstitial, or alveolar abnormalities. CT scanning (particularly high-resolution scanning) can assess for the presence of interstitial changes. Pulse oximetry and arterial blood gases are helpful to determine the degree of gas exchange abnormalities that may be present. Pulmonary function tests reveal a decrease in the FEV_1, FVC, and TLC with maintenance (or an increase) in the FEV_1/FVC ratio. A low diffusing capacity may be seen late in the disease course, particularly for patients with interstitial fibrosis. A reduction in the maximal expiratory and inspiratory pressures may be seen in patients with neuromuscular diseases. To determine the effects of the restrictive process during exertion, exercise testing must be performed. Measurements of pulse oximetry and expired gases can help assess the effects of the restrictive process. An abnormal response to exercise is noted in most patients with restrictive lung disease (22). The type of response may help determine the type of restrictive disease present. For example, a patient with interstitial fibrosis might be expected to primarily have gas exchange abnormalities, whereas a patient with neuromuscular weakness might be expected to primarily have abnormalities in the ability to increase ventilation with exercise.

EXERCISE LIMITATIONS ASSOCIATED WITH PATIENTS WITH RESTRICTIVE LUNG DISEASE

> **1.1.14-CES: Identify normal and abnormal respiratory responses during rest and exercise as assessed during a pulmonary function test (i.e., FVC, MVV, $FEV_{1.0}$, flow volume loop).**

The abnormality common to all of the restrictive lung diseases is a reduction in the TLC and FVC. This reduction in lung volume may lead to collapse of the smaller airway units with subsequent decrease in the functional alveolar–capillary interface and may lead to impaired gas exchange. A decrease in the diffusing capacity of the lungs may result in those who have disruption of this alveolar–capillary unit.

Interstitial lung disease is the best studied of the restrictive lung processes. Although there are a variety of causes for interstitial lung disease, the pathophysiologic and clinical characteristics for these diseases are similar. Chronic inflammation of the interstitium and alveoli

---

BOX 23-2	CAUSES OF INTERSTITIAL LUNG DISEASE

1. Occupational and environmental exposures
   Inorganic dusts (silica, asbestos, tin, coal, hard metals)
   Organic (hypersensitivity pneumonitis caused by bacteria, fungi, animal proteins)
2. Drugs or medications (chemotherapy agents, radiation exposure, oxygen)
3. Collagen vascular diseases (scleroderma, systemic lupus erythematosus, rheumatoid arthritis, polymyositis)
4. Neoplasm (bronchoalveolar carcinoma, lymphoma)
5. Unknown causes (interstitial pulmonary fibrosis, sarcoidosis, lymphangioleiomyomatosis, eosinophilic granuloma, nonspecific interstitial pneumonia, bronchiolitis obliterans organizing pneumonia)

BOX 23-3	ABNORMALITIES NOTED DURING EXERCISE IN PATIENTS WITH INTERSTITIAL LUNG DISEASE

Dyspnea

Reduced maximal oxygen consumption

Reduced work rate

Reduced V_T with increased respiratory rate at submaximal work rates

Increased dead space ventilation (V_D/V_T)

Arterial oxyhemoglobin desaturation during exercise

Unchanged $PaCO_2$ during exercise

VD, dead space; VT, tidal volume.

results in fibrosis of these structures. These changes reduce lung compliance and increase lung stiffness (23). A stiff lung requires more energy to stretch, requiring an increase in the transpulmonary pressure to achieve a given V_T. Not only are there changes in the lung capacity and stiffness, but the alveolar–capillary units are altered, as well as being replaced with fibrous tissue.

Gas exchange is often disrupted as a result of these pathologic changes and is the major factor in exercise limitation. In the early stages of the disease process, the resting arterial oxygen tension is normal but decreases during exercise, and the alveolar–arterial oxygen gradient increases (Box 23-3). As the disease progresses, resting hypoxemia with widening of the alveolar–arterial oxygen gradient occurs. Imbalance of ventilation and perfusion, shunting, and impaired oxygen diffusion all play a role in the development of the hypoxemia (14).

A characteristic ventilatory response to exercise occurs in patients with interstitial lung disease (54). The tidal volume is functionally limited because of the interstitial process, and an increase in minute ventilation occurs through an increase in the respiratory rate rather than the expected increase in V_T. Because of the constraints noted, the patient breathes with very rapid, shallow breaths in an attempt to reduce the work of breathing. This results in an increase in dead space ventilation (V_D/V_T) because of the decrease in V_T. Normally during exercise, V_D/V_T decreases because of the increase in V_T, but in patients with interstitial lung disease, the V_D/V_T remains constant or increases.

An increase in elastic recoil of the lung at functional residual capacity is present in patients with interstitial lung disease. In combination with the reduction in lung volumes, an adverse impact occurs on the ability of the respiratory system to adapt to the increasing ventilatory demands required during exercise.

Pulmonary hypertension may develop because of hypoxic vasoconstriction and obliteration of the pulmonary vascular bed by the underlying interstitial process. Most patients with interstitial lung disease develop significant pulmonary hypertension with exercise (61), and nearly all patients with interstitial lung disease have right ventricular hypertrophy. Pulmonary hypertension has been shown to significantly correlate with hypoxemia during exercise. Hypoxemia plays a more important role than does the abnormal ventilatory mechanics in the exercise limitation found in these patients. In fact, it has been suggested that the gas exchange abnormalities (secondary to this circulatory pathophysiology) are perhaps the most important factors in exercise limitation in patients with interstitial lung disease (14).

There are several other types of restrictive lung disease (e.g., neuromuscular, pleural, thoracic cage abnormality, or alveolar), and in each, a different pathophysiology in regards to the response to exercise occurs. For a patient with neuromuscular disease (e.g., myasthenia gravis), the ventilation and perfusion units of the lung are normal. In such an instance, the gas exchange of the lung is normal. Patients with neuromuscular disease will have limitation to exercise based on muscular limitations. Patients will not be able to increase tidal volume with exercise and will have a rapid increase in the ventilatory rate. Once the ventilation is limited by the underlying neuromuscular process, exercise will end. Patients with pleural disease or thoracic cage abnormalities will have a similar response to exercise. Patients with alveolar processes will have impairment in gas exchange, and exercise limitation is often secondary to hypoxemia.

In all of the various types of restrictive lung disease, gas exchange abnormalities can eventually occur secondary to loss of effective matching of ventilation and perfusion and diffusing abnormalities. As the diseases progress, hypoxemia and carbon dioxide retention results and exercise limitation occurs.

VASCULAR LUNG DISEASE

A variety of etiologies can result in **vascular lung disease**. These include diseases that involve the pulmonary veins and arteries and are generally characterized by obstruction of the pulmonary circulation and or disruption of the alveolar–capillary membrane. Both cause a decrease of the effective vascular bed, resulting in impairment of diffusion and gas exchange. Pulmonary hypertension and right ventricular failure ultimately develop.

Pulmonary hypertension is a mean pulmonary artery pressure at rest of <25 mm Hg or <30 mm Hg with exercise. It is often characterized as idiopathic or secondary. Idiopathic pulmonary hypertension is a disease, by definition, of uncertain etiology (7). Secondary pulmonary hypertension is a result of a specific disease process (e.g., severe COPD, interstitial lung disease, left ventricular [LV] dysfunction, mitral valvular stenosis, chronic thromboembolic disease [45], HIV infection [32], sleep-disordered breathing, connective tissue disease, medications, and portopulmonary hypertension).

CLINICAL ASSESSMENT AND LABORATORY EVALUATION OF PATIENTS WITH VASCULAR LUNG DISEASE

Patients with vascular lung disease present with the symptom of shortness of breath, often first noted during exercise. Typically, very few historical clues are present as to the cause of the patient's pulmonary hypertension. The clinical examination of the patient is often normal, with clear lung fields and normal mechanical movement of the chest and abdominal walls during inspiration and expiration. A cardiac murmur heard best at the base of the heart may suggest mitral stenosis. A gallop is suggestive of LV systolic dysfunction. A loud second heart sound, heard best over the second left intercostal space, can be present and is secondary to the accentuated closure of the pulmonary valve. With long-standing disease, right-sided heart failure may develop and hepatomegaly, peripheral edema, and jugular venous distention may be seen. Clubbing of the fingers can also be seen.

The laboratory evaluation of a patient with pulmonary hypertension should include a chest radiograph and ECG. The radiograph will show clear lung fields and an enlargement of the cardiac silhouette. An ECG will show a right ventricular strain pattern. Pulse oximetry determination of oxyhemoglobin saturation and arterial blood gas analysis are helpful to determine the presence of gas exchange abnormalities. The diagnosis is often first noted following an echocardiogram. Valvular heart abnormalities, LV systolic dysfunction, and RV dysfunction can be determined via echocardiography. An estimation of the systolic pulmonary artery pressure can be made. Ventilation perfusion scanning is helpful to determine the presence of chronic thromboembolic pulmonary hypertension. CT scanning and pulmonary angiography can help to assess the pulmonary parenchyma and the pulmonary vascular bed. Right heart catheterization with measurement of the right atrial, right ventricular, pulmonary artery, and left atrial pressures is necessary to confirm the diagnosis and to help direct therapy.

EXERCISE LIMITATION OF PATIENTS WITH VASCULAR LUNG DISEASE

> **1.1.14-CES: Identify normal and abnormal respiratory responses during rest and exercise as assessed during a pulmonary function test (i.e., FVC, MVV, FEV$_{1.0}$, flow volume loop).**

The pulmonary circulation is normally able to receive a five- to sixfold increase in blood flow with only a minimal resultant increase in pressure. Although pulmonary artery pressure increases during exercise, right atrial pressure increases only minimally. The pressure gradient increase across the pulmonary vascular bed occurring during exercise is less than the increase in cardiac output. This results in a decrease in the pulmonary vascular resistance and is felt to occur because of recruitment and distention of pulmonary capillaries. At peak exercise, improved efficiency of ventilation and perfusion and a decrease in the alveolar dead space occur (resulting in an increase in the V_D/V_T ratio).

The exercise limitation associated with pulmonary hypertension is primarily because of cardiac dysfunction (Box 23-4). Pulmonary vasoconstriction and remodeling of the vascular bed increase right ventricle afterload and limit stroke volume in response to exercise (22). As the right ventricle dilates over the course of the disease, a decrease in LV compliance and diastolic filling occurs. With exercise, an abnormal increase in right atrial and mean pulmonary artery pressure with a relatively normal pulmonary capillary wedge pressure is present (30). A decrease in the maximal cardiac output and arterial oxyhemoglobin desaturation occur, resulting in the production of lactic acidosis at a lower level of exercise. Underperfused and well-ventilated lung units cause an increase in V_D/V_T and the ventilatory requirements for exercise. These factors result in the production of lactic acidosis at a lower level of exercise (reduced anaerobic threshold) and a decrease in the maximal oxygen consumption. A normal breathing reserve is usually found because the ventilatory mechanisms themselves are usually intact (47,56).

BOX 23-4   ABNORMALITIES NOTED DURING EXERCISE IN PATIENTS WITH PULMONARY VASCULAR DISEASE (PULMONARY HYPERTENSION)

Reduced maximal oxygen consumption

Reduced work rate

Decreased anaerobic threshold

Arterial oxyhemoglobin desaturation

Elevation in pulmonary artery wedge pressure (>30 mm Hg)

Elevation in right atrial pressure (>14 mm Hg)

BOX 23-5	INDICATIONS FOR EXERCISE TESTING IN PATIENTS WITH LUNG DISEASE

Evaluation of exercise tolerance

Evaluation of undiagnosed exercise intolerance

Evaluation of patients with respiratory symptoms

Exercise evaluation and prescription for pulmonary rehabilitation

Evaluation of impairment or disability

Evaluation for lung transplantation

Evaluation for oxyhemoglobin desaturation

EXERCISE ASSESSMENT

> **1.3.2-CES: Knowledge of exercise testing procedures for various clinical populations, including those individuals with cardiovascular, pulmonary, and metabolic diseases in terms of exercise modality, protocol, physiologic measurements, and expected outcomes.**

Exercise testing is an important component of the evaluation and management of most patients with pulmonary disease (Box 23-5). It is important to determine the patient's ability to undergo exercise testing. Contraindications to exercise testing (also see GETP8 Box 3-5) include an unstable cardiac condition (e.g., unstable angina), severe hypoxemia, orthopedic impairment, neurologic impairment, psychiatric disorders, poor motivation, or inability to perform the test. Neither carbon dioxide retention nor age are contraindications to the performance of exercise testing.

MODE OF EXERCISE TESTING

The assessment of exercise capacity is an important component of the overall evaluation and management of patients with lung disease (also see GETP8 Chapter 10). A variety of exercise testing modalities are available to help with this evaluation. The selection of the exercise testing modality depends on the clinical question being asked and available equipment and facilities (Box 23-6). Exercise testing should be performed when further information (e.g., in addition to the history and physical examination, chest radiograph, pulmonary function tests, and ECG) is necessary regarding the patient's underlying disease process (33).

Stair Climbing

This simple and inexpensive test has been primarily used to assess postoperative risk for patients undergoing thoracic or upper abdominal surgery and is currently being used to assess functional capacity in patients with COPD (59). Although there is no standardized testing proce-

BOX 23-6	MODALITIES OF CLINICAL EXERCISE TESTING FOR PATIENTS WITH LUNG DISEASE

Stair climbing

Timed walk tests (6- or 12-minute walk)

Shuttle walk tests

Graded exercise tests

Cardiopulmonary exercise test

dure, the patient is asked to climb as many stairs as possible until needing to stop for symptoms (e.g., dizziness, shortness of breath, fatigue, chest pain). Measurements made during the test include the number of stairs walked, oxyhemoglobin saturation, level of dyspnea, and heart rate (HR). Variable reporting of the pace of the stair climbing and the actual number of stairs climbed (often referred to as "flights of stairs") adds to the nonuniform nature of the testing procedure.

A good correlation ($r = 0.7$) has been reported between the number of steps climbed and the maximal oxygen consumption (measured during cycle ergometry) in a study of 31 patients with COPD (51). The inability to walk two flights of stairs resulted in a significant increase in the number of postoperative complications (18,59). This test can provide a general assessment of the postoperative risk for patients with lung disease in a simple and low-cost manner (20,24,46).

Timed Walk Tests

> **1.3.34-CES: Ability to perform a 6-minute walk test and appropriately utilize the results to assess prognosis, fitness, and/or improvement.**

The **timed walk tests** (6-minute walk [6 MWT], shuttle walk) are practical and simple to perform (33). They do not require advanced training or specialized equipment and provide an objective assessment of exercise tolerance or functional capacity in a manner that is comfortable for most patients to perform. The 6 MWT is the most commonly used test. A standardized protocol for the performance of the test exists (1), and guidelines have been recently developed to include a track size and length, patient preparation, monitoring, protocol, measurements, and practice testing. The track should be 30 meters in length and clearly marked every 3 meters. Comfortable shoes should be worn by the patient, and the test should be performed each time at the same time of day with the patient taking his or her usual medication regimen. Monitoring equipment should include a stopwatch, a pulse oximeter, and a sphygmomanometer. Before beginning the test, baseline HR and blood pressure (BP) measurements should be made, as well as a measure of the patient's level of dyspnea (see GETP8 Figure 5-4) and oxyhemoglobin saturation. Standardized instructions should be read to the patient, and the words for encouragement and notification of time elapsed should be consistent for all patients. At the end of the testing, immediate measurements of oxyhemoglobin saturation, pulse, BP, perceived exertion (e.g., using a Borg scale) (5), level of dyspnea (ACSM dyspnea scale [GETP8 Figure 5-4]), and length of walk should be made. Because there may be a training effect noted with such testing, it is important to perform several tests (up to three) on the same day (with 1 hour of rest in between tests), with reporting of the longest distance walked. Reference values for healthy adults have been reported (17).

The 6 MWT has good reproducibility and correlation with other measures of functional capacity and, thus, has been used in lieu of cardiopulmonary exercise test (CPET) when this testing modality is not available. A good correlation between the 6 MWT and maximal oxygen consumption ($r = 0.73$) has been shown in patients with COPD (9). The 6 MWT test represents a submaximal and motivational alternative compared with the CPET. It also represents a test for which patients are familiar with the testing modality (i.e., walking).

The 6 MWT test has been usefully applied to the evaluation of functional capacity (e.g., patients with COPD, interstitial lung disease) (12), medical interventions (40), response to pulmonary rehabilitation (15), and prediction of morbidity (27). It has also been used successfully in the evaluation and management of patients with congestive heart failure (8).

There are some concerns about the actual performance of the test and the comparisons that are made from one testing site to another, but the 6 MWT has been used in large multicenter trials (36). There is a statistically significant improvement (averaging 7%) in distance walked when the test is repeated on a second day. The shape of the walking course (continuous versus straight) appears to be more a determinant of the distance walked than does the length of a straight course (53). The minimally clinically important difference (MCID) for the 6 MWT is estimated to be 54 meters (60).

Shuttle Walk Tests

The incremental shuttle walk test (ISWT) is a symptom-limited, maximal exercise test (55). Subjects are instructed to walk around a 10-m course at a speed indicated by beeps played from a CD player. The speed increases incrementally until the patient is unable to continue or maintain the required speed. The total time walked is recorded. Performance in the ISWT is predictive of peak oxygen consumption, and the test is reproducible after a single practice walk.

The endurance shuttle walk test (ESWT) is a constant work rate exercise test. After a 2-minute warm-up period, the subject is asked to walk around a 10-m course. The

speed is constant and is set at an equivalent of 85% of the predicted peak maximal oxygen consumption achieved during the ISWT. The total time walked is recorded (49). These tests are externally paced tests of maximal and submaximal exercise performance, respectively. Each may be used to compare the distance walked before and after an intervention (e.g., response to pulmonary rehabilitation). There are no established minimal clinically important distances for either the shuttle walk or the endurance shuttle walk tests (60).

Cardiopulmonary Exercise Test

1.1.9-CES: Plot the normal resting and exercise values associated with increasing exercise intensity (and how they may differ for cardiac, pulmonary, and metabolic diseased populations) for the following: heart rate, stroke volume, cardiac output, double product, arteriovenous O_2 difference, O_2 consumption, systolic and diastolic blood pressure, minute ventilation, tidal volume, breathing frequency, Vd/Vt, V_E/VO_2, and V_E/VCO_2, $FEV_{1.0}$, SaO_2, blood glucose.

1.1.14-CES: Identify normal and abnormal respiratory responses during rest and exercise as assessed during a pulmonary function test (i.e., FVC, MVV, $FEV_{1.0}$, flow volume loop).

1.2.7-CES: Describe the resting and exercise cardiorespiratory and metabolic responses in those with pulmonary disease.

1.3.25-CES: Compare and contrast obstructive and restrictive lung diseases and their effect on exercise testing and training.

1.3.28-CES: Describe the aerobic and anaerobic metabolic demands of exercise testing and training in individuals with cardiovascular, pulmonary, and/or metabolic diseases undergoing exercise testing or training.

1.3.29-CES: Identify the variables measured during cardiopulmonary exercise testing (e.g., heart rate, blood pressure, rate of perceived exertion, ventilation, oxygen consumption, ventilatory threshold, pulmonary circulation) and their potential relationship to cardiovascular, pulmonary, and metabolic disease.

1.4.11-CES: Identify resting and exercise ECG changes associated with cardiovascular disease, hypertensive heart disease, cardiac chamber enlargement, pericarditis, pulmonary disease, and metabolic disorders.

1.5.2-CES: Describe mechanisms and actions of medications that may affect exercise testing and prescription (i.e., β-blockers, nitrates, calcium channel blockers, digitalis, diuretics, vasodilators, anitarrhythmic

agents, bronchodilators, antilipemics, psychotropics, nicotine, antihistamines, over-the-counter [OTC] cold medications, thyroid medications, alcohol, hypoglycemic agents, blood modifiers, pentoxifylline, antigout medications, and anorexiants/diet pills).

 1.5.3-CES: Recognize medications associated in the clinical setting, their indications for care, and their effects at rest and during exercise (i.e., β-blockers, nitrates, calcium channel blockers, digitalis, diuretics, vasodilators, anitarrhythmic agents, bronchodilators, antilipemics, psychotropics, nicotine, antihistamines, OTC cold medications, thyroid medications, alcohol, hypoglycemic agents, blood modifiers, pentoxifylline, antigout medications, and anorexiants/diet pills).

1.5.7-CES: Manage patients on oxygen therapy as needed during exercise testing or training.

1.5.14-CES: Ability to perform pulse-oximetry and blood glucose evaluations and appropriately interpret the data in a given clinical situation.

1.5.1-HFS: Knowledge of common drugs from each of the following classes of medications and describe the principal action and the effects on exercise testing and prescription, including antianginals, antihypertensives, antiarrhythmics, anticoagulants, bronchodilators, hypoglycemics, psychotropics, and vasodilators.

Cardiopulmonary exercise testing (CPET) is a traditional symptom-limited graded exercise test with the addition of a metabolic cart that collects and analyzes expired gases, thereby assessing the integration of the cardiovascular, pulmonary, and muscular systems during exercise performance. This type of testing allows an evaluation of the patient's ability to perform exercise and of the system responsible for the exercise impairment. Modalities for CPET can include the treadmill or cycle ergometer and are performed in a continuous ramp-type protocol until fatigue, dyspnea, or other indications for stopping an exercise test are evident (GETP8, chapter 5). Expired gases from the patient are collected using a metabolic cart that has the capability to determine the tidal volume, respiratory rate, rate of oxygen consumption, and rate of carbon dioxide elimination. Measurements of HR and oxyhemoglobin saturation (via pulse oximetry) are also made. All measurements are on a continuous basis, thus allowing for interpretation at various levels of exercise. Regarding the KSAs for this section these are more detailed then possible for this text to present. The reader is referred to the Selected References for Further Reading for complete information for KSAs.

Interpretation of CPET can be daunting given the significant amount of information obtained with each study (2,58,62). The use of gas collection spirometry and pulse oximetry provides for a comprehensive interpretation of CPET data. To organize the data to make functional and diagnostic assessments, several questions need to be evaluated (58,62).

1. Is exercise capacity normal? Maximal oxygen consumption, maximal work rate, functional aerobic impairment, and respiratory exchange ratio can be utilized to assess exercise capacity.
2. Is cardiovascular function normal? ECG responses, double product, oxygen pulse, and anaerobic threshold can be used to evaluate cardiovascular function.
3. Is ventilatory function normal? Maximal respiratory rate and ventilatory reserve can assess ventilatory function.
4. Is gas exchange normal? Oxygen saturation and dead space ventilation can evaluate gas exchange.

The various disease states discussed in this chapter have major distinguishing features in regard to the measurements obtained during CPET. Patients with COPD have a reduced exercise capacity (reduced maximal oxygen consumption), ventilatory limitation (reduced or absent ventilatory reserve, hypercapnia, hypoxemia), and a normal cardiovascular response (normal oxygen pulse) with exercise. However, the heart rate response may be blunted secondary to pulmonary limitations and dyspnea. Patients with interstitial lung disease have a reduced exercise capacity (reduced maximal oxygen consumption), ventilatory limitation (high maximum respiratory rate and low tidal volume at end exercise, elevated dead space ventilation with an abnormal reduction during exercise), and a normal cardiovascular response with exercise. Patients with vascular lung disease have a reduced exercise capacity (reduced maximal oxygen consumption), no ventilatory limitation, and an abnormal cardiovascular response (early onset of anaerobic threshold, early plateau of the oxygen pulse with a low maximum value) with exercise (Table 23-2).

During any type of exercise testing, a complete knowledge of the patient's comorbid illnesses and medication usage are of vital importance. The effects of various types of medications on the response to exercise must also be considered. Although most medications will not limit exercise endurance per se over the limitations associated

TABLE 23-2. DISTINGUISHING FEATURES NOTED AT END EXERCISE

DISEASE	COPD	INTERSTITIAL LUNG DISEASE	VASCULAR LUNG
Exercise capacity	↓	↓	↓
Oxygen consumption	↓	↓	↓
Ventilatory limitation	Yes	Yes	No
Cardiovascular response	Normal	Normal	Abnormal

↓, decreased; COPD, chronic pulmonary obstructive disease.

with the disease state itself, in some instances (e.g., β-blocker use), the exercise response may be limited.

Maintenance of an adequate level of oxyhemoglobin saturation during exercise is important. Oxyhemogloblin desaturation (usually below a level of 90%) will limit exercise performance. During all exercise testing, measurement of the oxyhemoglobin saturation by pulse oximetry should be made. If the oxyhemoglobin level falls below 88%, the administration of supplemental oxygen (usually via a nasal cannula) should be afforded to the patient. An oxyhemoglobin level >88% should be maintained throughout exercise with increase in the level of oxygen delivery as so needed.

SUMMARY

Shortness of breath is a common presenting symptom for a patient with lung disease. There are three general types of lung disease: obstructive, restrictive, and vascular. Patients with obstructive lung disease have airflow limitation, primarily during expiration. Those with restrictive lung disease have reduction in lung volumes, and those with vascular lung disease have alterations of the pulmonary vascular bed. Each disease process has a specific pathophysiology, both at rest and during exercise. Appropriate assessment of patients with lung disease includes performance of a thorough history and physical examination, laboratory studies (including chest radiograph, ECG, arterial blood gas, pulse oximetry, complete blood count, and pulmonary function tests), and, in some instances, a CT scan of the chest or a ventilation–perfusion scan. Exercise testing is helpful to confirm the disease's pathophysiology and to help direct treatment.

REFERENCES

1. American Thoracic Society. Guidelines for the six-minute walk test. *Am J Respir Crit Care Med.* 2002;166:111–117.
2. American Thoracic Society/American College of Chest Physicians. ATS/ACCP Statement on Cardiopulmonary Exercise Testing. *Am J Respir Crit Care Med.* 2003;167:211–217.
3. American Thoracic Society. Standards for the diagnosis and care of patients with chronic obstructive pulmonary disease. *Am J Respir Crit Care Med.* 1995;152:S77–S152.
4. Barnes PJ, Chung KF, Page CP. Inflammatory mediators of asthma: an update. *Pharmacol Rev.* 1998;50:515–596.
5. Borg GAV. Psychophysical bases of perceived exertion. *Med Sci Sports Exerc.* 1982;14:377–381.
6. Brines R, Thorne M. Clinical consensus of COPD. *Respir Med.* 2007;3:42–48.
7. Broekhuizen R, Wouters EF, Creutzberg EC, et al. Raised CRP levels mark metabolic and functional impairment in advanced COPD. *Thorax.* 2006;61:17–22.
8. Cahalin L, Mathier MA, Semigran MJ, et al. The six-minute walk test predicts peak oxygen uptake and survival in patients with advanced heart failure. *Chest.* 1996;110:325–332.
9. Cahalin L, Pappagionopolous P, Prevost S, et al. The relationship of the 6-minute walk test to maximal oxygen consumption in transplant candidates with end-stage lung disease. *Chest.* 1995;108:452–459.
10. Calverley PMA. Exercise and dyspnea in COPD. *Eur Respir J.* 2006;15:72–79.
11. Casaburi R. Skeletal muscle dysfunction in chronic obstructive pulmonary disease. *Med Sci Sports Exerc.* 2001;33:662–670.
12. Chang JA, Curtis JR, Patrick DL, Raghu G. Assessment of health-related quality of life in patients with interstitial lung disease. *Chest.* 1994;105:163–167.
13. Chen Y, Horne SL, Dosman JA. Increased susceptibility to lung dysfunction in female smokers. *Am Rev Respir Dis.* 1991;143:1224–1230.
14. Debigare R, Cote CH, Maltais F. Peripheral muscle wasting in chronic obstructive pulmonary disease. *Am J Respir Crit Care Med.* 2001;164:1712–1717.
15. DeTorres JP, Pinto-Plata V, Ingenito E, et al. Power of outcome measurements to detect clinically significant changes in pulmonary rehabilitation of patients with COPD. *Chest.* 2002;121:1091–1098.
16. Diaz O, Villanfranco C, Ghezzo H, et al. Exercise tolerance in COPD patients with and without tidal expiratory flow limitation at rest. *Eur Respir J.* 2000;16:269–275.
17. Enright PL, Sherrill DL. Reference equations for the six-minute walk in healthy adults. *Am J Respir Crit Care Med.* 1998;158:1384–1387.
18. Fedullo P, Auger W, Channick R, et al. Chronic thromboembolic pulmonary hypertension. *Clin Chest Med.* 2001;22:561–581.
19. Ferguson GT, Enright PL, Buist AS, Higgins MW. Office spirometry for lung health assessment in adults. *Chest.* 2000;117:1146–1161.
20. Girish M, Trayner E Jr, Dammann O, et al. Symptom-limited stair climbing as a predictor of postoperative cardiopulmonary complications after high-risk surgery. *Chest.* 2001;120:1147–1151.
21. Gold DR, Wang X, Wypij D, et al. Effects of cigarette smoking on pulmonary function in adolescent boys and girls. *N Engl J Med.* 1996;335:931–937.
22. Hansen JE, Wasserman K. Pathophysiology of activity limitation in patients with interstitial lung disease. *Chest.* 1996;109:1566–1576.
23. Hill AT, Bayley D, Stockley RA. The interrelationship of sputum inflammatory markers in patients with chronic bronchitis. *Am J Respir Crit Care Med.* 1999;160:893–898.
24. Holden DA, Rice TW, Stelmach K, Meeker DP. Exercise testing, 6-minute walk, and stair climb in the evaluation of patients at high risk for pulmonary resection. *Chest.* 1992;102:1774–1779.
25. Holgate ST. The cellular and mediator basis of asthma in relation to natural history. *Lancet.* 1997;350(suppl II):5–9.
26. Keatings VM, Collins PD, Scott DM, Barnes PJ. Differences in interleukin-8 and tumor necrosis factor-alpha in induced sputum from patients with chronic obstructive pulmonary disease or asthma. *Am J Respir Crit Care Med.* 1996;153:530–534.
27. Kessler R, Faller M, Fourgaut G, et al. Predictive factors of hospitalizations for acute exacerbations in a series of 64 patients with chronic obstructive pulmonary disease. *Am J Respir Crit Care Med.* 1999;159:158–164.
28. MacNee W. Pathophysiology of cor pulmonale in chronic obstructive pulmonary disease. Part II. *Am J Respir Crit Care Med.* 1994;150:1158–1168.
29. Maltais FA, Simard A, Simard C, et al. Oxidative capacity of the skeletal muscle and lactic acid kinetics during exercise in normal subjects and in patients with COPD. *Am J Respir Crit Care Med.* 1994;154:442–447.
30. Markovitz GH, Cooper CB. Exercise and interstitial lung disease. *Curr Opin Pulm Med.* 1998;4:272–280.
31. McFadden ER Jr, Gilbert FA. Exercise induced asthma. *N Engl J Med.* 1994;330:1362–1367.
32. Mehta JN, Khan IA, Mehta RN, Sepkowitz DA. HIV-related pulmonary hypertension. *Chest.* 2000;118:1133–1141.
33. Montes de Oca M, Ortega Balza M, Lezama J, Lopez JM. Chronic obstructive pulmonary disease: evaluation of exercise tolerance using three different exercise tests. *Arch Bronchopneumol.* 2001;37:69–74.

34. Mueller R, Changez P, Campbell AM, et al. Different cytokine patterns in bronchial biopsies in asthma and chronic bronchitis. *Respir Med.* 1996;90:79–85.

35. Mullen JB, Wright JL, Wiggs BR, et al. Reassessment of inflammation of airways in chronic bronchitis. *BMJ.* 1985;291:1235–1239.

36. National Emphysema Treatment Trial. A randomized trial comparing lung-volume-reduction surgery with medical therapy for severe emphysema. *N Engl J Med.* 2003;348:2059–2073.

37. Niewoehner DE, Kleinerman J, Rice DB. Pathologic changes in the peripheral airways of young cigarette smokers. *N Engl J Med.* 1974;291:755–758.

38. O'Donnell DE, Laveneziana P. Physiology and consequences of lung hyperinflation in COPD. *Eur Respir J.* 2006;15:61–67.

39. O'Donnell DE, Revill S, Webb KA. Dynamic hyperinflation and exercise intolerance in COPD. *Am J Respir Crit Care Med.* 2001;164:770–777.

40. Oga T, Nishimura K, Tsukino M, et al. The effects of oxitropium bromide on exercise performance in patients with stable chronic obstructive pulmonary disease: a comparison of three different exercise tests. *Am J Respir Crit Care Med.* 2000;161:1897–1901.

41. Pauwels RA, Buist SA, Calverley PMA, et al. Global strategy for the diagnosis, management, and prevention of chronic obstructive pulmonary disease. *Am J Respir Crit Care Med.* 2001;163:1256–1276.

42. Peinado VI, Barbera JA, Abate P, et al. Inflammatory reaction in pulmonary muscular arteries of patients with mild chronic obstructive pulmonary disease. *Am J Respir Crit Care Med.* 1999;159:1605–1611.

43. Petty TL. Strategies in preserving lung health and preventing COPD and associated diseases. The National Lung Health Education Program. *Chest.* 2000;117:1146–1161.

44. Petty TL, Weinmann GG. Building a national strategy for the prevention and management of and research in chronic obstructive pulmonary disease. National Heart, Lung, and Blood Institute Workshop Summary. *JAMA.* 1997;277:246–253.

45. Pinto-Plata V, Mullerova H, Roso JF, et al. C-reactive protein in patients with COPD, control smokers, and non-smokers. *Thorax.* 2006;61:23–28.

46. Pollock M, Roa J, Benditt J, Celli B. Estimation of ventilatory reserve by stair climbing: a study in patients with chronic airflow obstruction. *Chest.* 1993;104:1378–1383.

47. Raeside DA, Smith A, Brown A, et al. Pulmonary artery pressure measurement during exercise testing in patients with suspected pulmonary hypertension. *Eur Respir J.* 2000;16:282–287.

48. Repine JE, Bast A, Lankhorst I. Oxidative stress in chronic obstructive pulmonary disease. Oxidative Stress Study Group. *Am J Respir Crit Care Med.* 1997;156:341–357.

49. Revill SM, Morgan MD, Singh SJ, et al. The endurance shuttle walk: a new field test for the assessment of endurance capacity in chronic obstructive pulmonary disease. *Thorax.* 1999;54:213–222.

50. Roche WR, Beasley R, Williams JH, Holgate ST. Subepithelial fibrosis in the bronchi of asthmatics. *Lancet.* 1989;1(7965):882–884.

51. Rubin LJ. Primary pulmonary hypertension. *N Engl J Med.* 1997;336:111–117.

52. Saetta M, Di Stefano A, Turato G, et al. CD8+ T-lymphocytes in peripheral airways of smokers with chronic obstructive pulmonary disease. *Am J Respir Crit Care Med.* 1998;157:822–826.

53. Sciurba F, Criner GJ, Lee SM, et al. Six-minute walk distance in chronic obstructive pulmonary disease. *Am J Respir Crit Care Med.* 2003;167:1522–1527.

54. Sin DD, Man SFP. Skeletal muscle weakness, reduced exercise tolerance, and COPD: Is systemic inflammation the missing link? *Thorax.* 2006;61;1–3.

55. Singh SJ, Morgan MD, Hardman AE, et al. Comparison of oxygen uptake during a conventional treadmill test and the shuttle walking test in chronic airflow limitation. *Eur Respir J.* 1994;7:2016–2020.

56. Sun XG, Hansen JE, Oudiz RJ, Wasserman K. Exercise pathophysiology in patients with primary pulmonary hypertension. *Circulation.* 2001;104:429–435.

57. Vernoy JH, Kucukaycan M, Jacobs JA, et al. Local and system inflammation in patients with chronic obstructive pulmonary disease: soluble tumor necrosis factor receptors are increased in sputum. *Am J Respir Crit Care Med.* 2002;166:1240–1247.

58. Weisman IM, Zeballos RJ, eds. Clinical exercise testing. *Clin Chest Med.* 1994;15:173–451.

59. Widimsky J, Riedel M, Stanek V. Central haemodynamics during exercise in patients with restrictive pulmonary disease. *Bull Eur Physiopathol Respir.* 1997;13:369–379.

60. Wise RA, Brown CD. Minimally clinically important differences in the six-minute walk test and the incremental shuttle walking test. *J Chron Obstr Pulm Dis.* 2005;2:125–129.

61. Yende S, Waterer GW, Tolley EA, et al. Inflammatory markers are associated with ventilatory limitation and muscle dysfunction in obstructive lung disease in well functioning elderly subjects. *Thorax.* 2006;61:10–16.

62. Younes M. Interpretation of clinical exercise testing in respiratory disease. *Clin Chest Med.* 1984;5:189–206.

SELECTED REFERENCES FOR FURTHER READING

Swank AM, Berry MS, Woodward CM. Chronic obstructive pulmonary disease. In: Ehrman JK, Gordon PM, Visich PS, Keteyian SJ, editors. *Clinical Exercise Physiology* 2nd ed. Champaign (IL): Human Kinetics; 2008. p. 371–390.

Cherniak NS, Altose MD, Homma I. *Rehabilitation of the Patient with Respiratory Disease.* New York: McGraw Hill; 1999.

Myers JM. *Essentials of Cardiopulmonary Exercise Testing.* Champaign (IL): Human Kinetics; 1996.

Wasserman K, Hansen JE, Sue DY, Stringer WW, Whip BJ. Principles of Exercise Testing and Interpretation 4th ed. Baltimore: Lipincott, Williams & Wilkins 2004.

Weisman IM, Zeballos RJ. *Clinical Exercise Testing.* Basel, Switzerland: Karger; 2002.

INTERNET RESOURCES

- AACVPR: American Association of Cardiovascular and Pulmonary Rehabilitation: www.aacvpr.org
- American College of Chest Physicians: www.chestnet.org
- American Thoracic Society: www.thoracic.org
- National Lung Health Education Program: www.nlhep.org
- U.S. COPD Coalition: www.uscopd.org

Diagnostic Procedures in Patients with Metabolic Disease

> **1.3.2-CES:** Knowledge of exercise testing procedures for various clinical populations, including those individuals with cardiovascular, pulmonary, and metabolic diseases in terms of exercise modality, protocol, physiologic measurements, and expected outcomes.

The American Diabetes Association (ADA) reports that 20.8 million children and adults in the United States have diabetes (4) and that almost one third (6.2 million) of these individuals are unaware of having the disease (4). Of concern is that there is a greater increase in the incidence of diabetes in younger age groups than what is seen in older groups. Between 1990 and 1998, the incidence rate of diabetes increased 70% for the age group 30 to 39, 40% for the age group 40 to 49, and 31% for the age group 50 to 59 (47).

Individuals with diabetes have a higher incidence and prevalence of symptomatic as well as asymptomatic coronary artery disease (CAD) than nondiabetic individuals and as result are at higher risk for cardiovascular events (2,14,22,30,31,34,36,37,42,46,51,52,54,64,78). Women with diabetes are at greater risk for cardiovascular events as compared with women without diabetes (40,64), especially

> > > KEY TERMS

Autonomic nervous dysfunction: Abnormal function of the nerve fibers that belong or relate to the autonomic nervous system.

Blood glucose (sugar): *Blood sugar* is a common term used to refer to the amount of glucose in the blood.

Compensatory hyperinsulinemia: As a result of insulin resistance, the pancreas will compensate by producing more insulin, leading to excessive blood insulin levels.

Diabetic neuropathy: A generic term for diabetes-related disorder of the peripheral or autonomic nervous system and some cranial nerves.

Fasting blood glucose: Measurement of blood glucose after at least 8 hours with no caloric intake.

Glucagon: Released when the blood glucose levels are low (hypoglycemia), causing glucogenesis (production of glucose from stored glycogen) and thus increasing glucose levels.

Glucose tolerance: Capability to maintain normal blood glucose levels after consuming a high load of carbohydrate.

Glycosolated hemoglobin (Hb$_{A1c}$): Glycosylation (or glycation) is the process or result of the addition of sugars (i.e., saccharides) to proteins and lipids. This test is used as a tool to monitor diabetic control, but not to diagnose diabetes.

Hyperglycemia: High levels of glucose in the blood.

Insulin: Insulin is an anabolic hormone with a primary action to control (promote) carbohydrate metabolism and blood glucose disposal that acts to lower blood glucose levels.

Insulin receptor: Sits on cell surface and when activated acts to increase glucose uptake by stimulating the glucose transporters in muscle and adipose tissues.

Insulin resistance/insulin sensitivity: A condition in which normal amounts of insulin are not adequate to produce a normal insulin response from fat, muscle, and liver cells.

Oral glucose tolerance test (OGTT): Specific test to assess the ability to regulate blood glucose and to screen or diagnose patients for diabetes mellitus.

Pancreatic beta cells: Cells that respond to elevations in blood glucose to make and release insulin.

Radionuclide ventriculography: The display, by means of a stationary scintillation cameral device, of the passage of a bolus of a rapidly injected radiopharmaceutical through the heart.

Silent ischemia: Ischemia of the heart that does not result in anginal symptoms experienced by the patient. In diabetes, this is because of the dysfunction of the peripheral nerves.

if other risk factors are present (17). Asymptomatic individuals with diabetes have a higher prevalence of silent myocardial ischemia and associated autonomic nerve dysfunction than those without diabetes (37).

In addition, patients on insulin therapy or who have retinopathy have nearly a threefold higher prevalence of silent myocardial ischemia compared with those not taking insulin or without retinopathy (49). Wackers et al. (84) reported that 22% of all asymptomatic diabetes patients had a positive myocardial perfusion imaging scan and that the same positive test incidence rate occurred whether or not the group had traditional risk factors for CAD.

Routine exercise testing is an important diagnostic and prognostic procedure for individuals with diabetes (65,73). Because of the risk of exercise-related sudden death (33,76), it is recommended that adults with a long history of diabetes and those with one or more additional cardiovascular risk factors undergo exercise testing before beginning a vigorous exercise program (2,3,16,50,83).

The metabolic syndrome (MetSyn) has gained much attention since the 1980s as a condition that not only predicts a future diagnosis of diabetes, but is also shown to cause significant increases in risk for premature cardiovascular disease. Insulin resistance is a primary characteristic of MetSyn, and the pancreas responds with an excessive pancreatic β-cell production of insulin, resulting in compensatory hyperinsulinemia to successfully control glycemia (61). Hyperglycemia is initially controlled by insulin, but at the cost of hyperinsulinemia; and compensatory hyperinsulinemia is an area of great suspicion as a root cause for a variety of known cardiovascular risk factors. In addition, insulin resistance within fat tissue is thought to promote poor lipid metabolism, elevated cholesterol levels, and increase risk of type 2 diabetes. Hyperinsulinemia also increases various inflammatory markers and cytokines known to promote vascular inflammation and atherosclerosis references.

This chapter will address the diagnostic differences for type 1 and type 2 diabetes, and gestational diabetes mellitus. Additionally, MetSyn will be examined as an emerging condition that precedes type 2 diabetes, has a very high prevalence, and displays significant elevations in cardiovascular risk.

DIAGNOSIS OF METABOLIC SYNDROME

> **1.8.2-HFS: Knowledge of the following terms: obesity, overweight, percent fat, body mass index (BMI), lean body mass, anorexia nervosa, bulimia, metabolic syndrome, and body fat distribution.**

The term *metabolic syndrome* dates back to at least the late 1950s, but throughout the last several decades, there has been much revision, as well as increasing interest, in the constellation of conditions that make up the syndrome. This history MetSyn is reviewed in Chapter 8. Table 24-1

provides a comparison of the current definitions of metabolic syndrome as provided by several organizations (28). The following is summary of the primary factors identified for risk of developing MetSyn as produced by the American College of Endocrinology from the Conference on the Insulin Resistance Syndrome in 2002(1).

> **1.2.14-CES: Identify the contributing factors to metabolic syndrome, their pathologic sequalae, and their affect on the primary or secondary risk of cardiovascular disease.**

1. Overweight: BMI ≥ 25 kg $\cdot$ m^{-2}; waist circumference of >40 inches in men or >35 inches in women
2. A sedentary lifestyle
3. Non-Caucasian ethnicity (e.g., Latino/Hispanic American, African and Native American, Asian American, Pacific Islander)
4. Age 40 or older, with family history of type 2 diabetes, hypertension, or cardiovascular disease
5. A history of glucose intolerance or gestational diabetes
6. A diagnosis of hypertension, elevated triglycerides and/or low high-density lipoprotein (HDL) cholesterol, or cardiovascular disease
7. Acanthosis nigricans, which is an eruption of velvet warty benign growths and hyperpigmentation occurring in the skin of the axillae, neck, anogenital area, and groin
8. Polycystic ovary syndrome (PCOS)
9. Nonalcoholic fatty liver disease
10. Cancer

> **1.2.5-CES: Examine the role of lifestyle on cardiovascular risk factors, such as hypertension, blood lipids, glucose tolerance, and body weight.**

> **4.2.1-HFS: Knowledge of metabolic risk factors or conditions that may require consultation with medical personnel before testing or training, including obesity, metabolic syndrome, thyroid disease, kidney disease, diabetes or glucose intolerance, and hypoglycemia.**

Individuals with these risks should be evaluated for MetSyn (28). The diagnosis of MetSyn lies in the evaluation of each of the individual components (i.e., blood glucose, overweight/obesity, blood lipid values, blood pressure) using routine diagnostic assessments found elsewhere in this chapter and text (see Chapter 8). The diagnosis also relies on the recognition of the constellation of conditions of MetSyn and treating them appropriately with both medical and lifestyle interventions (28). If a diagnosis is made, then the individual should be assessed for safety for exercise before beginning any moderate- to high-intensity exercise training program. Treatment is very important because of the high risk of atherosclerosis that accompanies MetSyn. Because of this, it is often indicated to assess patients with MetSyn for CAD. This is

TABLE 24-1. A COMPARISON OF THE VARIOUS ORGANIZATIONAL DEFINITIONS FOR METABOLIC SYNDROME (28)

CLINICAL MEASURE	WHO (1998)	EGIR	ATP III (2001)	AACE (2003)	IDF (2005)
Insulin resistance	IGT, IFG, T2DM, or lowered insulin sensitivity* plus any 2 of the following	Plasma insulin >75th percentile plus any 2 of the following	None, but any 3 of the following 5 features	IGT or IFG plus any of the following based on clinical judgment	None
Body weight	Men: waist-to-hip ratio >0.90; women: waist-to-hip ratio >0.85 and/or BMI >30 kg/m²	WC ≥94 cm in men or ≥80 cm in women†	WC ≥102 cm in men or ≥88 cm in women†	BMI ≥25 kg/m²	Increased WC (population specific) plus any 2 of the following
Lipid	TG ≥150 mg/dL and/or HDL-C <35 mg/dL in men or <39 mg/dL in women	TG ≥150 mg/dL and/or HDL-C <39 mg/dL in men or women	TG ≥ 150 mg/dL HDL-C <40 mg/dL in men or <50 mg/dL in women	TG ≥150 mg/dL and HDL-C <40 mg/dL in men or <50 mg/dL in women	TG ≥150 mg/dL or on TG Rx HDL-C <40 mg/dL in men or <50 mg/dL in women or on HDL-C Rx
Blood pressure	≥140/90 mm Hg	≥140/90 mm Hg or on hypertension Rx	≥130/85 mm Hg	≥130/85 mm Hg	≥130 mm Hg systolic or ≥85 mm Hg diastolic or on hypertension Rx
Glucose	IGT, IFG, or T2DM	IGT or IFG (but not diabetes)	>110 mg/dL (includes diabetes)‡	IGT or IFG (but not diabetes)	≥100 mg/dL (includes diabetes)
Other	Microalbuminuria			Other features of insulin resistance§	

T2DM indicates type 2 diabetes mellitus; WC, waist circumference; BMI, body mass index; and TG, triglycerides; Rx, prescription. All other abbreviations as in text.

*Insulin sensitivity measured under hyperinsulinemic euglycemic conditions, glucose uptake below lowest quartile for background population under investigation.

†Some male patients can develop multiple metabolic risk factors when the waist circumference is only marginally increased (eg, 94 to 102 cm [37 to 39 in]). Such patients may have a strong genetic contribution to insulin resistance. They should benefit from changes in lifestyle habits, similar to men with categorical increases in waist circumference.

‡The 2001 definition identified fasting plasma glucose of ≥110 mg/dL (6.1 mmol/L) as elevated. This was modified in 2004 to be ≥100 mg/dL (5.6 mmol/L), in accordance with the American Diabetes Association's updated definition of IFG.[46,47,77]

§Includes family history of type 2 diabetes mellitus, polycystic ovary syndrome, sedentary lifestyle, advancing age, and ethnic groups susceptible to type 2 diabetes mellitus.

TABLE 24-2. FASTING PLASMA GLUCOSE TEST INTERPRETATION OF RESULTS

PLASMA GLUCOSA RESULT (mg · dL^{-1})	DIAGNOSIS
99 and below	Normal
100–125	Prediabetes (impaired fasting glucose)
126 and above	Diabetes[a]

[a]Confirmed by repeating the test on a different day.

TABLE 24-4. GESTATIONAL DIABETES: ABOVE-NORMAL RESULTS FOR THE ORAL GLUCOSE TOLERANCE TEST

WHEN	PLASMA GLUCOSE RESULT (mg · dL^{-1})
Fasting	95 or higher
At 1 hour	180 or higher
At 2 hours	155 or higher
At 3 hours	140 or higher

often initially done by exercise stress testing, as discussed later in this chapter.

DIAGNOSIS OF DIABETES MELLITUS

The following tests are used for the diagnosis of diabetes mellitus (2):

- A fasting plasma glucose (FPG) test measures blood glucose after at least 8 hours without eating. The FPG is convenient and most reliable when done in the morning. It simply requires the assessment of plasma glucose following an at-least-8-hour fast. If the blood glucose values following an FPG are ≥100 to ≤125 mg · dL^{-1}, a diagnosis of prediabetes, termed *impaired fasting glucose* (IFG), is suggested. When the value is 126 mg · dL^{-1} or greater and is confirmed by repeating the test on another day, the diagnostic criteria for diabetes mellitus is met. See Table 24-2 for a summary.
- An oral glucose tolerance test (OGTT) measures blood glucose after at least 8 hours without eating and 2 hours after consumption of a beverage of 75 g of carbohydrate. The OGTT is more sensitive than the FPG test for diagnosing diabetes but is less convenient to administer. If the blood glucose level is between 140 and 199 mg · dL^{-1} 2 hours after drinking the glucose solution, impaired glucose tolerance (IGT) is present. These individuals should begin aggressive treatment to reduce the risk of developing diabetes. Values >200 mg · dL^{-1} are considered diagnostic for diabetes. See Table 24-3 for a summary.
- A random plasma glucose test is interpreted without regard to the timing of the subject's last meal or caloric

intake. This test, along with an assessment of symptoms, is used to screen for diabetes.

Positive test results must be confirmed by repeating the FPG test or the OGTT on a different day. Additional diagnostic criteria and testing information is provided in Chapter 8.

Gestational diabetes is also diagnosed based on plasma glucose values measured during the OGTT, although the criteria differ. For women who are pregnant, the blood glucose levels are checked three times following the glucose ingestion, at 1, 2 and 3 hours. If blood glucose levels are above normal (>180, 144, and 140 mg · dL^{-1}, respectively) at least twice during the test, the patient is considered to have gestational diabetes. See Table 24-4 for a summary.

WHO SHOULD BE TESTED FOR DIABETES MELLITUS?

> **4.2.1-HFS: Knowledge of metabolic risk factors or conditions that may require consultation with medical personnel before testing or training, including obesity, metabolic syndrome, thyroid disease, kidney disease, diabetes or glucose intolerance, and hypoglycemia.**

The initial "diagnosis" of diabetes is often made through ordinary health screening and through new signs and symptoms that result from the diabetes, such as vision changes or unexplainable fatigue. The diagnosis of type 1 diabetes, and many cases of type 2, is prompted by recent-onset symptoms of excessive urination (polyuria) and excessive thirst (polydipsia), often accompanied by weight loss. These symptoms typically worsen over days to weeks. Diabetes screening is recommended for many people at various stages of life, and for those with cardiovascular risk factors such as hypertension, obesity, and abnormal lipid values. Generally, anyone 45 years of age or older should be considered for initial and routine diabetes testing, especially if they have the aforementioned risk factors or overt CAD (6). Assessment for diabetes is especially important in those who not only have the general risks for diabetes, but also wish to begin an exercise training program, in particular one that is of moderate or high intensity.

TABLE 24-3. ORAL GLUCOSE TOLERANCE TEST: INTERPRETATION OF RESULTS

2-HOUR PLASMA GLUCOSE RESULT (mg · dL^{-1})	DIAGNOSIS
139 and below	Normal
140–199	Prediabetes (impaired glucose tolerance)
200 and above	Diabetes[a]

[a]Confirmed by repeating the test on a different day.

CLINICAL EVALUATION

> **1.2.13-CES: Recognize and describe the pathophysiology of diabetes mellitus (prediabetes, type I and II, gestational) including blood glucose, Hb_{A1c}, insulin sensitivity, and the risk and affect on comorbid conditions.**

> **1.2.2-HFS: Knowledge of cardiovascular, pulmonary, metabolic, and musculoskeletal risk factors that may require further evaluation by medical or allied health professionals before participation in physical activity.**

The ADA recommends assessment of cardiovascular risk factors on an annual basis, including dyslipidemia, hypertension, smoking, family history, and micro- or macroalbuminuria for those with established diabetes (6). Patients with diabetes should undergo both a detailed history and thorough physical examination with a focus on determining the presence of macro- and microvascular disease, a neuropathic assessment for both peripheral and autonomic dysfunction, and, if appropriate, diagnostic studies before embarking on an exercise program (2,5,6,19). The 1998 Consensus Development Conference of the American Diabetes Association proposed that patients with multiple risk factors for cardiovascular disease might have the highest yield of positive results from cardiac testing, and this is a basis for criteria for selection of patients who should undergo routine and pre-exercise stress testing (2). However, recent studies have shown that the burden of traditional risk factors did not predict inducible ischemia with myocardial perfusion imaging (69) and demonstrated similar rates of ischemia in asymptomatic diabetic patients with or without traditional risk factors (84).

In the absence of symptomatic CAD, clinical features that help to identify the patient at increased risk for myocardial infarction (MI) or cardiac death include evidence of other atherosclerotic vascular disease (e.g., heart, carotid, peripheral); renal disease; abnormal resting electrocardiogram (ECG); and diabetes complications, including autonomic neuropathy, retinopathy, hypertension, and dyslipidemia. Although these factors do not indicate the presence or absence of inducible ischemia, they still warrant careful consideration for identifying patients at risk for events.

A resting 12-lead ECG is useful to identify evidence of ischemic heart disease, a previous MI, or even an unknown cardiac rhythm disturbance (9,64). These include the presence of nonspecific ST-T wave changes, which may be a predictor of inducible ischemia in asymptomatic diabetic patients (59). However, a resting ECG is insufficient for diagnosing ischemic cardiac conditions that often require a high degree of myocardial work, as during exercise, to invoke an ischemic response (48,72). Thus, there is a need for exercise testing in these individuals before beginning exercise training.

Microalbuminuria is predictive for vascular disease complications as well as progression to overt nephropathy (67). Patients with type 2 diabetes and chronic kidney disease as a result of diabetic nephropathy display a very high risk for acute MI and cardiac death. This is reported to be as high as 40% over a 5-year period and thus indicates another marker of vascular disease in this population (39).

Autonomic neuropathy is associated with a poor overall prognosis in patients with type 1 and type 2 diabetes. The mechanisms that confer the high risk are poorly understood but may include impairment in ischemia awareness, delaying the diagnosis of CAD, or hemodynamic dysfunction as a result of blunted parasympathetic activation. Autonomic neuropathy was a major predictor of inducible ischemia in the DIAD (Detection of Ischemia in Asymptomatic Diabetics) study and is associated with abnormal cardiac test findings in other studies (9,84).

The ADA recently recommended screening for cardiac autonomic neuropathy for patients with indications of autonomic dysfunction, beginning at the diagnosis of type 2 diabetes and 5 years after the diagnosis of type 1 diabetes (6). The possibility of cardiac autonomic neuropathy should be considered in the presence of unexplained tachycardia, orthostatic hypertension and/or hypotension, and other autonomic or peripheral neuropathies. Autonomic dysfunction may affect the ability to regulate blood pressure during exercise and make it difficult to use heart rate (HR) to guide exercise intensity.

Retinopathy is a manifestation of microvascular disease and a risk for CAD in both type 1 and type 2 diabetes. In clinical studies, retinopathy is associated with inducible ischemia in some, but not all, screening studies (9). Patients with diabetes should be regularly screened for retinopathy, and when present, limitations in lifting (i.e., resistance training) and any other activity that increases intraocular pressure may be indicated.

A consistently elevated and uncontrolled blood glucose value, as indicated by an Hb_{A1c} value >7.0 mg %, is a strong predictor of microvascular disease (74). Interventions to improve glycemic control are shown to reduce coronary events in the type 1 and type 2 diabetes populations. Hence, chronic uncontrolled hyperglycemia is a risk factor for cardiovascular disease (75). On the contrary, patients with diabetes are also at risk of hypoglycemia associated with exercise. This is especially true for those who use insulin. It may be wise to assess blood glucose values before and after exercise, including exercise testing, in those patients who use insulin.

Given these comorbid circumstances, routine stress testing with standard electrocardiography is valuable to assess the cardiovascular status of the diabetic patient and to prescribe exercise training. Additionally, several important developments in cardiovascular imaging

---

BOX 24-1 | **CLINICAL CHARACTERISTICS OF INDIVIDUALS WITH DIABETES: GUIDELINES FOR EXERCISE TESTING**

1. Previously sedentary individual with diabetes aged >35 years; or sedentary at any age and having diabetes >10 years
2. Having type 1 diabetes >15 years or type 2 diabetes >10 years (32)
3. Having additional major risk factors for coronary artery disease, such as the presence of smoking, hyperlipidemia, obesity, and being sedentary (51)
4. Displaying clinically advanced peripheral vascular or renal disease, microvascular disease, cardiomegaly, or congestive heart failure (17,34,51,56)
5. Presence of advanced autonomic, renal, or cerebrovascular disease (24)
6. Patients with known advanced coronary artery or carotid occlusive disease

---

technology have evolved to assist in detecting CAD in asymptomatic patients with risk factors, including diabetes. Moreover, professional societies have updated their recommendations for the use of computed tomography imaging (27,29).

PRACTICAL CONSIDERATIONS OF ROUTINE EXERCISE TESTING

> **1.10.5-CES: Describe the effects of cardiovascular and pulmonary disease, and the diseases of the metabolic syndrome on performance of and safety during exercise testing and training.**

As CAD is the major cause of morbidity, mortality, and medical costs in the diabetic population, early detection and intervention have significant prognostic appeal. More than 10 years ago, the ADA convened an expert panel and developed the consensus statement on the diagnosis of coronary heart disease in patients with diabetes (2). This document focused on a burden of risk factors and the duration of the diabetes in the patient to determine the need for stress testing. Since that time, new technologies of noninvasive cardiac imaging have demonstrated a high incidence of unknown cardiac ischemia in diabetes patients who do not have the traditional risk factors indicated in the 1998 consensus statement. The DIAD study reported that silent ischemia was found by single-photo emission computed tomography (SPECT) in 22% of asymptomatic diabetic subjects and stated that if the 1998 guidelines were applied, that CAD would have remained undetected in as many as 41% of type 2 diabetic patients (84).

The sensitivity and specificity of exercise testing in an asymptomatic individual may result in minimal diagnostic value depending on many variables, including the type and severity of diabetes, as well as the duration that a patient has had diabetes. One major concern is that exercise testing can be costly for routine screening, and with the significant number of individuals with type 2 diabetes, exercise testing such a large cohort would place a large financial burden on the healthcare system. Further-

more, in an asymptomatic population, exercise testing may result in a false-positive diagnosis and may be a poor predictor for major cardiac events (66).

Diagnostic cardiac stress testing is suggested by the ADA for those with typical or atypical cardiac symptoms or an abnormal resting electrocardiogram (6). Screening stress testing is suggested by the ADA for those with (a) history of peripheral or carotid occlusive disease, (b) sedentary lifestyle (<35 years of age with plans to start a vigorous exercise program), or (c) two or more risk factors (dyslipidemia, hypertension, smoking, family history of premature coronary disease, and micro- or macroalbuminuria) (6).

Before a patient with diabetes undergoes an exercise test, absolute and relative contraindications to exercise testing (see GETP8, Chapter 3, Box 3.5) should be evaluated to determine appropriateness and safety of testing (5). Box 24.1 summarizes clinical guidelines to help determine if an individual with diabetes should undergo a graded exercise test to evaluate his or her cardiac health status before beginning a moderate- to high-intensity exercise program (2,3,5). Whether a patient with diabetes should undergo an exercise test when beginning a light-intensity exercise program requires clinical judgment (Box 24.2). Generally, for patients planning to participate in very light (<20% $\dot{V}O_{2max}$, <50% max HR) or light (20%–39% $\dot{V}O_{2max}$, 50%–63% of max HR) exercise for 60 minutes (5), particularly in those without medical conditions that are contraindicative to regular exercise, an exercise test may not be warranted before starting an exercise program (3,5). However, it is recommended that an individual with typical or atypical cardiac symptoms or an abnormal resting ECG result have a diagnostic exercise test, even when beginning light exercise (5).

Individuals with diabetes are recommended to undergo an exercise test before engaging in moderate (40%–59 % $\dot{V}O_{2max}$, 64%–76% of max HR) to hard (60%–84% $\dot{V}O_{2max}$, 77%–93% max HR) exercise (5). Individuals with diabetes and advanced disease states, even those diseases not commonly associated with risks for CAD, should undergo exercise testing, as microvascular and neuropathic complications (e.g., diabetic retinopathy, nephropathy, and autonomic neuropathy) are often

BOX 24-2	CLINICAL CHARACTERISTICS OF AN INDIVIDUAL WITH DIABETES BEGINNING A VERY-LIGHT TO LIGHT-INTENSITY EXERCISE PROGRAM

1. Anticipating exercise activity level approximately equal to his or her walking pace ($<40\%$ $\dot{V}O_2$max, $<63\%$ max HR)
2. Age <35 years
3. Without additional major risk factors for coronary artery disease
4. Without additional risk factors for sudden death

5. Normal resting electrocardiogram

It is highly recommend that diabetic patients, especially those having diabetes for more than 10 years, have their physician thoroughly evaluate them before embarking on an exercise training program, even if at a low-intensity of effort. Those planning a moderate- to high-intensity exercise program should be evaluated by exercise testing.

HR, heart rate.

seen in these individuals, and they demonstrate an increased prevalence of sudden death (84).

To date, there are no recommendations pertaining to the exercise testing for individuals with MetSyn. Although recommendations do not currently exist, on a case-by-case basis, it may be indicated to assess those with MetSyn for CAD by exercise testing. The following recommendations pertain to those with diabetes only.

CARDIAC COMPLICATIONS SPECIFIC TO INDIVIDUALS WITH DIABETES

> **1.10.5-CES: Describe the effects of cardiovascular and pulmonary disease, and the diseases of MetSyn on performance of and safety during exercise testing and training.**

> **1.10.11-HFS: Knowledge of potential musculoskeletal injuries (e.g., contusions, sprains, strains, fractures), cardiovascular/pulmonary complications (e.g., tachycardia, bradycardia, hypotension/hypertension, tachypnea), and metabolic abnormalities (e.g., fainting/syncope, hypoglycemia/hyperglycemia, hypothermia/hyperthermia).**

Silent myocardial ischemia in asymptomatic men with diabetes occurs frequently (51,52,84), especially in those on long-term insulin treatment and with long-term uncontrolled hyperglycemia. These individuals often have autonomic neuropathy (43), which is associated with an increased risk of sudden death (21). Individuals with diabetes often show an early loss of parasympathetic function with later progression to sympathetic dysfunction. Additionally, cardiac autonomic control is frequently altered with diabetes, resulting in reduced HR variability (65), a condition related to chronic hyperglycemia (71), an elevated resting HR, and a reduced exercise HR response. Table 24-5 summarizes clinical issues during exercise in patients with diabetes and autonomic dysfunction.

EXERCISE TESTING MODALITIES

> **1.3.5-CES: Select an appropriate test protocol according to the age, functional capacity, physical ability, and health status of the individual.**

> **1.3.22-CES: Describe the differences in the physiologic responses to various modes of ergometry (e.g., treadmill, cycle and arm ergometers) as they relate to exercise testing and training.**

> **1.7.18-CES: Determine appropriate testing and training modalities according to the age, functional capacity, physical ability, and health status of the individual.**

Different testing modalities may be used in individuals with diabetes for detecting underlying CAD. Certain exercise testing modalities may be suited for persons with diabetes who may have peripheral artery disease or peripheral neuropathy. Specifically, those with foot ulcerations or a tendency for ulceration may consider avoiding exercise that involves foot impact, such as walking. For some, cycling may also be contraindicated. Supportive shoes should be used for stability and for protection, especially in those with peripheral neuropathy and loss of sensation in their feet (35). The room should be kept at a comfortable, cool temperature, and adequate hydration should be given after the test as some patients may have inhibited ability to regulate body temperature because of autonomic dysfunction. Before testing, vision and neurologic problems should be assessed, as these complications may interfere with exercise testing protocols. Chapter 22 provides further information regarding the selection of testing modalities in certain patients.

EXERCISE TESTING WITH ELECTROCARDIOGRAPHY

> **1.3.29-CES: Identify the variables measured during cardiopulmonary exercise testing (e.g., heart rate, blood pressure, rate of perceived exertion, ventilation, oxygen consumption, ventilatory threshold, pulmonary**

TABLE 24-5. ABNORMAL EXERCISE-INDUCED CARDIOVASCULAR PARAMETERS IN PATIENTS WITH DIABETES HAVING AUTONOMIC NEUROPATHY

PARAMETERS	ABNORMALITIES OR POSSIBLE ETIOLOGIES
Nervous system	Impaired sympathetic
	Impaired parasympathetic
Electrocardiogram	Resting tachycardia (>100 bpm)
	Reduced resting heart rate variability
	Prolonged QT intervals
	Attenuated chronotropic response
	ST-T wave abnormalities
Arrhythmia	Potentially secondary to exercise-induced hypoglycemia and its stimulation of the sympathetic nervous system
Diastolic function	Abnormal
Left ventricular ejection fraction	Impaired, both at rest and with exercise
Rate-pressure product	Higher resting; lower at maximum exercise
Blood pressure	Hypertension with exercise
	Hypotension with exercise
Orthostasis (↓ SBP >20 mmHg upon standing)	Decreased release of catecholamines with increased vasoconstrictive effect
Silent ischemia	Advanced coronary artery disease

circulation) and their potential relationship to cardiovascular, pulmonary, and metabolic disease.

A standard method to evaluate diabetic patients' cardiac status in response to exercise is through observation of their ECG response during and after progressive stages of treadmill or cycle ergometry exercise testing. This type of exercise testing is relatively easy to administer and less costly than other stress testing modalities utilizing echocardiography or radionuclide imaging. Symptom-limited testing, rather than HR-limited testing procedures, provides the best prognostic value, although test administrators should be aware of the increased possibility of chronotropic incompetence in individuals with diabetes.

Although exercise stress ECG testing is the most common stress testing modality for diagnosing underlying CAD, it may not be an adequate diagnostic testing method for women with diabetes (40). Women with diabetes may need to undergo exercise testing that includes radionuclide imaging to diagnose myocardial ischemia because of an increased frequency of false-positive exercise stress tests and because of their lower pretest likelihood of having advanced CAD as compared with men (79). The diagnostic accuracy obtained from a meta-analysis using exercise stress ECG testing results from patients without a prior MI showed the mean sensitivity to be 68% and the mean specificity of 77% for detecting underlying CAD (26).

STRESS ECHOCARDIOGRAPHIC TESTING

> **1.3.29-CES: Identify the variables measured during cardiopulmonary exercise testing (e.g., heart rate, blood pressure, rate of perceived exertion, ventilation, oxygen consumption, ventilatory threshold, pulmonary circulation) and their potential relationship to cardiovascular, pulmonary, and metabolic disease.**

Patients with diabetes who have an abnormal resting ECG, result or a slightly positive ECG response to exercise stress (1.0–1.5 mm ST-T depression at a moderate to high exercise-induced HR), or who are asymptomatic for CAD may be further evaluated using other tests, such as stress echocardiography. A stress echocardiography assessment identifies positive findings in 12% to 31% of asymptomatic diabetic patients and is an effective prognostic tool in diabetic patients with known or suspected CAD (11,58). Dobutamine stress echocardiography is equivalent to thallium-201 SPECT in detecting asymptomatic CAD in patients with diabetes, making it a good testing modality for facilities without nuclear scanning equipment (56).

RADIONUCLIDE STRESS IMAGING

Radionuclide Ventriculography

> **1.3.29-CES: Identify the variables measured during cardiopulmonary exercise testing (e.g., heart rate, blood pressure, rate of perceived exertion, ventilation, oxygen consumption, ventilatory threshold, pulmonary circulation) and their potential relationship to cardiovascular, pulmonary, and metabolic disease.**

Patients with diabetes who have an abnormal resting ECG result or a slightly positive ECG response to exercise stress may be further evaluated using stress SPECT myocardial perfusion imaging. Those with nonspecific ST-segment and T-wave changes on a resting ECG, or who have exercise-induced nonspecific ECG changes may need to be further tested using radionuclide or radiotracer imaging. Radionuclide ventriculography studies are also useful in patients needing an evaluation for exercise-induced ischemia who have abnormalities such as resting ST-segment depression >1 mm, left bundle branch block (LBBB), or electronically paced rhythm. Of the different noninvasive imaging tests used to diagnose occlusive coronary disease, stress nuclear imaging has established itself as one of the most reliable and informative tools (18,31).

A myocardial perfusion image showing a small fixed defect (30,46) should not restrict an individual with diabetes from exercising. However, imaging suggesting a large perfusion abnormality in a patient with diabetes with symptomatic or silent ischemia places him or her at risk for an adverse cardiac event (55).

Radionuclide Imaging in Combination with Pharmacologic Stress

> **1.3.29-CES: Identify the variables measured during cardiopulmonary exercise testing (e.g., heart rate, blood pressure, rate of perceived exertion, ventilation, oxygen consumption, ventilatory threshold, pulmonary circulation) and their potential relationship to cardiovascular, pulmonary, and metabolic disease.**

Individuals who are unable to undergo exercise testing may be assessed via pharmacologic stress testing using dobutamine, adenosine, or dipyridamole (Persantine), to cause myocardial hyperemia when performing thallium-201 myocardial perfusion imaging. This is covered in more detail in Chapter 22.

OTHER EXERCISE TESTING CONSIDERATIONS

> **1.3.20-CES: Describe and conduct immediate postexercise procedures and various approaches to cool-down and recognize normal and abnormal responses.**

> **1.5.2-CES: Describe mechanisms and actions of medications that may affect exercise testing and prescription (i.e., β-blockers, nitrates, calcium channel blockers, digitalis, diuretics, vasodilators, antiarrhythmic agents, bronchodilators, antilipemics, psychotropics, nicotine, antihistamines, over-the-counter (OTC) cold medications, thyroid medications, alcohol, hypoglycemic agents, blood modifiers, pentoxifylline, antigout medications, and anorexiants/diet pills).**

> **1.5.3-CES: Recognize medications associated in the clinical setting, their indications for care, and their effects at rest and during exercise (i.e., β-blockers, nitrates, calcium channel blockers, digitalis, diuretics, vasodilators, antiarrhythmic agents, bronchodilators, antilipemics, psychotropics, nicotine, antihistamines, over-the-counter (OTC) cold medications, thyroid medications, alcohol, hypoglycemic agents, blood modifiers, pentoxifylline, antigout medications, and anorexiants/diet pills).**

> **1.7.23-CES: Identify procedures for pre-exercise assessment of blood glucose, determining safety for exercise, and avoidance of exercise-induced hypoglycemia in patients with diabetes. Also, manage postexercise hypoglycemia when it occurs.**

> **1.10.11-HFS: Knowledge of potential musculoskeletal injuries (e.g., contusions, sprains, strains, fractures), cardiovascular/pulmonary complications (e.g., tachycardia, bradycardia, hypotension/hypertension, tachypnea), and metabolic abnormalities (e.g., fainting/syncope, hypoglycemia/hyperglycemia, hypothermia/hyperthermia).**

A review of diabetes medications should be completed before stress testing. This review is needed to predict the blood glucose changes to an upcoming exercise bout or a stress test. Excessive insulin levels during exercise is the primary cause of reduced blood glucose after exercise. Patients taking supplemental (exogenous) insulin are at risk of exercise-induced hypoglycemia (EIH), as are patients who are taking oral antiglycemic drugs that cause the pancreas to produce more insulin. These drugs are referred to as insulin secretagogues and are found in the sulfonylurea and meglitinide drug classes. Patients taking other oral antihyperglycemic drugs (biguinide or thiazolidinediones, DPP-IV inhibitors) are not at great risk of EIH, and supplemental feedings may not be required.

Ideally, the time of day individuals with diabetes undergo an exercise test should coincide with the time they would normally exercise if they plan to begin an exercise program, and the time should be coordinated with meals and insulin or oral antihyperglycemic agent doses. These individuals should be tested while taking their usual medications if test results are to be used for planning a systematic, individualized exercise program. Testing should be avoided if the patient's glucose levels are >250 mg $\cdot$ dL^{-1} and ketosis is present, or if glucose levels are >300 mg $\cdot$ dL^{-1} and ketosis is not present. If glucose levels are <100 mg $\cdot$ dL^{-1} and the patient is taking insulin or oral insulin secretogogue drugs then glucose ($\sim$ 20–30 g) should be ingested before exercise testing to prevent a hypoglycemic response. It is helpful to have patients monitor their blood glucose levels before and after exercise testing, especially in patients taking insulin or oral insulin secretogogue drugs, as these drugs cause the risk of EIH. Guidance during the exercise test can include beneficial information for the patients about maintaining their glycemic control when they are balancing their medications, meals, and exercise. Having patients self-monitor their blood glucose also provides the healthcare team the opportunity to ensure that patients are correct in their glucose monitoring methods. Some clinic facilities, however, may have their own testing equipment and require any testing performed for the purpose of guiding treatment to be performed using the facilities equipment.

After exercise testing, patients taking medications that cause vasodilatation may experience postexercise hypotension requiring an extended cool-down period, during which they should be closely monitored. This is especially true in patients with autonomic neuropathy, as sympathetic control may be impaired. Those being exercise tested while using an insulin pump should be advised to reduce or stop their insulin infusion rate, as indicated, during the stress test to prevent EIH.

SENSITIVITY AND SPECIFICITY OF STRESS TESTS

> **1.3.20-HFS: Ability to analyze and interpret information obtained from the cardiorespiratory fitness test and the muscular strength and endurance, flexibility, and body composition assessments for apparently healthy individuals and those with controlled chronic disease.**

The value of stress testing for detecting underlying CAD depends on good clinical judgment to determine the best method of testing. One consideration to determine an appropriate diagnostic testing modality depends on the patient's pretest probability of CAD, which is influenced by factors such as age, sex, symptoms, and medical history. Examples regarding the sensitivity and specificity values for diagnosing CAD using different myocardial testing modalities can be found in Chapter 22 (Table 22.1). Pooled data of different patient populations or single laboratory studies are provided (7,12,23,24,62) and, when indicated, reports for individuals with diabetes (7,8,10,51,77) are available.

PROGNOSTIC ASSESSMENT WITH EXERCISE TESTING

> **1.3.29-CES: Identify the variables measured during cardiopulmonary exercise testing (e.g., heart rate, blood pressure, rate of perceived exertion, ventilation, oxygen consumption, ventilatory threshold, pulmonary circulation) and their potential relationship to cardiovascular, pulmonary, and metabolic disease.**

> **1.10.6-CES: Risk stratify individuals with cardiovascular, pulmonary, and metabolic diseases, using appropriate risk stratification methods and understanding the prognostic indicators for high-risk individuals.**

> **1.3.20-HFS: Ability to analyze and interpret information obtained from the cardiorespiratory fitness test and the muscular strength and endurance, flexibility, and body composition assessments for apparently healthy individuals and those with controlled chronic disease.**

Both the resting and exercise test ECG can help predict mortality in individuals with diabetes. A prolonged QT interval (corrected for HR [QTc] and calculated as QT/QTc) can show a lengthening over time in those with diabetes (20). Those with either type 1 or type 2 diabetes have a high prevalence of QT prolongation, and this abnormality is associated with ischemic heart disease in population-based studies (38,80,81). Along with associated cardiac ischemia, those with type 2 diabetes and a prolonged QT dispersion have other cardiac complications, such as left ventricular hypertrophy and autonomic dysfunction (60). This abnormal electrophysiologic finding is also an independent predictor of mortality in those with type I diabetes (63,82).

The presence of poor prognostic signs during exercise testing can also be helpful in evaluating the risk stratification of the patient, influencing medical therapy, and providing valuable guidelines for an exercise prescription. A predictor of mortality associated with exercise testing includes frequent ventricular ectopy during and immediately after exercise (25). Another independent predictor of death for older patients (patients studied included those with diabetes) is impaired functional capacity (44).

> **1.3.20-CES: Describe and conduct immediate postexercise procedures and various approaches to cool-down, and recognize normal and abnormal responses.**

Heart rate recovery after exercise testing is an independent predictor of cardiovascular and all-cause death (13). Using the criteria that a decrease in HR of <12 bpm at 1-minute postexercise is considered abnormal, it is reported that this attenuated HR recovery after exercise is a predictor of mortality (15,53). Patients with diabetes show an increased likelihood of having an abnormal HR recovery (decrease ≤12 bpm), and hyperglycemia is inversely associated with a postexercise attenuated HR recovery (70). This information emphasizes the clinical value of monitoring postexercise testing HR recovery in individuals with diabetes.

When either exercise or dobutamine stress echocardiograms were used to assess for cardiac ischemia to predict mortality in predominantly type 2 patients with known or suspected CAD, abnormal stress echocardiography results were independent predictors of death, and myocardial ischemia proved to be an independent predictor of mortality, incremental to the clinical risks for CAD and left ventricular dysfunction (41). Even with a negative stress echocardiogram result, patients with diabetes, compared with those without diabetes, are at higher risk for major cardiac events secondary to a higher prevalence of CAD (28).

Major cardiac event rates in 1,271 patients with diabetes undergoing rest thallium-201/stress technetium-99m sestamibi scanning dual-isotope myocardial perfusion SPECT with exercise or adenosine pharmacologic testing have been reported (31) (Table 24-6). Results of this study show increased myocardial events in those with diabetes as compared with those without diabetes.

TABLE 24-6. ONE-YEAR FOLLOW-UP RATES FOR CARDIAC DEATH OR NONFATAL MYOCARDIAL INFARCTION FOR PATIENTS WITH DIABETES

NUCLIDE SCAN RESULTS	MYOCARDIAL EVENT RATES
Normal	1%–2%
Mildly abnormal	3%–4%
Moderate to abnormal	>7%

From Kang X, Berman DS, Lewin HC, et al. Incremental prognostic value of myocardial perfusion single photon emission computed tomography in patients with diabetes mellitus. *Am Heart J.* 1999; 138(6 Pt 1):1025–1032.

CORONARY ARTERY CALCIFICATION IMAGING

Those with diabetes tend to have larger amounts of coronary artery calcium (CAC) deposits than nondiabetic patients (45). A similar CAC score is also found in asymptomatic diabetic patients compared to nondiabetic patients with symptomatic CAD. No difference of CAC amounts are found between men and women with diabetes (32). An excessive CAC amount (i.e., coronary calcium score of >400) is found in 26% of asymptomatic patients, and for every increase in coronary calcium score, there is a greater increase in mortality for diabetic subjects compared with nondiabetic subjects (57,68).

SUMMARY

Individuals at risk for diabetes should be routinely screened. Because the risk of heart disease increases greatly once diagnosed with diabetes, it is important to appropriately screen for cardiovascular disease. The use of exercise testing for the diagnosis of underlying CAD is clinically important for individuals with diabetes. Because routine exercise is an important component in the management of diabetes, exercise testing can assist with the identification of ischemia during increased myocardial demands, such as those caused by exercise training. Although exercise test results can be used for diagnostic and prognostic purposes, an additional important use of test results is to prescribe a systematic, individualized exercise prescription. Chapter 37 reviews the development and implementation of the exercise prescription in those with diabetes.

REFERENCES

1. American College of Endocrinology. Position Statement on the Insulin Resistance Syndrome. *Endocrine Practice.* 2002;9(3): 236–239.
2. American Diabetes Association. Consensus development conference on the diagnosis of coronary heart disease in people with diabetes. *Diabetes Care.* 1998;21:1551–1559.
3. American Diabetes Association. Position stand: Diabetes mellitus and exercise. *Diabetes Care.* 2001;24(suppl 1):S51–S55.
4. American Diabetes Association Web site [Internet]. American Diabetes Association; Available from: www.diabetes.org/about-diabetes.jsp. Accessed February 2, 2007.
5. American Diabetes Association. Physical activity/exercise and diabetes. *Diabetes Care.* 2004;27:S58–S62.
6. American Diabetes Association. Standards of medical care in diabetes. *Diabetes Care.* 2008;31:S12–S54.
7. Bacci S, Villella M, Villella A, et al. Screening for silent myocardial ischaemia in type 2 diabetic patients with additional atherogenic risk factors: applicability and accuracy of the exercise stress test. *Eur J Endocrinol.* 2002;147:649–654.
8. Bar-Or O, Rowland TW. *Pediatric Exercise Medicine: From Physiologic Principles to Health Care Application.* Champaign (IL): Human Kinetics; 2004.
9. **Bax JJ, Bonow RO, Young LH, Steinberg HO, Frye RL, Barrett EJ. Consensus Statement: Screening for coronary artery disease in patients with diabetes. *Diabetes Care.* 2007;30(10):2729–2736.**
10. Bell DS, Yumuk VD. Low incidence of false-positive exercise thallium 201 scintigraphy in a diabetic population. *Diabetes Care.* 1996;19:185–186.
11. Bigi R, Desideri A, Cortigiani L, Bax JJ, Celegon L, Fiorentini C. Stress echocardiography for risk stratification of diabetic patients with known or suspected coronary artery disease. *Diabetes Care.* 2001;24:1596–1601.
12. **Cheitlin MD, Alpert JS, Armstrong WF, et al. ACC/AHA Guidelines for the Clinical Application of Echocardiography: a report of the American College of Cardiology/American Heart Association Task Force on Practice Guidelines (Committee on Clinical Application of Echocardiography). Developed in collaboration with the American Society of Echocardiography. *Circulation.* 1997;95:1686–1744.**
13. Cheng YJ, Lauer MS, Earnest CP, et al. Heart rate recovery following maximal exercise testing as a predictor of cardiovascular disease and all-cause mortality in men with diabetes. *Diabetes Care.* 2003; 26:2052–2057.
14. Chiariello M, Indolfi C, Cotecchia MR, et al. Asymptomatic transient ST changes during ambulatory ECG monitoring in diabetic patients. *Am Heart J.* 1985;110:529–534.
15. Cole CR, Blackstone EH, Pashkow FJ, et al. Heart-rate recovery immediately after exercise as a predictor of mortality. *N Engl J Med.* 1999;341:1351–1357.
16. Cosson E, Paycha F, Paries J, et al. Detecting silent coronary stenoses and stratifying cardiac risk in patients with diabetes: ECG stress test or exercise myocardial scintigraphy? *Diabet Med.* 2004; 21:342–348.
17. De S, Searles G, Haddad H. The prevalence of cardiac risk factors in women 45 years of age or younger undergoing angiography for evaluation of undiagnosed chest pain. *Can J Cardiol.* 2002;18: 945–948.
18. De Lorenzo A, Lima RS, Siqueira-Filho AG, Pantoja MR. Prevalence and prognostic value of perfusion defects detected by stress technetium-99m sestamibi myocardial perfusion single-photon emission computed tomography in asymptomatic patients with diabetes mellitus and no known coronary artery disease. *Am J Cardiol.* 2002;90:827–832.
19. Devlin JT, Ruderman N. Diabetes and exercise: the risk-benefit profile revisited. In: Ruderman N, Devlin JT, Schneider SH, Kriska A, editors. *Handbook of Exercise in Diabetes.* Alexandria (VA): American Diabetes Association; 2002.
20. Elming H, Brendorp B, Kober L, et al. QTc interval in the assessment of cardiac risk. *Card Electrophysiol Rev.* 2002:6:289–294.
21. Ewing DJ, Campbell IW, Clarke BF. The natural history of diabetic autonomic neuropathy. *QJM.* 1980;49:95–108.
22. Fazzini PF, Prati PL, Rovelli F, et al. Epidemiology of silent myocardial ischemia in asymptomatic middle-aged men (the ECCIS Project). *Am J Cardiol.* 1993;72:1383–1388.
23. Fleg JL. Stress testing in the elderly. *Am J Geriatr Cardiol.* 2001;10(6):308–315.
24. Fleischmann KE, Hunink MG, Kuntz KM. Exercise echocardiography or exercise SPECT imaging? A meta-analysis of diagnostic test performance. *JAMA.* 1998;280:913–920.

25. Frolkis JP, Pothier CE, Blackstone EH, et al. Frequent ventricular ectopy after exercise as a predictor of death. *N Engl J Med.* 2003;348:781–790.

26. Gibbons RJ, Smith Jr SC, Antman E American College of Cardiology/American Heart Association clinical practice guidelines: Part II. Evolutionary changes in a continuous quality improvement project. *Circulation.* 2003;107:3101–3107.

27. Greenland P, Bonow RO, Brundage BH, et al. ACCF/AHA 2007 clinical expert consensus document on coronary artery calcium scoring by computed tomography in global cardiovascular risk assessment and in evaluation of patients with chest pain: a report of the American College of Cardiology Foundation Clinical Expert Consensus Task Force (ACCF/AHA Writing Committee to Update the 2000 Expert Consensus Document on Electron Beam Computed Tomography). *Circulation.* 2007;115:402–426.

28. Grundy SM, Cleeman JI, Daniels SR, et al. AHA/NHLBI Scientific Statement: Diagnosis and management of the metabolic syndrome. *Circulation.* 2005;112:2735–2752.

29. Hendel RC, Patel MR, Kramer CM, et al. ACCF/ACR/SCCT/SCMR/ASNC/NASCI/SCAI/SIR 2006 appropriateness criteria for cardiac computed tomography and cardiac magnetic resonance imaging: a report of the American College of Cardiology Foundation Quality Strategic Directions Committee Appropriateness Criteria Working Group, American College of Radiology, Society of Cardiovascular Computed Tomography, Society for Cardiovascular Magnetic Resonance, American Society of Nuclear Cardiology, North American Society for Cardiac Imaging, Society for Cardiovascular Angiography and Interventions, and Society of Interventional Radiology. *J Am Coll Cardiol.* 2006;48:1475–1497.

30. Janand-Delenne B, Savin B, Habib G, et al. Silent myocardial ischemia in patients with diabetes: who to screen. *Diabetes Care.* 1999;22:1396–1400.

31. Kang X, Berman DS, Lewin HC, et al. Incremental prognostic value of myocardial perfusion single photon emission computed tomography in patients with diabetes mellitus. *Am Heart J.* 1999; 138(6 Pt 1):1025–1032.

32. Khaleeli E, Peters SR, Bobrowsky K, Oudiz RJ, Ko JY, Budoff MJ. Diabetes and the associated incidence of subclinical atherosclerosis and coronary artery disease: implications for management. *Am Heart J.* 2001;141:637–644.

33. Kohl HW 3rd, Powell KE, Gordon NF, et al. Physical activity, physical fitness, and sudden cardiac death. *Epidemiol Rev.* 1992;14:37–58.

34. Koistinen MJ. Prevalence of asymptomatic myocardial ischaemia in diabetic subjects. *BMJ.* 1990;301:92–95.

35. Lampman RM. Musculoskeletal disorders and sports injuries. In: Ruderman N, editor. *Handbook of Exercise in Diabetes.* Alexandria (VA): American Diabetes Association; 2001. p. 497–507.

36. Lane SE, Lewis SM, Pippin JJ, et al. Predictive value of quantitative dipyridamole-thallium scintigraphy in assessing cardiovascular risk after vascular surgery in diabetes mellitus. *Am J Cardiol.* 1989;64:1275–1279.

37. Langer A, Freeman MR, Josse RG, et al. Detection of silent myocardial ischemia in diabetes mellitus. *Am J Cardiol.* 1991;67:1073–1078.

38. Linnemann B, Janka HU. Prolonged QTc interval and elevated heart rate identify the type 2 diabetic patient at high risk for cardiovascular death. The Bremen Diabetes Study. *Exp Clin Endocrinol Diabetes.* 2003;111:215–222.

39. Mann JF, Gerstein HC, Pogue J, Bosch J, Yusuf S. Renal insufficiency as a predictor of cardiovascular outcomes and the impact of ramipril: the HOPE randomized trial. *Ann Intern Med.* 2001;134:629–636.

40. Manson JE, Colditz GA, Stampfer MJ, et al. A prospective study of maturity-onset diabetes mellitus and risk of coronary heart disease and stroke in women. *Arch Intern Med.* 1991;151:1141–1147.

41. Mark DB, Hlatky MA, Harrell FE, Lee KL, Califf RM, Pryor DB. Exercise treadmill score for predicting prognosis in coronary artery disease. *Ann Intern Med.* 1987;106:793–800.

42. May O, Arilsen H, Damsgaard EM, et al. Prevalence and prediction of silent ischemia in diabetes mellitus: population based study. *Cardiovasc Res.* 1997;34:241–247.

43. May O, Arilsen H, Damsgaard EM, et al. Cardiovascular autonomic neuropathy in insulin-dependent diabetes mellitus: prevalence and estimated risk of coronary heart disease in the general population. *J Intern Med.* 2000;248:483–491.

44. Messinger-Rapport B, Pothier Snader CE, Blackstone EH. Value of exercise capacity and heart rate recovery in older people. *J Am Geriatr Soc.* 2003;51:63–68.

45. Mielke CH, Shields JP, Broemeling LD. Coronary artery calcium, coronary artery disease, and diabetes. *Diabetes Res Clin Pract.* 2001;53:55–61.

46. Milan Study on Atherosclerosis and Diabetes (MiSAD) Group. Prevalence of unrecognized silent myocardial ischemia and its association with atherosclerotic risk factors in noninsulin-dependent diabetes mellitus. *Am J Cardiol.* 1997;79:134–139.

47. Mokad AH, Ford ES, Bowman BA. Diabetes trends in the U.S.: 1990–1998. *Diabetes Care.* 2000;23:1273–1278.

48. Nabel EG, Rocco MB, Selwyn AB. Characteristics and significance of ischemia detected by ambulatory electrocardiographic monitoring. *Circulation.*1987;75(6 Pt 2):V74–V83.

49. Naka M, Hiramatsu K, Aizawa T, et al. Silent myocardial ischemia in patients with non-insulin-dependent diabetes mellitus as judged by treadmill exercise testing and coronary angiography. *Am Heart J.* 1992;123:46–53.

50. Nesto RW. Screening for asymptomatic coronary artery disease in diabetes. *Diabetes Care.* 1999;9:1393–1395.

51. Nesto RW, Watson FS, Kowalchuk GJ, et al. Silent myocardial ischemia and infarction in diabetics with peripheral vascular disease: assessment by dipyridamole thallium-201 scintigraphy. *Am Heart J.* 1990;120:1073–1077.

52. Nesto RW, Phillips RT, Kett KG, et al. Angina and exertional myocardial ischemia in diabetic and nondiabetic patients: assessment by exercise thallium scintigraphy. *Ann Intern Med.* 1988;108:170–175.

53. Nishime EO, Cole CR, Blackstone EH. Heart rate recovery and treadmill exercise score as predictors of mortality in patients referred for exercise ECG. *JAMA.* 2000;284:1392–1398.

54. Paillole C, Passa P, Paycha F, et al. Non-invasive identification of severe coronary artery disease in patients with long-standing diabetes mellitus. *Eur J Med.* 1992;1:464–468.

55. Pancholy SB, Schalet B, Kuhlmeier V, et al. Prognostic significance of silent ischemia. *J Nucl Cardiol.* 1994;1:434–440.

56. Penfornis A, Zimmermann C, Boumal B, et al. Use of dobutamine stress echocardiography in detecting silent myocardial ischaemia in asymptomatic diabetic patients: a comparison with thallium scintigraphy and exercise testing. *Diabet Med.* 2001;18:900–905.

57. Raggi P, Shaw LJ, Berman DS, Callister TQ. Prognostic value of coronary artery calcium screening in subjects with and without diabetes. *J Am Coll Cardiol.* 2004;43:1663–1669.

58. Raggi P, Bellasi A, Rattie C. Ischemia imaging and plaque imaging in diabetes: complementary tools to improve cardiovascular risk management. *Diabetes Care.* 2005;28(11):2787–2794.

59. Rajagopalan N, Miller TD, Hodge DO, Frye RL, Gibbons RJ. Identifying high risk asymptomatic diabetic patients who are candidates for screening stress single-photon emission computed tomography imaging. *J Am Coll Cardiol.* 2005;45:43–49.

60. Rana BS, Band MM, Ogston S, et al. Relation of OT interval dispersion to the number of different cardiac abnormalities in diabetes mellitus. *Am J Cardiol.* 2002;90:483–487.

61. Reaven, G. The metabolic syndrome or the insulin resistance syndrome? Different names, different concepts, and different goals. *Endocrinol Metab Clin North Am.* 2004;33:283–303.

62. **Ritchie JL, Bateman TM, Bonow RO, et al. Guidelines for clinical use of cardiac radionuclide imaging. Report of the American College of Cardiology/American Heart Association Task Force on Assessment of Diagnostic and Therapeutic Cardiovascular Procedures (Committee on Radionuclide Imaging). Developed in**

collaboration with the American Society of Nuclear Cardiology. *J Am Coll Cardiol*. 1995;25:521–547.

63. Rossing P, Breum L, Major-Pedersen A, et al. Prolonged QTc interval predicts mortality in patients with type 1 diabetes mellitus. *Diabet Med*. 2001;18:199–205.

64. Scheidt-Nave C, Barrett-Connor E, Wingard DL. Resting electrocardiographic abnormalities suggestive of asymptomatic ischemic heart disease associated with non-insulin-dependent diabetes mellitus in a defined population. *Circulation*. 1990;81:899–906.

65. Schneider SH, Khachadurian AK, Amorosa LF, et al. Ten-year experience with an exercise-based outpatient life-style modification program in the treatment of diabetes mellitus. *Diabetes Care*. 1992;15:1800–1810.

66. Schneider SH, Shindler D. Application of the American Diabetes Association's guidelines for the evaluation of the diabetic patient before recommending an exercise program. In: Devline JT, Schneider SH, editors. *Handbook of Exercise in Diabetes*. Alexandria (VA): American Diabetes Association; 2001. p. 253–268.

67. Schuijf JD, Pundziute G, Jukema JW, et al. Diagnostic accuracy of 64-slice multislice computed tomography in the noninvasive evaluation of significant coronary artery disease. *Am J Cardiol*. 2006;98:145–148.

68. Schurgin S, Rich S, Mazzone T. Increased prevalence of significant coronary artery calcification in patients with diabetes. *Diabetes Care*. 2001;24:335–338.

69. Scognamiglio R, Negut C, Ramondo A, Tiengo A, Avogaro A. Detection of coronary artery disease in asymptomatic patients with type 2 diabetes mellitus. *J Am Coll Cardiol*. 2006;47:65–71.

70. Seshadri N, Acharya N, Lauer MS. Association of diabetes mellitus with abnormal heart rate recovery in patients without known coronary artery disease. *Am J Cardiol*. 2003;91:108–111.

71. Singh JP, Larson MG, O'Donnell CJ, et al. Association of hyperglycemia with reduced heart rate variability (the Framingham Heart Study). *Am J Cardiol*. 2000;86:309–312.

72. Siscovick DS, Ekelund LG, Johnson JL, et al. Sensitivity of exercise electrocardiography for acute cardiac events during moderate and strenuous physical activity. The Lipid Research Clinics Coronary Primary Prevention Trial. *Arch Intern Med*. 1991;151:325–330.

73. **Smith SC, Blair SN, Bonow RO, et al. AHA/ACC Guidelines for preventing heart attack and death in patients with atherosclerotic cardiovascular disease: 2001 update. A statement for healthcare professionals from the American Heart Association and the American College of Cardiology. *Circulation*. 2001;104:1577–1579.**

74. Sniderman AD. Intensive blood-glucose control with sulphonylureas or insulin compared with conventional treatment and risk of complications in patients with type 2 diabetes (UKPDS 33): UK Prospective Diabetes Study (UKPDS) Group. *Lancet*. 1999;354:602.

75. The Diabetes Control and Complications Trial Research Group. The effect of intensive treatment of diabetes on the development and progression of long-term complications in insulin-dependent diabetes mellitus. *N Engl J Med*. 1993;329:977–986.

76. Thompson PD, Klocke FJ, Levine BD, et al. 26th Bethesda conference: Recommendations for determining eligibility for competition in athletes with cardiovascular abnormalities. Task Force 5: Coronary artery disease. *Med Sci Sports Exerc*. 1994;26(10 Suppl):S271–S571.

77. Tomassoni TL. Conducting the pediatric exercise test. In: Rowland TW, editor. *Pediatric Laboratory Exercise Testing: Clinical Guidelines*. Champaign (IL): Human Kinetics; 1993.

78. Valensi P, Sachs RN, Lormeau B, et al. Silent myocardial ischaemia and left ventricle hypertrophy in diabetic patients. *Diabetes Metab*. 1997;23:409–416.

79. Vanzetto G, Halimi S, Hammoud T, et al. Prediction of cardiovascular events in clinically selected high-risk NIDDM patients. *Diabetes Care*. 1999;22:19–26.

80. Veglio M, Chinaglia A, Cavallo-Perin P. The clinical utility of QT interval assessment in diabetes. *Diabetes Nutr Metab*. 2000;13:356–365.

81. Veglio M, Bruno G, Borra M, et al. Prevalence of increased QT interval duration and dispersion in type 2 diabetic patients and its relationship with coronary heart disease: a population-based cohort. *J Intern Med*. 2002;251:317–324.

82. Veglio M, Sivieri R, Chinaglia A, et al. QT interval prolongation and mortality in type 1 diabetic patients: a 5-year cohort prospective study. Neuropathy Study Group of the Italian Society of the Study of Diabetes, Piemonte Affiliate. *Diabetes Care*. 2000;23:1381–1383.

83. Viviani V, Valensi P, Paycha F, et al. The stress test should be the first test performed when assessing silent myocardial ischemia in diabetic subjects. *Diabetes*. 1998;47:119A.

84. Wackers FJ, Young LH, Inzucchi SE, et al. Detection of silent myocardial ischemia in asymptomatic diabetic subjects: the DIAD study. *Diabetes Care*. 2004;27:1954–1961.

SELECTED REFERENCES FOR FURTHER READING

American Diabetes Association. Standards of medical care in diabetes. *Diabetes Care*. 2008;31:S12–S54.

American Heart Association Conference Proceedings: Prevention Conference VI: Diabetes and Cardiovascular Disease. Writing Group III: Risk assessment in persons with diabetes. *Circulation*. 2002;105:e144.

Ruderman N, Devlin JT, Schneider SH, Kriska A, editors. *Handbook of Exercise in Diabetes*. 2nd ed. Alexandria (VA): American Diabetes Association; 2001.

INTERNET RESOURCES

- American Diabetes Association: www.diabetes.org
- CDC Diabetes Public Health Resource: www.cdc.gov/diabetes
- National Diabetes Education Program: http//:ndep.nih.gov
- National Institute of Diabetes and Digestive and Kidney Disease: www.niddk.nih.gov
- WebMD: www.emedicine.com/med/topic2961.htm

Healthcare professionals can play an important role in optimizing vocational and nonvocational activity-related decisions for many patients, especially during the early recovery period after a major cardiac event. The focus of this chapter is on assessment and rehabilitative procedures that may promote optimal short-term as well as long-term activity decisions for those with known heart disease.

OCCUPATIONAL ASSESSMENT

Employment-related decisions in cardiac patients can be complex. In addition to the patient and employer, work-related decisions involve various professional agencies, including medical, disability, insurance, or legal (40,49). Several factors may influence the return-to-work process, including the patient's desire to return to work, job satisfaction, perception of disability, previous employment record, age, education level, work tolerance in relation to job demands, disease severity, family concerns, coworkers, supervisor's attitudes or restrictions, support mechanisms, psychological variables, available financial resources (e.g., disability income, insurance, savings), or other work incentives/disincentives (2,7,11,13,22,28,40,42,49,54). For those who resume work, employment can produce positive psychosocial, physical, and material benefits.

Because of the variety of factors that can influence work-related decisions, a significant percentage of patients do not resume work after a cardiac event or do not remain employed until a normal retirement age (7,11,30,49). Some of these individuals are granted disability benefits despite relatively good functional work reserve. In a study of 175 men who were receiving Social Security Disability Insurance (SSDI) secondary to is-

chemic heart disease, 65% were found to have a work capacity ≥5 METs and 12% a work capacity ≥7 METs (42). In this study, peak MET levels were determined with measurement of oxygen uptake. Based on their responses to an activity questionnaire, these men were fairly active with home or leisure-time physical activities, with approximately 20% to 30% of them performing relatively demanding home tasks, such as gardening, mowing (walking), and snow removal (blowing or shoveling). It is possible that greater reliance on functional work reserve in relation to expected job demands may lead to more optimal decisions regarding return to work and granting of disability benefits.

Premature loss of employment has significant societal economic implications and may also affect the social well-being of patients. In the United States, coronary heart disease (CHD) is a leading cause of disability under the Social Security Administration (SSA) program (2). In Canada, a Health Canada report indicated that cardiovascular disease is the highest cost in terms of burden of illness, equaling $18.5 billion annually, with long-term disability costs being $3.1 billion per year (25,66). Procedures that may help to optimize work resumption are reviewed in this chapter. Primary topics include clinical assessment, early intervention, job analysis, work tolerance testing, counseling, and early rehabilitation.

CLINICAL ASSESSMENT

> **1.5.8-CES: Recognize patient clinical need for referral to other (non-CES) allied health professionals (e.g., behavioralist, physical therapist, diabetes educator, nurse, etc.).**

> **1.9.2-CES: Describe signs and symptoms of mal-adjustment and/or failure to cope during an illness crisis and/or personal adjustment crisis (e.g., job loss) that might prompt a psychological consult or referral to other professional services.**

> **1.9.7-HFS: Knowledge of signs and symptoms of mental health states (e.g., anxiety, depression, eating disorders) that may necessitate referral to a medical or mental health professional.**

Information gathered from several sources can be used to assess a patient's current medical status and future prognosis in terms of morbidity and mortality secondary to heart disease. Risk stratification of cardiac patients into low-, moderate-, and high-risk categories for future events can be helpful in counseling patients on resuming physical activity (4) (see GETP8 Boxes 2.2 and 2.3). Most jobs today are not physically demanding, so unnecessary delays in work resumption beyond the normal convalescent period should be avoided. This includes avoiding delays specifically to permit completion of a cardiac rehabilitation program or waiting for results from nonessential diagnostic tests before providing medical clearance for work resumption. Individuals who have physically demanding jobs, especially those in moderate and high clinical risk categories, may require further diagnostic evaluation or intervention before work resumption. Identification of signs of depression and other psychological disorders may be beneficial because psychological issues can have a negative influence on work-related decisions in some patients (2,54). Lewin indicated that 40% to 50% of individuals who do not return to work have reasons other than physical illness (31). An easily administered brief depression scale, the Depression Subscale, part of the Hospital Anxiety and Depression Scale, can help identify depressed patients who are less likely to return to work (34). Various methods can be used to help identify and treat psychological disorders (5).

EARLY INTERVENTION AND COUNSELING

Return to work should be discussed as early as possible with patients. In some situations, work resumption can be discussed while the patient is in hospital. Some possible factors to consider in discussing work-related issues with patients are listed in Box 25-1. Ignoring work-related matters early in the recovery process may cause patients to inappropriately perceive their event as leading to an inability to resume work. Patients can generally be given a positive message regarding work resumption along with a tentative timetable for resuming work before discharge. For some patients, particularly women, it is important to receive positive affirmations about domestic and social responsibilities (26). The actual timing for

| **BOX 25-1** | **CHECKLIST FOR POSSIBLE WORK RETURN INTERVENTIONS** |

- Assess disease severity and prognosis of patient after event.
- Ask the patient about preadmission employment status.
- Discuss expected recovery course with the patient, including return to work.
- Establish a tentative timetable for work resumption, when appropriate.
- Ask the patient about any work return concerns.
- Be prepared to discuss qualifying criteria for disability benefits.
- Determine if a job analysis, including an employer contact/work-site visit, is warranted.
- Suggest that the patient contact the employer to maintain contact and, if appropriate, discuss return to work.
- Encourage participation in a progressive exercise program to enhance work resumption potential.
- Consider referrals for procedures or treatments that may assist patients in returning to work.

return to work can vary with several factors, such as the cardiac event, disease severity, prognosis, job requirements, safety regulations, and employer attitudes or concerns. Most individuals can resume their jobs within 1 to 12 weeks after a major cardiac event. A study conducted by Kovoor et al. showed that patients following an acute myocardial infarction and stratified as low risk were able to safely return to full normal activities, including work, at 2 weeks postevent (27). Early return can be especially useful for individuals who are self-employed or lack the financial resources to remain off work. Some, especially those who work in jobs that may place coworkers and/or the public at risk, such as firefighters, commercial drivers, and airline pilots, may have greater delays or restrictions on returning to work, including meeting specific medical criteria to maintain a license to work (6,21,53).

JOB ANALYSIS

> **1.1.5-CES: Identify the metabolic equivalent (MET) requirements of various occupational, household, sport/exercise, and leisure time activities.**

> **1.3.13-HFS: Ability to obtain a health history and risk appraisal that includes past and current medical history, family history of cardiac disease, orthopedic limitations, prescribed medications, activity patterns,**

nutritional habits, stress and anxiety levels, and smoking and alcohol use.

 1.7.14-HFS: Knowledge of approximate METs for various sport, recreational, and work tasks.

A job analysis performed soon after a major cardiac event can serve as a basis for (a) delineating expected physical and psychological demands of the patient's job, thus determining if an individual will be safe on the job; (b) identifying the patient's concerns regarding work resumption; (c) establishing a tentative timeline for work resumption; and (d) individualizing assessment or rehabilitation procedures that may be undertaken during the early recovery period to optimize return-to-work decisions and capability (12,49,58). Generally, job titles provide little or, in some cases, misleading information about the work demands. Some of the factors that can be assessed in a job analysis include determination of specific job tasks from which expected energy cost requirements can be estimated: weight lifting, stacking, carrying, pushing, and pulling requirements; environmental conditions, including exposure to potentially hazardous materials; and psychological stressors. This information can be obtained by interviewing the patient; with the patient's permission, an employer contact and work-site visit can provide a wealth of information. The work demands from the employer's perspective, the employer's expectations, the return-to-work policy, sick leave, worker's compensation, the possibilities for a gradual return to work in terms of hours and duties or modifications, and specific job/union regulations (30,49,56,57,58,59,67) can be obtained utilizing a standard questionnaire, such as the job analysis questionnaire designed by Sheldahl, Wilke, and Tristani (49).

In estimating the average and peak physical demands of work for patients, various resources can be used. Employers may be able to provide specific work requirements that relate directly to their work sites. Increasingly, written physical demands analyses are available. If the employer can not be contacted, then *The Dictionary of Occupational Titles* (57), *The National Occupational Classification-Career Handbook in Canada* (36), and *Occupational Outlook Handbook* (56) provide general information regarding work requirements under specific job titles. MET tables (see GETP8, Table 1.1) provide approximations for average energy demands of various job and other activity tasks in units of multiples of resting energy expenditure (3,23). It should be emphasized that the values listed in MET tables are only approximations and that expected energy demands listed for some activities are estimated based on their similarity to other types of activities. The actual MET demands can vary with pace of work, worker efficiency, orthopedic disabilities, automation, assistive devices, protective equipment, body size, terrain, and temperature. A study on lawn mowing, for example, showed that the mean MET levels for lawn mowing using a walk-behind mower varied from 3 to 10 METs, depending on the type of mower (push, power push, or self-propelled), walking speed, lawn terrain, and subject characteristics (48). In using MET energy cost tables, it should be noted that most on-the-job energy expenditure studies were completed before 1960 (16,38). Sheldahl, Wilke, and others performed several energy expenditure studies in work simulation settings and at occupational work sites (14,15,19,41,43–45,47,50,51,62–64). In the job site studies (44), oxygen uptake was measured for 20 minutes with a portable device in workers at a variety of physical labor work settings. The on-the-job studies indicated that the average energy expenditure of most jobs requiring physical labor corresponds to <4 METs. Higher demands were required in some tasks, such as chain sawing or chipping, power push mowing, barn cleaning, air hammering, drywall and masonry, and weight carrying and repetitive lifting tasks. In addition to the influence of energy expenditure on myocardial oxygen requirements, it is important to assess whether other work-related conditions (e.g., adverse temperature stress, psychological stress, awkward body positioning, static work) may increase myocardial oxygen demands (49). The influence of selected environmental factors on myocardial oxygen requirements is discussed later in the chapter.

TRADITIONAL EXERCISE TESTING

 1.3.19-CES: Select and perform appropriate procedures and protocols for the exercise test, including modes of exercise, starting levels, increments of work, ramping versus incremental protocols, length of stages, and frequency of data collection.

 1.3.21-CES: Record, organize, perform, and interpret necessary calculations of test data.

 1.5.3-CES: Recognize medications associated in the clinical setting, their indications for care, and their effects at rest and during exercise (i.e., β-blockers, nitrates, calcium channel blockers, digitalis, diuretics, vasodilators, anitarrhythmic agents, bronchodilators, antilipemics, psychotropics, nicotine, antihistamines, over-the-counter (OTC) cold medications, thyroid medications, alcohol, hypoglycemic agents, blood modifiers, pentoxifylline, antigout medications, and anorexiants/diet pills).

The traditional symptom-limited graded exercise test (GXT) on a treadmill or cycle ergometer can be very helpful in providing realistic vocational recommendations (17,23,49). Information on work tolerance along with submaximal and maximal exercise-induced hemodynamic responses, electrocardiographic responses, and possible symptoms can help assess the ability of patients to resume work within a reasonable period and identify areas that need better management or further assessment.

Exercise testing may also reassure the patient, patient's family, and employer regarding the patient's ability to safely handle the job demands (GETP8 Chapter 5).

An important exercise test measurement is determination of functional MET capacity. In the clinical setting, functional MET capacity is typically estimated based on the peak workload achieved. GXTs using protocols with smaller increments, such as the Naughton or Balke, are more useful (see GETP8 Chapter 5). The patient should undergo the GXT while on usual medications to evaluate functional capacity in his/her "normal state." Ideally, oxygen uptake can be measured with a cardiopulmonary exercise (stress) test using a metabolic cart, thus assessing if a maximal effort has been made, determining any respiratory problems and the workload equivalent to the anaerobic threshold (11). After functional MET capacity is determined, it can be compared with the estimated average and peak METs of the individual's job. Work requirements should not induce myocardial ischemia or produce excessive fatigue. Over an 8-hour day, fatigue is more likely to occur when the average energy expenditure rate exceeds 50% of the individual's peak aerobic capacity. The appropriate upper-intensity level to recommend for short-term (e.g., <60 min) occupational work tasks should be individualized based on patient characteristics (e.g., severity of disease, serious arrhythmias), tolerance for physical work, type of work performed, duration and frequency of work tasks, and work environment. Most patients should be able to use the same physical activity guidelines that are individualized for them for home and leisure-time physical activities or for an unsupervised exercise program.

SIMULATED WORK TESTING

> **1.1.6-CES: Knowledge of the unique hemodynamic responses of arm versus leg exercise, combined arm and leg exercise, and of static versus dynamic exercise.**

For most people with heart disease, the only exercise test needed to assess functional tolerance for work resumption is the traditional GXT. There are limitations in advising some on work resumption based only on graded dynamic exercise testing. One limitation is that although the traditional GXT evaluates dynamic exercise tolerance, certain jobs may require a significant static workload (e.g., lift, carry, push, pull). This can result in questions regarding the patient's ability to tolerate the greater myocardial afterload stress expected with static work, along with potential questions regarding the appropriate upper static load to recommend. For some patients who have performed work that has mainly involved arm work (for example: operating heavy equipment), their arms may be better conditioned than their legs; thus, the exercise test results would underestimate their ability to perform upper-extremity work. Another limitation is that in contrast

to the traditional exercise test, work sites may have less-than-ideal work conditions (e.g., hot or cold climates, air pollution, intermittent heavy work tasks).

It is impractical and unnecessary to evaluate workers under all the various stressors encountered in the course of a typical work routine, although some of the more demanding work tasks can be evaluated in select patients using work simulation testing. Patients most likely to benefit from simulated work testing are those whose ability to return to work remain in question despite traditional exercise testing, perhaps because of lower aerobic capacity (<7 METs), left ventricular dysfunction, ischemia at submaximal levels, significant arrhythmias, or apprehension about resuming a physically demanding job (23,49,61). Simple, inexpensive work simulation tests can be set up. In terms of protocols, a weight-carrying test protocol and a repetitive weight-lifting test protocol have been published for evaluating tolerance for static work combined with light to moderate dynamic work (49). Both of these test protocols are graded and designed to be applicable to several types of work tasks requiring a static component. In some instances—for example, when there are sudden high demands on the job—it is preferable to design the test to simulate the work demands more closely, perhaps having an individual immediately lift the required weight without a warm-up.

The weight-carrying test protocol (Table 25-1) is designed to evaluate tolerance for light to heavy static effort combined with light dynamic work. In one protocol, the patient walks on a treadmill at a slow pace while carrying specified weight loads (e.g., dumbbell weights) in one or

TABLE 25-1. DYNAMIC-STATIC WORK SIMULATION TEST PROTOCOLS

WEIGHT-CARRYING TEST EXAMPLE[a] PROTOCOL

Stage[b]	Duration (min)	Speed (mph)	Load[c] (lb)	Predicted METs[d]
1	3	2.0	0	2.4
2	3	2.0	20	3.0
3	3	2.0	30	4.2
4	3	2.0	40	5.0
5	2	2.0	50	4.8[e]

REPETITIVE LIFTING TEST EXAMPLE[a] PROTOCOL

Stage[b]	Duration (min)	Lift Rate	Load[c] (lb)	Predicted METs[d]
1	6	Self-paced	30	3.8
2	6	Self-paced	40	4.2
3	6	Self-paced	50	4.5
4	6	Self-paced	30, 40, 50	4.2

METs, metabolic equivalents with 1 MET = oxygen uptake of $3.5 \text{ mL} \cdot \text{kg}^{-1} \cdot \text{min}^{-1}$.

[a]Test protocols can be modified to meet specific work conditions.

[b]A seated rest period of 1 to 3 minutes follows each stage.

[c]Weight load in weight-carrying test (e.g., dumbbell) can be carried in one or both hands; weight load in repetitive test can be lifted from floor or pallet to work bench.

[d]METs are based on tests using the specific protocol listed.

[e]The slightly lower MET level for carrying 50 lbs versus 40 lbs is likely because of the shorter walk time and the inability to achieve steady-state conditions.

Adapted with permission from American College of Sports Medicine. *Guidelines for Exercise Testing and Prescription.* 6th ed. Philadelphia: Lippincott Williams & Wilkins; 2000.

both hands. The repetitive weight-lifting test protocol (Table 25-1) is designed to evaluate tolerance for intermittent static work combined with a dynamic work component. In this protocol, the patient repetitively lifts specified weight loads, typically from the floor or pallet to a table or bench for a set period. Patients can be instructed to lift at a set pace or select a rate that simulates or somewhat exceeds their job requirement.

In assessing blood pressure (BP) responses to static or static–dynamic work, it is important to measure the BP in the nonexercising arm just before lifting and just before releasing the weight. BP decreases rapidly upon release of the static load. Electrocardiographic monitoring can be the same as for the traditional exercise test, or telemetry can be used if ischemia is not expected based on prior traditional exercise testing. Specialized work simulators (e.g., Baltimore Therapeutic and Valpar work simulators) are available for simulating various tasks, although the energy cost with some stations may be less than when performing tasks in the work setting (62).

ON-THE-JOB MONITORING

Ambulatory electrocardiographic monitoring can be considered for patients in whom concerns exist regarding potential for serious arrhythmias or ischemia on the job despite laboratory testing. Heart rate (HR) responses to work can also be evaluated with this procedure, although inexpensive HR monitors can be used or patients can be instructed to check their pulse rates during their more demanding work tasks. Some of the HR monitors can be programmed to emit a sound when a preprogrammed HR is exceeded or to provide average and peak HR information over a period of time. On-the-job HR monitoring can help evaluate the combined effects of the physical work and work-related factors (e.g., environmental) or work conditions that can increase myocardial demands. Patients may also be assured that their jobs are not causing an excessive myocardial demand by simply checking their pulse rate.

EARLY REHABILITATION

> **1.3.30-CES: Discuss the appropriate use of static and dynamic resistance exercise for individuals with cardiovascular, pulmonary, and metabolic disease.**

> **1.9.8-CES: Recognize and implement methods of stress management for patients with chronic disease.**

> **1.1.37-HFS: Knowledge of and skill to demonstrate exercises designed to enhance muscular strength and/or endurance of specific major muscle groups.**

> **1.7.11-HFS: Knowledge of and the ability to describe exercises designed to enhance muscular strength and/or endurance of specific major muscle groups.**

Participation in cardiac rehabilitation supervised exercise programs after a cardiac event (see GETP8 Chapter 9) has shown mixed results in terms of enhancing work resumption outcomes (2). Failure to find a positive impact in several studies may stem from the complexity of factors reported to influence work-related decisions. Tailoring of cardiac rehabilitation programs in the early phase of recovery to address the work-related concerns of patients resuming work may enhance work resumption potential (34,49). There may be a benefit from early intervention focusing on improving psychological parameters, as previously discussed, and encouraging use of exercise modes designed to enhance resumption of specific types of work (for example: arm exercise, resistive exercise) (see GETP 8 Chapter 9 and Box 9.9). Enrollment in a stress management program may improve confidence for return to work. For patients who will need to resume work in a hot environment, a gradual exposure to outdoor exercise may be more beneficial than only exercising in a climate-controlled facility.

DISABILITY

A small percentage of cardiac patients who were previously working will not be able to resume paid employment because of their disease severity. These patients may qualify for disability income through programs such as Social Security Disability Insurance (SSDI) in the United States and Canada Pension Plan-Disability (CPP-D) benefits in Canada, private long-term disability insurance, or Veterans Administration service- and nonservice-related pensions. Some patients may inappropriately think they will qualify for disability income. If they are not informed about the stringent qualifying criteria, some of them may unnecessarily go through the long process of applying for SSDI or CPP-D only to be rejected. In discussing return-to-work matters with patients, it is helpful to have a good understanding of the rules and regulations regarding common disability plans such as SSDI (60) and CPP-D (10).

In the SSDI program, Social Security pays benefits for individuals who can not work because they have a medical condition that is expected to last at least 1 year or result in death. The patient needs to have worked enough years to qualify (60). Eligibility for CPP-D is similar, requiring that an individual be between ages 18 and 65; has made contributions to CPP for a minimum qualifying period; and has a disability that is prolonged and severe, thus the person is incapable regularly of pursuing any substantially gainful occupation.

In some states, uniformed police officers or firefighters are covered under "accidental disability" (often referred to as "Heart Laws") (32,40,49). Under these programs, workers may be able to establish the existence of a disabling cardiac disease or hypertension without proving that the job caused the disabling condition. Considerable variability exists among states in terms of the coverage provided under "accidental disability." Contacting the public employee state retirement agency may help to inform/advise patients. In Canada, if the cardiac event can be directly attributed to the job, there may be eligibility for compensation through the Worker's Safety and Insurance Board (66). An example is an individual with no known coronary artery disease (CAD) chopping ice at work and suffering a myocardial infarction while working.

NEW EMPLOYMENT

Some patients may need to find employment after a cardiac event because they are unemployed or cannot return to their previous employment. Importantly, the Americans with Disabilities Act (ADA) "prohibits private sector employers who employ 15 or more individuals and all State and local government employers from discriminating against qualified individuals with disabilities in all aspects of employment" (58). The Canadian Human Rights Commission ensures that the principles of equal opportunity and nondiscrimination are followed in all areas of federal jurisdiction (9). State or provincial vocational services may be available for individuals who need retraining for employment. The extent of vocational services varies widely.

NONVOCATIONAL ACTIVITIES

> **1.2.8-CES: Describe the influence of exercise on cardiovascular, pulmonary, and metabolic risk factors.**

> **1.7.4-CES: Design, implement, and supervise individualized exercise prescriptions for people with chronic disease and disabling conditions, or who are young or elderly.**

> **1.7.6-CES: Knowledge of the concept of activities of daily living (ADLs) and its importance in the overall rehabilitation of the individual.**

> **1.2.2-HFS: Knowledge of cardiovascular, pulmonary, metabolic, and musculoskeletal risk factors that may require further evaluation by medical or allied health professionals before participation in physical activity.**

> **1.2.3-HFS: Knowledge of risk factors that may be favorably modified by physical activity habits.**

> **1.7.3-HFS: Knowledge of the benefits and precautions associated with exercise training across the lifespan (from youth to the elderly).**

> **1.7.5-HFS: Knowledge of how to select and/or modify appropriate exercise programs according the age, functional capacity, and limitations of the individual.**

> **1.7.20-HFS: Knowledge of and ability to describe activities of daily living (ADLs) and its importance in the overall health of the individual.**

An important goal after a cardiac event is for patients to maintain as active a lifestyle as possible considering the magnitude of the disease, which includes encouraging patients to participate in appropriate home and leisure-time activities. Maintaining an active daily routine with home and leisure-time activities can help those with heart disease meet secondary prevention guidelines as recommended by The American Heart Association & American College of Cardiology in 2006 (52). These guidelines suggest 30 to 60 minutes of moderate-intensity aerobic activity on most or preferably all days of the week, supplemented by an increase in daily lifestyle activities. Leisure-time activities that raise the HR into an aerobic zone can provide some individuals with an enjoyable way to participate in a regular aerobic-type exercise program. Importantly, regular exercise and good physical fitness provide many benefits in terms of prevention of disease progression and quality of life (29). Maintaining physical fitness may help to reduce cardiac events stemming from strenuous activity (55). Investigators (35,65) have shown that the risk of an acute myocardial infarction (MI) is temporarily increased during high-intensity physical activity, especially in those who are habitually sedentary. People who exercise regularly have a much lower relative risk associated with strenuous exercise. Plus they have the protective preventive effect associated with a regular program of exercise.

Most of the same procedures used for optimizing occupational work decisions are also applicable to advising patients on resumption of home and leisure-time activities, including medical assessment, early intervention, activity analysis, counseling, work tolerance testing, and exercise conditioning.

A major risk factor for CHD is age and, thus CHD is more common in elderly persons than within other age groups. Just as resumption of occupational work can have important individual and societal ramifications, so can resumption of independent living in the elderly population. In addition to the economic cost associated with assisted living, maintenance of an independent lifestyle affects the quality of life in elderly individuals. In a study of people with CHD >65 years of age, peak aerobic capacity and depression were shown to be predictors of physical functioning (1). Encouraging elderly patients to participate in supervised exercise programs, as well as resuming their home and leisure-time activities after a cardiac event, may promote greater tolerance and confidence among the elderly in performing activities important for independence. Because of the comorbidities common in elderly individuals, their exercise programs may need special tailoring to meet specific needs. Psychosocial counseling may help those with depression maintain a more positive outlook on life and thus engage in a more active lifestyle.

INFLUENCE OF ENVIRONMENTAL CONDITIONS

> **1.1.12-CES:** Describe the effects of variation in environmental factors (e.g. temperature, humidity, altitude) for normal individuals and those with cardiovascular, pulmonary, and metabolic diseases.

> **1.7.3-CES:** Design appropriate exercise prescription in environmental extremes for those with cardiovascular, pulmonary, and metabolic diseases.

> **1.7.16-HFS:** Knowledge of special precautions and modifications of exercise programming for participation at altitude, different ambient temperatures, humidity, and environmental pollution.

> **1.10.6-HFS:** Knowledge of the effects of temperature, humidity, altitude, and pollution on the physiologic response to exercise and the ability to modify the exercise prescription to accommodate for these environmental conditions.

Many home, leisure-time, and job activities are performed in less-than-ideal environmental conditions, which can alter myocardial oxygen uptake requirements and work tolerance.

HEAT STRESS

During sustained work in a hot environment, circulatory demand typically is increased to meet the dual blood flow demands for metabolism (muscle) and thermoregulation (skin) (18,46). A common characteristic of work combined with heat stress is a more progressive drift upward in HR and drift downward in stroke volume with work time compared with the same type of work performed in a thermoneutral environment. The addition of a humid environment produces an even greater drift. This cardiovascular drift represents an increase in myocardial oxygen requirements.

Most studies involving exercise in a hot environment have been performed on healthy individuals. In a study of asymptomatic men with heart disease, a similar cardiovascular drift response was seen with sustained moderate-intensity work (46). Left ventricular ejection fraction (LVEF) and cardiac output were maintained, and the incidence of arrhythmias was not increased with heat stress. The effect of work or exercise combined with heat stress in symptomatic patients or those at high risk is not known.

Encouraging individuals to monitor their pulse rate during work in a hot environment provides a useful means for adjusting work rate downward to avoid excessive myocardial demand. Individuals should also be informed about the importance of gradual exposure to exercise combined with heat stress after a period of cool or cold weather exposure to permit heat acclimation. Heat acclimation results in improved capacity to dissipate heat, which, in turn, reduces the magnitude of the cardiovascular drift and thereby myocardial oxygen demands. Heat acclimation can occur within a few days (3–10 days) of undertaking mild, sustained (up to 90 min) physical activity in a warm environment (see GETP8, Chapter 8 for guidelines).

COLD STRESS

Work in a cold environment may add to myocardial oxygen requirements by increasing myocardial afterload (e.g., BP, vascular resistance) and/or energy expenditure as a result of wearing heavier clothing, walking through snow, and perhaps shivering (15,43,45). Some CHD patients report angina at a lower work level in a cold environment (2). Mortality is increased in the winter months, but it remains uncertain how much of this is related to physical activity performed in a cold environment.

One of the more demanding wintertime physical activities is snow removal (15,20,43,45). Anecdotal reports of death from MI related to snow removal have raised questions regarding the ability of CHD patients to safely perform static–dynamic work tasks in a cold environment. In a study (20) of younger men shoveling wet snow, mean relative work intensity corresponded to 97% of peak HR. In view of the anecdotal reports and work requirements of snow removal, it seems prudent to advise moderate- and high-risk CHD patients and those with a work capacity <6.5 METs not to remove snow, especially with more physically demanding snow removal conditions (e.g., >2 inches of wet snow). Some patients continue to remove snow despite being advised against it. For those who plan to remove snow, precautions should be emphasized, such as the importance of regular exercise (including resistive training) before and during the winter season, working within appropriate limits, avoiding heavy static loads, dressing appropriately, limiting sustained work time to less than 30 to 45 minutes, stopping at onset of any symptoms, avoiding time pressure conditions, performing warm-up and cool-down exercises, and avoiding taking a hot shower immediately after removing snow.

ALTITUDE

Those traveling to the mountains for skiing or other physical activities should understand that hypoxia at altitude can significantly lower their work tolerance (37,68). The impact on work tolerance is greatest during the first few days at a high altitude. Over a few days (up to 5–10) of altitude exposure, tolerance for physical activities improves through acclimatization. Wyss et al. (68) reported that patients with CAD showed a significant decrease in coronary flow reserve (CFR) when evaluated immediately after supine cycle exercise under acute hypoxic conditions comparable to 2,500-m altitude. These patients also showed greater electrocardiographic and symptomatic evidence of exercise-induced ischemia with simulated altitude. In contrast, healthy control subjects did not show an exercise-induced decrease in CFR with hypoxic conditions at altitude simulations of 2,500 and 4,500 m. The investigators concluded that CAD patients with reduced CFR should be cautioned about performing physical activity at moderate or higher altitudes. Another environment factor that needs to be considered at altitude is exposure to less-than-ideal temperature conditions (38,50) (see GETP8, Chapter 8 for guidelines).

POLLUTANTS

Air pollutants should be taken into consideration in advising those on resuming work in certain affected communities or work sites, especially in those who have cardiopulmonary disease or are expected to work at relatively high work intensities. Recent reports indicate that both short- and long-term exposure to air pollutants results in an increased risk for cardiopulmonary events (8,18,25,39).

SUMMARY

Enabling cardiac patients to resume as active and productive a lifestyle as possible for their disease state is an important goal. This includes helping patients resume employment, when appropriate, as well as home and leisure-time activities. Various techniques can be used to help optimize work and activity resumption for patients, including a job or activity analysis, exercise testing, simulated work testing, and activity monitoring. Exercise training programs can also be tailored to enhance the potential of patients to resume specific types of work. To help optimize the return-to-work process for patients, healthcare professionals should have a basic understanding of job requirements and governmental policies and procedures that can influence work resumption and work conditions for patients.

REFERENCES

1. Ades PA, Savage PD, Tischler MD, et al. Determinants of disability in older coronary patients. *Am Heart J.* 2002;143:151–156.
2. **Agency for Health Care Policy and Research. Cardiac rehabilitation. Clinical Practice Guideline, No. 17. AHCPR Publication No. 96-0672. Rockville (MD): U.S. Department of Health and Human Services; 1995.**
3. Ainsworth BE, Haskell WL, Whitt MC, et al. Compendium of physical activities: an update of activity codes and MET intensities. *Med Sci Sports Exerc.* 2000;32(Suppl):S498–S516.
4. **American Association of Cardiovascular and Pulmonary Rehabilitation. *Guidelines for Cardiac Rehabilitation and Secondary Prevention Programs.* 4th ed. Champaign (IL): Human Kinetics; 2004.**
5. Blumenthal JA, Babyak MA, Carney RM, et al. Exercise, depression, and mortality after myocardial infarction in the ENRICHD Trial. *Med Sci Sports Exerc.* 2004;36:746–755.
6. **Blumenthal R, Braunstein J, Connolly H, et al. Cardiovascular advisory panel guidelines for the medical examination of commercial**

motor vehicle drivers. Available from: www.fmcsa.dot.gov/rules-regulations/administration/medical.htm . Accessed May 25, 2007.
7. Boudrez H, De Backer G. Recent findings on return to work after an acute myocardial infarction or coronary artery bypass grafting. *Acta Cardiol.* 2000;55:341–349.
8. Brook RD, Franklin B, Cascio W, et al. Air pollution and cardiovascular disease: a statement for healthcare professionals from the Expert Panel on Population and Prevention Science of the American Heart Association. *Circulation.* 2004;109:2655–2671.
9. Canadian Human Rights Commission. Canadian Human Rights Act. Available from: www.chrc-ccdp.gc.ca/. Accessed Nov 7, 2008.
10. Canada Pension Plan: Disability. Updated 2007 April 27. Available from: www.servicecanada.gc.ca/en/sc/cpp/disability/disabilitypension.shtml. Accessed May 30, 2007.
11. Dafoe W. Employment and insurability. In: Crawford MH, DiMarco JP, Paulus WJ, editors. *Cardiology.* 2nd ed. London: Elsevier; 2003. p. 1625–1634.
12. Dennis C, Houston-Miller N, Schwartz RG, et al. Early return to work after uncomplicated myocardial infarction: results of a randomized trial. *JAMA.* 1988; 260:214–220.
13. Dougherty CM. The natural history of recovery following sudden cardiac arrest and internal cardioverter-defibrillator implantation. *Prog Cardiovasc Nurs.* 2001;16:163–168.
14. Dougherty S, Sheldahl L, Wilke N, et al. Metabolic and hemodynamic responses to gardening in men with and without ischemic heart disease [abstract]. *J Cardiopulm Rehabil.* 1991;11:321.
15. Dougherty SM, Sheldahl LM, Wilke NA, et al. Physiologic responses to shoveling and thermal stress in men with cardiac disease. *Med Sci Sports Exerc.* 1993;25:790–795.
16. Durham JVGA, Passmore R. *Energy, Work and Leisure.* London: Heinemann Educational Books Ltd; 1967. p. 47–95.
17. **Fletcher GF, Balady G, Froelicher VF, et al. Exercise standards: a statement for healthcare professionals from the American Heart Association. *Circulation.* 1995;91:580–615.**
18. Folinsbee LJ. Heat and air pollution. In: Pollock MLL, Schmidt DH, editors. *Heart Disease and Rehabilitation.* 3rd ed. Champaign (IL): Human Kinetics; 1995, p.327–342.
19. Foss-Campbell B, Sheldahl L, Wilke N, et al. Effects of upper extremity load distribution on weight-carrying in men with ischemic heart disease. *J Cardiopulm Rehabil.* 1993;13:37–42.
20. Franklin BA, Hogan P, Bonzheim K, et al. Cardiac demands of heavy snow shoveling. *JAMA.* 1995;273:880–882.
21. **Transport Canada. Guidelines for the assessment of cardiovascular fitness in licenced aviation personnel 2003. Updated June 2, 2006. Available from: www.tc.gc.ca/CivilAviation/Cam/TP13312-2/cardiovascular/menu.htm. Accessed May 31, 2007.**
22. Gutmann MC, Sheldahl LM, Tristani FE, Wilke NA. Returning the patient to work. In: Pollock M, Schmidt D, editors. *Heart Disease and Rehabilitation.* 3rd ed. Champaign (IL): Human Kinetics; 1994. p. 405–422.
23. Haskell WL, Bradfeld N, Bruce RA, et al. Task Force II: Determination of occupational working capacity in patients with ischemic heart disease. *J Am Coll Cardiol.* 1989;14:1025–1034.
24. Health Canada. *Economic Burden of Illness in Canada, 1998.* Catalogue #H21-136/1998 E. Ottawa: Public Works and Government Services Canada; 2002. p. 6–7.
25. Johnson RL Jr. Relative effects of air pollution on lungs and heart. *Circulation.* 2004;109:5–7.
26. King K, Collins-Nakai R. Short term recovery from cardiac surgery in women: suggestions for practice. *Can J Cardiol.* 1998;14:1367–1371.
27. Kovoor P, Lee AK, Carrozzi F et al. Return to full normal activities including work at two weeks after acute myocardial infarction. *Am J Cardiol.* 2006;97(7):952–958.
28. Kushnir T, Luria O. Supervisors' attitudes toward return to work after myocardial infarction or coronary artery bypass graft. *J Occup Environ Med.* 2002;44:331–337.

29. Lakka TA, Venalainen JM, Raurama R, et al. Relation of leisure-time physical activity and cardiorespiratory fitness to the risk of acute myocardial infarction in men. *N Engl J Med.* 1994;330:1549–1554.

30. Leopold RS. *A Year in the Life of a Million American Workers.* New York: Metlife Group Disability; 2003.

31. Lewin R. Return to work after MI, the roles of depression, health beliefs and rehabilitation. *Int J Cardiol.* 1999;72:49–51.

32. Massachusetts Public Employee Retirement Administration Commission. Updated September 2001. Available from: www.mass.gov/perac/forms/01PhysicianStatement.pdf. Accessed June 1, 2007.

33. McGee HM, Doyle F, Conan RM, et al. Impact of briefly-assessed depression on secondary prevention outcomes after acute coronary syndrome: a one year longitudinal survey. *BMC Health Serv Res.* 2006 Feb 13;6:9.

34. Mital A, Shrey DE, Govindaraju M, et al. Accelerating the return to work (RTW) chances of coronary heart disease (CHD) patients: Part 1—development and validation of a training program. *Disabil Rehabil.* 2000;22:604–620.

35. Mittleman MA, Maclure M, Tofler GH, et al. Triggering of acute myocardial infarction by heavy physical exertion: protection against triggering by regular exertion. *N Engl J Med.* 1993;329:1677–1683.

36. National Occupational Classification. Updated February 20, 2007. Available from: www23.hrdc-drhc.gc.ca./2001/e/generic/welcome.shtml. Accessed May 30, 2007.

37. Pandolf KB, Young AJ. Altitude and cold. In: Pollock MLL, Schmidt DH, editors. *Heart Disease and Rehabilitation.* 3rd ed. Champaign (IL): Human Kinetics; 1995. p. 309–326.

38. Passmore R, Durnin JVGA. Human energy expenditure. *Physiol Rev.* 1955;35:801–840.

39. Pope III CA, Burnett RT, Thurston GD, et al. Cardiovascular mortality and long-term exposure to particulate air pollution: epidemiological evidence of general pathophysiological pathways of disease. *Circulation.* 2004;109:71–77.

40. Sagall EL, Nash IS. Cardiac evaluations for legal purposes. In: Fuster V, Alexander RW, O'Rourke RA, et al., editors. *Hurst's The Heart.* 10th ed. New York: McGraw-Hill; 2001. p. 2519–2532.

41. Sheldahl LM, Levandoski SG, Wilke NA, et al. Responses of patients with coronary artery disease to common carpentry tasks. *J Cardiopulm Rehabil.* 1993;13:283–290.

42. Sheldahl LM, Wilke NA, Dougherty SM, et al. Work capacity of men on disability for heart disease [abstract]. *Circulation.* 1992;86(suppl I):400.

43. Sheldahl LM, Wilke NA, Dougherty SM, et al. Effect of age and coronary artery disease on response to snow shoveling. *J Am Coll Cardiol.* 1992; 20:1111–1117.

44. Sheldahl LM, Wilke NA, Dougherty SM, Tristani FE. Energy cost of occupational work [abstract]. *J Am Coll Cardiol.* 1995;25:173A.

45. Sheldahl LM, Wilke NA, Dougherty S, Tristani FE. Snow blowing and shoveling in normal and asymptomatic coronary artery diseased men. *Int J Cardiol.* 1994;43:233–238.

46. Sheldahl LM, Wilke NA, Dougherty S, Tristani FE. Cardiac response to combined moderate heat and exercise in men with coronary artery disease. *Am J Cardiol.* 1992;70:186–191.

47. Sheldahl LM, Wilke NA, Dougherty SM, Tristani FE. Responses of women to snow shoveling and snow blowing [abstract]. *Circulation.* 1993;88:I-612.

48. Sheldahl LM, Wilke NA, Hanna RD, et al. Responses of people with coronary artery disease to common lawn-care tasks. *Eur J Appl Physiol.* 1996;72:357–364.

49. Sheldahl LM, Wilke NA, Tristani FE. Evaluation and training for resumption of occupational and leisure-time physical activities in patients after a major cardiac event. *Med Exerc Nutr Health.* 1995;4:273–289.

50. Sheldahl LM, Wilke NA, Tristani FE, Kalbfleisch JH. Response of patients after myocardial infarction to carrying a graded series of weight loads. *Am J Cardiol.* 1983;52:698–703.

51. Sheldahl LM, Wilke NA, Tristani FE, Kalbfleisch JH. Response to repetitive static-dynamic exercise in patients with coronary artery disease. *J Cardiac Rehabil.* 1985;5:139–145.

52. **Smith, SC, Allen J, Blair SN, et al. American Heart Association/American College of Cardiology. AHA/ACC Guidelines for secondary prevention for patients with coronary and other atherosclerotic vascular disease: 2006 update. *Circulation.* 2006;113(19): 2363–2372.**

53. Smith TW. Driving after ventricular arrhythmias [editorial]. *N Engl J Med.* 2001;345:451–452.

54. Soderman E, Lisspers J, Sundin O. Depression as a predictor of return to work in patients with coronary artery disease. *Soc Sci Med* (England). 2003;56:193–202.

55. Thompson D, Franklin BA, Balady GJ, et al. Exercise and acute cardiovascular events placing the risks into perspective. *Circulation.* 2007;115(17):2358–2368.

56. **U.S. Department of Labor, Bureau of Labor Statistics. *Occupational Outlook Handbook, 2006–07 Edition.* Available from: www.bls.gov/oco/home.htm. Accessed May 30, 2007.**

57. **U.S. Department of Labor. *Dictionary of Occupational Titles.* 4th ed, revised. Indianapolis (IN): JIST Works Inc; 1991.**

58. **U.S. Department of Labor, Office of Disability Employment Policy. Available from: www.dol.gov/odep/faqs/odep.htm. Accessed May 30, 2007.**

59. **U.S. Department of Labor. Workers' Compensation. Available from: www.dol.gov/dol/topic/workcomp/index.htm. Accessed May 25, 2007.**

60. **U.S. Social Security Administration. Updated June 1, 2007. Available from: www.ssa.gov. Accessed June 1, 2007.**

61. Vona M, Capodaglio P, Iannessa A, et al. The role of work simulation tests in a comprehensive cardiac rehabilitation program. *Monaldi Arch Chest Dis.* 2002;58:26–34.

62. Wilke NA, Sheldahl LM, Dougherty SM, et al. Baltimore Therapeutic Equipment work simulator: energy expenditure of work activities in cardiac patients. *Arch Phys Med.* 1993;74:419–424.

63. Wilke NA, Sheldahl LM, Dougherty SM, et al. Energy expenditure during household tasks in women with coronary artery disease. *Am J Cardiol.* 1995;75:670–674.

64. Wilke NA, Sheldahl LM, Dougherty SM, et al. Metabolic cost of wood splitting in men with and without ischemic heart disease [abstract]. *J Cardiopulm Rehabil.* 1990;10:382.

65. Willich SN, Lewis M, Lowel H, et al. Physical exertion as a trigger of acute myocardial infarction. *N Engl J Med.* 1993;329:1684–1690.

66. WSIB Ontario and CPAAT (Workplace Safety and Insurance Board and La Commission de la sécurité professionnelle et de l'assurance contre les accidents du travail). Available from: www.wsib.on.ca/wsib/wsibsite.nsf/public/home_e. Accessed May 30, 2007.

67. Wyman DO. Evaluating patients for return to work. *Am Fam Physician.* 1999;59:844–848.

68. Wyss CA, Koepfli P, Fretz G, et al. Influence of altitude exposure on coronary flow reserve. *Circulation.* 2003;108:1202–1207.

SELECTED REFERENCES FOR FURTHER READING

Leopold RS. *A Year in the Life of a Million American Workers.* New York: Metlife Group Disability; 2003.

Ranavaya MI, LeFevre P, Denniston PL Jr. Evidence-based disability duration guidelines. *J Disabil Med.* 2002;2:75–78.

Sagall EL, Nash IS. Cardiac evaluations for legal purposes. In: Fuster V, Alexander RW, O'Rourke RA, et al., editors. *Hurst's The Heart.* 10th ed, New York: McGraw-Hill; 2001. p. 2519–2532.

Sheldahl LM, Wilke NA, Tristani FE. Evaluation and training for resumption of occupational and leisure-time physical activities in patients after a major cardiac event. *Med Exerc Nutr Health.* 1995;4:273–289.

Wyman DO. Evaluating patients for return to work. *Am Fam Physician.* 1999;59:844–848.

INTERNET RESOURCES

- Disability Duration Guidelines: www.rgl.net/pdfs/Disability DurationGuidelinesBrochure.pdf
- Social Security Online: Employment Support for People with Disabilities: www.ssa.gov/work
- Social Security Online: Medical/Professional Relations: www.socialsecurity.gov/disability/professionals/bluebook
- Social Security Online: 2008 Red Book: www.ssa.gov/work/ ResourcesToolkit/redbook.html
- U.S. Department of Labor: Occupational Outlook Handbook, 2008–09 Edition: www.bls.gov/oco
- U.S. Department of Labor, Office of Disability Employment Policy: www.dol.gov/odep

CHAPTER 26

Exercise Assessment in Special Populations

General principles of exercise testing apply to all individuals, but in some special populations, additional factors may need to be considered. The focus of this chapter will be to provide additional information on how the general principles of exercise testing, as described previously in Chapter 21, may be applied. Specifically, this chapter will include considerations in exercise testing for pregnant women, the elderly, and children.

PREGNANCY

The safety of physical activity during pregnancy is a significant question for clinicians and researchers. In addition to maternal safety, fetal responses to strenuous maternal exercise are of concern. Fetal heart rates have been examined with no changes suggestive of fetal distress or changes in behavior (51). Investigations regarding compromise of uterine blood flow if blood flow is redistributed to working skeletal muscle have not been conclusive (63), although uterine contractions have been found to increase in frequency during exercise, with rapid recovery after exercise (51). In general, it appears the physiologic reserve of mother and fetus allow for short periods of exercise to be tolerated (63).

The American College of Obstetricians and Gynecologists (ACOG) suggests that pregnant women without medical or obstetric complications can follow the American College of Sports Medicine (ACSM) and Surgeon General's recommendation to accumulate 30 or more minutes of moderate exercise on most, if not all, days of the week (1). The benefits of physical activity during pregnancy related to chronic disease risk have been outlined in a roundtable consensus statement (41)

and recent literature review (61) and include benefits related to preeclampsia (risk may be reduced with physical activity), gestational diabetes (research is still needed to determine the optimal exercise program), and mental health. For more detailed information on these issues, as well as the relationship of physical activity to postpartum musculoskeletal conditions, breastfeeding, postpartum weight loss, and offspring health, please refer to the published statements (41,61).

As outlined in the ACSM *Guidelines for Exercise Testing and Prescription* (2), many physiologic changes occur during pregnancy that may alter the responses to exercise (Table 26-1). Guidelines set forth by ACOG (1) as well as the Joint Committee of the Society of Obstetricians and Gynecologists of Canada and the Canadian Society for Exercise Physiology (12) are endorsed by ACSM and will serve as the foundation for the recommendations in this section.

PRETESTING SCREENING

> **2.2.1-HFS: Knowledge of cardiovascular risk factors or conditions that may require consultation with medical personnel before testing or training, including inappropriate changes of resting or exercise heart rate and blood pressure, new onset discomfort in chest, neck, shoulder, or arm, changes in the pattern of discomfort during rest or exercise, fainting or dizzy spells, and claudication.**

Before beginning an exercise program, overall health and obstetric and medical risks should be reviewed (5). The Physical Activity Readiness Questionnaire (PAR-Q) is a frequently used instrument to determine an individual's

TABLE 26-1. PHYSIOLOGIC RESPONSES TO ACUTE EXERCISE DURING PREGNANCY COMPARED WITH PREPREGNANCY

OXYGEN UPTAKE (DURING WEIGHT DEPENDENT EXERCISE)	INCREASE V̇O$_2$
Heart rate	Increase
Stroke volume	Increase
Cardiac output	Increase
Tidal volume	Increase
Minute ventilation (V̇E)	Increase
Ventilatory equivalent for oxygen V̇E/V̇O$_2$	Increase
Ventilatory equivalent for carbon dioxide V̇E/V̇CO$_2$	Increase
Systolic blood pressure (SBP)	No change/decrease
Diastolic blood pressure (DBP)	No change/decrease

Adapted from Wolfe LA. Differences between children and adults for exercise testing and prescription. In: Skinner JS, editor. *Exercise Testing and Exercise Prescription for Special Cases.* 2nd ed. Philadelphia (PA): Lippincott Williams & Wilkins; 2005. p.377–91.

readiness to start an exercise program. The Canadian Society for Exercise Physiology has taken a step beyond the PAR-Q for pregnant women with their development of the Physical Activity Readiness Medical Examination, termed the PARmed-X for Pregnancy (7). This instrument includes a pre-exercise health checklist as well as contraindications for exercise. As stated within the instrument: "The safety of prenatal exercise programs depends on an adequate level of maternal-fetal physiological reserve. PARmed-X for Pregnancy is a convenient checklist and prescription for use by healthcare providers to evaluate pregnant patients who want to enter a prenatal fitness program and for on-going medical surveillance of exercising pregnant patients" (see PARmed-X for Pregnancy in Fig. 26-1).

EXERCISE TESTING

> **1.3.5-CES: Select an appropriate test protocol according to the age, functional capacity, physical ability, and health status of the individual.**

> **1.10.11-HFS: Knowledge of potential musculoskeletal injuries (e.g., contusions, sprains, strains, fractures), cardiovascular/pulmonary complications (e.g., tachycardia, bradycardia, hypotension/hypertension, tachypnea) and metabolic abnormalities (e.g., fainting/syncope, hypoglycemia/hyperglycemia, hypothermia/hyperthermia).**

In general, physician clearance is recommended for women who have been sedentary before pregnancy or who have a medical condition. In any exercise situation, which would include exercise testing, ACOG highlights warning signs to terminate exercise (Box 26-1).

> **1.3.23-HFS: Ability to identify individuals for whom physician supervision is recommended during maximal and submaximal exercise testing.**

Typically maximal exercise testing is not recommended for pregnant women. If a maximal exercise test is warranted because of a medical situation, the test should only be per-

formed with physician supervision. Maximal responses for weight-supported activity (cycle ergometer) have been found to be similar between a matched group of pregnant and nonpregnant women, although carbohydrate use appeared to be blunted at maximal exercise levels (21). The lower respiratory exchange ratio observed in pregnant women may be a protective mechanism with regard to glucose sparing for the fetus or to resist changes in pH (21). Fetal responses to maximal exercise are an ongoing area of research interest. Brief maximal exertion, as done during a maximal exercise test, has been suggested to be safe in active women with uncomplicated pregnancies (62). Pregnant women who exercised on a cycle ergometer had minor electrocardiographic changes (e.g., T-wave inversion in V2, shorter onset to maximal ST depression) at rest and during exercise compared with a control group of nonpregnant women, although the changes were considered normal unless symptoms were reported (35).

When a metabolic cart is not available, it is possible to predict V̇O$_{2peak}$. Recently, the following equation was developed using a modified Balke protocol (to volitional fatigue) to predict V̇O$_{2peak}$ for those without access to a metabolic cart [NOTE: Peak heart rate (HR) is in bpm, incline is in percent, speed is in mph, body mass index (BMI) (kg · m^{-1})] (41):

$$\dot{V}O_{2peak} \text{ (predicted)} = (0.055 \times \text{peak HR}) + (0.381 \times \text{incline}) + (5.541 \times \text{speed}) + (-0.090 \times \text{BMI}) - 6.846$$

> **1.3.22-CES: Describe the differences in the physiologic responses to various modes of ergometry (e.g., treadmill, cycle and arm ergometers) as they relate to exercise testing and training.**

> **1.7.8-CES: Demonstrate exercise equipment adaptations necessary for different age groups, physical abilities, and other potential contributing factors.**

In place of a maximal test, typically a submaximal exercise test [i.e., <75% heart rate reserve (HRR)] is used to predict maximum oxygen uptake (V̇O$_{2max}$). Most research studies have selected cycle ergometry for testing. Given the changes in posture and center of gravity during pregnancy, cycle ergometry would appear to provide a safe and secure exercise mode. Information on submaximal testing is found in the GETP8 and, although not specific for pregnant women, provides guidance on testing procedures.

SUMMARY

Benefits of physical activity during pregnancy have been well documented. Exercise, even brief maximal exercise, appears safe for women with uncomplicated pregnancy. Maximal exercise testing during pregnancy is not routinely recommended unless a medical condition warrants. In such situations, a physician should be present. More commonly, submaximal testing is conducted. Contraindications to

PARmed-X for PREGNANCY
PHYSICAL ACTIVITY READINESS MEDICAL EXAMINATION

PARmed-X for PREGNANCY is a guideline for health screening prior to participation in a prenatal fitness class or other exercise.

Healthy women with uncomplicated pregnancies can integrate physical activity into their daily living and can participate without significant risks either to themselves or to their unborn child. Postulated benefits of such programs include improved aerobic and muscular fitness, promotion of appropriate weight gain, and facilitation of labour. Regular exercise may also help to prevent gestational glucose intolerance and pregnancy-induced hypertension.

The safety of prenatal exercise programs depends on an adequate level of maternal-fetal physiological reserve. PARmed-X for PREGNANCY is a convenient checklist and prescription for use by health care providers to evaluate pregnant patients who want to enter a prenatal fitness program and for ongoing medical surveillance of exercising pregnant patients.

Instructions for use of the 4-page PARmed-X for PREGNANCY are the following:

1. The patient should fill out the section on PATIENT INFORMATION and the PRE-EXERCISE HEALTH CHECKLIST (PART 1, 2, 3, and 4 on p. 1) and give the form to the health care provider monitoring her pregnancy.

2. The health care provider should check the information provided by the patient for accuracy and fill out SECTION C on CONTRAINDICATIONS (p. 2) based on current medical information.

3. If no exercise contraindications exist, the HEALTH EVALUATION FORM (p. 3) should be completed, signed by the health care provider, and given by the patient to her prenatal fitness professional.

In addition to prudent medical care, participation in appropriate types, intensities and amounts of exercise is recommended to increase the likelihood of a beneficial pregnancy outcome. PARmed-X for PREGNANCY provides recommendations for individualized exercise prescription (p. 3) and program safety (p. 4).

NOTE: Sections A and B should be completed by the patient before the appointment with the health care provider.

A PATIENT INFORMATION

NAME _____

ADDRESS _____

TELEPHONE_____ BIRTHDATE _____ HEALTH INSURANCE No. _____

NAME OF
PRENATAL FITNESS PROFESSIONAL _____

PRENATAL FITNESS
PROFESSIONAL?S PHONE NUMBER _____

B PRE-EXERCISE HEALTH CHECKLIST

PART 1: GENERAL HEALTH STATUS

In the past, have you experienced (check YES or NO):

		YES	NO
1.	Miscarriage in an earlier pregnancy?	❏	❏
2.	Other pregnancy complications?	❏	❏
3.	I have completed a PAR-Q within the last 30 days.	❏	❏

If you answered YES to question 1 or 2, please explain:

_____

Number of previous pregnancies? _____

PART 2: STATUS OF CURRENT PREGNANCY

Due Date: _____

During this pregnancy, have you experienced:

		YES	NO
1.	Marked fatigue?	❏	❏
2.	Bleeding from the vagina ("spotting")?	❏	❏
3.	Unexplained faintness or dizziness?	❏	❏
4.	Unexplained abdominal pain?	❏	❏
5.	Sudden swelling of ankles, hands or face?	❏	❏
6.	Persistent headaches or problems with headaches?	❏	❏
7.	Swelling, pain or redness in the calf of one leg?	❏	❏
8.	Absence of fetal movement after 6th month?	❏	❏
9.	Failure to gain weight after 5th month?	❏	❏

If you answered YES to any of the above questions, please explain:

_____

PART 3: ACTIVITY HABITS DURING THE PAST MONTH

1. List only regular fitness/recreational activities:

_____

_____

INTENSITY	FREQUENCY (times/week)			TIME (minutes/day)		
	1-2	2-4	4+	<20	20-40	40+
Heavy	___	___	___	___	___	___
Medium	___	___	___	___	___	___
Light	___	___	___	___	___	___

2. Does your regular occupation (job/home) activity involve:

	YES	NO
Heavy Lifting?	❏	❏
Frequent walking/stair climbing?	❏	❏
Occasional walking (>once/hr)?	❏	❏
Prolonged standing?	❏	❏
Mainly sitting?	❏	❏
Normal daily activity?	❏	❏

3.	Do you currently smoke tobacco?*	❏	❏
4.	Do you consume alcohol?*	❏	❏

PART 4: PHYSICAL ACTIVITY INTENTIONS

What physical activity do you intend to do?

_____

Is this a change from what you currently do?   ❏ YES   ❏ NO

*NOTE: PREGNANT WOMEN ARE STRONGLY ADVISED NOT TO SMOKE OR CONSUME ALCOHOL DURING PREGNANCY AND DURING LACTATION.

C CONTRAINDICATIONS TO EXERCISE: to be completed by your health care provider

Absolute Contraindications			Relative Contraindications		
Does the patient have:	YES	NO	*Does the patient have:*	YES	NO
1. Ruptured membranes, premature labour?	❏	❏	1. History of spontaneous abortion or premature labour in previous pregnancies?	❏	❏
2. Persistent second or third trimester bleeding/placenta previa?	❏	❏	2. Mild/moderate cardiovascular or respiratory disease (e.g., chronic hypertension, asthma)?	❏	❏
3. Pregnancy-induced hypertension or pre-eclampsia?	❏	❏	3. Anemia or iron deficiency? (Hb < 100 g/L)?	❏	❏
4. Incompetent cervix?	❏	❏	4. Malnutrition or eating disorder (anorexia, bulimia)?	❏	❏
5. Evidence of intrauterine growth restriction?	❏	❏	5. Twin pregnancy after 28th week?	❏	❏
6. High-order pregnancy (e.g., triplets)?	❏	❏	6. Other significant medical condition?	❏	❏
7. Uncontrolled Type I diabetes, hypertension or thyroid disease, other serious cardiovascular, respiratory or systemic disorder?	❏	❏	Please specify: _____		

NOTE: Risk may exceed benefits of regular physical activity. The decision to be physically active or not should be made with qualified medical advice.

PHYSICAL ACTIVITY RECOMMENDATION: ❏ Recommended/Approved   ❏ Contraindicated

CSEP SCPE   © Canadian Society for Exercise Physiology
Société canadienne de physiologie de l'exercice

Supported by: 🍁 Health   Santé
Canada   Canada

FIGURE 26-1. PARmed-X for Pregnancy. Source: Physical Activity Readiness Medical Examination for Pregnancy (PARmed-X for Pregnancy), © 2002. Reprinted with permission of the Canadian Society for Exercise Physiology, www.csep.ca.

BOX 26-1	EXERCISE AND PREGNANCY: MEDICAL AND SAFETY CONCERNS FOR THE MOTHER AND FETUS		

MOTHER		**FETUS**	
Concern	**Solution**	**Concern**	**Solution or Effect**
Poor balance while running or jogging because of shifts in weight distribution and center of gravity.	Slow down, run cautiously and never alone.	Direct fetal trauma. Tissue and fluid surrounding fetus provides protection.	No scientific data.
Overheating and dehydration. Pregnancy elevates body core temperature by approximately 0.5°C, elevating resting metabolic rate by 15%–20%. Excessive sweating might reduce blood volume.	Drink plenty of fluids before, during, and after exercise. Use appropriate exercise clothing and/or avoid exercise during extremely hot and humid weather.	Hyperthermia and reduced fetal blood flow.	Might cause neural tube defects, growth retardation, reduced birth weight, and/or fetal abnormalities.
Leg, hip, and abdominal pain. Reduced circulation to lower extremities during late pregnancy, extra weight to carry.	Never forget to stretch and warm up before any exercise session. Wear cushioned and comfortable shoes.	Reduced fetal blood flow.	No scientific data.
Nutrient availability. Pregnancy increases energy requirements by approximately 300 kcal/day.	It is expected for pregnant women to gain 25–40 lbs.	Substrate availability and hypoxia: reduced fetal glucose and oxygen availability.	Might cause growth retardation, reduced birth weight, and/or fetal abnormalities.
Reduced oxygen availability for aerobic exercise. Cardiovascular drift: added blood circulation to placenta.	Modify exercise intensity. Never exercise to the point of fatigue or exhaustion. Avoid intense and prolonged exercise. Monitor heart rate and rates of perceived exertion.	Reduced fetal blood flow. Intense exercise causes a redistribution of blood flow. More to muscles, less to other areas, including the placenta.	Light to moderate physical activities are considered safe for mother and fetus.
Musculoskeletal injury. Ballistic movements, sudden postural changes can increase the risk of injury. However, the risk of injury for fit pregnant women should be lower.	Continuous/aerobic exercises are more acceptable than intermittent/anaerobic exercises.	Umbilical cord entanglement. Can cause reduced blood flow to important fetal organs.	No scientific data.

Note: A physician with background in exercise physiology should be consulted before any exercise program is considered during pregnancy. Ask about contraindications to exercise and a list of "high risk" sports to avoid during pregnancy.
From: American College of Obstetricians and Gynecologists. Exercise during pregnancy and the postpartum period. ACOG Committee Opinion No. 267. *Obstet Gynecol*. 2002;99:171–173.

exercise as well as warning signs to terminate exercise should be considered to ensure safety of mother and fetus (1).

ELDERLY

The term *older adult* includes individuals ≥65 years of age and those between 50 and 64 years of age with clinically significant chronic conditions or physical limitations that affect movement, physical fitness, or physical activity (2). Because of many factors, differences between chronologic age and physiologic age exist. As a result, exercise testing for this group must be individualized.

In the 2000 U.S. Census, almost 35 million people were older than age 65 (12.4% of the population) (55). In the coming years, as baby boomers age, the number of indi-

viduals in this group will increase. Understanding the age-associated changes in cardiovascular response to exercise allows clinicians and researchers to fully understand and appreciate stress test results (13). Between the ages of 20 and 80, reductions have been observed in the following parameters: oxygen consumption (50%), arteriovenous oxygen difference (25%), cardiac output (25%), heart rate (25%), stroke volume (0%–15%), and ejection fraction (15%) (31). Other changes include increases in end-diastolic volume (30%) and end-systolic volume (150%) (13).

CLINICAL EVALUATION

> **1.3.23-HFS: Ability to identify individuals for whom physician supervision is recommended during maximal and submaximal exercise testing.**

2.2.1-HFS: Knowledge of cardiovascular risk factors or conditions that may require consultation with medical personnel before testing or training, including inappropriate changes of resting or exercise heart rate and blood pressure; new onset discomfort in chest, neck, shoulder, or arm; changes in the pattern of discomfort during rest or exercise; fainting or dizzy spells; and claudication.

Age is considered a positive risk factor for atherosclerotic cardiovascular disease (2), specifically ≥45 years of age for men and ≥55 years of age for women. It is recommended that these individuals undergo a medical examination and a medically supervised exercise test before engaging in vigorous activity [>60% $\dot{V}O_{2max}$ or >6 metabolic equivalents (METs)], especially if other risk factors are present. For moderate activity (40%–60% $\dot{V}O_{2max}$ or 3–6 METs), a medical examination and medically supervised exercise test are not considered essential, although either would not be considered inappropriate (2).

PRACTICAL CONSIDERATIONS OF ROUTINE EXERCISE TESTING

1.3.2-CES: Knowledge of exercise testing procedures for various clinical populations, including those individuals with cardiovascular, pulmonary, and metabolic diseases in terms of exercise modality, protocol, physiologic measurements, and expected outcomes.

The use of exercise testing has value for both diagnosis and prognosis in the elderly (29). The sensitivity and specificity of exercise testing in asymptomatic individuals has been reviewed (14). The pretest probability of coronary artery disease (CAD) has been reported for men and women in the 60 to 69 age range and indicates a high probability (>90%) for those with typical/definite angina pectoris, intermediate pretest probability (10%–90%) for those with atypical/probable angina pectoris as well as nonanginal chest pain, and low probability (<10%) for those who are asymptomatic (14). No data are available for individuals beyond 69 years of age, although the assumption is that CAD risk increases with age (14).

EXERCISE TESTING CONSIDERATIONS

1.5.11-CES: Address exercise testing and training needs of elderly and young patients.

1.7.18-CES: Determine appropriate testing and training modalities according to the age, functional capacity, physical ability, and health status of the individual.

Understanding potential compromise of functional capacity in the elderly is important when selecting an appropriate stress test (i.e., exercise or pharmacologic) (14,58). Many test protocols result in fatigue within the first or second stage before maximal effort is achieved (58). Use of tests with shorter intervals and increased treadmill grade may be a viable alternative for those who cannot walk briskly (58). If steady state is desired during each stage, longer intervals may be warranted (49).

1.7.8-CES: Demonstrate exercise equipment adaptations necessary for different age groups, physical abilities, and other potential contributing factors.

Test modality appears to be an important factor to consider with regard to prognostic markers, as suggested by a recent study of patients with known or suspected CAD (42). Patients in this study had a higher peak heart rate but slower drop in heart rate in recovery with a treadmill exercise test compared with a bicycle test. Duke treadmill scores were significantly higher on the treadmill than bicycle because of the higher sensitivity in determining ST-segment deviations that result from exercise (42). [Note: The Duke treadmill score is determined by the following calculation: exercise time − (5 × ST deviation) − (4 × angina index). Time is in minutes, ST deviation is in mm, and angina index is coded 0–2 (33)]. Bicycle ergometry could result in a low-risk classification when a treadmill test may result in a higher-risk classification. Thus, it is not recommended to use chronotropic index or Duke treadmill scores for risk classification with bicycle exercise tests (42).

Selection of exercise mode must be made considering the benefits and potential shortcoming of each. Although bicycle exercise may be preferred to accommodate for gait or coordination concerns (58), many elderly are not familiar with cycle ergometry; because mainly leg muscles are used, systolic blood pressure tends to be higher (42), and localized leg fatigue may be an impediment to achieving maximal effort (32). Cycle ergometry does, however, allow for better stability, and thus electrocardiogram (ECG) tracings may be of better quality (32), although most current systems produce high-quality tracings regardless of modality (49). When a treadmill is used, the stress placed on the cardiovascular system will be greater because of the use of a larger muscle mass (58). Arm ergometry is typically used for those with severe orthopedic, neurologic, or peripheral vascular disease (58).

Several factors can influence exercise testing in the elderly and may warrant a modification of the test to produce an optimal evaluation. Table 26-2 outlines some common characteristics of the elderly, along with suggested test adaptations (37,49).

PROGNOSTIC ASSESSMENT WITH EXERCISE TESTING

Exercise ECG and exercise echocardiogram have been found to be superior to resting tests for predicting cardiac death and cardiac events (4,10). Of particular interest is the value of workload achieved in predicting both cardiac events and cardiac death (10,44). The Duke treadmill score has been found to be an independent predictor of

TABLE 26-2. EXERCISE TESTING FOR THE ELDERLY

 1.5.11-CES: Address exercise testing and training needs of elderly and young patients.

 1.3.22-HFS: Ability to modify protocols and procedures for cardiorespiratory fitness tests in children, adolescents, and older adults.

CHARACTERISTIC	SUGGESTED TEST MODIFICATION
Low $\dot{V}O_{2max}$	Start at a low intensity (2–3 METs)
More time required to reach a steady state	Long warm-up (3+ min); small rise in power output (0.5–1 MET) and/or 2–3 min at each stage
Increased fatigability	Reduce total test time to 12–15 min or use an intermittent protocol
Increased need to monitor ECG, BP, and HR	Bike > treadmill > step test
Poor balance	Bike > treadmill > step test; use treadmill built into the floor
Poor strength (especially upper thighs)	Treadmill > bike or step test
Less ambulatory ability	Increase treadmill grade rather than speed (maximum of 3–3.5 mph)
Poor neuromuscular coordination	Increase amount of practice; may require more than one test
Difficulty holding mouthpiece with dentures	Add support or use face mask to measure $\dot{V}O_2$
Impaired vision	Bike > treadmill or step test
Impaired hearing	Treadmill > bike or step test, if person needs to follow a cadence; difficulty understanding and responding in a noisy environment (use electronic bike)
Senile gait patterns and foot problems (e.g., bunions and calluses)	Bike > treadmill or step test

ECG, electrocardiogram; BP, blood pressure; HR, heart rate.

From Tanner CS, Heise CT, Barber G. Correlation of the physiologic parameters of a continuous ramp verus an incremental James exercise protocol in normal children. *Am J Cardiol.* 1991;67:309–312.

cardiac mortality and mortality in a group of asymptomatic women because of the exercise capacity component of the score (18). The prognostic value of workload achieved on a treadmill exercise test was found to be similar between individuals <65 years of age compared with those ≥65 years of age (17,50).

For those with intermediate Duke treadmill scores, the use of exercise echocardiogram may be helpful in predicting mortality (34). Similarly, exercise echocardiography was found to be helpful in stratifying those with intermediate, as well as low, Duke treadmill scores into risk categories, although the cost-effectiveness of the low-score subgroup is questionable because of low absolute risk (40). The use of multiple tests [Duke treadmill score, first-pass radionuclide angiography with ejection fraction calculation, and perfusion single-photon emission computed tomography (SPECT)] resulted in optimal risk stratification, as each was a significant predictor of cardiovascular events in a group of high-risk patients with a median age of 60 years (30). Dobutamine stress ^{99m}Tc-tetrofosmin SPECT provided incremental prognostic information for prediction of all-cause mortality and cardiac events in a group of elderly patients ≥65 years of age (48).

In older men (>75 years of age), no exercise test responses were found to be predictive of either all-cause or cardiovascular death (64), nor was the Duke treadmill score (28), although high cycling power was strongly and independently associated with decreased death risk for 75-year-old men and women in a population-based study (24). Other more sophisticated tests, such as the exercise SPECT, may provide additional ability to accurately predict risk level as found in an older (≥75 years of age) population capable of exercise (57).

EXERCISE PROTOCOLS

 1.3.5-CES: Select an appropriate test protocol according to the age, functional capacity, physical ability, and health status of the individual.

 1.3.15-CES: Ability to provide testing procedures and protocol for children and the elderly with or without various clinical conditions.

 1.3.22-HFS: Ability to modify protocols and procedures for cardiorespiratory fitness tests in children, adolescents, and older adults.

Specific protocols for testing are outlined in the ACSM GETP8 (2). Considerations for protocol selection include:

- The purpose of the evaluation
- The specific outcomes desired
- The characteristics of the individual being tested

Realize that additional practice may be needed to allow individuals to feel comfortable with the testing protocol.

 1.3.22-CES: Recognize the emergence of new imaging techniques for the assessment of heart disease [e.g., computed tomography (CT) angiography].

Treadmill testing requires some special considerations because older individuals will often have poor balance and muscular strength. Allowing individuals to hold the treadmill handrail may allow them to feel more comfortable but can also alter the energy cost of the activity. If $\dot{V}O_2$ is being measured, rather than predicted from work capacity or heart rate, this may not be an issue. Conversely, if prediction of maximal work capacity or $\dot{V}O_2$ is made from heart rate responses during such testing, error will be introduced (49).

Although the Bruce treadmill test remains one of the most commonly used protocols, it may not be appropriate for all elderly patients because of its longer stages (3 minutes) and relatively large and unequal workload increases with each stage (2–3 METs). Older individuals may benefit from protocols such as the Naughton or Balke-Ware, in which workload increments between stages are smaller (≤ 1 MET). Consider protocols in which the grade increases rather than speed. The initial workload should be low (i.e., ≤ 3 METs). Increases in treadmill grade of 1% to 3% per minute with constant belt speeds of 1.5 to 2.5 mph (2.4 to 4.0 kph) have been recommended for older populations (2). Ramp protocols are another option in which work rate increases in a series of small but constant increments. Ramp protocols are most common for cycle ergometry testing, but many treadmills now also have this capacity.

Cycle ergometry may be prefered over a treadmill for those with poor balance, poor neuromuscular coordination, impaired vision, impaired gait patterns, weight-bearing limitations, and/or foot problems (49). However, a lack of familiarity with cycling activity may be a limitation in this population (14). Increments of 10 to 15 watts ($1\ W = 6.12\ kg \cdot m \cdot min^{-1}$) per minute can be used on the cycle ergometer for elderly persons (2).

Although fatigue may become an issue when conducting exercise testing with the elderly, no unique test termination criteria for older individuals have been published. Recommended termination criteria established for adults should be used (see GETP8, Chapter 5) (2).

Special Considerations for Those Older Than 75 Years

In those older than 75 years, potential chronic medical conditions, increased physical limitations, and higher prevalence of asymptomatic CAD may necesitate a different approach (15). Exercise testing in this age group will often require pharmocologic stress testing with radionuclide imaging to detect myocardial ischemia in asymptomactic patients because of the inability of most to achieve maximal effort on an exercise test (15). In a community-based study including individuals >75 years with no known cardiovascular disease or other medical contraindication, only 12.2% were able to achieve a maximal effort on a treadmill test (defined as a respiratory exchange ratio of >1.10 and at least 2 minutes on the Cornell treadmill protocol) in the 75- to 79-year-old group. The ability to attain maximal effort continued to decrease with advancing age (7.1% in the 80–84-year-old age group and 1.7% in the >85-year-old age group) (22).

In addition, individuals in the 75+ age range are unlikely to engage in vigorous exercise (one indication for an exercise test). Promoting physical activity should be encouraged, and the benefits of physical activity should not be lost because of the expense or fear of exercise testing. Thus, a complete medical history and physical examination may be sufficient to identify potential cardiac issues related to exercise (15).

Those with cardiovascular disease or overt symptoms should be treated according to published guidelines (see GETP8, Chapter 2) prior to beginning in exercise program, (2), whereas those without symptoms or disease should be able to initiate a low-intensity (≤ 3 METs) exercise program without undue risk. Functional fitness testing examining aspects related to health (including flexiblity, endurance, strength, balance, and body composition) have been highlighted for emphasis in the elderly (49), and specific suggestions are available for those older than age 75 years (8).

MEDICATION USE

Commonly, elderly individuals will be taking medication(s), both over-the-counter (OTC) and prescribed. In the Slone Survey, 91% of men and 94% of women >65 years of age reported using a medication (prescription, OTC, vitamin/mineral, herbal/supplement) in the previous week (26). When only prescription medications were considered, 71% of men and 81% of women reported usage, whereas 19% of men and 23% of women reported taking more than five prescription medications (26). Many medications influence the ECG, blood pressure, or heart rate responses to exercise. Understanding the influence of medications is vital in any testing situation, especially with the elderly.

SUMMARY

Stress testing in the elderly has both a diagnostic and prognostic value. Understanding the potential benefits and limitations of various testing methods will allow for optimal test outcomes and appropriate test interpretation. Physiologic limitations and medication use must also be considered with this population.

CHILDREN

Indications for exercise testing of children have been described and include the following: (a) evaluating cardiac and pulmonary functional capacity, (b) detecting myocardial ischemia, (c) evaluating cardiac rhythm and rate, (d) determining blood pressure response, (e) assessing symptoms with exercise, (f) detecting and managing exercise-induced asthma, (g) assessing physical fitness, (h) charting the course of a progressive disease and evaluating therapy, and (i) assessing the success of rehabilitation programs (46). Although this list could apply to other

TABLE 26-3. HEMODYNAMIC AND RESPIRATORY CHARACTERISTICS OF CHILDREN'S RESPONSES TO EXERCISE

FUNCTION	TYPICAL FOR CHILDREN (COMPARED WITH ADULTS)
HR at submaximal intensity	Higher, especially at first decade
HR max	Higher
Stroke volume (submax and max)	Lower
$\dot{Q}$ at given $\dot{V}O_2$	Somewhat lower
AV difference for O_2 at given $\dot{V}O_2$	Somewhat higher
Blood flow to active muscle	Higher
SBP, DBP submax and max	Lower
$\dot{V}E$ at given $\dot{V}O_2$	Higher
$\dot{V}E$ "breaking point"	Similar
Respiratory rate	Higher
Vt/VC	Lower

HR, heart rate; AV, arteriovenous; SBP, systolic blood pressure; DBP, diastolic blood pressure; $\dot{Q}$, cardiac output; $\dot{V}E$, minute ventilation; $\dot{V}O_2$, oxygen consumption; Vt, tidal volume; VC, vital capacity.

From James FW, Kaplan S, Glueck CJ, Tsay JY, Knight MJ, Sarwar CJ. Responses of normal children and young adults to controlled bicycle exercise. *Circulation*. 1980;61:902–912.

populations, the following section will focus on aspects unique to pediatric exercise testing.

Children present a greater challenge in exercise testing because of their smaller body size (when compared with testing equipment), relatively poor peak performance (in contrast to the work rate increments possible with exercise equipment), potentially shorter attention span, and reduced motivation (19). Hemodynamic and respiratory characteristics of children's responses to exercise are shown in Table 26-3 (20).

EXERCISE TESTING CONSIDERATIONS

 1.3.15-CES: Ability to provide testing procedures and protocol for children and the elderly with or without various clinical conditions.

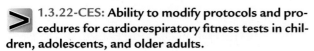 **1.5.11-CES: Address exercise testing and training needs of elderly and young patients.**

1.3.22-CES: Ability to modify protocols and procedures for cardiorespiratory fitness tests in children, adolescents, and older adults.

Whether to allow a parent(s) or guardian(s) into the room during testing should be determined on an individual basis with consideration for the relationship between the adult and child and also the child's temperament (54). If a parent/guardian is allowed into the testing room, the person must not distract the child or interfere with the test (54). Maintaining a space at the back of the testing room for the parent is suggested (38).

The testing procedure must be explained clearly to both the parent/guardian and the child. All questions must be answered completely but in simple terms. The child must understand what is being asked of him/her so he/she can communicate with the tester when he/she is unable to continue. Once both parent/guardian and the

child are comfortable with the testing procedure, the informed consent should be signed by the parent (54), and verbal assent should be obtained from the child if older than 7 or 8 years (38).

1.3.23-HFS: Ability to identify individuals for whom physician supervision is recommended during maximal and submaximal exercise testing.

Primary oversight of the exercise test should be by a physician trained in exercise testing and exercise physiology (38). The presence of the physician for direct supervision of the test depends on the risk to the patient (38). Laboratory personal should include at least two trained individuals, at least one of whom should be trained in pediatric advanced life support (38).

EQUIPMENT USED IN TESTING

1.7.8-CES: Demonstrate exercise equipment adaptations necessary for different age groups, physical abilities, and other potential contributing factors.

1.3.22-HFS: Ability to modify protocols and procedures for cardiorespiratory fitness tests in children, adolescents, and older adults.

2.2.1-HFS: Knowledge of cardiovascular risk factors or conditions that may require consultation with medical personnel before testing or training, including inappropriate changes of resting or exercise heart rate and blood pressure; new onset discomfort in chest, neck, shoulder, or arm; changes in the pattern of discomfort during rest or exercise; fainting or dizzy spells; and claudication.

The American Heart Association (AHA) notes three purposes of ECG recording for children, including to (a) accurately assess heart rate as related to exercise effort and test end point, (b) diagnose and evaluate arrhythmia, and (c) assess conduction abnormalities, ST-segment, and T-wave changes consistent with myocardial ischemia and QT interval (38). AHA recommendations for ECG recording equipment are listed in Box 26-2.

Blood pressure is another important variable. AHA recommends that the blood pressure be measured before the exercise test (rest), during the exercise test, and in recovery (38). Typically, the exercise and recovery measures are taken every 3 minutes (38). Various devices are available (e.g., aneroid, automated), each with limitations. Because mercury-based devices are no longer commonly used, it is important to realize the importance of frequent calibration of aneroid devices. Automated (oscillometric) devices are sensitive to movement and vibration and thus may be problematic in exercise testing. The cuff must completely surround the arm, and the width of the cuff bladder should be least 40% of the arm circumference (38). Potentially the most important factor in attaining accurate and reliable blood pressures

BOX 26-2	EQUIPMENT RECOMMENDATIONS FOR ELECTROCARDIOGRAM (ECG) RECORDING EQUIPMENT (AMERICAN HEART ASSOCIATION)

- Real-time display screen of adequate size to see easily during testing
  - Display at least three leads
- Printer to create copies
  - Able to print immediate copies of real-time ECG and continuous ECG rhythm strips
  - Helpful to print median ECG complexes at each stage
- Analogue recording is acceptable but digital is preferred
- Computer-based recording system can provide review of tracings at a later time

Paridon SM, Alpert BS, Boas SR, et al. Clinical stress testing in the pediatric age group: A statement from the American Heart Associate Council on Cardiovascular Disease in the Young, Committee on Atherosclerosis,Hypertension, and Obesity in Youth. *Circulation* 113:1905–1920, 2006.

measures is the person taking the measurement, and thus periodic retraining and technique evaluation is recommended (38).

The metabolic cart is another piece of valuable equipment when assessing children. Various carts are available and have been reviewed elsewhere (38). No matter the particular cart used, collection of expired air must be made with care to avoid leaks. For children who do not easily handle a mouthpiece and nose clip, the use of a mask with sealant gel may be more appropriate (38).

Other devices potentially used in testing include echocardiography, nuclear myocardial blood flow imaging, and spirometry (38). Equipment related to safety should include a defibrillator, oxygen, suction system, and emergency drugs (38).

EXERCISE EQUIPMENT

> **1.7.8-CES: Demonstrate exercise equipment adaptations necessary for different age groups, physical abilities, and other potential contributing factors.**

> **1.7.18-CES: Determine appropriate testing and training modalities according to the age, functional capacity, physical ability, and health status of the individual.**

> **1.3.22-HFS: Ability to modify protocols and procedures for cardiorespiratory fitness tests in children, adolescents, and older adults.**

Cycle ergometers and treadmills are the two most common exercise modes used in pediatric exercise testing (6). The equipment used must be appropriate for the child's age and size (38). Treadmills should have side and front handrails at appropriate heights (38). Ideally, cycle ergometers used in testing will have adjustable leg cranks and handlebars. If not available, use of blocks to increase pedal height may be necessary for smaller children to allow for 10 to 15 degrees of knee flexion at the bottom of the pedal stroke (38). Realize that with both exercise modes, however, children may need additional time to practice (38). Treadmill exercise is typically preferred, especially for younger children, to avoid limitations because of undeveloped thigh musculature, resulting in early fatigue when cycling (20). Addi-

TABLE 26-4. COMPARISON OF TREADMILL VERSUS CYCLE ERGOMETER FOR PEDIATRIC EXERCISE TESTING

VARIABLE	TREADMILL	CYCLE ERGOMETER
Expense	More expensive	Less expensive
Noise	Louder	Quieter
Safety	More dangerous	Less dangerous
Workload adjustments	Easy to adjust workload by speed and grade changes	Easy to adjust work rate
Determination of work efficiency	More difficult to quantify work rate because of influence of body size, weight, gait, and stride length	Electronically braked ergometers provide a more accurate measurement of mechanical power output than mechanically braked ergometers
Measurement ease	More difficult to obtain blood pressure because of movement artifact	Easier to obtain blood pressure and measures of gas exchange
Space	Require more laboratory space	Require less laboratory space
Other	Easier to calibrate than either mechanically braked or electronically braked cycle ergometers	More difficult to maintain workload as younger children may not maintain a steady cadence

Paridon SM, Alpert BS, Boas SR, et al. Clinical stress testing in the pediatric age group: A statement from the American Heart Associate Council on Cardiovascular Disease in the Young, Committee on Atherosclerosis,Hypertension, and Obesity in Youth. *Circulation* 113:1905–1920, 2006.

tionally, treadmill exercise involves a greater muscle mass and thus allows for higher $\dot{V}O_{2max}$ (6).

Advantages and disadvantages of each mode of exercise are shown in Table 26-4 as adapted from the 2006 Statement form the American Heart Association on Clinical Stress Testing in the Pediatric Age Group (38).

MAXIMAL EFFORT CRITERIA AND OTHER MEASURES

Criteria commonly used to verify maximal effort in children include (a) respiratory exchange ratio of >1.1, (b) peak heart rate approaching 200, and (c) subjective observation of experienced testers (38). Attainment of a

plateau in $\dot{V}O_2$ despite increasing workload (an adult criterion) is not typically observed in children (38,45).

Use of rating of perceived exertion (RPE) scales is possible in children, in particular, the children's OMNI scale of perceived exertion, which has been validated for cycling exercise and walking/running (43,56). See Figure 26-2 for these two visual scales.

INDICATIONS AND CONTRAINDICATIONS FOR STRESS TESTING

> **2.2.1-HFS: Knowledge of cardiovascular risk factors or conditions that may require consultation with medical personnel before testing or training,**

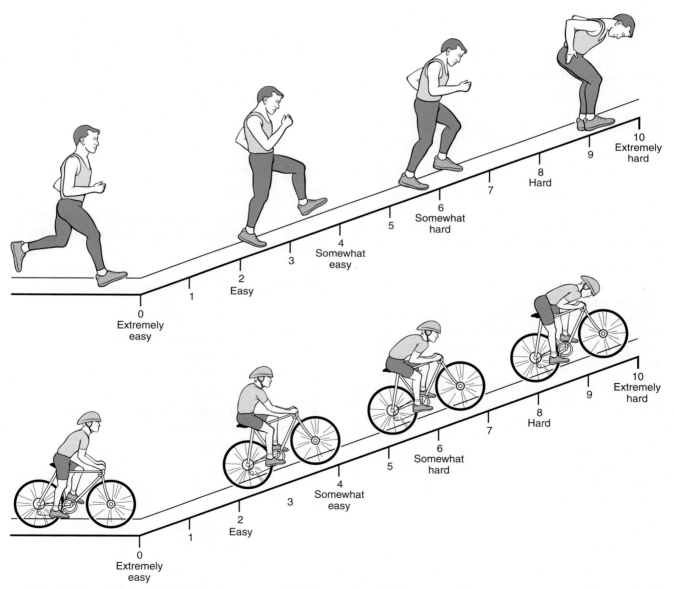

FIGURE 26-2. OMNI scales of perceived exertion for cycling and walking/running. From: Robertson RJ, Goss FL, Boer NR, et al. Children's OMNI Scale of Perceived Exertion: mixed gender and race validation. *Med Sci Sports Exerc.* 2000;32(3):452–458 and Utter AC, Roberston RJ, Nieman DC, Kang J. Children's OMNI Scale of Perceived Exertion: walking/running evaluation. *Med Sci Sports Exerc.* 2002;34(1):139–144.

TABLE 26-5. RELATIVE RISKS FOR STRESS TESTING

LOWER RISK	HIGHER RISK
Symptoms during exercise in an otherwise healthy child who has a normal cardiovascular exam and ECG	Patients with pulmonary hypertension
Exercise-induced bronchospasm studies in the absence of severe resting airway obstruction	Patients with documented long-QTc syndrome
Asymptomatic patients undergoing evaluation for possible long-QTc syndrome	Patients with dilated/restrictive cardiomyopathy with congestive heart failure or arrhythmia
Asymptomatic ventricular ectopy in patients with structurally normal hearts	Patients with a history of a hemodynamically unstable arrhythmia
Patients with unrepaired or residual congenital lesions who are asymptomatic at rest (including left to right shunts, obstructive right heart lesions without severe resting obstruction, obstructive left heart lesions with severe resting obstruction, regurgitation lesions regardless of severity)	Patients with hypertrophic cardiomyopathy who have symptoms, greater than mild left ventricular outflow tract obstruction, and documented arrhythmia
Routine follow-up of asymptomatic patients at risk for myocardial ischemia, including Kawasaki disease without giant aneurysm or known coronary stenosis, after repair of anomalous left coronary artery, after arterial switch procedure	Patients with greater than moderate airway obstruction on baseline pulmonary function tests
Routine monitoring in cardiac transplant patients not currently experiencing rejection	Patients with Marfan syndrome and activity-related chest pain in whom a noncardiac cause of chest pain is suspected
Patients with palliated cardiac lesions without uncompensated congestive heart failure, arrhythmia, or extreme cyanosis	Patients suspected to have myocardial ischemia with exertion
Patients with a history of hemodynamically stable supraventricular tachycardia	Routine testing of patients with Marfan syndrome
Patients with stable dilated cardiomyopathy without uncompensated congestive heart failure or documented arrhythmia	Unexplained syncope with exercise

ECG, electrocardiogram.

Paridon SM, Alpert BS, Boas SR, et al. Clinical stress testing in the pediatric age group: A statement from the American Heart Associate Council on cardiovascular disease in the young. Committee on Atherosclerosis, Hypertension, and Obesity in Youth, *Circulation*. 2006;113:1905–1920.

including inappropriate changes of resting or exercise heart rate and blood pressure; new onset discomfort in chest, neck, shoulder, or arm; changes in the pattern of discomfort during rest or exercise; fainting or dizzy spells; and claudication.

> **3.2.1-HFS: Knowledge of pulmonary risk factors or conditions that may require consultation with medical personnel before testing or training, including asthma, exercise-induced asthma/bronchospasm, extreme breathlessness at rest or during exercise, bronchitis, and emphysema.**

Generally, children with acute myocardial or pericardial inflammatory disease or those with severe outflow obstruction requiring surgery should not be tested. Other than these situations, general safety of testing has been established. Understanding risk level helps to ensure safety and minimizes risk. Table 26-5 includes relative risks for exercise testing (38).

Because the goal of most stress testing is to elicit symptoms and access cardiopulmonary reserves, maximal effort is desired. Test termination is typically indicated when diagnostic findings are established, monitoring equipment fails, or when signs/symptoms indicate a compromise to the child's well-being (38). Specifically, see Box 26-3 for a listing of usual indications for test termination made in light of clinical judgment (these should not be seen as rigid guidelines) (38).

EXERCISE PROTOCOLS

> **1.3.15-CES: Ability to provide testing procedures and protocol for children and the elderly with or without various clinical conditions.**

> **1.3.22-CES: Describe the differences in the physiologic responses to various modes of ergometry (e.g., treadmill, cycle and arm ergometers) as they relate to exercise testing and training.**

> **1.7.18-CES: Knowledge of the advantages and disadvantages of implementation of interval, continuous, and circuit training programs.**

> **1.3.22-HFS: Ability to modify protocols and procedures for cardiorespiratory fitness tests in children, adolescents, and older adults.**

Protocol selection is based on the individual being tested and the purpose of the test (52). In general, to obtain $\dot{V}O_{2max}$, the child should reach his/her tolerance limit in 10 ± 2 minutes (38). In the United States, treadmills are more frequently used than cycle ergometers (9). Multistage incremental protocols commonly used include the Bruce and Balke treadmill protocols and the James and McMaster cycle protocols. Incremental protocols (ramps and 1-minute stages), such as the Godfrey test, have been used as well. Individualized protocols (based on predicted $\dot{V}O_{2max}$ and basal $\dot{V}O_2$) are also well tolerated by children (25).

1.3.2-CES: Knowledge of exercise testing procedures for various clinical populations including those individuals with cardiovascular, pulmonary, and metabolic diseases in terms of exercise modality, protocol, physiologic measurements, and expected outcomes.

BOX 26-3	USUAL INDICATIONS FOR TEST TERMINATION

1. Decrease in ventricular rate with increasing workload associated with extreme fatigue, dizziness, or other symptoms suggestive of insufficient cardiac output
2. Failure of heart rate to increase with exercise and extreme fatigue, dizziness, or other symptoms suggestive of insufficient cardiac output
3. Progressive fall in systolic blood pressure with increasing workload
4. Severe hypertension, >250 mm Hg systolic or 115 mm Hg diastolic, or blood pressures higher than can be measured by laboratory equipment
5. Dyspnea that the patient finds intolerable
6. Symptomatic tachycardia that the patient finds intolerable
7. Progressive fall in oxygen saturation to <90% or a 10-point drop from resting saturation in a patient who is symptomatic
8. Presence of ≥3 mm flat or downward sloping ST-segment depression
9. Increasing ventricular ectopy with increasing workload, including a >3-beat run
10. Patient requests termination of the study

Paridon SM, Alpert BS, Boas SR, et al. Clinical stress testing in the pediatric age group: A statement from the American Heart Associate Council on cardiovascular disease in the young. Committee on Atherosclerosis, Hypertension, and Obesity in Youth, *Circulation*. 2006;113:1905–1920.

The Bruce protocol has been used on subjects of all ages, and normative data are available for children (11). Advantages of the Bruce protocol include the ability to track a person over time and that $\dot{V}O_{2max}$ can be estimated from test duration (38). Disadvantages of the Bruce protocol include the larger work increments leading to potential premature termination within the first minute of the stage, boredom with the initial low-intensity stages, boredom with the 3-minute stages, and steep grades that encourage excessive handrail holding (38).

The Balke protocol involves a constant speed with increasing grade. The Balke protocol has been modified in various ways, including use of a faster speed and starting at a higher grade (3,47). Faster speeds (jogging, running) compared with slower (walking) have been found to be appropriate for $\dot{V}O_{2max}$ determination (39).

The James cycle ergometer protocol includes three exercise protocols (predetermined work rates based on body surface area) using three 3-minute stages followed by work rate increase each minute until volitional fatigue (23). An advantage of this protocol is the availability of normative data (23,60). A disadvantage is the possibility of early test termination by younger or less fit children. Another cycle testing protocol, the McMaster cycle ergometer protocol, also includes three predetermined work rates (based on height). This protocol, however, utilizes 2-minute stages (6).

The Godfrey test is a 1-minute incremental test that includes three protocols (predetermined by height) in which the work rate increments are 10 to 20 watts. Normative data are available for this protocol (16). Ramp protocols have also been used in this patient population with similar maximal responses (36,53,65). Although selection of work

rate increment is made on a case-by-case basis, typical increases of 20 to 25 watts/min are appropriate for fit children and 10 watts/min for younger and unfit children (38).

PHARMACOLOGIC STRESS TESTING

 1.3.22-HFS: Ability to modify protocols and procedures for cardiorespiratory fitness tests in children, adolescents, and older adults.

 1.7.34-HFS: Ability to modify exercises based on age, physical condition and cognitive status.

In situations in which exercise testing is inappropriate, pharmacologic stress testing may be used (e.g., patients who are too young or are unable to perform exercise, or when exercise may interfere with data collection, including some echocardiographic studies) (38). The two main types of pharmacologic agents include those that increase oxygen consumption of the heart (e.g., dobutamine, isoproterenol) and those that cause vasodilatation of the coronary arteries (e.g., adenosine, dipyridamole) (38). The rate of adverse reactions to pharmacologic stress testing in children is not known, although it appears low (38).

ECHOCARDIOGRAPHY

Echocardiography allows for assessment of regional wall motion abnormalities when evaluating myocardial perfusion or gradients and/or function when assessing issues related to the coronary arteries (25,27). Conditions related to coronary artery pathology for which echocardiography are appropriate include Kawasaki disease, transplant graft vasculopathy, arterial switch operation for transposition of the great arteries, anomalous coronary artery origins or pathways, pulmonary atresia with intact ventricular septum, hyperlipidemia, insulin-dependent diabetes mellitus, and supravalvular aortic stenosis (27). Other aspects, which can be examined under stress, include gradients (e.g., for conditions like hypertropic cardiomyopathy or aortic and pulmonic stenosis), cardiac pressures (e.g., in pulmonary hypertension), and ventricular function (e.g., in dilated cardiomyopathy or mitral and aortic regurgitation) (25).

Pharmacologic or exercise stress can be used with echocardiography. Typically with treadmill exercise and upright cycling, echocardiography is done before and immediately after the exercise. With supine cycling, echocardiography is done before and then during each stage of the test (38). Pharmacologic stressors include dobutamine, isoproterenol, adenosine, and dipyridamole (the latter two for ischemic evaluation only) (25).

SUMMARY

Exercise testing in children can present unique challenges related to ensuring complete understanding of the stress test, adaptability of equipment for smaller size, protocol selection to avoid boredom and elicit maximal effort, and exercise modality selection to ensure patient comfort with the activity. Staffing of pediatric testing requires individuals with an appropriate knowledge base, as well as the experience and skill to work with children.

REFERENCES

1. American College of Obstetricians and Gynecologists. Exercise during pregnancy and the postpartum period. ACOG Committee Opinion No. 267. *Obstet Gynecol*. 2002;99:171–173.
2. American College of Sports Medicine. *Guidelines for Exercise Testing and Prescription*. 8th ed. Philadelphia: Lippincott Williams & Wilkins; 2008.
3. Armstrong H, Balding J, Gentle P, Williams J, Kirby B. Peak oxygen uptake and physical capacity in 11- to 16-year olds. *Pediatr Exerc Sci*. 1990;2:349–358.
4. Arruda AM, Das MK, Roger VL, Klarich KW, Mahoney DW, Pellikka PA. Prognostic value of exercise echocardiography in 2,632 patients >65 years of age. *J Am Coll Cardiol*. 2001;37:1036–1041.
5. Artal R, O'Toole M. Guidelines of the American College of Obstetricians and Gynecologists for exercise during pregnancy and the postpartum period. *Br J Sports Med*. 2003;37:6–12.
6. Bar-Or O, Rowland TW. *Pediatric Exercise Medicine: From Physiologic Principles to Health Care Application*. Champaign (IL): Human Kinetics; 2004.
7. Canadian Society for Exercise Physiology. *PARmed-X for Pregnancy*. Gloucester, Ontario: Canadian Society for Exercise Physiology; 2002.
8. Carr K, Emes C, Rogerson C. Exercise testing protocols for different abilities in the older population. *Activities, Adaptation & Aging*. 2003;28(1):49–66.
9. Chang RKR, Gurvitz M, Rodriguez S, Hong E, Klitzner TS. Current practice of exercise stress testing among pediatric cardiology and pulmonary centers in the United Stated. *Pediatr Cardiol*. 2006;27:110–116.
10. Chuah S, Pellikka PA, Roger VL, McCully RB, Seward JB. Role of dobutamine stress echocardiography in predicting outcome in 860

11. Cummings GR, Everatt D, Hastman L. Bruce treadmill test in children: normal values in a clinic population. *Am J Cardiol*. 1978;41: 69–75.
12. Davies GA, Wolfe LA, Mottola MF, MacKinnon C. Society of Obstetricians and Gynecologists of Canada, SOGC Clinical Practice Obstetrics Committee. Joint SOGC/CSEP Clinical Practice Guideline: Exercise in pregnancy and the postpartum period. *Can J Appl Physiol*. 2003;28:330–341.
13. Fleg, JL. Stress testing in the elderly. *Am J Geriatr Cardiol*. 2001; 10(6):308–315.
14. Gibbons RJ, Balady GJ, Bricker JT, et al. ACC/AHA 2002 guideline update for exercise testing: a report of the American College of Cardiology/American Heart Association Task Force on Practice Guidelines (Committee on Exercise Testing), *Circulation*. 2002; 106:1883–1892.
15. Gill TM, DiPietro L, Krumholz HM. Role of exercise stress testing and safety monitoring for older persons starting an exercise program. *JAMA*. 2000;284(3):342–349.
16. Godfrey S, Davies CT, Wozniak E, Barnes CA. Cardio-respiratory response to exercise in normal children. *Clin Sci*. 1971;40:419–431.
17. Goraya TY, Jacobsen SJ, Pellikka PA, et al. Prognostic value of treadmill exercise testing in elderly persons. *Ann Intern Med*. 2000;132:862–870.
18. Gulati J, Arnsdorft MF, Shaw LJ, et al. Prognostic value of the Duke treadmill score in asymptomatic women. *Am J Cardiol*. 2005;96: 369–375.
19. Hebestreit H. Exercise testing in children: What works, what doesn't, and where to go? *Paediatr Respir Rev*. 2004;5(suppl A):S11–S14.
20. Hebestreit HU, Bar-Or O. Differences between children and adults for exercise testing and exercise prescription. In: Skinner JS, editor. *Exercise Testing and Exercise Prescription for Special Cases*. 2nd ed. Philadelphia: Lippincott Williams & Wilkins; 2005 p.68–84.
21. Heenan AP, Wolfe LA, Davies GAL. Maximal exercise testing in late gestation: maternal responses. *Obstet Gynecol*. 2001;97(1):127–134.
22. Hollenberg M, Ngo LH, Turner D, Tager IB. Treadmill exercise testing in an epidemiologic study of elderly subjects. *J Gerontol*. 1998;53A(4):B259–B267.
23. James FW, Kaplan S, Glueck CJ, Tsay JY, Knight MJ, Sarwar CJ. Responses of normal children and young adults to controlled bicycle exercise. *Circulation*. 1980;61:902–912.
24. Kallinen M, Kauppinen M, Era P, Heikkinen E. The predictive value of exercise testing for survival among 75-year-old men and women. *Scand J Med Sci Sports*. 2006;16:237–244.
25. Karila C, de Blic J, Waernessycle S, Benoist M-R, Scheinmann P. Cardiopulmonary exercise testing in children: an individualized protocol for workload increases. *Chest*. 2001;120:81–87.
26. Kaufman DW, Kelly JP, Rosenberg L, Anderson TE, Mitchell AA. Recent patterns of medication use in the ambulatory adult population of the United States: the Slone Survey. *JAMA*. 2002;287:337–344.
27. Kimball, TR. Pediatric stress echocardiography. *Pediatr Cardiol*. 2002;23:347–357.
28. Kwok JMF, Miller TD, Hodge DO, Gibbons RJ. Prognostic value of the Duke treadmill score in the elderly. *J Am Coll Cardiol*. 2002; 39:1475–1481.
29. Lai S, Kaykha A, Yamazaki T, et al. Treadmill scores in elderly men. *J Am Coll Cardiol*. 2004;43:606–615.
30. Liao L, Smith IV WT, Tuttle RH, Shaw LK, Coleman RE, Borges-Neto S. Prediction of death and nonfatal myocardial infarction in high-risk patients: a comparison between the Duke treadmill scores, peak exercise radionuclide angiography, and SPECT perfusion imaging. *J Nucl Med*. 2005;46:5–11.
31. MacPhail A, Davies GAL, Victory R, Wolfe LA. Maximal exercise testing in late gestation: fetal responses. *Obstet Gynecol*. 2000; 96(4):565–570.
32. Martinez-Caro D, Alegria E, Lorente D, Azpilicueta J, Calabuig J, Ancin R. Diagnostic value of stress testing in the elderly. *Eur Heart J*. 1984;5(suppl E):63–67.

patients with known or suspected coronary artery disease. *Circulation*. 1998;97:1474–1480.

33. Marwick TH, Case C, Sawada S, et al. Use of stress echocardiography to predict mortality in patients with diabetes and known or suspected coronary artery disease. *Diabetes Care.* 2002;25:1042–1048.

34. Marwick TH, Case C, Vasey C, Allen S, Short L, Thomas JD. Prediction of mortality by exercise echocardiography: a strategy for combination with the Duke treadmill score. *Circulation.* 2001;103: 2566–2571.

35. Mottola MF, Davenport MH, Brun CR, Inglis SD, Charlesworth S, Sopper MM. VO$_{2max}$ prediction and exercise prescription for pregnant women. *Med Sci Sports Exerc.* 2006;8: 1389–1395.

36. Myers J, Buchanan N, Walsh D, et al. Comparison of the ramp versus standard exercise protocols. *J Am Coll Cardiol.* 1991;17:1334–1342.

37. Paillole C, Ruiz J, Juliard JM, et al. Detection of coronary artery disease in diabetic patients. *Diabetologia.* 1995;38:726–731.

38. **Paridon SM, Alpert BS, Boas SR, et al. Clinical stress testing in the pediatric age group: a statement from the American Heart Associate Council on Cardiovascular Disease in the Young, Committee on Atherosclerosis, Hypertension, and Obesity in Youth. Circulation. 2006;113:1905–1920.**

39. Paterson DH, Cunningham DA, Donner A. The effect of different treadmill speeds on the variability of VO$_{2\,max}$ in children. *Eur J Appl Physiol Occup Physiol.* 1981;47:113–122.

40. Peteiro J, Monserrrat L, Pineiro M, et al. Comparison of exercise echocardiography and the Duke treadmill score for risk stratification in patients with known or suspected coronary artery disease and normal resting electrocardiogram. *Am Heart J.* 2006;151:1324. e1–10.

41. Pivarnik JM, Chambliss HO, Clapp JF, et al. Impart of physical activity during pregnancy and postpartum on chronic disease risk. *Med Sci Sports Exerc.* 2006;38(5):989–1006.

42. Rahimi K, Thomas A, Adam M, Hayerizadeh B-F, Schuler G, Secknus M-A. Implications of exercise test modality on modern prognostic markers in patients with known or suspected coronary artery disease: treadmill versus bicycle. *Eur J Cardiovasc Prev Rehabil.* 2006;13:45–50.

43. Robertson RJ, Goss FL, Boer NF, et al. Children's OMNI Scale of Perceived Exertion: mixed gender and race validation. *Med Sci Sports Exerc.* 2000;32(3):452–458.

44. Roger VL, Jacobsen SJ, Pellikka PA, Miller TD, Bailey KR, Gersh BJ. Prognostic value of treadmill exercise testing: a population-based study in Olmsted County, Minnesota. *Circulation.* 1998;98: 2836–2841.

45. Rowland TW. Does peak VO$_2$ reflect VO$_{2max}$ in children? Evidence from supramaximal testing. *Med Sci Sports Exerc.* 1993;25(6): 689–693.

46. Rowland TW In: Rowland TW, editor. *Pediatric Laboratory Exercise Testing: Clinical Guidelines.* Champaign (IL): Human Kinetics; 1993 p. 19–42.

47. Rowland TW, Varzeas MR, Walsh CA. Aerobic responses to walking training in sedentary adolescents. *J Adolesc Health.* 1991; 12:30–34.

48. Schinkel AFL, Elhendy A, Biagini E, et al. Prognostic stratification using dobutamine stress ^{99m}Tc-Tetrofosmin myocardial perfusion SPECT in elderly patients usable to perform exercise testing. *J Nucl Med.* 2005;46(1):12–18.

49. Skinner JS. Aging for exercise testing and prescription. In: Skinner JS, editor. *Exercise Testing and Exercise Prescription for Special Cases.* 2nd ed. Philadelphia: Lippincott Williams & Wilkins; 2005, p. 85–99.

50. Spin JM, Prakash M, Froelicher VF, et al. The prognostic value of exercise testing in elderly men. *Am J Med.* 2002;112:453–459.

51. Spinnewijn WEM, Lotgering FK, Struijk PC, Wallenburg HCS. Fetal heart rate and uterine contractility during maternal exercise at term. *Am J Obstet Gynecol.* 1996;174(1):43–48.

52. Stephens P, Paridon SM. Exercise testing in pediatrics. *Pediatr Clin North Am.* 2004;51:1569–1587.

53. Tanner CS, Heise CT, Barber G. Correlation of the physiologic parameters of a continuous ramp verus an incremental James exercise protocol in normal children. *Am J Cardiol.* 1991;67:309–312.

54. Tomassoni TL. Conducting the pediatric exercise test. In: Rowland TW, editor. *Pediatric Laboratory Exercise Testing: Clinical Guidelines.* Champaign (IL): Human Kinetics; 1993 p. 1–17.

55. United States Census Bureau [Internet]. Available from: www.census.gov. Accessed May 2007.

56. Utter AC, Roberston RJ, Nieman DC, Kang J. Children's OMNI Scale of Perceived Exertion: walking/running evaluation. *Med Sci Sports Exerc.* 2002;34(1):139–144.

57. Valeti US, Miller TD, Hodge DO, Gibbons RJ. Exercise single-photon emission computed tomography provides effective risk stratification of elderly men and elderly women. *Circulation.* 2005;111: 1771–1776.

58. Vasilomanolakis EC. Geriatric cardiology: when exercise stress testing is justified. *Geriatrics.* 1985;40(12):47–57.

59. Veille J-C, Kitzman DW, Bacevice AE. Effects of pregnancy on the electrocardiogram in healthy subjects during strenuous exercise. *Am J Obstet Gynecol.* 1996;175:1360–1364.

60. Washington RL, van Gundy JC, Cohen C, Sondheimer HM, Wolfe RR. Normal aerobic and anaerobic exercise data for North American school-age children. *J Pediatr.* 1988;112:223–233.

61. Weissgerber TL, Wolfe LA, Davies GAL, Mottla MF. Exercise in the prevention and treatment of maternal-fetal disease: a review of the literature. *Appl Physiol Nutr Metab.* 2006;31:661–676.

62. Wolfe LA. Pregnancy. In: Skinner JS, editor. *Exercise Testing and Exercise Prescription for Special Cases.* 2nd ed. Philadelphia: Lippincott Williams & Wilkins; 2005. p. 377–391.

63. Wolfe LA, Charlesworth SA, Glenn NM, Heenan AP, Davies GAL. Effects of pregnancy on maternal work tolerance. *Can J Appl Physiol.* 2005;30(2):212–232.

64. Yamazaki T, Myers J, Froelicher VF. Effect of age and end point on the prognostic value of the exercise test. *Chest.* 2004;125: 1920–1928.

65. Zhang YY, Johnson II MC, Chow N, Wasserman K. Effect of exercise testing protocol on parameters of aerobic function. *Med Sci Sports Exerc.* 1991;23:625–630.

Electrocardiography

Electrocardiography is the clinical representation and study of the electrical activity of the myocardium. The electrocardiogram (ECG) gives basic information about rate, rhythm, impulse conduction through the myocardium, pathology of the myocardium, and previous heart disease and/or damage, as well as yielding information about current physiologic status of the myocardium.

The ECG is one of the most basic, commonly used tools in diagnostic cardiology. Careful interpretation of the ECG is necessary because abnormal ECGs are not uncommon in healthy individuals, and they may be present without obvious heart disease. Use of exercise ECG has changed considerably, and it is now rare that an exercise test, using solely exercise ECG, is performed without some additional diagnostic modality. The most common modalities include pharmacologic, nuclear, or echocardiographic exercise testing, all of which significantly improve both specificity and sensitivity of the test.

> > > KEY TERMS

Acute pericarditis: Infected or inflamed pericardium.

Antiarrhythmic agent: A pharmacologic agent that acts physiologically to decrease dysrhythmias. These agents are subdivided into classes (I through V) by mechanism of action.

Atrioventricular block: An obstruction or delay in electrical conduction that occurs in the normal conduction pathways between the sinus node and the Purkinje fibers.

Automaticity: The ability of specialized cells in the heart (normally in the sinus node) to spontaneously depolarize and initiate a new electrical impulse.

Bigeminy: A conduction pattern in which a premature beat (either supraventricular or ventricular) follows every normal sinus beat.

Bundle branch blocks: Conduction block in either the left or right bundle branch; results in a wider (>0.12 sec) than normal QRS and a QRS configuration that is different for a left versus a right bundle branch block.

Digitalis: A drug in a class called *cardiac glycosides* that increases the force of myocardial contraction and decreases heart rate.

Dysrhythmia: Any cardiac rhythm that is not a regular sinus rhythm; it may be a single beat or a sustained rhythm.

Fascicular block: A conduction block that occurs in one or more of the fascicles of the intraventricular Purkinje system.

False-positive: A test result that indicates the presence of disease when no disease is present.

Left ventricular hypertrophy: An increase in thickness of the left ventricular wall that results in increased amplitude of the R wave in leads over the left ventricle (V_5, V_6) and increased amplitude in the S wave in leads over the right ventricle (V_1, V_2).

Pathologic Q waves: Q waves that have a longer duration (>0.04 sec) than normal and greater amplitude ($\geq$ one third the amplitude of the R wave in the same QRS complex).

R waves: The first upward deflection in the QRS complex.

ST segment: The line in the electrocardiogram connecting the end of the QRS to the beginning of the T wave; a measure of time from the end of ventricular depolarization to the start of ventricular repolarization.

T waves: The wave or deflection on the electrocardiogram that reflects repolarization of the ventricles.

Ventricular aneurysm: Thinning of the ventricular wall, resulting in a paradoxical bulging in that area during ventricular contraction.

Depolarization of myocardial cells is normally a very orderly process. The *normal* ECG is consistent and relatively easy to discern because there are predictable waveforms, as well as time intervals for those waveforms. Abnormalities of myocardial anatomy and physiology, pathology of various cardiovascular diseases and many other influences can cause or influence abnormal waveform and/or rhythm. The most common of these abnormal ECGs, as well as the normal ECG, will be discussed in this chapter.

BASIC ELECTROCARDIOGRAPHY

EQUIPMENT

> **1.3.11-CES: Describe the importance of accurate and calibrated testing equipment (e.g., treadmill, ergometers, electrocardiograph, gas analysis systems, and sphygmomanometers) and ability to recognize and remediate equipment that is no longer properly calibrated.**

All equipment used in both resting and exercise electrocardiography must be maintained and calibrated on a regular basis. Ongoing maintenance of such equipment should include electronic and mechanical checks by qualified biomedical engineers or technicians. ECG equipment is standardized with respect to paper speed and waveform deflection, and normally the documentation of this standardization is part of the warm-up routines on all ECG equipment. Treadmill calibration with respect to both speed and elevation should be checked on a regular

basis. Other equipment utilized in exercise and resting electrocardiography must be regularly maintained and checked at least quarterly. All such quality checks must be documented and records retained. Equipment that does not meet standards and that cannot be brought to standard calibration and operation should be discarded.

LEAD PLACEMENT AND PREPARATION FOR THE ELECTROCARDIOGRAM

> **1.3.3-CES: Describe anatomic landmarks as they relate to exercise testing and programming (e.g., electrode placement, blood pressure).**

> **1.4.13-CES: Locate the appropriate sites for the limb and chest leads for resting, standard, and exercise (Mason Likar) ECGs, as well as commonly used bipolar systems (e.g., CM-5).**

> **1.4.15-CES: Ability to minimize ECG artifact.**

> **1.4.14-CES: Obtain and interpret a pre-exercise standard and modified (Mason-Likar) 12-lead ECG on a participant in the supine and upright position.**

Surface electrodes are placed on the chest, wrists, and ankles for a standard 12-lead ECG. The limb leads, one on each wrist and ankle, are modified for exercise testing (the Mason Likar lead system) by placing these leads in the subclavicular and suprailiac areas. See Box 27-1 and Figure 27-1 for details on lead placement in the Mason-Likar leads.

BOX 27-1   MASON-LIKAR 12-LEAD SYSTEM

The Mason-Likar 10 electrode placement allows for conventional 12-lead exercise ECG tracings. The location of these electrodes are described below:

Right arm: upper right arm-chest region immediately below the mid-point of the clavicle.

Left arm: upper left arm-chest region immediately below the mid-point of the clavicle.

Right leg: lower right abdominal region, at the midclavicular line, at the level of the last rib

Left leg: lower left abdominal region, at the midclavicular line, at the level of the last rib

V1: on the right sternal border in the 4th intercostal space.

NOTE: the 4th intercostal space can be found by locating the sternoclavicular joint and placing the index finger in the space immediately below the first rib. This is the 1st intercostal space. Proceed down the sternum until the 4th space is found.

V2: on the left sternal border in the 4th intercostal space

V3: at the midpoint on a straight line between V2 and V4

V4: on the fifth intercostal space at the midclavicular line

V5: on the anterior axillary line, horizontal to V4

V6: on the midaxillary line, horizontal to both V4 and V5

The leg electrodes may also be placed at the level of the navel. However, there may be excessive motion artifact with this placement. Placement on the last rib at the mid-clavicular line tends to be more stable with no effect on the ECG tracing.

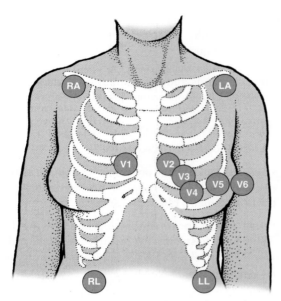

FIGURE 27-1. The Mason-Likar simulated 12-lead ECG electrode placement for exercise testing.

By combining these electrodes in various configurations, the ECG gives electrical views of the heart from all three planes: horizontal, frontal, and vertical. Figure 27-2 shows the anatomy of the heart along with the conduction system. Figure 27-3 shows a normal ECG complex with associated representation of the anatomic correlates for each wave. By examining the ECG in more than one plane and lead, normal and abnormal function of the myocardium can be determined. Table 27-1 shows the ECG wave associated with the corresponding electrical event in the myocardium.

Artifact from movement, environmental (electrical) interference, and poor skin preparation can significantly affect both resting and especially exercise ECG. It is extremely important to minimize all such artifact through proper and careful skin preparation, precise electrode placement, and standardized operating conditions within ECG and exercise testing facilities.

THE CONDUCTION SYSTEM

> **1.4.5-CES: Identify resting and exercise ECG changes associated with the following abnormalities: axis; bundle branch blocks and bifascicular blocks; atrioventricular blocks; sinus bradycardia and tachycardia; sinus arrest; supraventricular premature contractions and tachycardia; ventricular premature contractions (including frequency, form, couplets, salvos, tachycardia); atrial flutter and fibrillation; ventricular fibrillation; and myocardial ischemia, injury, and infarction.**

> **1.4.3-HFS: Knowledge of the basic properties of cardiac muscle and the normal pathways of conduction in the heart.**

The anatomy of the conduction system is depicted in Figure 27-2. Electrical depolarization originates in the sinoatrial (SA) node, located in the right atrium near the superior vena cava. The wave of depolarization subsequently spreads through the right atrium into the left atrium and to the atrioventricular (AV) node. The impulse next proceeds through the AV node and depolarizes the bundle of His, which extends into the intraventricular septum, then into the right and left bundle branches. The right bundle branch travels down the right side of the septum and into the right ventricle (RV). The left bundle branch divides into anterior and posterior branches as it proceeds through the left ventricle (LV). The bundle branches terminate in Purkinje fibers, which are diffuse throughout the LV.

The SA node is responsible for initiating depolarization of the myocardium. However, in people with both normal and abnormal hearts, abnormal depolarization sequences can and do occur. These abnormalities are called dysrhythmias and/or blocks. Dysrhythmias are often classified as brady- or tachydysrhythmias (slow or fast).

SINUS RHYTHMS

"Normal sinus rhythm" is indicative of a normal ECG waveform at rates between 60 and 100 beats per minute (bpm). Rates slower than 60 bpm are termed **bradycardia**, and rates faster than 100 bpm are termed **tachycardia**. Whether these two conditions are normal depends on the situation and the individual. For example, sinus tachycardia at rates in excess of 150 to 200 may be entirely normal in the context of exercise, but not in an individual with coronary artery disease (CAD) who is at rest. Likewise, bradycardia at rates lower than 50—and even 40 in some cases—may occur asymptomatically and without problem in highly trained endurance athletes; however, in an individual with significant myocardial pathology, this rate may merit serious medical therapy.

BRADYCARDIAS

> **1.4.5-CES: Identify resting and exercise ECG changes associated with the following abnormalities: axis; bundle branch blocks and bifascicular blocks; atrioventricular blocks; sinus bradycardia and tachycardia; sinus arrest; supraventricular premature contractions and tachycardia; ventricular premature contractions (including frequency, form, couplets, salvos, tachycardia); atrial flutter and fibrillation; ventricular fibrillation; and myocardial ischemia, injury, and infarction.**

Most bradycardia is related to physiologic or neurogenic factors, including increased vagal tone related to physical fitness (e.g., the slow, resting heart rate of many endurance athletes) or to other mechanisms that affect

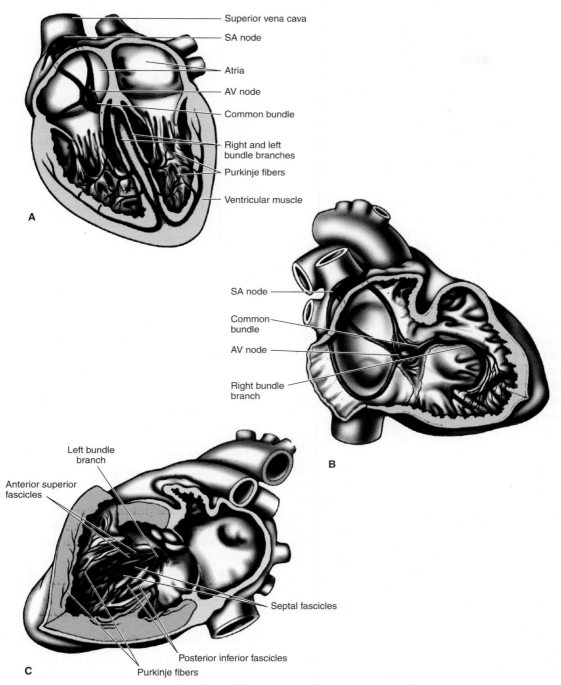

FIGURE 27-2. The anatomy of the conduction system from three different views: (a) anterior, (b) right, (c) left. AV, atrioventricular; SA, sinoatrial.

parasympathetic/sympathetic tone. Sinus bradycardia is defined as having sinus rate <60 bpm. These bradycardias are rarely clinically significant in the absence of heart disease or other myocardial pathology.

Other bradycardias related to sinus or other pacemaker nodal dysfunction, vasovagal reactions, or other pathologic entities can be more problematic. Pathologic pacemaker failure (sometimes called "sick sinus syndrome"), for example, usually requires pacemaker im-

plant. SA block and frequent sinus pauses are other examples of (likely) pathologic bradycardias that may or may not require therapeutic intervention.

SINUS TACHYCARDIA

> **1.4.5-CES: Identify resting and exercise ECG changes associated with the following abnormalities: axis; bundle branch blocks and bifascicular blocks;**

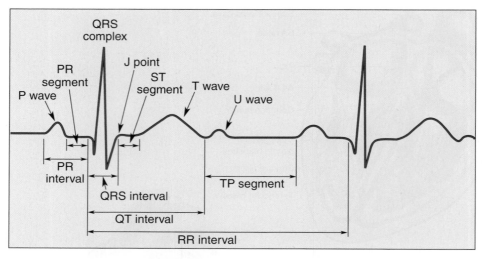

FIGURE 27-3. A normal ECG waveform.

atrioventricular blocks; sinus bradycardia and tachycardia; sinus arrest; supraventricular premature contractions and tachycardia; ventricular premature contractions (including frequency, form, couplets, salvos, tachycardia); atrial flutter and fibrillation; ventricular fibrillation; and myocardial ischemia, injury, and infarction.

Sinus tachycardia is defined by a rate >100 bpm and is the result of an enhanced firing rate of the sinus node. Sinus tachycardia results when increased activity of the sympathetic nervous system is present, including during times of fear, exercise, fever, hypovolemia, bleeding, hypoxia, and other acute illness. Decreased stroke volume in severe LV dysfunction may also result in sinus tachycardia because the sympathetic nervous system is activated in an attempt to preserve adequate cardiac output.

Three key features of sinus tachycardia are important. First, patients typically exhibit a gradual increase in heart rate (i.e., sudden acceleration from 80 to 150 bpm does not occur). Second, although exceptions occur, the sinus rate typically does not exceed the maximum heart rate. Finally, the P-wave must be normal.

Sinus bradycardia occurs when the impulse originates from the sinus node at a rate <60 bpm. This may be pres-

ent in trained individuals with high parasympathetic (vagal) tone, in patients who are receiving drugs that slow the heart rate (e.g., β-blockers), or in individuals who have disease of the sinus node (e.g., sick sinus syndrome).

MECHANISMS OF TACHYDYSRHYTHMIAS

 1.4.8-CES: Describe potential causes of various cardiac arrhythmias.

Three mechanisms are primarily responsible for most cardiac tachydysrhythmias: (a) circus re-entry, (b) enhanced **automaticity**, and (c) triggered activity. Brief explanations of these appear in Box 27-2, but the interested reader is referred to additional recommended reading for more complete explanations.

ATRIAL DYSRHYTHMIAS

 1.4.5-CES: Identify resting and exercise ECG changes associated with the following abnormalities: axis; bundle branch blocks and bifascicular blocks; atrioventricular blocks; sinus bradycardia and tachycardia; sinus arrest; supraventricular premature contractions and tachycardia; ventricular premature contractions (including frequency, form, couplets, salvos, tachycardia); atrial flutter and fibrillation; ventricular fibrillation; and myocardial ischemia, injury, and infarction.

 1.4.1-HFS: Knowledge of how each of the following arrhythmias differs from the normal condition: premature atrial contractions and premature ventricular contractions.

TABLE 27-1. NORMAL SEQUENCE OF DEPOLARIZATION AND THE ECG CORRELATION

Sinoatrial node	Flat
Atrial depolarization	P wave
Atrioventricular node	PR interval
His bundle	PR interval
Purkinje fibers	PR interval
Ventricular muscle depolarization	QRS complex
Ventricular isoelectric period	ST segment
Ventricular muscle repolarization	T wave

> **1.4.8-CES: Describe potential causes and pathophysiology of various cardiac arrhythmias.**

BOX 27-2   MECHANISMS OF TACHYDYSRHYTHMIAS

Enhanced automaticity: An increased rate of depolarization of a single myocardial cell occurs, and the threshold potential is reached rapidly. The cell depolarizes, and that impulse depolarizes the remainder of the myocardium.

Re-entry: The substrate for re-entry requires two pathways. If an impulse arrives at a time when the slow pathway has recovered but the fast pathway is refractory (not recovered from the previous depolarization), the impulse conducts over the slow pathway.

If the slow pathway has recovered, depolarization of the slow path occurs, and a re-entrant loop occurs.

Triggered activity: Triggered activity exhibits features of both re-entry and automaticity. After-depolarization or increases in the membrane potential occur during the repolarization phase of the action potential. If the magnitude of these after-depolarizations is great enough, depolarization may be triggered.

PREMATURE ATRIAL COMPLEXES

Many people experience premature atrial complexes (PACs) or premature ventricular complexes (PVCs) during exercise or other periods when catecholamine levels are increased. PACs occur when an atrial site other than the sinus node depolarizes prematurely. The impulse proceeds through the AV node and the ventricles (in the absence of bundle branch block or myocardial disease) and generates a narrow QRS complex. A series of normal sinus beats alternating with PACs is called atrial bigeminy.

ATRIAL TACHYCARDIA

Atrial tachycardia may be the result of rapid firing of an automatic or triggered atrial focus or re-entry within the atrium (Box 27-2). The ventricular rate depends on the atrial rate and the refractory period of the AV node. The P wave has altered waveform shape, and the PR interval is often short.

ATRIAL FIBRILLATION

Atrial fibrillation (Fig. 27-4) is a relatively common **dysrhythmia** that results from multiple re-entrant waves of depolarization in the atria. These waves are not organized and do not cause contraction of the atria. The characteristics of atrial fibrillation are an irregular ventricular rhythm and rate, often tachycardic. This rhythm may have important consequences, including decreased cardiac output, which can be clinically significant in the presence of compromised left ventricular function, often impairing one's ability to perform physical activities and causing symptoms. Atrial fibrillation increases risk for developing atrial thrombus, which may cause stroke or other embolic events.

Treatment of atrial fibrillation centers on normalizing the ventricular rate with pharmacologic agents, such as digitalis, calcium channel blockers, β-blockers and antiarrhythmic agents. Anticoagulation may also be necessary. Synchronized electrical cardioversion (delivery of a timed electrical shock to the myocardium) may be required if the rhythm persists. Most patients with atrial fibrillation have underlying cardiac disease.

ATRIAL FLUTTER

Atrial flutter (Fig. 27-5) results from a re-entrant circuit in the atria that generates flutter waves, usually at a rate of 250 to 350 per minute. The atrial waves are best visualized in inferior leads (II, III, aVF) or lead V_1. The ventricular rate may or may not be accelerated during atrial flutter, and rhythm may be regular or irregular. Flutter waves typically have a classic "sawtooth" shape and

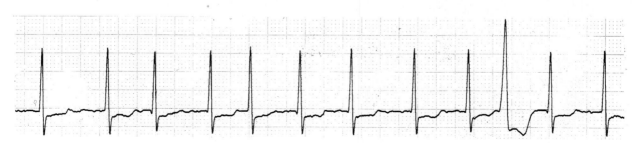

FIGURE 27-4. Atrial fibrillation with rapid ventricular response, along with a single PVC.

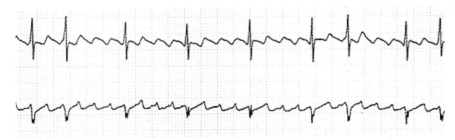

FIGURE 27-5. Atrial flutter with 2:1 atrioventricular conduction.

appearance in inferior leads. There is often 2:1 block (two flutter waves for each ventricular complex), and if the ventricular rate is near 150 bpm, atrial flutter should be considered. This rhythm may convert to sinus rhythm but more often degenerates into atrial fibrillation. Treatment may include pharmacologic agents or radiofrequency catheter ablation.

SUPRAVENTRICULAR TACHYCARDIA

Supraventricular tachycardia (SVT) is any arrhythmia that originates above the AV node. Atrial fibrillation and atrial flutter are types of SVTs. However, there are other mechanisms of SVT including, AV node re-entrant tachycardias, Wolf-Parkinson-White syndrome (WPW), and concealed accessory pathways.

VENTRICULAR DYSRHYTHMIAS

> **1.4.8-CES: Describe potential causes and pathophysiology of various cardiac arrhythmias.**

> **1.4.9-CES: Identify potentially hazardous arrhythmias or conduction defects observed on the ECG at rest, during exercise, and during recovery.**

> **1.4.10-CES: Describe the diagnostic and prognostic significance of ischemic ECG responses and arrhythmias at rest, during exercise, and during recovery.**

> **1.4.1-HFS: Knowledge of how each of the following arrhythmias differs from the normal condition: premature atrial contractions and premature ventricular contractions.**

Unlike many of the atrial dysrhythmias, ventricular dysrhythmias can be serious and even life threatening. Recognition and understanding of these ventricular dysrhythmias is essential to patient safety in ECG and during exercise testing. The exercise professional must be prepared for emergencies, and the presence of ventricular dysrhythmias can be precursors for such emergent situations.

PREMATURE VENTRICULAR COMPLEXES

Premature ventricular complexes (Fig. 27-6) occur when a site in the ventricle fires before the next wave of depolarization from the sinus node reaches the ventricle. PVCs are usually wide QRS complexes and may occur singly, in groups, in runs, or even alternating with sinus beats. The various combinations are defined and named in Box 27-3.

VENTRICULAR TACHYCARDIA

Ventricular tachycardia (Figs. 27-7 and 27-8) is typically seen in patients with underlying heart disease, most commonly CAD or cardiomyopathy. Ventricular tachycardia is defined as three or more consecutive ventricular beats at 100 bpm or faster. Nonsustained ventricular tachycardia lasts <30 seconds, and sustained ventricular tachycardia is generally said to last >30 seconds.

People with ventricular tachycardia can have normal blood pressure and few symptoms if the hemodynamics of the left ventricle are relatively normal and the ventricular rate is low. More commonly, ventricular tachycardia

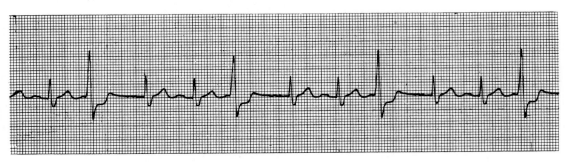

FIGURE 27-6. Normal sinus rhythm with premature ventricular complexes.

BOX 27-3   TYPES OF DYSRHYTHMIC PREMATURE VENTRICULAR COMPLEXES

Couplet: Two consecutive PVCs without intervening sinus beats.

Triplet: Three consecutive PVCs without intervening sinus beats.

Multiform: The PVC waveform changes from beat to beat, indicating that the PVC may emanate from more than one foci in the ventricle or may be the

result of more than a single physiologic or pathologic process.

Bigeminy: A single PVC alternating with single sinus beats.

Trigeminy: Single PVCs alternating with two consecutive sinus beats.

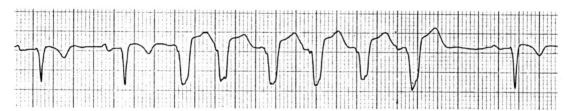

FIGURE 27-7. Normal sinus rhythm with a run of nonsustained ventricular tachycardia.

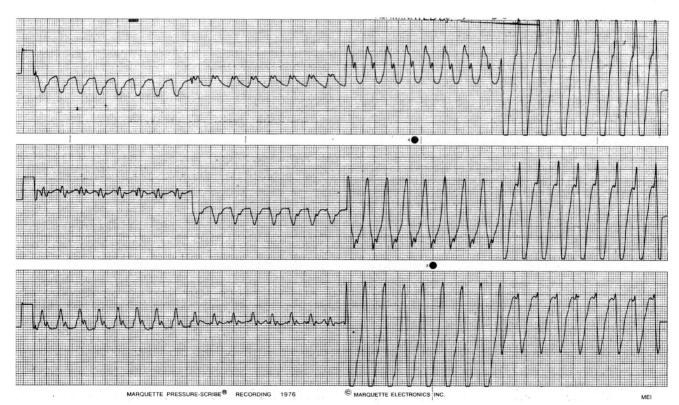

MARQUETTE PRESSURE-SCRIBE® RECORDING 1976   © MARQUETTE ELECTRONICS INC.   MEI

FIGURE 27-8. Sustained ventricular tachycardia as seen in different leads.

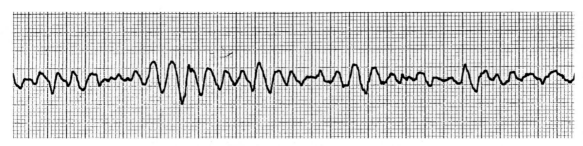

FIGURE 27-9. Ventricular fibrillation (coarse).

compromises hemodynamic status and is associated with sudden death and cardiac arrest. It usually requires emergency measures to resolve.

TORSADE DE POINTES

Torsade de pointes is a type of ventricular tachycardia in which the appearance of the complexes are somewhat "twisted"—thus the name *torsade*. This rhythm is also usually lethal and requires immediate emergent measures to resolve and insure patient safety.

VENTRICULAR FIBRILLATION

Ventricular fibrillation (Fig. 27-9) is a life-threatening rhythm that must be treated with immediate electrical defibrillation per advanced cardiac life support protocol (see Chapter 50 and GETP8 Appendix B).

ATRIOVENTRICULAR (AV) BLOCKS

> **1.4.5-CES: Identify resting and exercise ECG changes associated with the following abnormalities: axis; bundle branch blocks and bifascicular blocks; atrioventricular blocks; sinus bradycardia and tachycardia; sinus arrest; supraventricular premature contractions and tachycardia; ventricular premature contractions (including frequency, form, couplets,**

salvos, tachycardia); atrial flutter and fibrillation; ventricular fibrillation; and myocardial ischemia, injury, and infarction.

> **1.4.9-CES: Identify potentially hazardous arrhythmias or conduction defects observed on the ECG at rest, during exercise, and during recovery.**

There are generally three accepted classifications of AV block. **First-degree** AV block is a prolongation of the PR interval. This may be the result of intra- or interatrial conduction delay, delayed conduction through the AV node, impaired conduction through the His–Purkinje system, or a combination thereof.

Second-degree AV block (Figs. 27-10, 27-11) may be divided into type I and type II. Type I is also known as Wenckebach. The PR interval progressively lengthens until a P wave is not conducted to the ventricles. Type II is characterized by a fixed PR interval until a P wave is not conducted. Type II block is often associated with a wide QRS complex. A rhythm disorder that may cause interpretive confusion is called *2:1 AV block*. Typically, in AV block, the pathology is present below the AV node.

Third-degree or complete heart block (Figure 27-12) occurs when the atrial activity is not conducted through the AV junction to generate a QRS complex, thus atrial and ventricular depolarizations (and, therefore, contractions) are unrelated. The atrial rate is faster than the

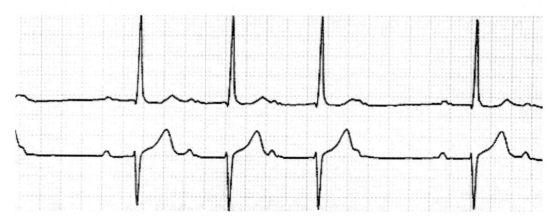

FIGURE 27-10. Second-degree, type I atrioventricular block (Wenckebach).

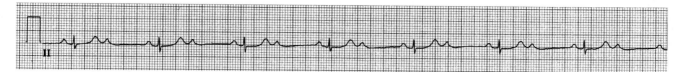

FIGURE 27-11. Second-degree, type II atrioventricular block.

ventricular rate, and the P waves have no influence on the QRS complexes. QRS complexes may be narrow or wide.

BUNDLE BRANCH BLOCKS

Bundle branch blocks are characterized by a wide QRS complex ($\geq$120 ms). Wide QRS complexes usually result from disease in the bundle branches or ventricular abnormalities but may also be related to the effects of drugs, electrolyte, or metabolic disorders. These blocks are classified as right bundle branch block (RBBB), left bundle branch block (LBBB), or nonspecific intraventricular conduction defects (IVCDs). A QRS $\geq$120 ms without the morphology of RBBB or LBBB is best termed a *nonspecific IVCD*.

In RBBB (Fig. 27-13), activation of the LV occurs before that of the RV. After the septum is depolarized, the impulse travels through the LV, generating the initial portion of the QRS complex. After the LV has been partially depolarized, the RV depolarizes, resulting in a triphasic complex in lead V_1, (and often also in V_2) sometimes described as a "rabbit ears" or an RSR complex. RBBB does not prohibit ECG interpretation of ST changes in leads other than V_1, V_2, and V_3.

In LBBB (Fig. 27-14), the initial force travels across the septum from right to left, altering the initial QRS deflection. This results in an initial negative deflection in lead V_1 and an initial upright deflection in lead V_6. The depolarization of the RV is obscured by the LV. The repolarization pattern is altered in LBBB, thus the ECG may not be used to ascertain ischemic ST-T changes during exercise.

FASCICULAR BLOCKS

Fascicular block, also known as *hemiblocks*, are recognized by their effects on the frontal plane axis. Disease in the left bundle branch results in minimal prolongation of the QRS complex. Left anterior **fascicular block** causes significant left axis deviation, resulting in small Q waves in lead I and aVL and small R waves in leads II, III, and aVF. Left posterior fascicular block produces right axis deviation with small Q waves in leads II, III, and aVF and small R waves in leads I and aVL. Unlike left bundle branch, these entities have no adverse effect on the ability to interpret ECG changes during exercise testing. A fascicular block plus a bundle branch block is known as a bifascicular block.

MYOCARDIAL ISCHEMIA

> **1.4.2-CES: Describe myocardial ischemia and identify ischemic indicators of various cardiovascular diagnostic tests.**

> **1.4.7-CES: Identify ECG changes that correspond to ischemia in various myocardial regions.**

> **1.4.10-CES: Describe the diagnostic and prognostic significance of ischemic ECG responses and arrhythmias at rest, during exercise, or during recovery.**

Myocardial ischemia is the result of inadequate supply of oxygen to the myocardium. It is usually a reversible phenomenon. Myocardial infarction (MI) occurs when a portion of the myocardium receives inadequate oxygen supply for several minutes or longer, resulting in the death of myocardial cells in the affected area. Certain ECG changes are associated with both of these events.

Myocardial ischemia is reflected by ECG changes, including ST-segment depression or inversion of the T waves. ECG changes are normally considered as part of the entire clinical picture when diagnosing myocardial ischemia. The location of the ischemia may be determined

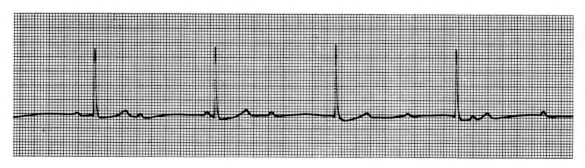

FIGURE 27-12. Complete heart block.

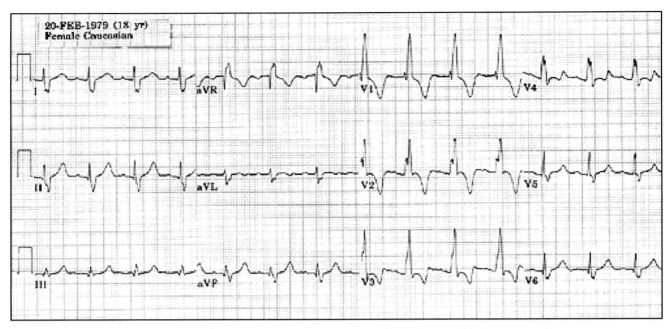

FIGURE 27-13. Normal sinus rhythm with right bundle branch block.

by noting the leads in which the ST or T-wave changes occur (Table 27-2). Resting ST-T segment changes, especially ST segment elevation, are associated with transmural myocardial ischemia, are termed a *current of injury,* and are associated with acute MI.

MYOCARDIAL INFARCTION

> **1.4.2-CES: Describe myocardial ischemia, and identify ischemic indicators of various cardiovascular diagnostic tests.**

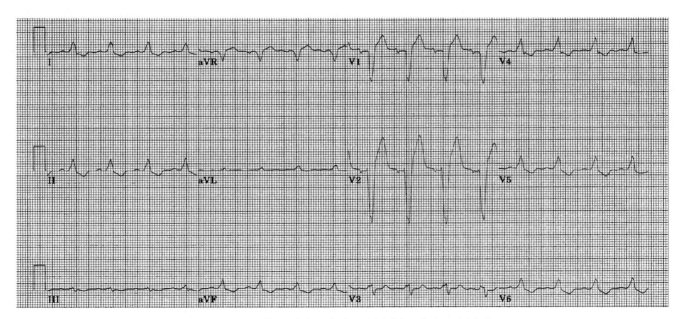

FIGURE 27-14. Normal sinus rhythm with left bundle branch block.

1.4.7-CES: Identify ECG changes that correspond to ischemia in various myocardial regions.

TABLE 27-2. LOCATIONS OF MYOCARDIAL INFARCTION AND ISCHEMIA

LOCATION	LEADS AFFECTED
Anteroseptal	V_1, V_2
Anterior	V_1–V_4
Extensive anterior	V_1–V_6, I, aVL
Anterolateral	V_3–V_6, I, aVL
High lateral	I, aVL
Inferior	II, III, aVF
Posterior	V_1, V_2 (ST depression, tall R waves noted)

 1.4.3-CES: Describe the differences between Q-wave and non-Q-wave infarction, and ST elevation (STEMI) and non-ST elevation myocardial infarction (non-STEMI).

 1.4.7-CES: Identify ECG changes that correspond to ischemia in various myocardial regions.

 1.4.10-CES: Describe the diagnostic and prognostic significance of ischemic ECG responses and arrhythmias at rest, during exercise, or during recovery.

Myocardial infarction results from the near-total or total occlusion of a coronary artery, blocking blood flow to an area of the myocardium. ECG changes may include ST-T segment changes; peaked T waves; various types of blocks and ventricular dysrhythmias, including single and multiple PVCs; ventricular tachycardia; and ventricular fibrillation. The magnitude of ischemia is usually considered to be proportional to the degree of ST-segment depression, the number of ECG leads involved, and the duration of ST-segment depression in recovery (Figs. 27-15 and 27-16).

In the days and weeks following an MI, T waves often invert, and ST segments gradually return to baseline. Depending on the location and extent of myocardial damage, Q waves and/or loss of R waves may also develop. MIs that are not accompanied by Q waves or ST-segment elevation are called non-ST elevation myocardial infarction (non-STEMI), whereas MIs that are accompanied by the aforementioned ST-T changes are called ST elevation myocardial infarction (STEMI). Patients with non-STEMI infarcts have a better short-term but a worse long-term prognosis than patients with STEMI.

Acute injury or infarct is often diagnosed by the presence of ST elevation or hyperacute T waves. Q waves, baseline ST segments, and inverted T waves indicate recent MI (2 weeks to 1 year) or are often read as "of indeterminate age." If only Q waves with no ST- or T-wave changes are present, the infarction is considered "remote." Specific combinations or configurations of leads with abnormalities (Q waves, loss of R wave amplitude, etc.) indicate the region of the ischemia and infarction (see Table 27-2).

Causes of ST-segment elevation other than myocardial injury and infarction are common. **Acute pericarditis** (Fig. 27-17) causes generalized ST-segment elevation (usually a concave appearance) in all ECG leads, whereas acute injury and infarction caused by CAD usually affects adjacent leads.

Benign or early repolarization variants are another common cause of ST-segment elevation. These variants are most commonly seen in young African-American men but may be seen in other patients as well. Elevation of the J point is present, and the ST segments are elevated but exhibit a concave upward appearance (Fig. 27-18).

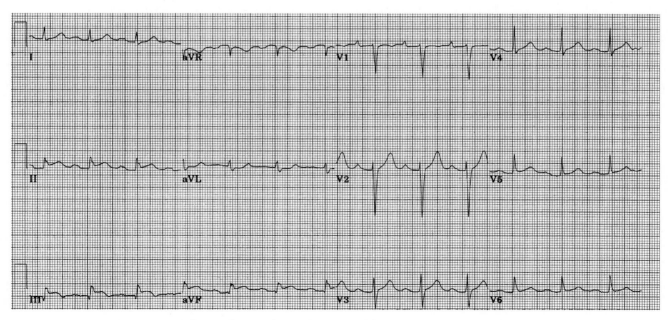

FIGURE 27-15. Acute inferior wall injury. Abnormal P waves and first-degree atrioventricular block are also evident.

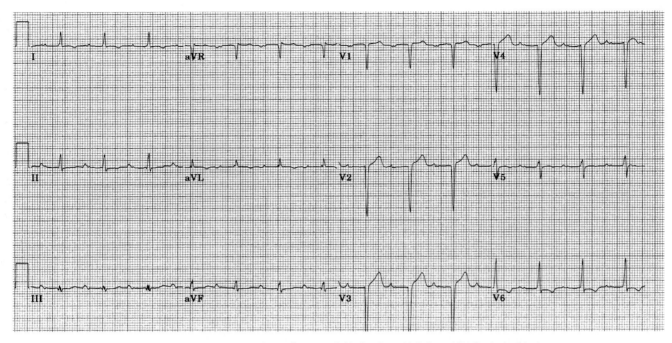

FIGURE 27-16. Recent anterior wall myocardial infarction with left anterior fascicular block.

PACEMAKERS AND INTERNAL DEFIBRILLATORS

> **1.4.4-CES: Identify the ECG patterns at rest and responses to exercise in patients with pacemakers and implantable cardioverter defibrillators. In addition, recognize the ability of biventricular pacing and possibility of pacemaker malfunction (e.g., failure to sense and failure to pace).**

Pacemakers (PMs), implantable cardioverter defibrillators (ICDs), and other electronic devices used for therapy of dysrhythmias exhibit ECG "signatures" that indicate their presence. They are implanted for treatment of sudden death and dangerous ventricular dysrhythmias, sinus node dysfunction, certain AV blocks, severe bradycardias associated with diseases of the conduction system, and most recently, for chronic congestive heart failure (CHF). These biventricular PMs deliver an inno-

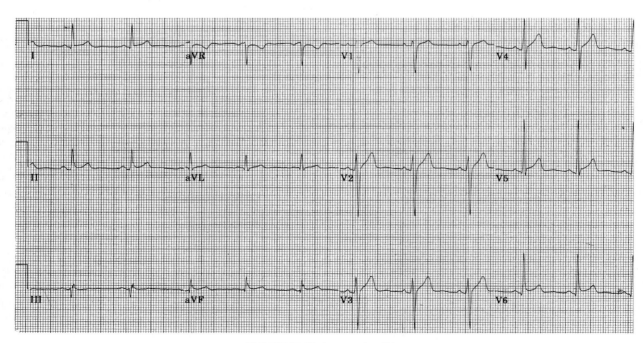

FIGURE 27-17. Acute pericarditis.

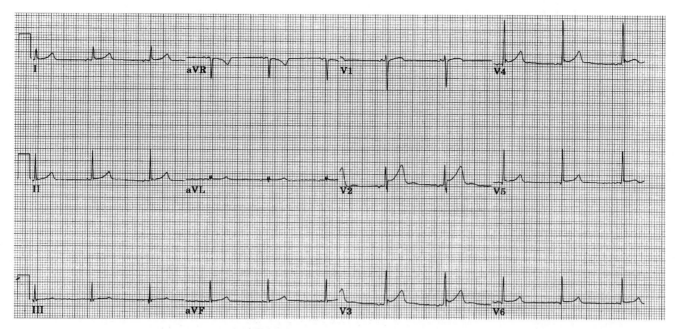

FIGURE 27-18. Benign repolarization variant.

vative therapy called cardiac resynchronization therapy, which, in specific subpopulations of people with CHF, is very effective at decreasing symptoms and increasing functional capacity.

The usual indicator of such devices is a "pacemaker" spike that precedes either the P wave or the QRS complex, depending on the type and role of the PM implanted. The ECG is not necessarily abnormal or altered by the PM, other than the presence of the spike, but may be abnormal because of the inherent pathology that required the PM. Figure 27-19 is an example of a 12-lead ECG with PM spikes. Pacemakers are "coded" according to a five-letter system. The convention for the system is, in the order of the letter:

1. Chamber paced (A = atrium; V = ventricle; D = dual or A + V)
2. Chamber sensed (A = atrium; V = ventricle; D = dual or A + V)
3. Response to sensing (T = triggered; I = inhibited; D = dual)
4. Rate modulation (R = rate modulation)
5. Multisite pacing (A = atrium; V = ventricle; D = dual or A + V)

A pacemaker-coded *DDDV* would, therefore, be one that paces both atria and ventricles, that senses both, that responds to both chambers, and that paces only ventricles.

EXERCISE ELECTROCARDIOGRAPHY

> **1.4.9-CES: Identify potentially hazardous arrhythmias or conduction defects observed on the ECG at rest, during exercise, and during recovery.**

> **1.4.10-CES: Describe the diagnostic and prognostic significance of ischemic ECG responses and arrhythmias at rest, during exercise, or during recovery.**

> **1.4.16-CES: Describe the diagnostic and prognostic implications of the exercise test ECG and hemodynamic responses.**

MYOCARDIAL ISCHEMIA

Electrocardiogram exercise testing can detect **dysrhythmias** and ischemic changes precipitated by or associated with exercise, but in the absence of additional diagnostic tools, such as echocardiography or nuclear imaging, it may be less sensitive and specific than necessary for proper diagnosis of CAD. Dysrhythmias, discussed above, are sometimes elicited and appear during exercise or postexercise. Individuals performing exercise testing, particularly in those who are at moderate to high risk for disease, should be comfortable with interpretation of dysrhythmias and with advanced cardiac life support (ACLS).

Ischemia may induce ST-segment depression during exercise testing, but if baseline ST-T changes are present, the test becomes less specific (see definition of specificity and sensitivity in Chapters 21 and 22 of this resource manual). Both the magnitude and the character of the ST depression are important. Horizontal or downsloping ST depression is more specific for CAD than upsloping ST depression. The subendocardial area of the left ventricular apex is most often rendered ischemic during exercise, therefore the ST segment shifts in V_4, V_5, and V_6 are the most sensitive for detection of ischemia.

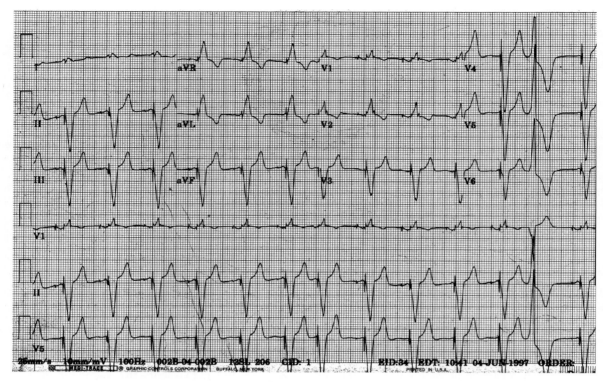

FIGURE 27-19. DDD pacemaker with pacing spikes present before the P waves and QRS complexes.

Criteria for terminating an exercise test are found in Table 27-3 and in Chapter 5 (Box 5-2) of ACSM's Guidelines for Exercise Testing and Prescription, 8th edition (Table 27-3).

Persistent ST-segment elevation after an infarction may suggest **ventricular aneurysm** formation. This typically involves the anterior wall of the left ventricle and occurs after large infarcts. The presence of Q waves in the involved leads in a patient after MI suggests this diagnosis.

FACTORS AFFECTING INTERPRETATION OF THE ST SEGMENT

 1.4.8-CES: Describe potential causes of various cardiac arrhythmias.

Digitalis is a medication that interferes with the interpretation of ST-T segment changes for myocardial ischemia. Digitalis is often used to treat patients with congestive heart failure or atrial dysrhythmias. Digitalis may cause

 1.4.6-CES: Define the ECG criteria for initiating and/or terminating exercise testing or training.

TABLE 27-3. INDICATIONS FOR TERMINATING EXERCISE TESTING

ABSOLUTE INDICATIONS

- Drop in systolic blood pressure of >10 mm Hg from baseline[a] blood pressure despite an increase in workload when accompanied by other evidence of ischemia
- Moderately severe angina (defined as 3 on standard scale)
- Increasing nervous system symptoms (e.g., ataxia, dizziness, or near syncope)
- Signs of poor perfusion (cyanosis or pallor)
- Technical difficulties monitoring the ECG or systolic blood pressure
- Subject's desire to stop
- Sustained ventricular tachycardia
- ST elevation (+1.0 mm) in leads without diagnostic Q waves (other than V_1 or aVR)

RELATIVE INDICATIONS

- Drop in systolic blood pressure of >10 mm Hg from baseline[a] blood pressure despite an increase in workload in the absence of other evidence of ischemia
- ST or QRS changes, such as excessive ST depression (>2 mm horizontal or downsloping ST-segment depression) or marked axis shift
- Arrhythmias other than sustained ventricular tachycardia, including multifocal PVCs, triplets of PVCs, supraventricular tachycardia, heart block, or bradyarrhythmias
- Fatigue, shortness of breath, wheezing, leg cramps, or claudication
- Development of bundle branch block or intraventricular conduction delay that cannot be distinguished from ventricular tachycardia
- Increasing chest pain
- Hypertensive response (systolic blood pressure of >250 mm Hg and/or a diastolic blood pressure of >115 mm Hg)

ECG, electrocardiogram; PVC, premature ventricular complex.

[a]*Baseline* refers to a measurement obtained immediately before the test and in the same posture as the test is being performed.

Modified from Gibbons RJ, Balady GJ, Bricker JT, et al. ACC/AHA 2002 Guideline Update for Exercise Testing: a report of the American College of Cardiology/American Heart Association Task Force on Practice Guidelines Committee on Exercise Testing, 2002. Available at: www.acc.org/clinical/guidelines/exercise/dirIndex.htm. Accessed on June 15, 2007.

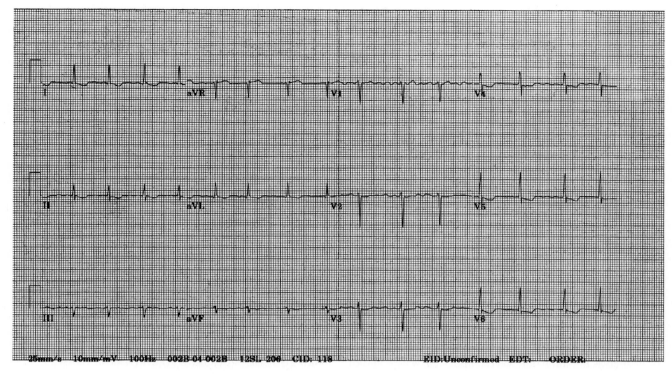

FIGURE 27-20. ST depression caused by digitalis. The rhythm is atrial fibrillation.

false-positive stress ECG findings by depressing the ST segment (Fig. 27-20). Additional imaging modalities may be required to increase the specificity of the study.

Electrolyte disorders are associated with ECG changes that may also interfere with ST-T segment interpretation. Hyperkalemia can cause prolonged QRS interval, peaked T waves, and even disappearance of P waves. Hypokalemia can be associated with diminished T waves, prolonged QT interval, and prominent U waves. Hypocalcemia can prolong QT interval, whereas hypercalcemia can shorten QT interval. Note that prolonged QT interval can predispose individuals to malignant ventricular tachycardias. Those individuals with prolonged QT should be referred to a cardiologist or an electrophysiologist for further assessment before exercise testing.

CHAMBER ENLARGEMENT

> **1.4.11-CES: Identify resting and exercise ECG changes associated with cardiovascular disease, hypertensive heart disease, cardiac chamber enlargement, pericarditis, pulmonary disease, and metabolic disorders.**

VENTRICULAR HYPERTROPHY

All four chambers can be physiologically enlarged as a result of several common pathologic conditions, including pulmonary disease, valvular disease, ischemic disease, and congenital heart disease. The ECG can be used as one diagnostic tool for evaluating chamber enlargement, but other diagnostic tools, including echocardiography and angiography, are considered gold standards for these diagnoses. Although some specific criteria for chamber enlargement exist, they should be considered within the entire clinical picture and should direct further diagnostic assessment.

Ventricular hypertrophy (right or left) can be either hypertrophic (increased ventricular mass and wall thickness) or dilated (decreased ventricular mass and wall thickness).

Increased voltages in R waves across the myocardium are usual indicators of left ventricular hypertrophy (LVH). There are several ECG systems (scoring systems) that assist in this diagnosis. One of these systems, Estes criteria for LVH, is illustrated in Table 27-4. **Left ventricular hypertrophy** (Fig. 27-21) can be a cause of ST-segment changes without the presence of ischemia. Long-standing hypertension (especially untreated) is often associated with LVH. The presence of LVH on the baseline tracing may result in an indeterminate or false-positive stress ECG result. **Right ventricular hypertrophy** (RVH) is less common than LVH and is usually associated with pulmonary disease. Table 27-5 outlines the requisites for ECG manifestations of RVH.

TABLE 27-4. ESTES ELECTROCARDIOGRAM CRITERIA FOR THE DETERMINATION OF LEFT VENTRICULAR ENLARGEMENT

	POINTS
1. Any of the following	
R or S in limb lead ≥20 mm	
S wave in V1, V2, V3, ≥25 mm	
R wave in V4, V5, V6 ≥25 mm	3
2. Any ST shift	3
Typical strain ST-T changes:	1
3. LAD >15 degrees	2
4. QRS interval >0.09 sec	1
5. Intrisicoid deflection >0.04 sec	1
6. P- terminal force V1 >0.04	3
Total (LVH >5 points, probable LVH >4 points)	13

Adapted with permission from Wagner GS. Marriott's Practical Electrocardiography, 9th ed. Baltimore: Williams & Wilkins, 1994.

ATRIAL ENLARGEMENT

Atrial enlargement may or may not be associated with ventricular hypertrophy. Atrial hypertrophy (both right and left) is associated with changes in P-wave morphology. Features such as notching of P waves, biphasic P waves, and/or tall, peaked P waves are often seen in atrial enlargement.

METABOLIC DISORDERS

Metabolic disorders, such as thyroid disorders and obesity, as well as other conditions, such as hypothermia, are associated with ECG changes. See Table 27-6 for examples of those changes.

TABLE 27-5. ELECTROCARDIOGRAPHIC MANIFESTATIONS OF RIGHT VENTRICULAR HYPERTROPHY

Right axis deviation
R wave in V1 >than 7 mm
R in V1 + 5 in V5 or V6 >10 mm
R:S ratio in V1 >1.0
S:R in V6 >1.0
Right intraventricular conduction defect
Right ventricular strain pattern in V1, V2, or II, III, and aVF

Adapted with permission from Wagner GS. Marriott's Practical Electrocardiography, 9th ed. Baltimore: Williams & Wilkins, 1994.

> **1.4.11-CES: Identify resting and exercise ECG changes associated with cardiovascular disease, hypertensive heart disease, cardiac chamber enlargement, pericarditis, pulmonary disease, and metabolic disorders.**

TABLE 27-6. METABOLIC DISEASE AND ELECTROCARDIOGRAM

METABOLIC DISORDERS AND ELECTROCARDIOGRAM CHANGES

Thyroid conditions	
Hypothyroid	• Decreased sinus rate
Hyperthyroid	• Increased sinus rate
Obesity	• Increased sinus rate
	• Increased PR, QRS, and QTc interval
Hypothermia	• Lengthened PR, RR, QRS, and QT intervals
	• J point deflection (called *Osborn waves*)

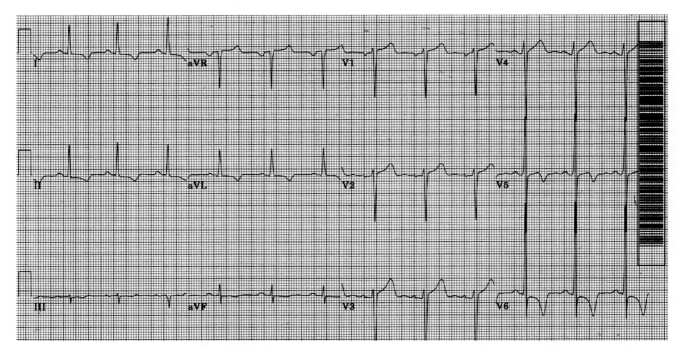

FIGURE 27-21. Left ventricular hypertrophy with left atrial enlargement.

SUMMARY

Electrocardiography and exercise electrocardiography, as well as associated diagnostic procedures, are basic and fundamental methods of evaluation in cardiovascular disease and health assessment. To provide safe and effective care for patients, exercise professionals must have knowledge of both normal and abnormal cardiovascular physiology and pathophysiology that can lead to changes in the ECG, as well as the waveforms and patterns that are associated with the pathophysiology. This chapter attempts to provide the basic principles and information for ECG.

SELECTED REFERENCES FOR FURTHER READING

Atwood S, Stanton C, Storey-Davenport J. *Introduction to Basic Dysrhythmias.* 3rd ed. St. Louis: Mosby; 2003.

Dubin D. *Rapid Interpretation of EKGs: An Interactive Course.* Tampa (FL): Cover Publishing Company; 2001.

Ellenbogen KA, Kay GN, Lau C, Wilkoff BL. *Clinical Cardiac Pacing, Defibrillation and Resynchronization Therapy.* Philadelphia: Saunders-Elsevier Pub; 2007.

ECG Interpretation: An Incredibly Easy! Pocket Guide. 4th ed. Philadelphia: Lippincott/Springhouse Nursing Collection; 2007.

Huff J. *ECG Workout: Exercises in Arrhythmia Interpretation.* 4th ed. Philadelphia: JB Lippincott; 2002.

Huzar RJ. *Basic Dysrhythmias: Interpretation and Management,* 3rd ed. St. Louis: Mosby; 2002.

Lip GYH, Godtfredsen J. *Cardiac Arrhythmias.* St. Louis: Mosby; 2003.

Thaler MS. *The Only EKG Book You'll Ever Need.* 4th ed. Philadelphia: Lippincott Williams & Wilkins; 2003.

Wagner GS. *Marriott's Practical Electrocardiography.* 11th ed. Philadelphia: Lippincott Williams & Wilkins; 2007.

INTERNET RESOURCES

- The Alan E. Lindsay ECG Learning Center: http://medstat.med.utah.edu/kw/ecg
- ECG Library: www.ecglibrary.com

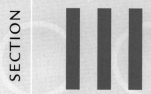

III

Exercise Prescription

DAVID SWAIN, PhD, FACSM
and
JONATHAN K. EHRMAN, PhD, FACSM, *Section Editors*

Cardiorespiratory capacity is the maximum ability to perform large muscle, dynamic exercise through the use of oxygen—i.e., maximum oxygen consumption ($\dot{V}O_{2max}$). Cardiorespiratory capacity is the best indicator of the fitness of the heart, vasculature, and pulmonary system. Attaining a high level of cardiorespiratory capacity requires the development of a large cardiac output (via a large stroke volume), vascular adaptations to deliver blood flow to the working muscles without excessive increases in systemic arterial blood pressure, tissue adaptations to increase the utilization of oxygen, and sufficient alveolar ventilation and gas exchange to support the body's demand for oxygen. **Cardiorespiratory endurance** is the ability to perform a given intensity of large muscle, dynamic exercise—i.e., aerobic exercise—for prolonged periods of time. Cardiorespiratory endurance is related, in part, to the ability to effectively process substrates for energy while avoiding or postponing glycogen depletion and also avoiding an excessive buildup of lactic acid in the blood. The lactate and ventilatory thresholds are useful indicators of cardiorespiratory endurance. Cardiorespiratory capacity and endurance, along with muscle strength, muscle endurance, flexibility, body composition, balance, and agility, are two of the components of physical fitness.

Both physical activity (31,48) and cardiorespiratory capacity (3) have been found to produce significant health benefits. However, cardiorespiratory capacity is more strongly correlated with a reduced risk of heart disease than is physical activity (50). **Physical activity** is defined as any bodily movement produced by skeletal muscles that results in energy expenditure (48). The physiologic adaptations resulting from cardiorespiratory exercise are described in Chapter 30, and the health benefits from physical activity and exercise are summarized in GETP8 Chapter 1. This chapter addresses the prescription of cardiorespiratory exercise to achieve health and physical fitness benefits for apparently healthy adults, as presented in GETP8 Chapter 7. Cardiorespiratory exercise prescription to treat or rehabilitate individuals with chronic disease, and for other special populations, is covered in other chapters of this Resource Manual.

PRINCIPLES OF TRAINING

Exercise training is defined as planned, structured, and repetitive bodily movement done to improve or maintain one or more components of physical fitness. The principles of training apply more to exercise training and exercise

> > > **KEY TERMS**

Cardiorespiratory capacity: The maximum ability to perform aerobic exercise ($\dot{V}O_{2max}$).

Cardiorespiratory endurance: The ability to perform submaximal aerobic exercise for prolonged periods of time.

Exercise prescription: Individualized exercise design based on specific assessment information.

Exercise training: Planned, structured, and repetitive bodily movement done to improve or maintain one or more components of physical fitness.

FITT principle: A method of prescribing exercise that incorporates *Frequency*, *Intensity*, *Time* (duration), and *Type* (mode).

Heart rate reserve (HRR): The range of heart rate from rest to maximum; a percentage of this range is typically used to establish target heart rates in training, as %HRR provides similar intensities as equivalent values of %$\dot{V}O_2$R.

Physical activity: Any bodily movement produced by skeletal muscles that results in energy expenditure.

$\dot{V}O_2$ reserve ($\dot{V}O_2$R): The range of oxygen consumption from rest to maximum; a percentage of this range is used to establish cardiorespiratory exercise intensity.

therapy than to physical activity. A basic assumption in exercise programming is that something useful or beneficial occurs as a result of repeated bouts of exercise. This assumption is predicated on several physiologic principles. The most central of these is the *principle of adaptation*, which states that if a specific physiologic capacity is taxed by a physical training stimulus within a certain range and on a regular basis, this physiologic capacity usually expands. Adaptation also depends on two correlated physiologic principles: *threshold* and *overload*. To elicit an adaptation, the physiologic capacity must be challenged beyond a certain minimal intensity called the *training threshold*. If the training stimulus exceeds this threshold, it is a training *overload*, and the process of physiologic adaptation will occur. As the physiologic capacities of the body expand, the initial training stimulus may be rendered subthreshold, and the workload must increase (*progression*) to maintain overload. The concept of progression also encompasses the practice of using very modest intensities of work during the initial sessions of an exercise program. *Detraining* refers to a cessation or diminution of training that results in a decrease in physiologic capacity—i.e., the loss of previous adaptations. *Overtraining* is a when the overload is excessive relative to the amount of time allotted for recovery, resulting in a chronic overtaxing of physiologic systems and a decrease in performance. The term *overreaching* is sometimes used to refer to a brief period of excessive overload that may overtax the body but does not result in overt decreases in ability.

A final principle of central importance in exercise programming is the concept of *specificity*. Specific physiologic capacities expand only if they are stressed in the course of an exercise program. For example, swimmers have an 11% increase in swim ergometry performance over the course of a training season but show no change in run time to exhaustion on a treadmill (25).

Each of these principles guides the design of an exercise program. In exercise training, the mode of exercise—as well as the frequency, duration, and intensity of training—are critical in achieving fitness, athletic, or health outcomes. The mode must be specific to the targeted component of fitness, and the frequency, duration, and intensity must be combined in a systematic overload that will result in physiologic adaptations.

DESIGNING AN EXERCISE PRESCRIPTION

> **1.7.27-HFS: Ability to differentiate between the amount of physical activity required for health benefits and/or for fitness development.**

The process of **exercise prescription** can be divided into three steps, which are illustrated in Figure 28-1. The first step is assessing health and fitness information. The second step is to interpret that information. The third step is to formulate an exercise prescription based on the interpreted information and the goals of the client.

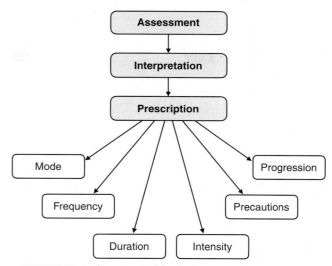

FIGURE 28-1. The process of developing an exercise prescription.

Exercise training spans a broad continuum from improving and maintaining physical fitness, including athletic performance, to disease prevention, treatment, and rehabilitation. Exercise prescription is a means of using the principles of training along with assessment to provide an effective exercise training regimen. The nature of the assessments (see Chapter 12) may vary by setting (clinical vs. health or fitness), program goals (weight loss vs. athletic performance), and clientele (low fit vs. high fit).

An example of exercise prescription in the commercial health and fitness industry is when an exercise professional uses information from a health and medical history, anthropometric estimation of body fat, one-repetition maximum, and submaximal cycle ergometer test with heart rate (HR) monitoring to develop an exercise program for a client. On the opposite end of the spectrum, for exercise prescription in the clinical setting, medical records, blood reports, pulmonary function tests, and symptom-limited maximal exercise testing with the analysis of expired gases and electrocardiography (ECG) may be incorporated to develop an exercise prescription to treat a patient with chronic obstructive pulmonary disease.

One of the most common uses of exercise training in the health and fitness setting has been to improve physical fitness. As stated earlier, the mode is selected specific to the targeted fitness component, whether it is muscle strength, muscle endurance, cardiorespiratory capacity, cardiorespiratory endurance, or flexibility. Intensity, duration, and frequency combine to create the overload. After fitness is achieved, exercise training can be modified to maintain physical fitness. Most often, the overload duration or frequency can be reduced to maintain the physical fitness. Athletic performance requires similar but more intensive exercise training. In addition to the higher levels of physical fitness, skill practice and strategic development combine to develop athletic performance. Exercise therapy is the use of exercise training to treat modern chronic diseases and associated comorbidities. Certain health benefits, including a reduced risk of coronary heart disease, accrue from a general increase in physical activity. The Surgeon General recommends at least 30 minutes of moderate-intensity physical activity on most days of the week to obtain these benefits (48). The Surgeon General also states that greater levels of duration and intensity result in additional health benefits (48). Current evidence suggests that the best reductions in cardiovascular risk occur when a prescribed program of exercise training aimed at improving cardiorespiratory fitness is employed (43).

ELEMENTS OF THE EXERCISE PRESCRIPTION

Although the purpose of exercise may range from the training of athletes to the treatment of disease, the exercise prescription can be expressed with the *FITT* principle, incorporating *F*requency, *I*ntensity, *T*ime (i.e., duration), and *T*ype (i.e., mode). Of these four elements, the *type*, or mode of exercise, should be selected first, using the specificity principle of training to choose a type of exercise that will stimulate the desired outcome. *Frequency* is typically the number of exercise sessions per week or, in some cases, per day. *Intensity* is the level of effort, which may be expressed relative to the client's maximum ability, specifically as a percentage of oxygen consumption reserve ($\dot{V}O_2R$), the difference between resting $\dot{V}O_2$ and maximum $\dot{V}O_2$. Once selected, the intensity can be translated to a heart rate, workload, or subjective level of perceived exertion. *Time* is the duration of each session, not including warm-up and cool-down, generally expressed in minutes. As stated earlier, frequency, intensity, and time combine to produce an overload.

The total *volume* of exercise is determined by the product of frequency, intensity, and duration. If the $\dot{V}O_2$ or workload of the exercise is known, then this volume can be expressed as the number of kilocalories expended per week through exercise (i.e., the net value above resting energy expenditure; see below for calculations). This net energy expenditure can be used to estimate expected fat weight loss.

Progression of the absolute intensity must occur as the client's fitness improves to maintain an overload. However, the relative intensity may remain the same. For example, if a patient initially walks at 3 mph (4.8 kph) to achieve 50% HRR, in a few weeks the patient may need to walk at 4 mph (5.4 kph) to attain the same heart rate. Of course, the relative intensity can also be increased. For example, a new target of 60% HRR may be prescribed to further develop the client's aerobic capacity. Although progression of intensity is important, progression is also applied to duration and frequency, especially in the case of weight loss prescription.

Precautions for exercise are the modifications in the prescription or the additional concerns that must be addressed for each disease process, comorbidity, or disability to make exercise safe (see Chapters 34–41). For example, individuals with diabetes who exercise should be given several precautions for the timing of meals, insulin injections, and glucose monitoring that are not given to individuals without diabetes who exercise (see Chapter 37 and GETP8 Chapter 10). Precautions given to individuals with angina are not the same as those given to individuals with low back pain. Each chronic disease and disability has a specific set of precautions.

DEVELOPING CARDIORESPIRATORY FITNESS

> **1.7.10-HFS: Knowledge of the recommended intensity, duration, frequency, and type of physical activity necessary for development of cardiorespiratory fitness in an apparently healthy population.**

The 1998 American College of Sports Medicine (ACSM) position stand on the recommended quantity and quality of exercise for developing and maintaining cardiorespiratory fitness in healthy adults (33) provided the following recommendations for developing cardiorespiratory fitness:

- **Frequency:** 3 to 5 days per week
- **Intensity:** 40%/50% to 85% of $\dot{V}O_2R$
- **Time (duration):** 20 to 60 min
- **Type (mode):** Continuous, rhythmic exercise using large muscle groups

These recommendations were used in the 6th and 7th editions of GTEP and have been modified as follows in the 8th edition:

- **Frequency:** If only performing moderate intensity, at least 5 days per week
  If only performing vigorous intensity, at least 3 days per week
  If performing a combination of moderate and vigorous, 3 to 5 days per week
- **Intensity:** Moderate, defined as 40% to 59% of $\dot{V}O_2R$
  Vigorous, defined as $\geq$60% of $\dot{V}O_2R$
- **Time (duration):** 20 to 60 min
- **Type (mode):** Continuous, rhythmic exercise using large muscle groups
- **Volume:** A minimum of 1,000 kcal·wk^{-1}; 2,000 to 4,000 kcal·wk^{-1} may be optimal

An exercise program that follows these guidelines will result in an increase in both cardiorespiratory capacity and cardiorespiratory endurance. Higher-intensity training places more emphasis on the development of capacity, whereas longer duration training places more emphasis on the development of endurance and also allows one to accumulate a large volume of energy expenditure for purposes of weight loss.

PRESCRIBING MODE

In accordance with the principle of specificity, cardiorespiratory (i.e., aerobic) exercises should be used to improve cardiorespiratory fitness. Cardiorespiratory exercises are continuous, rhythmic exercises that use a large amount of muscle mass and require aerobic metabolic pathways to sustain the activity. The requirement of a large amount of muscle mass is to cause a sufficient increase in total body oxygen consumption to result in adaptations of the central cardiopulmonary system, not just adaptations in the locally active muscle. Examples of these exercises include walking, jogging, cycling, swimming, rowing, dancing, in-line skating, and cross-country skiing.

Cardiorespiratory activities can be classified by skill and energy expenditure, as listed in Table 28-1. Group A&B activities are recommended for exercise programs in which it is important to regulate and maintain the intensity of effort. Group A and B activities provide predictable levels of energy expenditure that are not significantly affected by age, sex, or skill and are affected by body weight in a predictable manner. For example, walking and jogging require the same relative oxygen consumption (expressed in $mL \cdot kg^{-1} \cdot min^{-1}$) from individuals of different sizes, whereas the absolute oxygen consumption ($L \cdot min^{-1}$) of stationary cycling is largely unaffected by body weight (except for a small effect of moving the mass of the legs, as described below). Group A exercises are commonly used with beginners so that their intensity of exercise can be closely controlled. Similarly, group A exercises are used in rehabilitation programs in which the control of exercise intensity is vital to the safety of the exercise program. Group B simply refers to higher intensities of exercise using the same modes as in Group A.

As individuals progress to higher fitness levels, exercises from groups C and D may provide more variation in the types of activities. To determine the intensity of exercise when performing group C and D activities, one relies on the heart rate response or subjective ratings of perceived exertion. Alternatively, a rough estimate of the metabolic demand of the activities can be obtained from the Compendium of Physical Activities (1). However, it should be noted that metabolic equivalent (MET) values (where 1 MET is equivalent to oxygen consumption at rest—i.e., $3.5 \, mL \cdot kg^{-1} \cdot min^{-1}$) for many of the activities in the compendium vary not just with skill, but also with an individual's chosen level of effort.

Classifying cardiovascular exercise by body-weight dependency is a different classification system than by skill and energy expenditure. Weight-dependent exercises, or weight-bearing activities, are those in which the body weight is moved throughout the exercise. Examples of weight-bearing exercise are walking, jogging, running, and hiking. On the other hand, in weight-independent exercise, or non–weight-bearing activity, the body weight is supported by the implement or media and may contribute minimally to the energy demand. Examples of non–weight-bearing exercise are cycling and swimming. (Note that larger individuals do require more energy to swim or to cycle outdoors than smaller individuals; but the difference is proportional to surface area, which varies less between individuals than body mass) (41). Non–weight-bearing exercise may be more effective in preventing lower-limb overuse injuries associated with exercise, but this advantage must be balanced by the lack of bone stimulation. Non–weight-bearing exercise is good for minimizing orthopedic stress, but not for reducing the risk of osteoporosis.

The mode of exercise that is effective in producing the desired outcome must be the first consideration in choosing the mode of exercise. However, modifications and variations can be made in mode to promote adherence if

TABLE 28-1. GROUPING OF CARDIORESPIRATORY EXERCISES AND ACTIVITIES

	GROUP A	GROUP B	GROUP C	GROUP D
Definition	Ease of maintaining constant intensity	Ease of maintaining constant intensity	Ease of maintaining constant intensity	Energy expenditure highly variable
	Low interindividual variation in energy expenditure	Low interindividual variation in energy expenditure	Energy expenditure is related to skill	Skill highly variable
	Low to moderate intensity can be prescribed	Vigorous intensity can be prescribed		
Use	Desirable for precise control of exercise intensity, as in beginning of program	Desirable for continued improvement in fitness	Acceptable for beginner, but difficult to prescribe intensity	Good for group interactions social support
				Good for program variation
Examples	Treadmill walking	Treadmill walking	Swimming	Racquet sports
	Cycle ergometry	Cycle ergometry	Cross-country skiing	Outdoor bicycling
		Running		Basketball
				Soccer

Modified from GETP8, Table 7.3. Groups A and B are identical, except that B refers to higher intensities.

needed. Varying the mode of exercise among the weekly workouts and substituting recreational activities may be strategies that promote a higher adherence to the program.

PRESCRIBING FREQUENCY AND DURATION

Frequency is prescribed in sessions per day and in days per week. To improve cardiorespiratory fitness for apparently healthy adults, the range of frequency is from 3 to 7 days per week. If only moderate-intensity exercise (40%–59% $\dot{V}O_2R$) is being performed, then the frequency should be fairly high: 5 to 7 days per week. If only vigorous-intensity exercise ($\geq$60% $\dot{V}O_2R$) is being performed, it should be done at least 3 days per week. Depending on the orthopedic stress of the mode of exercise chosen, vigorous exercise should be performed on alternate days, not on consecutive days. For many patients, the best approach is to do moderate-intensity exercise on some days and vigorous-intensity exercise on others, for a total of 3 to 5 days per week. When sedentary individuals begin an exercise program, the intensity should be moderate and the frequency 3 alternating days per week. As the patient adapts to the stress of the exercise, and as the patient's fitness increases, greater frequency and duration of exercise, and the addition of vigorous intensity, may be incorporated to reach the patient's goals for weekly energy expenditure and increased aerobic capacity. In some rehabilitation settings, patients with very low initial fitness may be prescribed a frequency as high as several times per day (e.g., in phase I cardiac rehabilitation). However, the intensity and the duration will be very low.

Exercise duration ranges typically from 20 to 60 minutes. A minimum duration of 20 minutes is recommended to achieve improvement in cardiorespiratory fitness (33). Sedentary patients should begin with 20 minutes per session and increase gradually. It is not necessary that the entire duration for a given day be completed in one session. Multiple, shorter sessions performed throughout the day may be added to attain the desired duration, but each mini-session should entail at least 10 minutes of exercise at the prescribed intensity (although shorter bouts may be used in rehabilitation for specific patient groups). Prescribed exercise duration rarely exceeds 60 minutes. However, for weight loss a duration of up to 90 minutes may be needed to achieve the necessary total volume of exercise per week (13,17); that is, the combination of frequency, duration, and intensity should be at least 2,000 kcal per week for weight loss (13,17). Overweight individuals, who may not be capable of vigorous-intensity exercise, may need to gradually increase duration up to 90 minutes to achieve this targeted volume of energy expenditure. Endurance athletes often exercise for longer than 90 minutes in a given session, but the guidelines presented in GETP8 and here are aimed primarily at the general public.

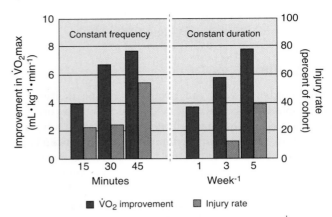

FIGURE 28-2. The influence of overload on improvement in $\dot{V}O_{2max}$ and subsequent injury rates. Adapted from Pollock MJ, Gettman L, Milesis C, et al. Effects of frequency and duration of training on attrition and incidence of injury. *Med Sci Sports*. 1977;9:31–37.

The combination of exercise frequency and duration should be viewed with caution. Pollock et al. exercised six groups of men with various combinations of frequency and duration (34). Intensity was the same for all groups. Three groups exercised for 15, 30, or 45 minutes per session for 3 days a week. Three other groups exercised for 30 minutes per session, but with frequencies of one, three, or five times per week. As expected, the improvements in fitness were related to the overload (Fig. 28-2). However, high overloads were also related to higher injury rates. The group with the highest duration and the group with the highest frequency experienced the highest injury rates. Therefore, caution should be taken in determining the optimal duration and frequency to improve fitness without causing overuse injuries.

PRESCRIBING INTENSITY

Intensity of cardiorespiratory exercise is measured as a percent of maximal capacity or, more specifically, as a percent of $\dot{V}O_2$ reserve (%$\dot{V}O_2R$). Two steps are involved in prescribing exercise intensity for cardiorespiratory exercise:

- Select a target intensity range based on %$\dot{V}O_2R$.
- Provide the client with a means of monitoring the intensity, such as by HR, workload, or a subjective rating of perceived exertion.

The translation of intensity into HR, workload, or perceived exertion will be presented in a later section. First, the selection of a target intensity will be discussed.

Threshold Intensity for Improving Cardiorespiratory Fitness

The classic study of Karvonen et al. in 1957 is well known for introducing the use of heart rate reserve (HRR) as a

TABLE 28-2. THRESHOLD INTENSITIES FOR INCREASING $\dot{V}O_{2MAX}$ BASED ON INITIAL FITNESS

INITIAL FITNESS	INITIAL $\dot{V}O_{2MAX}$ (mL·kg^{-1}·min^{-1})	RECOMMENDED MINIMUM INTENSITY[a]
Low to moderate	<40	30% $\dot{V}O_2R$ or HRR
Average to good	40–51	45% $\dot{V}O_2R$ or HRR
High	52–59	75% $\dot{V}O_2R$ or HRR
Very high	≥60	90%–100% $\dot{V}O_2R$ or HRR

HRR, heart rate reserve.

[a]These intensities are the minimum for obtaining further increases in $\dot{V}O_{2max}$. Other benefits, such as caloric expenditure for weight loss, may be obtained at lower intensities.

means of prescribing exercise intensity (18). The study's purpose, however, was to determine if a threshold intensity was required to improve aerobic fitness; i.e., is there a minimum intensity of exercise below which no improvement in aerobic fitness will occur? Karvonen et al. studied six young adult men and found that an intensity of 60% HRR was not sufficient to increase aerobic fitness, but an intensity of 71% to 75% HRR was. Since 1957, other studies provided further insight on a possible threshold, and in its 1998 position stand, ACSM concluded that deconditioned individuals need to use an intensity of at least 40% $\dot{V}O_2R$ or HRR, whereas more active individuals needed an intensity of at least 50% $\dot{V}O_2R$ or HRR (33). In 2002, Swain and Franklin (42) did an extensive review of past training studies and found that studies using subjects with mean initial $\dot{V}O_{2max}$ values below 40 mL·kg^{-1}·min^{-1} (range 13–39 mL·kg^{-1}·min^{-1}) were always successful in increasing $\dot{V}O_{2max}$, with intensities ranging as low as 30% $\dot{V}O_2R$. However, subjects with mean initial $\dot{V}O_{2max}$ values of 41 to 51 mL·kg^{-1}·min^{-1} demonstrated a threshold. These moderately fit subjects failed to achieve any increase in $\dot{V}O_{2max}$ when using intensities of approximately 45% $\dot{V}O_2R$ or less, but always succeeded in raising $\dot{V}O_{2max}$ in studies using intensities higher than approximately 45% $\dot{V}O_2R$. In the study of Karvonen et al., $\dot{V}O_{2max}$ was not measured, but HR and workload data provided about the subjects allows one to estimate their mean initial $\dot{V}O_{2max}$ as 54 mL·kg^{-1}·min^{-1}. They had a threshold at approximately 70% HRR or $\dot{V}O_{2max}$. A recent study by Helgerud et al. (14) failed to obtain increases in $\dot{V}O_{2max}$ using either 70% or 85% HR$_{max}$ (approximately 47% and 72% of $\dot{V}O_2R$) in subjects with an initial mean $\dot{V}O_{2max}$ of 58 mL·kg^{-1}·min^{-1}, but did increase $\dot{V}O_{2max}$ using intervals at approximately 85% of $\dot{V}O_2R$ (90%–95% HR$_{max}$). As the upper limit of one's genetic potential is reached, as in highly trained athletes, training with aerobic intervals may be the only means of obtaining any remaining available improvement in $\dot{V}O_{2max}$. Smith et al. (38) obtained a 5% increase in $\dot{V}O_{2max}$ of runners with a mean initial value of 62 mL·kg^{-1}·min^{-1}, whereas Billat et al. (2) obtained no increase with athletes starting at 71 mL·kg^{-1}·min^{-1}.

Therefore, when selecting an exercise intensity for clients, knowledge of their initial fitness is important. The higher the initial aerobic capacity, the higher is the minimum intensity required to further increase that capacity (Table 28-2). The basic guidelines on intensity in GETP8, as listed above under the heading "Developing Cardiorespiratory Fitness," prescribe intensities of 40% to 59% $\dot{V}O_2R$ (moderate) and ≥60% $\dot{V}O_2R$ (vigorous). But this is expanded in GETP8 Table 7.4 to include intensities as low as 30% $\dot{V}O_2R$ for sedentary patients, with increasing intensities for those with higher initial fitness.

The Value of Higher Intensities

Although the previous section described the *minimum* intensity needed to increase cardiorespiratory fitness, intensities above the threshold are more effective at increasing fitness—i.e., $\dot{V}O_{2max}$—and may also be more effective for reducing the risk of coronary heart disease (43). Several research studies have compared two or more groups of subjects who trained at different intensities while the total volume of exercise (i.e., energy expenditure) was held constant across groups. Of nine such studies identified previously (42), all nine found a greater increase in $\dot{V}O_{2max}$ in the higher- versus lower-intensity groups, with three of the nine studies reaching statistical significance. Given the generally low sample size in the individual studies, the combined evidence points to greater increases in $\dot{V}O_{2max}$ with higher-intensity training. The initial fitness of the subjects plays a role in the training response, as illustrated in Figure 28-3 (40). Most recently, a study by Gormley et al. compared continuous training at a moderate intensity (50% $\dot{V}O_2R$), continuous training at a vigorous intensity (75% $\dot{V}O_2R$),

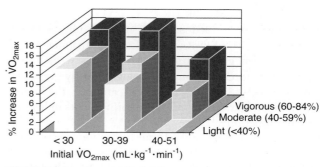

FIGURE 28-3. Influence of initial fitness and intensity of training on increase in $\dot{V}O_{2max}$. Reprinted with permission from Swain DP. *Prev Cardiol*, 2005.

and interval training at near maximal intensity (95% $\dot{V}O_2R$) (12). The final intensities were maintained for the last 4 weeks of the study, with interval training performed three times per week and continuous training four times per week, and with total volume of exercise equalized between groups. $\dot{V}O_{2max}$ increased significantly by 10%, 14%, and 21% in the three groups, respectively, with the vigorous group's increase significantly greater than the moderate group's, and the interval group's increase significantly greater than the vigorous group's.

> **1.7.13-HFS: Knowledge of the various types of interval, continuous, and circuit training programs.**

> **1.7.18-HFS: Knowledge of the advantages and disadvantages of implementation of interval, continuous, and circuit training programs.**

Interval training, once confined to the training of athletes, has been increasingly studied in other populations. Gormley et al.'s subjects were young adult women and men with a mean initial $\dot{V}O_{2max}$ of 35 mL·kg^{-1}·min^{-1} (12). They performed five sets of 5-min intervals three times per week for 4 weeks. Helgerud et al.'s subjects were young adult men with a mean initial $\dot{V}O_{2max}$ of 58 mL·kg^{-1}·min^{-1} (14). They performed four sets of 4-min intervals three times per week for 8 weeks. In 2005, Warburton et al. looked at male cardiac patients with an average age of 56 years and mean initial $\dot{V}O_{2max}$ of 32 mL·kg^{-1}·min^{-1} to compare continuous training at 65% $\dot{V}O_2R$ 5 days per week for 16 weeks, with an isocaloric program that combined 3 days of continuous training with 2 days of interval training at 90% $\dot{V}O_2R$ (49). Seven 2-min intervals were performed in each training session. The combination group increased $\dot{V}O_{2max}$ by 18% compared with 13% in the continuous training only group. Although the increases in $\dot{V}O_{2max}$ were not significantly different from each other, the combination group did have significantly greater increases in ventilatory threshold and time to exhaustion. In 2007, Wisloff et al. trained male and female congestive heart failure patients with an average age of 76 years and mean initial $\dot{V}O_{2max}$ of 13 mL·kg^{-1}·min^{-1} (51). One group performed continuous training at 70% of peak HR (~47% $\dot{V}O_2R$), whereas another group performed isocaloric interval training at 95% peak HR (~90% $\dot{V}O_2R$), using four 4-min intervals per session. Both groups trained 3 days per week for 12 weeks. The interval group had a significantly greater increase in $\dot{V}O_{2max}$ (46% versus 14%), and only the interval group demonstrated significant improvements in left ventricular function.

These studies of interval training using near-maximal aerobic intensity demonstrate that such training can be safely and effectively used in a wide range of clients, and that it results in greater improvements in fitness than does lower-intensity training utilizing the same volume of energy expenditure. Therefore, such training should be considered as an adjunct to continuous training at moderate or vigorous intensities. For example, sedentary individuals who begin a training program using moderate intensity (40%–59% $\dot{V}O_2R$) for 20 to 30 minutes three times per week will normally be progressed in duration and frequency for a period of 2 to 3 months. During this time, intensity may be progressed within the 40% to 59% $\dot{V}O_2R$ window. After this initial training period, the incorporation of continuous vigorous training and/or aerobic interval training two to three times per week into the overall program should be considered to maximize gains in both fitness and health.

> **1.7.44-HFS: Ability to design training programs using interval, continuous, and circuit training programs.**

Interval training is typically done in the following manner. A 10-min warm-up is performed, then a near-maximal effort (≥90% $\dot{V}O_2R$) for 2 to 5 minutes, which is immediately followed by an equal period at a low to moderate intensity. The work/recovery periods are repeated for a total of four to six intervals. Although interval training has been successfully used for as long as 12 to 16 weeks at a time (49,51), one should consider using this high-intensity exercise training intermittently in a program to avoid excessive orthopedic stress.

One additional caution with the use of vigorous-intensity exercise and near-maximal intensity interval training is the elevated risk of cardiac events in those with underlying disease (28). Although interval training has been used safely with cardiac patients (49,51), the patients must be medically stable. Vigorous and higher intensities should not be used in the fitness setting with moderate-risk or high-risk clients, even though they may have no *known* disease, unless clearance is obtained by a physician (see Chapter 2 of GETP8).

TRANSLATING INTENSITY INTO PRACTICAL TERMS

> **1.7.24-HFS: Skill in the use of various methods for establishing and monitoring levels of exercise intensity, including heart rate, rating of perceived exertion, and oxygen cost.**

> **1.7.25-HFS: Ability to identify and apply methods used to monitor exercise intensity, including heart rate and rating of perceived exertion.**

> **1.7.28-HFS: Knowledge of and ability to determine target heart rates using two methods: percent of age-predicted maximum heart rate and heart rate reserve (Karvonen).**

After assessing a client, the fitness professional chooses a range of exercise intensity based on the client's goals and current level of fitness. For example, a sedentary client interested in improving fitness and reducing risk of heart disease might begin with 30% to 45% $\dot{V}O_2R$ (see GETP8 Table 7.4). However, unless the client is going to perform his or her training while attached to a metabolic cart, this intensity range must be translated into practical indicators that the client and professional can monitor. This is done in one of the following ways:

- Target heart rate, based on either %HRR or %HR_{max}
- Target workload, calculated from %$\dot{V}O_2R$ or %$\dot{V}O_{2max}$, or from MET tables
- Subjective rating, based on the talk test or a rating scale

TARGET HEART RATE USING PERCENTAGE OF HEART RATE RESERVE

The heart rate reserve method (also known as the Karvonen method) is the most accurate way of establishing a target heart rate for two reasons. First, percentages of HRR have been shown to accurately reflect the same percentages of $\dot{V}O_2$ reserve. This was first demonstrated by Swain and Leutholtz in 1997 (44), prompting the ACSM to adopt $\dot{V}O_2R$ and HRR as the primary means of establishing exercise intensity in its 1998 position stand (33). Swain and Leutholtz studied young adults who performed cycle ergometry and confirmed the finding in young adults performing treadmill exercise (45). The one-to-one relationship of %$\dot{V}O_2R$ and %HRR has subsequently been confirmed in a variety of studies in a wide range of populations, including cardiac patients with or without β-blocker medication (5), diabetic patients with or without autonomic neuropathy (7), obese individuals (6), young adults exercising on an elliptical machine (8), and elite competitive cyclists (24).

The second advantage of using %HRR is that it takes into account resting heart rates of different clients, which can vary over a wide range. If resting HR is not accounted for, as in prescriptions calculated from %HR_{max}, two individuals prescribed the same intensity may actually be exercising at different relative levels of effort (see below).

To prescribe exercise intensity using %HRR, select the desired intensity based on %$\dot{V}O_2R$, and express this value as a fraction in the Karvonen equation:

$$\text{Target HR} = (\text{fractional intensity})(\text{HR}_{max} - \text{HR}_{rest}) + \text{HR}_{rest}$$

For example, what is the target HR at 60% to 75% of $\dot{V}O_2R$ for a client with a maximal HR of 175 bpm and a resting HR of 64 bpm? At the lower limit (60%):

$$\text{Target HR} = 0.60(175 - 64) + 64$$
$$\text{Target HR} = 0.60(111) + 64$$
$$\text{Target HR} = 67 + 64 = 131 \text{ bpm}$$

Repeating the process at the upper limit (75%) yields 147 bpm.

Resting HR should be measured after at least 5 minutes of quiet rest, preferably with the client in a similar position as in the prescribed exercise mode. Maximal HR would best be obtained from an incremental exercise test. If that information is not available, it may be estimated from the following equation:

$$\text{Estimated HR}_{max} = 200 - \text{age}$$

A more accurate equation, especially for older clients is $207 - 0.7$ (age), based on cross-sectional research by Tanaka et al. (46) and longitudinal research by Gellish et al. (11). Regardless of which equation is used to estimated HR_{max}, one must recognize that true HR_{max} varies widely among individuals of a given age and that the resulting target HRs are also only estimates.

TARGET HEART RATE USING PERCENTAGE OF MAXIMAL HEART RATE

As mentioned above, the %HR_{max} method is less accurate than the %HRR method because of variation of resting HR within the population. For example, consider two clients who have the same maximal HR of 160 bpm but have resting HRs of 55 and 85 bpm. If both are placed at an intensity of 64% HR_{max}, they would both be instructed to exercise at 102 bpm. However, the client with the lower resting HR would be raising his HR by 47 bpm (to 45% of HRR or $\dot{V}O_2R$), whereas the other raises his HR by only 17 bpm (to 23% of HRR or $\dot{V}O_2R$). The relative intensity is actually twice as great for one client.

Another consideration with the %HR_{max} method is that the desired percentages of $\dot{V}O_2R$ must be adjusted upward to obtain relatively appropriate intensities, as seen in Table 28-3 (15). Nonetheless, %HR_{max} is a simpler calculation than %HRR, does not require the measurement of resting HR, and is convenient for use in group exercise classes, when individual prescriptions for each client are not feasible. To use this method, first select a desired intensity range in %$\dot{V}O_2R$ units, and then identify the appropriate intensity in %HR_{max} units from Table 28-3. Then enter that value as a fraction in the following equation:

$$\text{Target HR} = (\text{intensity fraction})\text{HR}_{max}$$

For example, what is the target HR at 50% $\dot{V}O_2R$ for a 62-year-old client? From Table 28-3, 50% $\dot{V}O_2R$ corresponds to approximately 70% HR_{max}. From the Tanaka equation, HR_{max} is calculated as:

$$\text{HR}_{max} = 208 - 0.7(62) = 165 \text{ bpm}$$

Therefore,

$$\text{Target HR} = 0.70(165) = 116 \text{ bpm}$$

TABLE 28-3. CARDIORESPIRATORY EXERCISE INTENSITY: COMPARISON OF METHODS

%HRR OR $\dot{V}O_2R$	%HR_{MAX}[a]	RPE*	20 MET %$\dot{V}O_{2MAX}$	10 MET %$\dot{V}O_{2MAX}$	5 MET %$\dot{V}O_{2MAX}$
30	57	10	34	37	44
40	64	12	43	46	52
50	70	13	53	55	60
60	77	14	62	64	68
70	84	16	72	73	76
80	91	17	81	82	84
90	96	19	91	91	92
100	100	20	100	100	100

HRR, heart rate reserve; $\dot{V}O_2R$, oxygen consumption reserve; HR_{max}, maximum heart rate; RPE, rating of perceived exertion, 6–20 scale (4); $\dot{V}O_{2max}$, maximum oxygen consumption. Adapted from Howley ET. Type of activity: resistance, aerobic and leisure versus occupational physical activity. *Med Sci Sports Exerc.* 2001;33:S364–369; and GETP8 Table 1.2.

[a]Values for %HR_{max} are approximate and vary with resting HR. Values for RPE are crude and should be confirmed during supervised exercise.

TARGET WORKLOAD USING PERCENTAGE OF OXYGEN CONSUMPTION RESERVE

The intensity of exercise may be expressed as an absolute workload, such as a running speed outdoors, a treadmill walking speed and grade, or a power setting on a cycle ergometer. This method is especially useful for individuals whose HR is affected by medications or who find monitoring of HR difficult. In the case of β-blocker medication, if a stress test is performed while the patient is on the medication, the test results can still be used to establish intensity with HR (5); however, daily variations in the HR response to the medication may be problematic.

There are three steps in establishing the target workload:

- Select the desired intensity in %$\dot{V}O_2R$ units.
- Calculate the target $\dot{V}O_2$.
- Convert the target $\dot{V}O_2$ to a workload using the ACSM metabolic equations.

To calculate the target $\dot{V}O_2$, use the $\dot{V}O_2R$ formula, which is similar to the HRR formula:

$$\text{Target } \dot{V}O_2 = (\text{intensity fraction})(\dot{V}O_{2max} - \dot{V}O_{2rest}) + \dot{V}O_{2rest}$$

Substituting 3.5 mL $\cdot$ kg^{-1} $\cdot$ min^{-1} for resting $\dot{V}O_2$, this becomes:

$$\text{Target } \dot{V}O_2 = (\text{intensity fraction}) (\dot{V}O_{2max} - 3.5) + 3.5$$

For example, what is the target $\dot{V}O_2$ at 40% $\dot{V}O_2R$ for a client with a $\dot{V}O_{2max}$ of 26 mL $\cdot$ kg^{-1} $\cdot$ min^{-1}?

$$\text{Target } \dot{V}O_2 = (0.40)(26 - 3.5) + 3.5$$
$$\text{Target } \dot{V}O_2 = (0.40)(22.5) + 3.5$$
$$\text{Target } \dot{V}O_2 = 9.0 + 3.5 = 12.5 \text{ mL} \cdot \text{kg}^{-1} \cdot \text{min}^{-1}$$

This $\dot{V}O_2$ would then be entered into a metabolic equation to determine the workload for a desired mode of exercise, as described below.

TARGET WORKLOAD USING PERCENTAGE OF MAXIMUM OXYGEN CONSUMPTION

Before the publication of the ACSM's 1998 position stand (33), the primary basis for establishing exercise intensity was %$\dot{V}O_{2max}$, not %$\dot{V}O_2R$. %$\dot{V}O_{2max}$ is a viable means of prescribing intensity that some practitioners may still use. However, %$\dot{V}O_{2max}$ has two drawbacks. First, it does not translate directly into %HRR units. A discrepancy exists between %HRR and %$\dot{V}O_{2max}$ units that is most noticeable with low-fit clients exercising at low intensities (44). However, even elite athletes obtain more accurate prescriptions using %$\dot{V}O_2R$ than %$\dot{V}O_{2max}$ (24). The second shortcoming using %$\dot{V}O_{2max}$ is that it does not provide equivalent relative intensities for individuals with different fitness levels. Consider a prescribed intensity of 40% $\dot{V}O_{2max}$ in three clients, one deconditioned (5 MET capacity, or 17.5 mL $\cdot$ kg^{-1} $\cdot$ min^{-1}), one average (10 METs; 35 mL $\cdot$ kg^{-1} $\cdot$ min^{-1}) and one highly trained (20 METs; 70 mL $\cdot$ kg^{-1} $\cdot$ min^{-1}). An intensity of 40% $\dot{V}O_{2max}$ yields target $\dot{V}O_2$s of 7.0, 14.0, and 28.0 mL $\cdot$ kg^{-1} $\cdot$ min^{-1}, respectively. As percentages of $\dot{V}O_2R$, these translate to 25%, 33%, and 37%, respectively. Therefore, the deconditioned client would be asked to use a much smaller portion of his or her exercise capacity than the other clients. To accurately establish relative intensities, %$\dot{V}O_2R$ is preferred.

For those choosing to use %$\dot{V}O_{2max}$, the calculation is simpler than for %$\dot{V}O_2R$:

$$\text{Target } \dot{V}O_2 = (\text{intensity fraction}) \dot{V}O_{2max}$$

As a starting point, the same intensity fractions designated for %$\dot{V}O_2R$ may be selected, but these should be adjusted upward. The amount of adjustment is greater for lower versus higher intensities of prescribed exercise and is greater for low-fit clients than for higher-fit clients (Table 28-3). As with the %$\dot{V}O_2R$ method, the resulting target $\dot{V}O_2$ would then be converted to a workload using the ACSM metabolic equations. Note that %$\dot{V}O_{2max}$ values do not match up with %HRR values, so one should not attempt to use a target HR based on %$\dot{V}O_{2max}$.

TARGET WORKLOAD USING METABOLIC EQUIVALENTS

 1.7.14-HFS: Knowledge of approximate METs for various sport, recreational, and work tasks.

As mentioned previously, the Compendium of Physical Activities provides rough intensity ranges for various activities in METs (1). First, select the desired intensity in $\%\dot{V}O_2R$ units, then determine the target intensity using a modified Karvonen equation for METs:

$$\text{Target METs} = (\text{intensity fraction})[(\dot{V}O_{2max} \text{ in METs}) - 1] + 1$$

$\dot{V}O_{2max}$ in METs is found by dividing the value in $mL \cdot kg^{-1} \cdot min^{-1}$ by 3.5. For example, what is the target MET level at 60% of $\dot{V}O_2R$ for a client with a $\dot{V}O_{2max}$ of 22 $mL \cdot kg^{-1} \cdot min^{-1}$?

$$\text{Maximum MET value} = (22 \text{ mL} \cdot kg^{-1} \cdot min^{-1})/(3.5 \text{ mL} \cdot kg^{-1} \cdot min^{-1} \text{ per MET}) = 6.3 \text{ METs}$$
$$\text{Target METs} = (0.60)(6.3 - 1) + 1$$
$$\text{Target METs} = (0.60)(5.3) + 1$$
$$\text{Target METs} = 3.2 + 1 = 4.2 \text{ METs}$$

Then, the Compendium is consulted to identify activities with an appropriate MET intensity range. However, caution must be used to discuss the appropriate subjective level of effort the client will use during the activity.

TARGET INTENSITY USING PERCEIVED EXERTION

Many individuals are able to regulate the intensity of exercise based on how hard it feels. Well-trained athletes can easily establish a pace that they feel is light or moderate or hard and pace themselves for a given distance or duration. Novice exercisers may be taught to subjectively regulate their intensity through a variety of methods, including the talk test and various scales for rating one's perceived level of exertion.

The Talk Test

The talk test can establish a moderate exercise intensity. The client is asked to work at a level that causes a sensation of increased breathing, but that still allows comfortable speaking in complete sentences. When asked "Can you still speak comfortably?", answering "yes" is consistently associated with an intensity below the ventilatory threshold (32). The intensity when a patient provides an equivocal answer is approximately at the ventilatory threshold, whereas intensities at which the patient says "no" are above the ventilatory threshold.

Ratings of Perceived Exertion

The original, linear, Borg scale (see GETP8, Table 4.7) is mostly widely used (4), although a newer "category-ratio" Borg scale is also available (30). The original Borg scale ranges from 6 to 20, with 6 being rest and 20 being maximal effort. Descriptors such as "very light" and "somewhat hard" are associated with every other number. The scale was designed to correspond to HRs of 60 to 200 bpm in young adults, but may be used by individuals of any age to subjectively rate their level of effort. Clients should be instructed to report the overall sensation of effort and not localize their rating to how the legs feel or how difficult the breathing is.

The OMNI scale has been recently reported (35,47), which uses pictures illustrating varying levels of exertion along with short descriptors and numbers from 0 to 10 and has been used to differentiate feelings of exertion in the legs and chest. The Borg scales (4,30) and OMNI scale (16,35,47) have been validated against physiologic measures, such as $\dot{V}O_2$, HR, and serum lactate concentration during incremental exercise. However, when a client is asked to report increasing numbers on a scale as the intensity of exercise is increased, strong correlations with physiologic measures that also increase must occur. The ability of subjective scales to place a client at a desired intensity during a prescribed exercise session is less certain. To maximize the utility of these scales, clients should be familiarized with them during an incremental exercise test, and the levels corresponding to desired exercise intensity should be pointed out.

DETERMINING WORKLOAD FROM THE ACSM METABOLIC EQUATIONS

> **1.7.35-HFS:** Ability to apply energy cost, $\dot{V}O_2$, METs, and target heart rates to an exercise prescription.

> **1.7.36-HFS:** Ability to convert between the U.S. and metric systems for length/height (inches to centimeters), weight (pounds to kilograms) and speed (miles per hour to meters per minute).

> **1.7.37-HFS:** Ability to convert between absolute ($mL \cdot min^{-1}$ or $L \cdot min^{-1}$) and relative oxygen costs ($mL \cdot kg^{-1} \cdot min^{-1}$ and/or METs).

> **1.7.38-HFS:** Ability to determine the energy cost for given exercise intensities during horizontal and graded walking and running, stepping exercise, cycle ergometry, arm ergometry, and stepping.

> **1.7.39-HFS:** Ability to prescribe exercise intensity based on $\dot{V}O_2$ data for different modes of exercise, including graded and horizontal running and walking, cycling, and stepping exercise.

When using the $\%\dot{V}O_2R$ method to establish the exercise intensity as a target $\dot{V}O_2$, the $\dot{V}O_2$ must be translated into a workload with a given mode of exercise. Table 7.2 in GETP8 provides the equations for determining $\dot{V}O_2$ (in $mL \cdot kg^{-1} \cdot min^{-1}$) during walking, running, leg cycle ergometry, arm cycle ergometry, and stepping. The derivations of the equations are discussed briefly below (39). The values are gross, including both the $\dot{V}O_2$ needed for rest (i.e., 3.5 $mL \cdot kg^{-1} \cdot min^{-1}$) and the net value needed to perform the exercise.

The equations may be used to prescribe a workload, and may also be used to determine the $\dot{V}O_2$ and energy expenditure associated with a self-selected workload. To convert oxygen consumption to energy expenditure, the $\dot{V}O_2$ must first be expressed in absolute terms, $L \cdot min^{-1}$. This is done by multiplying the relative $\dot{V}O_2$, in $mL \cdot kg^{-1} \cdot min^{-1}$, by the client's body mass and then dividing by 1,000 (i.e., 1,000 mL per L). Approximately 5 kcal of energy are expended when 1 L of O_2 is consumed (slightly more when using only carbohydrates, slightly less when using only fats). When determining the energy expenditure for weight loss purposes, it is essential that the net value, not the gross value, be used (see below).

OXYGEN CONSUMPTION OF WALKING

Walking requires 0.1 mL of O_2 for each m of horizontal motion for each kg of body mass—i.e., 0.1 mL per $kg \cdot m$ (9). Vertical ascent requires 1.8 mL of O_2 for each m climbed for each kg of mass raised, i.e., 1.8 mL per $kg \cdot m$ (9). The oxygen demand of downhill walking is complex, as it decreases as the slope becomes steeper up to a point (−10% grade), and then increases with greater steepness, surpassing the cost of level walking at grades steeper than −20% (27). Therefore, the ACSM equation is not valid for downhill walking. The gross $\dot{V}O_2$ of level or uphill walking can be expressed as:

$$\dot{V}O_2 \text{ of walking} = 3.5 + 0.1(\text{speed}) + 1.8(\text{speed})(\text{grade})$$

where speed is in $m \cdot min^{-1}$, and grade is expressed as a fraction.

For example, what is the gross $\dot{V}O_2$ and net energy expenditure of a 70-kg client walking at 3 mph up a 5% grade? The conversion factor for speed is 1 mph = 26.8 $m \cdot min^{-1}$. Therefore, speed is (3 mph)(26.8 $m \cdot min^{-1}$/mph) = 80.4 $m \cdot min^{-1}$.

$$\dot{V}O_2 = 3.5 + 0.1(80.4) + 1.8(80.4)(0.05)$$
$$\dot{V}O_2 = 3.5 + 8.04 + 7.236 = 18.8 \ mL \cdot kg^{-1} \cdot min^{-1}$$

The gross $\dot{V}O_2$ is 18.8 $mL \cdot kg^{-1} \cdot min^{-1}$, whereas the net $\dot{V}O_2$ is 3.5 less—i.e., 15.3 $mL \cdot kg^{-1} \cdot min^{-1}$. To determine the net energy expenditure, first convert the net $\dot{V}O_2$ from relative units to absolute units: (15.3 $mL \cdot kg^{-1} \cdot min^{-1}$) (70 kg)/(1,000 mL/L) = approximately 1.1 $L \cdot min^{-1}$.

Now convert the $L \cdot min^{-1}$ of $\dot{V}O_2$ to $kcal \cdot min^{-1}$ of energy expenditure: (1.1 $L \cdot min^{-1}$)(5 kcal/L) = 5.5 $kcal \cdot min^{-1}$.

OXYGEN CONSUMPTION OF RUNNING

Running requires exactly twice as much oxygen or energy for horizontal movement as does walking—i.e., 0.2 mL per $kg \cdot m$ (9,26)—because of the work of jumping off the ground between steps. When running uphill, some of the vertical work of jumping between steps can be applied to the ascent, and the coefficient for uphill running is reduced from that of walking (i.e., 0.9 mL per $kg \cdot m$) (9,26).

As with walking, the energy cost of downhill running is complex (27) and not covered in the ACSM equation:

$$\dot{V}O_2 \text{ of running} = 3.5 + 0.2(\text{speed}) + 0.9(\text{speed})(\text{grade})$$

For example, if a client runs comfortably at 6 mph (161 $m \cdot min^{-1}$), what treadmill grade would be needed to exercise at a target $\dot{V}O_2$ of 50 $mL \cdot kg^{-1} \cdot min^{-1}$? Enter the known values into the running equation, and solve for the unknown grade.

$$50 = 3.5 + 0.2(161) + 0.9(161)(\text{grade})$$
$$50 = 3.5 + 32.2 + 144.9(\text{grade})$$
$$50 = 35.7 + 144.9(\text{grade})$$
$$50 - 35.7 = 144.9(\text{grade})$$
$$14.3 = 144.9(\text{grade})$$
$$14.3/144.9 = \text{grade}$$
$$0.099 = \text{grade, or approximately } 10\%$$

What is the net energy expenditure of walking or running 1 mile on level ground for a 136-lb (62-kg) client? One mile is 1,609 m. The oxygen cost of horizontal walking is 0.1 mL per $kg \cdot m$, thus the O_2 consumed over 1 mile (above resting needs) would be (0.1 $mL/kg \cdot m$)(1,609 m)(62 kg) = approximately 10,000 mL, or 10 L. The oxygen cost of running would be (0.2 $mL/kg \cdot m$)(1,609 m)(62 kg) = 20,000 mL or 20 L. Given 5 kcal per L of O_2, the energy expenditure would be 10 L × 5 kcal/L = 50 kcal for walking and 20 L × 5 kcal/L = 100 kcal for running. This is the derivation of the often cited "100 kcal for running a mile." However, the energy cost of walking a mile is exactly half that. Patients who are heavier (or lighter) than 62 kg would have proportionally more (or less) energy expenditure.

OXYGEN CONSUMPTION OF LEG CYCLING

In addition to the resting component, stationary cycling requires approximately 3.5 $mL \cdot kg^{-1} \cdot min^{-1}$ just to spin the legs at 50 to 60 rpm without any resistance (39). To overcome resistance, an additional 1.8 mL of O_2 is needed for each $kg \cdot m$ of work (as in the vertical component of the walking equation) (19,20,23). Thus, the leg cycling equation is:

$$\dot{V}O_2 \text{ of leg cycling} = 3.5 + 3.5 + 1.8(\text{workload})/(\text{body mass})$$

where the workload is expressed in $kg \cdot m \cdot min^{-1}$. If power is measured in watts, note that 1 W equals approximately 6 $kg \cdot m \cdot min^{-1}$ (if greater accuracy is desired, use 6.12).

For example, what is the gross $\dot{V}O_2$ of a 62-kg client cycling at 100 W? First, convert the power to workload as (100 W)(6 $kg \cdot m \cdot min^{-1}$/W) = 600 $kg \cdot m \cdot min^{-1}$. Then use the leg cycling equation:

$$\dot{V}O_2 = 3.5 + 3.5 + 1.8(600)/62$$
$$\dot{V}O_2 = 7 + 17.4 = 24.4 \ mL \cdot kg^{-1} \cdot min^{-1}$$

OXYGEN CONSUMPTION OF ARM CYCLING

The arm cycling equation includes the resting component and a component to account for the resistance of the ergometer. The latter is 3 mL of O_2 per kg · m, as opposed to 1.8 for the legs (10). The higher value is apparently because of lower efficiency with the smaller muscle mass of the arms and also because the oxygen cost of unloaded cycling is incorporated within the term.

$$\dot{V}O_2 \text{ of arm cycling} = 3.5 + 3(\text{workload})/(\text{body mass})$$

OXYGEN CONSUMPTION OF STEPPING

In addition to the resting component, stepping requires a term for the forward and backward motion of the person, as well as a term for raising and then lowering the body on and off the step. The horizontal term is 0.2 mL of O_2 times the stepping rate. The vertical term is 1.8 mL per kg · m (as in the walking and leg cycling equations), plus one third of that for lowering the body back down (29).

$$\dot{V}O_2 \text{ of stepping} = 3.5 + 0.2(\text{rate}) + 2.4(\text{rate})(H)$$

where the stepping rate is in complete four-cycle steps per minute, and H is the height of the step in m.

A complete four-cycle step involves (a) lifting the first leg and placing the foot on the step; (b) extending the first leg to raise the body, placing the foot of the second leg on the step; (c) moving the foot of the first leg back to the floor by lowering the body with the second leg; and (d) placing the foot of the second leg on the floor. In this sequence, the first leg does virtually all of the concentric work, and the second leg does virtually all of the eccentric work. The client should vary this by occasionally switching legs on the fourth beat. This is done by tapping the foot of the second leg on the ground and lifting it on the first beat of the next cycle.

THE CALORIC COST OF EXERCISE

The caloric cost of exercise can be determined from the metabolic equations above, as illustrated in the walking example. This should be expressed in net terms and must be for weight-loss calculations. Resting oxygen consumption of 3.5 mL · kg^{-1} · min^{-1} (i.e., 1 MET) translates to 1 kcal · kg^{-1} · hr^{-1}. Consider a 70-kg client with a resting energy expenditure of (1 kcal · kg^{-1} · hr^{-1})(70 kg)(24 hr) = 1,680 kcal per day. If the client walks for 1 hour at 3 mph (80 m · min^{-1}), gross $\dot{V}O_2$ will be 11.5 mL · kg^{-1} · min^{-1}, or 0.8 L · min^{-1}, for a gross energy expenditure of 4 kcal · min^{-1} or 240 kcal for the entire 1-hour session. What is the total energy expenditure for the day? During the 1 hour of walking, the client used 70 kcal for existing resting metabolic needs and 170 kcal for walking itself. Thus, the total energy expenditure for the day is not 1,680 + 240, as the resting component for the hour of walking would be counted twice. Rather, the total is 1,680 + 170 = 1,850 kcal.

If the client did 1 hour of walking 5 days per week, how much fat weight loss could be expected, assuming this is a new program for the client and diet is not changed? Five hours per week times the net energy expenditure of 170 kcal per hour = 850 kcal per week expended above rest. One pound (0.45 kg) of fat contains 3,500 kcal. Thus, 850/3,500 = 0.24 lb. The client would lose about 1/4 lb per week. Thus, a greater volume of exercise and a reduction in caloric intake would be needed to reach a weight loss of 1 to 2 lb weekly.

The ACSM recommends that a minimum of 1,000 kcal be expended per week in physical activity and exercise, which is associated with a significant 20% to 30% reduction in risk of all-cause mortality (13,21), and this should be the initial goal for previously sedentary individuals. Based on the dose–response relationships between physical activity and health and fitness, individuals should be encouraged to move toward attainment of 2,000 to 4,000 kcal per week as their fitness improves during the training program. For the purposes of weight loss, the minimum exercise dose should reach 2,000 kcal per week (17). Energy expenditure in excess of 2,000 kcal · wk^{-1} have been successful for both short- and long-term weight control (36,37).

An alternative to calculating the energy expenditure of exercise from the metabolic equations is to use the following equation based on the MET level of the activity:

$$(\text{METs} \times 3.5 \times \text{body mass in kg})/200 = \text{kcal·min}^{-1}$$

This formula (derived from conversions listed above) helps an individual understand the components of the exercise prescription and the volume of exercise necessary to achieve the caloric goals of the program.

Consider the following example. The weekly goal of the exercise program has been set at 1,000 kcal for an individual who weighs 70 kg, and the MET level of the prescribed activity is 6 METs. In this example, the *net* caloric expenditure from the exercise would be 5 METs because 1 MET of the activity represents resting metabolic rate. Therefore, the *net* caloric expenditure from the exercise is $(5 \times 3.5 \times 70)/200 = 6.1$ kcal·min^{-1}, which requires 164 minutes per week to attain the 1,000 kilocalorie threshold. Given a 4-d · wk^{-1} program, the individual would require approximately 41 minutes per day to achieve the 1,000 kcal goal (or 33 minutes per day, 5 d · wk^{-1}). Working backward from the caloric goal to determine the volume of exercise needed to reach the goal is useful in determining the appropriate exercise prescription components. If the goal was a more aggressive 2,000 kcal · week^{-1}, the net caloric expenditure of 6.1 kcal · min^{-1} would require 328 minutes·wk^{-1} or approximately 47 min·day^{-1} on all days of the week.

EXERCISE PROGRESSION

> **1.7.15-HFS: Knowledge of the components incorporated into an exercise session and the proper sequence (i.e., pre-exercise evaluation, warm-up,**

aerobic stimulus phase, cool-down, muscular strength and/or endurance, and flexibility).

> **1.7.17-HFS: Knowledge of the importance of recording exercise sessions and performing periodic evaluations to assess changes in fitness status.**

> **1.7.21-HFS: Skill to teach and demonstrate the components of an exercise session (i.e., warm-up, aerobic stimulus phase, cool-down, muscular strength/endurance, flexibility).**

The rate of progression of exercise depends on $\dot{V}O_{2max}$, health status, age, activity preferences, and goals, as well as the tolerance to training. Exercise progression is essential for sedentary individuals beginning exercise programs and is important for all populations. Most training programs feature three progressive stages: initiation, improvement, and maintenance.

INITIATION STAGE

The goal of the initial stage of training is to allow time to begin the adaptive process. Typically, this is accomplished by working at a lower intensity and shorter duration and with careful attention to signs of intolerance, particularly musculoskeletal or cardiopulmonary. The initial stage is the time to develop the habit of exercise with minimal discomfort and soreness. It is also a time to allow the exercise professional to instruct the individual as to proper exercise form. Every cardiorespiratory exercise session should be preceded by a 5- to 10-minute warm-up, performing the mode of exercise prescribed for the work phase at a low intensity to allow the cardiopulmonary system to adjust to the new demand and to allow the temperature of the muscles to increase. Stretching may be performed at the end of the warm-up if desired and should be performed at the end of the cool-down. Following the work phase, the low-intensity cool-down is performed for 5 to 10 minutes to prevent blood pooling and to promote the clearance of lactic acid. If resistance training is to be performed in the same exercise session, it is best performed at the conclusion of the aerobic cool-down and before the stretching. See Chapter 29 for additional information on resistance and flexibility exercise.

Suitable initial intensities may range from 30% $\dot{V}O_2R$ for very deconditioned individuals, 40% of $\dot{V}O_2R$ for other beginners, to more than 50% of $\dot{V}O_2R$ for individuals with higher aerobic capacities or experienced exercisers returning from time off regular exercise. Appropriate initial duration of exercise ranges from 20 to 30 minutes per session. Older, obese, and profoundly sedentary individuals may start with as little as 10 minutes of continuous exercise. In such situations, intermittent exercise or multiple daily sessions may be helpful. If intensity is kept low to moderate, sedentary but otherwise healthy adults may be able to start with sessions of 20 to 30 minutes.

The exercise session itself may be modified during the initial stage of training by expanding the warm-up period, using it to inventory possible signs of injury or soreness, providing information, and answering questions. The initial stage of training generally lasts 4 weeks but may be expanded for those requiring additional time to adapt. Monitoring exercise HRs may also be an indication for progression. If exercise or recovery HRs are lower for the same amount of work, the intensity or duration can be increased.

IMPROVEMENT STAGE

The goal of this stage of training is to provide a gradual increase in the overall exercise stimulus to allow for significant improvements in cardiorespiratory fitness. In the improvement stage, expanding physiologic capacities are further challenged. This stage is typified by the phrase *progressive overload*. Small increments in intensity and duration may occur nearly every week. The challenge of the improvement stage is to increase training at a rate that continues to stimulate further advancement without causing overtraining.

Failure to complete an exercise session, lack of normal interest in training, increased HR or rating of perceived exertion at the same rate of external work, and an increase in minor aches and pains are all signs that progression may be too rapid (22). In an appropriately incremented improvement stage, interest and appetite for exercise normally increase in tandem with the subjective and objective impressions that progress is being made. In general, frequency, intensity, and duration should not be increased together in any single week, and total weekly training volume should not be advanced by more than 10%. Increasing duration by 5 to 10 minutes per session on a weekly basis is usually well tolerated, as is building intensity gradually through the range of 40% to 59% of aerobic capacity and eventually adding sessions of more vigorous intensity. Progression of both intensity and duration in a single session is not recommended.

Competitive athletes who train intensively and those encountering musculoskeletal or other physical obstacles impeding progress may benefit from the early incorporation of techniques such as cross-training, which are more typical of the maintenance stage.

The adaptive potential of physiologic function is finite, and large increments in fitness, typical in the improvement stage, always taper at some point. Aerobic capacity can be expected to expand by approximately 10% to 30% in the course of a program following ACSM guidelines. Improvements of more than 30% rarely occur unless accompanied by a large reduction in body weight and fat. If training is discontinued, gains in fitness regress by approximately 50% within 4 to 12 weeks (33). After approximately 6 months of training, most individuals make the transition from improvement to maintenance.

MAINTENANCE STAGE

The goal of this stage of training is the long-term maintenance of cardiorespiratory fitness developed in the previous stage. The maintenance stage is typified by diversification of the training program and purposeful attempts to rotate and reduce the stresses of continued training. Diversification may take the form of using several modes of exercise to maintain enjoyment and explore new capabilities. This may be particularly important to lifelong programs with goals such as weight management and general health.

For those using the maintenance phase as a sustained period of performance or competition, diversification may be used as a means of reducing the potential for overuse injuries, particularly in programs with high training volumes or for participants with musculoskeletal limitations. *Cross-training*, as this approach is often called, refers to using a variety of modes of cardiorespiratory endurance exercise (e.g., swimming, running, biking) to maintain a high training stimulus for central aerobic adaptations, such as enhanced stroke volume and expanded blood volume. This approach allows rotation of local fatigue and musculoskeletal stresses across a range of muscle groups.

Cognitively, the maintenance stage is a time for enjoyment, surveillance, and reappraisal. It is a time for enjoying the fruits of labor by competing, engaging in new activities, or reducing the demands of weekly training. Surveillance for overuse injury must continue during the maintenance phase. Equipment and footwear should be re-evaluated. Finally, the goals of the program may be re-examined, physiologic or performance testing may be repeated, and new goals may be established, triggering the start of a new improvement stage. Further advancing performance and cardiorespiratory fitness often requires special techniques such as periodization, in which volume and intensity of exercise are varied in a systematic way over several months.

SUMMARY

The proper application of frequency, intensity, time (duration), and type (mode) in an exercise prescription will result in improved cardiorespiratory fitness, reduced risk of cardiovascular disease, and weight loss or maintenance. Intensity of exercise should be prescribed judiciously. Low to moderate intensities are appropriate for beginners. Higher intensities should be considered as fitness improves, provided the client is not at risk for cardiovascular events. Care should be taken in all programs to avoid excessive orthopedic stress and overtraining.

REFERENCES

1. **Ainsworth BE, Haskell WL, Whitt MC, et al. Compendium of physical activities: an update of activity codes and MET intensities. *Med Sci Sports Exerc.* 2000;32(9 Suppl):S498–504.**

2. Billat VL, Flechet B, Petit B, et al. Interval training at $\dot{V}O_{2max}$: effects of aerobic performance and overtraining markers. *Med Sci Sports Exerc.* 1999;31:156–163.

3. Blair SN, Kohl HWI, Paffenbarger RS, et al. Physical fitness and all-cause mortality: a prospective study of healthy men and women. *JAMA.* 1989;262:2395–2401.

4. Borg GA. Perceived exertion. *Exerc Sports Sci Rev.* 1974;2:131–153.

5. Brawner CA, Keteyian SJ, Ehrman JK. The relationship of heart rate reserve to $\dot{V}O_2$ reserve in patients with heart disease. *Med Sci Sports Exerc.* 2002;34:418–422.

6. Byrne NM, Hills AP. Relationships between HR and $\dot{V}O_2$ in the obese. *Med Sci Sports Exerc.* 2002;34:1419–1427.

7. Colberg SR, Swain DP, Vinik A. Use of heart rate reserve and rating of perceived exertion to prescribe exercise intensity in diabetic autonomic neuropathy. *Diabetes Care.* 2003;26:986–990.

8. Dalleck LC, Kravitz L. Relationship between % heart rate reserve and %$\dot{V}O_2$ reserve during elliptical crosstrainer exercise. *J Sports Sci Med.* 2006;5:662–671.

9. Dill DB. Oxygen cost of horizontal and grade walking and running on the treadmill. *J Appl Physiol.* 1965;20:19–22.

10. Franklin BA. Exercise testing, training and arm ergometry. *Sports Med.* 1985;2:100–119.

11. Gellish RL, Goslin BR, Olson RE, McDonald A, Russi GD, Moudgil VK. Longitudinal modeling of the relationship between age and maximal heart rate. *Med Sci Sports Exerc.* 2007;39:822–829.

12. Gormley SE, Swain DP, Huff R, et al. The effect of intensity of aerobic training on $\dot{V}O_{2max}$.

13. **Haskell WL, Lee I-M, Pate RR, et al. Physical activity and public health: updated recommendations from the American College of Sports Medicine and the American Heart Association. *Med Sci Sports Exerc.* 2007;39:1423–1434.**

14. Helgerud J, Hoydal K, Wang E, et al. Aerobic high-intensity intervals improve $\dot{V}O_{2max}$ more than moderate training. *Med Sci Sports Exerc.* 2007;39:665–671.

15. Howley ET. Type of activity: resistance, aerobic and leisure versus occupational physical activity. *Med Sci Sports Exerc.* 2001;33:S364–369.

16. Irving BA, Rutkowski J, Brock DW, et al. Comparison of Borg- and OMNI-RPE as markers of the blood lactate response to exercise. *Med Sci Sports Exerc.* 2006;38:1348–1352.

17. **Jakicic JM, Clark K, Coleman E, et al. American College of Sports Medicine position stand. Appropriate intervention strategies for weight loss and prevention of weight regain for adults. *Med Sci Sports Exerc.* 2001;33:2145–2156.**

18. Karvonen M, Kentala K, Musta O. The effects of training on heart rate: a longitudinal study. *Ann Med Exp Biol Fenn.* 1957;35: 307–315.

19. Lang PB, Latin RW, Berg KE, et al. The accuracy of the ACSM cycle ergometry equation. *Med Sci Sports Exerc.* 1992;24:272–276.

20. Latin RW, Berg KE. The accuracy of the ACSM and a new cycle ergometry equation for young women. *Med Sci Sports Exerc.* 1994;26:642–646.

21. Lee IM, Skerrett PJ. Physical activity and all-cause mortality: What is the dose-response relation? *Med Sci Sports Exerc.* 2001;33:S459–S471, S493–S494.

22. Lehmann MJ, Lormes W, Opitz-Gress A, et al. Training and overtraining: an overview and experimental results in endurance sports. *J Sports Med Phys Fitness.* 1997;37:7–17.

23. Londeree BR, Moffitt-Gerstenberger J, Padfield JA, et al. Oxygen consumption of cycle ergometry is nonlinearly related to work rate and pedal rate. *Med Sci Sports Exerc.* 1997;29:775–780.

24. Lounana J, Campion F, Noakes TD, Medelli J. Relationship between %HR_{max}, %HR reserve, %$\dot{V}O_{2max}$ and %$\dot{V}O_2$ reserve in elite cyclists. *Med Sci Sports Exerc.* 2007;39:350–357.

25. Magel JR, Foglia GF, McArdle WD. Specificity of swim training on maximum oxygen uptake. *J Appl Physiol.* 1975;38:151.

26. Margaria R, Cerretelli P, Aghemo P. Energy cost of running. *J Appl Physiol.* 1963;18:367–370.

27. Minetti AE, Moia C, Roi GS, Susta D, Ferretti G. Energy cost of walking and running at extreme uphill and downhill slopes. *J Appl Physiol*. 2002;93:1039–1046.

28. Mittleman MA, MaClure M, Tofler GH, Sherwood JB, Goldberg RJ, Muller JE. Triggering of acute myocardial infarction by heavy physical exertion. *N Engl J Med*. 1993;329:1677–1683.

29. Nagle FJ, Balke B, Naughton JP. Gradational step tests for assessing work capacity. *J Appl Physiol*. 1965;20:745–748.

30. Noble BJ, Borg GA, Jacobs I, Ceci R, Kaiser P. A category-ratio perceived exertion scale: relationship to blood and muscle lactates and heart rate. *Med Sci Sports Exerc*. 1983;15:523–528.

31. **Pate RR, Pratt M, Blair SN, et al. Physical activity and public health: a recommendation from the Centers for Disease Control and Prevention and the American College of Sports Medicine. *JAMA*. 1995;273:402–407.**

32. Persinger R, Foster C, Gobson M, Fater DC, Porcari JP. Consistency of the talk test for exercise prescription. *Med Sci Sports Exerc*. 2004;36:1632–1636.

33. **Pollock ML, Gaesser GA, Butcher JD, et al. The recommended quantity and quality of exercise for developing and maintaining cardiorespiratory and muscular fitness, and flexibility in healthy adults. *Med Sci Sports Exerc*. 1998;30:975–991.**

34. Pollock MJ, Gettman L, Milesis C, et al. Effects of frequency and duration of training on attrition and incidence of injury. *Med Sci Sports*. 1977;9:31–37.

35. Robertson RJ, Goss FL, Dube J, et al. Validation of the adult OMNI scale of perceived exertion for cycle ergometer exercise. *Med Sci Sports Exerc*. 2004;36:102–108.

36. Ross R, Janssen I. Physical activity, total and regional obesity: dose-response considerations. *Med Sci Sports Exerc*. 2001;33:S521–S529.

37. **Saris W, Blair SN, van Baak M, et al. How much physical activity is enough to prevent unhealthy weight gain? Outcome of the IASO 1st Stock Conference and consensus statement. *Obesity Rev*. 2003;4:101–114.**

38. Smith TP, McNaughton LR, Marshall KJ. Effects of 4-wk training using V_{max}/T_{max} on $\dot{V}O_{2max}$ and performance in athletes. *Med Sci Sports Exerc*. 1999;31:892–896.

39. Swain DP. Energy cost calculations for exercise prescription: an update. *Sports Med*. 2000;30:17–22.

40. Swain DP. Moderate or vigorous intensity exercise: Which is better for improving aerobic fitness? *Prev Cardiol*. 2005;8:55–58.

41. Swain DP, Coast JR, Clifford PS, Milliken MC, Stray-Gundersen J. The influence of body size on oxygen consumption during bicycling. *J Appl Physiol*. 1987;62:668–672.

42. Swain DP, Franklin BA. $\dot{V}O_2$ reserve and the minimal intensity for improving cardiorespiratory fitness. *Med Sci Sports Exerc*. 2002;34:152–157.

43. Swain DP, Franklin BA. Comparative cardioprotective benefits of vigorous vs. moderate intensity aerobic exercise. *Am J Cardiol*. 2006;97:141–147.

44. Swain DP, Leutholtz BC. Heart rate reserve is equivalent to $\%\dot{V}O_2$ reserve, not to $\%\dot{V}O_{2max}$. *Med Sci Sports Exerc*. 1997;29:410–414.

45. Swain DP, Leutholtz BC, King ME, Haas LA, Branch JD. Relationship of % heart rate reserve and $\%\dot{V}O_2$ reserve in treadmill exercise. *Med Sci Sports Exerc*. 1998;30:318–321.

46. Tanaka H, Monahan KD, Seals DR. Age-predicted maximal heart rate revisited. *J Am Coll Cardiol*. 2001;37:153–156.

47. Utter AC, Robertson RJ, Green JM, Suminski RR, McAnulty SR, Nieman DC. Validation of the adult OMNI scale of perceived exertion for walking/running exercise. *Med Sci Sports Exerc*. 2004;36:1776–1780.

48. **U.S. Department of Health and Human Services. *Physical Activity and Health: A Report of the Surgeon General*. Washington (DC): U.S. Department of Health and Human Services, Centers for Disease Control and Prevention, National Center for Chronic Disease Prevention and Health Promotion; 1996.**

49. Warburton DER, McKenzie DC, Haykowsky MJ, et al. Effectiveness of high-intensity interval training for the rehabilitation of patients with coronary artery disease. *Am J Cardiol*. 2005;95:1080–1084.

50. Williams PT. Physical fitness and activity as separate heart disease risk factors: a meta-analysis. *Med Sci Sports Exerc*. 2001;33:754–761.

51. Wisloff U, Stoylen A, Loennechen JP, et al. Superior cardiovascular effect of aerobic interval training versus moderate continuous training in heart failure patients. *Circulation*. 2007;115:3086–3094.

SELECTED REFERENCES FOR FURTHER READING

ACSM's Metabolic Calculations Tutorial CD-ROM. Philadelphia: Lippincott Williams & Wilkins; 2000.

Haskell WL, Lee I-M, Pate RR, et al. Physical activity and public health: updated recommendations from the American College of Sports Medicine and the American Heart Association. *Med Sci Sports Exerc*. 2007;39:1423–1434.

Pollock ML, Gaesser GA, Butcher JD, et al. The recommended quantity and quality of exercise for developing and maintaining cardiorespiratory and muscular fitness, and flexibility in healthy adults. *Med Sci Sports Exerc*. 1998;30:975–991.

Swain DP, Leutholtz BC. *Exercise Prescription: A Case Study Approach to the ACSM Guidelines*. 2nd ed. Champaign (IL): Human Kinetics; 2007.

U.S. Department of Health and Human Services. *Physical Activity and Health: A Report of the Surgeon General*. Washington (DC): U.S. Department of Health and Human Services, Centers for Disease Control and Prevention, National Center for Chronic Disease Prevention and Health Promotion; 1996.

INTERNET RESOURCES

- American College of Sports Medicine: www.acsm.org
- Centers for Disease Control and Prevention: www.cdc.gov
- United States Department of Health and Human Services Physical Activity Guidelines for Americans. Available at http://www.health.gov/PAGuidlines/pdf/paguide.pdf. Accessed 10/7/08.

Musculoskeletal Exercise Prescription

Individualization and proper exercise prescription of resistance training are vital for gaining needed physiologic adaptations. Perhaps the best-known benefit of resistance training is increased strength, although increases in power and local muscular endurance are also very important characteristics of a resistance-training program. Along with this comes an increase in muscle size, which is vital for men and women to offset any sarcopenia—significant muscular atrophy with disease or the aging process. Increased strength is important to athletes for performance improvement, but it is also important to each of us for the performance of many activities of daily living (ADLs), such as shoveling snow or climbing stairs. As we age, a lack of strength may eventually prevent us from performing many ADLs needed for basic independence, from walking to getting out of a chair. Lack of strength may eventually also prevent us from performing recreational activities at a level that is safe and enjoyable, such as basketball, softball, golf, or hiking. Resistance training brings about strength increases in both men and women no matter what their age. It is important to increase or maintain strength as we age so that we can comfortably perform recreational as well as ADLs.

> > > KEY TERMS

Accommodating resistance: Maximum resistance throughout the whole range of motion is maintained by controlling the speed of the movement.

Atrophy: The wasting or loss of muscle tissue resulting from disease or lack of use.

Classic (linear) periodization: A type of periodization using a systematic increase in the intensity and decrease in the volume of training over the course of a training program.

Concentric: A muscular action in which a muscle develops force and shortens, creating movement at a joint.

Constant resistance: Absolute (external) resistance remains constant throughout the range of motion.

Eccentric: A muscular action in which a muscle develops force but is lengthened by a greater opposing force.

Hyperplasia: Formation of new muscle cells.

Hypertrophy: Growth of individual muscle fibers and of whole muscle.

Isometric: A muscular action in which a muscle develops force against a fixed resistance and no limb or joint angle movement occurs.

Isotonic: A muscular action in which muscular force is constant throughout the movement; this term technically applies to the contractions of isolated muscles in laboratory experiments. Although sometimes used to denote dynamic (concentric and eccentric) contractions, normal movements are not isotonic, as intact muscles vary their force throughout the range of motion to compensate for changes in joint angle.

Nonlinear periodization: A type of periodization employing variation in the intensity and volume of training within each week over the course of the training program.

Periodization: Systematic manipulation of acute program variables over time with planned rest periods used to provide recovery.

Progressive resistance: A principle of training in which the stress on the muscle is increased over time as it becomes capable of producing greater force (a specific example of the overload principle).

Valsalva maneuver: Contracting the muscles of exhalation but not allowing air to escape. Performed as breath holding during muscular effort.

Variable resistance: Absolute (external) resistance changes during the range of motion.

> **1.1.36-HFS: Knowledge of the following terms: progressive resistance, isotonic/isometric, concentric, eccentric, atrophy, hyperplasia, hypertrophy, sets, repetitions, plyometrics, Valsalva maneuver.**

HISTORY OF RESISTANCE TRAINING

Resistance training can be traced through much of recorded history for more than 5,000 years. Interestingly, the training practices of the twentieth century were shaped by the three competitive sports of weightlifting, power lifting, and bodybuilding. In the twentieth century, Bob Hoffman at York Barbell Company in York, Pennsylvania, promoted weightlifting and was the epicenter for some of the world's strongest men well into the 1950s, dominating world weightlifting competitions. He also promoted weight training for bodybuilding and physical development for health. In the famous meeting in 1940 of Peter Karpovich, a founder of the *American College of Sports Medicine,* and Bob Hoffman at Springfield College, one of Hoffman's body builders, John Grimek, demonstrated with feats of flexibility that bodybuilders and weightlifters did not have to be inflexible or muscle bound. This changed the minds of many that there was some merit in weight training beyond that of a spectacle. Also part of the development of weight-training programs in the twentieth century was Joe Weider, who promoted bodybuilding with such notables as Arnold Schwarzenegger.

Thomas Delorme might be considered the father of modern resistance training from the perspective of its study in medicine and science. His research as a captain in the U.S. Army and then as an orthopedic surgeon at the Massachusetts General Hospital in Boston provided medical evidence that resistance training could improve not only strength but also performance in the rehabilitation of injured soldiers from World War II (2). In a conversation with his wife over dinner one night, she came up with the term *progressive resistance training* to describe his use of different percentage loads of the 10-repetition maximum (RM) Delorme Method to elicit changes in muscular strength with resistance training (personal communication, Dr. Terry Todd). By the late 1970s into the early 1980s, the use of an expanded arsenal of laboratory techniques quickly extended our understanding of resistance exercise. During the 1980s, there was an exponential rise in the number of investigations on resistance training and on the multitude of physiologic systems studied: dramatic discoveries in the areas of muscle fiber subtype transitions, sex differences in adaptations, training compatibility (i.e., simultaneous heavy resistance training and high-intensity endurance training), as well as opening up a whole new venue for resistance training with the elderly in the fight against sarcopenia. The exponential increase in the study of resistance exercise continued during the 1990s, culminating with a progressions model position stand by the American College of Sports Medicine (ACSM) in 2002 (10).

BASIC PRINCIPLES OF RESISTANCE TRAINING

> **1.7.12-HFS: Knowledge of the principles of overload, specificity, and progression and how they relate to exercise programming.**

It is important to understand some of the basic principles of resistance training to optimize the exercise prescription and the programs developed. When undertaking a needs analysis for a training program, there a few underlying principles to consider.

PROGRESSIVE OVERLOAD

Progressive overload is a universal training principle stipulating that one needs to continually increase the exercise demands to see progression in a performance variable, as defined within the construct of the variable being trained (i.e., strength, power, or local muscular endurance). As a muscle becomes capable of producing greater force or greater power, or has more local muscular endurance, the stress needs to be increased to maintain an overload and have further gains. Consider an individual whose 3RM (the maximal amount of weight that can be lifted three times without rest) for the bench press is 250 lb. Training with this weight is a sufficient stimulus to produce an increase in strength. Later in the training program, if the individual's strength has increased, 250 lb is no longer the 3RM or a sufficient stimulus to further increase strength. If the training stimulus is not increased at this point, no further gains in strength will occur.

Several methods can be utilized to progressively overload the muscle. The resistance (amount of weight utilized) to perform a certain number of repetitions can be increased. The use of RMs automatically provides progressive overload because as the muscle's strength increases, the amount of resistance necessary to perform a true RM also increases. For example, a 3RM may increase from 250 lb to 260 lb after several weeks of training. Another method of progressively overloading the muscle is to increase the volume of training performed (i.e., the number of sets and repetitions of a particular exercise) or decrease the rest period between sets. (However, if increasing strength, per se, is the goal, then increasing the resistance appears to be the most important variable.) An important corollary is that progression must be varied as directed by the periodization principle of resistance training (see below), so that overtraining (see Chapter 31) is minimized or eliminated in an exercise prescription.

SPECIFICITY OF TRAINING

This is very much the underlying principle of any exercise program. Training is specific to the type of program utilized, and only those muscles that are trained will adapt and change in response to a resistance-training program. For example, light resistance will not activate many motor units; therefore, the muscle fibers contained in other motor units will not be trained nor adapt to the loading (3). In addition, training the upper body only will not influence the lower-body muscle fibers (14,15). Thus, resistance training is specific to the motor units that are activated and their influence on physiologic systems to support their homeostasis, repair, and remodeling.

SAID PRINCIPLE

SAID is the acronym for *Specific Adaptations to Imposed Demands*. The SAID principle states that the adaptations to resistance exercise are specific to the demands of the program (which, in turn, are determined by the acute program variables). This principle is an extension of the concept of specificity and underscores the importance of the exercise prescription in targeting those features of adaptation that are influenced by a specific resistance-training program. These adaptations depend on the exercise range of motion and specific mode. For instance, isometric exercise may increase strength, but only at the specific angle the exercise is performed.

PERIODIZATION OF TRAINING

Overtraining is a decrease in performance despite continued training. To eliminate the potential for overtraining and boredom in resistance training, variation in the exercise stimuli is vital. Periodization of training involves the systematic manipulation of the acute program variables over time with planned rest periods used to provide recovery, as opposed to the standard progressive overload method, in which the repetition range remains constant for several weeks while the weight is increased as strength allows. Unloading or lighter cycles of workouts also provide the body with recovery periods needed for optimal training. Both the classical linear periodization program (which manipulates workout protocols over each week within 4-week microcycles) and the nonlinear method (which manipulates intensity, volume, and other acute program variables within a week) have been shown superior to standard progression programs (11,16,25,27).

PRIORITIZATION OF TRAINING

With any total conditioning program, one has to prioritize the training goals. Even within a periodized program, the trainable goals for resistance training are maximal strength, power, local muscular endurance, and muscle hypertrophy. As discussed in Chapter 31, many of the other systems adapt as well in support of these training goals (e.g., connective tissue). Thus, each training cycle needs to have a training priority based on the goals of the individual.

NEEDS ANALYSIS

> **1.1.23-HFS: Knowledge of the principles involved in promoting gains in muscular strength and endurance.**

> **1.1.37-HFS: Knowledge of and skill to demonstrate exercises designed to enhance muscular strength and/or endurance of specific major muscle groups.**

> **1.7.42-HFS: Ability to design resistive exercise programs to increase or maintain muscular strength and/or endurance.**

> **1.7.11-HFS: Knowledge of and the ability to describe exercises designed to enhance muscular strength and/or endurance of specific major muscle groups.**

Before designing a resistance-training program, a thorough needs analysis must take place (10). To ensure the program is individualized, assessment should focus on goals and needs, such as the intended time frame for achieving these goals, targeted areas or muscle groups, health issues (e.g., hypertension, asthma, diabetes), musculoskeletal limitations, recent surgeries, chronic injuries, and sites of pain. The needs analysis will dictate the prescription of the acute program variables, and determine what energy systems and muscle actions are to be trained. Baseline fitness assessment, consisting of anthropometric measurements (e.g., height, weight, circumferences), body composition, and tests of muscular strength and endurance may assist in this by determining the level of the different fitness variables. In addition, follow-up assessments using these tools will provide feedback on progress. Designing an optimal resistance-training program depends heavily on the individual strengths, weaknesses, and goals of the patient (3).

METABOLIC DEMANDS

Each resistance-training workout can be designed to give a very different metabolic response, ranging from short-rest-period workouts that are physiologically very demanding to heavy resistance workouts with long rest periods that focus on maximal force development (12,13). The metabolic demands of a resistance-training program should match the goals of the individual. For example, short-rest, circuit-type programs help to develop acid-base tolerance and local muscular endurance, whereas heavy resistance-training programs enhance maximal force production with little impact on local muscular endurance.

BIOMECHANICAL ACTIONS

Because of the principles of training specificity and SAID, fitness professionals must first conduct a thorough analysis of the movements performed by their patients during sport and ADLs before commencing with resistance-training program design. Most training programs will include whole-body exercises to promote intramuscular coordination, exercises inclusive to both the upper- and lower-body musculature, and exercises that utilize all the muscles around each joint. Including these integral movements will ensure proper muscular development and transferability to the desired activity(s) performed by the client. Like acute program variables, the biomechanical portion of the needs analysis will be helpful in prescribing exercises and resistance levels that will best transfer to the primary sport or activity for which an individual trains.

INJURY POTENTIAL

Resistance exercises chosen should not predispose participants to injury. Rather, careful planning of the resistance-training program can efficiently address the concept of "prehabilitation," or prevention of injury through planned, progressive improvements in strength and motor control of that strength. Further, exercises that address prior sites of injury are also important to eliminate the potential for tissue weakness and vulnerability in sport or recreational activities. For example, a client with a unilateral, injury-induced strength deficit may benefit from exercises that emphasize unilateral movements using dumbbells as opposed to bilateral movements using a barbell. With unilateral movements, the stronger muscle group is discouraged from "cheating" for the weaker muscle group.

ACUTE PROGRAM VARIABLES

Once the needs analysis is completed, resistance-training program design can occur. In program design, one has specific "tools" to work with, referred to as acute program variables. Examples of acute program variables include choice of exercises, order of exercises, split routines, number of sets, intensity of exercise, and the rest periods between sets and between exercises. Without an appreciation of how to properly implement and manipulate acute program variables, two fundamental flaws will occur: (a) all programs will look the same and thus not meet the specific needs of the individual and (b) the individual will not progress and training plateaus will ensue. Therefore, understanding the acute program variables and their influence on the effectiveness of a resistance training program is vital to optimal exercise prescription.

CHOICE OF EXERCISES

The choice of exercise is related to the biomechanical characteristics of the goals targeted for improvement. The number of possible joint angles and exercises are almost as limitless as the body's functional movements. Because muscle tissue that is not activated will not benefit from resistance training, the exercises should be selected so they stress the muscles, joints, and joint angles specified by the client's needs analysis.

Exercises are designated as primary or assistance exercises. Primary exercises train the prime movers in a particular movement and are typically major muscle group exercises (e.g., leg press, bench press, hang pulls). Assistance exercises train predominantly a single muscle group (e.g., triceps press, bicep curls) that aid (synergists) in the movement produced by the prime movers.

Exercises may also be classified as multijoint or single-joint exercises. Multijoint exercises require the coordinated action of several muscle groups and joints. Power cleans, hang power cleans, power snatches, dead lifts, and squats are good examples of whole-body multijoint exercises. The bench press, which involves movement of both the elbow and shoulder joints, is also a multijoint, multimuscle group exercise, although it only involves movement in the upper body. Other examples of multijoint exercises are the lateral pull-down and military press.

Exercises that attempt to isolate the particular muscle group movement of a single joint are single-joint and/or single-muscle-group exercises. Bicep curls, knee extensions, and knee curls are examples of isolated single-joint, single-muscle-group exercises. Many assistance exercises are classified as single-muscle-group or single-joint exercises.

Multijoint exercises require neural coordination among muscles and thus promote coordinated multijoint and multimuscle-group movements. Multijoint exercises require a longer initial learning or neural phase compared with single-joint exercises; however, it is very important to include multijoint exercises in a resistance-training program because most sports and functional activities in everyday life (e.g., climbing stairs) depend on structural multijoint movements. For most sports, whole-body strength/power movements are the basis for success. Running and jumping—as well as activities such as tackling in American football, a take down in wrestling, or hitting a baseball—all depend on whole-body strength/power movements. Thus, incorporating multijoint exercises in a resistance-training program is important for both athletes and nonathletes. A basic program will include eight to ten different exercises (primarily multijoint) that work all the major muscle groups.

Many multijoint exercises, especially those with an explosive component, involve the need for advanced-lifting techniques (e.g., power cleans, power snatches). An important advantage to multijoint exercises is that they are time efficient, because several different muscle groups are activated at the same time. In addition, they allow for intramuscular coordination between joints. Multijoint exercises—in terms of muscle tissue activated, hormonal response, and metabolic demands—far outweigh the benefits of single-joint exercises, and most workouts should revolve around these exercises. Of course, because they involve more complex movements and larger muscle groups, the fitness professional must incorporate multijoint exercises into a training program judiciously and always with the abilities and disabilities of the client in focus.

ORDER OF EXERCISES

Sequencing of specific exercises within a session significantly affects force production and fatigue rate during a resistance exercise session (4). As already discussed (Choice of Exercises), multijoint exercises are more effective for increasing muscular strength than single-joint exercises. Therefore, these exercises should be given priority within the training session (i.e., placed early in the training sessions when fatigue is minimal). Experts have made the following recommendations regarding exercise order (10):

When training all major muscle groups in a workout:

- Perform large muscle group exercises before small muscle group exercises.
- Perform multijoint exercises before single-joint exercises.
- Rotate upper- and lower-body exercises.

Also, for power training, perform total-body exercises (from most to least complex) before basic exercises. For example, perform power cleans before back squats (15). This is especially important when teaching new exercises.

When training individual muscle groups:

- Perform multijoint exercises before single-joint exercises.
- Perform higher-intensity exercises (i.e., those that require a greater percentage of one's 1RM) before lower-intensity exercises.
- An alternative technique sometimes used by bodybuilders is to perform single-joint exercises (i.e., triceps) before multijoint exercises (i.e., bench press) to prefatigue the assistance muscles, thus increasing the overload on the primary muscles.

It is especially important to check for proper exercise technique anytime a change is made in the program design (e.g., changing the order of exercise, changing the rest period lengths). Changes in the program design could have an impact on the skills of a particular lift. Complex multijoint exercises (e.g., power cleans) are more sensitive to such program alterations because of the higher technique demands.

Split Routines

Advanced lifters often use split routines, in which a portion of the body is trained two or three nonconsecutive days per week and a separate portion is trained on alternate days. This practice allows the lifter to perform a greater total volume of training without becoming overly fatigued in a given lifting session. Guidelines for the order of exercises are similar as for training the entire body in one workout. For example, when training upper-body exercises on one day and lower-body exercises on a separate day:

- Perform large muscle group exercises before small muscle group exercises.
- Perform multijoint exercises before single-joint exercises.
- Rotate opposing (agonist and antagonist) exercises.

NUMBER OF SETS

This variable has received much attention, as the number of sets for an exercise is part of the total work equation. When progression is desired for a given exercise, more work is needed (10,26). One set of an exercise is a starting point for beginners because of limited toleration of the exercise stress (33).

The number of sets performed for each exercise is a factor in what is referred to as the *volume* of exercise (i.e., sets × reps × resistance). As such, one of the major roles of the number of sets performed is to regulate the volume performed during a particular exercise protocol or training program. In studies examining resistance-trained individuals, multiple-set programs have been found to be superior for strength, power, hypertrophy, and high-intensity endurance improvements (16). These findings have prompted the recommendation from ACSM (2002) for periodized multiple-set programs when long-term progression (not maintenance) is the goal (10). No study has shown single-set training superior to multiple-set training in either trained or untrained individuals. Thus, it appears that both single- and multiset programs can be effective in increasing strength in untrained clients during short-term training periods (i.e., 6–12 weeks). However, some short-term and all long-term studies support the contention that the greater training stimulus associated with the higher volume from multiple sets is needed to create further improvement and progression in physical adaptation and performance (10,31).

Variation in training stimuli, as will be discussed in detail later, is also critical for continued improvement, and this variation often includes a reduction in training volume during certain phases of the overall training program. The determining factor here is in the "periodization" of training volume rather than in the number of sets, as sets is only one of the components in volume. Once initial fitness has been achieved, a multiple presentation of the exercise stimulus (typically two to four sets, but as many as six in the training of athletes), with specific rest periods between sets allowing for the use of the desired resistance, is superior to a single presentation of the training stimulus (2). Some advocates of single-set programs believe that a muscle or muscle group can only perform maximal exercise for a single set; however, this has not been demonstrated. On the contrary, studies have found that with sufficient rest between sets, trained individuals can produce the same maximal effort during multiple sets (10).

Exercise volume is a vital concept in resistance-training progression, especially for those who have already achieved a basic level of training or strength fitness. As mentioned earlier, the principle of variation in training—or, more specifically, "periodized training"—involves the number of sets and repetitions performed. Because the use of a constant volume program can lead to staleness and lack of adherence to training, variations in training volume (i.e., both low- and high-volume exercise protocols) are important during a long-term training program to provide adequate rest and recovery periods. This concept is addressed later in the chapter under "Periodization."

INTENSITY OF EXERCISE

The amount of resistance used for a specific exercise is one of the key variables in any resistance-training program (31). It is the major stimulus related to changes observed in measures of strength and local muscular endurance. When designing a resistance-training program, the resistance for each exercise must be chosen in accordance with the abilities, disabilities, and goals of the participant. The **repetition maximum** is often used to designate intensity, defined as the greatest weight that can be lifted for a given number of repetitions with proper form. For example, the 10RM is a weight that can be lifted 10 times, but not 11 times. Typically, a single training RM target (e.g., 10RM) or an RM target range (e.g., 3–5RM) is used. Throughout the training program, the absolute resistance is then adjusted to match the changes in strength so a true RM target or RM target resistance range continues to be used. Performing every set until failure occurs can be stressful on the joints, but it is important to ensure that the resistance used corresponds to the targeted number of repetitions. This is because performing four to five repetitions with a resistance that allows for only four to five repetitions compared with a resistance that would allow 14 or 15 repetitions produces quite different training results.

Another method of determining resistances for an exercise involves using a percentage of the 1RM (e.g., 70% or 85% of the 1RM). If the client's 1RM for an exercise is 200 pounds (90.9 kg), a 70% resistance would be 140 pounds (63.6 kg). This method requires that the maximal strength in all exercises used in the training program be evaluated regularly. Without regular 1RM testing (e.g., each week initially, or each month later in a program), the percentage of the true 1RM used during training will decrease as the individual becomes stronger, and the rela-

tive training intensity will consequently fall. This is especially true at the beginning of a program, when strength gains may be rapid. From a practical perspective, use of percentages of 1RM as the resistance for many exercises may not be administratively effective because of the amount of testing time required. In addition, for beginners, the reliability of a 1RM test can be poor. It is therefore recommended that the RM target or RM target range be used as it allows the trainer to alter the resistance in response to changes in the number of repetitions that can be performed at a given absolute resistance. For general conditioning, lifting to the point of muscular fatigue (not complete failure) in 8 to 12 repetitions is recommended (corresponding to approximately 60%–80% of the 1RM) (10). Lifting to the point of muscular fatigue may be described as stopping the set when the lifter feels he or she is unlikely to complete an additional repetition, whereas lifting to the point of complete failure refers to continuing to attempt additional repetitions until the lifter is unable to move through the full range of motion and must be spotted.

As is the case for all the acute program variables, the loading intensity should depend on the goal and training status of the client. The intensity of the loading (as a percentage of 1RM) has an effect on the number of repetitions that can be performed and vice versa. It is ultimately the number of repetitions that can be performed at a given intensity that will determine the effects of training on strength development (7,8). If a given absolute resistance allows for a specific number of repetitions (defined as the repetition maximum), then any reductions in the number of repetitions without an increase in the resistance will cause a change in the training stimulus. In this case, the change in the stimulus will lead to a change in the motor units recruited to perform the exercise and thus the neuromuscular adaptations.

Specific neuromuscular adaptations to resistance training depend in large part on the resistance used. These adaptations follow the principle of specificity presented earlier in this chapter. Heavier resistances will produce lower numbers of repetitions (one to six) and have been found to lead to greater improvements in maximal strength (10,31). Thus, if development of maximal strength is desired, higher loads should be used. Alternately, if muscular endurance is the goal, a lower load should be used, which will in turn allow a greater number of repetitions (e.g., 15–25) to be performed. Muscular hypertrophy appears to be optimized by moderate loading and a moderate repetition range (10,31).

REST BETWEEN SETS AND EXERCISES

The rest periods play an important role in dictating the metabolic stress of the workout and influence the amount of resistance that can be used during each set or exercise. A major reason for this is that the primary energy system used during resistance exercise, the ATP-creatine phosphate system, needs to be replenished, and this process takes time. Therefore, the duration of the rest period significantly influences the metabolic, hormonal, and cardiovascular responses to an acute bout of resistance exercise, as well as the performance of subsequent sets. For advanced training emphasizing absolute strength or power (few repetitions and maximal or near-maximal resistance), rest periods of 3 to 5 minutes are recommended for large muscle mass multijoint exercises (such as squat, power clean, or dead lift), whereas shorter rest periods (1–2 min) may be sufficient for smaller muscle mass exercises or single-joint movements (10). For a novice-to-intermediate resistance exercise protocol, rest periods of 2 to 3 minutes may suffice for large muscle mass multijoint exercises because the lower absolute resistance used at this training level seems to be less stressful to the neuromuscular system. Performance of maximal resistance exercises requires maximal energy substrate availability at the onset of the exercise and a minimum fatigue level and thus requires relatively long rest periods between sets and exercises. Resistance training that stresses both the glycolytic and ATP-creatine phosphate energy systems appears to be superior in enhancing muscle hypertrophy (e.g., body building), thus less rest (1–2 min) between sets appears to be more effective in promoting hypertrophy. If the goal is to optimize both strength and muscle mass, both types of protocols should be used. However, short-rest resistance-training programs can cause greater psychological anxiety and fatigue (32), potentially because of the greater discomfort, muscle fatigue, and high metabolic demands of the program. Therefore, psychological ramifications of using short-rest workouts must be carefully considered and potentially discussed with the patient before the training program is designed. The increase in anxiety appears to be associated with the high metabolic demands found with short-rest exercise protocols (i.e., 1 min or less). Despite the high psychological demands, the changes in mood states do not constitute abnormal psychological changes and may be a part of the normal arousal process before a demanding workout.

CHRONIC PROGRAMMING

Progressive resistance training programs often increase the absolute resistance over time (i.e., the weight increases), whereas the relative resistance (the RM range) does not vary. Such programs are considered constant in their approach to progression. However, greater variation in resistance training variables over time is vital for optimal results and has been shown to be superior to training programs that progress in a constant manner (10,31). Periodization is a type of chronic programming that allows for optimal variation of training.

PERIODIZATION OF TRAINING

Periodization of training has evolved into two specific models: classic (or linear) and nonlinear periodization. Classic periodization typically involves 2- to 4-week periods called *microcycles* in which the workouts within each microcycle are similar, and intensity is increased from one microcycle to the next. Nonlinear periodization utilizes great variation within each microcycle, such as having four or five distinct workouts in a 7- to 10-day period (11,23). Both are effective and are superior over time to constant relative resistance-training programs (e.g., three sets of 8–10RM) (18,34).

Classic (Linear) Periodization

Classic periodization methods utilize a progressive increase in the intensity with only small variations in each 2- to 4-week microcycle (19,23). An example of a classic four-cycle linear periodized program (using 4 weeks for each cycle) is given in Box 29-1. The group of four microcycles is termed a *mesocycle*. A long-term training program consisting of several mesocycles is termed a *macrocycle* (e.g., a 1-year training plan).

There is some variation within each microcycle as the lifter progresses from the low end to the high end of the designated repetition range (and then increases the absolute resistance to return to the lower end of the repetition range). Still, the general trend for this example 16-week program is a steady linear increase in the intensity of the training program (lower RM range in each succeeding microcycle) with a decrease in the volume of exercise (lower combination of sets × repetitions × weight in each microcyle, despite the increase in weight). Because of the straight-line increase in the intensity of the program, it has been termed *linear periodized training*.

It is important to point out that one must be careful not to progress too quickly to train with high volumes of heavy weights. Pushing too hard can potentially lead to a serious overtraining syndrome. Overtraining can compromise progress for months. Although it takes a great deal of excessive work to produce such an overtraining

BOX 29-1	SAMPLE CLASSIC (LINEAR) PERIODIZED PROGRAM

Microcycle 1	**Microcycle 2**
3–5 sets of 12–15RM	4–5 sets of 8–10RM
Microcycle 3	**Microcycle 4**
3–4 sets of 4–6RM	3–5 sets of 1–3RM

Each microcycle lasts 4 weeks in this example. The group of four microcycles is a mesocycle. The next mesocycle would repeat the pattern with higher absolute resistance.

effect, highly motivated trainees can easily make the mistake out of sheer desire to make gains and see progress in their training. Thus, it is important to monitor for signs of overtraining, such as decreased performance and undue fatigue.

High volume exercise in the early microcycles has been thought to promote the muscle hypertrophy needed to eventually enhance strength in the later phases of training (30). Thus, the late cycles of training are linked to the early cycles of training and enhance each other, as strength gains are related to size changes in the muscle. Programs that attempt to gain strength without increasing muscle tissue are limited in their potential.

The increases in the intensity of the periodized program develop the needed nervous system adaptations for enhanced motor unit recruitment. This happens as the program progresses and heavier resistances are used. Heavier weights demand high threshold motor units to become involved in the force production process. The associated increase in muscle protein in the muscles from the early cycle training enhances the force production of the motor units. Here again, one sees an integration of the different parts of the 16-week training program.

The 16-week program in the example provided is the mesocycle; a 1-year training program, the macrocycle, is made up of several mesocycles (3). In classic periodization, each mesocycle in a single macrocycle uses the same pattern of sets and RM ranges, but the absolute resistance increases as the lifter improves. Each mesocycle attempts to progress the body's muscle hypertrophy, strength, and/or power upward toward one's theoretical genetic maximum. Thus, the theoretical basis for a linear method of periodization consists of developing hypertrophy followed by improved nerve function and strength (23). This is then repeated with each mesocycle, with a new resistance for each RM load, and progress is made in the training program.

Nonlinear Periodization

More recently, the concept of nonlinear periodized training programs has been developed to maintain variation in the training stimulus (11). The nonlinear program allows for variation in the intensity and volume within each microcycle (typically 7–10 days) over the course of the training program (e.g., a 16-week mesocycle). An example of a nonlinear periodized training program is given in Box 29-2.

In the nonlinear example, variation in training is much greater within the 7- to 10-day microcycle than in the 4-week microcycle in the linear example described earlier. One can easily see that intensity spans over a maximum of a 14RM range (possible 1RM sets versus 15RM sets in the 1-week cycle). This span in training variation appears to be as effective as linear programs. One can also add a "power" training day when loads may

---

BOX 29-2 SAMPLE NONLINEAR PERIODIZED PROGRAM

Monday (Day 1)	**Wednesday (Day 2)**
4 sets 12–15RM	3–4 sets of 4–6RM
Friday (Day 3)	**Monday (Day 4)**
4 sets of 8–10RM	4–5 sets of 1–3 RM

Wednesday (Day 5)

Power day: 3–5 sets of 3 at 30%–45% of 1RM

This protocol uses a 5-day rotation with 1 day of rest between each workout to create a 10-day microcycle. A mesocycle of, for example, 16 weeks could be completed by increasing the absolute resistance in subsequent microcycles.

---

be from 30% to 45% of 1RM and the light resistance allows for explosive movement. Exercise choice is vital as only power-type exercises should be used (e.g., squat jumps, bench throws, hang power cleans, hang pulls). Exercises in which one holds onto the mass have a great deal of joint deceleration (e.g., bench press) because of the mass not being released at the end of the range of motion to protect the joint (22). In essence, muscle activation in such situations is also inhibited; thus, they are not optimal exercises for increasing power output.

Different from the linear methods, nonlinear programs attempt to train both the hypertrophy and neural aspects of strength within the same week. Thus, one is working on two different physiologic adaptations within the same 7- to 10-day period of the 16-week mesocycle. This appears possible and may be more conducive to many individuals' schedules, especially when competitions, travel, or other schedule conflicts can make the traditional linear method difficult to adhere to.

In the nonlinear program, one rotates through the different protocols. The workout rotates between very heavy, heavy, moderate, power, and/or light training sessions. If one misses a given workout, the rotation order is just pushed forward, meaning one performs the missed workout on the next training day. For example, if the light (12–15RM) workout was scheduled for Monday and it is missed, the lifter performs it on Wednesday and continues with the rotation sequence. In this way, no workout stimulus is missed in the training program. One can also say that a mesocycle will be completed when a certain number of workouts are completed (e.g., 48) and not use training weeks to set the program length.

Again, the primary exercises are typically periodized, but one can also use a two-cycle program to vary the small muscle group exercises. For example, in the triceps push-down, one could rotate between the moderate (8–10RM) and the heavy (4–6RM) cycle intensities.

This would provide the hypertrophy needed for such isolated muscles of a joint, but also provide the strength needed to support heavier workouts of the large muscle groups.

In conclusion, two different approaches can be used to periodize a training program: linear and nonlinear. The programs appear to produce similar benefits but are superior to constant training programs (1). It appears that this is accomplished by training either the hypertrophy component first and the neural strength component second in the linear method, or both components within a 7- to 10-day period in the nonlinear method. The key to workout success is variation, and different approaches can be used over the year to accomplish this training need.

BASIC TECHNIQUES IN RESISTANCE TRAINING

Basic understanding of various aspects of resistance training is vital to provide a safe environment for training. These techniques can include breathing, range of motion, repetition speed, and warm-up.

BREATHING

The lifter should inhale just before and during the eccentric (lowering) phase of the repetition and exhale during the concentric (lifting) phase. During isometric training, the lifter should breathe throughout the muscular contraction. Although there is a tendency for lifters to hold breath during the last repetition of a set or during heavy lifts (e.g., 1–6RM), one should not allow breath holding throughout a complete repetition. When a lifter holds his or her breath during effort and contracts the muscles of exhalation without allowing air to escape, intrathoracic pressure rises, resulting in a large increase in systemic arterial blood pressure. This is known as the Valsalva maneuver, and the increased arterial blood pressure can pose a hazard to individuals with underlying cardiovascular disease and may also result in damage to blood vessels (e.g., in the eye, resulting in Valsalva retinopathy). The increased intrathoracic pressure limits venous return to the heart. If the Valsalva maneuver is held for several seconds (as during a maximal effort lift), the decreased venous return reduces cardiac output, arterial pressure falls, and blood flow to the brain is reduced. This can cause light-headedness and even fainting, which can result in loss of control of the weight and possible injury. This problem is especially true during maximal lifting and when going to failure in a set. One can limit the negative effects by using an RM zone and lifting to the point of muscular fatigue versus complete failure. If one exhales continuously through the concentric phase of the lift, the problem can be avoided.

FULL RANGE OF MOVEMENT

Each exercise should be performed through a full range of motion in order for each part of the muscle to gain the benefits of the resistance used. With some resistance training machines, range of motion can be a concern if the machine poorly fits individual users. Many machines are designed to fit adult men. In smaller individuals, including prepubescent children, the limbs are too short for a proper fit, which makes correct technique and full range of motion of the exercise virtually impossible.

With some machines, simple alterations can be made to allow a child to safely use the machine; for example, use additional seat pads on a knee extension machine or use blocks under a bench for the child to place his or her feet. Simply adjusting seat height often is not enough to make a machine fit the child. One may also need to adjust for proper positioning of the arms and legs on the contact points of the machine. In addition, raising the seat height may make it impossible for the child's feet to reach the floor. In many exercises, the feet need to touch the floor to aid in balance. Therefore, if the seat is raised, one may also need to place blocks under the child's feet.

MOVEMENT SPEED

When using maximal loads, movement speed will necessarily be slow. With submaximal loads, a lifter can choose to move the weight at various speeds. Maximal speed is used to move the weight explosively for power training. Slower speeds provide greater control over the weight. The speed of movement will often become slower during a set as fatigue occurs. This phenomenon was demonstrated in a study examining repetition velocity during a 5RM bench-press set. It was shown that the first three repetitions were 1.2 to 1.6 seconds in duration, whereas the last two repetitions were 2.5 and 3.3 seconds in duration, respectively (20).

Intentional use of a very slow velocity [10-s CON (concentric action); 5-s ECC (eccentric action)] compared with a slow velocity (2-s CON; 4-s ECC) has been shown to result in significantly less strength gains over a 10-week training program (9). Compared with slow velocities, moderate and fast velocities have been shown to be more effective for increasing the number of repetitions performed, work and power output, and total volume of training (17,21), and for increasing the rate of strength gains (6).

WARM-UP

At the beginning of a resistance training session, a period of time should be devoted to warming up the muscles and preparing them for the intensity of the upcoming exercise. This may be accomplished by first performing 5 to 10 minutes of a general cardiorespiratory warm-up through such exercises as treadmill walking or stationary cycling. The general warm-up is followed by 5 to 10 minutes of specifically warming up the muscles to be targeted in the resistance-training session. This may involve dynamic stretching movements (see below) and the use of a light load on a preliminary set of each resistance exercise.

MACHINE AND FREE-WEIGHT EXERCISES

> **1.7.29-HFS: Ability to identify proper and improper technique in the use of resistive equipment, such as stability balls, weights, bands, resistance bars, and water exercise equipment.**

> **1.7.45-HFS: Ability to describe the advantages and disadvantages of various commercial exercise equipment in developing cardiorespiratory fitness, muscular strength, and muscular endurance.**

The use of free-weight versus machine resistance exercises is a topic of debate. Below are some points of comparison between the two modalities.

1. Machines are not always designed to fit the proportions of all individuals. Individuals who are obese, have special physical considerations or disabilities, or are shorter, taller, or wider than the norm may not be able to fit comfortably in the machines and use them with ease. Free-weight exercises can easily be adapted to fit most clients' physical size or special requirements.

2. Machines utilize a fixed range of motion, thus the individual must conform to the movement limitations of the machine. Often, these movements do not mimic functional or athletic movements. Free weights allow for full range of motion, and the transfer to real-world movements is greater than for machines.

3. Most machines isolate a muscle or muscle group, thus negating the need for other muscles to act as assistant movers and stabilizers. Free-weight exercises almost always involve assisting and stabilizing muscles. On the other hand, if the goal is to isolate a specific muscle or muscle group, as in some rehabilitation settings or because of physical disabilities, machine exercises can more easily accomplish this.

4. Although it is never advisable to perform resistance exercise alone, machines do allow for greater independence as the need for a spotter or helper is usually diminished once the individual has learned the technique of the exercise. Moreover, it is simpler and easier to change the weight between sets when using machines. However, the perception of extra safety may lead to a lack of attention being paid to the exercise. It is still possible to become injured when using machines.

5. Machine exercises may be more useful than free-weight exercises in some special populations. One reason for this is that machines are often perceived to be less intimidating to a beginner. As the resistance-training skill and experience level increases, free-weight

exercise can gradually be introduced if desired. However, it is important to inform clients of the benefits that free weights have compared with machines (e.g., increased musculoskeletal loading that reduces risk of developing osteoporosis) (10).

6. Some muscle groups can more easily be trained with specialized machines than with free weights (e.g., training the latissimus dorsi with a lateral pull-down machine).

7. Some machines are designed to provide a variable resistance through the range of motion, providing less resistance when the joint angle is disadvantageous and more resistance when the joint angle is optimal. These variable resistance machines may be useful for providing a more consistent training stimulus through the range of motion, although their applicability to real-world movements is limited compared with free weights.

From the comparison above, it is clear that there are advantages and disadvantages to both machines and free weights. In many cases, free weights are a superior training tool, but machine exercises can still be useful in resistance training when used appropriately. For midlevel and advanced clients and athletes, machines are best used as an adjunct to free-weight training. However, for beginners and some special populations, the ease of use may be an advantage when introducing an individual to resistance training. Table 29-1 lists the common weight-training modalities and gives some examples and advantages and disadvantages of each.

SPOTTING REQUIREMENTS

Good spotting technique is vital for a safe resistance training program. Spotters should be cognizant of the following points:

1. Know proper exercise technique.
2. Know proper spotting technique for free weights or machines.
3. Be sure the spotter is strong enough to assist the lifter with the resistance he or she is using in a free-weight exercise.
4. Know how many repetitions the lifter intends to do.
5. Be attentive to the lifter at all times.
6. Stop the exercise if a movement technique is wrong. Have the lifter practice the exercise with little or no resistance.
7. Know the plan of action if a serious injury occurs.
8. Be prepared to assist the lifter with racking and unracking of the weights.
9. Do not assist the lifter with each repetition; rather, be prepared to assist if the lifter loses control or is unable to complete a repetition.
10. Use proper body mechanics as the spotter.

The goal of correct spotting is to prevent injury. A lifter should always have access to a spotter.

TABLE 29-1. WEIGHT-TRAINING MODALITIES

MODALITY	DEFINITION	EXAMPLES	ADVANTAGES	DISADVANTAGES
Variable resistance devices	Absolute resistance changes during the range of motion	– Machines with a cam or roll bar – Elastic bands	Increase the absolute resistance at the point in the range of motion where the musculoskeletal system is at a biomechanical advantage	At the beginning of a muscle contraction, the resistance is low and not offering a maximal tissue stimulus
Constant resistance devices	Absolute resistance remains constant throughout the range of motion	– Dumbbells – Barbells – Machines with a fixed pivot point or that use cables and pulleys – Medicine balls	Low or no limitation in the range of motion allowed Exercise can easily be adapted to accommodate for the size of an individual	Does not stimulate the neuromuscular systems involved maximally throughout the entire range of motion
Static resistance devices	Involve isometric muscle action	– Pushing against an immovable object, such as a wall	May be used for an athlete to overcome a sticking point	Not practical for most sports or for everyday functioning
Accommodating resistance devices	Maximum resistance throughout the whole range of motion is maintained by controlling the speed of the movement	– Hydraulic machines – Isokinetic devices	No real advantage over variable or constant resistive devices outside of a rehabilitation setting	Hydraulic machines typically have no eccentric movement Impractical Expensive

SUPPLEMENTAL EQUIPMENT

The three most commonly used strength-training accessories are a weight-training belt, gloves, and shoes. Although not absolutely necessary for a safe and effective strength-training program, all three do offer some benefits.

Weight-Training Belts

A weight-training belt has a wide back and is designed to help support the lower back. Although weight-training belts come in many sizes, a belt small enough to fit small children is not commonly available. A belt is not necessary for resistance training but is merely an aid to counteract a lack of strong abdominal and lower-back musculature. Weight-training belts do help support the lower spine but not from the back as is commonly thought. The belt gives the abdominal muscles an object to push against, allowing a buildup of intra-abdominal pressure, which pushes against the lower spine from the front.

Wearing a tightly cinched belt during activity causes a higher blood pressure than if the activity is performed without a belt (5,24). This makes the pumping of blood by the heart more difficult and may cause undue cardiovascular stress. Thus, wearing a belt during resistance exercises in which the lower back is not heavily involved is not recommended. A belt can be worn during lifts involving the lower back, particularly when maximal or near-maximal loads are used, but it should not be used to alleviate technique problems that are due to weak lower-back and abdominal muscles. Rather than allowing a lifter to rely on a belt, incorporate exercises into the program to strengthen the abdominal and lower-back muscles. This can help eliminate chronic lower-back weakness, which could otherwise lead to poor exercise technique. In addition, strong abdominals and lower-back muscles can help prevent injury to the lower back during all physical activity.

Weight-Training Gloves and Shoes

Specially designed resistance training gloves do not cover the fingers but only the palms. They protect the palms somewhat from such things as the knurling on many barbells, dumbbells, and equipment handles, and they may help prevent the formation of blisters or the ripping of calluses on the hands. However, gloves are typically not necessary for safe resistance training.

Weight-training shoes are mainly designed to provide good arch support, a tight fit, and a nonskid surface on the sole. In addition, weight-training shoes offer little or no shock absorbance in the soles; thus any force or power that the lifter develops by extending the leg or hip is not used to compress the sole of the shoe and is available to lift the weight in such exercises as the squat or clean. A lifter should wear a shoe with a nonskid surface on the sole and good arch support, but it does not have to be a shoe specifically designed for power or Olympic weightlifting.

FLEXIBILITY TRAINING

Flexibility training can be done as part of the total conditioning program. Resistance training itself will help with this, but as one ages, additional flexibility training can cause greater augmentation. Flexibility is an important component of physical fitness and needs to be addressed in the context of both resistance and cardiorespiratory training programs.

TYPES OF FLEXIBILITY

Stretching can be performed in both the warm-up and cool-down phases of a training session. Dynamic stretching is recommended in the warm-up phase before resistance training because of possible negative influences of static stretching on muscle contractile forces (28). There are four basic types of stretching techniques:

- Static stretching
- Dynamic or ballistic stretching
- Slow movements
- Proprioceptive neuromuscular facilitation (PNF) techniques

Static Stretching

The most common type of stretching is the static stretching technique. Use of this form of stretching involves a voluntary passive relaxation of the muscle while it is elongated. This technique has become popular because it is easy to learn, effective, and accompanied by minimal incidence of soreness. Static stretching is still one of the most effective and desirable techniques to use when comfort and limited training time are major factors in the implementation of a stretching program. This technique involves holding the muscle in a static position at the desired length. Many variations of this technique have been proposed with stretch time ranging from 15 to 60 seconds. Up to four repetitions of the stretch may be performed.

Dynamic or Ballistic Stretching

Dynamic stretching involves a swinging, bouncing, or bobbing movement during the stretch as the final position in the movement is not held. Dynamic stretching has become popular before maximal effort events or training, as this type of stretching has no negative effects on performance. Delayed muscle soreness in beginners who have no prior resistance-training experience is possible with dynamic stretching.

Slow Movements

Slow movements of a muscle(s)—such as neck rotations, arm rotations, and trunk rotations—are also a type of dynamic stretching activity. The value of using this type of stretching technique may be more important to warm-up activities than to achieving increases in flexibility.

Proprioceptive Neuromuscular Facilitation Techniques

Proprioceptive neuromuscular facilitation (PNF) stretching techniques have increased in popularity as a method of improving flexibility. There are several variations of PNF techniques described in research literature and, unfortunately, the terminology is often overlapping or contradictory. Two basic techniques will be described here (29).

- Hold-relax (sometimes called contract-relax): After an initial passive stretch, the muscle being stretched is isometrically contracted for 6 seconds against resistance, subsequently relaxed, and passively moved into a greater stretch that is held for 10 to 30 seconds. For example, a client lies supine, and a trainer lifts one extended leg until the hamstrings are put in a position of stretch. Then the client forcefully contracts the hamstrings as if to return the leg to the floor, but no movement occurs as the trainer applies resistance. Following 6 seconds of this isometric contraction, the client relaxes the hamstrings, the trainer pushes the leg into a greater position of stretch, and this new position is held for up to 30 seconds.
- Agonist contract-relax: The procedure is the same as the hold-relax, with one addition. During the second stretch of the targeted muscle (e.g., hamstrings as described above), the client contracts the opposing muscle group (quadriceps and hip flexors in this case; termed the *agonist* as this muscle contracts concentrically) to assist the trainer in creating a greater range of motion.

The theoretic basis of these techniques is twofold (29). First, the isometric contraction of the muscle being stretched stimulates its own Golgi tendon organs, resulting in an autogenic inhibition of the stretched muscle, potentially increasing its subsequent stretch. Second, if the opposing muscle is contracted, this results in reciprocal inhibition of the muscle being stretched.

WHEN TO TRAIN FLEXIBILITY

Stretching to improve range of motion is typically performed after a cardiorespiratory or resistance-training session and as a part of the cool-down. This has the advantage of exercising a neuromuscular system that is warm and physiologically more pliable to changes in the range of motion because of prior activity. A flexibility regimen of at least 10 minutes should be performed after other training sessions, with a minimum frequency of twice per week.

SUMMARY

Program design should be specific to training goals, but the potential for creating new resistance-training programs is nearly unlimited. Via manipulation of acute program variables, it is easy to design many distinctly different programs. Further, any training systems, especially popular or faddish ones, should be evaluated in terms of their acute program variables and their ability to address the needs of an individual or sport. Determining which training system or systems to use depends on the goals of the program, time constraints, available training tools, and how the goals of the resistance-training program relate to the goals of the individual's entire fitness program. However, the major goal of any program is to bring about physiologic adaptations (see Chapter 31) while providing the needed rest and recovery to avoid overtraining.

REFERENCES

1. Campos GE, Luecke TJ, Wendeln HK, et al. Muscular adaptations in response to three different resistance-training regimens: specificity of repetition maximum training zones. *Eur J Appl Physiol.* 2002;88(1-2):50–60.
2. DeLorme TL, Watkins AL. Techniques of progressive resistance exercise. *Arch Phys Med.* 1948;29:263–273.
3. Fleck SJ, Kraemer WJ. *Designing Resistance Training Programs.* 3rd ed. Champaign (IL): Human Kinetics; 2004.
4. Hakkinen K, Komi PV, Alen M. Effect of explosive type strength training on isometric force- and relaxation-time, electromyographic and muscle fibre characteristics of leg extensor muscles. *Acta Physiol Scand.* 1985;125(4):587–600.
5. Harman EA, Rosenstein RM, Frykman PN, Nigro GA. Effects of a belt on intra-abdominal pressure during weight lifting. *Med Sci Sports Exerc.* 1989;21(2):186–190.
6. Hay JG, Andrews JG, Vaughan CL. Effects of lifting rate on elbow torques exerted during arm curl exercises. *Med Sci Sports Exerc.* 1983;15(1):63–71.
7. Hoeger WWK, Barette SL, Hale DF, Hopkins DR. Relationship between repetitions and selected percentages of one repetition maximum. *J Appl Sport Sci Res.* 1990;4(2):47–54.
8. Hoeger WWK, Hopkins DR, Barette SL, Hale DF. Relationship between repetitions and selected percentages of one repetition maximum: a comparison between untrained and trained males and females. *J Appl Sport Sci Res.* 1987;1(1):11–13.
9. Keeler LK, Finkelstein LH, Miller W, Fernhall B. Early-phase adaptations of traditional-speed vs. superslow resistance training on strength and aerobic capacity in sedentary individuals. *J Strength Cond Res.* 2001;15(3):309–314.
10. **Kraemer WJ, Adams K, Cafarelli E, et al. American College of Sports Medicine position stand. Progression models in resistance training for healthy adults. *Med Sci Sports Exerc.* 2002;34(2): 364–380.**
11. Kraemer WJ, Fleck SJ. *Optimizing Strength Training: Designing Nonlinear Periodization Workouts.* Champaign (IL): Human Kinetics Publishers Inc.; 2007.
12. Kraemer WJ, Marchitelli L, Gordon SE, et al. Hormonal and growth factor responses to heavy resistance exercise protocols. *J Appl Physiol.* 1990;69(4):1442–1450.
13. Kraemer WJ, Noble BJ, Clark MJ, Culver BW. Physiologic responses to heavy-resistance exercise with very short rest periods. *Int J Sports Med.* 1987;8(4):247–252.
14. Kraemer WJ, Patton JF, Gordon SE, et al. Compatibility of high-intensity strength and endurance training on hormonal and skeletal muscle adaptations. *J Appl Physiol.* 1995;78(3):976–989.
15. Kraemer WJ, Ratamess NA. Fundamentals of resistance training: progression and exercise prescription. *Med Sci Sports Exerc.* 2004;36(4):674–688.
16. Kraemer WJ, Ratamess N, Fry AC, et al. Influence of resistance training volume and periodization on physiological and performance adaptations in collegiate women tennis players. *Am J Sports Med.* 2000;28(5):626–633.
17. Lachance PF, Hortobagyi T. Influence of cadence on muscular performance during push-up and pull-up exercises. *J Strength Cond Res.* 1994;8:76–79.
18. Marx JO, Ratamess NA, Nindl BC, et al. Low-volume circuit versus high-volume periodized resistance training in women. *Med Sci Sports Exerc.* 2001;33(4):635–643.
19. Medvedyev AS. Several bases on the methodics of training weightlifters. *Soviet Sports Reviews.* 1988;22(4):203–206.
20. Mookerjee S, Ratamess NA. Comparison of strength differences and joint action durations between full and partial range-of-motion bench press exercise. *J Strength Cond Res.* 1999;13:76–81.
21. Morrissey MC, Harman EA, Frykman PN, Han KH. Early phase differential effects of slow and fast barbell squat training. *Am J Sports Med.* 1998;26(2):221–230.
22. Newton RU, Murphy AJ, Humphries BJ, Wilson GJ, Kraemer WJ, Hakkinen K. Influence of load and stretch shortening cycle on the kinematics, kinetics and muscle activation that occurs during explosive upper-body movements. *Eur J Appl Physiol Occup Physiol.* 1997;75(4):333–342.
23. Plisk SS, Stone MH. Periodization strategies. *Strength and Conditioning Journal.* 2003;25:19–37.
24. Rafacz W, McGill SM. Wearing an abdominal belt increases diastolic blood pressure. *J Occup Environ Med.* 1996;38(9):925–927.
25. Rhea MR, Alderman BL. A meta-analysis of periodized versus nonperiodized strength and power training programs. *Res Q Exerc Sport.* 2004;75(4):413–422.
26. Rhea MR, Alvar BA, Burkett LN. Single versus multiple sets for strength: a meta-analysis to address the controversy. *Res Q Exerc Sport.* 2002;73(4):485–488.
27. Rhea MR, Phillips WT, Burkett LN, et al. A comparison of linear and daily undulating periodized programs with equated volume and intensity for local muscular endurance. *J Strength Cond Res.* 2003;17(1):82–87.
28. Rubini EC, Costa AL, Gomes PS. The effects of stretching on strength performance. *Sports Med.* 2007;37(3):213–224.
29. Sharman MJ, Cresswell AG, Riek S. Proprioceptive neuromuscular facilitation stretching: mechanisms and clinical implications. *Sports Med.* 2006;36(11):929–939.
30. Stone MH, O'Bryant H, Garhammer J. A hypothetical model for strength training. *J Sports Med Phys Fitness.* 1981;21(4):342–351.
31. Tan B. Manipulating resistance training program variables to optimize maximum strength in men: a review. *J Strength Cond Res.* 1999;13(3):289–304.
32. Tharion W, Harman E, Kraemer W, Rauch T. Effects of different weight training routines on mood states. *J Strength Cond Res.* 1991;5(2):60–65.
33. **Williams MA, Haskell WL, Ades PA, et al. Resistance exercise in individuals with and without cardiovascular disease: 2007 update: a scientific statement from the American Heart Association Council on Clinical Cardiology and Council on Nutrition, Physical Activity, and Metabolism. *Circulation.* 2007;116(5):572–584.**
34. Willoughby D. The effects of mesocycle-length weight training programs involving periodization and partially equated volumes on upper and lower body strength. *J Strength Cond Res.* 1993;7(1):2–8.

SELECTED REFERENCES FOR FURTHER READING

Fleck SJ, Kraemer WJ. *Designing Resistance Training Programs.* 3rd ed. Champaign (IL): Human Kinetics Publishers Inc.; 2004.

Kraemer WJ, Fleck SJ. *Optimizing Strength: Designing Non-Linear Periodization Workouts.* Champaign (IL): Human Kinetics; 2007.

Kraemer WJ, Häkkinen K, editors. *Handbook of Sports Medicine and Science: Strength Training for Sport.* IOC Medical Commission Publication. Oxford, UK: Blackwell Science Ltd.; 2002.

Zatsiorsky VM, Kraemer WJ. *Science and Practice of Strength Training.* 2nd ed. Champaign (IL): Human Kinetics; 2006.

INTERNET RESOURCES

- American College of Sports Medicine: www.acsm.org
- National Strength and Conditioning Association: www.nsca-lift.org

30 Adaptations to Cardiorespiratory Exercise Training

Each day we engage in various types and intensities of physical activity. It may be carrying groceries, going for a 3-mile walk, playing soccer, or running an 800-m race. In each case, the cardiovascular, endocrine, pulmonary, blood (hematologic), and skeletal muscle systems must alter their function in a manner that allows the body to complete the activity. Additionally, repeated and regular exposure to physical activity or sports stimulates the body to develop long-term adaptations. It does this in a manner that is favorable for both exercise performance and health.

This chapter summarizes the chronic adaptations (training effects) that develop in the cardiovascular and pulmonary systems (collectively referred to as the cardiorespiratory or cardiopulmonary system) when an individual participates in cardiorespiratory (aerobic) exercise training. It also describes the loss of these training adaptations that occurs when an individual stops training. Whenever possible, the chapter provides examples and data comparing healthy but untrained (sedentary) individuals with well-trained athletes to demonstrate how the cardiac and pulmonary systems adjust to exercise training.

CARDIORESPIRATORY FITNESS

Physical inactivity is a major contributing risk factor for cardiovascular disease, with an overall, independent risk that is similar to dyslipidemia, cigarette smoking, and hypertension (22). Furthermore, longitudinal studies show that higher levels of aerobic or **cardiorespiratory fitness**, as well as physical activity, are associated with a lower rate of mortality from heart disease, even after statistical adjustments for other disease-related risk factors (4). This holds true for those with known heart disease (37).

Cardiorespiratory fitness is best described by maximal oxygen consumption ($\dot{V}O_{2max}$). Cardiorespiratory fitness is the ability of the body to transport and utilize oxygen. It relies on the effective integration of the cardiovascular, pulmonary, hematologic, and skeletal muscle systems. To appreciate the effect of exercise training on $\dot{V}O_{2max}$, it is important to understand the factors that contribute to $\dot{V}O_{2max}$. Physiologically, it can be defined by rearranging the Fick equation (Adolph Fick, circa 1870):

$$\dot{V}O_2 = \dot{Q} \times a\text{-}\overline{v}O_2 \text{ diff (Also note that } \dot{Q} = HR \times SV)$$

Where: $\dot{V}O_2$ = oxygen consumption; volume of O_2 consumed per minute

$\dot{Q}$ = cardiac output; volume of blood ejected from the left ventricle per minute

SV = stroke volume; volume of blood ejected from the left ventricle per heart beat

> > > **KEY TERMS**

Cardiac hypertrophy: Increase in the size of the heart; this may be an increase in the size of the ventricular chambers or an increase in the ventricular wall thickness.

Cardiorespiratory fitness: The ability to engage in physical activities that rely on oxygen consumption as the primary source of energy; best indicated by the body's ability to transport and utilize oxygen, i.e., maximal oxygen consumption ($\dot{V}O_{2max}$).

Detraining: Changes in body structure or function caused by reduction or cessation of regular physical training.

Dyspnea: Labored breathing; shortness of breath disproportionate to the work being performed.

Myocardial oxygen consumption: The amount of oxygen used by the heart.

Overtraining: State in which there is altered mood and reduced exercise performance despite ongoing exercise training.

Rate-pressure product: Product of heart rate and systolic blood pressure; serves as an estimate of myocardial oxygen demand.

HR = heart rate; cardiac contractions per minute
a - $\bar{v}O_2$ diff = arteriovenous O_2 difference; volume of O_2 extracted per liter of blood

Based on this equation, it should be clear that cardiorespiratory fitness (i.e., $\dot{V}O_{2max}$) is the product of the body's ability to transport oxygen (i.e., cardiac output, stroke volume, heart rate, blood volume, hemoglobin) and to utilize oxygen (i.e., myoglobin, aerobic capacity of muscle, a - $\bar{v}O_2$ diff). Each of these components can affect the magnitude of $\dot{V}O_{2max}$ and can be influenced by age, sex, genetics, the volume and intensity of physical activity or inactivity, the environment (e.g., hypobaria, microgravity), medications, and illness. For example, someone with chronic heart failure has a reduced peak cardiac output, which results in a lower $\dot{V}O_{2max}$ (<50% of normal). On the other hand, a healthy person will have a lower $\dot{V}O_{2max}$ at 14,000 ft (4,300 m) than at sea level because of the reduced ambient pressure that reduces the diffusion gradient for oxygen from the alveoli to hemoglobin in the blood. In each example, $\dot{V}O_{2max}$ is reduced for different reasons, but the end result is a lower cardiorespiratory reserve (peak exercise minus rest) and increased physiologic responses (e.g., heart rate, respiratory rate) and therefore greater perceived effort at submaximal exercise.

PHYSIOLOGIC ADAPTATIONS TO CARDIORESPIRATORY (AEROBIC) EXERCISE TRAINING

> **1.1.17-HFS: Describe knowledge of the physiologic adaptations that occur at rest and during submaximal and maximal exercise following chronic aerobic and anaerobic exercise training.**

OXYGEN CONSUMPTION

$$\dot{V}O_2 = \dot{Q} \times a\text{ - }\bar{v}O_2 \text{ diff}$$

Improving cardiorespiratory fitness depends, in part, on the ability of the cardiovascular and pulmonary systems to adapt to a stimulus of regular bouts of physical activity. Many exercise studies involving healthy people demonstrate 10% to 30% increase in $\dot{V}O_{2max}$ following 12 to 24 weeks of exercise training, with the greatest percent improvement from baseline occurring among the least fit (47). The upper limit of $\dot{V}O_{2max}$ in humans is likely ~85 mL·kg^{-1}·min^{-1} in men and ~75 mL·kg^{-1}·min^{-1} in women, but may be <15 mL·kg^{-1}·min^{-1} in patients with congestive heart failure.

Factors contributing to the exercise training response of $\dot{V}O_{2max}$ have been elucidated through several reports from data obtained in the Heritage Family Study. The Heritage Family Study is a consortium of five institutions that have studied the variability in responses to 20 weeks of exercise training among a heterogeneous group of

more than 700 subjects (www.pbrc.edu/Heritage/index.html). Based on these data, researchers have concluded that there are high, medium, and low responders to exercise training and that the *absolute change* in $\dot{V}O_{2max}$ is not related to age, sex, race, or initial fitness level. Initial fitness level is related to *percent change* in $\dot{V}O_{2max}$, in that those with initially low $\dot{V}O_{2max}$ experience greater proportional increases in $\dot{V}O_{2max}$ following training (58). In addition, data from the Heritage Family Study have also shown heritability (e.g., genetic contribution) for $\dot{V}O_{2max}$ of about 50% (6).

An absolute submaximal work rate, such as walking at 3 mph (4.8 kph), requires a fixed aerobic or oxygen requirement that is similar between humans. Activities like this will be perceived as easier and require less relative effort for individuals with higher cardiorespiratory fitness. A greater cardiorespiratory reserve allows individuals with a higher fitness level to work at a lower percentage of $\dot{V}O_{2max}$. On the other hand, activities of daily living, such as vacuuming, are perceived more difficult by those with lower $\dot{V}O_{2max}$ and therefore decreased cardiorespiratory reserve.

Enhanced oxygen transport, particularly increased maximal stroke volume and cardiac output, is the primary mechanism underlying the increase in $\dot{V}O_{2max}$ with training. Other exercise training responses during submaximal or peak exercise that reflect improved cardiorespiratory fitness include changes in heart rate, a - $\bar{v}O_2$ diff, peripheral resistance, blood volume, blood lactate, and ventilation. Table 30-1 summarizes the physiologic responses to cardiorespiratory exercise training in previously unconditioned persons. Similar changes occur among moderately trained individuals who increase their exercise training, but the greatest relative changes occur in those that are initially sedentary.

It is important to point out that the above-mentioned increases in $\dot{V}O_{2max}$ are associated with repeated participation in an aerobic or large motor activity, such as walking/jogging, swimming, cycling, skating, or Nordic skiing. Resistance training, both dynamic (sometimes referred to as *isotonic*) and isometric, can have a small effect on improving cardiorespiratory fitness, but the magnitude of change is small compared with aerobic exercise training. This is not to say resistance-exercise training is not important. A balanced conditioning program that incorporates both aerobic and resistance training is preferred to help clients improve all aspects of fitness.

Regular aerobic exercise training in previously sedentary, apparently healthy people is associated with improved stamina, an improved ability to tolerate routine activities of daily living, and less fatigue during the day, often occurring within just weeks after starting a program. These changes in healthy people are largely caused by an improved cardiac or central response to exercise.

Modest levels of exercise volume (the product of intensity, duration, and frequency per week) can increase

TABLE 30-1. NORMAL PHYSIOLOGIC ADAPTATIONS TO CARDIORESPIRATORY EXERCISE TRAINING

VARIABLE	REST	SUBMAXIMAL EXERCISE[a]	MAXIMAL EXERCISE
Workload	—	—	↑
Oxygen consumption	↔	↔	↑
Cardiac output	↔	↔	↑
Stroke volume	↑	↑	↑
Heart rate	↓	↓	↔ (or slight ↓)
Blood pressure	↓	↓	↔
a-$\bar{v}O_2$ diff	↔	↔	↑
Minute ventilation	↔	↓ or ↔	↑
Blood volume	↑		—
Blood lactate	↔	↓	↑

↑, increase; ↓, decrease; ↔, no change; —, not applicable.

[a]Submaximal exercise refers to a standardized submaximal work rate, such as 100 watts or walking at 2 mph (3.2 kph).

$\dot{V}O_{2max}$. This is illustrated in the study by Church et al. (8), in which they reported on more than 460 sedentary, low-fit, overweight/obese, postmenopausal women during 6 months of aerobic exercise training of different exercise volumes. The lowest-volume group exercised at just 50% of their peak $\dot{V}O_2$ for about 72 minutes per week, yet showed a 4% increase in peak $\dot{V}O_2$. Study groups assigned to increased duration of exercise, but also at 50% peak $\dot{V}O_2$, incrementally showed larger increases in peak $\dot{V}O_2$.

Patients with coronary artery disease who undergo aerobic training also experience improved function, and those who are symptomatic often experience a decrease in angina symptoms (56). In fact, until the late 1980s, when evidence was presented that regular exercise in these patients improved clinical outcomes (e.g., mortality), the primary reasons for referring these patients to cardiac rehabilitation programs were symptom management and improved exercise tolerance. These reasons, along with the fact that most patients with clinically manifest coronary artery disease have cardiorespiratory fitness levels that are markedly below normal (50%–70% of age and sex predicted) (1), support the use of cardiac rehabilitation.

CARDIAC OUTPUT

$$\dot{V}O_2 = \dot{Q} \times a\text{-}\bar{v}O_2 \text{ diff}$$

Maximum cardiac output is significantly higher in trained than in untrained individuals, primarily because of the ability to increase stroke volume (23,50). Among endurance-trained male subjects, maximal cardiac output can exceed $30 \text{ L} \cdot \text{min}^{-1}$, which represents a five- to sixfold increase over resting values. Among elite class endurance athletes, it is not uncommon to observe maximal cardiac outputs near $40 \text{ L} \cdot \text{min}^{-1}$ (eightfold increase). Generally, the higher the maximal cardiac output, the higher the maximal aerobic power or $\dot{V}O_{2max}$. However, cardiac output is essentially the same at any fixed submaximal work rate in both conditioned and unconditioned individuals (50). Among well-conditioned athletes, a small decrease

may be observed over time, along with a decrease in $\dot{V}O_2$, because of improved economy of effort; however, these changes may not be observed in the average person. Although cardiac output during submaximal exercise may not change following exercise training, the ability to increase maximal cardiac output does, which results in improved exercise capacity and $\dot{V}O_{2max}$.

STROKE VOLUME

$$\dot{V}O_2 = HR \times SV \times a\text{-}\bar{v}O_2 \text{ diff}$$

Heart rate and stroke volume both contribute to increases in cardiac output during acute exercise. Stroke volume increases during exercise secondary to (a) increased venous return (Frank-Starling mechanism), which allows left ventricular end-diastolic volume to remain unchanged or increase slightly; and (b) increased contractile state (perhaps by neurohormonal influences) (3,39,40). Regular aerobic exercise training also leads to **cardiac hypertrophy**, characterized by an enlarged ventricular chamber that does not exceed the upper limits of normal (<56 mm) and a proportionally increased wall thickness; considered together, the ratio of wall thickness to chamber diameter remains constant. For example, left ventricular end-diastolic diameter may approach 55 mm in highly trained endurance athletes versus <45 mm in nonactive, age-matched unconditioned people (23). One important factor contributing to this adaptation of the left ventricle is the 10% to 15% increase in blood volume that develops soon (days) after starting an exercise training program. Intensive exercise training usually results in blood volume increasing by approximately 500 mL through the expansion of plasma volume (11,28). Finally, another contributing factor induced by training is that it likely strengthens myocardial tissue and enables more forceful contractions (21,44,50,57). The result is an augmented ejection of end-diastolic volume (i.e., increased ejection fraction). However, in patients with heart disease, this effect is much less appreciated. In these patients, an improvement in exercise capacity is primarily mediated by improved peripheral oxygen utilization (discussed later in this chapter) and not increases in stroke volume and cardiac output. However, using exercise intensities that exceed current recommendations, some studies have shown increases in stroke volume following exercise training in patients with heart disease (20).

As a result of aerobic exercise training, conditioned individuals are able to increase ejection fraction to a greater degree than their sedentary counterparts; hence, stroke volume is higher in conditioned individuals at any fixed or relative submaximal work rate. The increased stroke volume caused by training allows conditioned individuals to exercise at similar absolute work rates with a lower heart rate, thus decreasing the myocardial oxygen demand of submaximal exercise (39,40). The increase in ejection fraction is generally quite modest—approximately 5% to 10% during maximal exercise. The above-mentioned cardiovascular morphologic characteristics, along with increases in central blood volume and total hemoglobin, are closely correlated with the $\dot{V}O_{2max}$.

HEART RATE

$$\dot{V}O_2 = HR \times SV \times a\text{-}\overline{v}O_2 \text{ diff}$$

Heart rate is the second factor contributing to cardiac output. Among deconditioned persons, exercise causes a proportionally greater increase in heart rate from rest to any fixed submaximal work rate compared with better-conditioned persons. Therefore, because of an attenuated stroke volume response in untrained persons, heart rate plays a greater role in increasing cardiac output during exercise of increasing intensity (52), such as during an exercise stress test.

In a meta-analysis by Cornelissen and Fagard (12), among 72 studies, exercise training resulted in a reduction in resting heart rate of 7 beats $\cdot$ min^{-1}. The reduced heart rate may be caused by altered autonomic function (reduced sympathetic drive and increased parasympathetic drive) and an increase in blood volume. The increased blood volume results in a greater stroke volume via the Frank-Starling mechanism. Maximal heart rate is unchanged or slightly decreased (3–10 beats $\cdot$ min^{-1}) after aerobic exercise training (23).

Although cardiac output at rest or at a given submaximal intensity of exercise (e.g., walking at 2 mph) does not change after an exercise training program, the cardiac output is attained with a lower heart rate and greater stroke volume. A lower heart rate (and, therefore, lower rate-pressure product; see below) requires less myocardial oxygen demand, which may mean delayed onset of angina for the person with exercise-induced angina or less shortness of breath during submaximal activities, such as typical activities of daily living.

ARTERIOVENOUS OXYGEN DIFFERENCE

$$\dot{V}O_2 = \dot{Q} \times a\text{-}\overline{v}O_2 \cdot \text{diff}$$

A final major contributor to the training-induced increase in $\dot{V}O_{2max}$ is an improved a-$\overline{v}O_2$ diff. The difference between arterial and venous content of oxygen in blood reflects the ability of skeletal muscle tissue to extract and use oxygen (46,50). Regular aerobic exercise training increases the number of capillaries surrounding each muscle fiber (23) and enhances the activity of mitochondrial enzymes used in aerobic metabolism, thereby enhancing the ability to extract and utilize the oxygen that is transported in circulating blood. This increased ability to transport oxygen to the working skeletal muscle and to remove and use it to generate energy is a hallmark adaptation of aerobic exercise training.

As was the case for cardiac output, a-$\overline{v}O_2$ diff is similar in trained and untrained persons at submaximal levels of exercise. However, at $\dot{V}O_{2max}$, a-$\overline{v}O_2$ diff is greater in trained than untrained persons (e.g., 155 mL $\cdot$ L^{-1} vs. 135 mL $\cdot$ L^{-1}, respectively). Regular aerobic exercise training enhances the ability to increase a-$\overline{v}O_2$ diff, which contributes to increased exercise capacity.

BLOOD PRESSURE AND BLOOD FLOW

Mean arterial blood pressure (P_{mean}) increases in a relatively linear fashion with cardiac output and, therefore, with $\dot{V}O_2$ and work rate during exercise. Mean arterial blood pressure can be expressed as follows:

$$P_{mean} = 1/3 \text{ (systolic BP} - \text{diastolic BP)} + \text{diastolic BP}$$

Note: At higher heart rates,

$$P_{mean} = 1/2 \text{ (systolic BP} - \text{diastolic BP)} + \text{diastolic BP}$$

$$P_{mean} = \dot{Q} \times T_S P_R$$

Where: $\dot{Q}$ = cardiac output
  BP = blood pressure
  $T_S P_R$ = total systemic peripheral resistance

Primary control of blood pressure (BP) is regulated by alterations in total systemic peripheral resistance, which is accomplished by (a) neural mechanisms affecting peripheral arterioles, (b) locally released substances called endothelial-derived relaxing factors (the most studied is nitric oxide), and (c) changes in local chemistry (e.g., temperature, hydrogen and potassium ions, adenosine) within the metabolically more active skeletal muscles (35,42). There is vasoconstriction in some areas (e.g., splanchnic areas) during exercise and vasodilation in others (e.g., skeletal muscle and myocardium). The overall effect is a decreased total peripheral resistance (23,57). These changes in vasomotor tone allow for a 15-fold or more increase in blood flow to the metabolically active skeletal muscles, a reduction of blood flow to the splanchnic areas, an increase in blood flow to the heart, and maintenance of blood flow to the central nervous system.

Mean arterial BP increases during an acute bout of progressively increasing exercise (such as during an exercise stress test) in healthy individuals because the magnitude of the increase in cardiac output is greater than the decrease in total systemic peripheral resistance. Because diastolic BP remains constant or may decrease slightly in both conditioned and unconditioned individuals, the increase in mean arterial BP is mostly because of increased systolic BP.

Relative to pretraining, after an exercise training program, mean arterial and systolic BP at a fixed submaximal work rate (e.g., walking at 2 mph) will be reduced, with no change in maximum BP. The greater maximum cardiac output following training despite no change in maximum BP indicates that training increases the maximum vasodilatory capacity of the trained muscles. Greater vasodilation leads to a greater reduction in total systemic peripheral resistance, allowing a greater volume of blood to be pumped without requiring higher BPs. Systolic BP at rest and at a fixed work rate is generally lower in trained than untrained people. It is frequently reported that in individuals with known mild or moderate hypertension, regular exercise training lowers resting systolic BP by 4 to 9 mm Hg (7). In a meta-analysis involving 72 studies of exercise training, Cornelissen and Fagard (12) concluded that exercise training among persons without hypertension lowered resting BP by 3.0 mm Hg and 2.4 mm Hg for systolic and diastolic BP, respectively. The training effect was greater among those with hypertension, where resting systolic and diastolic BP were reduced 6.9 mm Hg and 4.9 mm Hg, respectively. Proposed mechanisms responsible for this decrease include neurohumoral, vascular, and structural adaptations. A decrease in plasma catecholamines, improved insulin sensitivity, and favorable changes in endogenous vasoconstricting and vasodilating agents have also been postulated as responsible for the antihypertensive effects of regular exercise training.

After a single bout of exercise, resting systolic BP will be reduced and will remain below pre-exercise values for up to 24 hours. However, although instructive for patients, it is important to understand that this effect is likely a result of reduced total systemic peripheral resistance that occurs during exercise and not a result of permanent biologic adaptations that occur following a program of aerobic exercise training.

RATE–PRESSURE PRODUCT

At rest, the heart consumes about 70% of the oxygen it receives from blood flowing through the coronary arteries, which is almost three times that of skeletal muscle. As a result, the heart responds to increased demand for oxygen by increasing blood flow. In fact, coronary blood flow can increase fourfold from rest to maximal exercise in an adult without coronary artery disease, from 250 $mL \cdot min^{-1}$ to approximately 1,000 $mL \cdot min^{-1}$.

The main factors that influence **myocardial oxygen demand** are heart rate, left ventricular size, and myocardial contractility. However, except for heart rate, it is difficult to gather these measures in most exercise physiology laboratories. The product of heart rate and systolic BP provides a reasonable estimate of myocardial oxygen demand, called the **rate–pressure product** (also known as double product). Rate-pressure product is defined as:

$$RPP = HR \times SBP$$

Where: RPP = rate-pressure product
   HR = heart rate
   SBP = systolic blood pressure

After a program of aerobic exercise training, the magnitude of increase in RPP from rest to a given submaximal work rate is less compared with pretraining values. This attenuated increase is attributable to the previously mentioned chronic adaptations in heart rate and BP, both of which increase less after training and translate to a lesser increase in RPP and myocardial oxygen demand. Collectively, this results in improved efficiency of the heart, pumping a given cardiac output with less oxygen demand.

PULMONARY FUNCTION

> **1.1.29-HFS: Knowledge of and ability to describe the physiologic adaptations of the pulmonary system that occur at rest and during submaximal and maximal exercise following chronic aerobic and anaerobic training.**

Because of the pulmonary system's ability to respond quickly to acute exercise and the fact that it does not normally limit maximal exercise, the demand for pulmonary system adaptations to exercise training is less than other systems (e.g., cardiovascular, skeletal muscle). However, there are several pulmonary-related adaptations that result from a program of aerobic exercise training.

Before discussing these adaptations, it is important to point out that among patients with pulmonary diseases—such as those with chronic bronchitis, emphysema, or asthma—limitations in pulmonary function caused by the disease often minimize expected physiologic gains attributable to exercise training. Also, the **dyspnea** or labored breathing that is associated with most pulmonary disorders often causes individuals to avoid being active, which leads to a vicious circle of further self-imposed activity restriction. This does not mean that these patients do not improve exercise tolerance as a result of participating in an exercise or pulmonary rehabilitation program. Both submaximal endurance and total walking time are usually improved, but typically with little change in $\dot{V}O_{2max}$.

MINUTE VENTILATION

Minute ventilation during exercise is augmented by increasing tidal volume and breathing frequency. Ventilation is controlled by neural and chemical factors, and by sensory mechanisms within the lungs and respiratory muscles. Although ventilation generally does not limit exercise performance in apparently healthy individuals, the limits of ventilation may be reached at maximal exercise in elite aerobic trained athletes (23). Minute ventilation can be defined as:

$$\dot{V}_E = V_T \times f_B$$

Where: $\dot{V}_E$ = minute ventilation; volume of air expired per minute

V_T = tidal volume; volume of air expired per breath

f_B = breathing frequency; breaths per minute

Following a program of exercise training, minute ventilation is unchanged at rest ($\sim$6 L $\cdot$ min^{-1}; tidal volume $\sim$500 mL $\cdot$ breath^{-1}; breathing frequency $\sim$12 breaths $\cdot$ min^{-1}). However, minute ventilation at maximal exercise is increased after training, with the increase attributable to increases in both maximal tidal volume and breathing frequency. Tidal volume and breathing frequency may approach 3,000 mL $\cdot$ breath^{-1} and 55 breaths $\cdot$ min^{-1}, respectively.

Whereas untrained college-aged individuals may achieve a peak ventilation of 120 L $\cdot$ min^{-1}, a 60-year-old patient with heart disease might only achieve a peak value of 60 to 80 L $\cdot$ min^{-1}. In both cases, it is reasonable to assume that an aerobic exercise training program will increase maximal minute ventilation by 15% to 25%. In contrast, well-conditioned male and female athletes may achieve maximal ventilation that approaches 200 L $\cdot$ min^{-1} and 150 L $\cdot$ min^{-1}, respectively. Although exercise training may increase maximal ventilatory capacity, it is unclear that this provides any advantage except at peak exercise. Higher peak ventilatory capacity might increase the buffering capacity for lactate (via increased expiration of CO_2) and allow the partial pressure of O_2 in the alveoli to be maintained in the face of increased pulmonary blood flow to keep hemoglobin saturated. Because ventilation does not limit the ability to perform maximal exercise in apparently healthy persons, increased maximal ventilation following exercise training is likely a consequence of the increased peak workload and $\dot{V}O_{2max}$.

Minute ventilation at a standardized submaximal work rate decreases or is unchanged following exercise training. This is likely because of improved pulmonary diffusion. Ventilation changes in tandem with CO_2 because of neural feedback mechanisms that control ventilation in response to changes in blood pH (i.e., hydrogen ion concentrations). Therefore, if following exercise training lactate threshold is delayed (e.g., occurs at a higher work rate), then ventilation will also be lower. This will also be seen in an increased ventilatory efficiency, as evidenced by a reduced ventilatory equivalent for oxygen ($\dot{V}_E/\dot{V}O_2$) in trained, compared with untrained, individuals.

PULMONARY DIFFUSION CAPACITY

Diffusion capacity is defined as the volume of gas that diffuses through a membrane each minute for a partial pressure difference (i.e., gas concentration difference) of 1 mm Hg. During exercise, diffusion capacity increases in a near linear manner before leveling off near peak exercise. This pattern is observed in trained and untrained individuals, regardless of sex.

At rest and during submaximal and peak exercise, diffusion capacity is greater in endurance-trained individuals. Functionally, this means that O_2 and CO_2 will pass between blood and alveoli more easily in trained persons. Among untrained and trained individuals, maximal diffusion capacity may approach 54 and 74 mL $O_2 \cdot$ min$^{-1} \cdot$ mm Hg^{-1}, respectively (23). It is common to note that the resting diffusion capacity of well-trained runners may approach the values observed at maximal exercise in unconditioned individuals, which may contribute to decreased ventilation at rest and submaximal exercise. The precise mechanism responsible for the increase in diffusion capacity with exercise training is not known.

LACTATE AND VENTILATORY THRESHOLDS

> **1.1.28-HFS: Knowledge of and ability to describe the implications of ventilatory threshold (anaerobic threshold) as it relates to exercise training and cardiorespiratory assessment.**

The lactate threshold is the exercise intensity or oxygen consumption during incremental exercise when the blood lactate concentration rises abruptly (see Chapter 3). Blood lactate concentrations throughout submaximal exercise are reduced as a result of exercise training (Fig. 30-1). Conversely, following exercise training, the intensity of exercise (e.g., speed of running, swimming, cycling) at the lactate threshold is increased, reflecting an improved ability to perform at a higher absolute workload (and $\dot{V}O_2$). Among athletes, it is common to guide training intensity

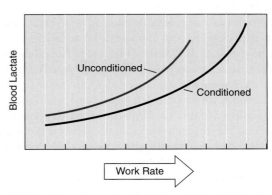

FIGURE 30-1. Blood lactate at increasing exercise intensities in conditioned versus unconditioned persons. The conditioned person typically exhibits lower lactate concentrations at any given work rate than the unconditioned person, but reaches a higher maximum lactate.

using lactate threshold. For example, among elite male rowers, swimmers, and cyclists, the heart rate or work rate corresponding to their individual lactate threshold is identified and then used to guide training intensity at, below, or above their lactate threshold.

Although the precise physiologic adaptations responsible for the above-mentioned decrease in blood lactate during submaximal exercise are not known, there are several possibilities. These include a smaller oxygen deficit incurred at the beginning of exercise attributable to a faster adjustment of oxygen uptake (oxygen kinetics) relative to energy demand; a greater clearance of lactate from the blood produced during exercise, as it is metabolized via the Cori cycle in the liver and also used as an energy source by other organs; and exercise training–induced increases in the size of skeletal muscle mitochondria and in the concentration of enzymes involved in fatty acid oxidation. Concerning the last point, the net result is an improved ability of the skeletal muscle to use fatty acids and to operate aerobically during prolonged exercise versus having to rely as much on anaerobic glycolysis to generate adenosine trisphosphate (ATP).

As discussed in Chapter 3, lactate threshold can be noninvasively identified using ventilatory gas exchange data (i.e., ventilatory threshold) collected during a progressive exercise test. Changes in ventilatory threshold will parallel expected changes in lactate threshold.

DETRAINING AND BED REST

 1.1.32-HFS: Knowledge of the concept of detraining or reversibility of conditioning and its implications in exercise programs.

Although exercise training promotes a variety of physiologic adaptations, long periods of inactivity (i.e., **detraining**) are associated with a reversal of many of these favorable chronic changes. This detraining concept implies that when physical training is stopped or reduced, the organ systems readjust in accordance with the diminished physiologic stimuli.

An extreme example of detraining is bed rest, such as when a person suffers a myocardial infarction and is then confined to bed rest while in the hospital. In the 1960s, such a person may have been ordered to bed rest for up to 3 weeks in the hospital. Upon arriving home, these people often reported being easily fatigued and having a loss of stamina throughout the day, much of it caused by the marked effect that occurred during bed rest (53). Bed rest results in significant deconditioning and also causes central circulatory changes associated with remaining horizontal for a prolonged period of time (e.g., orthostatic hypotension will occur when attempting to become upright).

Today, patients who suffer an uncomplicated myocardial infarction are encouraged to ambulate within 48 to 72 hours of their event and usually find themselves discharged for home within 3 to 5 days. People who suffer a myocardial infarction today spend much less time in bed, which means much less detraining and preserved exercise tolerance and $\dot{V}O_{2max}$.

MAXIMAL OXYGEN CONSUMPTION

Moderate endurance training increases $\dot{V}O_{2max}$ by 10% to 30%, mostly attributable to increases in cardiac output and stroke volume (5,52). Conversely, prolonged detraining (8–10 weeks or more) has been reported to result in a complete return of $\dot{V}O_{2max}$ to pretraining levels (45). Generally, $\dot{V}O_{2max}$ values decline rapidly during the first month of inactivity, with a slower decline to untrained levels occurring during the second and third months of detraining (19,23,26,38). Therefore, the available evidence suggests that increases in $\dot{V}O_{2max}$ produced by endurance training involving exercise of low to moderate intensities and durations are totally reversed after several months of detraining and adoption of a more sedentary lifestyle.

Whether an extended history of intensive endurance training results in a more persistent maintenance of $\dot{V}O_{2max}$ after subsequent inactivity than shorter periods of less intensive training has also been studied (16). Figure 30-2 illustrates the time course of the decline in $\dot{V}O_{2max}$ and related variables (stroke volume, heart rate and a - $\bar{v}O_{2diff}$) when subjects become sedentary after training intensively for approximately 10 years (15). Note the rapid decline in $\dot{V}O_{2max}$ in the first 12 to 21 days and its association with a marked decline in maximal stroke volume. Table 30-2 compares a sedentary group with an athletic group and the changes associated with detraining at the central and peripheral levels (13,15,16).

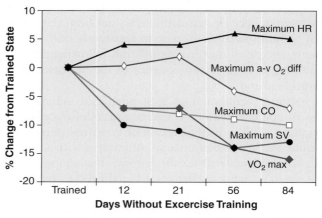

FIGURE 30-2. Effects of detraining on changes in heart rate (HR), arteriovenous oxygen difference (a- $\bar{v}O_2$ diff), stroke volume (SV), and oxygen consumption ($\dot{V}O_2$) at maximum exercise. Adapted from Coyle EF, Martin WH 3rd, Sinacore DR, et al. Time course of loss of adaptations after stopping prolonged intense endurance training. *J Appl Physiol.* 1984;57:1857–1864.

TABLE 30-2. DATA FOR SEDENTARY SUBJECTS (n = 8) COMPARED WITH HIGHLY TRAINED ATHLETES (n = 6) BEFORE AND AFTER 3 MONTHS OF DETRAINING

	SEDENTARY GROUP	ATHLETE GROUP	
		TRAINED	DETRAINED
$\dot{V}O_{2max}$ (mL·kg^{-1}·min^{-1})	43.3	62.1[a]	50.8[a,b]
Maximum stroke volume (mL·beat^{-1})	128	148[a]	129[b]
Maximum a-$\bar{v}O_2$ diff (mL O_2·1 L blood^{-1})	12.6	15.1[a]	14.1[a,b]
$\dot{V}O_2$ at lactate threshold (mL·kg^{-1}·min^{-1})	26.9	49.2[a]	37.6[a,b]
Submaximal $\dot{V}_E$ (L·min^{-1})	—	70.5	90.0[b]
Submaximal heart rate (beats·min^{-1})	—	158	184[b]

[a] $p < 0.05$ for trained athletes or detrained athletes versus sedentary group.

[b] $p < 0.05$ for trained athletes versus detrained athletes.

Adapted from Coyle EF, Martin WH 3rd, Bloomfield SA, et al. Effects of detraining on responses to submaximal exercise. *J Appl Physiol.* 1985;59:853–859; and Coyle EF, Martin WH 3rd, Sinacore DR, et al. Time course of loss of adaptations after stopping prolonged intense endurance training. *J Appl Physiol.* 1984;57:1857–1864.

STROKE VOLUME

Whereas prolonged intensive endurance training promotes increased heart mass (i.e., cardiac hypertrophy), detraining typically results in decreased heart mass (21,32,42), although not all studies report a decrease (17,48). It is not clear whether training-induced increases in left ventricular dimension and myocardial contractility regress totally with inactivity. Athletes who become sedentary have larger hearts and higher $\dot{V}O_{2max}$ than those of people who have never trained (54).

One of the most striking effects of detraining in endurance-trained individuals is the rapid decline in stroke volume. Martin et al. (41) measured stroke volume during exercise in trained subjects in both the upright and supine positions and again after 21 and 56 days of inactivity (Fig. 30-3). The large decline in stroke volume during upright cycling was associated with parallel reductions in left ventricular end-diastolic diameter. However, when the subjects exercised in the supine position, which usually augments ventricular filling because of increased venous return from elevated lower extremities, reduction in left ventricular end-diastolic diameter was minimal. As a result, stroke volume during exercise in the supine position was maintained within a few percent of trained levels during the 56-day detraining period. These observations indicate that cardiac filling is an important factor in establishing stroke volume during exercise and that when it declines, perhaps as a result of reductions in blood volume, stroke volume also declines.

BLOOD VOLUME

It appears that the rapid detraining-induced reduction of stroke volume during exercise in the upright position is related to a decrease in blood volume (14). Blood volume increases within the first few days of an exercise training program, but quickly reverses when training ceases. Therefore, the decline in stroke volume and the increase

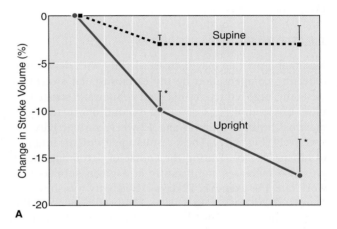

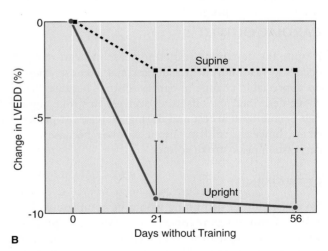

FIGURE 30-3. Percent decline in exercise stroke volume (**A**) and left ventricular end-diastolic diameter (LVEDD) (**B**) during exercise in the upright and supine positions when trained and after 21 and 56 days of inactivity (solid line indicates upright, dashed line indicates supine). *Responses in upright position are significantly ($p < 0.05$) lower than in supine position and lower than when trained. Reprinted with permission from Costill DL, Fink WJ, Hargreaves M, et al. Metabolic characteristics of skeletal muscle during detraining from competitive swimming. *Med Sci Sports Exerc.* 1985;17:339–343.

in heart rate during submaximal exercise, which normally accompany several weeks of detraining, can be reversed, returning to near-trained levels when the blood volume is artificially expanded to a level similar to that of trained subjects (14).

Because stroke volume during exercise is maintained close to trained levels when blood volume is high, the ability of the heart to fill with blood is not significantly altered by detraining. If ventricular mass does decrease, then thinning of ventricular walls, not decreased left ventricle end-diastole diameter, may be responsible (41). Thus, decreased intrinsic cardiovascular function, at least during submaximal exercise, is apparently minimal after several weeks of inactivity in men who had been training intensively for several years (14). The large reduction in stroke volume during exercise in the upright position is largely a result of reduced blood volume, not deterioration of heart function.

HEART RATE

Maximal heart rate may increase slightly with detraining, reflecting compensation by the cardiovascular system to offset the large reductions in blood volume and stroke volume. Coyle et al. (16) observed 4% and 6% increases in maximal heart rate after 3 and 12 weeks of inactivity, respectively (Fig. 30-2). These results agree with the findings of others (17,36). During the course of detraining, heart rate also increases significantly at a given submaximal work rate. For example, 12 days of inactivity was shown to increase heart rate from 158 to 170 beats $\cdot$ min^{-1} at the same absolute intensity, then to 184 beats $\cdot$ min^{-1} after 84 days of detraining (15).

CARDIAC OUTPUT

Despite the detraining-related increase in heart rate that occurs at rest and during submaximal exercise, there is no appreciable change in cardiac output because of the above-described and offsetting decrease in stroke volume that occurs both at rest and during exercise. At peak exercise, however, cardiac output is lower because of the decrease in peak stroke volume.

RETRAINING

No discussion of detraining would be complete without at least mentioning the concept of retraining. Popular belief once held that the training effects one achieved via endurance training could be increased if the athlete had previously undergone training and detraining periods. However, scientific evidence does not support this concept. We now know that prior endurance training does not, in itself, positively influence the gains made through a subsequent retraining period (23). What is more important to remember is that a relatively brief layoff can significantly decrease exercise capacity.

MAINTENANCE OF TRAINING EFFECT

Discussion thus far has primarily focused on adaptations to both high-level endurance training and inactivity. However, most humans live the majority of life somewhere in between these two extremes, and it is unlikely one can be in "race shape" all of the time. Therefore, one would want to preserve, as much as possible, previously obtained fitness gains during the off-season or those periods of time associated with a reduced amount of exercise training. This begs the question: What level of exercise is required to maintain cardiorespiratory fitness once achieved by a high level of endurance training?

A series of papers by Hickson et al. provides insight into this question. In one study, $\dot{V}O_{2max}$ was maintained following a 15-week period of decreased training frequency (from 6 to 2 days per week) by keeping intensity and duration constant (34). In a subsequent study (33), $\dot{V}O_{2max}$ was maintained following a 15-week period of decreased training duration (from 40 to both 26 and 13 minutes per session) by keeping intensity and frequency constant. However, endurance performance (time to exhaustion at 80% $\dot{V}O_{2max}$) was reduced 10% in the 13 minutes per session group. In yet a third study (31), $\dot{V}O_{2max}$ and endurance performance were significantly reduced by 5% to 10% and 20% to 30%, respectively, following a 15-week period of decreased training intensity (by both one third and two thirds of initial intensity), even though frequency and duration remained constant. Collectively, these studies suggest that after periods of intensive training, $\dot{V}O_{2max}$ can be maintained for up to 15 weeks of reduced training frequency or duration as long as intensity is maintained.

Over a shorter period (4 weeks), McConell et al. (43) showed that $\dot{V}O_{2max}$ was maintained despite reductions in training intensity, frequency, and time; however, endurance performance (5-km run time) was reduced. This suggests $\dot{V}O_{2max}$ can be maintained for a shortened period (4 weeks versus 15 weeks) despite a reduction in all training parameters (intensity, frequency, and time).

EXERCISE TRAINING WITH ARM ERGOMETRY

Upper-body exercise modes, such as arm ergometry, are widely accepted as an integral part of a comprehensive exercise training program in persons with and without heart disease. Franklin et al. (25) reported the effects of a 6-week training program involving upper- and lower-extremity exercise devices in patients with a history of myocardial infarction. Following exercise training, rate–pressure product during submaximal arm and leg exercise were similarly decreased, and exercise capacity measured during arm and leg ergometry increased 13% and 11%, respectively (Fig. 30-4). These findings indicated that the upper extremities respond to aerobic exercise training in a similar manner as the lower extremities.

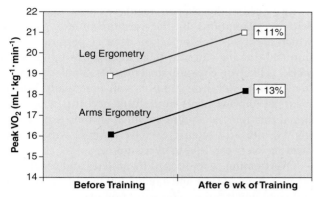

FIGURE 30-4. Peak $\dot{V}O_2$ during arm and leg ergometry before and after exercise training in men (n = 13) with previous myocardial infarction. Adapted from Franklin BA, Vander L, Wrisley D, Rubenfire M. Trainability of arms versus legs in men with previous myocardial infarction. *Chest*. 1994;105:262–264.

EXERCISE MODE AND SPECIFICITY OF TRAINING

> **1.1.31-HFS: Knowledge of how the principles of specificity and progressive overload relate to the components of exercise programming.**

To improve one's ability to perform a given physical activity, whether it is walking up two flights of stairs or swimming 100 m, involves training specific muscles or organ systems with increasing volume (duration, frequency, or intensity). This concept emphasizes the principles of specificity of training and progressive overload. Regarding specificity of training, numerous studies of normal subjects and patients with heart disease have investigated the cardiorespiratory adaptations of trained versus untrained muscle to physical conditioning. Results generally demonstrate little or no crossover of arm and leg training. After endurance training of one limb or set of limbs, several investigators report increased $\dot{V}O_{2max}$ and ventilatory threshold, and decreased heart rate, blood lactate, pulmonary ventilation, ventilatory equivalent for $\dot{V}O_{2max}$, BP, and perceived exertion during submaximal exercise with the trained but not the untrained limbs (10,49). These limb-specific training effects imply that a substantial portion of the conditioning response is attributed to peripheral factors, such as alterations in blood flow and cellular and enzymatic adaptations in the trained limbs alone (18,30,55).

Conversely, studies in both normal subjects and patients with heart disease indicate some crossover of training effects (i.e., increased $\dot{V}O_{2max}$ or reduced submaximal exercise heart rate in untrained limbs), providing evidence for central circulatory adaptations to endurance training (9,59). Although the conditions under which the crossover between arm and leg training may vary, evidence suggests that the initial fitness level—as well as the intensity, frequency, and duration of training, —may be important variables in determining the extent of cross-training benefits from arms to legs and vice versa.

The limited degree of cardiorespiratory and metabolic crossover from one set of limbs to another appears to discount the general practice of restricting aerobic conditioning to the lower extremities. Several recreational activities and many occupational tasks require sustained arm work to a greater extent than leg work. Consequently, individuals who rely on their upper extremities for vocational or leisure-time pursuits should train their arms as well as their legs, with the expectation of improved cardiorespiratory, hemodynamic, and perceived exertion responses to both forms of effort. Arm ergometers or combined arm–leg ergometers are particularly beneficial for upper-extremity training. Other various factors affecting the response to exercise training are summarized in Table 30-3.

TABLE 30-3. FACTORS INFLUENCING THE PHYSIOLOGIC ADAPTATIONS TO CARDIORESPIRATORY EXERCISE TRAINING

VARIABLE(S)	COMMENTS
Age, habitual physical activity, and initial $\dot{V}O_{2max}$	Improvement generally demonstrates an inverse relationship with these variables; however, recent studies suggest that older and younger adults demonstrate similar response.
Genetics	Heritability may account for 50%.
Volume of training (combination of intensity, frequency and duration)	Improvement in aerobic capacity generally demonstrates a positive correlation to training volume.
Intensity of training	Improvement in aerobic capacity is positively correlated with intensity, even with total volume held constant.
Adherence to the exercise prescription	Parallels the magnitude of improvement in cardiorespiratory function.
Detraining and prolonged bed rest	When physical conditioning is stopped or reduced, training-induced cardiorespiratory adaptations are reversed over time.
Beta-adrenergic blockade therapy	Despite an attenuated heart rate response, patients on β-blockers can derive similar adaptations from exercise training.
Heart disease, including coronary artery disease or chronic heart failure	Exercise training is generally safe and effective in improving cardiorespiratory function; however, the severity or progression of disease may limit the magnitude of improvement.

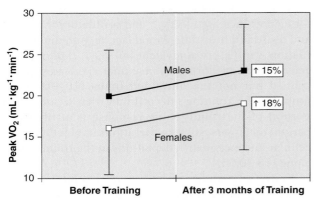

FIGURE 30-5. Peak $\dot{V}O_2$ before and after 20 weeks of exercise training in men (n = 287) and women (n = 346). Adapted from Skinner JS, Jaskólski A, Jaskólska A, et al. Age, sex, race, initial fitness, and response to training: the HERITAGE Family Study. *J Appl Physiol.* 2001;90:1770–1776.

SEX-SPECIFIC IMPROVEMENT AND TRAINABILITY

For many years, the majority of studies on the effects of aerobic exercise training involved men. However, numerous studies also provide ample data on $\dot{V}O_{2max}$, cardiovascular hemodynamics, body composition, and serum lipids in younger, middle-aged, and older women who undergo exercise training. The results demonstrate that women respond to aerobic exercise training in much the same way as men when subjected to comparable programs in terms of frequency, intensity, and duration of exercise (2, 27) (Fig. 30-5). Improvement in cardiorespiratory fitness is inversely correlated with age, habitual physical activity, and initial $\dot{V}O_{2max}$ (which is generally lower in women than men), and positively correlated with exercise frequency, intensity, and duration (24). It is important to note that when comparing similar groups of athletes or apparently healthy persons, $\dot{V}O_{2max}$ expressed per kilogram of body weight is generally 15% to 25% lower in women than men. This difference is caused by sex-specific biologic differences, including a slightly greater amount of essential body fat, a smaller peak stroke volume attributable to smaller left ventricular dimension, and a lower hemoglobin concentration (23).

In general, an average increase in $\dot{V}O_{2max}$ of between 10% and 30% is anticipated for college-age men and women after an 8- to 12-week endurance training program. When gain in $\dot{V}O_{2max}$ is expressed per kilogram of body weight, the values achieved for men and women are similar. However, because the initial $\dot{V}O_{2max}$ of women is generally lower than men, the percent increase is often greater among women.

OVERTRAINING

> **1.1.33-HFS: Knowledge of the physical and psychological signs of overreaching/overtraining and to provide recommendations for these problems.**

As discussed in this chapter, regular exercise training can lead to adaptations in the cardiorespiratory system, which has a positive impact on exercise performance. A minimal training stimulus (e.g., intensity or minutes per week) is likely to elicit minimal benefits. Similarly, a maximal training level or stimulus will potentially lead to maximal improvements in performance. It is widely believed that there is a point at which chronic exposure to high volumes of intense exercise training with insufficient recovery can lead to **overtraining**.

Overtraining, as described by athletes and coaches, is an altered mood state and a reduction in performance despite ongoing training. This condition may require weeks to months and maybe years to resolve. However, as discussed by Halson and Jeukendrup (29), researchers have had difficulty describing and detecting overtraining. This is, in part, because of a lack of consistent terminology, differences in diagnostic tools, differences in performance measures and training regimens, and individual differences in athletes and sporting activities. Overtraining is generally a diagnosis by exclusion of other causes for decreased performance and altered mood. The cause of overtraining is not fully understood, but is likely related to both training (e.g., exercise volume, recovery) and nontraining (e.g., psychological stress, sleep, nutrition) factors (51). Several markers of overtraining have been investigated, including performance, mood state, cardiovascular physiology (e.g., stroke volume, heart rate), lactate, glycogen depletion, immune system function, hormone imbalances, and changes in autonomic nervous system function (29). Currently there is no agreed-upon constellation of signs or symptoms characterizing overtraining.

SUMMARY

When exposed to repeated bouts of exercise (i.e., exercise training), both the cardiac and pulmonary systems show measurable changes (adaptations) consistent with a training effect. Generally, these changes are associated with improved exercise performance and health. The adaptations that take place are organ system or tissue specific and generally occur similarly in men and women. Consistent with the above, periods of detraining, lesser training, and bed rest are associated with loss of exercise performance, and many, if not all, of the previously attained training effects.

REFERENCES

1. Ades PA, Savage PD, Brawner CA, et al. Aerobic capacity in patients entering cardiac rehabilitation. *Circulation.* 2006;113:2706–2712.
2. Ades PA, Waldmann ML, Polk DM, Coflesky JT. Referral patterns and exercise response in the rehabilitation of female coronary patients aged greater than or equal to 62 years. *Am J Cardiol.* 1992;69:1422–1425.
3. Bevegard BS, Shepherd JT. Regulation of the circulation during exercise in man. *Physiol Rev.* 1967;47:178–213.

4. Blair SN, Kohl HW III, Paffenbarger RS, et al. Physical fitness and all-cause mortality: a prospective study of healthy men and women. *JAMA*. 1989;262:2395–2401.

5. Blomqvist CG, Saltin B. Cardiovascular adaptations to physical training. *Annu Rev Physiol*. 1983;45:169–189.

6. Bouchard C, Daw EW, Rice T, et al. Familial resemblance for VO₂max in the sedentary state: the HERITAGE family study. *Med Sci Sports Exerc*. 1998;30:252–258.

7. **Chobanian AV, Bakris GL, Black HR, et al. The seventh report of the joint national committee on prevention, detection, evaluation, and treatment of high blood pressure: the JNC 7 report. *JAMA*. 2003; 289:2560–2572.**

8. Church TS, Earnest CP, Skinner JS, Blair SN. Effects of different doses of physical activity on cardiorespiratory fitness among sedentary, overweight or obese postmenopausal women with elevated blood pressure. *JAMA*. 2007;297:2081–2091.

9. Clausen JP, Klausen K, Rasmussen B, Trap-Jensen J. Central and peripheral circulatory changes after training of the arms or legs. *Am J Physiol*. 1973;225:675–682.

10. Clausen JP, Trap-Jensen J, Lassen NA. The effects of training on the heart rate during arm and leg exercise. *Scand J Clin Lab Invest*. 1970;26:295–301.

11. Convertino VA, Brock PJ, Keil LC, et al. Exercise training-induced hypervolemia: role of plasma albumin, renin, and vasopressin. *J Appl Physiol*. 1980;48:665–669.

12. Cornelissen VA, Fagard RH. Effects of endurance training on blood pressure, blood pressure-regulating mechanisms and cardiovascular risk factors. *Hypertension*. 2005;46:667–675.

13. Costill DL, Fink WJ, Hargreaves M, et al. Metabolic characteristics of skeletal muscle during detraining from competitive swimming. *Med Sci Sports Exerc*. 1985;17:339–343.

14. Coyle EF, Hemmert MK, Coggan AR. Effects of detraining on cardiovascular responses to exercise: role of blood volume. *J Appl Physiol*. 1986;60:95–99.

15. Coyle EF, Martin WH 3rd, Bloomfield SA, et al. Effects of detraining on responses to submaximal exercise. *J Appl Physiol*. 1985;59: 853–859.

16. Coyle EF, Martin WH 3rd, Sinacore DR, et al. Time course of loss of adaptations after stopping prolonged intense endurance training. *J Appl Physiol*. 1984;57:1857–1864.

17. Cullinane EM, Sady SP, Vadeboncoeur L, et al. Cardiac size and do not decrease after short-term exercise cessation. *Med Sci Sports Exerc*. 1986;18:420–424.

18. Davies CT, Sargeant AJ. Effects of training on the physiological responses to one- and two-leg work. *J Appl Physiol*. 1975;38:377–385.

19. Drinkwater BL, Horvath SM. Detraining effects on young women. *Med Sci Sports*. 1972;4:91–95.

20. Ehrman JK. Myocardial infarction. In: Ehrman JK, Gordon PM, Visich PS. Keteyian SJ, editors.*Clinical Exercise Physiology*. Champaign (IL): Human Kinetics; 2003. p. 212.

21. Ehsani AA, Hagberg JM, Hickson RC. Rapid changes in left ventricular dimensions and mass in response to physical conditioning and deconditioning. *Am J Cardiol*. 1978;42:52–56.

22. **Fletcher GF, Balady G, Blair SN, et al. Statement on exercise: benefits and recommendations for physical activity programs for all Americans. A statement for health professionals by the Committee on Exercise and Cardiac Rehabilitation of the Council on Clinical Cardiology, American Heart Association. *Circulation*. 1996;94: 857–862.**

23. Foss ML, Keteyian SJ. *Fox's Physiological Basis for Exercise and Sport*. 6th ed. New York: WCB McGraw-Hill; 1998. p. 294–336.

24. Franklin BA, Bonzheim K, Berg T. Gender differences in rehabilitation. In: Julian DG, Wenger NK, editors. *Women and Heart Disease*. London: Martin Dunitz; 1997. p. 151–171.

25. Franklin BA, Vander L, Wrisley D, Rubenfire M. Trainability of arms versus legs in men with previous myocardial infarction. *Chest*. 1994;105:262–264.

26. Fringer MN, Stull GA. Changes in cardiorespiratory parameters during periods of training and detraining in young adult females. *Med Sci Sports*. 1974;6:20–25.

27. Getchell LH, Moore JC. Physical training: comparative responses of middle-aged adults. *Arch Phys Med Rehabil*. 1975;56:250–254.

28. Green HJ, Thomson JA, Ball ME, et al. Alterations in blood volume following short-term supramaximal exercise. *J Appl Physiol*. 1984;56:145–149.

29. Halson SL, Jeukendrup AE. Does overtraining exist? An analysis of overreaching and overtraining research. *Sports Med*. 2004;34: 967–981.

30. Henriksson J, Reitman JS. Time course of changes in human skeletal muscle succinate dehydrogenase and cytochrome oxidase activities and maximal oxygen uptake with physical activity and inactivity. *Acta Physiol Scand*. 1977;99:91–97.

31. Hickson RC, Foster C, Pollock ML, Galassi TM, Rich S. Reduced training intensities and loss of aerobic power, endurance, and cardiac growth. *J Appl Physiol*. 1985;58:492–499.

32. Hickson RC, Hammons GT, Holloszy JO. Development and regression of exercise-induced cardiac hypertrophy in rats. *Am J Physiol*. 1979;236:H268–H272.

33. Hickson RC, Kanakis C, Davis JR, Moore AM, Rich S. Reduced training duration effects on aerobic power, endurance, and cardiac growth. *J Appl Physiol*. 1982;53:225–259.

34. Hickson RC, Rosenkoetter MA. Reduced training frequencies and maintenance of increased aerobic power. *Med Sci Sports Exerc*. 1981;13:13–16.

35. Holloszy JO. Adaptations of skeletal muscle to endurance exercise. *Med Sci Sports*. 1975;7:155–164.

36. Houston ME, Bentzen H, Larsen H. Interrelationships between skeletal muscle adaptations and performance as studied by detraining and retraining. *Acta Physiol Scand*. 1979;105:163–170.

37. Keteyian SJ, Brawner CA, Savage PD, et al. Peak aerobic capacity predicts prognosis in patients with coronary heart disease.

38. Klausen K, Andersen LB, Pelle I. Adaptive changes in work capacity, skeletal muscle capillarization and enzyme levels during training and detraining. *Acta Physiol Scand*. 1981;113:9–16.

39. Levine BD, Lane LD, Buckey JC, et al. Left ventricular pressure-volume and Frank-Starling relations in endurance athletes: implications for orthostatic tolerance and exercise performance. *Circulation*. 1991;84:1016–1023.

40. Longhurst JC, Kelly AR, Gonyea WJ, Mitchell JH. Chronic training with static and dynamic exercise: cardiovascular adaptation, and response to exercise. *Circ Res*. 1981;48(6 Pt 2):I171–I178.

41. Martin WH 3rd, Coyle EF, Bloomfield SA, Ehsani AA. Effects of physical deconditioning after intense endurance training on left ventricular dimensions and stroke volume. *J Am Coll Cardiol*. 1986;7:982–989.

42. McAllister RM. Endothelial-mediated control of coronary and skeletal muscle blood flow during exercise: introduction. *Med Sci Sports Exerc*. 1995;27:1122–1124.

43. McConell GK, Costill DL, Widrick JJ, Hickey MS, Tanaka H, Gastin PB. Reduced training volume and intensity maintain aerobic capacity but not performance in distance runners. *Int J Sports Med*. 1993;14:33–37.

44. Michielli DW, Stein RA, Krasnow N, Diamond JR, Horwitz B. Effects of exercise training on ventricular dimensions at rest and during exercise. *Med Sci Sports*. 1979;11:82.

45. Orlander J, Kiessling KH, Karlsson J, Ekblom B. Low intensity training, inactivity and resumed training in sedentary men. *Acta Physiol Scand*. 1977;101:351–362.

46. Oscai LB, Williams BT, Hertig BA. Effect of exercise on blood volume. *J Appl Physiol*. 1968;24:622–624.

47. **Pate RR, Pratt M, Blair SN, et al. Physical activity and public health: a recommendation from the Centers for Disease Control and Prevention and the American College of Sports Medicine. *JAMA*. 1995;273:402–407.**

48. Pavlik G, Bachl N, Wollein W, et al. Resting echocardiographic parameters after cessation of regular endurance training. *Int J Sports Med.* 1986;7:226–231.

49. Rasmussen B, Klausen K, Clausen JP, Trap-Jensen J. Pulmonary ventilation, blood gases, and blood pH after training of the arms or the legs. *J Appl Physiol.* 1975;38:250–256.

50. Rerych SK, Scholz PM, Sabiston DC Jr, Jones RH. Effects of exercise training on left ventricular function in normal subjects: a longitudinal study by radionuclide angiography. *Am J Cardiol.* 1980;45:244–252.

51. Robergs RA, Keteyian SJ. *Fundamentals of Exercise Physiology for Fitness, Performance, and Health.* 2nd ed. New York: McGraw Hill; 2003. p. 212–213.

52. Rowell LB. Human cardiovascular adjustments to exercise and thermal stress. *Physiol Rev.* 1974;54:75–159.

53. Saltin B, Grimby G. Physiological analysis of middle-aged and old former athletes: comparison with still active athletes of the same ages. *Circulation.* 1968;38:1104–1115.

54. Saltin B, Nazar K, Costill DL, et al. The nature of the training response; peripheral and central adaptations of one-legged exercise. *Acta Physiol Scand.* 1976;96:289–305.

55. Saltin B, Blomqvist G, Mitchell JH, Johnson RL, Wildenthal K, Chapman CB. Response to exercise after bed rest and after training. *Circulation.* 1968;37(suppl VII):1–78.

56. Schairer JR, Keteyian SJ. Exercise in patients with cardiovascular disease. In: Kraus WE, Keteyian SJ, editors. *Cardiac Rehabilitation.* Totowa (NJ): Humana Press; 2007. p. 177.

57. Schairer JR, Stein PD, Keteyian S, et al. Left ventricular response to submaximal exercise in endurance-trained athletes and sedentary adults. *Am J Cardiol.* 1992;70:930–933.

58. Skinner JS, Jaskólski A, Jaskólska A, et al. Age, sex, race, initial fitness, and response to training: the HERITAGE Family Study. *J Appl Physiol.* 2001;90:1770–1776.

59. Thompson PD, Cullinane E, Lazarus B, Carleton RA. Effect of exercise training on the untrained limb exercise performance of men with angina pectoris. *Am J Cardiol.* 1981;48:844–850.

SELECTED REFERENCES FOR FURTHER READING

Robergs RA, Keteyian SJ. *Fundamentals of Exercise Physiology for Fitness, Performance, and Health.* 2nd ed. New York: McGraw-Hill; 2003.

Rowell LB, Shephard JT. *Handbook of Physiology. Exercise: Regulation and Integration of Multiple Organ Systems.* New York: Oxford University Press; 1996.

INTERNET RESOURCES

- Centers for Disease Control and Prevention, Division of Nutrition and Physical Activity: www.cdc.gov/nccdphp/dnpa/index.htm
- HERITAGE Family Study: www.pbrc.edu/Heritage/index.html
- SPORTSCIENCE: www.sportsci.org/
- Exercise performance and training adaptations: home.hia.no/~stephens/exphys.htm

Adaptations to Resistance Training

The key factor in resistance exercise and its subsequent repeated exposure with resistance training is the activation of *motor units* (the alpha motor neuron and its associated muscle fibers). If muscle tissue is not activated, then it will not adapt. The amount of muscle tissue activated dictates the magnitude of the support systems needed to maintain homeostasis during and after exercise. The act of resistance training itself does not necessitate that adaptations will take place. Rather, the progressive overloading of the musculoskeletal system is needed for subsequent adaptations to take place beyond the initial phase of training (78–80). Each individual has a threshold level of conditioning for all health- and skill-related components of muscular fitness, and the human body will only adapt favorably if the resistance-training stimulus is at or above this threshold point. Thus, challenging workouts are needed for progression to take place (68,78–80).

The *size principle* is a key concept needed to understand muscle tissue activation and the adaptations associated with resistance training. The size principle conceptually developed by Henneman hypothesized that motor units are recruited in order by different "sizing factors" (e.g., the size of the soma of motor neurons located within the spinal cord; those associated with type I, slow twitch, muscle fibers being smaller than those associated with type II, fast twitch, muscle fibers) to produce the needed amount of force to meet the external demands or to lift a weight (50). For example, low-threshold motor units produce low levels of force. As the activation stimulus increases, higher-threshold motor units are recruited, and more force is produced. Higher-threshold motor units may contain larger muscle fibers, a higher number of muscle fibers, or type II (fast twitch) muscle fibers. Essentially, some "sizing factor" will mediate greater force capabilities until the maximal amount of force is produced when all available motor units are recruited in a specific movement. In addition, *selective recruitment* of fast-twitch motor units may occur under certain circumstances (ballistic or explosive resistance training), enabling inhibition of lower-threshold motor units in lieu of activating the higher-threshold motor units for maximal strength and power performance (110). Activated fast-twitch motor units may stay facilitated for some time afterward, thereby enabling enhanced power performance, i.e.,

> > > KEY TERMS

DOMS: Delayed onset muscle soreness, which typically occurs 24 to 48 hours following resistance training, particularly when eccentric actions are emphasized.

Hyperplasia: An increase in the number of muscle fibers within a given muscle.

Hypertrophy: An increase in the size of individual muscle fibers; also, an increase in the size of an entire muscle.

Motor unit: A motor neuron and the muscle fibers that it innervates; the basic unit of muscular contraction.

Neuromuscular junction: The site where a motor neuron axon terminal connects with the sarcolemma of a muscle fiber (separated by a small space, the synaptic cleft); also known as a *motor endplate*.

Overtraining: A decrease in performance despite a maintenance or progressive increase in training.

Size principle: The concept by which motor units with smaller motor neuron somas (cell bodies, located in the spinal cord) are more easily recruited by central motor command than are motor units with larger motor neuron somas. Type I (slow-twitch) motor units have smaller motor neuron somas than type II (fast-twitch) motor units.

postactivation potentiation (135). It is important to understand that not all individuals have the same complement of motor units in a specific muscle, nor does every muscle in a given individual have the same complement of motor units. Finally, the joint angle of a resistance exercise will dictate a different combination of motor units needed for movement. Exercise choices, resistance loading, metabolic demands, and fatigue state of the muscle all influence what muscle tissue is activated and what adaptations will occur.

Finally, although the activation of muscle is the key event in resistance training, the specific resistance exercise stimulus or the type of workout performed will determine the number of physiologic systems that are needed to support the exercise stress and allow for recovery, repair, and remodeling of tissue after the workout. The basis of any adaptation is the exercise stimulus created by the workout. The quality of the exercise stimulus is governed by the principles of *specificity, progressive overload,* and *variation* (78–80). How the workout is designed and changed over time (manipulation of intensity, volume, exercise selection and order, rest intervals, frequency, and velocity of muscle action) dictates the success in achieving a targeted training goal and the level of adaptations attained. For example, a whole-body workout will demand more physiologic system involvement and support than one set of an arm curl exercise using 50% of a one repetition maximum (1RM) load. Thus, adaptations in the musculoskeletal system can carry over to other physiologic systems, depending on the specific demands of the exercise protocol.

RESISTANCE TRAINING

> **1.1.23-HFS: Knowledge of the principles involved in promoting gains in muscular strength and endurance.**

> **1.1.31-HFS: Knowledge of how the principles of specificity and progressive overload relate to the components of exercise programming.**

Resistance training can encompass a wide range of workout protocols. Typical protocols involve upper-, lower-, and total-body exercises, and ones for each side of the joints (agonist and antagonist pairs) and for the front and back of the body. This typically ranges from eight to ten exercises for a whole-body workout. Resistances can range from light to heavy and are varied over time (periodized) to effectively stimulate the neuromuscular system and provide for recovery. Adaptations are then related to the principle of specificity and are dictated by the type of workouts used to address program goals and requirements of the individual. Chapter 29 addresses the basic techniques and programming in resistance training.

RESPONSES VERSUS ADAPTATIONS

Training is typically thought of as repeated and systematic exposure of the body to an exercise stimulus. Some adaptations take place within one or two workouts. A *response* is the human body's acute change in physiologic function to the stress of resistance exercise. Thus, training adaptations may be viewed as the quantification of consistent individual responses to the stress of resistance exercise. The human body may adapt to resistance exercise and training by altering its homeostatic balance or by modifying the acute responses to a workout. If one looks at it from a temporal perspective, or as adaptations taking place on a time continuum, the changes can range from early- and late-phase adaptations up to (potentially) an individual's genetic maximum for the phenotypic expression of a trait. For example, when a resistance exercise workout is performed over the first week, changes occur within two to four workouts for the type of myosin protein, yet few changes have been observed for many other morphologic characteristics, such as muscle fiber size, until a few weeks later (143). Thus, neurologic adaptations and changes in the "quality of muscle proteins" dominate the early-phase adaptations in skeletal muscle and are part of the adaptational continuum. If training is stopped, then detraining occurs, and over time phenotypic expression of the change reverts back to near-baseline physiologic status. The physiologic adaptations to critical bodily systems—such as the neuromuscular, connective tissue, endocrine, metabolic, cardiovascular, and immune systems—are discussed in this chapter and summarized in Table 31-1.

NEUROMUSCULAR ADAPTATIONS

Several neural mechanisms are responsible for the adaptations in strength and power observed with resistance training. Resistance training may elicit adaptations along the neuromuscular chain, initiating in the higher brain centers and continuing down to the level of individual muscle fibers. Interestingly, not all mechanisms are operational in every muscle or exercise; therefore, the mediators of neural adaptations are a complex set of mechanisms working to produce greater force. These include increased neural drive, in which the amount of electromyographic (EMG) activity is lower for a given resistance lifted; increased synchronization, in which a greater number of motor units are activated nearly simultaneously for a given lifting effort; increased time of neural activation, which might allow more higher-threshold motor units to become activated; and reduction in central and local inhibitory reflexes, which limit neural activation (136). The combinations of mechanisms that can mediate such changes are debatable, but changes in force production occur rapidly with no changes in the cross-sectional area of muscle, arguing for a strong neural component in the adaptational effects.

TABLE 31-1. ADAPTATIONS TO RESISTANCE TRAINING

ADAPTATION	SIGNIFICANCE
Neural Adaptations	
↑ Motor cortex activity	↑ Muscle force production, rate of force development, power, "cross education," improved resistance exercise technique, and reduced bilateral deficit
↑ Motor unit recruitment	
↑ Motor unit firing rate	
↑ Motor unit synchronization	
↑ Fast-twitch fiber selective recruitment	
↑ Postactivation potentiation	
↑ Reflex potentiation	
↓ Golgi tendon organ inhibition	
↓ Antagonist muscle coactivation	
Neuromuscular Junction	
↑ Terminal branching, asymmetry, area	↑ Neurotransmitter release, force, and power production
Muscle Adaptations	
↑ Muscle cross sectional area—mostly in type II fibers	↑ Muscle growth, strength, power, recovery, and endurance
↑ Hyperplasia (primarily because of neural sprouting)	
↑ Up-regulation of factors in myogenesis (Myo D, myogenin)	
↓ Myostatin	
↑ Expression of ~70 genes	
↑ Net protein accretion via multiple pathways (contractile and noncontractile proteins)	
↑ Myofibrillar volume	
↑ SR- and T-tubule volume	
↑ Na+/K+ ATPase activity	
↑ Up-regulation (transient) of muscle growth factors (e.g., mechano growth factor and calcineurin)	
↑ Pennation angle and fascicle length	
↑ Fiber type and myosin heavy chain transitions IIX–IIAX–IIA	
↓ Muscle damage with repeated RE exposure	
↑ Buffer capacity	
Metabolic Adaptations	
↑, ↓, ↔ ATP-CP, glycolytic enzymes	↑ Energy liberation, force, and power
↑ ATP, CP, and glycogen storage	↓ Oxidative capacity
↓ Capillary density (↑ # capillaries)	
↓ Mitochondrial density (↑ # mitochondria)	
↓ Myoglobin	
Endocrine Adaptations	
Hormonal response (see Table 31-2)	↑ Acute and chronic force, power, and endurance enhancement, muscle hypertrophy
↑ Up-regulation of androgen receptors	
Connective Tissue Adaptations	
↑ Bone mineral density	↑ Skeletal strength, force transmission, and ability to sustain muscle hypertrophy
↑ Blood markers of bone osteogenesis	
↑ Tendon and ligament cross-sectional area	
↑ Tendon stiffness	
↑ Collagen synthesis	
Cardiovascular Adaptations	
↑ Stroke volume	Improved cardiovascular disease risk factors and health, ↑ tolerance to pressure overload, ↓ cardiovascular demand to submaximal exercise
↑ Left ventricular wall thickness	
↑ Septal wall thickness	
↓, ↔ Resting heart rate	
↓, ↔ Blood pressure	
↓ Cardiovascular response to acute exercise of similar workload or intensity, low-density lipoproteins	
↑, ↔ Blood high-density lipoproteins	
Immune Adaptations	
↑ Leukocyte and cytokine response to resistance exercise	Tissue remodeling, inflammation, and repair
↔ Resting immune cell concentrations	

(continued)

TABLE 31-1. ADAPTATIONS TO RESISTANCE TRAINING (*Continued*)

ADAPTATION	SIGNIFICANCE
Performance Adaptations	
↑ Muscle strength	↑ Performance
↑ Muscle power	
↑ Balance and coordination	
↑, ↔ Flexibility	
↑ Lean tissue mass	
↑ Muscle endurance	
↑ Motor performance	
↑, ↔ VO$_{2max}$	
Health and Fitness Adaptations	
↓ Percent body fat	↑ Health and wellness
↑ Insulin sensitivity	
↓ Insulin concentrations and response to glucose challenge	
↓ Sarcopenia and osteoporosis	
↓ Low back pain	
↑ Basal metabolic rate	

↑, increase; ↓, decrease; ↔, no change; RE, resistance exercise; ATP-CP, adenosine phosphate-creatine phosphate; CP, creatine phosphate; VO$_{2max}$, maximal oxygen consumption.

EARLY-PHASE ADAPTATIONS

The ability to increase neural drive begins in the motor cortex with the intent to produce maximal levels of muscular force and power. A substantial proportion of the neural changes that occur during resistance training take place in the spinal cord along the descending corticospinal tracts. A classic study by Moritani and DeVries demonstrated the quintessential early-phase adaptations of the neural system (108). In examining an 8-week resistance-training program, they found that for a given level of force, less EMG activity was required following training. This indicated that a greater neural drive with training apparently mediated the adaptations in strength, and such early-phase improvements could not be accounted for by muscle hypertrophy. This and other subsequent research supports the idea that an increase in neural drive to a muscle results in greater strength. Neural factors related to strength gain include increased neural drive (i.e., recruitment and rate of firing) to the muscle, increased synchronization of the motor units, increased activation of agonists, decreased activation of antagonists, coordination of motor units and muscle(s) involved in a movement, and inhibition of the protective mechanisms of the muscle (i.e., Golgi tendon organs) (136). This is evident in untrained or moderately trained individuals, for whom it has been shown that untrained individuals may only activate 71% of their muscle cross-sectional area (CSA) during maximal effort (3). However, training reduces this deficit greatly, thereby demonstrating a greater potential to recruit fast-twitch motor units during the early phase of training adaptation (2).

Studies have revealed some other interesting neural adaptations/responses to resistance exercise and training. Resistance training may enhance the reflex (i.e., muscle spindle or stretch reflex) response by 15% to 55%, thereby enhancing the magnitude and rate of force development (2,53,137). In fact, positive correlations have been shown between enhanced stretch reflex and increased rate of force development during resistance training (53). In untrained individuals, the force produced when both limbs are contracting together is less than the sum of each limb contracting unilaterally (*bilateral deficit*). Research has shown that the corresponding EMG is lower during bilateral contractions, and the bilateral deficit is reduced with bilateral training (37). *Cross-education*, training one limb only, can result in an increase in strength in the untrained limb up to 22%, with the average strength increase about 8% (109). The increase in strength in the untrained limb is accompanied by greater EMG. Lastly, the level of tissue activation that takes place during resistance training when muscle hypertrophy takes place is important. A larger muscle does not require as much neural activation to lift a standard weight as it did before the growth took place, thereby demonstrating the importance of progressive overload during resistance training to continually recruit an optimal amount of muscle tissue (120).

Neural factors and quality of protein changes (e.g., alterations in the type of myosin heavy chains and type of myosin ATPase enzymes) may explain some part of early (2–8 weeks) strength gains. It is during this time that strength gains are much greater than what can be explained by muscle hypertrophy. The specific type of program utilized may be one of the most important factors in initial strength gains as a result of neural factors, because programs that are of very high intensity (>90% of 1RM) but low in total exercise volume may not be optimal for muscle tissue growth. Therefore, strength gains may be more dependent on neural factors with these types of programs (136). Neural adaptations are also prominent during power training, when moderate loads are lifted at maximal velocities (80). In general, muscle fiber hypertrophy has been shown to require more than 16 workouts to show significant increases (143). Thus, it may be possible that various types of training might be able to more quickly enhance the hypertrophy of muscle in the early phases (1–8 weeks) of training, thereby enhancing the hypertrophic contribution to strength and power gains (15,16). The majority of studies have demonstrated that in the early phases of a heavy resistance training program, increased voluntary activation of muscle is the largest contributor to strength increases (136). After this period, muscle hypertrophy becomes the predominant factor in strength increases, especially for younger men. On the basis of this kind of evidence, scientists have concluded that neural factors have a profound influence on muscular force production.

LATE-PHASE ADAPTATIONS

The classic curve developed by Sale shows that neural factors predominate in the early phase of strength-training adaptations until muscle protein accretion catches up with the process after about 2 to 3 months (136). A theoretical interaction of neural and muscle fiber hypertrophic components is presented in Figure 31-1. Neural factors mediate the strength-training adaptations in the early phase. As training time continues, a larger amount of the strength increase is explained by increases in muscle hypertrophy. Thus, with advancing training, there appears to be an interaction of neural and hypertrophic mechanisms mediating strength and power gains depending on the manipulation of the acute program variables. For example, training phases characterized by heavy loading (low volume) or explosive, ballistic repetitions may stimulate the nervous system to a higher degree, whereas moderate-to-high intensity protocols with higher volumes may stimulate greater muscle growth (80). If one's current level of muscle size is capable of withstanding the training stimulus, then there is little need for neural adaptations to take place as well. As Ploutz et al. have shown, less fiber

recruitment is needed to lift a given load when hypertrophy occurs (120). Progressive overload during consistent resistance training is critical for neural adaptations to continue to take place, and it has been suggested that neural adaptations may precede hypertrophy in advanced training (80). This might be best seen in advanced competitive weightlifters, in whom little or no hypertrophy may take place. In a classic study by Häkkinen et al., minimal changes in muscle fiber size were observed in competitive Olympic weightlifters, but strength and power increased over 2 years of training (47). EMG data demonstrated that voluntary activation of muscle was enhanced over the training period. Thus, even in advanced resistance-trained athletes, the mechanisms of strength and power improvement may be related to neural factors. It must be kept in mind that competitive weightlifters who compete in body mass classification groups were studied, and gains in muscle mass may not necessarily enhance their competitive advantage. Furthermore, the types of programs used by Olympic weightlifters are primarily related to strength and power development (73). Other types of programs for bodybuilders or other athletes may have some similar characteristics related to power development, but must also be designed to meet muscle mass and/or specific sport performance needs. Thus, training goals and specific protocols play a key role in the neural adaptations to resistance training.

ADAPTATIONS IN SKELETAL MUSCLE

 1.1.14-HFS: Knowledge of the anatomic and physiologic adaptations associated with strength training.

The primary target of resistance exercise is skeletal muscle. In addition, connective tissue will be stimulated, as well as the many physiologic systems needed to support tissue repair and recovery. Skeletal muscle is a heterogeneous mixture of several types of muscle fibers that potentially grow in size. The process of hypertrophy involves a proportionate increase in the net accretion of the contractile proteins actin and myosin, as well as other structural proteins (91). Mechanical loading leads to a series of intracellular signaling processes that ultimately regulate gene expression and subsequent protein synthesis. Several proteins have recently been identified that are responsive to mechanical stress and increase in activity before hypertrophy (64). Recent studies have shown that resistance training has the potential to alter the activity of nearly 70 genes, up-regulate factors involved with *myogenesis* (e.g., myogenin, MyoD), and down-regulate inhibitory growth factors (e.g., myostatin) (67,132,133). Skeletal muscle is multinucleated, with each nucleus governing a domain of protein (57). It has been postulated that the number of nuclei in part limit the amount of muscle hypertrophy and, after about a 26% increase in fiber size, the addition of more myonuclei are needed to

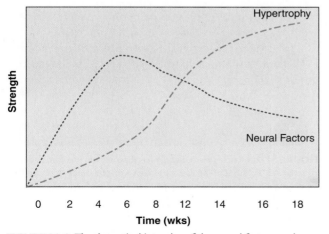

FIGURE 31-1. The theoretical interplay of the neural factors and hypertrophic factors over time with resistance training.

mediate effective sizes of nuclear domains. A major adaptation in skeletal muscle fibers is the increase in the number of myonuclei through mitotic division of activated satellite cells stimulated in the damage-repair cycle (57,94). Optimal muscle growth may comprise maximizing the combination of mechanical (use of heavy weights, inclusion of eccentric muscle actions, and low-to-moderate volume) and metabolic (metabolite formation) stimuli via training periodization (80). Thus, one must consider a host of different mechanisms that may have regulatory control of function and adaptational abilities.

MUSCLE FIBER TYPES AND ADAPTATIONS

Quantification of different biochemical and physical characteristics of different muscle fibers has led to the development of several muscle fiber histochemical classifications (119). Most scientists use the myosin ATPase or myosin heavy chain (MHC) analyses to classify muscle fiber types of a given muscle. The major fiber types in humans are types I (slow-twitch) and II (fast-twitch), with each having muscle fiber subtypes: type I, IC, IIC, IIAC, IIA, IIAX, and IIX. Although genetics predominantly determines proportions of type I and II fibers in the human body, transitions within each fiber type may occur. Heavy resistance training (i.e., loads >80%–85% of the 1RM) is needed to activate high-threshold motor units (IIX), as these fibers appear to be "reservoir" fibers and are mostly activated when high levels of force or power are needed (77). With such progressive programs, as stipulated in the American College of Sports Medicine (ACSM) position stand on progression, there is a transition in the percentage distribution from type IIX to IIA with little or no movement to IIC, with concomitant changes in MHC content (4,68,77). Thus, a major training adaptation is a shift to the more oxidative type IIA fiber type, via an up-regulation of type IIA protein synthesis and down-regulation of type IIX protein synthesis. Further, an early study compared kayakers with runners and found that type I predominated in the arms of the kayakers (but not legs) and the legs of the runners (but not arms), suggesting some training effect on type I–II conversion (148).

There is a progressive increase in muscle fiber CSA via the addition of myofibrillar proteins to the periphery during resistance training. Fiber CSA increases in both type I and II fibers, but to a greater extent in type II fibers (98). Muscle activation translates to whole-muscle hypertrophy. Interestingly, simultaneous use of high-intensity aerobic training with heavy resistance training can create some incompatibility of adaptation. Minimal or no hypertrophy may occur in type I fibers, with most taking place in type II fibers (12,43,77,123). Thus, care must be taken at the higher levels of simultaneous training with both endurance and resistance training, and some prioritization of training is needed to optimize each element

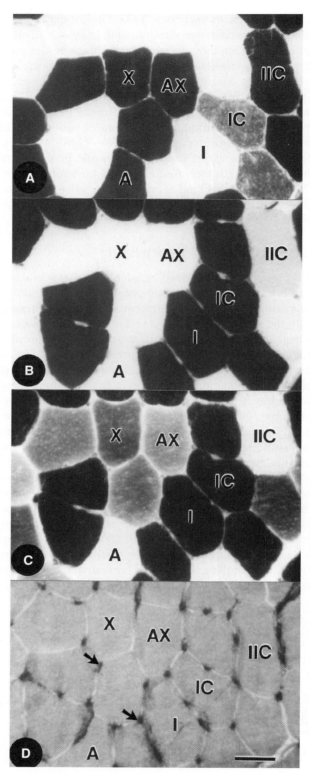

FIGURE 31-2. Muscle fiber types under different pH incubations **A:** 10.4. **B:** 4.3. **C:** 4.6. **D:** The capillary stain with the black dots capillaries. X- and AX-marked fibers are type II. (Courtesy of Dr. Robert Staron, Ohio University, Athens, Ohio)

over the entire training cycle. Figure 31-2 shows the different muscle fiber types and the MHC in humans.

HYPERTROPHY VERSUS HYPERPLASIA

Whole-muscle growth occurs predominantly because of an increase in the net amount of protein deposition within muscle fibers, or *hypertrophy*. Resistance training results in an increase in protein synthesis rate, a decrease in protein breakdown rate, or both, resulting in a net increase in muscle proteins. Muscle fiber *hyperplasia* or an increase in the number of muscle fibers has also been one possible mechanism for increasing the size of muscle. The mechanism for hyperplasia appears to be related to satellite cell involvement in myogenesis (i.e., creating new fibers) or longitudinal splitting of existing fibers when a ceiling limit of cell size is reached. Although shown in animals, the concept of hyperplasia following resistance training in humans has not been directly proven because of methodological difficulties (e.g., one cannot take out the whole muscle for examination). Cross-sectional studies of strength-trained athletes show greater muscle fiber number compared with untrained individuals; however, genetics cannot be ruled out as an explanation. In a 12-week training study of men, McCall et al. using both magnetic resonance imaging and biopsy techniques to examine hypertrophy, and the possible increase in cell number after a heavy resistance program showed some evidence for hyperplasia in the biceps muscle despite hypertrophy accounting for the greatest portion of muscle enlargement (101). It can be postulated that hyperplasia might account for approximately 5% of the adaptational response to resistance training, possibly in response to fibers reaching a theoretic upper limit in size.

Neuromuscular Junction

Neural sprouting may occur where new fibers are added to motor units. At the neuromuscular junction (NMJ), high-intensity training has been shown to produce more dispersed, irregularly shaped synapses, high terminal branching, increased endplate perimeter length and area, and greater dispersion of acetylcholine receptors within the endplate region (24,25). Thus, changes in the NMJ with larger surface areas, higher amounts of neurotransmitters, and neuronal sprouting all may affect the adaptations to resistance training.

MUSCLE ARCHITECTURE

Muscle architecture refers to the geometric arrangement of muscle fibers in *pennate* muscles (I). Changes in muscle architecture occur during resistance training, accommodating muscle hypertrophy. Resistance training increases the angle of pennation in pennate muscles. Although during acute muscle contraction, an increase in pennation angle may result in force loss, the additional

packing of contractile tissue with hypertrophy is compensatory, thereby allowing the muscle to produce more force and power. In addition, fascicle length has been shown to increase in some studies but not all (7,59,60,140). These architectural changes affect the manner in which force is transmitted to tendons and bones.

ENZYMATIC ADAPTATIONS

Increases in energy enzyme activity can lead to greater adenosine triphosphate (ATP) production and increases in physical performance. However, there have been conflicting reports regarding enzymatic changes during resistance training. Enzyme activity of the adenosine energy source (e.g., creatine phosphokinase and myokinase) has been shown to increase in humans during isokinetic and traditional resistance training (22,66). However, little or no change, or a decrease in creatine phosphokinase and myokinase have also been observed as a result of resistance training (89,146,149). Myosin ATPase has shown only minor changes in pooled muscle fibers (147). Resistance-training programs that primarily stress the phosphagens (i.e., readily available ATP CP) demonstrate reductions in glycolytic enzyme concentrations with pronounced hypertrophy, whereas intermittent high-intensity training, such as bodybuilding, may enhance glycolytic enzyme activity primarily in type II fibers. Phosphorylase activity has been shown to increase following resistance training (41,66). Phosphofructokinase (PFK) activity has been shown to increase or not change (or slightly decrease) (22,149). Lactate dehydrogenase (LDH) activity has been shown to increase, whereas no changes have been observed in hexokinase and malate dehydrogenase (22,41). Some increases in aerobic enzymes have been reported but are not typical, as traditional resistance training poses little stress to aerobic metabolism (22). Aerobic enzyme activity has been shown to be lower in lifters compared with untrained individuals (150). Bodybuilders using high-volume programs, short rest periods between sets and exercises, and moderate-intensity training resistances have been shown to have higher citrate synthase activity in type II fibers than other types of lifters who train with heavier loads and longer rest periods between sets (147). However, it should be noted that bodybuilders typically perform aerobic exercise as well as resistance training, thus cross-sectional data should be viewed with caution. Therefore, most studies showing no change or a decrease in enzyme activity also reported significant muscle hypertrophy. Initially, enzyme activity may increase in response to resistance training, but may not change or even decrease with subsequent training that produces significant muscle hypertrophy because of *protein dilution* (i.e., a reduction in concentration per unit of muscle weight that is due to increased muscle cross-sectional area). It appears that enzymatic changes associated with resistance training depend on the energy system demand, which is a composite of the interaction between intensity, volume, rest interval length, and muscle mass involvement. Traditional heavy resistance training will have minimal effects on enzyme activity, whereas a training program that minimizes hypertrophy and targets specific energy systems will most likely result in greater enzyme activities.

MUSCLE SUBSTRATE STORES

Anaerobic energy source substrates are enhanced with resistance training. Repeated bouts of resistance exercise acutely reduce ATP and CP concentrations, and can increase storage of these compounds via a "supercompensation" effect. Five months of resistance training has been shown to increase resting intramuscular concentrations of CP and ATP by 28% and 18%, respectively; however, normal concentrations of CP and ATP have been reported in athletes having a significant amount of muscular hypertrophy (93,147). A 66% increase in intramuscular glycogen stores was shown after resistance training for 5 months (93). Bodybuilders have been shown to have approximately a 50% greater concentration of glycogen than untrained individuals (147). However, muscle glycogen content has also been shown to not change with resistance training (147). Whether an increase in CP and ATP occurs with resistance training may depend on pre-training status, muscle group examined, and type of program performed. Lastly, a change in muscle triglyceride stores with resistance training remains equivocal, as lower and no difference from normal triglyceride content in the muscles of trained lifters have been reported (147). Although dietary practices and type of program may affect triglyceride concentrations, it can be hypothesized that intramuscular triglyceride concentrations are minimally affected by resistance training unless accompanied by significant weight loss.

CAPILLARY AND MYOGLOBIN ADAPTATIONS

A larger number of capillaries in muscle supports metabolism by increasing blood supply to the muscle. McCall et al. observed significant increases in numbers of capillaries (*capillarization*) per type I and II fibers following 12 weeks of resistance training (101). However, no changes in *capillary density* (number of capillaries per fiber area) were observed as a result of fiber hypertrophy. Improved capillarization has been observed with resistance training in untrained subjects (144,147). Power lifters and weightlifters exhibit no change in capillary number and a decrease in capillary density when compared with nonathletic individuals; however, bodybuilders display greater capillarization and capillary density (56,139,151). Thus, it appears high-intensity/low-volume resistance training decreases capillary density, whereas low-intensity/high-volume resistance training with short rest intervals may

increase capillary density, depending on the magnitude of hypertrophy. These workouts result in large elevations in blood lactate, and higher capillary density may facilitate lactate removal from the muscle to the blood (76). To conclude, capillarization can increase with resistance training, but this is typically, though not always, associated with a reduction in capillary density that is due to muscle hypertrophy. The time required for capillarization to take place may be >12 weeks. Lastly, muscle myoglobin content following strength training may be decreased (50), which may decrease the ability of the muscle fibers to extract oxygen.

MITOCHONDRIAL DENSITY

In a manner similar to capillary density, mitochondrial density has been shown to decrease with resistance training because of the dilution effects of muscle hypertrophy (92). Decreased mitochondrial density is consistent with the minimal demands for oxidative metabolism placed on the musculature during most resistance-training programs. Chilibeck et al. reported reduced mitochondrial density of regionally distributed mitochondria (i.e., subsarcolemmal and intermyofibrillar mitochondrial density decreased similarly) following resistance training (18). Thus, mitochondrial density appears to decrease in response to resistance training.

ENDOCRINE ADAPTATIONS

Hormones play a multitude of important regulatory roles in adaptation to resistance training. Neuroendocrine responses to resistance exercise take place in a unique physiologic environment and are a result of increased secretion, reduced hepatic clearance, plasma volume reductions, and/or reduced degradation rates (81). Acute elevations in circulating blood hormone concentrations observed during and immediately following a resistance exercise session increase the molar exposure of a hormone to its receptor on either the target tissue cell membrane (e.g., peptides) or with nuclear/cytoplasmic receptors located within the target tissue (e.g., steroid receptors), and increase receptor availability for binding and subsequent cellular changes. Receptor response from this interaction initiates events (through signaling cascades), ultimately leading to a specific cellular response, such as an increase in muscle protein synthesis or the use of a particular metabolic substrate. Endocrine release of hormones into the blood, paracrine release of hormones locally to affect other cells, and autocrine release of hormones to interact with the same cell are all involved with the hormonal control of cellular metabolism, repair, and remodeling.

The primary anabolic hormones are testosterone (T), growth hormone (GH), insulinlike growth factors (IGF), and insulin, whereas cortisol is a catabolic hormone. *Testosterone* is a steroid hormone produced by the testes that increases protein synthesis, growth, strength, and power, and controls secondary sex characteristics. It can also be produced in the adrenal gland via conversion from prohormones, which is the major way in which women produce T. The acidophilic cells of the anterior pituitary secrete the superfamily of *growth hormone* polypeptides. The most commonly studied GH isoform, the 22 kD molecule, consists of 191 amino acids. Other biologically active spliced fragments are released, such as a 20 kD isoform missing residues 32 to 46, a 5-kD isoform consisting of residues 1 to 43, and a 17-kD isoform consisting of residues 44 to 191. In addition, other monomeric, dimeric, protein-bound GH, and aggregates of GH have been identified that are included in this GH superfamily. GH is essential for promoting tissue anabolism. Many of the effects of GH are mediated by the anabolic protein hormone produced in the liver, *insulinlike growth factor-1* (IGF-1). *Insulin* has a potent up-regulating effect on muscle protein synthesis when adequate amino acids are available. Insulin concentrations parallel changes in blood glucose, and its response is enhanced by protein/carbohydrates ingestion before, during, or immediately following the workout. Without such ingestion before exercise, serum insulin concentrations have been shown to decrease or show no change during an acute bout of resistance exercise (156). *Catecholamines* (epinephrine, norepinephrine, dopamine) reflect the acute demands of resistance exercise and are important for increasing force production, muscle contraction rate, and energy availability, and augmenting other hormones, such as T. The adrenal cortex releases *cortisol,* which stimulates lipolysis in adipose cells, increases protein degradation (breakdown), and decreases protein synthesis in muscle cells. Cortisol may have a negative influence on mTOR signaling cues and negatively affects protein synthesis. It is possible that the effects of cortisol may be greater in fast-twitch compared with slow-twitch muscle fibers, and the disinhibition of cortisol effects may occur with training in which the intensity of receptor interactions may decrease.

ACUTE HORMONAL RESPONSE

Hormonal adaptations are governed by their acute response to a workout, chronic changes in resting concentrations, and chronic changes in the acute response (Table 31-2) (52). Resistance exercise has been shown to result in elevated T (total and free) and GH and its molecular variants during and for up to 15 to 30 minutes postexercise in men (70,71,72,84). Testosterone elevations are most prominent in men, although some studies have shown slight T elevations in women despite women having 10- to 30-fold lower T concentrations than men (115). The magnitude of T, cortisol, and GH elevation is greatest when large muscle mass exercises are performed

TABLE 31-2. HORMONAL ADAPTATIONS TO RESISTANCE TRAINING

HORMONE	ACUTE RESPONSE TO RE	CHRONIC RESTING ADAPTATIONS	CHRONIC CHANGES TO ACUTE RESPONSE
Testosterone	May ↑ or ↔; an ↑ is likely with high-intensity, high-volume programs with short rest intervals Most critical for recovery and adaptation	Typically ↔ unless there are substantial changes in volume and intensity May ↓ with overtraining	May ↑ slightly if individual can train at higher levels
Growth Hormone	↑ or ↔ with low-volume, low-intensity workouts ↑ is related to anaerobic nature of workout and to blood lactate when high-intensity and -volume programs with short rest elicit large response	↔; however, overnight "bursts" may ↑ if workout is strenuous enough	Acute ↑ can be higher when individuals train harder over time
Insulin	↔, response related to diet or plasma volume ↓	↔	↔
IGF-1	Delayed response based on GH secretion patterns	Related to GH changes, ↔ or ↑ IGF-1 in muscle ↑	Related to GH
Cortisol	↑ or ↔ with low-volume, low-intensity workouts ↑ is related to anaerobic nature of workout when high-intensity and -volume programs with short rest elicit large response	↔; ↓; may ↑ with overtraining	May not change
Catecholamines	↑ during workout and before in anticipation	↔	↔

↑, increase; ↓, decrease; ↔, no change; RE, resistance exercise; GH, growth hormone; IGF-1, insulinlike growth factor-1.

Modified from Hoffman JR, Ratamess NA. *A Practical Guide to Developing Resistance-Training Programs.* Monterey (CA): Coaches Choice Books; 2006.

and during workouts moderate to high in intensity and volume with short rest intervals (81). High correlations between blood lactate and GH concentrations have been reported, and it is thought that H+ accumulation may be the primary factor influencing GH and cortisol release (45). When large muscle mass exercises are performed early in a workout, they have a positive effect (i.e., greater strength and hypertrophy) on smaller muscle mass exercises performed later because, in part, of an enhanced T response (48). These data provide support for the ACSM's recommendation of performing large muscle mass exercises before small mass exercises for resistance exercise sequencing (68). Resistance exercise increases concentrations of epinephrine, norepinephrine, and dopamine, and the catecholamine concentrations are elevated before resistance exercise in anticipation (32,72,76). The magnitude may be dependent on the force of muscle contraction, amount of muscle stimulated, volume of resistance exercise, and rest interval length. In addition, the acute hormonal response to resistance exercise is attenuated when carbohydrates or protein are consumed before the workout (128).

CHRONIC CHANGES IN RESTING CONCENTRATIONS

Reported changes in resting T concentrations during resistance training have been inconsistent, with elevations, no differences, and reductions reported (81). It appears that resting concentrations reflect the muscle tissue's current state relative to changes in training volume and intensity. Substantial changes in volume and intensity may elicit transient changes in resting T concentrations, and values may return to baseline when the individual returns to "normal" training. Chronic elevations in T may not be desirable in the sense that androgen receptor desensitization can occur; thus, the acute response may be most critical for tissue remodeling. Resistance training does not appear to affect resting concentrations of 22 kD GH in men and women (75). This contention is supported by data showing similar resting concentrations of GH in elite Olympic weightlifters/strength athletes compared with lesser-trained individuals (5). These findings are consistent with dynamic feedback mechanisms of GH and its roles in the homeostatic control of other variables, e.g., glucose. This may be because of the lack of regulatory roles for the 22 kD monomer. One theory is that the larger molecular variants and binding proteins are more responsive to training adaptations. In a study by Kraemer et al., it was shown that different resistance training programs displayed different training effects based on the assay used to determine GH concentrations (74). Interestingly, the large aggregate GH isoforms were sensitive to training, and these affect muscle and connective tissue signaling and adaptations. Chronic exercise induces no consistent changes in immunoassayable GH variants, whereas bioassayable GH may increase across all fractions and training regimens.

Short-term resistance training does not appear to change resting levels of IGF-1, but long-term training may elicit some elevations. Resting IGF-1 concentrations have been shown to be higher in trained than untrained men and during high-volume multiple set training (99,134). Borst et al. reported significant elevations in resting serum IGF-1 following 13 weeks of resistance training (13). However, these elevations were similar between single-set and multiple-set training groups, despite a significantly larger increase in strength for the multiple-set group. Thus, it appears that the intensity and volume of training significantly affects the chronic long-term IGF-1 adaptations. Resting cortisol concentrations generally reflect long-term training stress. Resting cortisol concentrations do not appear to produce consistent patterns, as elevations, reductions, and no change have been found (81). Thus, the acute cortisol response may reflect metabolic stress, whereas chronic changes (or lack of change) may be important to tissue homeostasis involving protein metabolism.

CHRONIC CHANGES IN THE ACUTE HORMONAL RESPONSE

As a result of consistent resistance training, the acute hormonal response to a resistance exercise bout may improve as the individual exerts him- or herself to a greater extent. This has been shown predominantly with GH (81). The exercise-induced elevation has been correlated with type I and type II muscle fiber hypertrophy (102). Thus, progressive overload is critical for potentially enhancing the acute hormonal response. It appears that a potentiated hormonal response takes several weeks to months of resistance training to occur; it has recently been shown that the short-term acute hormonal response to a standard resistance exercise protocol was not augmented, despite slightly higher resistance exercise volume in strength and power athletes (128).

AUTOCRINE/PARACRINE ACTIONS

Insulinlike growth factor-1 has autocrine/paracrine functions within muscle cells. Two nonhepatic isoforms, IGF-1EA (similar to the circulating hepatic IGF-1) and *mechano growth factor* (MGF), appear to increase protein synthesis, promote satellite cell activation, and are sensitive to the mechanical overload of resistance training. Bamman et al. found significant elevations in muscle IGF-1 mRNA following resistance exercise (10). Thus, it appears that overloaded muscle and subsequent mechanical damage associated with resistance training is a prominent stimulus for muscle IGF-1 isoform production/release.

ANDROGEN RECEPTOR ADAPTATIONS

Androgen receptors (ARs) mediate the effects of androgens and are found in most tissues. Content depends on several factors, including muscle fiber type, contractile activity, and the concentrations of T. Resistance training has been shown to up-regulate AR mRNA (10,55). The resistance exercise stimulus appears to mediate the magnitude of acute AR modifications. Ratamess et al. compared two protocols (one vs. six sets of 10 repetitions of squats) and reported no differences in AR content 1 hour following the single-set protocol (130). However, the higher-volume protocol elicited significant down-regulation of AR content, demonstrating that, like other proteins, initial down-regulation may occur when sufficient volume is reached before the up-regulation that has been observed in other studies (10). It has also been discovered that ingestion of a protein/carbohydrate supplement before and after the workout attenuates the AR down-regulation, with higher-volume resistance exercise observed 1 hour postexercise (85). Thus, nutritional intervention plays a critical role in AR modification post–resistance exercise. In addition, significant correlations between baseline AR content in the vastus lateralis and 1RM squat suggest that AR content, in part, assists in mediating strength changes during resistance training (130).

CONNECTIVE TISSUE ADAPTATIONS

BONE

Bone is sensitive to intensity, compression, strain, and strain rate. Greater muscle strength increases the mechanical stress on bone, forcing bone to adapt by increasing mass and strength (an increase in *bone mineral density* [BMD]). Such forces are common in resistance training and relate to the type of exercise utilized, intensity of the resistance, number of sets, rate of loading, direction of forces, and frequency of training. It has been generally recommended that three to six sets of 1- to 10RM loads for multiple-joint exercises be used, with 1 to 4 minutes of rest between sets for optimal bone loading (20). BMD increases during resistance training, provided that sufficient intensity and volume are utilized (62). Strength athletes—i.e., weightlifters and power lifters—have been shown to have very high BMD values (hip, femur, lumbar spine, whole body) compared with untrained individuals (21,26,152). In a later investigation, Tsuzuku et al. reported significantly greater BMD in men resistance training with high versus low intensity, thus showing that heavy loading is needed to see improvements in BMD (153). Recent research has indicated power training (light to moderate loads, high velocity) to be as or more effective than traditional resistance training for maintaining BMD in postmenopausal women (157).

Resistance training is effective for increasing BMD in men and women of all ages; however, the time course is rather long (i.e., ~6 months or longer) and depends on the structure of the program (17,63,112). Cussler et al. reported that the amount of weight lifted during 1 year of resistance training was correlated to changes in BMD in

postmenopausal women (23). In particular, weight lifted for the squat correlated highly to femur BMD, and the weighted march exercise (i.e., hiking with a weighted backpack) correlated highly to total BMD. This study, as well as others, demonstrated the importance of intensity of resistance training for eliciting increases in BMD and osteoporosis risk reduction (153). Of significance have been recent studies demonstrating that many men and women resistance training in health clubs self-select intensities far below 60% of their respective 1RM (31,39,125). Ratamess et al. have shown that women who trained on their own self-selected intensities of 38% to 48% of their 1RM, whereas women who were trained by a personal trainer self-selected intensities of 43% to 57% of their 1RM (125). Only 7% of the women tested self-selected at least 75% of 1RM on at least one of the four exercises tested (125). These studies demonstrate that many individuals fail to adequately overload the skeletal system. Therefore, it appears that only high-intensity resistance training may be effective for long-term progression in BMD enhancement.

Although increases in BMD accompanying resistance training take at least several months to be observed, the process of adaptation begins within the first few workouts, as evidenced by blood elevations of two markers of bone anabolism: *bone alkaline phosphatase* and *osteocalcin* (58). Several studies have shown elevated serum osteocalcin (or bone alkaline phosphatase) concentrations during 1 to 18 months of resistance training, and the magnitude of change has been shown to be affected by protein intake in some studies (9,36,103,127). Thus, the mechanisms of bone osteogenesis are engaged within the first few workouts, but it takes several months before measurable changes in BMD can be shown.

CARTILAGE, LIGAMENTS, TENDONS, AND FASCIA

Connective tissue is abundantly distributed throughout the body. As skeletal muscle strength increases, tendons, ligaments, cartilage, and fascia must also adapt to support greater loading. The primary stimulus for growth of connective tissue is the mechanical forces created during resistance exercise. Signals from mechanical loading initiate a cascade of events ultimately leading from gene expression to greater protein synthesis incorporated into connective tissue. As with bone, the magnitude of connective tissue adaptation appears to be proportional to resistance-exercise intensity. Changes in collagen size, number, and packing density within a tendon contribute to its size and strength. Exercise increases the size and strength of tendons and ligaments (145). Increased strength of the ligaments and tendons is a necessary adaptation to aid in preventing possible injury. It also appears that these structures hypertrophy somewhat slower than muscle, as increases in *tendon stiffness* (force transmission per unit of strain), without changes in tendon CSA, have been reported, despite increases in muscle strength and hypertrophy (86–88). Critical is the intensity, as heavy loads (80% of 1RM) increase tendon stiffness but light loads (20% of 1RM) do not (87). Thus, structural changes (e.g., mechanical quality of collagen) may precede tendon hypertrophy. Connective tissue hypertrophy appears to occur in proportion to muscle size increases. This contention is supported by reports that bodybuilders do not differ from control subjects in the relative amount of connective tissue in the biceps brachii, and men and women bodybuilders possess similar relative amounts of connective tissue (9.7% vs. 10.7%, respectively) (8,90).

CARDIORESPIRATORY ADAPTATIONS

ACUTE RESPONSES TO RESISTANCE EXERCISE

Resistance exercise poses a high acute stress to the cardiovascular system. Heart rate, stroke volume, cardiac output, and blood pressure increase significantly to meet the demands of resistance exercise (29). The blood pressure response increases nonlinearly with the magnitude of active muscle mass (29). Although large elevations in blood pressure may occur, no negative effects on resting blood pressure have been reported. During each set of resistance exercise, stroke volume and cardiac output increase, especially when a *Valsalva maneuver* (see Chapter 29) is used (28). In addition, ventilation is significantly elevated during each set, but this elevation quickly decreases to normal during the first minute of recovery (126). Ventilations in excess of 60 L/min during resistance exercise have been observed with short rest intervals (126). Overall, the magnitude of the acute cardiovascular responses depends on the intensity and volume of exercise, muscle mass involvement, rest intervals used, and contraction velocity (78,80). However, resistance training does not significantly affect maximal aerobic capacity (see below).

RESTING ADAPTATIONS

Decreased resting heart rate, or *bradycardia*, and blood pressure are positive cardiovascular adaptations that reduce cardiac workload and decrease the risk of myocardial infarction. Resistance training may reduce or not change resting heart rate, depending on one's level of fitness (as unfit individuals are most responsive). Highly resistance-trained athletes have an average or slightly below average resting heart rate (29). Resistance training has shown small significant decreases in resting heart rate of 5% to 12% (29). Decreases in resting heart rate are much more prominent during aerobic training. Resting systolic and diastolic blood pressure of strength-trained athletes is average or slightly below average (29). A meta-analysis of studies in which individuals performed weight training for 4 weeks or more showed that resistance training decreases resting systolic and diastolic blood pressure

approximately 2% and 4%, respectively (61). Stroke volume has been shown to increase in absolute magnitude, but not relative to body surface area or lean body mass (29). In addition, resistance training may either not change or slightly decrease total cholesterol and low-density-lipoprotein (LDL) cholesterol, and increase high-density-lipoprotein (HDL) cholesterol (54). High-volume, short rest interval programs (e.g., bodybuilding, circuit training) with high continuity appear most effective at eliciting cardiovascular adaptations at rest but still are inferior to aerobic training. Lastly, resistance training has been shown to increase left ventricular and intraventricular septal wall thicknesses, which are critical to tolerating greater cardiac pressure overload during resistance exercise (29). Increased wall thicknesses are also observed in several conditions that produce chronic elevations in afterload (systolic blood pressure), such as hypertension.

CHRONIC CHANGES TO THE ACUTE RESISTANCE EXERCISE RESPONSE

Resistance training reduces the cardiovascular response to an acute bout of resistance exercise of similar absolute intensity or workload. Resistance training has been shown to reduce the acute increases in heart rate and blood pressure during a workout of similar level of effort (138). In addition, resistance training leads to faster recovery of heart rate to resting values after a work bout (138). The decreases in heart rate and blood pressure during submaximal work are viewed as positive adaptations and reduce cardiovascular stress.

MAXIMAL OXYGEN CONSUMPTION

Resistance training does not significantly affect maximal oxygen consumption ($\dot{V}O_{2max}$) in fit individuals, although deconditioned individuals may see improvements. The lack of continuity during resistance exercise (i.e., rest periods between sets) appears to pose limitations for potential improvements in $\dot{V}O_{2max}$. Large muscle mass workouts have been shown to elicit responses peaking at 60% of $\dot{V}O_{2max}$, which may not reach the critical threshold needed for improvement (147). Circuit training and high-volume, short rest period programs have been shown to improve $\dot{V}O_{2max}$, but the effects are considerably less than aerobic training (38).

It is important to note that some studies have shown combining high-intensity resistance and aerobic training may interfere primarily with strength and power gains if the aerobic training is high in intensity and volume/frequency (77). In contrast, most studies have shown no adverse effects on $\dot{V}O_{2max}$ from heavy resistance exercise despite the expected physiologic changes caused by resistance training, although a study has shown the addition of strength training can hinder $\dot{V}O_{2max}$ improvements (40). The physiologic mechanisms involved in the incompatibility may be related to alterations in neural recruitment patterns, attenuation of muscle hypertrophy, overtraining, inadequate recovery in between workouts, hormonal environment, and residual fatigue from aerobic workouts during resistance exercise. It is important to note that incompatibility may be seen at higher levels of training and may not be expected in a general health and fitness setting.

IMMUNE SYSTEM RESPONSES AND ADAPTATIONS

The overload associated with resistance exercise causes trauma to skeletal muscle. The immune system responds with a series of reactions leading to an inflammatory response that contains and repairs the damage, removes debris from the injured area, and ultimately plays a key role in skeletal muscle hypertrophy. The immune system responds to infection, injury, and inflammation, and contains many types of cells, including leukocytes (e.g., neutrophils, monocytes, eosinophils, basophils, lymphocytes, and subsets), immunoglobulins, and cytokines (116). Along with monocytes/macrophages, *neutrophils* are the first line of immune defense localized to the injury/inflammation site, especially with damaged skeletal muscle induced by exercise. *Monocytes* are involved in phagocytosis, antigen presentation, cytokine production, and cytotoxicity; differentiate into macrophages; and produce interleukin (IL)-1, IL-6, and tumor necrosis factor-alpha (TNF-α). Macrophages move to the injury site and secrete cytokines, growth factors, and other substances. *Lymphocytes* are involved with cytokine production, antigen recognition, antibody production, and cytotoxicity, and give rise to subpopulations of *T-cells* (CD3+, CD8+, and CD4+), *B-cells* (CD19+), and *natural killer (NK) cells* (CD16+ and CD56+). *Immunoglobulins* (e.g., IgA, IgG, IgE, and IgM) are antibodies that react with antigens and are involved in phagocytosis. *Cytokines* are polypeptides involved in communication between lymphoid and other cells, and perform virtually all immune functions. They are responsible for protein breakdown, removal of damaged muscle cells, and an increased production of prostaglandins (hormonelike substances that help to control the inflammation). Some major anti-inflammatory cytokines include IL-1 receptor antagonist, IL-4, IL-10, IL-11, IL-12, and IL-13. The cytokines IL-1, TNF-α, and IL-6 function as proinflammatory cytokines. Because of the mechanical stress to the neuromuscular system, it has been of interest to examine whether resistance training (i.e., because of soreness, damage, etc.) could suppress immune function during the postworkout period. Interestingly, most studies have shown that resistance exercise does not lead to immunosuppression in young or elderly individuals unless overtraining is present (30,65,95,141).

LEUKOCYTES

Leukocyte concentrations increase during and after exercise for several hours, with the magnitude related to exercise intensity and volume (95). The increase is mostly attributed to neutrophils, although lymphocyte and monocyte counts also increase. During resistance exercise, total leukocytes significantly increase in a similar pattern to endurance exercise (30,69). However, the response is less pronounced in basophils and eosinophils (95). Following resistance exercise that causes muscle damage, the leukocyte response in skeletal muscle appears to be biphasic: There is an 8% to 10% elevation in the first 8 hours after the workout, but a 14% elevation between the eighth and twenty-first hours postexercise, which corresponded to a period of halted recovery (124). The magnitude of increase appears to be similar between athletes and nonathletes. Resting leukocyte counts typically do not change unless the athlete is overtrained, then reductions may occur. A substantial portion of the exercise-induced changes in leukocyte number may be mediated by the endocrine system, in which hormones such as catecholamines, cortisol, GH, T, and estrogen have been shown to affect lymphocyte subpopulations and proliferation, NK cell activity, and the neutrophils response (118).

Lymphocytes and subsets increase in response to all types of exercise. Moderate and intense interval exercise results in 50% to 200% increases, whereas long and prolonged exercise results in 25% to 100% increases (95,96). Miles et al. have shown acute resistance exercise results in elevations in CD4+, CD8+, NK, and B cells by 42% to 242%, with the response highest when blood lactates were high (105). Lymphocyte proliferation was studied during acute resistance exercise between women with high (~72 kg) and low (~40 kg) 1RM squats; an increase was observed in the low-strength group, whereas a decrease was observed in the high-strength group, thereby demonstrating the potential factor of maximal strength and loading on the immune response (27). At rest, no differences have been observed between resistance-trained women and controls; however, male weightlifters have been shown to have higher values based on the training cycle (65,105,106). Resistance exercise may increase B cells and T-cell subsets (106,114). However, NK cell cytotoxic activity has been shown to be decreased by 40% at 2 hours following intensive resistance exercise (114). Resting concentrations of lymphocytes do not differ between athletes (endurance and power) and nonathletes, and long-term training does not alter resting subset distribution (95). However, Miles et al. reported that after 3 months of resistance training in previously untrained women, resting NK concentrations were higher but returned to baseline after 6 months of training (105). Monocytes increase during resistance exercise by approximately 15% to 50%, whereas prolonged endurance exercise results in a 50% to 250% increase (95). Resting concentrations typically do not change. Interestingly, rest interval length may play a role. Mayhew et al. have recently shown that lymphocytosis and monocytosis are significantly greater 1.5 hours postexercise by 32% to 67% when 1-min versus 3-min rest intervals were used for 10 sets of 10 repetitions of the leg press, thus showing the acute response depends on the program used (100).

IMMUNOGLOBULINS

Resting concentrations of IgA, IgG, IgE, and IgM are similar between athletes unless the athlete is overtrained (i.e., reductions may be observed) (104). Acute exercise has been shown to produce small increases (8%–12%) of some immunoglobulins, but many studies show no effect (95). The combination of resistance and endurance training in the elderly has been shown to increase IgA at rest (6).

CYTOKINES

Cytokines are released in response to exercise (118). Proinflammatory cytokines increase significantly, as do anti-inflammatory cytokines during exercise, especially when there is a strong eccentric component. It is thought that the rise in anti-inflammatory cytokines restrict the magnitude and duration of the inflammatory response (118). Acute resistance exercise has been shown to increase plasma concentrations of IL-6, IL-8, IL-10, and IL-1 receptor antagonist (113). In addition, muscle mRNA for IL-1β, IL-6, IL-8, and TNF-α increase following resistance exercise (113). IL-1 (α and β) may increase two- to fivefold days after heavy eccentric exercise in skeletal muscle. IL-6 and TNF-α have been shown to increase significantly following resistance exercise (117). In the elderly, high levels of IL-6 and TNF-α were associated with low muscle size and strength (155). Greiwe et al. reported that 3 months of resistance training in the elderly reduced skeletal muscle TNF-α mRNA and protein levels, and protein synthesis rate was inversely related to levels of TNF-α (42). Thus, down-regulation of proinflammatory cytokines may be another mechanism by which resistance training elicits muscle growth. It has been shown that IL-15 is found in high concentrations in muscle and has anabolic and angiogenic properties. Riechman et al. examined 10 weeks of resistance training and reported that plasma IL-15 concentrations were elevated following a workout and that the acute response was not enhanced over 10 weeks (131). However, IL-15 protein was not associated with gains in muscle size. In addition, a polymorphism in the IL-15 receptor α gene was associated with greater amounts of muscle hypertrophy.

DELAYED ONSET MUSCLE SORENESS

> **1.1.16-HFS: Knowledge of the common theories of muscle fatigue and delayed onset muscle soreness (DOMS).**

Delayed onset muscle soreness (DOMS) is the pain or discomfort experienced 24 to 72 hours after resistance exercising, which subsides within 2 to 3 days. DOMS is associated with localized pain in the exercised muscles, reduced range of motion, loss of muscle strength and power, greater muscle stiffness, and swelling. Resistance exercise with a strong eccentric component leads to the most substantial magnitude of muscle damage, as measured directly via muscle biopsies or indirectly via blood markers, such as creatine kinase (CK), myoglobin, lactate dehydrogenase, troponin I, and myosin heavy chain fragments (116). The extent of muscle damage depends on the intensity, volume, and type of muscle actions used and the training status of the individual. In fact, resistance-trained individuals have shown significantly less elevation in CK and myoglobin concentrations and less muscle damage 12 to 120 hours following an acute resistance-exercise protocol compared with untrained individuals (154). Repeated bouts of resistance exercise exert a protective effect on skeletal muscle, thereby making it less susceptible to damage and accelerating the rate of repair in young and elderly individuals (97,121). In addition, the extent of muscle damage has been attenuated, and recovery has been enhanced by amino acid and L-carnitine L-tartrate supplementation (83,142).

Several mechanisms have been proposed to explain DOMS. DOMS may result from mechanical stress via heavy resistance exercise or from metabolic stress characteristic of low-to-moderate–intensity resistance exercise coupled with high volume or short rest intervals. Different (novel) muscle recruitment patterns (e.g., performing an unfamiliar exercise) may lead to unaccustomed stress placed on muscles, ligaments, and tendons. Mechanical traumas to contractile proteins and cytoskeleton, acute inflammation, local ischemia, muscle spasm, connective tissue damage, and free radical proliferation have all been implicated in DOMS. It is likely that DOMS is multifactorial and a result of multiple conditions. Treatments for DOMS are limited. For example, stretching, nonsteroidal anti-inflammatory agents, hyperbaric oxygen therapy, cryotherapy, massage, ultrasound, and nutritional supplementation (vitamins C and E) have shown limited effectiveness (19). Thus, it appears that the cascade of events leading to muscle damage and DOMS (i.e., swelling, inflammatory response, prostaglandin E_2 release, leukotriene synthesis, immune response) may be critical to the tissue remodeling process.

HEALTH AND FITNESS ADAPTATIONS

As mentioned previously, resistance training elicits positive cardiovascular adaptations related to pressure overload. $\dot{V}O_{2max}$ may improve only slightly, and this effect is greatest in unfit individuals. In addition, blood lipid profiles (decreased triglycerides, increased HDLs, decreased LDLs) may not change or improve (although aerobic exercise and diet have more substantial effects). However, resistance training may elicit other adaptations that benefit general health and fitness. Flexibility may improve, as well as muscular strength, endurance, and power (82). Resistance training has been shown to reduce percent body fat; increase insulin sensitivity; decrease basal insulin levels and insulin response to a glucose challenge; increase basal metabolic rate; attenuate muscle sarcopenia; reduce the risk of osteoporosis, colon cancer, and low back pain; and maintain long-term independence and functional capacity (82,158). These benefits, as well as the performance-related benefits, have been shown to improve the quality of life in the elderly and clinical populations such as those with low-back pain, osteoarthritis, cardiovascular disease, stroke, HIV (human immunodeficiency virus), neuromuscular disease (e.g., myasthenia gravis, myotonic dystrophy), obesity, renal failure, chronic obstructive pulmonary disease, and type 2 diabetes mellitus (82).

OVERTRAINING

> **1.1.33-HFS: Knowledge of the physical and psychological signs of overreaching/overtraining and to provide recommendations for these problems.**

Overtraining is long-term excessive frequency, volume, or intensity of training resulting in prolonged fatigue and decreased performance. Short-term excessive training is called *overreaching*. The rationale is to overwork and then taper (reduce the training stimulus) to "rebound" in performance. Short-term overreaching followed by a tapering period has been shown to result in substantial strength and power gains, and this effect has been shown to be enhanced with creatine or amino acid supplementation (35,83,129). However, overreaching can become overtraining syndrome if it continues beyond a reasonable period of time. Overtraining syndrome may include a plateau or reduction in performance. The progression in the overtraining continuum follows: the *overload stimulus* to *acute fatigue* to *overreaching* to *overtraining*. Resistance or anaerobic overtraining is not the same as aerobic overtraining, and the signs and symptoms may differ. Overtraining is associated with greater damage or negative physiologic alterations in the neuromuscular system. Overtraining classically was thought to be a function of either chronic use of high intensity, high volume, or a combination of both. Training periodization consists of careful planning to avoid overtraining. Overreaching has been shown to decrease resting concentrations of T and IGF-1 (46). If the source of overtraining is volume related, elevations in cortisol and reductions in resting luteinizing hormone (LH), total, and free T concentrations have been reported (33,34). Intensity-related overtraining does not appear to alter resting concentrations of hormones (33,34). However, desensitization to the sympathetic response (i.e., the ratio of epinephrine to the

density of β2 adrenergic receptors) occurs, which can contribute to performance reductions (35). Other symptoms of overtraining include mood disturbances; decreased vigor, motivation, and confidence; higher levels of tension, depression, anger, fatigue, confusion, anxiety, and irritability; and impaired concentration.

DETRAINING

> **1.1.32-HFS: Knowledge of the concept of detraining or reversibility of conditioning and its implications in exercise programs**

Detraining is the decrease in performance and loss of some physiologic adaptations that result from cessation of resistance training or a substantial reduction in its frequency, volume, or intensity. The magnitude of strength loss depends on the length of the detraining period and the training status of the individuals. Decrements may occur in as little as 2 weeks and possibly sooner in highly strength-trained individuals, but little to no reductions may be seen in recreationally trained men within 6 weeks of detraining (74). Strength loss appears related to neural mechanisms initially, with muscle atrophy predominating as the detraining period extends; however, the magnitude of strength lost rarely exceeds the strength gained through training (74). That is, residual resistance training effects are shown, as maximal strength after detraining is still higher than maximal strength assessed before beginning a weight-training program. The high strength retainment suggests "muscle memory."

AGING INFLUENCES ON THE NEUROMUSCULAR SYSTEM

Physiologic limitations in endocrine and immune function, cell regeneration, cell water, neuronal death, and a host of other underlying changes are related to aging. Ultimately, this leads to *sarcopenia*, a loss of muscle tissue (whether by reduced fiber size or number), which leads to reduced performance capacity. Strength is an important factor for functional abilities. Muscle weakness can advance to a stage at which an elderly individual cannot do common activities of daily living, such as getting out of a chair, sweeping the floor, or taking out the trash. Reduced functional ability may lead to a loss of independence. Thus, muscle strength is vital to our health, functional abilities, and independent living. Under normal conditions, strength performances appear to peak between the ages of 20 and 30 years, after which changes in strength remain relatively stable or slightly decrease over the next 20 years, depending on an individual's activity level. Large dramatic decreases are observed in the sixth decade of life, and this decrease may be more dramatic in women. In fact, Bassey and Harries reported a loss of grip strength of 3% per year for men and nearly 5% for women

BOX 31-1	NEUROMUSCULAR FACTORS ASSOCIATED WITH AGE-RELATED DECREASES IN STRENGTH AND POWER

- Change in resting hormone levels
- Blunted acute hormonal response to exercise
- Decrease in muscular energy substrate content
- Decrease in anaerobic enzyme concentration and activity
- Decrease in mitochondrial mass
- Denervation or death of muscle cells
- Decreased muscle mass (atrophy of muscle fibers, particularly of type II)

- Decreased ability to develop force rapidly
- Antagonistic coactivation
- Changes in ability to maximally activate a muscle
- Changes at the neuromuscular junction
- Decreased firing rate of motor units
- Decreased insulin sensitivity and tolerance

over a 4-year period (11). The muscle's ability to exert force rapidly (power) diminishes with age and may be more sensitive to reduction than maximal strength. Adequate muscle power may serve as a protective mechanism against falling in the elderly, which is one of the leading causes of injury and may lead to death. Thus, loss of power significantly reduces functional capacity. Box 31-1 overviews some basic changes with aging.

Resistance training can offset the magnitude of strength loss; however, some reductions may occur even in individuals who have strength trained most of their lives. The loss of strength in the lower extremities has been shown to be greater than that of the upper extremities. It appears that muscle strength losses are most dramatic after the age of 70 years. Cross-sectional as well as longitudinal data indicate that muscle strength declines by approximately 15% per decade in the sixth and seventh decade and about 30% thereafter (49). Muscle power trainability in seniors has received limited study but may be even more important for performance of activities of daily living (walking, climbing stairs, and lifting objects). Bassey et al. reported that leg extensor power was significantly correlated with chair-rising speed, stair-climbing speed, and power, and walking speed in elderly men and women (11). Recent studies have investigated power training in the elderly and have revealed positive results. Integration of power exercises into resistance training has shown to be effective for improving performance (44,111). Henwood and Taaffe examined 8 weeks of power training (three sets of eight repetitions with 35%–75% of 1RM at maximal concentric velocity) and reported 21% to 82% increases in muscle strength, 16% to 33% increases in muscle power, and significant enhancement of stair-climbing ability, 6-m walk, and ability to rise from a chair and the floor (51). Bottaro et al. compared 10 weeks of power training with traditional resistance training and reported similar increases in strength between groups; however, the power training group improved up-and-go and 30-s chair stand performance by 15% to 43%, whereas the traditional group did not improve functional capacity (14). Similar findings were reported by Miszko

et al., who reported power training to be more effective than traditional resistance training for improving functional performance (107). Other studies have shown similar findings (122). Thus, resistance training programs for the elderly also should address the need for power.

REFERENCES

1. Aagaard P, Andersen JL, Dyhre-Poulsen P, et al. A mechanism for increased contractile strength of human pennate muscle in response to strength training: changes in muscle architecture. *J Physiol*. 2001;534(Pt. 2):613–623.
2. Aagaard P, Simonsen EB, Andersen JL, Magnusson P, Dyhre-Poulsen P. Neural adaptation to resistance training: changes in evoked V-wave and H-reflex responses. *J Appl Physiol*. 2002;92(6): 2309–2318.
3. Adams GR, Harris RT, Woodard D, Dudley GA. Mapping of electrical muscle stimulation using MRI. *J Appl Physiol*. 1993;74(2):532–537.
4. Adams GR, Hather BM, Baldwin KM, Dudley GA. Skeletal muscle myosin heavy chain composition and resistance training. *J Appl Physiol*. 1993;74(2):911–915.
5. Ahtiainen JP, Pakarinen A, Kraemer WJ, Hakkinen K. Acute hormonal responses to heavy resistance exercise in strength athletes versus nonathletes. *Can J Appl Physiol*. 2004;29(5):527–543.
6. Akimoto T, Kumai Y, Akama T, et al. Effects of 12 months of exercise training on salivary secretory IgA levels in elderly subjects. *Br J Sports Med*. 2003;37(1):76–79.
7. Alegre LM, Jimenez F, Gonzalo-Orden JM, Martin-Acero R, Aguado X. Effects of dynamic resistance training on fascicle length and isometric strength. *J Sports Sci*. 2006;24(5):501–508.
8. Alway SE, Grumbt WH, Gonyea WJ, Stray-Gundersen J. Contrasts in muscle and myofibers of elite male and female bodybuilders. *J Appl Physiol*. 1989;67(1):24–31.
9. Ballard TL, Clapper JA, Specker BL, Binkley TL, Vukovich MD. Effect of protein supplementation during a 6-mo strength and conditioning program on insulin-like growth factor I and markers of bone turnover in young adults. *Am J Clin Nutr*. 2005;81(6): 1442–1448.
10. Bamman MM, Shipp JR, Jiang J, et al. Mechanical load increases muscle IGF-I and androgen receptor mRNA concentrations in humans. *Am J Physiol Endocrinol Metab*. 2001;280(3):E383–390.
11. Bassey EJ, Fiatarone MA, O'Neill EF, Kelly M, Evans WJ, Lipsitz LA. Leg extensor power and functional performance in very old men and women. *Clin Sci (Lond)*. 1992;82(3):321–327.
12. Bell GJ, Syrotuik D, Martin TP, Burnham R, Quinney HA. Effect of concurrent strength and endurance training on skeletal muscle properties and hormone concentrations in humans. *Eur J Appl Physiol*. 2000;81(5):418–427.

13. Borst SE, De Hoyos DV, Garzarella L, et al. Effects of resistance training on insulin-like growth factor-I and IGF binding proteins. *Med Sci Sports Exerc.* 2001;33(4):648–653.

14. Bottaro M, Machado SN, Nogueira W, Scales R, Veloso J. Effect of high versus low-velocity resistance training on muscular fitness and functional performance in older men. *Eur J Appl Physiol.* 2007;99(3):257–264.

15. Cannon RJ, Cafarelli E. Neuromuscular adaptations to training. *J Appl Physiol.* 1987;63(6):2396–2402.

16. Carolan B, Cafarelli E. Adaptations in coactivation after isometric resistance training. *J Appl Physiol.* 1992;73(3):911–917.

17. Chilibeck PD, Calder A, Sale DG, Webber CE. Twenty weeks of weight training increases lean tissue mass but not bone mineral mass or density in healthy, active young women. *Can J Physiol Pharmacol.* 1996;74(10):1180–1185.

18. Chilibeck PD, Syrotuik DG, Bell GJ. The effect of strength training on estimates of mitochondrial density and distribution throughout muscle fibres. *Eur J Appl Physiol Occup Physiol.* 1999;80(6):604–609.

19. Connolly DA, Sayers SP, McHugh MP. Treatment and prevention of delayed onset muscle soreness. *J Strength Cond Res.* 2003;17(1):197–208.

20. Conroy BP, Earle RW. Bone, muscle, and connective tissue adaptations to physical activity. In: Baechle TR, Earle RW, editors. *Essentials of Strength Training and Conditioning.* Champaign (IL): Human Kinetics; 2000, p. 57–72.

21. Conroy BP, Kraemer WJ, Maresh CM, et al. Bone mineral density in elite junior Olympic weightlifters. *Med Sci Sports Exerc.* 1993;25(10):1103–1109.

22. Costill DL, Coyle EF, Fink WF, Lesmes GR, Witzmann FA. Adaptations in skeletal muscle following strength training. *J Appl Physiol.* 1979;46(1):96–99.

23. Cussler EC, Lohman TG, Going SB, et al. Weight lifted in strength training predicts bone change in postmenopausal women. *Med Sci Sports Exerc.* 2003;35(1):10–17.

24. Deschenes MR, Judelson DA, Kraemer WJ, et al. Effects of resistance training on neuromuscular junction morphology. *Muscle Nerve.* 2000;23(10):1576–1581.

25. Deschenes MR, Maresh CM, Crivello JF, Armstrong LE, Kraemer WJ, Covault J. The effects of exercise training of different intensities on neuromuscular junction morphology. *J Neurocytol.* 1993;22(8):603–615.

26. Dickerman RD, Pertusi R, Smith GH. The upper range of lumbar spine bone mineral density? An examination of the current world record holder in the squat lift. *Int J Sports Med.* 2000;21(7):469–470.

27. Dohi K, Mastro AM, Miles MP, et al. Lymphocyte proliferation in response to acute heavy resistance exercise in women: influence of muscle strength and total work. *Eur J Appl Physiol.* 2001;85(3-4):367–373.

28. Falkel JE, Fleck SJ, Murray TF. Comparison of central hemodynamics between power lifters and bodybuilders during exercise. *J Appl Sport Sci Res.* 1992;6:24–35.

29. Fleck SJ. Cardiovascular responses to strength training. In: Komi PV, editor. *Strength and Power in Sport.* Malden (MA): Blackwell Scientific Publications; 2003. p. 387–406.

30. Flynn MG, Fahlman M, Braun WA, et al. Effects of resistance training on selected indexes of immune function in elderly women. *J Appl Physiol.* 1999;86(6):1905–1913.

31. Focht BC. Perceived exertion and training load during self-selected and imposed-intensity resistance exercise in untrained women. *J Strength Cond Res.* 2007;21(1):183–187.

32. French DN, Kraemer WJ, Volek JS, et al. Anticipatory responses of catecholamines on muscle force production. *J Appl Physiol.* 2007;102(1):94–102.

33. Fry AC, Kraemer WJ. Resistance exercise overtraining and overreaching: neuroendocrine responses. *Sports Med.* 1997;23(2):106–129.

34. Fry AC, Kraemer WJ, Ramsey LT. Pituitary-adrenal-gonadal responses to high-intensity resistance exercise overtraining. *J Appl Physiol.* 1998;85(6):2352–2359.

35. Fry AC, Schilling BK, Weiss LW, Chiu LZ. beta2-Adrenergic receptor downregulation and performance decrements during high-intensity resistance exercise overtraining. *J Appl Physiol.* 2006;101(6):1664–1672.

36. Fujimura R, Ashizawa N, Watanabe M, et al. Effect of resistance exercise training on bone formation and resorption in young male subjects assessed by biomarkers of bone metabolism. *J Bone Miner Res.* 1997;12(4):656–662.

37. Gabriel DA, Kamen G, Frost G. Neural adaptations to resistive exercise: mechanisms and recommendations for training practices. *Sports Med.* 2006;36(2):133–149.

38. Gettman LR, Culter LA, Strathman T. Physiological changes after 20 weeks of isotonic vs isokinetic circuit training. *J Sports Med Phys Fitness.* 1980:265–274.

39. Glass SC, Stanton DR. Self-selected resistance training intensity in novice weightlifters. *J Strength Cond Res.* 2004;18(2):324–327.

40. Glowacki SP, Martin SE, Maurer A, Baek W, Green JS, Crouse SF. Effects of resistance, endurance, and concurrent exercise on training outcomes in men. *Med Sci Sports Exerc.* 2004;36(12):2119–2127.

41. Green H, Dahly A, Shoemaker K, Goreham C, Bombardier E, Ball-Burnett M. Serial effects of high-resistance and prolonged endurance training on Na+-K+ pump concentration and enzymatic activities in human vastus lateralis. *Acta Physiol Scand.* 1999;165(2):177–184.

42. Greiwe JS, Cheng B, Rubin DC, Yarasheski KE, Semenkovich CF. Resistance exercise decreases skeletal muscle tumor necrosis factor alpha in frail elderly humans. *FASEB J.* 2001;15(2):475–482.

43. Hakkinen K, Alen M, Kraemer WJ, et al. Neuromuscular adaptations during concurrent strength and endurance training versus strength training. *Eur J Appl Physiol.* 2003;89(1):42–52.

44. Hakkinen K, Kraemer WJ, Pakarinen A, et al. Effects of heavy resistance/power training on maximal strength, muscle morphology, and hormonal response patterns in 60–75-year-old men and women. *Can J Appl Physiol.* 2002;27(3):213–231.

45. Hakkinen K, Pakarinen A. Acute hormonal responses to two different fatiguing heavy-resistance protocols in male athletes. *J Appl Physiol.* 1993;74(2):882–887.

46. Hakkinen K, Pakarinen A, Alen M, Kauhanen H, Komi PV. Daily hormonal and neuromuscular responses to intensive strength training in 1 week. *Int J Sports Med.* 1988;9(6):422–428.

47. Hakkinen K, Pakarinen A, Alen M, Kauhanen H, Komi PV. Neuromuscular and hormonal adaptations in athletes to strength training in two years. *J Appl Physiol.* 1988;65(6):2406–2412.

48. Hansen S, Kvorning T, Kjaer M, Sjogaard G. The effect of short-term strength training on human skeletal muscle: the importance of physiologically elevated hormone levels. *Scand J Med Sci Sports.* 2001;11(6):347–354.

49. Harries UJ, Bassey EJ. Torque-velocity relationships for the knee extensors in women in their 3rd and 7th decades. *Eur J Appl Physiol Occup Physiol.* 1990;60(3):187–190.

50. Henneman E. Relation between size of neurons and their susceptibility to discharge. *Science.* 1957;126(3287):1345–1347.

51. Henwood TR, Taaffe DR. Improved physical performance in older adults undertaking a short-term programme of high-velocity resistance training. *Gerontology.* 2005;51(2):108–115.

52. Hoffman JR, Ratamess NA. *A Practical Guide to Developing Resistance-Training Programs.* Monterey (CA): Coaches Choice Books; 2006.

53. Holtermann A, Roeleveld K, Engstrom M, Sand T. Enhanced H-reflex with resistance training is related to increased rate of force development. *Eur J Appl Physiol.* 2007;101(3):301–312.

54. Hurley BF. Effects of resistance training on lipoprotein-lipid profiles: a comparison to aerobic exercise training. *Med Sci Sports Exerc.* 1989;21:689–693.

55. Kadi F, Bonnerud P, Eriksson A, Thornell LE. The expression of androgen receptors in human neck and limb muscles: effects of training and self-administration of androgenic-anabolic steroids. *Histochem Cell Biol.* 2000;113(1):25–29.

56. Kadi F, Eriksson A, Holmner S, Butler-Browne GS, Thornell LE. Cellular adaptation of the trapezius muscle in strength-trained athletes. *Histochem Cell Biol.* 1999;111(3):189–195.

57. Kadi F, Schjerling P, Andersen LL, et al. The effects of heavy resistance training and detraining on satellite cells in human skeletal muscles. *J Physiol.* 2004;558(Pt 3):1005–1012.

58. Karlsson MK, Vergnaud P, Delmas PD, Obrant KJ. Indicators of bone formation in weight lifters. *Calcif Tissue Int.* 1995;56(3):177–180.

59. Kawakami Y, Abe T, Kuno SY, Fukunaga T. Training-induced changes in muscle architecture and specific tension. *Eur J Appl Physiol Occup Physiol.* 1995;72(1-2):37–43.

60. Kearns CF, Abe T, Brechue WF. Muscle enlargement in sumo wrestlers includes increased muscle fascicle length. *Eur J Appl Physiol.* 2000;83(4-5):289–296.

61. Kelley GA, Kelley KS. Progressive resistance exercise and resting blood pressure: a meta-analysis of randomized controlled trials. *Hypertension.* 2000;35(3):838–843.

62. Kelley GA, Kelley KS, Tran ZV. Exercise and bone mineral density in men: a meta-analysis. *J Appl Physiol.* 2000;88(5):1730–1736.

63. Kelley GA, Kelley KS, Tran ZV. Resistance training and bone mineral density in women: a meta-analysis of controlled trials. *Am J Phys Med Rehabil.* 2001;80(1):65–77.

64. Kemp TJ, Sadusky TJ, Saltisi F, et al. Identification of Ankrd2, a novel skeletal muscle gene coding for a stretch-responsive ankyrin-repeat protein. *Genomics.* 2000;66(3):229–241.

65. Kilgore JL, Pendlay GW, Reeves JS, Kilgore TG. Serum chemistry and hematological adaptations to 6 weeks of moderate to intense resistance training. *J Strength Cond Res.* 2002;16(4):509–515.

66. Komi PV, Suominen H, Heikkinen E, Karlsson J, Tesch P. Effects of heavy resistance and explosive-type strength training methods on mechanical, functional, and metabolic aspects of performance. In: Komi PV, editor. *Exercise and Sport Biology.* Champaign (IL): Human Kinetics; 1982. p. 90–102.

67. Kosek DJ, Kim JS, Petrella JK, Cross JM, Bamman MM. Efficacy of 3 days/wk resistance training on myofiber hypertrophy and myogenic mechanisms in young vs. older adults. *J Appl Physiol.* 2006;101(2):531–544.

68. **Kraemer WJ, Adams K, Cafarelli E, et al. American College of Sports Medicine position stand. Progression models in resistance training for healthy adults. *Med Sci Sports Exerc.* 2002;34(2):364–380.**

69. Kraemer WJ, Clemson A, Triplett NT, Bush JA, Newton RU, Lynch JM. The effects of plasma cortisol elevation on total and differential leukocyte counts in response to heavy-resistance exercise. *Eur J Appl Physiol Occup Physiol.* 1996;73(1-2):93–97.

70. Kraemer WJ, Fleck SJ, Callister R, et al. Training responses of plasma beta-endorphin, adrenocorticotropin, and cortisol. *Med Sci Sports Exerc.* 1989;21(2):146–153.

71. Kraemer WJ, Fleck SJ, Dziados JE, et al. Changes in hormonal concentrations after different heavy-resistance exercise protocols in women. *J Appl Physiol.* 1993;75(2):594–604.

72. Kraemer WJ, Fleck SJ, Maresh CM, et al. Acute hormonal responses to a single bout of heavy resistance exercise in trained power lifters and untrained men. *Can J Appl Physiol.* 1999;24(6):524–537.

73. Kraemer WJ, Koziris LP. Olympic weightlifting and power lifting. In: Lamb DR, Knuttgen HG, Murray R, editors. *Physiology and Nutrition for Competitive Sport.* Carmel (IN): Cooper Publishing Group; 1994. p. 1–54.

74. Kraemer WJ, Koziris LP, Ratamess NA, et al. Detraining produces minimal changes in physical performance and hormonal variables in recreationally strength-trained men. *J Strength Cond Res.* 2002;16(3):373–382.

75. Kraemer WJ, Nindl BC, Marx JO, et al. Chronic resistance training in women potentiates growth hormone in vivo bioactivity: characterization of molecular mass variants. *Am J Physiol Endocrinol Metab.* 2006;291(6):E1177–1187.

76. Kraemer WJ, Noble BJ, Clark MJ, Culver BW. Physiologic responses to heavy-resistance exercise with very short rest periods. *Int J Sports Med.* 1987;8(4):247–252.

77. Kraemer WJ, Patton JF, Gordon SE, et al. Compatibility of high-intensity strength and endurance training on hormonal and skeletal muscle adaptations. *J Appl Physiol.* 1995;78(3):976–989.

78. Kraemer WJ, Ratamess NA. Physiology of resistance training: current issues. In: Hughes C, editor. *Orthopaedic Physical Therapy Clinics of North America: Exercise Technologies.* Philadelphia: WB Saunders; 2000.

79. Kraemer WJ, Ratamess NA. Endocrine responses and adaptations to strength and power training. In: Komi PV, editor. *Strength and Power in Sport.* Malden (MA): Blackwell Scientific Publications; 2003.

80. Kraemer WJ, Ratamess NA. Fundamentals of resistance training: progression and exercise prescription. *Med Sci Sports Exerc.* 2004;36(4):674–688.

81. Kraemer WJ, Ratamess NA. Hormonal responses and adaptations to resistance exercise and training. *Sports Med.* 2005;35(4):339–361.

82. Kraemer WJ, Ratamess NA, French DN. Resistance training for health and performance. *Curr Sports Med Rep.* 2002;1(3):165–171.

83. Kraemer WJ, Ratamess NA, Volek JS, et al. The effects of amino acid supplementation on hormonal responses to resistance training overreaching. *Metabolism.* 2006;55(3):282–291.

84. Kraemer WJ, Rubin MR, Hakkinen K, et al. Influence of muscle strength and total work on exercise-induced plasma growth hormone isoforms in women. *J Sci Med Sport.* 2003;6(3):295–306.

85. Kraemer WJ, Spiering BA, Volek JS, et al. Androgenic responses to resistance exercise: effects of feeding and L-carnitine. *Med Sci Sports Exerc.* 2006;38(7):1288–1296.

86. Kubo K, Kanehisa H, Fukunaga T. Effects of resistance and stretching training programmes on the viscoelastic properties of human tendon structures in vivo. *J Physiol.* 2002;538(Pt 1):219–226.

87. Kubo K, Komuro T, Ishiguro N, et al. Effects of low-load resistance training with vascular occlusion on the mechanical properties of muscle and tendon. *J Appl Biomech.* 2006;22(2):112–119.

88. Kubo K, Yata H, Kanehisa H, Fukunaga T. Effects of isometric squat training on the tendon stiffness and jump performance. *Eur J Appl Physiol.* 2006;96(3):305–314.

89. MacDougall JD. Adaptability of muscle to strength training: a cellular approach. In: Saltin B, editor. *Biochemistry of Exercise VI.* Champaign (IL): Human Kinetics; 1986. p. 501–513.

90. MacDougall JD, Sale DG, Alway SE, Sutton JR. Muscle fiber number in biceps brachii in bodybuilders and control subjects. *J Appl Physiol.* 1984;57(5):1399–1403.

91. MacDougall JD, Sale DG, Elder G, Sutton JR. Ultrastructural properties of human skeletal muscle following heavy resistance exercise and immobilization. *Med Sci Sports Exerc.* 1976;8(72).

92. MacDougall JD, Sale DG, Moroz JR, Elder GC, Sutton JR, Howald H. Mitochondrial volume density in human skeletal muscle following heavy resistance training. *Med Sci Sports.* 1979;11(2):164–166.

93. MacDougall JD, Ward GR, Sale DG, Sutton JR. Biochemical adaptation of human skeletal muscle to heavy resistance training and immobilization. *J Appl Physiol.* 1977;43(4):700–703.

94. Mackey AL, Esmarck B, Kadi F, et al. Enhanced satellite cell proliferation with resistance training in elderly men and women. *Scand J Med Sci Sports.* 2007;17(1):34–42.

95. MacKinnon L. Exercise and cytokines. In: MacKinnon L. *Advances in Exercise Immunology.* Champaign (IL): Human Kinetics, 1999.

96. Mackinnon LT. Chronic exercise training effects on immune function. *Med Sci Sports Exerc.* 2000;32(7 Suppl):S369–376.

97. Mair J, Mayr M, Muller E, et al. Rapid adaptation to eccentric exercise-induced muscle damage. *Int J Sports Med.* 1995;16(6):352–356.

98. Martel GF, Roth SM, Ivey FM, et al. Age and sex affect human muscle fibre adaptations to heavy-resistance strength training. *Exp Physiol.* 2006;91(2):457–464.

99. Marx JO, Ratamess NA, Nindl BC, et al. Low-volume circuit versus high-volume periodized resistance training in women. *Med Sci Sports Exerc.* 2001;33(4):635–643.

100. Mayhew DL, Thyfault JP, Koch AJ. Rest-interval length affects leukocyte levels during heavy resistance exercise. *J Strength Cond Res.* 2005;19(1):16–22.

101. McCall GE, Byrnes WC, Dickinson A, Pattany PM, Fleck SJ. Muscle fiber hypertrophy, hyperplasia, and capillary density in college men after resistance training. *J Appl Physiol.* 1996;81(5):2004–2012.

102. McCall GE, Byrnes WC, Fleck SJ, Dickinson A, Kraemer WJ. Acute and chronic hormonal responses to resistance training designed to promote muscle hypertrophy. *Can J Appl Physiol.* 1999;24(1):96–107.

103. Menkes A, Mazel S, Redmond RA, et al. Strength training increases regional bone mineral density and bone remodeling in middle-aged and older men. *J Appl Physiol.* 1993;74(5):2478–2484.

104. Mero A, Miikkulainen H, Riski J, Pakkanen R, Aalto J, Takala T. Effects of bovine colostrum supplementation on serum IGF-I, IgG, hormone, and saliva IgA during training. *J Appl Physiol.* 1997;83(4):1144–1151.

105. Miles MP, Kraemer WJ, Grove DS, et al. Effects of resistance training on resting immune parameters in women. *Eur J Appl Physiol.* 2002;87(6):506–508.

106. Miles MP, Kraemer WJ, Nindl BC, et al. Strength, workload, anaerobic intensity and the immune response to resistance exercise in women. *Acta Physiol Scand.* 2003;178(2):155–163.

107. Miszko TA, Cress ME, Slade JM, Covey CJ, Agrawal SK, Doerr CE. Effect of strength and power training on physical function in community-dwelling older adults. *J Gerontol A Biol Sci Med Sci.* 2003;58(2):171–175.

108. Moritani T, deVries HA. Neural factors versus hypertrophy in the time course of muscle strength gain. *Am J Phys Med.* 1979;58(3):115–130.

109. Munn J, Herbert RD, Gandevia SC. Contralateral effects of unilateral resistance training: a meta-analysis. *J Appl Physiol.* 2004;96(5):1861–1866.

110. Nardone A, Romano C, Schieppati M. Selective recruitment of high-threshold human motor units during voluntary isotonic lengthening of active muscles. *J Physiol.* 1989;409:451–471.

111. Newton RU, Hakkinen K, Hakkinen A, McCormick M, Volek J, Kraemer WJ. Mixed-methods resistance training increases power and strength of young and older men. *Med Sci Sports Exerc.* 2002;34(8):1367–1375.

112. Nichols DL, Sanborn CF, Love AM. Resistance training and bone mineral density in adolescent females. *J Pediatr.* 2001;139(4):494–500.

113. Nieman DC, Davis JM, Brown VA, et al. Influence of carbohydrate ingestion on immune changes after 2 h of intensive resistance training. *J Appl Physiol.* 2004;96(4):1292–1298.

114. Nieman DC, Henson DA, Sampson CS, et al. The acute immune response to exhaustive resistance exercise. *Int J Sports Med.* 1995;16(5):322–328.

115. Nindl BC, Hymer WC, Deaver DR, Kraemer WJ. Growth hormone pulsatility profile characteristics following acute heavy resistance exercise. *J Appl Physiol.* 2001;91(1):163–172.

116. Paul GL, DeLany JP, Snook JT, Seifert JG, Kirby TE. Serum and urinary markers of skeletal muscle tissue damage after weight lifting exercise. *Eur J Appl Physiol Occup Physiol.* 1989;58(7):786–790.

117. Peake JM, Nosaka K, Muthalib M, Suzuki K. Systemic inflammatory responses to maximal versus submaximal lengthening contractions of the elbow flexors. *Exerc Immunol Rev.* 2006;12:72–85.

118. Pedersen BK, Hoffman-Goetz L. Exercise and the immune system: regulation, integration, and adaptation. *Physiol Rev.* 2000;80(3):1055–1081.

119. Pette D, Staron RS. Mammalian skeletal muscle fiber type transitions. *Int Rev Cytol.* 1997;170:143–223.

120. Ploutz LL, Tesch PA, Biro RL, Dudley GA. Effect of resistance training on muscle use during exercise. *J Appl Physiol.* 1994;76(4):1675–1681.

121. Ploutz-Snyder LL, Giamis EL, Formikell M, Rosenbaum AE. Resistance training reduces susceptibility to eccentric exercise-induced muscle dysfunction in older women. *J Gerontol A Biol Sci Med Sci.* 2001;56(9):B384–390.

122. Porter MM. Power training for older adults. *Appl Physiol Nutr Metab.* 2006;31(2):87–94.

123. Putman CT, Xu X, Gillies E, MacLean IM, Bell GJ. Effects of strength, endurance and combined training on myosin heavy chain content and fibre-type distribution in humans. *Eur J Appl Physiol.* 2004;92(4-5):376–384.

124. Raastad T, Risoy BA, Benestad HB, Fjeld JG, Hallen J. Temporal relation between leukocyte accumulation in muscles and halted recovery 10-20 h after strength exercise. *J Appl Physiol.* 2003;95(6):2503–2509.

125. Ratamess NA, Faigenbaum AD, Hoffman JR, Kang J. Self-selected resistance training intensity in healthy women: the influence of a personal trainer. *J Strength Cond Res.* 2008;22:103–111.

126. Ratamess NA, Falvo MJ, Mangine GT, Hoffman JR, Faigenbaum AD, Kang J. The effect of rest interval length on metabolic responses to the bench press exercise. *Eur J Appl Physiol.* 2007;100(1):1–17.

127. Ratamess NA, Hoffman JR, Faigenbaum AD, Mangine G, Kang J. The combined effects of protein intake and resistance training on serum osteocalcin concentrations in division III collegiate football players. *J Strength Cond Res.* 2007;21:1197–1203.

128. Ratamess NA, Hoffman JR, Ross R. Effects of an amino acid/creatine/energy supplement on performance and the acute hormonal response to resistance exercise. *Int J Sport Nutr Exerc Metab.* 2007;17:608–623.

129. Ratamess NA, Kraemer WJ, Volek JS, et al. The effects of amino acid supplementation on muscular performance during resistance training overreaching. *J Strength Cond Res.* 2003;17(2):250–258.

130. Ratamess NA, Kraemer WJ, Volek JS, et al. Androgen receptor content following heavy resistance exercise in men. *J Steroid Biochem Mol Biol.* 2005;93(1):35–42.

131. Riechman SE, Balasekaran G, Roth SM, Ferrell RE. Association of interleukin-15 protein and interleukin-15 receptor genetic variation with resistance exercise training responses. *J Appl Physiol.* 2004;97(6):2214–2219.

132. Roth SM, Ferrell RE, Peters DG, Metter EJ, Hurley BF, Rogers MA. Influence of age, sex, and strength training on human muscle gene expression determined by microarray. *Physiol Genomics.* 2002;10(3):181–190.

133. Roth SM, Martel GF, Ferrell RE, Metter EJ, Hurley BF, Rogers MA. Myostatin gene expression is reduced in humans with heavy-resistance strength training: a brief communication. *Exp Biol Med (Maywood).* 2003;228(6):706–709.

134. Rubin MR, Kraemer WJ, Maresh CM, et al. High-affinity growth hormone binding protein and acute heavy resistance exercise. *Med Sci Sports Exerc.* 2005;37(3):395–403.

135. Sale DG. Postactivation potentiation: role in human performance. *Exerc Sport Sci Rev.* 2002;30(3):138–143.

136. Sale DG. Neural adaptations to strength training. In: Komi PV, editor. *Strength and Power in Sport.* Malden (MA): Blackwell Scientific Publications; 2003. p. 281–314.

137. Sale DG, MacDougall JD, Upton AR, McComas AJ. Effect of strength training upon motoneuron excitability in man. *Med Sci Sports Exerc.* 1983;15(1):57–62.

138. Sale DG, Moroz DE, McKelvie RS, MacDougall JD, McCartney N. Effect of training on the blood pressure response to weight lifting. *Can J Appl Physiol*. 1994;19(1):60–74.

139. Schantz P. Capillary supply in hypertrophied human skeletal muscle. *Acta Physiol Scand*. 1982;114(4):635–637.

140. Seynnes OR, de Boer M, Narici MV. Early skeletal muscle hypertrophy and architectural changes in response to high-intensity resistance training. *J Appl Physiol*. 2007;102(1):368–373.

141. Simonson SR, Jackson CG. Leukocytosis occurs in response to resistance exercise in men. *J Strength Cond Res*. 2004;18(2):266–271.

142. Spiering BA, Kraemer WJ, Vingren JL, et al. Responses of criterion variables to different supplemental doses of L-carnitine L-tartrate. *J Strength Cond Res*. 2007;21(1):259–264.

143. Staron RS, Karapondo DL, Kraemer WJ, et al. Skeletal muscle adaptations during early phase of heavy-resistance training in men and women. *J Appl Physiol*. 1994;76(3):1247–1255.

144. Staron RS, Malicky ES, Leonardi MJ, Falkel JE, Hagerman FC, Dudley GA. Muscle hypertrophy and fast fiber type conversions in heavy resistance-trained women. *Eur J Appl Physiol Occup Physiol*. 1990;60(1):71–79.

145. Stone MH, Karatzaferi C. Connective tissue and bone response to strength training. In: Komi PV, editor. *Strength and Power in Sport*. Malden (MA): Blackwell Scientific; 2003 p. 343–360.

146. Tesch PA. Skeletal muscle adaptations consequent to long-term heavy resistance exercise. *Med Sci Sports Exerc*. 1988;20(5 Suppl):S132–134.

147. Tesch PA, Alkner BA. Acute and chronic muscle metabolic adaptations to strength training. In: Komi PV, editor. *Strength and Power in Sport*. Malden (MA): Blackwell Scientific Publications; 2003 p. 265–280.

148. Tesch PA, Karlsson J. Muscle fiber types and size in trained and untrained muscles of elite athletes. *J Appl Physiol*. 1985;59(6):1716–1720.

149. Tesch PA, Komi PV, Hakkinen K. Enzymatic adaptations consequent to long-term strength training. *Int J Sports Med*. 1987;8(Suppl 1):66–69.

150. Tesch PA, Thorsson A, Essen-Gustavsson B. Enzyme activities of FT and ST muscle fibers in heavy-resistance trained athletes. *J Appl Physiol*. 1989;67(1):83–87.

151. Tesch PA, Thorsson A, Kaiser P. Muscle capillary supply and fiber type characteristics in weight and power lifters. *J Appl Physiol*. 1984;56(1):35–38.

152. Tsuzuku S, Ikegami Y, Yabe K. Effects of high-intensity resistance training on bone mineral density in young male powerlifters. *Calcif Tissue Int*. 1998;63(4):283–286.

153. Tsuzuku S, Shimokata H, Ikegami Y, Yabe K, Wasnich RD. Effects of high versus low-intensity resistance training on bone mineral density in young males. *Calcif Tissue Int*. 2001;68(6):342–347.

154. Vincent HK, Vincent KR. The effect of training status on the serum creatine kinase response, soreness and muscle function following resistance exercise. *Int J Sports Med*. 1997;18(6):431–437.

155. Visser M, Pahor M, Taaffe DR, et al. Relationship of interleukin-6 and tumor necrosis factor-alpha with muscle mass and muscle strength in elderly men and women: the Health ABC Study. *J Gerontol A Biol Sci Med Sci*. 2002;57(5):M326–332.

156. Volek JS. Influence of nutrition on responses to resistance training. *Med Sci Sports Exerc*. 2004;36(4):689–696.

157. von Stengel S, Kemmler W, Kalender WA, Engelke K, Lauber D. Differential effects of strength versus power training on bone mineral density in postmenopausal women: a 2-year longitudinal study. *Br J Sports Med*. 2007;41(10):649–655; discussion 655.

158. Williams MA, Haskell WL, Ades PA, et al. Resistance exercise in individuals with and without cardiovascular disease: 2007 update: a scientific statement from the American Heart Association Council on Clinical Cardiology and Council on Nutrition, Physical Activity, and Metabolism. *Circulation*. 2007;116(5): 572–584.

SELECTED REFERENCES FOR FURTHER READING

Baechle TR, Earle RW. *Essentials of Strength Training and Conditioning*. Champaign (IL): Human Kinetics: 2002.

Hoffman J. *Physiological Aspects of Sport Training and Performance*. Champaign (IL): Human Kinetics; 2002.

Kraemer WJ, Adams K, Cafarelli E, et al. American College of Sports Medicine position stand. Progression models in resistance training for healthy adults. *Med Sci Sports Exerc*. 2002;34(2):364–380.

Kraemer WJ, Ratamess NA. Fundamentals of resistance training: progression and exercise prescription. *Med Sci Sport Exerc*. 2004; 36:674–678.

Zatsiorsky VM, Kraemer WJ. *Science and Practice of Strength Training*. 2nd ed. Champaign (IL): Human Kinetics; 2006.

INTERNET RESOURCES

- American College of Sports Medicine: www.acsm.org
- National Strength and Conditioning Association: www.nsca-lift.org

Group Exercise Programming 32

As with any form of exercise, the purpose of group exercise programming is to help people enhance their quality of life. The underlying goal is to improve the health-related components of fitness, which include cardiorespiratory capacity and endurance, muscular strength and endurance, flexibility, and body composition. It has been shown that exercising in a group can enhance overall adherence to exercise (9). Group exercise has increased balance and postural stability in older adults (11), as well as improved functional and psychological well-being of overweight women (20). It is important that group exercise program design revolve around the health-related components of fitness.

Group exercise has grown from traditional high- and low-impact classes (hi/lo) in the late 1970s to include step, indoor cycling, martial arts, sports conditioning, water exercise, dance options like Zumba, use of portable strength and conditioning equipment, Pilates, mind/body classes such as yoga (Fig. 32-1), fusion classes that combine two or more formats, stretching-only classes, and more.

TRENDS IN GROUP EXERCISE

According to Tharrett and Peterson, future programs for group exercise include group classes in a box (body pump, body flow, body sculpt, etc.), fusion fitness (blend styles such as spin/yoga or step/strength), extreme fitness (boot camp, SWAT fitness), and core and functional fitness classes (48). The IDEA 2005 Fitness Trends survey lists core conditioning, indoor cycling, small group classes, dance, and combination (or fusion) classes as growing, although hi/lo and step classes are on the decline (35). The IDEA 2006 Fitness Trends survey reported that class duration length has increased, with more 60-minute classes being offered (36). What happens in surveys from health clubs may not always be what is best for the general public. As obesity continues to increase and fewer people participate in exercise in general, one may question why duration is increasing in health clubs when fewer people are participating in regular exercise (23). It is important that professionals remain in touch with the general public and tailor programming to improve the overall health and wellness of the population at large.

GROUP EXERCISE INSTRUCTOR RESPONSIBILITIES

> **1.7.4-HFS: Knowledge of specific group exercise leadership techniques appropriate for working with participants of all ages.**

Group fitness instructors need to balance being a motivator and an educator to being effective as a leader. The motivational/inspirational aspect of instructing includes having new moves, new music, and state-of-the-art equipment. The educational part of instructing includes having the knowledge of why certain moves are selected

> > > KEY TERMS

Fusion: Group exercise programs that utilize more than one format in the same class, such as step training plus resistance training or yoga plus stability balls.

Group exercise: A class format in which several people participate in a given exercise mode in unison, lead by an instructor; although patterns of movement are uniform among participants, intensity level varies individually.

Hi/lo impact: A group exercise format involving dancelike movements designed to stimulate the cardiorespiratory system (i.e., aerobic dance) and involving relatively high or low amounts of foot impact with the floor.

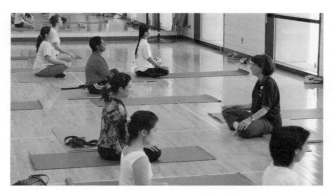

FIGURE 32-1. Group exercise has grown from a purely cardiorespiratory activity to include yoga and relaxation formats also.

and why some are contraindicated, making sure current research and knowledge are incorporated into the group exercise session, and making educated choices and decisions about the information given to participants. Each helps establish a professional and caring attitude. Learning to take responsibility for the health and well-being of participants starts with understanding the importance of establishing a positive attitude and atmosphere.

CREATING A HEALTHY EXERCISE ENVIRONMENT

Creating a comfortable and safe exercise environment involves establishing a healthy emotional outlook. Education and motivation alone may not suffice to keep participants coming back to group exercise. It is necessary to tap into the feelings and emotions of participants to affect adherence. Ornish believes that interpersonal interaction might be the single most important concept that breeds an accepting environment in a group exercise experience (32). One study concerning overweight women's perceptions of an exercise class revealed that the most powerful influences affecting their exercise behavior were concerns about embarrassment and judgment by others (2). Another author found that independent of body image concerns, women participating in rooms with mirrors felt worse after exercising than women in an environment without mirrors (19). Finally, it's noted that enjoyment during physical activity is optimized when a positive and supportive leadership style is coupled with an enriched and supportive group environment (15).

Instructors should realize that what they do and say has a major impact on the class atmosphere. Group exercise instructors affect exercise adherence and may be an important predictor of exercise behavior (5). Having social intelligence in any group setting dictates the success of the group experience. A specific example of social intelligence within a group exercise setting would be for an instructor to be located in the front of the class and talking only to those in the front row. The participants in the middle and back rows may not feel their presence is acknowledged. The instructor who knows everyone's name,

greets them when they come into class, and moves around the class throughout the workout will be creating a healthier emotional/social atmosphere for the participants.

It is important for all group exercise instructors to get out among the participants and observe and assist during the entire workout. Staying in one place gives only one frame of reference to participants. When the instructor is nearby and observing, the participants may improve their attention and their practicing of skills. The instructor as coach applies to all segments of the class format and needs to be evaluated throughout the class. It is important to allow participants to see that the group exercise instructor has empathy.

ROLE MODELING

Group exercise instructors should take care of themselves to be good role models for their students. Leg and foot pain as well as laryngeal discomfort are common overuse problems experienced by group exercise instructors (26). Instructors should model a reasonable level of fitness within the domains of cardiorespiratory, muscular, and body composition. Yet, instructors should also model a healthy body image and not fall prey to unrealistic, and frequently changing, societal views (14).

OVERALL CLASS FORMAT

> **1.7.15-HFS: Knowledge of the components incorporated into an exercise session and the proper sequence (i.e., pre-exercise evaluation, warm-up, aerobic stimulus phase, cool-down, muscular strength and/or endurance, and flexibility).**

> **1.7.21-HFS: Skill to teach and demonstrate the components of an exercise session (i.e., warm-up, aerobic stimulus phase, cool-down, muscular strength/endurance, flexibility).**

Group exercise classes may include segments such as preclass preparation, warm-up, cardiorespiratory training, resistance training, and flexibility/cool-down (24). Preclass preparation insures that all has been made ready for a safe and effective class. The warm-up incorporates movements, performed at a low-to-moderate intensity and range of motion, to increase the temperature and blood flow within the specific muscles to be targeted in the remainder of the class. The cardiorespiratory segment is aimed at improving cardiorespiratory capacity and endurance, as well as body composition, by keeping the heart rate (HR) elevated to a desired target range for 10 to 30 minutes typically, or even longer. Following the cardiorespiratory workout, a gradual cool-down reduces the HR toward resting levels and prevents pooling of blood in the lower extremities. A resistance-training segment, aimed at improving muscular strength and endurance, can be included either before, after, or in place of the

BOX 32-1 CLASS FORMAT SUMMARY

PRECLASS PREPARATION

- Know participants' health histories and survey new participants.
- Be available before class; orient new participants.
- Discuss and model appropriate attire and footwear.
- Have music cued up and equipment ready before class begins.
- Acknowledge class and introduce self.
- Preview class format and participant responsibilities.
- Encourage, participants to bring water to classes and provide breaks to drink.

WARM-UP SEGMENT

- Beginning segment includes an appropriate amount of dynamic movement.
- Focus on rehearsal moves as a large part of the movement selection.
- If stretching is used after the dynamic warm-up, hold briefly (5–10 sec).
- Verbal directions are clear, and volume and tempo of music are appropriate.

CARDIORESPIRATORY SEGMENT

- Promote independence and self-responsibility among participants.
- Gradually increase intensity.
- Provide options for varying impact and/or intensity.
- Build sequences logically and progressively.
- Utilize a variety of muscle groups.
- Use music to create a motivational atmosphere.
- Monitor intensity through heart rate and/or rating of perceived exertion checks.
- Incorporate a postcardio cool-down segment.

RESISTANCE TRAINING SEGMENT

- Muscle balance and functional fitness are encouraged.
- Instructor's form is appropriate, and instructor observes and corrects participants' form.
- Provide verbal, visual, and physical cues on posture and body mechanics.
- Describe adaptations for participants with injuries or special needs.
- Utilize equipment safely and effectively.
- Create a motivational/instructional atmosphere.

FLEXIBILITY SEGMENT

- Stretching of major muscle groups is performed in a safe and effective manner.
- Relaxation/visualization concludes the flexibility segment.

From Kennedy C, Yoke M. *Methods of Group Exercise Instruction*. Champaign (IL): Human Kinetics; 2005.

cardiorespiratory segment. If both are to be performed, the cardiorespiratory segment is usually performed before the resistance training segment, so that the former serves as a thorough warm-up for the latter. The class ends with a flexibility/cool-down component that includes stretching and relaxation exercises designed to further lower HR and enhance overall flexibility. In "fusion" classes, the segments might include, for example, 30 minutes of indoor cycling followed by 30 minutes of strength work (Fig. 32-2). The most important concept is to employ safe and effective programming to improve the health-related components of fitness regardless of the class format.

Individual segments of a group exercise class are described in detail below, and summarized in Box 32-1.

PRECLASS PREPARATION

There are a few common principles in the preclass preparation for any group exercise class, which will be reviewed in this section.

Know the Participants

Chapter 10 provides a review of acquiring health information. The information gathered from these sources needs to be transferred into making a safe and effective

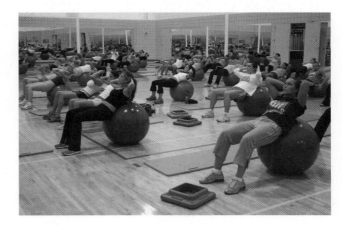

FIGURE 32-2. This group strength class was followed by a 30-minute cardio segment. This combination is an example of a "fusion class."

class. For example, if two participants say they have occasional lower-back pain, incorporating abdominal and low-back strengthening as well as hamstring stretching into the class format on a regular basis would help their conditions. Make sure participants are aware that the time they took to fill out the health information is useful by asking participants' questions and also letting them know about the modifications. Of course, some modifications will need to be explained directly to an individual participant if it is not appropriate to address the issue to the entire class.

Orient New Participants

A professional group exercise instructor takes the time to meet and orient new participants, and also makes him- or herself available if any participants have questions. This is a time when instructors get the most amount of feedback about the class in general. This is part of establishing a positive and comfortable class environment and may also enhance adherence of the participants.

Choose Appropriate Attire

The group exercise instructor's attire should be appropriate for the specific group exercise format. For certain class formats, such as indoor cycling, special attire is needed and should be modeled by the instructor. However, when teaching a senior class, it would not be appropriate to wear a midriff outfit, as it might be intimidating. In many group exercise classes, correct spinal alignment and form should be visible with each movement the instructor demonstrates, requiring the use of form-fitting clothing. The instructor must balance the comfort level of the class with functional wear.

Equipment Preparation

With the large variety of equipment available for group exercise (stability balls, handheld weights, resistance bands, balance devices, yoga blocks, etc.), it is important to be prepared ahead of time and inform participants about what will be used. If participants are expected to obtain individual items (such as from an equipment closet), posting a note ahead of class time would facilitate this. Equipment to be used by the instructor (exercise equipment, but also sound systems, etc.) must be ready before the class start time.

Use of Music

Many group exercise classes utilize music as a way to motivate participants and create more overall enjoyment in the experience. Research has validated the idea that music is beneficial from a motivational standpoint (4,18). In terms of utilizing music to create a beat to follow, research has found that external auditory cues, such as rhythmic music and percussion pulses, favorably affect coordinated walking and proprioceptive control (43).

Moving to the beat of music is not always necessary in a group exercise setting. Some yoga and outdoor group exercise sessions do not even use music. However, although using the beat is important in most kickboxing, step, and hi/lo classes, music is also used in cycling, boot camp, and water exercise as background sound to help motivate or set a mood. It is important to balance music and verbal cueing. If the music is so loud that the verbal cueing is not heard, that can be a problem for the participants. Seniors especially need to be asked about the volume of the music. IDEA published an opinion statement on the volume of music based on standards established by the United States Occupational Safety and Health Administration. IDEA stated that music intensity during group exercise classes should measure no more than 90 decibels (dB) and, because the instructor's voice needs to be about 10 dB louder than the music to be heard, the instructor's voice should measure no more than 100 dB (22). A study on voice problems with group exercise instructors found that 44% of instructors surveyed experienced partial or complete voice loss during and after instructing (28). They also had increased episodes of voice loss, hoarseness, and sore throat unrelated to illness since they began instructing. To protect the voice of instructors, it is important to have a microphone system available.

Always ask participants about their preference for music. Just as many personal trainers make the mistake of giving their own workout to potential clients, group fitness instructors often choose music that is personally motivating. Although it is important that music motivate the instructor, it is imperative that it motivate the participants (Fig. 32-3).

Acknowledge Class Participants

Creating a positive attitude and atmosphere begins with an instructor welcoming people before class begins and introducing himself/herself, especially when teaching in a facility where different people come to class every week and there is no set class roster. If participants are aware of the instructor's name, they will be more likely to come up and ask questions afterward. New people coming to a group exercise class are often afraid of asking questions or may feel out of place. Understanding this and asking for feedback will create a more open, safe environment for all participants, not just the regular participants. Also, approach all new participants individually at the end of each of their first few classes.

Preview Class Format

An overview of what the specific class format will be should accompany the instructor introduction. Make sure to introduce the class format before each class begins. After previewing the class format, it is also important that participants understand their individual responsibilities. Intensity is the responsibility of the participant, not the

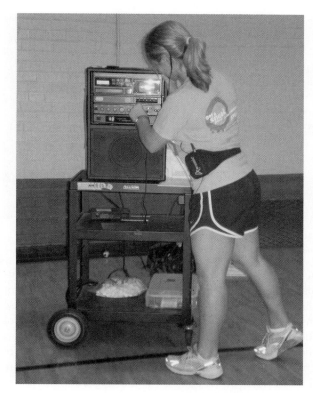

FIGURE 32-3. A group exercise instructor needs sufficient time to prepare the stereo system and microphone during the preclass preparation.

instructor. The instructor provides modifications for various intensities to allow participants to make a choice. Encourage, demonstrate, and promote various exercise choices so participants are comfortable working at their own pace.

WARM-UP

There are a few common principles in the warm-up for any group exercise class, which will be reviewed in this section.

Appropriate Dynamic Movement

The purpose of the warm-up is to prepare the body for the more rigorous demands of the cardiorespiratory and/or resistance training segments by raising the body temperature. The higher temperatures increase the metabolism of the muscles as well as the blood flow and release of oxygen. Because these effects allow more efficient energy production to fuel muscle contraction, the goal of an effective warm-up should be to elevate internal temperatures sufficiently to induce sweating. Appropriate dynamic movement involves the use of large muscle groups exercising at a low to moderate intensity, e.g., marching in place as preparation for a hi/lo aerobic dance class.

Rehearsal Moves

Rehearsal moves are a less intense version of the movement patterns that participants will perform during the

cardiorespiratory portion of class. Rehearsal moves should make up the majority of the warm-up, thus preparing participants mentally and physically for the challenges of the workout ahead. Examples of these would be utilizing the bench to warm up during a step class, teaching participants how to hill climb briefly in an indoor cycling class, or utilizing light weights in the warm-up to prepare for a muscle-conditioning class. The concept of rehearsal moves relates to the principle of specificity of training. This principle states that the body adapts specifically to whatever demands are placed on it. Specificity applies not only to energy systems and muscle groups, but also to movement patterns. In a group exercise session, participants may become frustrated if they are not able to perform the movements effectively. Introducing these movement patterns in the warm-up will assist with learning the proper technique. For example, in a hi/lo class in which a grapevine half-turn movement is used, utilize the warm-up to break down the move, identify the directional landmarks in the room, and name the specific move (Fig. 32-4).

Stretches, If Appropriate

Whether to stretch during the warm-up is a debated issue. A literature review found that insufficient evidence existed to conclude that pre-exercise stretching prevented injuries (47). However, the authors stated that "the evidence is not of sufficient strength, quality, and generalizability to

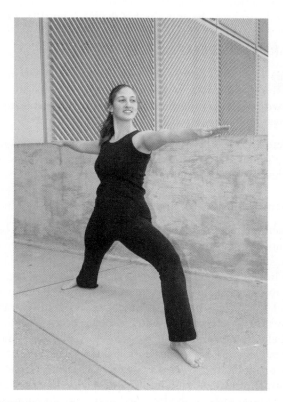

FIGURE 32-4. A rehearsal move for a yoga class might include practicing a new movement called a warrior pose in the warm-up segment in preparation for utilizing it in the class segment.

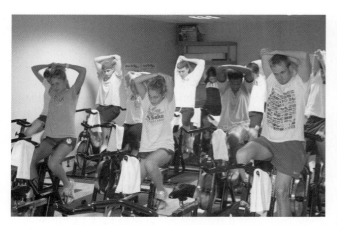

FIGURE 32-5. Enhancing flexibility in an indoor cycling group exercise class.

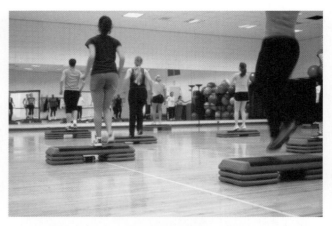

FIGURE 32-6. Participants are using different riser heights to make the intensity specific to their individual fitness levels and goals.

recommend altering or eliminating pre-exercise stretching" (47). Although there is no conclusive evidence showing any inherent benefit to stretching during the warm-up, there are no studies to show that it is dangerous. With this in mind, the warm-up should contain mostly dynamic warm-up activities. If static stretches are included, they should be held only briefly during the warm-up (e.g., 5–10 seconds) to lengthen the muscles in preparation for activity. The decision on how to go about warming up and stretching is an individual one. Flexibility is an important health-related component of fitness and should be included in the workout. However, optimum use of flexibility exercises may be at the end of the workout (Fig. 32-5).

CARDIORESPIRATORY SEGMENT

> **1.7.10-HFS: Knowledge of the recommended intensity, duration, frequency, and type of physical activity necessary for development of cardiorespiratory fitness in an apparently healthy population.**

There are a few common principles in the cardiorespiratory segment of most group exercise classes, which will be reviewed in this section.

Promote Self-Responsibility

Whether teaching yoga, group rowing, Zumba, or a boot camp class, it is impossible to be everywhere or help everyone simultaneously. Each participant is working at a different fitness level and has different goals. If participants try to exercise at the instructor's level or another participant's level, they may work too hard and sustain an injury, or they may not work hard enough to meet their goals. A few ways to help promote independence and self-responsibility are to encourage participants to work at their own pace, utilize HR or rating of perceived exertion (RPE) checks, and inform them how they should feel through common examples. Demonstrate high-, medium- and low-intensity options for individual movements or activities within a class. Group exercise instructors should help participants

achieve the level of effort they need to reach and continually remind them that intensity is their responsibility, not the instructor's. It is recommended that the group exercise instructor personally maintain a medium intensity most of the time, but also present other options and intensities as the need arises. Mastering this concept is the true "art" of group exercise and one reason why group exercise is more difficult than one-on-one instruction (Fig. 32-6).

Impact and/or Intensity Options

In most group exercise classes, movement selection can affect impact and/or intensity. For example, marching in place entails moderate impact, as some of the person's weight strikes the floor while some of the weight is supported by the other foot. Jumping activities are high impact in that the entire body weight leaves and then strikes the floor simultaneously. Impact is not an issue in an indoor cycling class, yet intensity options are still important. For example, a hill climb out of the saddle at a high resistance is considered a higher-intensity option, whereas seated at a lower-resistance (while maintaining a moderate cycling cadence) would be a lower-intensity option. All group exercise sessions have movements that can vary impact and intensity.

Building Sequences

In a hi/lo class, an example of building sequences logically would be teaching a group a grapevine move for the first time by breaking down the movement. Perform two step touches to the right followed by two step touches to the left. Then perform the same step touches, only this time, step behind to make a grapevine move. Progressing properly in a water exercise class would mean marking a specific move by performing it, then increasing the speed of movement, traveling with the move, and then resisting the movement. If sequences are logical and progressive, there is a certain "flow" to the class. Without such continuity, participants may end up standing and watching, feel confused while doing the movement, or execute it improperly.

Methods of Monitoring Cardiorespiratory Intensity

Monitoring exercise intensity within the cardiorespiratory segment is important. Heart rate is a common choice, but has limitations in certain forms of group exercise. During aerobic dance, for example, a given HR value is associated with a lower amount of oxygen consumption than the same HR during treadmill exercise (33). This may be because of the variety of intermittent movements using small amounts of muscle mass during aerobic dance as compared with continuous movement with a large amount of muscle mass (hips and thighs) during treadmill exercise. This HR discrepancy may be true for other similar forms of group exercise, such as kickboxing. During water exercise, HR values are lower than those observed in land exercise, likely because of a shift in blood volume caused by the water pressure (17). Although differences in HR between certain modes of exercise may make it difficult to accurately predict energy expenditure, HR can still be used as a relative indicator of changes in intensity within each mode. Indoor cycling classes utilize a mode of exercise involving an upright posture and continuous use of a large amount of muscle mass. Therefore, HR is an excellent means of monitoring intensity. The power readout in watts available on some cycling machines also provides an excellent means of monitoring intensity and provides nearly instantaneous feedback, whereas HR responds more slowly to changes in effort. When measuring HR, wearing a chest strap monitor greatly improves the accuracy and ease of use. If participants are to measure HR by palpation, they must be taught to do so accurately. RPE and the talk test are subjective means of monitoring exercise intensity. See Chapter 28 for more detail.

Application of Intensity Monitoring to the Group Exercise Setting

Whether using target HR, RPE, or the talk test to monitor exercise intensity, there are a few points of practical application within a group exercise setting:

- If using music, turn off the music during manual measurement of HR so the beats do not influence the counting.
- Palpation of the radial artery is preferred over the carotid pulse; if using the carotid pulse, press lightly to avoid slowing the HR through stimulation of the carotid baroreceptors.
- Check intensity several times during a workout so the intensity can be modified if needed.
- Keep participants moving to prevent blood from pooling in the lower extremities when checking HR.
- Use a brief counting period, such as 10 seconds, to facilitate ease and accuracy of HR measurement.

Postcardio Cool-down

If the cardiorespiratory segment is to be followed by a different segment, such as resistance training, a brief cool-down (e.g., 5 min) should be performed in between. Cooling down prevents blood from pooling in the lower extremities and allows the cardiopulmonary system to transition to less intense workloads. Encourage participants to relax, slow down, keep arms below the level of the heart, and put less effort into the movements. Using less driving music, changing one's tone of voice, and verbalizing the transition to the participants can create this atmosphere. If the cardiorespiratory segment is the last training segment of the workout, then a longer cool-down (5–10 min) should be performed, along with stretching. See below for more information in the section describing the flexibility segment of the group exercise class.

RESISTANCE-TRAINING SEGMENT

> **1.7.11-HFS: Knowledge of and the ability to describe exercises designed to enhance muscular strength and/or endurance of specific major muscle groups.**

A variety of group exercise formats involve resistance training for the development of muscular strength and endurance. Resistance can be provided by body weight, resistance bands and tubing, and handheld weights. Detailed information regarding the prescription of resistance training is provided in Chapter 29.

Progression in Programming

> **1.7.12-HFS: Knowledge of the principles of overload, specificity, and progression and how they relate to exercise programming.**

A method of exercise selection and progression has been described by Yoke and Kennedy that is tailored to the group exercise setting (54). This design progresses from simple to complex exercises in six steps, as described in Box 32-2 and illustrated in Figures 32-7 through 32-12.

Utilize Equipment Safely and Effectively

> **1.7.29-HFS: Ability to identify proper and improper technique in the use of resistive equipment, such as stability balls, weights, bands, resistance bars, and water exercise equipment.**

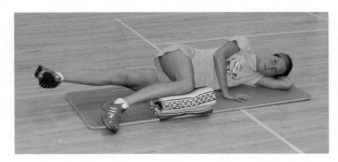

FIGURE 32-7. Level 1 adductor exercise that focuses on isolation and education in a side-lying position.

BOX 32-2 — SIX-STEP EXERCISE PROGRESSION MODEL FOR RESISTANCE TRAINING SEGMENT OF GROUP EXERCISE CLASSES

Level #1: Isolate and educate.

The participant is learning how to focus on the muscle and movement. Exercises in this level are often performed in the supine or prone position.

Level #2: Isolate and educate and add resistance.

Resistance is added to the exercise in Level #1.

Level #3: Add functional training position.

To better challenge the stabilizing muscles, an exercise in a seated or standing position (for the targeted muscles) is performed.

Level #4: Combine increasing function with resistance.

Some type of overload (e.g., weights, tubing, bands) is added to challenge the body's stabilizers in the functional position.

Level #5: Challenge multimuscle groups with increasing resistance and core challenge.

More complex exercises (e.g., squats and lunge variations) are added that combine muscular fitness, balance, coordination, and stability.

Level #6: Add balance, increased functional challenge, speed, or rotational movements.

The use of stability balls, Bosu balls (half stability balls), wobble boards, or spinal rotation to exercise movements is added. Some individuals may never reach this level because of their current fitness level, health history, or past or current musculoskeletal injury.

From Woodby-Brown S, Berg K, Latin RW. Oxygen cost of aerobic dance bench stepping at three heights. *J Strength Cond Res.* 1993;7:163–167.
From Yoke M, Kennedy C. Functional exercise progressions. Monterey (CA): Healthy Learning Publisher; 2004.

Portable resistance-training equipment, such as exercise bands, stability balls, handheld weights, and weighted bars are often utilized in a group exercise class. Research has shown that stability ball training (Fig. 32-13) helps improve spinal stability (10). One study concluded that the unstable nature of the ball elicits a greater neuromuscular response when compared with training on a stable surface (3).

It is important to separate resistance training from cardiorespiratory training. A study evaluated the effects of step-class training with and without the use of light handheld weights (27). Both groups improved aerobic fitness and strength, but the group using weights did not experience any greater improvement in aerobic fitness or strength compared with the group that did not use weights. Therefore, if the goal is to improve aerobic fitness, greater progression of aerobic activity within the cardiorespiratory segment of a class is needed. And similarly, if the goal is to improve strength or muscular endurance, greater progression within the resistance training segment is needed. Attempting to accomplish both goals simultaneously is not an effective technique.

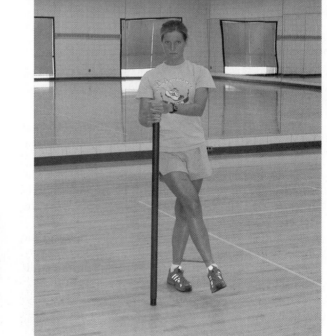

FIGURE 32-9. Level 3 adductor exercise that is performed in a standing position utilizing a body bar for stabilization and adding resistance to the hip adduction movement.

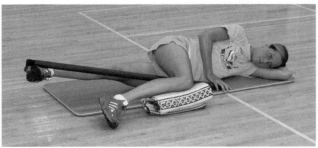

FIGURE 32-8. Level 2 adductor exercise that adds resistance to the Level 1 position using a weighted body bar.

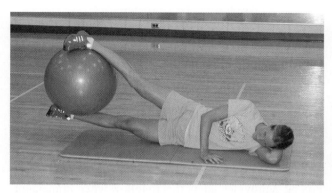

FIGURE 32-10. Level 4 adductor exercise that involves utilization of the stabilizer muscles to perform hip adduction.

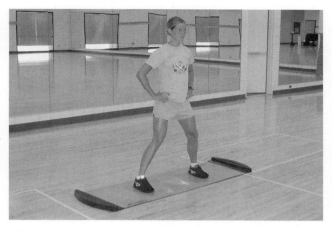

FIGURE 32-12. Level 6 adductor exercise using a slide board to destabilize the legs for increased functional challenge.

FLEXIBILITY SEGMENT

There are a few common principles in the flexibility segment of most group exercise classes. They will be reviewed in this section.

Stretching

It is important to stretch the muscle groups that have been used in the group exercise activity as well as muscles that are commonly tight. For instance, after an indoor cycling class, stretching the quadriceps, calves, and hamstrings is appropriate because they are major muscles used for cycling. In a kickboxing session, it is important to stretch the muscles that surround the hip. However, other muscle groups should not be ignored, as a balanced approach incorporates stretching all the major muscle groups (Fig 32-14). Chapter 29 provides detailed information regarding exercise prescription for flexibility.

Relaxation and Visualization

A popular activity to complete a group exercise class is meditation. This may be structured or free flowing. Guided imagery or creative visualization might help deepen the relaxation as, for example, the instructor describes quiet forests, gentle breezes, or a warm fire. Tightening and releasing muscle groups in a progression through the body is another meditative technique. One of the simplest techniques is for the participants to focus on their breathing. Complete silence, or the use of quiet music, may be used to set the appropriate mood for this aspect of the class session.

POPULAR GROUP EXERCISE PROGRAMS

> **1.7.19-HFS: Knowledge of the exercise programs that are available in the community and how these programs are appropriate for various populations.**

A diverse number of group exercise programs have emerged in an effort to meet the needs and interests of regular exercisers and to attract new fitness participants. Some of the popular group programs briefly highlighted in this section include hi/lo or mixed impact, step

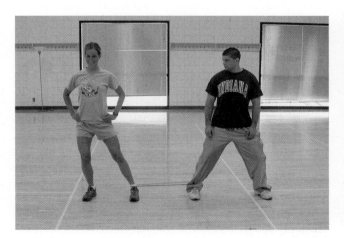

FIGURE 32-11. Level 5 adductor exercise where balance and stability are challenged by using a partner to perform hip adduction.

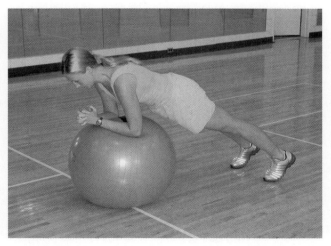

FIGURE 32-13. Stability balls can be used to enhance trunk stabilizer muscles.

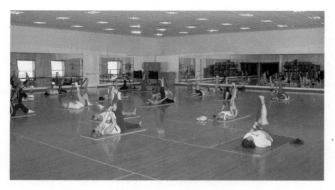

FIGURE 32-14. Flexibility can be enhanced in a group exercise setting using stretching bands.

training, martial arts exercise, water fitness, indoor cycling, yoga, stability ball workouts, and Pilates.

HI/LO OR MIXED-IMPACT GROUP EXERCISE CLASSES

Mixed-impact (or hi/lo) classes combine high-impact cardiorespiratory movements that are associated with greater stresses on the lower extremities (e.g., running, jumping, and hopping) with low-impact movements that provide minimal stress on the lower extremities (e.g., step touches and side lunges). Combinations and routines are choreographed to music and incorporate a variety of arm movements, leg movements, traveling patterns, and directional turns. An advantage of mixed-impact classes is the ability to modify the intensity of the exercise. A review of literature reveals a large difference in energy cost between low-impact ($4–5$ kcal·min^{-1}) and high-impact ($10–11$ kcal·min^{-1}) movement styles (52). Typically, the most common ways to modify any grouped exercise are to alter the speed of movement, modify the range of motion of the movement, vary the amount of traveling completed with a movement, and change the vertical component of the movement. A few considerations specific to mixed-impact classes are to not hop repeatedly on one foot (e.g., more than four times in a row) to avoid excessive impact-related stress, avoid twisting hop variations that may lead to spinal stress, and use a music tempo of 135 to 160 beats per minute.

STEP TRAINING

Step training has become a mainstay cardiorespiratory class format because of its widespread popularity and ease of administration to the multiple ability levels that are commonly seen in exercise classes (Fig.32-15). Step training has been described as a safe, low-impact exercise that may potentially provide high-intensity cardiorespiratory conditioning (37). The workouts can be as challenging as a rigorous jogging workout and yet produce impact forces as safe as walking. However, use of fast stepping cadences result in greater vertical ground reaction forces

on the body in less-experienced step enthusiasts (39). The cadence of step classes generally ranges from 118 to 128 bpm (38,42). Research demonstrates that changing bench height is the most consequential variable to alter step exercise intensity (16,34,37,50,53). The most widely used step platforms have adjustable heights from 4 to 12 inches (10–30 cm), with a stepping surface 14 inches wide by 42 inches long (36×107 cm). Instructors should instruct participants to use increasing step heights to accomplish progression of intensity. The typical riser increase allows for a 2-inch (5-cm) change in step height. Box 32-3 provides safety tips to follow when implementing a step-training program.

MARTIAL ARTS EXERCISE

Kickboxing and cardioboxing are two of the many martial arts exercise class formats that have become a staple component of the group fitness industry. Movements include kicks, punches, elbow strikes, jabs, knee strikes, and combinations thereof as used in boxing and martial arts. The athletic drills in these classes are mixed with recovery bouts of basic aerobic movements such as boxer-style rope skipping (with or without a rope), walking, and light jogging in place. Some kickboxing exercise classes involve boxing gloves, punching bags, and martial arts equipment, although other programs incorporate "shadow boxing," which involves no equipment (Fig. 32-16). The majority of these classes are driven by moderately paced music (approximately 120 to 135 bpm), although the music may be used only for motivation rather than to control the choreography.

A key concern with martial arts exercise classes is the preparation of instructors to properly teach the programs (51). Instructors need to have proper knowledge of correct punching techniques, as well as the progressive teaching skills to minimize joint-related injuries among class participants. Box 32-4 provides some safety guidelines to consider with martial arts exercise classes.

WATER FITNESS CLASSES

Water fitness classes are steadily growing in popularity (Fig. 32-17). However, there is a general lack of awareness about the benefits and special techniques associated with water fitness classes. Water exercise training programs have been shown to reduce percent body fat in overweight women (30), improve activities of daily living on land (46), and provide a variety of fitness and health-related benefits (7,12,45). A practical consideration is to progressively increase intensity by increasing speed of movement and by using equipment overload (surface area or buoyancy-resisted devices) to increase resistance to movement of the limbs through the water (29).

BOX 32-3   SAFETY CONSIDERATIONS FOR STEP-TRAINING CLASSES

- Step entirely on the top part of the platform with each step, not allowing any part of the foot to hang over an edge.
- Discourage flexing the knees more than 90 degrees; vary step height as needed. Avoid flexing the knees more than 60 degrees for participants predisposed to patellofemoral pain.
- Adding handheld weights to step training is not recommended because of a lack of additional gains in fitness (27).
- To lower the exercise intensity quickly, stop stepping and switch to marching in place on the ground.
- Use cross-training shoes or indoor fitness shoes for step workouts. Most running shoes doe not provide suitable support for step movements.

- Avoid step combinations that travel forward and down off the bench, which increase eccentric stress.
- Maintain an upright posture and bend at the knees for ascending and descending movements. Too much hip flexion while stepping may place unwanted stresses on the spine.
- Frequently change the leading foot when doing the step patterns to avoid overstressing one leg (e.g., at least once per minute).
- Avoid excessive repetition of movement patterns on one leg to avoid orthopedic stress.
- Include movement choices for a variety of muscle groups to include those that may not receive much use in activities of daily living (e.g., hamstrings, adductors, abductors).

Smith J. Injury prevention in step classes. *IDEA Health & Fitness Source.* 2000;18:36–45.

INDOOR CYCLING

Indoor group cycling classes are a unique group-led exercise format that has attracted many devoted supporters. Because of its non–weight-bearing nature, indoor cycling classes also offer some orthopedic advantages to special populations not able to perform traditional weight-bearing exercise. Also, for seasoned cyclists, indoor cycling offers a viable option to the hazards of wintertime weather cycling.

Instructors lead exercise enthusiasts through a "virtual" outdoor road ride, complete with valleys, hills, straightaways, and finish lines (6). Music for indoor cycling classes is selected for motivation and geared toward enhancing the mood during various portions of the class.

No beats-per-minute guidelines have been established with indoor cycling classes; however, faster and slower tempos are used in support of changes in exercise intensity (41). The success of an indoor cycling class depends heavily on the exercise program design knowledge of the instructor as well as the instructor's ability to motivate the fitness enthusiasts (25). Box 32-5 provides safety guidelines for indoor cycling.

YOGA

With origins in India, yoga has existed for at least 5,000 years. **Yoga** means *union*, and it refers to one of the symbolic systems of Hindu philosophy that strive to bring together and develop the body, mind, and spirit. Hatha yoga

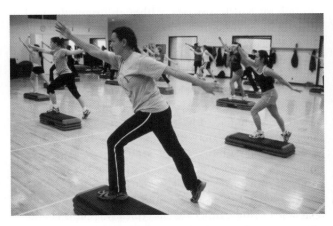

FIGURE 32-15. A group exercise step class.

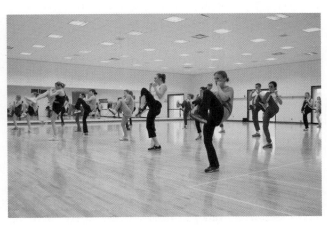

FIGURE 32-16. A group exercise kickboxing class.

BOX 32-4   SAFETY CONSIDERATIONS FOR KICKBOXING CLASSES

- Perform a satisfactory warm-up to properly prepare the muscles and joints for the ensuing challenge of the workout.
- With all upper-body strikes and jabs, make sure the elbow is not taken past its normal range of motion (ROM).
- To protect the supporting leg, execute no more than 10 kicks consecutively.
- Do not kick beyond the normal ROM. Control for any "snapping" movements during leg extension.
- Kicking and pivoting together may be contraindicated for many learners. Beginners should master the basic moves before progressing to advanced kickboxing movements.
- Use a music tempo of 120 to 135 bpm to discourage movements being performed incorrectly and hastily.
- Be aware that the novelty of martial arts movements may lead to delayed-onset muscle soreness in those just starting classes.
- To protect ligaments, turn out the toes slightly and flex the knee of the supporting leg when kicking.
- Deliver punches from the body as opposed to from the shoulders.

From Williams A. Injury prevention in kickboxing classes. *IDEA Health & Fitness Source*. 2000;18:58–67.

---

is the form with which Westerners are most familiar and is defined by a series of physical postures (*asanas*) and breathing patterns. There are several different forms of Hatha yoga that are popularly practiced. Some of the most popular forms of yoga are briefly described here. Iyengar yoga incorporates traditional Hatha techniques into fluid, dancelike sequences. It uses props such as chairs, pillows, blankets, and belts to accommodate persons with special needs (8). Ashtanga yoga is a fast-paced, athletic style that is the foundation for power-yoga classes (8,21). These classes are more vigorous workouts than other forms of yoga. Hot yoga, popularized as Bikram yoga, is done in a sauna-style room that is heated to approximately 100°F (38°C), so the muscles are warm for stretching (21). Kripalu yoga focuses on personal growth and self-improvement through the practice of meditation during poses (8,21). Kundalini yoga merges stretching, breathing, and meditation.

Some considerations for teaching yoga classes include the following (8,21):

- Consider the ability of the participants in a given class when selecting postures, as some postures require significant levels of strength or flexibility.
- Provide modifications of postures for participants who have muscle or joint problems, or whose strength and flexibility are below the class average.
- Avoid poses that place significant stress on the low back or the neck (e.g., the plow) unless working with advanced students.
- Participants with high blood pressure or glaucoma should not perform postures in which the head is positioned below the level of the heart, such as head stands.
- Always teach proper body alignment specific to each posture.

STABILITY BALL WORKOUTS

Originating in Europe, stability ball training is spreading throughout North America. Although originally used in rehabilitation, stability ball training is now used in group exercise classes. The unstable nature of the ball disturbs the position of one's body if the center of mass is not well controlled. Thus, the body's neuromuscular balance-regulating mechanisms are challenged when performing stability ball exercises, as opposed to performing the same movements on a solid base of support, such as a bench. Balls come in a variety of sizes. Proper ball size is observed when the individual is seated on the apex of the ball with the feet flat on the floor, and the hips and knees are bent at 90 degrees. Balls also come in a variety of shapes, such as "peanuts" and half balls, instead of spheres, and these other shapes typically are less challenging to one's balance, and more appropriate for beginners.

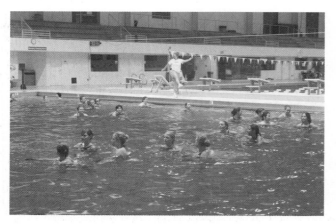

FIGURE 32-17. A group water exercise class.

BOX 32-5 SAFETY CONSIDERATIONS FOR INDOOR CYCLING CLASSES

- Seat height should be adjusted so that the knee is flexed 25-30 degrees as the pedal travels through the bottom of the stroke. (If the participant stops at the bottom of the stroke and lowers his or her heel so that the foot is parallel to the floor, knee flexion should be 5-10 degrees.)
- The front-to-back seat position should be set so that the front of the knee is directly above the center of the pedal halfway through the downstroke.
- Handlebar height is based on the comfort of the participant. Low handlebars that create a flat back position should only be used by those who are accustomed to such a posture, such as competitive road cyclists.
- Review the operation of the emergency brake with participants; suddenly stopping the pedaling action without using the brake can cause injury.
- Have participants wear correct cycling apparel. Cycling shorts with padded inserts help to lesson the discomfort of prolonged cycling. Hard-soled

cycling shoes are preferred to minimize the pressure on the feet when pedaling. Many cycling shoes have a cleat that can snap into the pedal, improving cycling mechanics and power transfer from the body.
- Because of the multiple fitness levels in a class, provide resistance or cadence options during the various class segments. In general, maintaining a relatively high cadence (such as 80-100 rpm) with a low resistance produces less stress on the knees than does a low cadence/high resistance combination.
- Encourage participants to bring water bottles to stay hydrated.
- Vary the riding position during the class to minimize lower back discomfort.
- To minimize wrist and upper body tension, instruct participants to not to place too much weight on the handlebars while in a standing position.

Information from Bryant CX, Wenson J, Peterson JA. Safe and enjoyable group cycling for your members. *Fitness Management* 2001;17:38–42. Kolovou T. Launching an indoor cycling program. *Fitness Management* 2000;16:40–42. Sherman RM. The indoor cycling revolution. *IDEA Today.* 1997;15:30–39. Vogel AE. Injury prevention in indoor cycling classes. *IDEA Health & Fitness Source.* 2000;18:48–57.

Many stability ball exercises are designed to work muscles of the trunk, but upper-body and lower-body exercises are performed as well.

Some considerations for teaching stability ball classes include the following (13,40):

- Initially, have the participants sit on the ball and become aware of their center of gravity on this unstable base of support. Progress with exercises once participants have mastered the sitting position.
- Less-skilled participants should place the ball close to a wall, with their back toward the wall or, preferably, be spotted.
- Individuals with advanced osteoporosis or with vestibular dysfunction (i.e., vertigo) should not use stability balls.
- Smooth floor surfaces (e.g., wood as opposed to carpet) are more difficult because of the reduced friction and should not be used with less-skilled participants (such as older adults).
- Bouncing one's body on the ball as a cardiorespiratory exercise is not recommended, as this action compromises balance.

PILATES

The historic roots of Pilates are from World War I, when Joseph Pilates (1880–1967) invented rehabilitation equipment and created a series of strength and flexibility exercises

for prisoners of war. Pilates eventually opened a training studio in New York, helping professional dancers with their conditioning. He wrote two books describing his training methods, *Return to Life through Contrology* and *Your Health*. Pilates-based programs today are popular in the United States. Pilates uses many different types of equipment, such as the reformer, trapeze table, and combo chair, as well as exercises on a mat. The common theme in Pilates programs is training of the deep abdominal and lower back muscles to improve postural control. It is not considered a cardiorespiratory form of exercise (1). A great variety of Pilates instructor certification courses are available (44), but there are no official standards, as use of the name *Pilates* is unrestricted.

SUMMARY

Group exercise is challenging because of the great variety of physical activities employed and the wide range of fitness and skill among participants. Effective group exercise instructors understand that modifications, variations, and individualized intensity monitoring are essential to ensure safe and enjoyable participation by all. Many group exercise classes involve some form of cardiovascular conditioning, along with strengthening exercises, flexibility activities, and proper warm-up and cool-down activities. For specialized group-led classes, it is recommended that instructors obtain additional training specific to the instructional method (Fig. 32-18).

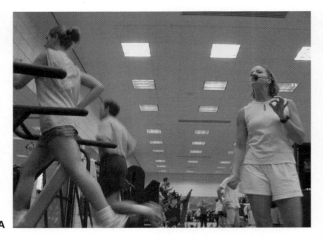 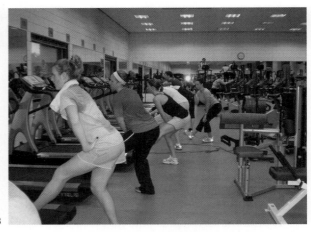

FIGURE 32-18. A and **B:** An instructor of this "trekking" group exercise class needs training in both group leadership and treadmill skills.

REFERENCES

1. American Council on Exercise. Can Pilates Do It All? *ACE Fitness Matters*. 2005;Nov/Dec:10–11.
2. Bain LL, Wilson T, Chaikind E. Participant perceptions of exercise programs for overweight women. *Res Q*. 1989;60(2):134–143.
3. Behm D, Anderson K. The role of instability with resistance training. *J Strength Cond Res*. 2006;20(3):716–722.
4. Boutche S, Trenske M. The effects of sensory deprivation and music on perceived exertion and affect during exercise. *J Sport Exerc Psychol*. 1990;12:167–176.
5. Bray S, Gyurcsik N, Culos-Reed S, Dawson K, Martin K. An exploratory investigation of the relationship between proxy efficacy, self-efficacy and exercise attendance. *J Health Psych*. 2001;6(4):425–434.
6. Bryant CX, Wenson J, Peterson JA. Safe and enjoyable group cycling for your members. *Fitness Management*. 2001;17:38–42.
7. Bushman B, Flynn M, Andres F, Lambert C, Taylor M, Braunl W. Effect of 2 weeks of deep water run training on running performance. *Med Sci Sports Exerc*. 1997;29(5):695–699.
8. Carrico M. Contraindications of yoga. *IDEA Health & Fitness Source*. 1998;16:34–43.
9. Carron A, Hausenblas H, Mack D. Social influence and exercise: a meta-analysis. *J Sport Exerc Psychol*. 1996;18:1–16.
10. Carter J, Beam WC, McMahan SG, Barr ML, Brown LE. The effects of stability ball training on spinal stability in sedentary individuals. *J Strength Cond Res*. 2006;20(2):429–435.
11. Clary S, Barnes C, Bemben D, Knehans A, Bemben M. Effects of ballates, step aerobics, and walking on balance in women aged 50–75 years. *J Sports Sci Med*. 2006;5:390–399.
12. Davidson K, McNaughton L. Deep water running training and road running training improve $\dot{V}O_{2max}$ in untrained women. *J Strength Cond*. 2000;14(2):191–195.
13. Eckmann TF. Older adults get on the ball. *IDEA Health & Fitness Source*. 1998;16:81–85.
14. Evans E, Kennedy C. The body image problem in the fitness industry. *IDEA Today*. 1993;May:50–56.
15. Fox L, Rejeski J, Gauvin L. Effects of leadership style and group dynamics on enjoyment of physical activity. *Am J Health Promot*. 2000;15(5):277–283.
16. Francis PR, Poliner J, Buono MJ, Francis LL. Effects of choreography, step height, fatigue and gender on metabolic cost of step training. *Med Sci Sports Exerc*. 1992;27:S69.
17. Frangolias D, Rhodes E. Maximal and ventilatory threshold responses to treadmill and water immersion running. *Med Sci Sports Exerc*. 1995;27(7):1007–1013.
18. Gfeller K. Musical components and styles preferred by young adults for aerobic fitness activities. *J Music Ther*. 1988;25:28–43.
19. Ginis M, Jung M, Gauvin L. To see or not to see: effects of exercising in mirrored environments on sedentary women's feeling states and self-efficacy. *Health Psychol*. 2003;22(4):354–361.
20. Grant SK, Todd T, Atchison P, Kelly P, Stoddart D. The effects of a 12 week group exercise program on physiological and psychological variables and function in overweight women. *Public Health*. 2004;118(1):31–34.
21. Hollingshead S. Yoga for sports performance. *IDEA Health & Fitness Source*. 2002;20:30–39.
22. IDEA. Recommendations for music volume in fitness classes. *IDEA Today*. 1997;June:50.
23. Jakicic J, Otto A. Physical activity considerations for the treatment and prevention of obesity. *Am J Clin Nutr*. 2005;82(1):2265–2295.
24. Kennedy C, Yoke M. *Methods of Group Exercise Instruction*. Champaign (IL): Human Kinetics; 2005.
25. Kolovou T. Launching an indoor cycling program. *Fitness Management*. 2000;16:40–42.
26. Komura Y, Inabab R, Fugita S, et al. Health conditions of female aerobic dance instructors: subjective symptoms and related factors. *Sangyo Igaku*. 1992;34(4):326–334.
27. Kravitz L, Heyward V, Stolarczyk L, Wilmerding V. Does step exercise with handweights enhance training effects? *J Strength Con. Res*. 1997;11(3):194–199.
28. Long J, Williford M, Olson M, Wolfe V. Voice problems and risk factors among aerobic instructors. *J Voice*. 1998;12(2):197–207.
29. Mayo J. Practical guidelines for the use of deep water running. *Strength Cond J*. 2000;22(1):26–29.
30. Nagle E, Robertson R, Jakicic J, et al. Effects of aquatic exercise and walking in sedentary obese women undergoing a behavioral weight-loss intervention. *Journal of Aquatic Research and Education*. 2007;1:43–56.
31. Olson MS, Williford HH. Martial arts exercise: A T.K.O. in studio fitness. *ACSM's Health & Fitness Journal*. 1999;3:6–13.
32. Ornish D. *Love and Survival*. New York: Harper Collins; 1998.
33. Parker S, Hurley B, Hanlon D, Vaccaro P. Failure of target heart rate to accurately monitor intensity during aerobic dance. *Med Sci Sports Exerc*. 1989;21(2):230–234.
34. Riker HA, Zabik RM, Dawson ML, Frye PA. The effect of step height and upper body involvement on oxygen consumption and energy expenditure during step aerobics. *Med Sci Sports Exerc*. 1998;30: S945.
35. Ryan P. Fitness trendlines. *October IDEA Fitness Manager*. 2005; 17(5):12.
36. Ryan P. Group exercise class participation. *October IDEA Fitness Manager*. 2006;5:14–15.

37. Scharff-Olson M, Williford HN, Blessing DL, Brown JA. The physiological effects of bench/step exercise. *Sports Med.* 1996;21:164–175.

38. Scharff-Olson M, Williford HN, Blessing DL, Greathouse R. The cardiovascular and metabolic effects of bench stepping exercise in females. *Med Sci Sports Exerc.* 1991;23:1311–1318.

39. Scharff-Olson M, Williford HN, Blessing DL, et al. Vertical impact forces during bench-step aerobics: exercise rate and experience. *Percept Mot Skills.* 1997;84:267–274.

40. Schlicht J. Stability balls: an injury risk for older adults. *ACSM's Health and Fitness Journal.* 2002;6:14–17.

41. Sherman RM. The indoor cycling revolution. *IDEA Today.* 1997;15:30–39.

42. Smith J. Injury prevention in step classes. *IDEA Health & Fitness Source.* 2000;18:36–45.

43. Staum M. Music and rhythmic stimuli in the rehabilitation of gait disorders. *J Music Ther.* 1983;20:69–87.

44. Stott M. How to start a Pilates-based program. *Fitness Management.* 2000;16:44–48.

45. Takeshima N, Rogers M, Watanebe E, et al. Water-based exercise improves health-related aspects of fitness in older women. *Med Sci Sports Exerc.* 2002;33(3):544–551.

46. Templeton MS, Booth DL, O'Kelly WD. Effects of aquatic therapy on joint flexibility and functional ability in subjects with rheumatic disease. *J Orthopedic Sports Ther.* 1997;23:376–381.

47. Thacker SB, Gilchrist J, Stroup DF, Kimsey Jr. CD. The impact of stretching on sports injury risk: a systematic review of the literature. *Med Sci Sports Exerc.* 2004;36(3):371–378.

48. Tharrett S, Peterson J. The health/fitness club industry: challenge and change. In: *Fitness Management.* Monterey (CA): Healthy Learning Publishers; 2006. p. 34.

49. Vogel AE. Injury prevention in indoor cycling classes. *IDEA Health & Fitness Source.* 2000;18:48–57.

50. Wang N, Scharff-Olson M, Williford HN. Energy cost and fuel utilization during step aerobics exercise. *Med Sci Sports Exerc.* 1993;25:S630.

51. Williams A. Injury prevention in kickboxing classes. *IDEA Health & Fitness Source.* 2000;18:58–67.

52. Williford HN, Scharff-Olson M, Blessing DL. The physiological effects of aerobic dance: a review. *Sports Med.* 1989;8:335–345.

53. Woodby-Brown S, Berg K, Latin RW. Oxygen cost of aerobic dance bench stepping at three heights. *J Strength Cond Res.* 1993;7:163–167.

54. Yoke M, Kennedy C. *Functional Exercise Progressions.* Monterey (CA): Healthy Learning Publisher; 2004.

SELECTED REFERENCES FOR FURTHER READING

Kennedy C, Yoke M. *Methods of Group Exercise Instruction.* Champaign (IL): Human Kinetics; 2005.

Yoke M, Kennedy C. *Functional Exercise Progressions.* Monterey (CA): Healthy Learning Publisher, 2004.

INTERNET RESOURCES

- Aerobics and Fitness Association of America: www.afaa.com
- American College of Sports Medicine: www.acsm.org
- American Council on Exercise: www.acefitness.org
- IDEA Health and Fitness Association: www.ideafit.com

1.8.4-CES: Describe the hypotheses related to diet, weight gain, and weight loss.

Obesity (body mass index [BMI] ≥30 kg·m^{-2}) and overweight (BMI = 25 to 29.9 kg·m^{-2}) are serious health issues in the United States. In 2004, 32% of U.S. adults were considered obese (44). The Centers for Disease Control and Prevention (CDC) report that individuals who are obese compose about 30% of the U.S. population, whereas obese and overweight combined are nearly 70% of the population (Fig. 33-1) (12). Obesity, which is considered a multifactorial condition, is related to many chronic diseases, such as coronary heart disease, hypertension, stroke, type 2 diabetes mellitus, dyslipidemia, gallbladder disease, and some cancers (1,42,55). Prevention of weight gain would likely decrease chronic disease, improve quality of life, and decrease healthcare costs in the United States.

As individuals age, they may lose their ability to regulate energy intake based on physiologic cues, leading to overeating and weight gain (6). These cues can be further ignored in an environment that promotes overeating by offering large portion sizes in restaurants (20) and in the home. In addition, many of the foods readily available are high-fat foods (20,26), which are high in energy density (26,64) but low in nutrient density. This inability to regulate energy intake, coupled with a sedentary lifestyle, are two major reasons why obesity has become increasingly more prevalent in the United States. Thus, it is imperative that both eating healthily and increased physical activity are promoted and encouraged. The primary goal of this chapter is to discuss the impact nutrition, exercise, behavioral interventions, and bariatric surgery have on weight management.

> > > KEY TERMS

1.8.2-HFI: Knowledge of the following terms: obesity, overweight, percent fat, BMI, lean body mass, anorexia nervosa, bulimia, metabolic syndrome, and body fat distribution.

Adipocyte: Fat cell.

Anorexia nervosa: A severe form of eating disorder, whereby the individual consumes little to no food energy each day and typically exercises excessively; this may or may not be coupled with use of other methods for decreasing intake (e.g., vomiting, diuretic use, laxative use); the individual is typically severely underweight.

Bariatrics: A branch of medicine that addresses the causes, prevention, and treatment of obesity.

Body fat distribution: An assessment of how body fat is distributed; android obesity ("apple shape"), in which more fat is stored in the abdominal area, is more strongly related to an increased risk of cardiovascular disease and type 2 diabetes mellitus than gynoid obesity ("pear shape"), in which more fat is stored in the hip area. A separate consideration of body-fat distribution is visceral (fat surrounding the internal organs) versus subcutaneous (fat directly beneath the skin); as with android obesity, visceral fat carries greater risk than subcutaneous fat.

Body mass index (BMI): A measure of a person's stockiness (body mass in kilograms divided by height in meters squared, kg·m^{-2}) used to assess if a person is underweight, of healthy weight, overweight, or obese.

Bulimia nervosa: A severe form of eating disorder, whereby the individual consumes normal or, more typically, much higher than needed amounts of food energy each day, followed by purging (e.g., vomiting, diuretic use, laxative use, overexercising); the individual is often of normal body weight.

Ergogenic aid: A substance that may (or claims to) improve performance, or may (or claims to) improve body weight or body composition.

Fat-free mass (FFM): Body mass minus the mass of all body fat, i.e., both essential fat (found within bone marrow, nervous tissue, and internal organs) and storage fat (visceral and subcutaneous adipose stores). Most body composition techniques estimate fat mass and FFM.

Lean body mass (LBM): Body mass minus the mass of storage fat. LBM and FFM are often erroneously used interchangeably, as FFM exceeds LBM.

Lipogenesis: The production ("creation") of fat.

Lipolysis: The breakdown of fat.

Metabolic syndrome: A condition conferring elevated risk for type 2 diabetes mellitus and cardiovascular disease, and defined (by the National Cholesterol Education Program—Adult Treatment Panel III [17], but modified for impaired fasting glucose as defined by the American Diabetes Association [23]) as having at least three of the following signs:

- Fasting plasma glucose ≥ 100 mg $\cdot$ dL^{-1}, or on medication for hyperglycemia
- Blood pressure $\geq 130/85$ mm Hg, or on medication for hypertension

- Fasting triglycerides ≥ 150 mg $\cdot$ dL^{-1}
- High-density lipoprotein (HDL) cholesterol <40 mg $\cdot$ dL^{-1} for men, <50 mg $\cdot$ dL^{-1} for women
- Abdominal obesity, waist circumference >102 cm (40 in) for men, >88 cm (35 in) for women

Obesity: Having a BMI ≥ 30.0 kg $\cdot$ m^{-2}.

Overweight: Having a BMI of 25.0 to 29.9 kg $\cdot$ m^{-2}.

Percent body fat: The percentage of an individual's mass that is fat. This can be measured by dual-energy x-ray absorptiometry (DEXA), plethysmography (e.g., Bod Pod™), hydrostatic weighing, skinfold assessment, or other methods (the first three methods listed are considered the most accurate).

Resting metabolic rate (RMR): The amount of energy needed to sustain life at rest, typically measured as kcal per day. RMR is usually measured after a person has fasted for at least 12 hours.

Thermogenesis: The production of heat, especially the increased heat production associated with digestion of a meal.

ESTABLISHING A HEALTHY BODY WEIGHT GOAL

 1.8.3-HFS: Knowledge of the relationship between body composition and health.

Several methods can be used to determine a person's "ideal body weight"; however, in many cases, especially for athletes, ideal body weight may be unrealistic. Thus,

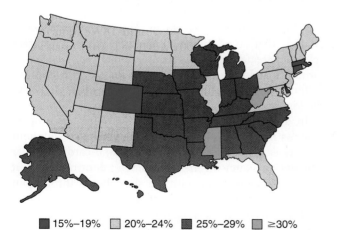

FIGURE 33-1. Percent of Obese Adults in the United States for 2006 (Body Mass Index >30 kg $\cdot$ m^{-2}). The data from this map show even more "new" colors from previous years, denoting a greater percentage of obesity in more states. (Adapted from: Centers for Disease Control and Prevention, 2007; www.cdc.gov/nccdphp/dnpa/obesity/trend/maps/).

Legend: 15%–19% | 20%–24% | 25%–29% | $\geq 30\%$

it is better to focus on a "healthy body weight" rather than an "ideal body weight." A healthy body weight is different for each individual, athlete or nonathlete, and is one that is relative to a person's overall health profile (e.g., serum lipid levels, glucose levels, blood pressure). The simplest method to determine a healthy body weight is by using the BMI. BMI is defined as a person's mass (in kilograms) divided by his or her height in meters squared (m^2). BMI is not perfect because it does not take into account body fat; thus, a muscular athlete may have a BMI that is considered "obese," whereas an individual with a narrow frame could have too much body fat and yet be considered of normal weight. BMI is a better indicator for determining the prevalence of overweight and obesity in a large population, rather than for determining body composition in an individual. Nonetheless, for the average sedentary person, BMI typically works well. For an overview of body composition measurement, refer to Chapter 17. Table 4.1 in the GETP8 lists the different BMI levels and how they match to overweight and obesity.

Note that a BMI between 18.5 and 24.9 kg $\cdot$ m^{-2} is considered healthy because individuals within this range are at the lowest risk for developing chronic disease. Although obesity increases the risk for major chronic diseases (such as type 2 diabetes mellitus and cardiovascular disease), a BMI of <18.5 kg $\cdot$ m^{-2} can place a person at risk for osteoporosis, gastrointestinal diseases, immune impairment, and diseases of the heart that are related to electrolyte imbalances. In addition, a low BMI may also be an indication of an eating disorder, which can also lead to the aforementioned risks. Aside from being overweight or obese, other risk factors to consider are hypertension, high levels of low-density lipoprotein cholesterol (LDL-C), low levels of HDL cholesterol (HDL-C), high serum triglyceride levels, high blood glucose levels, family history of heart disease, sedentary lifestyle, and cigarette smoking (see Table 2.3 in GETP8).

VARIOUS WEIGHT LOSS METHODS

> **1.5.6-CES: Direct patients actively attempting to lose weight in a formal or informal setting using behavioral, diet, exercise, or surgical methods.**

> **1.8.4-HFS: Knowledge of the effects of diet, exercise, and behavior modification as methods for modifying body composition.**

Although many individuals know that they should increase their physical activity levels, only about 25% of adults in the United States are moderately active for 30 minutes per day on most days of the week (12). By encouraging accumulated activity, this may allow for greater adherence to daily physical activity. In addition, accumulated activity is well documented to result in equal amounts of weight loss and improvement in cardiovascular fitness when compared with exercising for a single continuous bout (27,28,29,30,31). From 60% to 74% of U.S. adults are inactive or underactive (12,41). This lack of physical activity contributes to the increasing prevalence of obesity and, in turn, escalating healthcare costs. If this issue is not properly addressed, it is predicted that the majority of the U.S. population will be obese by the twenty-third century (19). Lifestyle interventions (diet and exercise programs) reduce body weight and lead to significant reductions in comorbidities (e.g., diabetes mellitus, coronary heart disease) (25). For example, Hamman et al. (25) reported that for every kilogram (kg) of weight lost, there was a 16% reduction in diabetes risk.

In conjunction with increasing physical activity levels, individuals need to decrease energy intake and consume healthier diets that will not only help with weight reduction/maintenance, but also provide positive effects to help stave off diseases such as cancer, diabetes mellitus, and coronary heart disease. In some cases, drastic dietary (i.e., very low calorie diets) and surgical approaches (i.e., **bariatric** surgery) may be used. In all cases, behavioral changes need to be made to ensure long-term success.

DIET, EXERCISE, AND A COMBINATION OF DIET PLUS EXERCISE

Researchers have assessed the effects of diet alone, exercise alone, and a combination of diet plus exercise on weight loss and the prevention of weight gain. Brinkworth et al. (9) reported that a 12-week exercise program led to reductions in body weight, cardiovascular risk factors, and risk factors for diabetes mellitus. In an attempt to evaluate the effects of a combined exercise and dietary weight loss strategy on serum LDL-C concentrations, Varady et al. (57) evaluated a low-fat diet combined with moderate endurance training on LDL particle size and distribution in 20 obese women who had hypercholesterolemia. They reported a significant mean weight loss of 14.8% with the combined low-fat diet (<30% fat, 50% to 60% carbohydrate, 20% protein) and endurance training program (>40 minutes moderate training, three times per week). In addition, serum total cholesterol, LDL-C, and triglyceride concentrations significantly decreased by 8.9%, 7.5%, and 27.1%, respectively, with a concomitant 9.9% increase (significant) in HDL-C concentrations.

Skender et al. (50) report that although their diet-plus-exercise and diet-only groups achieved the greatest weight loss at 1 year compared with exercise alone, the exercise group was able to maintain their weight loss at the 2-year mark, whereas the other groups gained weight (the diet-only group gained more weight, so that they weighed more than at baseline). Kraemer et al. (33,34) report that FFM was better maintained in their groups who included weight training as part of their exercise regimen. Nonetheless, these studies were only 12 weeks in duration and did not include an exercise-only group but did include control groups. Although Utter et al. (56) report significant weight loss in their diet-only and diet-plus-exercise groups compared with their control and exercise-only groups, their study was also only 12 weeks in duration. Both Kraemer et al. (33,34) and Utter et al. (56) report cardiorespiratory improvements in their exercise groups.

More recently (35), intensity of exercise was compared in men and women with a BMI of about 41 $kg \cdot m^{-2}$. Although body weight loss was equal between the low- and high-intensity exercise groups, the authors concluded that the higher-intensity exercise program achieved greater generalized improvement in muscle performance and physical fitness, as well as a stronger motivation for spontaneous physical activity compared with the low-intensity group (35).

In addition to exercise intensity, some researchers demonstrate that exercising in multiple bouts throughout the day is as effective for weight loss and cardiovascular benefits as exercising in for a single, continuous bout (30,31). Exercising in multiple short bouts throughout the day may provide greater adherence for some individuals who have erratic schedules. Jakicic et al. (31) also reported that weight loss is greatest if energy expended is >150 $min \cdot wk^{-1}$.

Furthermore, exercise appears to preserve muscle mass compared with diet alone. Weiss et al. (61) evaluated whether energy restriction decreases muscle mass and whether exercise preserves or improves muscle mass.

Healthy men and women, 50 to 60 years of age, with an average BMI of 23.5 to 29.9 $kg \cdot m^{-2}$, were evaluated before and after a 1-year energy restriction via weight loss (n = 18) or exercise (n = 16). They reported that muscle mass was decreased in response to energy restriction, but not in response to a similar weight loss induced by exercise.

Even though exercise preserves muscle mass, it may not provide the greatest weight loss over time; however, it does appear that exercise prevents weight gain and results in modest levels of weight loss (27). Nonetheless, with consistent exercise, the weight loss will be more likely to be maintained. However, combined with a lower energy intake, a greater weight loss will be achieved. Furthermore, with greater intensity exercise, greater improvements in physical fitness are observed. If weight loss or prevention of weight gain is the key, then the intensity of physical activity is not as important. However, if greater spontaneous exercise and, hence, greater energy expenditure will occur with higher-intensity exercise (and perhaps with multiple bouts of exercise), then these may be other motivational tools used with some individuals.

So what does this mean for exercise physiologists and other healthcare professionals working with the public? In the most basic sense, people need to get moving throughout their day, and the more minutes they are active, the more likely they will lose weight or prevent weight gain. The level of intensity and type of exercise need to be individualized based on the goals of particular patients, their likes and dislikes, and their overall health.

Perceived Barriers to Physical Activity and Healthier Eating

Although studies on combining diet and exercise have shown positive effects on weight loss and/or in the reduction of chronic disease risk (25,57), often they have not been able to maintain long-term weight loss, even with successful weight loss during the intervention trial (24).

The loss of social support from research personnel after the completion of diet and exercise interventions could be a reason for such high recidivism. Providing opportunities for increased physical activity and healthier eating are not the only issues that need to be addressed. Although facilities or time may be available, individuals will often not begin an exercise program and/or diet program because of their perceived barriers and lack of knowledge to initiate a program. Once an exercise and/or diet program is initiated, however, perceived benefits and barriers disappear (32). Kao et al. (32) found that providing an exercise program that assisted participants to develop individualized approaches significantly improved perceived exercise benefits and self-efficacy and decreased perceived barriers. Motivation and social support play primary roles in whether a person will begin an exercise program and/or diet. Counseling may be one avenue through which this goal can be achieved.

DIETARY COUNSELING AND WEIGHT LOSS

In an attempt to evaluate counseling people to exercise and eat within energy needs, Welty et al. (62) evaluated the effects of on-site dietitian counseling on weight loss and serum lipid concentrations in an outpatient physician's office. They assessed the effects of counseling 80 overweight or obese patients (average age = 55 ± 12 years; average BMI = 30.1 ± 6.4 $kg \cdot m^{-2}$) to exercise 30 minutes/day and eat an adapted Dietary Approaches to Stop Hypertension (DASH) diet. They reported a mean weight loss of 4.9 kg at 1.75 years follow-up. More importantly, 64 of the patients were able to maintain a significant weight loss of 5.3% at 2.6 years of follow-up. They also reported significantly improved serum lipid levels. Welty et al. (62) reported that a dietitian counseling patients to exercise and eat nutritiously in a physician outpatient setting is successful for weight loss, as well as for weight loss maintenance and improving coronary heart disease risk.

Dansinger et al. (14) conducted a meta-analysis of studies from 1980 through 2006 on the impact of dietary counseling on long-term weight loss. They reported that, compared with usual care, dietary counseling interventions resulted in modest weight loss that seemed to lessen over time. They added, however, that more studies are required that will focus on decreasing loss of participants to follow-up, as well as emphasizing factors that are most effective in weight loss.

DIFFERENT TYPES OF DIETS AND WEIGHT LOSS

> **1.8.2-CES: Compare and contrast dietary practices used for weight reduction and address the benefits, risks, and scientific support for each practice. Examples of dietary practices are high protein/low carbohydrate diets, Mediterranean diet, and low-fat diets, such as the American Heart Association–recommended diet.**

It is clear that energy balance is the key to weight maintenance and that altering energy balance through changes in intake and expenditure can result in weight loss (or weight gain). Although individual dietary needs differ, research on the effects of different types of diets continues. In addition, work on genetic predisposition to types of weight-loss treatments is also under way and in the near future may provide important information regarding the treatment most likely to be successful in a given individual based on genetic makeup.

The most popularly studied diets are the low-carbohydrate versus high-fat diets, or high-carbohydrate versus low-fat diets. Rankin and Turpyn (47) studied 29 overweight or obese women (BMI = 32 ± 5 $kg \cdot m^{-2}$) who were randomly assigned to a self-selected low-carbohydrate/high-fat diet or a high-carbohydrate/low-fat diet for

4 weeks. The two diets were similar in energy intake (about 1,360 kcals/day). A significantly greater weight loss was reported in the low-carbohydrate-diet group; however, there was a significant increase in C-reactive protein (a marker of inflammation) in the low-carbohydrate group compared with the high-carbohydrate group.

Although the aforementioned results are interesting, they are short term. A 12-year study on the long-term effects of a low -carbohydrate diet in Sweden (the Women's Lifestyle and Health cohort study that was initiated in 1991–1992) included 42,237 women, 30 to 49 years of age (36). Researchers reported that a low-carbohydrate/high-protein intake was related to increased total mortality, with a greater increase in cardiovascular disease, in this cohort of women. They stated, "Vigilance with respect to long-term adherence to such weight control regimes is advisable" (36). This is the first long-term study evaluating low-carbohydrate diets on disease risk.

Four popular diets (Atkins, Zone, LEARN, and Ornish) were compared in a study over a 1-year period in 311 overweight/obese premenopausal women (BMI ranged from 27 to 40 $kg \cdot m^{-2}$) (22). The women were randomly assigned to one of the above four diets. At one year, weight loss was greater for the Atkins group compared to the other diet groups (average weight loss: Atkins = 4.7 kg; Zone = 1.6 kg; LEARN = 2.6 kg; Ornish = 2.2 kg). Gardner et al. (22) stated, "While questions remain about long-term effects and mechanisms, a low-carbohydrate, high-protein, high-fat diet may be considered a feasible alternative recommendation for weight loss."

Aside from a low-carbohydrate or high-carbohydrate diet, the glycemic index may affect weight loss. Ebbeling et al. (16) examined if a low-glycemic-load diet (40% carbohydrate, 35% fat) fared better with weight loss and insulin secretion compared with a low-fat diet (55% carbohydrate, 20% fat). Their participants were 18 to 35 years of age and followed the respective diets for 6 months, with a 12-month follow-up. They found that plasma HDL-C and triglyceride concentrations improved more on the low-glycemic-load diet; however, LDL-C concentration improved more on the low-fat diet. They concluded that decreasing glycemic load may be particularly important to achieve weight loss amid individuals with high insulin secretion.

The Mediterranean diet is beneficial for heart disease and cancer prevention; however, it is not well studied with respect to weight loss. Recently Andreoli et al. (5) studied the effects of a moderately hypoenergetic Mediterranean diet and exercise program on body composition and cardiovascular disease risk factors in obese women. Of the 60 participants who began the study, 47 completed the entire study, resulting in a 22% attrition rate. Mean age of the subjects was 39.7 ± 13.2 years. Body weight, BMI, and fat mass were significantly decreased (p <0.001) at 2 and 4 months. Body weight decreased from 80.5 ± 15.8 to 75.2 ± 14.7 kg and BMI from 30.7 ± 6.0 to 28.7 ± 5.6 $kg \cdot m^{-2}$. In addition, cardiovascular risk factors were significantly improved (5).

Very-low-calorie diets (VLCDs) are often used for weight loss for morbidly obese individuals (BMI ≥35 or 30 $kg \cdot m^{-2}$ with comorbid conditions) (27). These diets routinely consist of highly engineered powdered supplements rich in protein and average in the range of 500 to 800 $kcal \cdot d^{-1}$. They are typically associated with hospitals or specialized clinics, and individuals undergoing these diets are monitored by physicians, as well as a team of other medical personnel, including registered dietitians, exercise physiologists, and registered nurses.

A potential value of the VLCD is the rapid weight loss that occurs, typically at the rate of 3 to 5 pounds per week. This rate of loss can be motivating to the individual and often allows him or her to lose very large amounts of weight. Individual programs report many who lose 50 to 100 pounds—occasionally those who lose more than 200 pounds—using a VLCD, and often a 20% group average weight loss for those engaged for at least 6 months. The length of a typical VLCD is 12 to 26 weeks; however, select individuals with careful monitoring have maintained a VLCD plan for more than a year to achieve very large amounts of weight loss. An individual who correctly implements a VLCD is typically not hungry despite taking in only 500 to 800 $kcal \cdot d^{-1}$. This is a result of the makeup of the food (high-quality protein, carbohydrates, and little fat) and the limited calories that produce a mild ketotic state (undetectable via urine dipstick assessment), which in turn curbs hunger. The allied health professional who counsels these patients often must request that they eat more supplements per day as they tend to eat fewer supplements because of not being hungry. This principle of VLCD (i.e., ketosis) is similar to the Atkins diet, which aims to deplete the liver and skeletal muscles of carbohydrate stores, which in turn requires the body to metabolize fat stores for energy production. The difference with the VLCD is its heart-healthy low-fat makeup.

The VLCD is often criticized as potentially dangerous. It is true that in the 1970s, there were several cardiac arrhythmic deaths linked to the VLCD, but increases in protein and micronutrients and careful medical monitoring have essentially eliminated this risk, and contemporary VLCD studies do not report significant dangers or side effects. Typical risks include dehydration and gallstones. Dehydration risk is minimized by requiring adequate water each day (64+ ounces), removing patients from diuretics as indicated, and adding a small amount of salt to the low-sodium VLCD. Gallstone risk can be minimized by eating a bolus of fat each day (~5–10 g) or by using the medication ursodiol.

The VLCD is also criticized for not being able to maintain the losses often achieved in the initial months of the diet. However, much of the research points to potential shortcomings in long-term maintenance planning. Leser et al. (39) reported that 3 years after weight loss using a VLCD, the women who were most successful were those who maintained physical activity and low-fat diets. Pekkarinen et al. (45) found that a 17-week VLCD program maintained 75% of the weight loss as measured at 1 year after the intervention. Additionally, they report continued reductions in blood pressure and continued positive effects on serum glucose, triglycerides, and HDL cholesterol. In a similar study, Pekkarinen et al. (46) report that at 1-year post-VLCD, 32% of patients maintained a >10% weight loss (i.e., successful patients), 42% maintained between 0% and 10% loss (i.e., partially successful patients), and the remainder were above their prestudy weight (i.e., unsuccessful). These types of success/nonsuccess rates are not different from more "traditional" diet regimens or other behavioral interventions, such as smoking cessation and exercise. Conversely, Wadden et al. (60) reported that women who were first placed on a VLCD ($420 \ kcal \cdot d^{-1}$ for 16 weeks) and then placed on a balanced deficit diet of 1,200 kcal/d lost the same amount of body weight (~11 kg) after 1 year compared with those individuals placed on the balanced deficit diet for the entire year.

Some are also concerned that using a VLCD will result in difficulty losing weight during subsequent diet attempts. Li et al. (40) assessed 480 patients who restarted a VLCD at least once, and some up to four times, to assess the ability to lose weight on subsequent attempts. During the initial attempt, the mean weight loss was 21.3 kg for women and 28.8 kg for men. In all subsequent weight loss attempts using VLCD, the rate of weight loss was not different from the initial attempt. Interestingly, the restart initial weight was lower than the first attempt weight, but the final weight was higher than the first attempt weight, on average. Patients also did not stay on the VLCD as long during subsequent attempts, potentially leading to not being able to achieve a lower final weight. An important part of a VLCD is variety of supplements used. Patients will get bored quickly simply drinking a vanilla or chocolate shake as some programs offer. A goal is to offer the patient variety. Recently, commercial supplement companies have developed a wide array of food types (shakes, puddings, soups, hot or cold drinks, bars, snacks, etc.) and flavors that reduces the boredom of previous iterations of the VLCD.

These high-protein supplements may also be used in a partial meal replacement diet strategy (often termed *low calorie diet* or LCD). These diets often are in the range of 1,000 to $1,200 \ kcal \cdot d^{-1}$ and are used for portion control along with some "regular" food. This type of plan is excellent for patients with diabetes. A report of the Look Ahead study, which is assessing patients with type 2 diabetes for the long-term (11 years) health effects of lifestyle intervention—including exercise and a low-calorie, low-fat diet with prescribed use of meal replacement products—found that attendance at meetings and the regular use of meal replacement supplements were associated with the best weight loss success in the 5,000 patients enrolled in this study (63). On average, patients in the intervention group achieved an 8.6% ± 6.9% weight loss at 1 year into the treatment protocol. Tsai and Wadden (52), using a meta-analysis approach, reported a similar long-term weight loss for a partial meal replacement (LCD) versus VLCD, thus suggesting the effectiveness of the partial meal replacement approach. This reference also provides an excellent overview of the history of the VLCD.

BEHAVIORAL APPROACHES TO WEIGHT LOSS

Behavioral change is the key to weight loss and maintenance. Certainly behavior/lifestyle counseling should be incorporated into any weight management program, including both the least and most aggressive methods. There have been several studies evaluating the effects of a combined behavioral, diet, exercise, and/or diet-plus-exercise approach to weight loss. Many have found positive results; however, recidivism usually occurs when the intervention is completed. In an interesting approach to using a behavioral treatment with weight loss, Ledikwe et al. (37) evaluated if energy density and energy intake changed with behavioral approaches to weight loss. They reported energy density and energy intake decreased, along with body weight with various behavioral interventions. In some cases, even if energy density was increased, energy intake was decreased.

Burke et al. (11) compared a standard (omnivorous) diet with a lacto-ovo vegetarian diet in 176 sedentary, overweight adults (average BMI = $34 \ kg \cdot m^{-2}$). The participants were either randomly assigned to one of the two diets or assigned to the diet of their preference, and the intervention included both exercise goals and 12 months of behavioral counseling. Seventy-five percent of the participants completed the study. The researchers reported that all groups significantly lost weight, ranging from 4% to 8%, with no difference between the two types of diets.

INTERNET-BASED APPROACHES TO WEIGHT LOSS

In the twenty-first century, it is rare to find people who have not or do not use a computer. Therefore, a tool for weight loss that cannot be ignored is the Internet. Because a complete review of this tool is beyond the scope of this chapter, a brief update on Internet-based weight-loss programs will be presented. Saperstein et al. (48) published a review article on the impact of the Internet for weight loss. They reported that the general public is definitely using the Internet for diet and fitness information. More importantly, they found that the Internet had affected behavior.

Successful Internet programs included the use of self-monitoring, altering energy balance, use of behavioral strategies, and providing feedback and support. It is important, therefore, to realize that patients may be obtaining other information (which may or may not be sound) from Internet-based weight loss sites. Also, the studies performed using Internet-based interventions typically used these in lieu of clinic visits with an allied health professional, such as a registered dietitian or exercise physiologist. Future investigations will likely focus on integrated models combining Internet technology and clinic visits.

SURGICAL METHODS OF WEIGHT LOSS

 1.6.4-CES: Describe and recognize bariatric surgery as a therapy for obesity.

Individuals who are morbidly obese (BMI ≥ 40 kg·m^{-2}) or have class II obesity (BMI 35–39.9 kg·m^{-2}) with comorbidities may be candidates for bariatric surgical techniques to induce weight loss. Such individuals should initially exhaust all attempts to lose weight through dietary and exercise interventions. However, for those who find it too difficult to lose weight successfully through standard methods, bariatric surgery is becoming increasing popular. The number of bariatric surgeries in the United States increased from 13,000 in 1998 to 121,000 in 2004 (65). Bariatric surgery is highly effective at inducing significant weight loss and has beneficial effects on type 2 diabetes mellitus, dyslipidemia, hypertension, and sleep apnea (10). Additionally, two important studies (2,49) recently reported significant long-term weight loss coupled with reductions in long-term mortality in patients who underwent bariatric surgery. These studies suggest not only that bariatric surgery is an effective treatment option in the morbidly obese, but also that long-term intentional weight loss definitively improves lifespan (8). And this positive effect is not thought to just be limited to bariatric surgery as the method for weight loss, but true for any method of intentional weight loss.

There are several bariatric surgical techniques. The two most common are Roux-en-Y gastric bypass and gastric banding (38). The Roux-en-Y procedure involves attaching the jejunum of the small intestine to a small portion of the proximal stomach. The lower portion of the stomach, the duodenum, and a short length of the jejunum are bypassed, but are reattached to the intact jejunum distal to the stomach pouch (forming one limb of the "Y" and allowing digestive enzymes from the duodenum to enter the distal jejunum). Weight loss is induced primarily by restricting the amount of food that can be eaten at one time, because of the very small size of the stomach pouch, and secondarily because of malabsorption caused by the stomach contents not passing through the duodenum. Gastric banding is a simpler procedure in which a band is placed around the proximal stomach and cinched to create a small pouch. As with gastric bypass, the small size of the stomach pouch restricts the amount of food that can be eaten. Unlike gastric bypass, gastric banding allows the contents of the pouch to enter the lower portion of the stomach and then proceed through the duodenum. Gastric banding is performed laparoscopically (through a small abdominal incision, guided with an endoscope) and thus has fewer surgical complications. Another advantage is that a greater percentage of weight loss is fat weight as opposed to fat-free weight following gastric banding as compared with gastric bypass and another bariatric technique, biliopancreatic diversion (13).

Both gastric bypass and gastric banding currently have relatively low surgical mortality, approximately 0.5% and 0.1%, respectively (38). However, there are several common postoperative complications, including vomiting (very prevalent and lasting up to 6 months), "dumping syndrome" (sweating, dizziness, and fatigue occurring after ingestion of sugar; very prevalent after gastric bypass), vitamin B$_{12}$ and iron deficiencies, and gallstone formation (21). Weight regain can also be an issue. Patients can adopt a habit of consuming multiple small meals and thus overcome the restrictive effect of the small stomach pouch. Bariatric surgery patients must be counseled regarding proper nutrition and caloric intake. It is important that behavior changes are adopted and continued after surgery. It has been reported that individuals with binge-eating disorder before bariatric surgery are likely to continue binge eating postsurgery (43).

Another common complication of bariatric surgery and subsequent weight loss is redundant skin that does not regress. The excessive skin is susceptible to rashes and infections, and may cause the patient significant psychological distress (51). The excess skin may be removed in circumferential abdominoplasty or other types of "body-contouring" plastic surgery. The incidence of such procedures in postbariatric surgery patients is rising rapidly, increasing from 56,000 in 2004 to 68,000 in 2005 (4).

Bariatric surgery is a very effective weight loss method for the morbidly obese with the potential to reduce mortality. However, patients must be encouraged to use diet and exercise as the first approach and, if choosing surgical intervention, be counseled regarding the lengthy period required to manage the postoperative complications.

IMPORTANCE OF AN ADEQUATE DAILY ENERGY INTAKE FOR HEALTHY WEIGHT MANAGEMENT

 1.8.5-HFS: Knowledge of the importance of an adequate daily energy intake for healthy weight management.

1.8.11-HFS: Knowledge of the number of kilocalories in 1 gram of carbohydrate, fat, protein, and alcohol.

1.8.12-HFS: Knowledge of the number of kilocalories equivalent to losing 1 pound of body fat and the ability to prescribe appropriate amount of exercise to achieve weight loss goals.

 1.8.3-CES: Calculate the effect of energy intake and energy expenditure on weight management.

The basic premise of weight maintenance is that energy intake equals energy expenditure. If weight loss is to be achieved, then energy intake must be less than energy expenditure (or energy expenditure must be greater than energy intake). It is important to maintain adequate energy intake because micronutrients (vitamins and minerals) are required for physiologic processes in the body. If micronutrients are not adequately consumed, other problems, such as impairment of the immune system, may occur.

Typically, a weight loss of no more than 2 lb (~1 kg) per week is often a goal for several reasons: (a) this smaller amount of weight loss may help to preserve lean body mass when a large amount of weight is lost; (b) although slower, this lower amount of weight loss may result in better adherence and better ability of the person to maintain that weight loss because, typically, the person has made lifestyle changes rather than drastic changes to his/her dietary intake; and (c) slower weight loss typically means less water loss and, thus, that a "false weight loss" has not occurred. However, in select individuals using properly designed aggressive weight loss methods (e.g., VLCD or surgery) that result in a greater per-week rate of weight loss, these issues can be overcome.

To lose 1 lb of body fat per week, a person should be in a 500-kcal deficit per day, because 1 lb of fat stores 3,500 kcal. It is important to note that not everyone loses 1 lb of fat with a 3,500-kcal deficit, but this is an average. Some individual variation occurs. Nonetheless, in general, a person can achieve this deficit by, for example, exercising enough to burn 250 kcal and decrease intake by 250 kcal daily. These values would need to be doubled if a 2-lb per week weight loss is desired. This level of deficit is moderate and increases compliance while also decreasing a person's likelihood of regaining the body weight lost. Although a combination of a moderate energy intake deficit and moderately increased energy expenditure may provide the best method to achieve weight loss, weight loss can be achieved by exercise alone. Donnelly et al. (15) reported that after 16 months, exercise alone prevented weight gain in women and resulted in a significant weight loss for men (~5.2 kg weight loss, on average) compared with a sedentary control group.

DETERMINING ENERGY NEEDS

Energy needs can be determined in several ways. Two important equations are the Harris-Benedict equation and the Mifflin-St. Jeor equation. These equations take into account a person's age, sex, weight, and height; however, the Harris-Benedict equation may overpredict a person's energy needs (7). Simply multiplying a person's body weight in pounds by 11 (providing a crude estimate of a person's resting metabolic rate [RMR]), then adding appropriate factors based on energy expenditure, is another way. The American College of Sports Medicine (ACSM) defines resting metabolism as 1 metabolic equivalent (MET), or an oxygen consumption of $3.5 \text{ mL} \cdot \text{min}^{-1} \cdot \text{kg}^{-1}$, which equals $1 \text{ kcal} \cdot \text{hour}^{-1} \cdot \text{kg}^{-1}$. This yields a daily value for resting metabolic rate of $24 \times$ body mass (kg) (or $10.9 \times$ body weight in pounds).

Determining a person's intake over time and assessing body weight is a more tedious method of assessing energy needs; however, this provides a more accurate estimate. Another more tedious but more accurate method is to assess an individual's RMR ($\text{kcal} \cdot \text{day}^{-1}$ used at rest), dietary-induced thermogenesis (energy expended after a meal; this must be conducted for up to 4 hours after a meal), and energy expended during exercise, all through indirect calorimetry (either using a metabolic cart or a whole-room calorimeter). These methods measure oxygen consumption and expiration of carbon dioxide, and then energy expenditure is calculated. Doubly labeled water provides the best estimate of a person's energy expenditure each day; however, it is expensive and does not partition how much energy is used for each activity.

Because many of these methods may not be practical, a useful tool for determining energy needs is to refer to the Food and Nutrition Board of the Institute of Medicine, National Academy of Sciences' (18) recommendations for energy intake based on energy expenditure.

ESTIMATING THE THERMIC EFFECT OF ACTIVITY

The thermic effect of activity varies based on an individual's activity patterns. The greater the duration and intensity of the exercise, the greater the energy expenditure. The Compendium of Physical Activities is a resource to estimate energy expenditure (3). The Compendium provides gross MET values (i.e., resting metabolism is included); therefore, RMR must be subtracted to avoid counting it twice. Also, the Compendium does not take into account factors such as the individual's body mass or the individual's personal choice of intensity for a given activity. For specific activities that have highly predictable energy expenditures, such as walking, running, and stationary cycling, the ACSM has developed metabolic equations that provide relatively accurate values (see Chapter 28).

THE MACRONUTRIENTS: CARBOHYDRATES, FAT, AND PROTEIN

 1.8.5-CES: Ability to differentiate and educate patients between nutritionally sound diets versus

fad diets and scientifically supported supplements and anecdotally supported supplements.

> **1.8.10-HFS: Knowledge of the myths and consequences associated with inappropriate weight loss methods (e.g., fad diets, dietary supplements, overexercising, starvation diets).**

Equally as important as consuming the proper amount of energy is the consumption of a proper balance of energy sources, macronutrients, and micronutrients (vitamins and minerals) (see Chapter 4). Although proper nutrition should be individualized, it is generally recommended that individuals consume about 45% to 65% of their total energy intake from carbohydrates (which provide $4 \text{ kcal} \cdot \text{g}^{-1}$) (18). These carbohydrates should consist mostly of whole grains (e.g., whole wheat products; brown rather than white rice). The consumption of whole grains provides more micronutrients as well as greater amounts of fiber, all of which can help to stave off cardiovascular disease and cancer. Protein is another macronutrient that is often perceived as the "building block" of muscle in the body. Although it is true that protein (which provides $4 \text{ kcal} \cdot \text{g}^{-1}$) is required for muscle growth, if protein intake is above what the body requires, much of it is stored as fat in **adipocytes**. In general, adults need about 0.8 g of protein per kg of body weight (sedentary healthy person), which is equal to about 0.4 g of protein per pound of body weight (18). For example, a 70-kg (150-lb) person requires, on average, about 56 g of protein per day. Each ounce of a protein food provides about 7 g of protein. A person who exercises strenuously may require slightly more protein per day (e.g., about 1.1 to 1.6 g per kg of body weight or 0.5 to $0.7 \text{ g} \cdot \text{lb}^{-1}$ body weight), especially if he or she is novice to the specific exercise program.

Fat, which is a nutrient that is often thought of as "bad," is required for proper bodily function. Fat provides $9 \text{ kcal} \cdot \text{g}^{-1}$ of energy. It is recommended that individuals consume about 20% to 35% of their total energy intake from fat (18); however, the type of fat consumed is most important. Monounsaturated fats (prevalent in olive oil, nuts, avocados) and polyunsaturated fats (e.g., safflower oil, sunflower oil) should be consumed in higher amounts than saturated fats (e.g., butter, lard, fat from meat) and hydrogenated fats. Hydrogenated fats are unsaturated fats that have been chemically altered to make them more stable. The hydrogenation process creates "trans" fats (referring to the molecular structure of double bonds within the fatty acid). Saturated and hydrogenated fats lead to increased risk of heart disease because they increase blood levels of LDL-C. Although alcohol provides energy ($7 \text{ kcal} \cdot \text{g}^{-1}$), it should be consumed in moderation because high consumption of alcohol can lead to malnutrition.

THE MICRONUTRIENTS

Vitamins and minerals are required for life, but they are required in much lower quantities than the macronutrients. Their functions are many, but they do *not* provide energy as do the macronutrients. However, many vitamins and minerals are required for energy metabolism and can affect exercise performance and overall health if they are not consumed in the right balance. It is beyond the scope of this chapter to review all the vitamins and minerals; therefore, the reader is referred to Chapter 4 and to an article in *ACSM's Health & Fitness Journal* (58).

INAPPROPRIATE WEIGHT-LOSS METHODS

Fad diets are promoted by television, newspaper, and magazine articles on a daily basis. The weight loss industry is a billion-dollar industry, and dieting books are among the top sellers. However, many times these fad diets are promoted by individuals who are not qualified or trained in any way to provide this information. Furthermore, because the weight loss may be unhealthy, these fad diets may be dangerous.

When assessing diet books, those that restrict certain food groups, especially fruits and vegetables, and state that their diets will cure everything, are not appropriate. Furthermore, exercise books that state that a person only needs to exercise 5 minutes per day to lose weight are greatly overstating the truth.

Other inappropriate weight loss methods that can be dangerous are use of saunas or steam rooms, exercising in the heat wearing heavy clothing to "sweat off the pounds," starvation diets, liquid diets that are not supervised by physicians and other healthcare professionals, diets that require megadosing of vitamin and mineral supplements (megadosing can be dangerous because many minerals compete for one another within the body if they share the same carrier), and diets that are only several weeks long, promising rapid weight loss. Often these rapid-weight-loss diets can be dangerous and can lead to loss of large amounts of muscle mass and water. If the claims seem too good to be true, they probably are, and that weight loss regimen should be avoided.

Furthermore, rapid weight loss that is not under medical supervision is not recommended because negative consequences can ensue. These consequences can be as serious as electrolyte imbalances leading to cardiac dysrhythmias. Individuals who lose weight rapidly also tend to lose more lean muscle mass, which can lead to an overall decline in RMR. This decline in RMR may make it more difficult for weight loss to occur in the future. In addition, if those who lose weight rapidly do not change the behavior that led to their obesity, their weight loss may not be maintained over time.

GENERAL GUIDELINES FOR PROPER WEIGHT LOSS

> **1.8.13-HFS: Knowledge of the guidelines for caloric intake for an individual desiring to lose or gain weight.**

> **1.8.16-HFS: Knowledge of the National Institutes of Health (NIH) Consensus statement regarding health risks of obesity, Nutrition for Physical Fitness Position Paper of the American Dietetic Association, and the ACSM Position Stand on proper and improper weight loss programs.**

The American College of Sports Medicine published a position stand on weight loss in 2001 (27). In brief, it stated that "the combination of reductions in energy intake and increases in energy expenditure, through structured exercise and other forms of physical activity, [should] be a component of weight loss intervention programs" (27). An energy deficit of 500 to 1,000 kcal per day was recommended by a combination of a reduction in energy intake and increases in energy expenditure. Furthermore, it was reported that although health benefits can be attained with a minimum of 150 min (2.5 hours) of moderate-intensity exercise per week, overweight and obese individuals may better maintain weight loss if they gradually increase exercise to 200 to 300 minutes (3.3 to 5.0 hours) of exercise per week (27). The incorporation of resistance training was also encouraged to increase strength and function, but it may not prevent the loss of FFM more than aerobic training when incorporated with a weight-loss program. Although weight loss via sensible exercise and healthy eating is promoted, the authors of the 2001 position stand state, "When medically indicated, pharmacotherapy may be used for weight loss, but pharmacotherapy appears to be most effective when used in combination with modifications of both eating and exercise behaviors" (27).

In 2005, the United States Department of Agriculture (USDA) replaced the Food Guide Pyramid with MyPyramid.gov (53). This Web site provides an excellent opportunity for individuals to participate in interactive learning about their energy intake and macro- and micronutrient needs.

The Dietary Guidelines for Americans (54) is also a helpful guide for eating more healthily. If people simply increase their fruit and vegetable intake, their overall energy intake usually decreases, and they are consuming products that provide a good deal of fiber and antioxidants, both of which help stave off some chronic diseases. In 2005, the sixth edition of the Dietary Guidelines for Americans (54) was published and stressed the importance of eating well and exercising. Box 33-1 lists the details of how to achieve each of these main guidelines. Recommendations related to weight-loss programs are summarized in Boxes 33-2, 33-3, and 33-4.

BOX 33-1 **DIETARY GUIDELINES FOR AMERICANS**

The following is a listing of the key points from the *Dietary Guidelines* that are pertinent to weight maintenance.

ADEQUATE NUTRIENTS WITHIN ENERGY (kcal) NEEDS

Key Recommendations

- Consume a variety of nutrient-dense foods and beverages within and among the basic food groups while choosing foods that limit the intake of saturated and *trans* fats, cholesterol, added sugars, salt, and alcohol.
- Meet recommended intakes within energy needs by adopting a balanced eating pattern, such as the USDA Food Guide or the DASH Eating Plan.

WEIGHT MANAGEMENT

Key Recommendations

- To maintain body weight in a healthy range, balance energy from foods and beverages with energy expended.
- To prevent gradual weight gain over time, make small decreases in food and beverage kcals, and increase physical activity.

PHYSICAL ACTIVITY

Key Recommendations

- Engage in regular physical activity and reduce sedentary activities to promote health, psychological well-being, and a healthy body weight.
- Achieve physical fitness by including cardiovascular conditioning, stretching exercises for flexibility, and resistance exercises or calisthenics for muscle strength and endurance.

*Adapted from U.S. Department of Health and Human Services. *Dietary Guidelines for Americans.* 6th edition. 2005. Available from: www.health.gov/dietaryguidelines/dga2005/document/default.htm. Accessed August 28, 2007.

SUMMARY

Proper weight loss takes time. People do not gain excess weight in a short period of time; therefore, they need to be reminded that weight loss will not take a short period of time. A small deficit in food consumption (e.g., 250 $kcal \cdot d^{-1}$), coupled with an increase in energy expenditure (e.g., 250 $kcal \cdot d^{-1}$), can lead to a weight loss of about 1 $lb \cdot wk^{-1}$. Properly designed aggressive weight-loss methods, such as surgery or a VLCD, can be very successful in

BOX 33-2 THINGS TO WATCH FOR WHEN CONSIDERING WEIGHT-LOSS PLANS

Be leery of weight loss plans that suggest any of the following:

- A diet that is drastically different from the recommendations given in the Dietary Guidelines for Americans and MyPyramid.gov, or other reputable sources such as the American Dietetic Association, the American College of Sports Medicine, the Centers for Disease Control and Prevention, and/or the National Institutes of Health.
- The diet plan promotes or stresses dietary supplements, herbal products, or other products sold by the company or person promoting the diet.
- The diet plan requires purchasing of special foods, especially if they are only available at a certain place and/or from the company or person promoting the diet.
- The diet plan is heavily endorsed through testimonials by famous people or even "everyday" people.
- The diet plan claims to be a cure-all for several medical conditions.
- The plan includes any catch phrases such as: "Lose weight while you sleep" or "Melt pounds away."
- The plan includes exercise gadgets that require the individual to do nothing (e.g., "If you wear this product, it will exercise your abs for you").

BOX 33-3 COMPONENTS OF GOOD WEIGHT-LOSS PROGRAMS

- The program should offer clear, scientific information about the success of their patients.
- The program has qualified individuals (e.g., registered dietitians, exercise physiologists, physicians) running it.
- A program should discuss with its patients the risk of disease. For example, a very-low-fat diet can lead to gallbladder disease in some individuals.
- A program should provide a realistic approach to the weight goal.
- A program should provide adequate energy for the person's needs. It is best to avoid diets of $<800 \text{ kcal} \cdot \text{d}^{-1}$ except under medical supervision.
- A dietary program needs to be coupled with an exercise program. This exercise program needs to be tailored to the individual.

Adapted from Food and Nutrition Board of the Institute of Medicine, National Academy of Sciences. *Dietary Reference Intakes for Energy, Carbohydrate, Fiber, Fat, Fatty Acids, Cholesterol, Protein, and Amino Acids.* Washington (DC): The National Academies Press; 2003.

BOX 33-4 COMPONENTS OF GOOD WEIGHT-LOSS PROGRAMS

- The program should satisfy all nutritional needs.
- The program should protect an individual from hunger between meals, provide a sense of well-being, and not result in fatigue.
- The program should have suitable alterations in energy intake and expenditure, and can be conducted throughout a lifetime.
- The program should be simple to maintain, whether at home or away.
- The program parallels normal eating habits and tastes as much as possible.
- The program uses foods readily available from the grocery store, not specially packaged foods.
- The program includes exercise or physical activities that are enjoyable and do not require a certain instrument to promote increased physical activity.

select individuals. It appears that individuals who are successful at maintaining weight loss consume a moderately lower energy intake, exercise on a daily basis, and have had some behavioral therapy to change their overall lifestyle. Wadden et al. (59) reported that long-term weight control included "continued patient-practitioner contact (whether on-site or by e-mail), high levels of physical activity, and the long-term use of pharmacotherapy [if warranted] combined with lifestyle modification." A lifestyle change is the key to successful weight loss. It is important that individuals understand inappropriate weight-loss methods to prevent any serious side effects from occurring.

REFERENCES

1. Adamo KB, Tesson F. Genotype-specific weight loss treatment advice: how close are we? *Appl Physiol Nutr Metab.* 2007;32(3): 351–366.
2. Adams TD, Gress RE, Smith SC, et al. Long-term mortality after gastric bypass surgery. *N Engl J Med.* 2007;357:753–761.
3. Ainsworth BE, Haskell WL, Whitt MC, et al. Compendium of physical activities: an update of activity codes and MET intensities. *Med Sci Sports Exerc.* 2000;32(9 Suppl):S498–504.
4. American Society of Plastic Surgeons. Body contouring after massive weight loss. Available at: www.plasticsurgery.org/media/statistics/loader.cfm?url=/commonspot/security/getfile.cfm&PageID=18093. Accessed March 8, 2008.
5. Andreoli A, Lauro S, Di Daniele N, Sorge R, Celi M, Volpe SL. Effect of a moderately hypoenergetic Mediterranean diet and exercise program on body cell mass and cardiovascular risk factors in obese women. *Eur J Clin Nutr.* 2008;62(7):892–897.
6. Birch LL, Davison KK. Family environmental factors influencing the developing behavioral controls of food intake and childhood overweight. *Child Adolesc Obesity.* 2001;48:893–907.
7. Boullata J, Williams J, Cottrell F, Hudson L, Compher C. Accurate determination of energy needs in hospitalized patients. *J Am Diet Assoc.* 2007;107(3):393–401.

8. Bray GA. The missing link: lose weight, live longer. *N Engl J Med.* 2007;357:818–820.

9. Brinkworth GD, Noakes M, Buckley JD, Clifton PM. Weight loss improves heart rate recovery in overweight and obese men with features of the metabolic syndrome. *Am Heart J.* 2006;152(4):693.e1–6.

10. Buchwald H, Avidor Y, Braunwald E, et al. Bariatric surgery: a systematic review and meta-analysis. *JAMA.* 2004;292:1724–1737.

11. Burke LE, Warziski M, Styn MA, Music E, Hudson AG, Sereika SM. A randomized clinical trial of a standard versus vegetarian diet for weight loss: the impact of treatment preference. *Int J Obes (Lond).* 2008;32(1):166–176.

12. Centers for Disease Control and Prevention. Physical activity trends—United States, 1990–1998. *MMWR Morb Mortal Wkly Rep.* 2001;50(9):166–169.

13. Chaston TB, Dixon JB, O'Brien PE. Changes in fat-free mass during significant weight loss: a systematic review. *Int J Obes (Lond).* 2007;31(5):743–750.

14. Dansinger ML, Tatsioni A, Wong JB, Chung M, Balk EM. Meta-analysis: the effect of dietary counseling for weight loss. *Ann Intern Med.* 2007;147(1):41–50.

15. Donnelly JE, Hill JO, Jacobsen DJ, et al. Effects of a 16-month randomized controlled exercise trial on body weight and composition in young overweight men and women: the Midwest exercise trial. *Arch Intern Med.* 2003;163:1343–1350.

16. Ebbeling CB, Leidig MM, Feldman HA, Lovesky MM, Ludwig DS. Effects of a low-glycemic load vs low-fat diet in obese young adults: a randomized trial. *JAMA.* 2007;297(19):2092–2102.

17. **Executive Summary of the Third Report of the National Cholesterol Education Program (NCEP) Expert Panel on Detection, Evaluation, and Treatment of High Blood Cholesterol in Adults (Adult Treatment Panel III). *JAMA.* 2001;285:2486–2497.**

18. **Food and Nutrition Board, Institute of Medicine, National Academy of Sciences. *Dietary Reference Intakes for Energy, Carbohydrate, Fiber, Fat, Fatty Acids, Cholesterol, Protein, and Amino Acids.* Washington (DC): The National Academies Press; 2003.**

19. Foreyt J, Goodrick K. The ultimate triumph of obesity. *Lancet.* 1995;15(346):134–135.

20. French SA, Jeffery RW, Story M, et al. A pricing strategy to promote low-fat snack choices through vending machines. *Am J Public Health.* 1997;87:849–851.

21. Fujioka K. Follow-up of nutritional and metabolic problems after bariatric surgery. *Diabetes Care.* 2005;28(2):481–484.

22. Gardner CD, Kiazand A, Alhassan S, et al. Comparison of the Atkins, Zone, Ornish, and LEARN diets for change in weight and related risk factors among overweight premenopausal women: the A to Z Weight Loss Study: a randomized trial. *JAMA.* 2007;297(9):969–977.

23. **Genuth S, Alberi KG, Bennett P, et al. The Expert Committee on the Diagnosis and Classification of Diabetes Mellitus: Follow-up report on the diagnosis of diabetes mellitus. *Diabetes Care.* 2003;26: 3160–3167.**

24. Gilden Tsai A, Wadden TA. The evolution of very-low-calorie diets: an update and meta-analysis. *Obesity (Silver Spring).* 2006;14(8):1283–1293.

25. Hamman RF, Wing RR, Edelstein SL, et al. Effect of weight loss with lifestyle intervention on risk of diabetes. *Diabetes Care.* 2006;29(9):2102–2107.

26. Hill JO, Peters JC. Environmental contributions to the obesity epidemic. *Science.* 1998;280:1371–1374.

27. **Jakicic JM, Clark K, Coleman E, et al. American College of Sports Medicine position stand: Appropriate intervention strategies for weight loss and prevention of weight regain for adults. *Med Sci Sports Exerc.* 2001;33:2145–2156.**

28. Jakicic JM, Wing RR, Butler BA, Anglin K. The effect of home visits versus clinic-based therapy on maintenance of weight loss. *Ann Behav Med.* 1996; International Congress Supplement: S113.

29. Jakicic JM, Wing RR, Butler BA, Jeffery RW. The relationship between the presence of exercise equipment and participation in physical activity. *Am J Health Promot.* 1997;11:363–365.

30. Jakicic JM, Wing RR, Butler BA, Robertson RJ. Prescribing exercise in multiple short bouts versus one continuous bout: effects on adherence, cardiorespiratory fitness, and weight loss in overweight women. *Int J Obes Relat Metab Disord.* 1995;19:893–901.

31. Jakicic JM, Winters C, Lang W, Wing RR. Effects of intermittent exercise and use of home exercise equipment on adherence, weight loss and fitness in overweight women: a randomized trial. *JAMA.* 1999;282:1554–1560.

32. Kao YH, Lu CM, Huang YC. Impact of transtheoretical model on the psychosocial factors affecting exercise among workers. *J Nurs Res.* 2002;10(4):303–310.

33. Kraemer WJ, Volek JS, Clark KL, et al. Influence of exercise training on physiological and performance changes in weight loss in men. *Med Sci Sports Exerc.* 1999;9:1320–1329.

34. Kraemer WJ, Volek JS, Clark KL, et al. Physiological adaptation to a weight-loss dietary regimen and exercise programs in women. *J Appl Physiol.* 1997;83:270–279.

35. Lafortuna CL, Resnik M, Galvani C, Sartorio A. Effects of non-specific vs individualized exercise training protocols on aerobic, anaerobic and strength performance in severely obese subjects during a short-term body mass reduction program. *J Endocrinol Invest.* 2003;26:197–205.

36. Lagiou P, Sandin S, Weiderpass E, et al. Low carbohydrate-high protein diet and mortality in a cohort of Swedish women. *J Intern Med.* 2007;261(4):366–374.

37. Ledikwe JH, Rolls BJ, Smiciklas-Wright H, et al. Reductions in dietary energy density are associated with weight loss in overweight and obese participants in the PREMIER trial. *Am J Clin Nutr.* 2007;85(5):1212–1221.

38. Lee CW, Kelly JJ, Wassef WY. Complications of bariatric surgery. *Curr Opin Gastroenterol.* 2007;23(6):636–643.

39. Leser MS, Yanovski SZ, Yanovski JA. A low-fat intake and greater activity level are associated with lower weight regain 3 years after completing a very-low-calorie diet. *J Am Diet Assoc.* 2003;102:1052–1056.

40. Li Z, Hong K, Wong E, Maxwell M, Heber D. Weight cycling in a very low-calorie diet programme has no effect on weight loss velocity, blood pressure and serum lipid profile. *Diabetes Obes Metab.* 2007;9:379–385.

41. Marcus BH, Forsyth LH. How are we doing? *Am J Health Promot.* 1999;14(2):118–124.

42. Must A, Anderson SE. Effects of obesity on morbidity in children and adolescents. *Nutr Clin Care.* 2003;6(1):4–12.

43. Niego SH, Kofman MD, Weiss JJ, Geliebter A. Binge eating in the bariatric surgery population: a review of the literature. *Int J Eat Disord.* 2007;40(4):349–359.

44. Ogden CL, Carroll MD, Curtin LR, McDowell MA, Tabak CJ, Flegal KM. Prevalence of overweight and obesity in the United States, 1999–2004. *JAMA.* 2006;295(13):1549–1555.

45. Pekkarinen T, Takala I, Mustajoki P. Two year maintenance of weight loss after a VLCD and behavioural therapy for obesity: correlation to the scores of questionnaires measuring eating behavior. *In J Obes Relat Disord.* 1996;20(4):332–337.

46. Pekkarinen T, Takala I, Mustajoki P. Weight loss with very-low-calorie diet and cardiovascular risk factors in moderately obese women: one-year follow-up study including ambulatory blood pressure monitoring. *Int J Obes Relat Metab Disord.* 1998;22(7):661–666.

47. Rankin JW, Turpyn AD. Low carbohydrate, high fat diet increases C-reactive protein during weight loss. *J Am Coll Nutr.* 2007;26(2):163–169.

48. Saperstein SL, Atkinson NL, Gold RS. The impact of Internet use for weight loss. *Obes Rev.* 2007;8(5):459–465.

49. Sjostrom L, Narbo K, Sjostrom CD, et al. Effects of bariatric surgery on mortality in Swedish obese subjects. *N Engl J Med.* 2007;357:741–752.

50. Skender ML, Goodrick KG, Del Junco DJ, et al. Comparison of 2-year weight loss trends in behavioral treatments of obesity: diet, exercise, and combination interventions. *J Am Diet Assoc.* 1996;4:342–346.

51. Song AY, Rubin JP, Thomas V, et al. Body image and quality of life in post massive weight loss body contouring patients. *Obesity.* 2006;14(9):1626–1636.

52. Tsai AG, Wadden TA. The evolution of very-low-calorie diets: an update and meta-analysis. *Obesity.* 2006;14:1283–1293.

53. **U.S. Department of Agriculture. MyPyramid.gov. Available at: http://mypyramid.gov. Accessed August 28, 2007.**

54. **U.S. Department of Health and Human Services.** *Dietary Guidelines for Americans.* **6ᵗʰ edition. 2005. Available from: www.health.gov/dietaryguidelines/dga2005/document/default.htm. Accessed August 28, 2007.**

55. **U.S. Department of Health and Human Services.** *Healthy People 2010,* **vol. 1. McLean (VA): International Medical Publishing; 2000. p. 28–29.**

56. Utter AC, Nieman DC, Shannonhouse EM, et al. Influence of diet and/or exercise on body composition and cardiorespiratory fitness in obese women. *Int J Sport Nutr.* 1998;8:213–222.

57. Varady KA, Lamarche B, Santosa S, Demonty I, Charest A, Jones PJ. Effect of weight loss resulting from a combined low-fat diet/exercise regimen on low-density lipoprotein particle size and distribution in obese women. *Metabolism.* 2006;55(10):1302–1307.

58. Volpe SL, Soolman J. Minerals for weight loss: fact or fiction? *ACSM's Health & Fitness Journal.* 2007;11(3):1–7.

59. Wadden TA, Butryn ML, Wilson C. Lifestyle modification for the management of obesity. *Gastroenterology.* 2007;132(6):2226–2238.

60. Wadden TA, Foster GD, Letizia KA. One-year behavioral treatment of obesity: comparison of moderate and severe caloric restriction and the effects of weight maintenance therapy. *J Consult Clin Psychol.* 1994;62:165–171.

61. Weiss EP, Racette SB, Villareal DT, et al. Washington University School of Medicine CALERIE Group. Lower extremity muscle size and strength and aerobic capacity decrease with caloric restriction but not with exercise-induced weight loss. *J Appl Physiol.* 2007; 102(2):634–640.

62. Welty FK, Nasca MM, Lew NS, et al. Effect of onsite dietitian counseling on weight loss and lipid levels in an outpatient physician office. *Am J Cardiol.* 2007;100(1):73–75.

63. Wing R, Wadden T, West D, et al. Factors associated with weight loss success in Look AHEAD intensive lifestyle intervention.

64. Yao M, Roberts SB. Dietary energy density and weight regulation. *Nutr Rev.* 2001;59:247–258.

65. Zhao Y, Encinosa W. Bariatric surgery utilization and outcomes in 1998 and 2004. *Healthcare Cost and Utilization Project. Statistical Brief #23.* Available at: www.hcup-us.ahrq.gov/reports/statbriefs/sb23.pdf. Accessed March 9, 2008.

SELECTED REFERENCES FOR FURTHER READING

Adamo KB, Tesson F. Genotype-specific weight loss treatment advice: how close are we? *Appl Physiol Nutr Metab.* 2007;32(3):351–366.

Bauchowitz A, Azarbad L, Day K, Gonder-Frederick L. Evaluation of expectations and knowledge in bariatric surgery patients. *Surg Obes Relat Dis.* 2007;3(5):554–558.

Boullata J, Williams J, Cottrell F, Hudson L, Compher C. Accurate determination of energy needs in hospitalized patients. *J Am Diet Assoc.* 2007;107(3):393–401.

Gardner CD, Kiazand A, Alhassan S, et al. Comparison of the Atkins, Zone, Ornish, and LEARN diets for change in weight and related risk factors among overweight premenopausal women: the A to Z Weight Loss Study: a randomized trial. *JAMA.* 2007; 297(9):969–977.

Gilden Tsai A, Wadden TA. The evolution of very-low-calorie diets: an update and meta-analysis. *Obesity (Silver Spring).* 2006;14(8): 1283–1293.

Hamman RF, Wing RR, Edelstein SL, et al. Effect of weight loss with lifestyle intervention on risk of diabetes. *Diabetes Care.* 2006;29(9): 2102–2107.

Hill JO, Wyatt HR, Reed GW, Peters JC. Obesity and the environment: Where do we go from here? *Science.* 2003;299:853–855.

Jakicic JM, Clark K, Coleman E, et al. American College of Sports Medicine position stand: Appropriate intervention strategies for weight loss and prevention of weight regain for adults. *Med Sci Sports Exerc.* 2001;33:2145–2156.

Kennedy MS. Making progress against childhood obesity. *Am J Nurs.* 2007;107(9):22.

National Institutes of Health. *Clinical Guidelines on the Identification, Evaluation, and Treatment of Overweight and Obesity in Adults: The Evidence Report.* NIH Publication No. 98–4083; September 1998.

Volpe SL, Sabelawski SB, Mohr CR. *Fitness Nutrition for Special Dietary Needs.* Champaign (IL): Human Kinetics; 2007.

Volpe SL, Soolman J. Minerals for weight loss: fact or fiction? *ACSM's Health & Fitness Journal.* 2007;11(3):1–7.

INTERNET RESOURCES

- American Dietetic Association: www.eatright.org/Public
- American Society for Metabolic and Bariatric Surgery: www.asbs.org/
- Centers for Disease Control and Prevention. Obesity and Overweight: www.cdc.gov/nccdphp/dnpa/obesity/resources.htm
- Medline Plus. Obesity: www.nlm.nih.gov/medlineplus/obesity.html
- National Heart, Lung, and Blood Institute. Clinical Guidelines on the Identification, Evaluation, and Treatment of Overweight and Obesity in Adults: www.nhlbi.nih.gov/guidelines/obesity/ob_home.htm
- North American Association for the Study of Obesity: www.naaso.org
- U.S. Department of Agriculture. Healthy School Meals Resource System: http://schoolmeals.nal.usda.gov/
- U.S. Department of Agriculture. MyPyramid.gov: http://mypyramid.gov/
- U.S. Department of Agriculture, Food and Nutrition Information Center. Childhood Obesity: A Food and Nutrition Resource List for Educators and Researchers: www.nal.usda.gov/fnic/pubs/bibs/topics/weight/childhoodobesity.html
- U.S. Department of Health and Human Services. Dietary Guidelines for Americans, 6ᵗʰ ed.: www.health.gov/dietaryguidelines/dga2005/document/default.htm
- U.S. Department of Health and Human Services. Overweight and Obesity: The Surgeon General's Call to Action to Prevent and Decrease Overweight and Obesity: www.surgeongeneral.gov/topics/obesity
- Weight-control Information Network: http://win.niddk.nih.gov/publications/prescription.htm

Exercise Prescription and Medical Considerations

Cardiovascular, pulmonary, and metabolic abnormalities sometimes arise during exercise testing and participation and may occasionally result in illness and death. In addition, musculoskeletal injuries are common in the physically active population. Such challenges and threats to personal health and safety must be met with increased levels of education and training. This chapter reviews the medical considerations of exercise testing and training. Pertinent information is presented concerning causes, recognition, care, and prevention of injuries and illnesses unique to exercise participation. In addition, environmental influences during exercise and their associated health risks are discussed.

PREPARTICIPATION SCREENING

> **1.7.2-CES:** Compare and contrast benefits and risks of exercise for individuals with risk factors for or established cardiovascular, pulmonary, and/or metabolic diseases.

> **1.5.2-CES:** Describe mechanisms and actions of medications that may affect exercise testing and prescription (i.e., β-blockers, nitrates, calcium channel blockers, digitalis, diuretics, vasodilators, antiarrhythmic agents, bronchodilators, antilipemics, psychotropics, nicotine, antihistamines, over-the-counter (OTC) cold medications, thyroid medications, alcohol, hypoglycemic agents, blood modifiers, pentoxifylline, antigout medications, and anorexiants/diet pills).

> **1.3.33-CES:** Recognition of the value of heart and lung sounds in the assessment of patients with cardiovascular and/or pulmonary disease.

> **1.5.15-CES:** Ability to assess for peripheral edema and other indicators of fluid retention and respond appropriately in a given clinical setting.

> **1.3.2-HFS:** Knowledge of the value of the health/medical history.

> **1.3.3-HFS:** Knowledge of the value of a medical clearance before exercise participation.

> **4.2.1-HFS:** Knowledge of metabolic risk factors or conditions that may require consultation with medical personnel before testing or training, including obesity, metabolic syndrome, thyroid disease, kidney disease, diabetes or glucose intolerance, and hypoglycemia.

The beneficial impact of exercise on many diseases is well known. Several laboratory studies as well as large-scale trials demonstrate an inverse relationship between physical activity and cardiovascular disease, hypertension, strokes, osteoporosis, type 2 diabetes mellitus, obesity, colon cancer, breast cancer, anxiety, and depression (34,42,46,47,49,56,60,68,72,73,77,81). As the goal of

> > > KEY TERMS

Air quality index: An index for reporting daily air quality that indicates how clean or polluted the air is and what associated health effects might be a concern.

Angina pectoris: Transient pain or discomfort in the chest (or adjacent areas) caused by myocardial ischemia.

Chondromalacia: Softening of any cartilage.

Musculotendinous degeneration: Deterioration of the muscle-tendon area.

Myocardial ischemia: Insufficient blood supply to the heart muscle.

Overtraining syndrome: A collection of emotional, behavioral, and physical symptoms caused by excess training and inadequate rest that leads to a decrease in exercise performance.

exercise is to preserve or improve fitness and overall health, participants should be screened for risk factors that could lead to injury or disease when starting a new exercise program or increasing the intensity of their current training.

When discussing risks from exercise, it is important to remember that as compared with sedentary adults, physically fit individuals have one quarter to one half of the risk of developing cardiac disease (6,79). Expanded exercise participation by a larger and older population potentiates the incidence of injury as the number of participants and volume of training increases. Additionally, it is well documented that acute exercise transiently increases the risk of sudden cardiac death. Exercise professionals are encouraged to perform health and fitness screenings before participants begin exercise programs (see Chapter 10). These screenings should be used to detect not only cardiopulmonary and metabolic abnormalities but also musculoskeletal problems that are a contraindication to exercise. The AHA (American Heart Association)/ACSM (American College of Sports Medicine) Health/Fitness Screening Questionnaire serves as a useful assessment form (Box 34-1) (14).

The screening process must document any history of cardiac, pulmonary, and/or metabolic disease, or musculoskeletal injury before the implementation of an exercise

---

| **BOX 34-1** | **AHA/ACSM HEALTH/FITNESS FACILITY PREPARTICIPATION SCREENING QUESTIONNAIRE** |

Assess your health needs by marking all true statements.

History

You have had:

___ A heart attack
___ Heart surgery
___ Cardiac catheterization
___ Coronary angioplasty (PTCA)
___ Pacemaker, implantable cardiac defibrillator, or rhythm disturbance
___ Heart valve disease
___ Heart failure
___ Heart transplantation
___ Congenital heart disease

Symptoms

___ You experience chest discomfort with exertion.
___ You experience unreasonable breathlessness.
___ You experience dizziness, fainting, blackouts.
___ You take heart medications.

Cardiovascular risk factors

___ You are a man ≥45 years.
___ You are a woman ≥55 years, you have had a hysterectomy, or you are postmenopausal.
___ You smoke.
___ Your BP is ≥140/90 mm Hg.
___ You don't know your BP.
___ You take BP medication.
___ Your blood cholesterol level is ≥200 mg·dL^{-1}.
___ You don't know your cholesterol level.
___ You have a close blood relative who had a heart attack before age 55 (father or brother) or age 65 (mother or sister).
___ You are diabetic or take medicine to control your blood sugar.
___ You are physically inactive (i.e., you get <30 minutes of physical activity on at least 3 days per week).
___ You are more than 20 pounds overweight.

___ None of the above is true.

If you marked any of the statements in this section, consult your healthcare provider before engaging in exercise. You may need to use a facility with a medically qualified staff member to guide your exercise program.

Other health issues:

___ You have musculoskeletal problems.
___ You have concerns about the safety of exercise.
___ You take prescription medication(s).
___ You are pregnant.

If you marked two or more of the statements in this section, you should consult your healthcare provider before engaging in exercise. You might benefit by using a facility with a professionally qualified exercise staff member to guide your exercise program.

You should be able to exercise safely without consulting your healthcare provider in almost any facility that meets your exercise program needs.

ACSM, American College of Sports Medicine; AHA, American Heart Association; BP, blood pressure; PTCA, percutaneous transluminal coronary angioplasty.

Reprinted with permission from Balady GJ, Chaitman B, Driscoll D, et al. American Heart Association/American College of Sports Medicine Joint Scientific Statement: Recommendations for cardiovascular screening, staffing, and emergency policies at health/fitness facilities. *Med Sci Sports Exerc.* 1998;30:1009–1018.

program. A focused exam should be performed, searching for signs necessitating further evaluation. This would include listening to heart and lung sounds, evaluating for edema, and a musculoskeletal exam. Examples that would require further examination and/or a more detailed medial history are a new or previously unknown heart murmur, which may signify hypertrophic cardiomyopathy or aortic stenosis, both of which could cause catastrophic consequences during an elevated level of activity; or wheezing, rales, or crackles heard in the lung fields, which may be a sign of bronchospasm or fluid accumulated in the airways from an acute or chronic disease process such as pulmonary disease, heart failure, kidney disease, cirrhosis, or cancer. Peripheral edema can also indicate an acute process, such as a deep venous thrombosis, in the setting of asymmetric lower-extremity edema, or a chronic disease that leads to fluid retention. A more complete list of the major signs and symptoms of cardiopulmonary and metabolic disease can be found in Box 34-2.

The musculoskeletal exam should be performed to identify the ranges of motion of major joints involving both the upper and lower extremities and the cervical and lumbar spines. It is important to determine previous orthopedic surgery history, particularly knee and hip replacements. In addition, muscle strength, motor control, and balance should be assessed, using functional activities for the purpose of determining the individual's ability to participate or perform specific activity (69).

In addition to assessing for risk factors by history and exam, a complete list of current medications, both prescription and OTC, and last dosage taken should be obtained for any individual wishing to undergo exercise testing or begin a new training program. Many common medications directly alter the physiologic response to exercise. For example, β-blockers, commonly used for heart failure, hypertension, or coronary artery disease, will decrease heart rates and blood pressures of exercising individuals, but may have varying effects on maximal exercise capacity. Some antidepressants can increase heart rates and lower blood pressure during rest or exercise. Alcohol, nicotine, and caffeine may have variable effects on exercise response. A more complete list of common medications and their effects on heart rate, blood pressure, electrocardiogram (ECG), and exercise capacity can be found in Table A-2 of the GETP8.

CONTRAINDICATIONS TO EXERCISE TESTING AND TRAINING

 1.7.11-CES: Describe relative and absolute contraindications to exercise training.

Through preparticipation screening, individuals may be found with contraindications to exercise such that the risks outweigh the benefits. The absolute and relative contraindications to exercise testing and training are listed in Box 34-3, which are equivalent to Box 3.5 in GETP8 (37).

These patients should be instructed to refrain from exercise until further medical evaluation can be performed. Those with absolute contraindications should be treated for their disease process and stabilized before exercise testing or training, whereas those with relative contraindications may only need further evaluation of the risk/benefit ratio before starting an exercise program. Also, see Chapter 3 of GETP8 for further information.

HEALTH CONSIDERATIONS

MUSCULOSKELETAL CONDITIONS

Most types of physical activities are beneficial because moderate exercise is an important element for general well-being (75). The risk of musculoskeletal injury increases for all levels of participation with increasing physical activity, intensity, and duration of training (58). Understanding the associated risks, preventive measures, and procedures of immediate care can reduce the incidence and severity of exercise-related musculoskeletal injuries.

INJURY RISK FACTORS

5.2.1-HFS: Knowledge of musculoskeletal risk factors or conditions that may require consultation with medical personnel before testing or training, including acute or chronic back pain, osteoarthritis, rheumatoid arthritis, osteoporosis, inflammation/pain, and low-back pain.

Musculoskeletal injuries are among the most common adverse effects of regular exercise and physical activity for individuals of all ages (11,12). Musculoskeletal injuries can be attributed to the complex interaction of intrinsic and extrinsic risk factors (Box 34-4) that predispose physically active individuals to specific types of injuries (64,65,70). Poor baseline physical fitness, excessive training, improper biomechanics, and improper training techniques also affect the incidence of injury. Helping exercise participants identify modifiable short- and long-term injury risks could assist in developing strategies to decrease injuries.

The annual injury rate for recreational adult fitness participants is between two and three injuries per participant per year (66). A majority of these injuries (76%) result in time lost from physical activity. The risk of musculoskeletal injury associated with various physical activities and cardiorespiratory fitness levels among recreationally active adults is also reported (39). The findings indicate that the moderate types and duration of physical activity promoted by the ACSM and national health organizations have lower injury risk than more vigorous types and longer durations of physical activity (5,75). The risk of physical activity–related injury among adults increases for runners, sports participants, persons engaging in more than 1.25 hours per week of physical activity, and individuals with moderate to high cardiores-

| BOX 34-2 | MAJOR SIGNS OR SYMPTOMS SUGGESTIVE OF CARDIOVASCULAR, PULMONARY, OR METABOLIC DISEASE[a,b] |

SIGN OR SYMPTOM	CLARIFICATION/SIGNIFICANCE
Pain, discomfort (or other anginal equivalent) in the chest, neck, jaw, arms, or other areas that may result from ischemia	One of the cardinal manifestations of cardiac disease, in particular coronary artery disease Key features *favoring an ischemic origin* include: • *Character:* Constricting, squeezing, burning, "heaviness" or "heavy feeling" • *Location:* Substernal, across midthorax, anteriorly; in both arms, shoulders; in neck, cheeks, teeth; in forearms, fingers; in interscapular region • *Provoking factors:* Exercise or exertion, excitement, other forms of stress, cold weather, occurrence after meals Key features *against an ischemic origin* include: • *Character:* Dull ache; "knifelike," sharp, stabbing; "jabs" aggravated by respiration • *Location:* In left submammary area; in left hemithorax • *Provoking factors:* After completion of exercise, provoked by a specific body motion
Shortness of breath at rest or with mild exertion	Dyspnea (defined as an abnormally uncomfortable awareness of breathing) is one of the principal symptoms of cardiac and pulmonary disease. It commonly occurs during strenuous exertion in healthy, well-trained persons and during moderate exertion in healthy, untrained persons. However, it should be regarded as abnormal when it occurs at a level of exertion that is not expected to evoke this symptom in a given individual. Abnormal exertional dyspnea suggests the presence of cardiopulmonary disorders, in particular left ventricular dysfunction or chronic obstructive pulmonary disease.
Dizziness or syncope	Syncope (defined as a loss of consciousness) is most commonly caused by a reduced perfusion of the brain. Dizziness and, in particular, syncope *during* exercise may result from cardiac disorders that prevent the normal rise (or an actual fall) in cardiac output. Such cardiac disorders are potentially life-threatening and include severe coronary artery disease, hypertrophic cardiomyopathy, aortic stenosis, and malignant ventricular dysrhythmias. Although dizziness or syncope shortly *after* cessation of exercise should not be ignored, these symptoms may occur even in healthy persons as a result of a reduction in venous return to the heart.
Orthopnea or paroxysmal nocturnal dyspnea	Orthopnea refers to dyspnea occurring at rest in the recumbent position that is relieved promptly by sitting upright or standing. Paroxysmal nocturnal dyspnea refers to dyspnea, beginning usually 2–5 h after the onset of sleep, which may be relieved by sitting on the side of the bed or getting out of bed. Both are symptoms of left ventricular dysfunction. Although nocturnal dyspnea may occur in persons with chronic obstructive pulmonary disease, it differs in that it is usually relieved after the person relieves himself or herself of secretions rather than specifically by sitting up.
Ankle edema	Bilateral ankle edema that is most evident at night is a characteristic sign of heart failure or bilateral chronic venous insufficiency. Unilateral edema of a limb often results from venous thrombosis or lymphatic blockage in the limb. Generalized edema (known as anasarca) occurs in persons with the nephrotic syndrome, severe heart failure, or hepatic cirrhosis.
Palpitations or tachycardia	Palpitations (defined as an unpleasant awareness of the forceful or rapid beating of the heart) may be induced by various disorders of cardiac rhythm. These include tachycardia, bradycardia of sudden onset, ectopic beats, compensatory pauses, and accentuated stroke volume resulting from valvular regurgitation. Palpitations also often result from anxiety states and high cardiac output (or hyperkinetic) states, such as anemia, fever, thyrotoxicosis, arteriovenous fistula, and the so-called idiopathic hyperkinetic heart syndrome.
Intermittent claudication	Intermittent claudication refers to the pain that occurs in a muscle with an inadequate blood supply (usually as a result of atherosclerosis) that is stressed by exercise. The pain does not occur with standing or sitting, is reproducible from day to day, is more severe when walking upstairs or up a hill, and is often described as a cramp, which disappears within 1–2 min minutes after stopping exercise. Coronary artery disease is more prevalent in persons with intermittent claudication. Patients with diabetes are at increased risk for this condition.
Known heart murmur	Although some may be innocent, heart murmurs may indicate valvular or other cardiovascular disease. From an exercise safety standpoint, it is especially important to exclude hypertrophic cardiomyopathy and aortic stenosis as underlying causes because these are among the more common causes of exertion-related sudden cardiac death.
Unusual fatigue or shortness of breath with usual activities	Although there may be benign origins for these symptoms, they also may signal the onset or change in the status of cardiovascular, pulmonary, or metabolic disease.

[a]Modified from Gordon SMBS. Health appraisal in the non-medical setting. In: Durstine JL, King AC, Painter PL, editors. *ACSM's Resource Manual for Guidelines for Exercise Testing and Prescription.* Philadelphia: Lea & Febiger; 1993. p. 219–28.

[b]These signs or symptoms must be interpreted within the clinical context in which they appear because they are not all specific for cardiovascular, pulmonary, or metabolic disease.

BOX 34-3 CONTRAINDICATIONS TO EXERCISE TESTING

ABSOLUTE

- A recent significant change in the resting electro-cardiogram suggesting significant ischemia, recent myocardial infarction (within 2 days), or other acute cardiac event
- Unstable angina
- Uncontrolled cardiac dysrhythmias causing symptoms or hemodynamic compromise
- Symptomatic severe aortic stenosis
- Uncontrolled symptomatic heart failure
- Acute pulmonary embolus or pulmonary infarction
- Acute myocarditis or pericarditis
- Suspected or known dissecting aneurysm
- Acute systemic infection, accompanied by fever, body aches, or swollen lymph glands

RELATIVE[a]

- Left main coronary stenosis
- Moderate stenotic valvular heart disease
- Electrolyte abnormalities (e.g., hypokalemia, hypomagnesemia)
- Severe arterial hypertension (i.e., systolic blood pressure of >200 mm Hg and/or a diastolic blood pressure of >110 mm Hg) at rest
- Tachydysrhythmia or bradydysrhythmia
- Hypertrophic cardiomyopathy and other forms of outflow tract obstruction
- Neuromuscular, musculoskeletal, or rheumatoid disorders that are exacerbated by exercise
- High-degree atrioventricular block
- Ventricular aneurysm
- Uncontrolled metabolic disease (e.g., diabetes, thyrotoxicosis, or myxedema)
- Chronic infectious disease (e.g., mononucleosis, hepatitis, AIDS)
- Mental or physical impairment leading to inability to exercise adequately

[a]Relative contraindications can be superseded if benefits outweigh risks of exercise. In some instances, these individuals can be exercised with caution and/or using low-level endpoints, especially if they are asymptomatic at rest.

Modifed from Gibbons RJ, Balady GJ, Bricker J, et al. ACC/AHA 2002 guideline update for exercise testing: a report of the American College of Cardiology/American Heart Association Task Force on Practice Guidelines (Committee on Exercise Testing). 2002. Available at: hwww.acc.org/qualityandscience/clinical/statements.htm.

BOX 34-4 INJURY RISK FACTORS

INTRINSIC RISK FACTORS

History of previous injury
Inadequate fitness or conditioning
Body composition
Bony alignment abnormalities
Strength or flexibility imbalances
Joint or ligamentous laxity
Predisposing musculoskeletal disease

EXTRINSIC RISK FACTORS

Excessive load on the body
Type of movement
Speed of movement
Number of repetitions
Footwear
Surface
Training errors
Excessive distances
Fast progression
High intensity
Running on hills
Poor technique
Fatigue
Adverse environmental conditions
Air quality
Darkness
Heat or cold
High humidity
Altitude
Wind
Worn or faulty equipment

Modified with permission from Renstrom P, Kannus P. Prevention of sports injuries. In: Strauss RH, editor. *Sports Medicine.* Philadelphia: WB Saunders; 1992.

piratory fitness levels. However, walking for exercise does not appear to be associated with a significant increased risk of activity-related injuries, even among walkers with the highest duration of activity per week. This low risk of musculoskeletal injury suggests that participation in walking can be safely recommended as a way to improve health and fitness for virtually any individual (24,39).

Comparisons of injury rates of athletes and exercise participants provide a perspective for understanding the magnitude of the problem of fitness-related injuries. The annual overall incidence of injury among distance runners is reported to range from 24% to 65% for heterogeneous populations of recreational and competitive runners (41). The cause of musculoskeletal running injuries is related to the runner, the running activity itself, and the environment (59). Training errors are reported in 60% to 80% of injuries to runners and are commonly caused by exceeding limits of duration and intensity, high rates of progression, and excessive hill running (43).

High-impact aerobics and dance are also associated with a substantial incidence of injury (36). The incidence of injury in aerobic dance is reported to be approximately 45% of students and 75% of instructors (53). Eighty percent of these injuries affect the lower legs and are related to frequency of exercise; improper footwear; or exercise on hard, nonresilient surfaces (67). Low-impact aerobics participation is now common and is used as an alternative to high-impact aerobics, which was primarily performed in earlier years. The injury rate is not known for low-impact aerobic dance because no comprehensive study has yet to be published. This includes more recent derivations, such as kickboxing, boot camp, and other intensive "floor routine"–based training programs.

The risk of acute injury from weight training and weight equipment is estimated to be from 2.4% to 7.6% of participants per year. A recent study showed a 35% increase in the number of emergency department injuries related to weight-training activities (40). Injuries reported included soft tissue injury, lacerations, concussions, and fractures and dislocations. Most weight-training injuries occur from excessive training, improper techniques, and the misuse of weight-training equipment, with the most important precipitating factor being inadequate recovery (19,63).

Overtraining is caused by excessive overload precipitated by poorly structured exercise programs. The consequences of overtraining involve complex interactions among biological and psychological factors that may lead to illness, musculoskeletal injury, or dramatic performance decreases in individuals of all training levels (44,51,62). The proper design of exercise training programs is essential to avoid overtraining. Proper periodization of training (planned variation), nutrition (glycogen replenishment and rehydration), and sufficient recovery time (recuperation from training) are important considerations to prevent the **overtraining syndrome** (19,62).

Overtraining can occur on a short-term basis, which is defined as overreaching (poor performance in training and competition) (35,62). Overtraining syndrome is untreated overreaching that results in long-term decreased performance, impaired ability to train, chronic fatigue, or other problems that may require medical attention (35,62). Two types of overtraining syndrome have been described: sympathetic overtraining syndrome (includes elevated sympathetic activity at rest, e.g., increased heart rate [HR] and blood pressure [BP], elevated basal metabolic rate) and parasympathetic overtraining syndrome (includes increased parasympathetic activity at rest, e.g., decreased resting HR and BP, and with exercise an early onset of fatigue or rapid HR recovery after exercise) (51). The symptoms of overtraining are highly individualized, with the presence of one or more of the symptoms of overtraining syndrome sufficient to identify the individual as overtrained. A review of common anaerobic and aerobic overtraining indicators is presented in Box 34-5.

Disorders of the musculoskeletal system may directly increase the risk of acute or chronic injury by interrupting normal structure and function of bone, joint, and soft tissue. The most common musculoskeletal risk factors include osteoarthritis, osteoporosis, **chondromalacia**, age-related **musculotendinous degeneration**, and malalignments of the lower extremities (55). Excessive body weight predisposes individuals to acute and overuse injuries, including osteoarthritic changes of the hip and knee with weight-bearing recreational activities (31,33). Weight loss reduces the risk of developing knee osteoarthritis, but its effect on the progression of the disease is unknown (32). In addition, vigorous physical activity may predispose participants to osteoarthritis by means of mechanical trauma to the joint (33). For example, there is an increased risk of osteoarthritis for competitive sports and running but not for recreational running (45).

Obesity, a poor sitting posture that duplicates the fully flexed standing posture, frequent back flexion, loss of back extension, and low physical activity are among proposed causative factors of low-back pain (20,38). Episodes of low-back pain are usually related to acute trauma or overuse. However, the individual's age, type of activity, and activity level are also risk factors for low-back pain. The incidence and recurrence of low-back pain are associated with muscle fatigue and movements such as a poor lifting technique (see Fig. 2.11) and failure to correctly position oneself before attempting lifts (38).

Concerns for Exercise Testing and Programming

Musculoskeletal injuries are a health burden because they may lead to permanent reductions in activity, thereby resulting in deconditioning. To reduce the incidence and severity of injury, it is important to identify predisposing risk factors through education and clinical intervention. Behavior modification with regard to early detection of symptoms of overuse is important for preventing injury. Participants should be encouraged to report injuries and symptoms because untreated muscu-

BOX 34-5 COMMON SIGNS AND SYMPTOMS OF THE OVERTRAINING SYNDROME

FUNCTIONAL INDICATORS

- Decline in physical performance and early onset of fatigue
- Decreased desire to train or decreased enjoyment from training or competition
- Loss of muscle strength, coordination, and maximal working capacity
- Increased submaximal HR
- Prolonged recovery from typical training sessions or competitive events
- Presence of tenderness and soreness in muscles and joints
- Overuse injuries

METABOLIC AND PSYCHOLOGIC INDICATORS

- Loss of appetite and body weight loss
- GI disturbances; occasional nausea
- Increased susceptibility to upper respiratory infections (altered immune function)
- Emotional instability characterized by general fatigue, apathy, depression, and irritability
- Sleep disturbances

PHYSIOLOGIC INDICATORS

- Decreased maximal oxygen uptake
- Increased creatine kinase
- Altered cortisol concentration
- Decreased total testosterone concentration
- Decreased ratio of total testosterone to cortisol
- Decreased ratio of total testosterone to sex hormone–binding globulin
- Decreased sympathetic tone (decreased nocturnal and resting catecholamines)
- Increased sympathetic stress response
- Altered resting HR and BP

BP, blood pressure; GI, gastrointestinal; HR, heart rate.

Information from American College of Sports Medicine. Recommended quantity and quality of exercise for developing and maintaining cardiorespiratory and muscular fitness, and flexibility in healthy adults. *Med Sci Sports Exerc.* 1998;30:975–991. Colbert LH, Hootman JM, Macera CA. Physical activity-related injuries in walkers and runners in the aerobics center longitudinal study. *Clin J Sports Med.* 2000;10:259–263. Kaufman KR, Brodine S, Shaffer R. Military training-related injuries: surveillance, research, and prevention. *Am J Prev Med.* 2000;18:54–63.

loskeletal injuries are likely to worsen the problem or predispose to future exercise-related injury (2). Strenuous exercise is contraindicated in the presence of acute joint injury, chronic joint inflammation (osteoarthritis), or uncontrolled systemic joint disease (rheumatoid arthritis). Under medical management, submaximal and symptom-limited fitness testing along with exercise program participation should be possible. The progression and level of physical activity must be pain free, individualized, and otherwise limited by precautions and contraindications associated with specific medical conditions (see Chapter 28). The goal of exercise programs for individuals after musculoskeletal injury or those with orthopedic disease and disability should be to prevent debilitation caused by inactivity and to improve endurance, exercise tolerance, strength, and flexibility (30).

Treatment Considerations

Most activity-related injuries result from either *macrotrauma* (tension, shear, or compression) or *microtrauma* (overuse or repetitive motion). Damage to tissue caused by trauma is defined as the primary injury. With the exception of controlling hemorrhage, initial treatment has little effect on the extent or severity of primary injury. Improper care or delay in treatment may cause additional pain, swelling, and tissue

damage of healthy tissues. Secondary hypoxic/inflammatory injury (the death of healthy cells caused by lack of oxygen or inflammation) is caused by the body's natural response to hemorrhage with a decrease in blood flow to the injured body segment. Secondary injury may continue even after bleeding is controlled, which necessitates that the initial treatment protocol consists of rest, ice, compression, elevation, and stabilization during the 24 to 72 hours after injury.

Exercise professionals are often asked for advice regarding the management of musculoskeletal problems or injuries. This may entail making recommendations about training and modifications in exercise programs, rendering immediate first aid, or referring participants to physicians. To help in decision-making, knowledge of common exercise injuries (Table 34-1) and their causative mechanisms (Table 34-2) is important. When injury occurs, the initial evaluation process for musculoskeletal injury should follow a logical sequence (Box 34-6). Evaluation using the HOPS (*History, Observation, Palpation, Special tests*) procedure is especially important for understanding the cause and severity of the injury (69).

Basic first aid procedures for common exercise-related musculoskeletal injuries are outlined in Table 34-3. The combination of *Rest, Ice, Compression, Elevation*, and *Stabilization* (RICES) is the appropriate treatment for immediate care of patients with acute injuries (61). When

TABLE 34-1. DESCRIPTIONS OF GENERAL EXERCISE INJURIES

CONDITION	DESCRIPTION	CHARACTERISTICS
Sprain	A stretch or tear to the ligaments and stabilizing connective tissues of a joint	Swelling, pain, joint instability, loss of function
Strain	A stretch or tear in the muscle or adjacent tissue, such as the fascia or muscle tendon	Movement pain, local tenderness, loss of strength and ROM
Contusion	A bruise that occurs from a sudden traumatic blow to soft or bony tissue	Soft tissue hemorrhage, hematoma, ecchymosis, movement restriction
Acute fracture	A sudden break of a bone	Deformity, bone point tenderness, swelling, ecchymosis
Stress fracture	Microscopic damage to the bone caused by repetitive stress	Insidious onset of pain that persists when attempting activity; tenderness
Bursitis	Inflammation of a bursa between bony prominences and muscle or tendon	Swelling, pain, some loss of function
Tendonitis	Inflammation of a tendon	Gradual onset, diffuse or local pain, tenderness, loss of strength
Plantar fasciitis	Inflammatory condition to the plantar surface of the foot	Inferior heel pain, pain increased with weight bearing
Shin splints	An overuse injury that indicates pain in the anteromedial shin	Pain occurring before, during, or after activity; bone tenderness
Patellar femoral pain syndrome	Knee pain caused by lateral deviation of the patella as it tracks in the femoral groove	Tenderness of the lateral patella, pain, swelling
Low-back pain	Condition resulting from trauma or multiple episodes of microtrauma resulting in muscular or joint pain	Pain accentuated by sudden flexion, extension, or rotation; muscle weakness
Rotator cuff tendonitis	Inflammation of the rotator cuff muscles or tendons	Diffuse pain, increased with overhead activities; muscle weakness in external rotation
Tennis elbow	Inflammation of the lateral epicondyle of the humerus	Pain in lateral elbow during and after activity; weakness of the wrist in extension

ROM, range of motion.

used properly, the RICES treatment regimen reduces the total amount of tissue damage, decreases swelling and pain, and aids in controlling the inflammatory response, which results in quicker rehabilitation and recovery. Rest allows time to control the effects of trauma and to avoid additional tissue damage. Rest is a continuum ranging from complete rest or immobilization to restricted activity (relative rest) of the involved body part. The application of ice or some form of cold application helps lower tissue temperature, thus slowing cell metabolism. Cold applications also are beneficial for reducing pain and muscle spasms that accompany musculoskeletal injuries. Both compression and elevation contribute to swelling control. Stabilization allows musculature around the injury to relax, which, along with the ice, aids in limiting the pain–spasm cycle (61).

Therapeutic treatments, such as heat modalities and exercise rehabilitation (e.g., physical therapy), are often prescribed after the initial treatment and are designed to promote healing and allow return to regular physical activity. It is recommended that a physician or sports medicine professional direct this follow-up treatment.

CARDIOVASCULAR CONDITIONS

> **1.2.6-HFS: Knowledge of the risk factor thresholds for ACSM risk stratification which includes genetic and lifestyle factors related to the development of coronary artery disease (CAD).**

> **1.3.4-HFS: Knowledge of and the ability to perform risk stratification and its implications toward medical clearance before administration of an exercise test or participation in an exercise program.**

> **1.7.40-HFS: Ability to explain and implement exercise prescription guidelines for apparently healthy patients, increased risk patients, and patients with controlled disease.**

> **1.7.41-HFS: Ability to adapt frequency, intensity, duration, mode, progression, level of supervision, and monitoring techniques in exercise programs for patients with controlled chronic disease (e.g., heart disease, diabetes mellitus, obesity, hypertension), musculoskeletal problems (including fatigue), pregnancy and/or postpartum, and exercise-induced asthma.**

> **2.2.1-HFS: Knowledge of cardiovascular risk factors or conditions that may require consultation with medical personnel before testing or training, including inappropriate changes of resting or exercise heart rate and blood pressure; new onset discomfort in chest, neck, shoulder, or arm; changes in the pattern of discomfort during rest or exercise; fainting or dizzy spells; and claudication.**

> **1.2.2-HFS: Knowledge of cardiovascular, pulmonary, metabolic, and musculoskeletal risk factors that may require further evaluation by medical or allied health professionals before participation in physical activity.**

TABLE 34-2. COMMON ACUTE AND CHRONIC EXERCISE INJURIES AND CAUSES

BODY REGION	INJURY	MECHANISM OF INJURY
Upper Extremities		
Shoulders	Rotator cuff strain	Throwing; swimming
	Rotator cuff tendonitis	Use of arm above horizontal; repetitive overhead activities
	Anterior glenohumeral dislocation	Forced horizontal abduction, external rotation
Upper arms	Bicipital tenosynovitis	Repeated forceful external rotation of the arm
Elbows	Lateral epicondylitis	Repeated forceful extension of the elbow (tennis elbow)
	Medial epicondylitis	Repeated forceful flexion of the elbow
Wrists and hands	Carpal tunnel syndrome	Activities that require repeated wrist flexion
	Strains and sprains	Falling on the wrist or outstretched hand
	Fractures	Falling on the outstretched hand
Lower Extremities		
Feet	Heel bruise	Contusion; sudden stop-and-go movements in running
	Plantar fasciitis	Unequal leg length; inflexible longitudinal arch; tight gastrocnemius–soleus muscle
	Metatarsalgia	Excessive pressure under the forefoot; fallen metatarsal arch
	Metatarsal stress fracture	Training overload; unequal leg length; hyperpronation of foot
Ankle, lower legs	Inversion ankle sprain	Foot forced into inversion-plantar flexion
	Achilles tendon strain	Sudden excessive dorsiflexion of foot
	Achilles tendonitis	Training errors; tight gastrocnemius–soleus muscle
	Anterior, posterior tibial tendonitis	Faulty posture alignment; falling arches; overuse stress
	Stress fracture of the tibia, fibula	Overuse stress; biomechanical foot problems
	Shin splints	Overtraining; running on hard surface; malaligned lower leg
Knees	Patellofemoral pain syndrome	Overuse (e.g., hill running); patellar compression
	Joint sprain	Direct straight-line or rotary forces
	Meniscal lesion	Excessive pressure (squatting); shear forces
	Patellar subluxation, dislocation	Alignment abnormalities; quadriceps weakness
	Chondromalacia patella	Abnormal patellar tracking; anatomic variation
	Degenerative arthritis	Overuse stress; obesity
	Patellar or quadriceps tendonitis	Sudden or repetitive forceful extension of knee
	Iliotibial band friction syndrome	Overuse stress associated with running, cycling
Upper legs	Quadriceps muscle strain	Weak muscles; sudden contraction, as during jumping
	Hamstring muscle strain	Strength imbalance; tightness; explosive movements
Hips	Trochanteric bursitis	Increased Q-angle; unequal leg length; faulty running form
Trunk		
Abdomen	Muscle strain	Sudden twisting of the trunk; reaching overhead
Spine	Lumbar strain and sprain	Poor posture; lumbar lordosis; sudden abrupt extension or contraction, sometimes with trunk rotation
	Low-back pain	Acute traumatic event; overuse; poor sitting posture; static or repeated flexion activities

 1.2.3-HFS: Knowledge of risk factors that may be favorably modified by physical activity habits.

 1.7.9-CES: Identify patients who require a symptom-limited exercise test before exercise training.

 1.4.2-CES: Describe myocardial ischemia and identify ischemic indicators of various cardiovascular diagnostic tests.

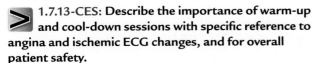 **1.7.13-CES: Describe the importance of warm-up and cool-down sessions with specific reference to angina and ischemic ECG changes, and for overall patient safety.**

In addition to the many musculoskeletal injuries that have been discussed, a variety of additional health-related conditions can potentially affect exercise participants. The stress of physical exertion during exercise, accompanied by pathologic risk factors or environmental condi-

tions, can increase the risk for cardiopulmonary or metabolic complications that affect the individual's health.

As above, the AHA/ACSM Health/Fitness Facility Preparticipation Screening Questionnaire uses history, symptoms, and risk-factor information to help direct people to either begin an exercise program or contact a physician before starting exercise (Box 34-1) (14). The AHA and ACSM have jointly published guidelines for classifying exercise participants according to disease risk (14). The recommendation states that participants should be classified into one of three risk strata: apparently healthy persons, persons at increased risk, and persons with known cardiovascular disease. After an individual has been stratified, decisions can be made regarding the need for and the types of medical examination and exercise testing. People at higher risk for coronary heart disease are directed to seek exercise facilities providing appropriate levels of staff supervision (Table 34-4) (3).

BOX 34-6   THE INJURY RECOGNITION PROCESS

1. Check vital signs and perform immediate first aid, if necessary.
2. Stabilize the individual.
3. Identify the injury.
   - **History:** Subjective statements by the injured person that include major symptoms and injury history (e.g., description of injury mechanism, functional impairments, pain, previous injury, training level and changes, equipment used, and rehabilitation).
   - **Observation:** Inspect or look at the individual and the injured part. Note variations in size, swelling, discoloration, posture, gait, limping, joint ROM, instability or deformity, and atrophy. Compare the injured part with the uninjured part.
   - **Palpation:** Using the fingers, carefully and gently feel the affected part, including soft and bony structures. Examine for edema, skin temperature variations, deformity, and point tenderness.
   - **Special tests:** Detect specific conditions, such as joint ROM and stability, muscle strength, neurologic status, and circulation.
4. Decide your course of action.
   - RICES
   - Referral to physician
   - Return to activity
5. Complete administrative procedures.
   - Record injury or incident in file.
   - Inform your immediate supervisor.

RICES, rest, ice, compression, elevation, and stabilization; ROM, range of motion.

TABLE 34-3. BASIC FIRST AID GUIDELINES FOR EXERCISE-RELATED MUSCULOSKELETAL AND SKIN INJURIES

CONDITION	FIRST AID PROCEDURES
Acute musculoskeletal injuries Contusion Sprain Strain	If no fracture, follow the RICES guidelines: set the area at rest (immobilize), apply an ice bag or cold pack with an elastic wrap for 20 to 30 minutes, and elevate the extremity above the heart. Reevaluate after initial first aid, support the injured area, and apply an elastic wrap to maintain compression, keeping the extremity elevated, if possible. Reapply ice or cold packs every 2 hours for 30 minutes and then continue to maintain compression and elevation during periods when cold is not being applied. Repeat these procedures for the first 24 to 72 hours, depending on the severity of injury and symptoms.
Fracture	Keep the individual still with the extremity in the position found, without moving the extremity or individual, if possible. Activate EMS or the facility's emergency response system to transport the individual to an ER. Do not apply a commercial or homemade splint unless the individual must be moved. Apply a cold pack. Calm and reassure the individual. Monitor the individual for signs and symptoms of shock, internal bleeding, and other life-threatening conditions. If splinting is warranted, proper splinting technique includes the following: (a) check distal pulse, skin temperature, color, and sensation for damage to nerves and blood vessels; (b) keep the individual still, and immobilize the joints above and below the suspected fracture site along with the broken bone ends with splinting materials, the ground, or other body part; and (c) recheck for circulation and sensation distal to the injury site.
Open skin wounds	With all open wounds, be sure to place a barrier (e.g., disposable latex gloves) between yourself and the individual's blood or body fluids and follow universal precautions to prevent the transfer of bloodborne pathogens. Be sure to wash your hands immediately after providing care. Minor wounds without significant bleeding (e.g., blisters, abrasions, lacerations, and incisions) should be cleaned with soap and water and treated with a germicide cream or solution, followed by the application of a sterile dressing (such as an adhesive plastic strip, gauze pad, or other commercial wound cover). The individual should be reminded to watch for signs of infection, keep the area clean and dry, and change the dressing as needed. Significant wounds that are bleeding severely should be treated by one or more of the following procedures: (a) apply direct pressure by applying a sterile dressing directly to the wound and applying pressure with the flat of the hand and fingers (if the dressing becomes saturated, apply additional dressings on top of the previous without removing the saturated dressing); (b) elevate the limb (if no fracture is suspected) while maintaining direct pressure elevate the wound above the individual's heart; (c) apply a bandage snugly over the dressing; or (d) if the preceding methods fail to stop the wound from bleeding, apply pressure to the brachial artery in the arm for upper-extremity wounds or femoral artery in the groin for lower-extremity wounds. Activate EMS or the facility's emergency response system.

EMS, emergency medical services; ER, emergency room; RICES, rest, ice, compression, elevation, and stabilization.

TABLE 34-4. EMERGENCY PLANS AND EQUIPMENT FOR HEALTH FITNESS FACILITIES

	LEVEL 1	LEVEL 2	LEVEL 3	LEVEL 4	LEVEL 5
Type of Facility	Unsupervised exercise room (e.g., hotel, commercial building)	Single exercise leader	Fitness center for general membership	Fitness center offering special programs for clinical populations	Medically supervised clinical exercise program (e.g., cardiac rehabilitation)
Personnel	None	Exercise leader; recommended: medical liaison	General manager; H/F instructor; exercise leader; recommended: medical liaison	General manager; exercise specialist; H/F instructor; medical liaison	General manager; exercise specialist; H/F instructor; exercise leader; medical liaison
Emergency Plan	Present	Present	Present	Present	Present
Emergency Equipment	Telephone in room Signs; encouraged: PAD plan with AED as part of the composite PAD plan in the host facility (hotel, commercial building)	Telephone; signs Encouraged: BP kit, stethoscope, PAD plan with AED	Telephone; signs Encouraged: BP kit, stethoscope, PAD plan with AED (the latter re strongly encouraged in facilities with membership >2,500 and those in which EMS response time is expected to be <5 min from recognition of arrest)	Telephone; signs BP kit stethoscope; strongly encouraged: PAD plan with AED	Telephone; signs BP kit, stethoscope, oxygen, crash cart defibrillator[a]

AED, automated external defibrillator; BP, blood pressure; EMS, emergency medical services; H/F, health and fitness; PAD, public access to defibrillation.

[a]Standard equipment in level 5 facilities includes a defibrillator (1,14).

Reprinted with permission from American College of Sports Medicine/American Heart Association Joint Position Statement (19).

With coronary artery disease (CAD), exercise participants may be unaware that disease is present or progressing to the point at which it could cause major health complications. Fewer than 10 of 100,000 men will have a heart attack during exercise (1). Of the millions of participants in high school, collegiate, and professional sports, fewer than 20 individuals die per year as a result of sudden death syndrome (50). When death during exercise occurs in people age 30 years or older, it usually results from cardiac arrhythmia caused by CAD. Those younger than age 30 years are most likely to die from hypertrophic cardiomyopathy, congenital aortic stenosis, or anomalous coronary artery anatomy. The examination of postexercise heart attack episodes in 1,228 men and women shows that the risk of heart attack is 5.9 times higher after heavy versus lighter or no physical exertion in those who usually exercise very little. Men may be more susceptible to sudden death because they may participate at higher levels of physical activity and ignore prodromal symptoms compared with women (50,76).

In those older than age 35 years who die during exercise, ischemia may manifest as a continuum of diastolic dysfunction, a decrease in left ventricular ejection fraction, abnormal BP responses, ECG abnormalities such ST segment changes or T-wave inversions, arrhythmias, or angina. Atrial and ventricular tachycardias are serious arrhythmias that can lead to ventricular fibrillation and sudden death (26). Unstable tachycardia exists when the heart beats too fast, resulting in reduced diastolic filling time and reduced stroke volume. This unstable tachycardia may lead to hemodynamic instability and signs and symptoms such as pain, myocardial infarction (MI), hypotension, or congestive heart failure (Table 34-5).

In untrained individuals, *bradycardia* (decreased resting HR) is usually the result of conduction abnormalities, such as complete heart block. However, a natural consequence of endurance training is a decreased resting HR. The actual mechanisms responsible for this decrease are not entirely known, but training appears to alter the intrinsic heart rate, probably as a function of structural remodeling, including enhance left ventricular dimension and stroke volume, and by increases in parasympathetic and reduced sympathetic activity (48). Therefore, it is necessary to distinguish between training-induced bradycardia and pathologic bradycardia, which can be a serious cause for concern. Both autonomic influences and the intrinsic pathology of the conducting system can lead to bradycardia. In particular, acute MI can lead to ischemic damage to the conducting system of the heart, producing bradycardias that range from sinus bradycardia to complete third-degree heart block (Table 34-5) (26). Typically, if a person is asymptomatic and is physically active or performing regular intentional exercise training, it is likely that the bradycardia is not pathologic.

TABLE 34-5. CARDIOPULMONARY AND METABOLIC CONDITIONS

CONDITION OR ABNORMALITY	DEFINITION	SIGNS AND SYMPTOMS
Hypertrophic cardiomyopathy	Hypertrophy of the myocardium	Cardiac palpitations, angina, syncope, vertigo; asymptomatic
Tachycardia	HR ≥100 bpm in adults at rest	Chest palpitations; difficulty breathing, severe chest pressure, chest pain, shortness of breath while exercising
Bradycardia	HR <60 bpm in adults at rest	Chest pain, shortness of breath, fatigue, exercise intolerance, hypotension, decrease in BP when standing
Tachypnea	Abnormal rapidity of respiration	Hyperventilation syndrome (aka behavioral breathlessness or psychogenic dyspnea)
Hypertension	Systolic BP ≥140 mm Hg Diastolic BP ≥90 mm Hg	Headache; most people are symptom free until complications arise
Hypotension	Decreased systolic and diastolic BP	Syncope and fatigue; occurs in shock, hemorrhage, and dehydration
Fainting	Feeling weak as though about to lose consciousness	Paleness; weakness; dizziness; weak, rapid, irregular pulse
Syncope	Transient loss of consciousness caused by inadequate blood flow to the brain	Peripheral circulatory failure; cardiac arrhythmia; hyperventilation
Hypoglycemia	Abnormal decreased blood glucose level	Headache; shakiness, confusion, faintness, blurred or double vision, tachycardia, pallor, convulsions, unconsciousness
Hyperglycemia	Abnormal increased blood glucose level	Nausea, dizziness when rising, polyuria, blurred vision, weight loss

BP, blood pressure; HR, heart rate.

Concerns for Exercise Testing and Programming

In patients with multiple coronary risk factors, exercise testing may provide important insight into exercise capacity as well as diagnostic and prognostic information. In patients with a recent myocardial infarction, submaximal exercise testing may be performed 4 to 6 days after the event, and symptom limited tests may be performed >14 days after the MI (37). Some of the indicators of poor prognosis during exercise testing are ST depression at a low workload, peak capacity <5 metabolic equivalents (METs), a hypotensive response to exercise, chronotropic incompetence (i.e., failure to achieve 80% to 85% of age-predicted peak HR during maximal exercise testing), and a low heart rate recovery response (i.e., failure of HR to decrease from peak exercise by at least 12 b · min^{-1}) at 2 minutes postexercise (37).

Although the general principles of exercise prescription hold for patients with cardiovascular disease, as outlined in Chapters 7 and 8 of GETP8, particular attention should be paid to the warm-up and cool-down phases, as well as resistance training. An adequate warm-up may aid in preventing ST-segment depression, arrhythmias, and transient left ventricular dysfunction (15,16). An adequate cool-down allows for HR and BP to return to baseline values, reducing postexercise hypotension, dizziness, and catecholamine surges (29). Other potential adverse health effects from exercise include cardiac dysfunction, ischemic arrhythmias, and an excessive hypertensive response (Table 34-5).

For individuals with cardiovascular disease, several forms of exercise (i.e., high intensity, resistance training) may prove harmful because of the acute hemodynamic effects caused by the pressor response associated with

Valsalva-type maneuvers (71). Although adequate study for the safety of resistance training in patients with moderate- to high-risk cardiovascular disease do not yet exist, there are data that show benefit in low-risk individuals. A low-risk individual is defined as no evidence of ischemia with exercise, no severe left ventricular dysfunction, and without complex ventricular arrhythmias.

It is generally recommended that low- to moderate-risk cardiac patients complete at least 2 to 4 weeks of an aerobic exercise program before initiating resistance training. The resistance training should be at low to moderate intensity with correct breathing and avoidance of the Valsalva maneuver. If prescribed, resistance training in patients with moderate- to high-risk disease should be closely monitored. ACSM endorses guidelines regarding resistance exercise in individuals with cardiovascular disease, including heart failure, set forth by the AHA (78).

Those with hypertension can benefit from exercise. Exercise programs that primarily include endurance activity, resistance training, or both are beneficial in preventing new hypertension or treating chronic hypertension. An exercise training program can decrease systolic blood pressure by 5 to 7 mm Hg in patients with hypertension (57). This is important, as a decrease of 2 mm Hg of systolic and diastolic pressures reduces the risk of stroke by 14% and 17%, and the risk of CAD by 9% and 6%, respectively (57).

There is emerging evidence that high-intensity exercise training at levels up to 95% of the age-predicted peak HR may be beneficial for patients with cardiac disease (80). A pilot study found that exercise intensity was an important factor for reversing left ventricular remodeling and improving aerobic capacity, endothelial function, and quality of life in patients with postinfarction heart failure. Currently, however, there are no guidelines recommending this type of exercise for patients with cardiac disease.

PULMONARY CONDITIONS

> **1.3.25-CES: Compare and contrast obstructive and restrictive lung diseases and their effect on exercise testing and training.**

> **3.2.1-HFS: Knowledge of pulmonary risk factors or conditions that may require consultation with medical personnel before testing or training, including asthma, exercise-induced asthma/bronchospasm, extreme breathlessness at rest or during exercise, bronchitis, and emphysema.**

Obstructive lung disease and restrictive pulmonary disease are two conditions that require special consideration for exercise prescription. Obstructive lung disease is characterized by air trapping and lung hyperinflation, often diagnosed as emphysema, chronic bronchitis, or small airway disease. Asthma is included in this category but is a clinical diagnosis; it is characterized by reversible airflow obstruction and may be induced by exercise. In obstructive lung disease, hypoxia can develop as a result of ventilation/perfusion mismatch caused by hyperventilation of emphysematous areas in the lung, leading to an increase in dead-space ventilation (23). However, dyspnea that is due to mechanical constraints and hyperinflation may occur without hypoxemia and may respond well to supplemental oxygen. During exercise, the goal is to optimize airflow by controlling inflammation, bronchospasm, airway mucus, and predisposing conditions (including tobacco use or triggers such as allergies and cold air).

Restrictive lung disease encompasses multiple disease processes that involve either the lung parenchyma, pleura, or chest wall and result in reduced filling of the lung. The incidence of restrictive lung disease is low compared with obstructive lung disease. Diagnosis is made by pulmonary function testing with a reduced total lung capacity. During exercise, the reduction in ventilation volume may lead to hypoxemia secondary to an increase in dead-space ventilation from a higher respiratory rate (rapid shallow breathing).

In general, exercise testing and training may be safely performed by patients with chronic lung disease, given that the subject's specific lung disease is accounted for and guidelines for pulmonary rehabilitation are followed. Pulmonary rehabilitation is a program used to progressively increase exercise capacity in patients with lung disease, but its role has not been well established in restrictive disease. Pulse oximetry and supplement oxygen may be needed during testing or training, depending on the severity of the subject's lung disease. See Chapter 36 for a more detailed description of pulmonary considerations in exercise and pulmonary rehabilitation.

METABOLIC CONDITIONS

> **4.2.1-HFS: Knowledge of metabolic risk factors or conditions that may require consultation with medical personnel before testing or training, including obesity, metabolic syndrome, thyroid disease, kidney disease, diabetes or glucose intolerance, and hypoglycemia.**

Diabetes mellitus (DM) is a chronic metabolic disorder marked by hyperglycemia. Diabetes mellitus results either from failure of the pancreas to produce insulin (type I DM) or from insulin resistance, with inadequate insulin secretion to sustain normal metabolism (type 2 DM). Type 1 DM usually presents as an acute illness with dehydration and often diabetic ketoacidosis. Type 2 DM is frequently asymptomatic in its early years and is, therefore, occult (8). Diagnosis is based on a fasting plasma glucose level of $126 \, mg \cdot dL^{-1}$ or higher on more than one occasion; a glucose level exceeding $200 \, mg \cdot dL^{-1}$ in a patient with excessive urinary volume (polyuria), excessive thirst (polydipsia), and excessive weight; or a glucose level $>200 \, mg \cdot dL^{-1}$ measured 2 hours after a 75-g oral glucose tolerance test (8).

If an individual with DM has any diabetic complications, consultation with the physician is warranted to determine appropriate exercise guidelines. These complications include heart disease, renal dysfunction, retinopathies, peripheral arterial disease, slowly healing lower-limb/foot ulcers, and an inability to control blood glucose with a propensity for hyper- or hypoglycemia. Some guidelines that are helpful in avoiding exercise-induced hypoglycemia in the diabetic population include those indicated in Box 34-7 (9). In patients with poorly controlled diabetes (i.e., a blood sugar $>300 \, mg \cdot dL^{-1}$),

---

BOX 34-7 GUIDELINES FOR AVOIDING EXERCISE-INDUCED HYPOGLYCEMIA

- Check blood glucose before exercise.
- If blood glucose $<100 \, mg \cdot dL^{-1}$, then eat 15 to 20 g carbohydrate 15 to 30 minutes before training.
- Recheck blood glucose after 30 minutes of training or sooner if symptoms are present.
- Exercise 1 to 2 hours after eating.
- Avoid exercise during insulin peak time.
- Avoid insulin injection into exercising limbs; suggest injection into abdominal tissue.
- Have fast-acting glucose available at all times (e.g., glucose tablets).
- Check blood glucose immediately after exercise; if blood glucose $<60 \, mg \cdot dL-1$, then eat 15 to 20 g carbohydrate (glucose preferred).

exercise may actually increase glucose levels because of counterregulatory hormones and should be avoided. Chapter 37 provides specifics for exercise training for persons with diabetes.

PREGNANCY

Pregnancy causes a multitude of changes to human physiology that affect the response to exercise. These changes depend on the stage of pregnancy but are related to weight gains, large increases in blood volume, and fetal/uterine growth that exerts upward pressure on the abdominal organs as well as the diaphragm. Box 34-8 lists contraindications to exercise in pregnant women; as such, each pregnancy should be evaluated for safety of both the mother and the baby. Healthy women without such contraindications should be encouraged to exercise throughout pregnancy because of the benefits to both the mother and child (4,28). ACSM endorses guidelines regarding exercise in pregnancy and the postpartum period set forth by the American College of Obstetricians and Gynecologists, the Joint Committee of the Society of Obstetricians and Gynecologists of Canada, and the Canadian Society for Exercise Physiology (4,13,27,52).

In general, exercise prescription for pregnant women is consistent with that for healthy adults. However, the intensity, efficacy, and safety of the exercise program should often be re-evaluated because of the constantly changing physiologic effects of pregnancy. See Chapter 41 for further discussion of exercise programming in pregnancy.

NEUROMUSCULAR CONDITIONS

> **1.3.27-CES: Identify basic neuromuscular disorders (e.g., Parkinson disease, multiple sclerosis) as they relate to modifications of exercise testing and programming.**

Often patients presenting to clinical exercise programs for treatment of cardiac, pulmonary, or metabolic disease have concomitant neuromuscular conditions. The following paragraphs briefly discuss some of these conditions.

Multiple sclerosis (MS) is a neuromuscular process that leads to dysfunction of the central nervous system. Current recommendations are for baseline fitness evaluation using a cycle ergometer. Common issues that affect patients with MS and should be considered in exercise prescription include lower-extremity muscle weakness, including foot drop; loss of sensation, balance, and muscle coordination; muscle spasticity; and visual disturbances. As such, low-impact exercises such as walking, cycling, and water aerobics may be necessary for safe training. Patients with MS are also known to have a greater sensitivity to heat with exacerbation of neural deficits and may benefit from precooling with water immersion as well as early-morning exercise training to control the rise in core body temperature. Regular stretching may enhance the effects of medications in the management of spasticity in patients with MS (18). See the ACSM's Resource Manual for Registered Clinical Exercise Physiologists (RCEP) for a more detailed description of MS and exercise considerations.

Parkinson disease is a progressive neuromuscular disease that affects the central nervous system, leading to resting tremors, bradykinesia, rigidity, and postural instability. In ambulatory patients, walking is the preferred method of exercise testing or endurance training, whereas a stationary, recumbent, or upper-extremity ergometer is more appropriate for those patients with postural instability. If a treadmill is used, a safety harness system may be necessary. See the ACSM's Resource Manual for Registered Clinical Exercise Physiologists (RCEP) for more information on Parkinson disease and exercise testing and training.

Patients with Parkinson disease or MS both benefit from adequate warm-up and flexibility activities, as they are often quite inflexible from their conditions and associated sedentary living. It would be wise to assess flexibility

---

BOX 34-8	**CONTRAINDICATIONS FOR EXERCISING DURING PREGNANCY[a]**

RELATIVE

- Severe anemia
- Unevaluated maternal cardiac dysrhythmia
- Chronic bronchitis
- Poorly controlled type 1 diabetes mellitus
- Extreme morbid obesity
- Extreme underweight
- History of extremely sedentary lifestyle
- Intrauterine growth restriction in current pregnancy
- Poorly controlled hypertension
- Orthopedic limitations
- Poorly controlled seizure disorder
- Poorly controlled hyperthyroidism
- Heavy smoker

ABSOLUTE

- Hemodynamically significant heart disease
- Restrictive lung disease
- Incompetent cervix/cerclage
- Multiple gestation at risk for premature labor
- Persistent second or third trimester bleeding
- Placenta previa after 26 weeks of gestation
- Premature labor during the current pregnancy
- Ruptured membranes
- Preeclampsia/pregnancy-induced hypertension

[a]Reprinted with permission from American College of Obstetricians and Gynecologists. Exercise during pregnancy and the postpartum period. ACOG Committee Opinion No. 267. *Obstet Gynecol.* 2002;99:171–173.

and begin a program to enhance range of motion as an adjunct to a cardiovascular and/or resistance-based exercise training program. This will likely assist to improve functional status and potentially allow some additional exercise modalities to be utilized that require a minimal amount of flexibility to use.

ENVIRONMENTAL CONSIDERATIONS

The human body experiences unique challenges and occasionally adverse health effects when performing physical activity in extreme environmental conditions (e.g., high temperature, high humidity, high altitude, and pollution). Special precautions and modifications of exercise programming are sometimes needed to reduce health risks related to the exercise environment (Table 34-6). It is vitally important that exercise professionals have knowledge about environmental factors to assist them in planning and conducting safe exercise programs. These environmental conditions are more important for some individuals than

for others, depending on their baseline status and specific disease(s) or condition(s). Chapter 3 provides detailed information on the physiologic effects of exercise in different environmental conditions.

Heat

The stress of physical exertion is often complicated by environmental thermal conditions that result in elevated body temperature above the normal range (i.e., hyperthermia). Heat stress is not always accurately reflected by air temperature alone. Humidity, air velocity (or wind), and thermal radiation also contribute to the total heat stress when exercising (Box 34-9). The human body regulates temperature by increasing skin blood flow, up to 12 to 15 liters per minute, which leads to increased sweat production as well as better cooling through convection and conduction mechanisms. During exercise, sweat evaporation becomes the most important avenue of heat loss. Because sweat must evaporate to provide cooling,

TABLE 34-6. BASIC FIRST AID GUIDELINES FOR ENVIRONMENTAL AND EXERCISE INTOLERANCE CONDITIONS

CONDITION	GUIDELINES
Environmental and exercise intolerance	Stop activity; calm and reassure the individual; monitor vital signs; activate EMS, if warranted.
Dizziness	Stop activity; position patient supine with legs elevated; monitor vital signs and seek medical attention if symptoms persist.
Fainting	Position patient in supine with the legs elevated, provided no injury is suspected; monitor vital signs and seek medical attention if symptoms persist. If individual has fallen, check for additional injuries before moving.
Syncope	Position patient in supine with the legs elevated, provided no injury is suspected; monitor vital signs; assess for heat stress or other conditions that may predispose syncope; maintain normal body temperature; seek medical attention if symptoms persist or worsen. If individual has fallen, check for additional injuries before moving.
Heat cramps	Stop activity; attempt to reduce muscular cramp by stretching, relaxation, and massage; replace lost salt and fluids with salty snacks and sodium-containing fluids; continue to monitor the individual's hydration status for the next few days.
Heat exhaustion	Stop activity and move the individual to a shaded or air-conditioned area; remove excess clothing and cool individual if body temperature is elevated; place the individual in a reclining position with the legs above the heart; if not nauseated, vomiting, or experiencing any CNS dysfunction, rehydrate with chilled water or sports drink; monitor vital signs, core temperature, and CNS status; activate EMS system if rapid improvement is absent.
Heat stroke	Aggressive and immediate whole-body cooling via cold-water immersion (35°–58°F or 1.67°–14.5°C) if constant monitoring of core temperature is possible; alternative cooling strategies include spraying body with cold water, using fans, placing ice or cold towels over as much of the body possible, or moving to shaded or air-conditioned facility; activate EMS and monitor ABCs, as core temperature, and CNS; cease cooling when core temperature reaches approximately 101°F (38.3°C).
Hyponatremia	Distinguish between hyponatremia, heat exhaustion, dehydration, and heat stroke; activate EMS and transfer to medical facility; individuals with suspected hyponatremia should not be administered fluids unless directed by a physician. Weight gain during exercise resulting in hyponatremia is because of overdrinking fluids.
Systemic hypothermia	Carefully move individual to a warm place; activate EMS; arrange rapid transport to emergency facility; monitor vital signs and provide care for shock; remove wet clothing and cover with blankets to retain body heat; provide external heat; encourage drinking hot liquids.
Local injury (frostbite, chilblain, frostnip)	Remove wet clothing; soak area in warm water (100°–105°F or 37.8°–40.5°C); cover the affected area with dry, sterile dressings; check ABCs, monitor vital signs, and care for shock; do not rewarm a frostbitten area if there is danger of refreezing; activate EMS or transport individual to an emergency medical facility.

ABC, airway, breathing, circulation; CNS, central nervous system; EMS, emergency medical services.

BOX 34-9   HEAT INDEX

					AIR TEMPERATURE (°F)						
RH	70	75	80	85	90	95	100	105	110	115	120
30	67	73	78	84	90	96	104	113	123	135	148
35	67	73	79	85	91	98	107	118	130	143	
40	68	74	79	86	93	101	110	123	137	151	
45	68	74	80	87	95	104	115	129	143		
50	69	75	81	88	96	107	120	135	150		
55	69	75	81	89	98	110	126	142			
60	70	76	82	90	100	114	132	149			
65	70	76	83	91	102	119	138				
70	70	77	85	93	106	124	144				
75	70	77	86	95	109	130					
80	71	78	86	97	113	136					
85	71	78	87	99	117						
90	71	79	88	102	122						
95	71	79	89	105							
100	72	80	91	108							

RH, relative humidity.

130 or above, heat stroke highly likely with continued exposure; 105–130, heat stroke likely with prolonged exposure; 90–105, heat stroke possible with prolonged exposure.

Adapted from the National Oceanic and Atmospheric Administration. Meteorological tables. Available at: www.erh.noaa.gov.

high humidity limits sweat evaporation and heat loss. Patients with diabetes and those with neuromuscular conditions, particularly MS, do not sweat normally and may be prone to hyperthermia. Care must be taken to assist them in maintaining a safe body temperature, such as exposing skin and using a fan to facilitate convective heat loss. Patients who have had gastric bypass surgery are also at risk for hyperthermia during exercise because of a reduced ability to drink large boluses of water. They must learn and practice continual sipping of water throughout the day, even during nonexercise time, to remain adequately hydrated and maintain their ability to sweat properly during exercise. Another particular concern is that body temperature regulation may be compromised in patients with heart failure who cannot generate an adequately high cardiac output to transfer excess body heat to the environment (25). Consequently, body temperature can increase to critical levels, seriously jeopardizing health (7,17).

Heat illnesses are more likely in hot, humid weather but can also occur in the absence of hot and humid conditions (Box 34-10). When the exercise session is conducted in hot, humid conditions or if the individual is not acclimated to exercise in the heat, special precautions and modifications of exercise programming for exertional heat illnesses must be undertaken. The most important factors in reducing heat illness are to limit the intensity and duration of activity, wear minimal clothing to allow heat dissipation from the body, increase the number and length of rest breaks, and encourage proper hydration. Several other factors important to preventing heat illnesses are listed in Box 34-11 (17,21).

Cold

Increasing year-round participation in such sporting activities as the triathlon, hiking, running, and cycling has created new concerns about exercise in the cold. The two major cold stressors, ambient temperature (air) and water, cause a loss of body heat that threatens homeostasis. *Hypothermia* occurs when body temperature falls below 36°C (97°F) and results when a person is exposed to wet or cold conditions or after trauma (7). Ambient temperature and wind influence the coldness of an environment. The windchill index determines the wind's cooling effect on exposed tissue and can be used as a guide to determine suitable outdoor exercise conditions (Box 34-12). When exposed to cold, the body attempts to increase internal heat production by increasing muscular activity, such as shivering, and by increasing the individual's basal metabolic rate. After the body temperature falls below 34.5°C (94°F), the hypothalamus begins to lose its ability to regulate body temperature. This ability is completely lost when the internal temperature falls to about 29.5°C (85°F). Predisposing factors to cold injury include inadequate insulation from wind and cold, restricted circulation because of arterial disease or tight clothing (including footwear), fatigue, and the body's shunting of blood away from the skin when exposed to the cold. Box 34-13 provides a list of characteristics increasing the risk of cold injury (22).

The hazards of excessive cold exposure include potential injury to both peripheral tissues and the life-supporting cardiovascular and respiratory systems. Considerable water

BOX 34-10 COMMON EXERTIONAL HEAT ILLNESSES

EXERCISE-ASSOCIATED MUSCLE (HEAT) CRAMPS

- Acute, painful, involuntary muscle contraction
- Present during or after intense exercise sessions
- Caused by fluid deficiencies (dehydration), electrolyte imbalances, neuromuscular fatigue

HEAT SYNCOPE (ORTHOSTATIC DIZZINESS)

- Occurs when exposed to high environmental temperatures or dehydration
- Individuals may be vulnerable during initial exercise sessions in the heat (unacclimated state)
- Caution for individuals with heart disease and those taking diuretics
- Can occur immediately after cessation of activity or after rapid assumption of upright posture after lying or sitting

EXERCISE (HEAT) EXHAUSTION

- The inability to continue exercise associated with any combination of heavy sweating, dehydration, sodium loss, and energy depletion
- Body core temperature generally ranges between 36°C (97°F) and 40°C (104°F); pallor, weakness, headache, dizziness, diarrhea
- Difficult to distinguish from exertional heat stroke without measuring rectal temperature

EXERTIONAL HEAT STROKE

- Elevated core temperature (usually > 40°C [104°F]) associated with signs of organ system failure caused by hyperthermia
- Tachycardia, hypotension, sweating (skin may be wet or dry at time of collapse), altered mental status, and vomiting
- Can result in death

EXERTIONAL HYPONATREMIA

- Relatively rare condition defined as a blood sodium level <130 mmol $\cdot$ L^{-1}, producing intracellular swelling that causes potentially fatal neurologic and physiologic dysfunction
- Disorientation, altered mental status, headache, vomiting, lethargy, swelling of hands and feet, pulmonary and cerebral edema
- Can result in death

BOX 34-11 RECOMMENDATIONS FOR PREVENTING HEAT ILLNESS

- Modify activity under high-risk conditions (Wet Bulb Globe Temperature >28°C [82°F]); consider rescheduling or delaying the session until safer conditions prevail.
- Schedule exercise sessions to avoid the hottest time of the day (10 a.m. to 5 p.m.).
- Avoid radiant heating from direct sunlight.
- Progressively increase the intensity and duration of work in the heat over days or weeks (i.e., acclimatization).
- Consume an adequate volume of fluids (water or sports drinks) to maintain hydration.
- Fluid replacement: Maintain proper hydration (educate the individual to match fluid intake with sweat and urine losses).
- Instruct individuals to drink sodium-containing fluids to keep their urine clear to light yellow to improve hydration.

- Individual should weigh themselves before and after exercise to estimate the amount of body water lost during exercise and to ensure a return to pre-exercise weight before the next exercise session.
- Consume approximately 1.00 to 1.25 L (16–20 oz) of fluid for each kg of body water lost during exercise.
- Wear loose-fitting, absorbent, light-colored clothing, mesh clothing, or new-generation cloth blends specially designed to allow effective cooling.
- Conduct warm-up and stretching sessions in the shade (for outdoor activities).
- Individuals who have lost 2% of body weight should be excluded from participation (as should those who exhibit heat illness symptoms).

BOX 34-12   WINDCHILL CHART

Wind (mph)

Calm	5	10	15	20	25	30	35	40	45	50	55	60
40	36	34	32	30	29	28	28	27	26	26	25	25
35	31	27	25	24	23	22	21	20	19	19	18	17
30	25	21	19	17	16	15	14	13	12	12	11	10
25	19	15	13	11	9	8	7	6	5	4	4	3
20	13	9	6	4	3	1	0	−1	−2	−3	−3	−4
15	7	3	0	−2	−4	−5	−7	−8	−9	−10	−11	−11
10	1	−4	−7	−9	−11	−12	−14	−15	−16	−17	−18	−19
5	−5	−10	−13	−15	−17	−19	−21	−22	−23	−24	−25	−26
0	−11	−16	−19	−22	−24	−26	−27	−29	−30	−31	−32	−33
−5	−16	−22	−26	−29	−31	−33	−34	−36	−37	−38	−39	−40
−10	−22	−28	−32	−35	−37	−39	−41	−43	−44	−45	−46	−48
−15	−28	−35	−39	−42	−44	−46	−48	−50	−51	−52	−54	−55
−20	−34	−41	−45	−48	−51	−53	−55	−57	−58	−60	−61	−62
−25	−40	−47	−51	−55	−58	−60	−62	−64	−65	−67	−68	−69
−30	−46	−53	−58	−61	−64	−67	−69	−71	−72	−74	−75	−76
−35	−52	−59	−64	−68	−71	−73	−76	−78	−79	−81	−82	−84
−40	−57	−66	−71	−74	−78	−80	−82	−84	−86	−88	−89	−91
−45	−63	−72	−77	−81	−84	−87	−89	−91	−93	−95	−97	−98

Temperature (°F)

Frostbite occurs in 15 minutes or less.

Windchill (°F) = $35.74 + 0.6215T − 35.75(V0.16) + 0.4275T(V0.16)$

where
T = Air Temperature (°F)
V = Wind Speed (mph)
Adapted from National Oceanic and Atmospheric Administration. Meteorological tables. Available at: www.erh.noaa.gov.

BOX 34-13   RISK FACTORS FOR COLD INJURY AND HYPOTHERMIA

- Exercising in water and rain significantly increases the risk for developing hypothermia.
- Individuals with lower combined values of subcutaneous fat thickness, % fat, and muscle mass may not maintain core temperature appropriately.
- Older individuals (>60 yr) are at an increased risk of hypothermia because of blunted physiologic and behavioral responses to cold.
- Children are at a greater risk of hypothermia than adults because of differences in body composition and anthropometry.

- Hypoglycemia impairs shivering and increases the risk for hypothermia.
- Winter athletes have a higher incidence of exercise-induced bronchospasm than the general population.
- Patients with coronary artery disease are at increased risk because of hemodynamic changes from cold stress.

loss from the respiratory passages can lead to dehydration during exercise on cold days (51). Inspired ambient air temperature generally does not pose a danger to the respiratory tract tissues. However, in some cases, cold air inhalation may exacerbate asthma symptoms or result in chest pain in those with coronary artery disease. The use of a scarf or mask to allow heating and humidifying of inspired cold air may help in these situations. But avoidance of cold air during exercise for these vulnerable individuals is always best.

The early warning signs of peripheral cold injury include tingling and numbness in the fingers and toes or a burning sensation in the nose and ears (10). Effects of cold on body function and local injury include:

1. Systemic hypothermia (both core and shell temperatures decrease)
   - Slowing of body functions
   - Cardiac arrhythmias
   - Cardiac arrest and possible death at very low core body temperatures
2. Local injury (core temperature is maintained, but shell [skin] temperature is decreased)
   - Frostnip: Mild cold injury resulting in reversible blanching of the skin
   - Chilblain: Mild cold injury marked by localized redness, burning, and swelling on exposed body parts
   - Frostbite: Severe tissue and cell damage caused by freezing a body part

The principles of care for cold injuries are to prevent further heat loss, rewarm as quickly as possible, and watch for complications. Specific prevention strategies include:

- Practice prevention through preparation (length of exposure, anticipating weather changes).
- Layer clothing properly.
- Have dry clothing available, if possible.
- Avoid overdressing (excessive sweating and poor evaporation of sweat can promote heat loss in the cold).
- Recognize individual's susceptible to cold injury.
- Be able to recognize the signs and symptoms of hypothermia, frost bite, and cold injury.

Altitude

Acute exercise or sports competition at high altitude is associated with performance impairment of about 1% for every 100 m above 1,500 m for nonathletic individuals. The lower barometric pressure of high altitude results in lower partial pressures of oxygen, which limits pulmonary diffusion and oxygen transport in the tissues (51). Hyperventilation and increased submaximal cardiac output via elevated HR are the primary immediate responses to altitude exposure.

Clinical problems associated with exercise at high altitude can include increased susceptibility to cold-related disorders and dehydration caused by colder and dryer air temperature as altitude increases. In addition, because the atmosphere is thinner and drier, solar radiation is more intense. Those with cardiac or pulmonary limitations with oxygen exchange at the lungs or transport to tissue may have a difficult time at altitude. Patients with CAD may precipitate indicators of ischemia at lower activity intensities at altitude than at sea level. If a person has obstructive pulmonary disease, he or she may experience hypoxemia as a result of the low oxygen partial pressures. Both of these types of patients should be advised to not exercise at altitude and may benefit also from not living at altitude. If exercise is performed at altitude, it should be of low intensity, and those with pulmonary limitations may require supplemental oxygen if their hemoglobin saturation falls below 88%.

Three medical problems resulting from exercising at moderate to high altitudes include (51):

1. Acute mountain sickness (headache, dyspnea on exertion, lightheadedness, fatigue, nausea, difficulty sleeping)
2. High-altitude pulmonary edema (severe fatigue and weakness, dyspnea, and cough)
3. High-altitude cerebral edema (severe headaches, nausea, vomiting, impaired mental processing, ataxia, and ashen skin color)

Exercise considerations when exercising at altitude include that:

- The length of time required for altitude acclimatization increases as altitude increases.
- Observable improvements in exercise tolerance occur within 5 to 7 days of initial altitude exposure. Full adaptations require about 2 weeks, although acclimatization to relatively high altitudes may require 4 to 6 weeks. Individuals with cardiac or pulmonary disease may require additional acclimation time, and those with severe disease may never fully acclimate.
- Aerobic and endurance-related exercise capacity is reduced because acclimatization does not fully compensate for reduced partial pressure of oxygen at altitude for any individual.

Pollution

The U.S. Environmental Protection Agency (EPA) is responsible for informing and alerting the general population about air quality (76). The EPA uses the **air quality index (AQI)** for five major pollutants: ground-level ozone, particulate matter, carbon monoxide, sulfur dioxide, and nitrogen dioxide. For each of these pollutants, the EPA has established national air quality standards to protect against harmful health effects. AQI levels can vary, depending on the time of day or from one season to the next. Table 34-7 provides a health advisory statement for the major pollutants and guidelines to follow that protect health and prevent unsafe exercise participation (74). As for altitude, patients with cardiac and pulmonary disease may be more adversely affected by pollutants than

TABLE 34-7. AIR QUALITY INDEX[a]

INDEX VALUES	LEVELS OF HEALTH CONCERN	HEALTH ADVISORY: OZONE	HEALTH ADVISORY: PM$_{2.5}$	HEALTH ADVISORY: CO	HEALTH ADVISORY: SO$_2$	HEALTH ADVISORY: NO$_2$
0–50	Good	None	None	None	None	None
51–100	Moderate	Unusually sensitive people should limit prolonged outdoor exertion	None	None	None	None
101–150	Unhealthy for sensitive groups	Active children and adults and people with respiratory disease such as asthma	None	People with CVD (e.g., such as angina) should limit heavy exertion and avoid sources of CO (e.g., heavy traffic)	People with asthma should consider limiting outdoor exertion.	None
151–200	Unhealthy	Active children and adults and people with respiratory disease (e.g., asthma; everyone else, especially children, should avoid prolonged outdoor exertion.	People with respiratory or heart disease, the elderly, and children should avoid prolonged exertion; everyone else should limit prolonged exertion.	People with CVD (e.g., angina) should limit moderate exertion and sources of CO, such as heavy traffic.	Children, asthmatics, and people with heart or lung disease should limit outdoor exertion.	None
201–300	Very unhealthy	Active children and adults and people with respiratory disease (e.g., asthma) should avoid all outdoor exertion; everyone else should limit outdoor exertion.	People with respiratory or heart disease, the elderly, and children should avoid any outdoor activity; everyone else should avoid prolonged exertion.	People with CVD (e.g., angina) should avoid exertion and sources of CO (e.g., heavy traffic).	Children, asthmatics, and people with heart or lung disease should avoid outdoor exertion; everyone else should limit outdoor exertion.	Children and people with respiratory disease (e.g., asthma) should limit heavy outdoor exertion.
301–500	Hazardous	Everyone should avoid all outdoor exertion.	Everyone should avoid any outdoor exertion; people with respiratory or heart disease, the elderly, and children should remain indoors.	People with CVD (e.g., angina) should avoid exertion and sources of CO (e.g., heavy traffic); everyone else should limit heavy exertion.	Children, asthmatics, and people with heart or lung disease should remain indoors; everyone else should avoid outdoor exertion.	Children and people with respiratory disease (e.g., asthma) should limit moderate and heavy outdoor exertion.

CVD, cardiovascular disease.

[a]Pollutants: ground-level ozone, particulate matter (PM$_{2.5}$), carbon monoxide (CO), sulfur dioxide (SO$_2$), and nitrogen dioxide (NO$_2$).

Adapted from the United States Environmental Protection Agency. EPA-454/K-03-002, August 2003. Available at: www.airnow.gov/.

healthy individuals. Avoiding outdoor exercise on ozone action/alert days is prudent in these instances.

SUMMARY

Musculoskeletal injuries and underlying cardiopulmonary or metabolic diseases may complicate exercise participation. Adequate screening and evaluation are important to identify and counsel individuals with underlying contraindications before beginning exercise. Health and fitness facility personnel involved in the management or delivery of exercise programs must possess the knowledge to prevent, recognize, and provide treatment for exercise-related injuries and illnesses.

REFERENCES

1. Albert CM, Mittleman MA, Chae CU, et al. Triggering of sudden death from cardiac causes by vigorous exertion. *N Engl J Med.* 2000;343:1355–1361.

2. Almeida SA, Trone DW, Leone DM, et al. Gender differences in musculoskeletal injury rates: a function of symptom reporting? *Med Sci Sports Exerc.* 1999;31:1807–1812.

3. American Association of Cardiovascular and Pulmonary Rehabilitation. *Guidelines for Cardiac Rehabilitation and Secondary Prevention Programs.* 4th ed. Champaign (IL): Human Kinetics; 2004.

4. American College of Obstetricians and Gynecologists. Exercise during pregnancy and the postpartum period. ACOG Committee Opinion No. 267. *Obstet Gynecol.* 2002;99:171–173.

5. American College of Sports Medicine. Recommended quantity and quality of exercise for developing and maintaining cardiorespiratory and muscular fitness, and flexibility in healthy adults. *Med Sci Sports Exerc.* 1998;30:975–991.

6. American College of Sports Medicine. *Guidelines for Exercise Testing and Prescription.* Philadelphia: Lippincott Williams and Wilkins; 2008.

7. American College of Sports Medicine. Heat and cold illnesses during distance running. *Med Sci Sports Exerc.* 1996;28:I–X.

8. American Diabetes Association. Diagnosis and classification of diabetes mellitus. *Diabetes Care.* 2006;29:S43–S48.

9. American Diabetes Association. Physical activity/exercise and diabetes. *Diabetes Care.* 2004;27:S58–S62.

10. American Red Cross. Community first aid and safety. Manasha (WI): Banta Printing; 2000.

11. Andrews JR. Overuse syndromes of the lower extremity. *Clin Sports Med.* 1983;2:137–148.

12. Arendt EA. Common musculoskeletal injuries in women. *Phys Sports Med.* 1996;7:39–48.

13. Artal R, O'Toole M. Guidelines of the American College of Obstetricians and Gynecologists for exercise during pregnancy and the postpartum period. *Br J Sports Med.* 2003;37:6–12.

14. Balady GJ, Chaitman B, Driscoll D, et al. American Heart Association/American College of Sports Medicine Joint Scientific Statement: Recommendations for cardiovascular screening, staffing, and emergency policies at health/fitness facilities. *Med Sci Sports Exerc.* 1998;30:1009–1018.

15. Barnard RJ, Gardner GW, Diaco NV, et al. Cardiovascular responses to sudden strenuous exercise: heart rate, blood pressure and EKG. *J Appl Physiol.* 1973;34:833–837.

16. Barnard RJ, MacAlpin R, Katus AA, et al. Ischemic response to sudden strenuous exercise in healthy men. *Circulation.* 1973;48:936–942.

17. Binkley HM, Beckett J, Casa DJ, et al. National Athletic Trainers' Association Position Statement: Exertional heat illnesses. *J Athl Train.* 2002;37:329–343.

18. Brar SP, Smith MB, Nelson LM, Franklin GM, Cobble ND. Evaluation of treatment protocols on minimal to moderate spasticity in multiple sclerosis. *Arch Phys Med Rehabil.* 1991;72:186–189.

19. Bruin G, Kuipers H, Keizer HA, Vander Vusse GJ. Adaptation and overtraining in horses subjected to increasing training loads. *J Appl Physiol.* 1994;76:1908–1913.

20. Carpenter DM, Nelson BW. Low back strengthening for the prevention and treatment of low back pain. *Med Sci Sports Exerc.* 1999;31:18–24.

21. Casa DJ, Armstrong LE, Hillman SK, et al. National Athletic Trainers' Association Position Statement: Fluid replacement for athletes. *J Athl Train.* 2000;35:212–224.

22. Castellani JW, Young AJ, Ducharme MB, Giesbrecht GG, Glickman E, Sallis RE. American College of Sports Medicine Position Stand: Prevention of cold injuries during exercise. *Med Sci Sports Exerc.* 2006;38(11):2012–2029.

23. Celli BR. Pathophysiology of chronic obstructive pulmonary disease. In: Hodgkins JE, Celli BR, Conners GL, editors. *Pulmonary Rehabilitation: Guidelines to Success.* 3rd ed. Philadelphia: Lippincott, Williams & Wilkins; 2000. p. 41–55.

24. Colbert LH, Hootman JM, Macera CA. Physical activity-related injuries in walkers and runners in the aerobics center longitudinal study. *Clin J Sports Med.* 2000;10:259–263.

25. Cui J, Arbab-Zadeh A, Prasad A, Durand S, Levine BD, Crandall CG. Effects of heat stress on thermoregulatory responses in congestive heart failure patients. *Circulation.* 2005;112:2286–2292.

26. Cummins RO, ed. *ACLS Provider Manual.* Dallas: American Heart Association; 2001.

27. Davies GA, Wolfe LA, Mottola MF, MacKinnon C. Society of Obstetricians and Gynecologists of Canada, SOGC Clinical Practice Obstetrics Committee. Joint SOGC/CSEP Clinical Practice Guideline: Exercise in pregnancy and the postpartum period. *Can J Appl Physiol.* 2003;28:330–341.

28. Dempsey FC, Butler FL, Williams FA. No need for a pregnant pause: physical activity may reduce the occurrence of gestational diabetes mellitus and preeclampsia. *Exerc Sports Sci Rev.* 2005; 3:141–149.

29. Dimsdale JE, Hartly H, Guiney T, et al. Postexercise peril: plasma catecholamines and exercise. *JAMA.* 1984;251:630–632.

30. Durstine JL, Moore GE, eds. *ACSM's Exercise Management for Persons with Chronic Diseases and Disabilities.* 2nd ed. Champaign (IL): Human Kinetics; 2003.

31. Ettinger WH, Burns R, Messier SP, et al. A randomized trial comparing aerobic exercise and resistance exercise with a health education program in older adults with knee osteoarthritis: the Fitness Arthritis and Seniors Trial (FAST). *JAMA.* 1997;277:25–31.

32. Felson DT, Zhang Y, Anthony JM, et al. Weight loss reduces the risk for symptomatic knee osteoarthritis in women. *Ann Intern Med.* 1992;116:535–539.

33. Felson DT, Zhang Y, Hannan MT, et al. Risk factors for incident radiographic knee osteoarthritis in the elderly: the Framingham Study. *Arthritis Rheum.* 1997;40:728–733.

34. Feskanich D, Willett W, Colditz G. Walking and leisure-time activity and risk of hip fracture in postmenopausal women. *JAMA.* 2002;288(18):2300–2306.

35. Fry AC, Kraemer WJ. Resistance exercise overtraining and overreaching. *Sports Med.* 1997;23:106–129.

36. Garrick JG, Gillien DM, Whiteside P. The epidemiology of aerobic dance injuries. *Am J Sports Med.* 1986;14:67–72.

37. Gibbons RJ, Balady GJ, Bricker J, et al. ACC/AHA 2002 guideline update for exercise testing: a report of the American College of Cardiology/American Heart Association Task Force on Practice Guidelines (Committee on Exercise Testing). 2002. Available at: hwww.acc.org/qualityandscience/clinical/statements.htm.

38. Heistaro SE, Vartiainen E, Heliovaara M, et al. Trends in back pain in eastern Finland, 1972–1992, in relation to socioeconomic status and behavioral risk factors. *Am J Epidemiol.* 1998;148:671–682.

39. Hootman JM, Macera CA, Ainsworth BE, et al. Association among physical activity level, cardiorespiratory fitness, and risk of musculoskeletal injury. *Am J Epidemiol.* 2001;154:251–258.

40. Jones CS, Christensen C, Young M. Weight training injury trends: a 20-year survey. *Phys Sports Med.* 2000;28:61–72.

41. Kaufman KR, Brodine S, Shaffer R. Military training-related injuries: surveillance, research, and prevention. *Am J Prev Med.* 2000;18:54–63.

42. Kesaniemi YK, Danforth E Jr, Jensen MD, Kopelman PG, Lefebvre P, Reeder BA. Dose-response issues concerning physical activity and health: an evidence-based symposium. *Med Sci Sports Exerc.* 2001; 33(6 Suppl):S351–S358.

43. Kopland JP, Rothenberg RB, Jones EL. The natural history of exercise: a 10-yr follow-up of a cohort of runners. *Med Sci Sports Exerc.* 1995;27:1180–1184.

44. Kreider RB, Fry AC, O'Toole ML, eds. *Overtraining in Sport.* Champaign (IL): Human Kinetics; 1998.

45. Lane NE. Physical activity at leisure and risk of osteoarthritis. *Ann Rheum Dis.* 1996;55:682–684.

46. Lee IM, Rexrode KM, Cook NR, Manson JE, Buring JE. Physical activity and coronary heart disease in women: is "no pain, no gain" passe? *JAMA*. 2001;285(11):1447–1454.

47. Leitzmann MF, Rimm EB, Willett WC, et al. Recreational physical activity and the risk of cholecystectomy in women. *N Engl J Med*. 1999;341(11):777–784.

48. Lewis SF, Nylander E, Gad P, Areskog NH. Non-autonomic component in bradycardia of endurance trained men at rest and during exercise. *Acta Physiol Scand*. 1980;109(3):297–305.

49. Manson JE, Greenland P, LaCroix AZ, et al. Walking compared with vigorous exercise for the prevention of cardiovascular events in women. *N Engl J Med*. 2002;347(10):716–725.

50. Marron BJ, Shirani J, Poliac LC, et al. Sudden death in young competitive athletes. *JAMA*. 1996;276:199–204.

51. Mcardle WD, Katch FI, Katch VL. *Exercise Physiology: Energy, Nutrition, and Human Performance*. 5th ed. Philadelphia: Lippincott Williams & Wilkins; 2001.

52. Mottola MF, Davenport MH, Brun CR, Inglis SD, Charlesworth S, Sopper MM. VO$_{2max}$ prediction and exercise prescription for pregnant women. *Med Sci Sports Exerc*. 2006;38:1389–1395.

53. Mutoh Y, Sawai S, Takanashi Y, et al. Aerobic dance injuries among instructors and students. *Phys Sports Med*. 1988;16:81–88.

54. National Oceanic and Atmospheric Administration. Meteorological tables. Available at: www.erh.noaa.gov.

55. Nieman DC. *Exercise Testing and Prescription*. 5th ed. Boston: McGraw Hill; 2003.

56. Paffenbarger RS Jr, Hyde RT, Wing AL, Lee IM, Jung DL, Kampert JB. The association of changes in physical-activity level and other lifestyle characteristics with mortality among men. *N Engl J Med*. 1993;328(8):538–545.

57. **Pescatello LS, Franklin BA, Fagard R, Farquhar WB, Kelley GA, Ray CA. American College of Sports Medicine position stand. Exercise and hypertension. *Med Sci Sports Exerc*. 2004;36(3):533–553.**

58. Powell KE, Heath GW, Kresnow M-J, et al. Injury rates from walking, gardening, weightlifting, outdoor bicycling, and aerobics. *Med Sci Sports Exerc*. 1998;30:1246–1249.

59. Powell KE, Kohl HW, Caspersen CJ, et al. An epidemiologic perspective on the causes of running injuries. *Phys Sports Med*. 1986; 14:100–114.

60. Powell KE, Thompson PD, Caspersen CJ, Kendrick JS. Physical activity and the incidence of coronary heart disease. *Annu Rev Public Health*. 1987;8:253–287.

61. Prentice WE. *Arnheim's Principles of Athletic Training*. 11th ed. Boston: McGraw Hill; 2003.

62. Raglin J, Audrius B, editors. Overtraining in athletes: the challenge of prevention. A Consensus Statement. *ACSM's Health & Fitness Journal*. 1999;3:27–31.

63. Reeves RK, Laskowski ER, Smith J. Weight training injuries. Part 2: Diagnosing and managing chronic conditions. *Phys Sports Med*. 1998;26:54–63.

64. Renstrom P, editor. *The Encyclopedia of Sports Medicine: Sports Injuries*. Oxford: Blackwell Scientific Publications; 1993.

65. Renstrom P, Kannus P. Prevention of sports injuries. In: Strauss RH, editor. *Sports Medicine*. Philadelphia: WB Saunders; 1992.

66. Requa RK, De Avilla LN, Garrick JG. Injuries in recreational adult fitness activities. *Am J Sports Med*. 1993;21:461–467.

67. Richie DH, Kelso SF, Bellucci PA. Aerobic dance injuries: a retrospective study of instructors and participants. *Phys Sports Med*. 1985;13:130–140.

68. Rockhill B, Willett WC, Manson JE, et al. Physical activity and mortality: a prospective study among women. *Am J Public Health*. 2001;91(4):578–583.

69. Schenck RC, editor. American Academy of Orthopaedic Surgeons. *Athletic Training and Sports Medicine*. 3rd ed. Park Ridge (IL): American Academy of Orthopaedic Surgeons; 1999.

70. Shephard RJ, Astrand PO, eds. *The Encyclopedia of Sports Medicine: Endurance in Sport*. Oxford: Blackwell Scientific Publications; 1992.

71. Soukup JT, Maynard TS, Kovaleski JE. Resistance training guidelines for individuals with diabetes mellitus. *Diabetes Educ*. 1994; 20:129–137.

72. Tanasescu M, Leitzmann MF, Rimm EB, Willett WC, Stampfer MJ, Hu FB. Exercise type and intensity in relation to coronary heart disease in men. *JAMA*. 2002;288(16):1994–2000.

73. **United States Department of Health and Human Services. Physical activity and health: a report of the Surgeon General. Atlanta: US DHHS, Centers for Disease Control and Prevention, National Center for Chronic Disease Prevention and Health Promotion; 1996.**

74. **United States Environmental Protection Agency. EPA-454/K-03-002, August 2003. Available at: www.airnow.gov/.**

75. **United States Department of Health and Human Services. Physical Activity and Health: A Report of the Surgeon General. Atlanta: US DHHS, Centers for Disease Control and Prevention, National Center for Chronic Disease Prevention and Health Promotion; 1996.**

76. Van Camp SP, Bloor CM, Mueller FU, et al. Nontraumatic sports deaths in high school and college athletes. *Med Sci Sports Exerc*. 1995;27:641–647.

77. **Wenger NK, Froelicher ES, Smith LK, et al. Cardiac rehabilitation as secondary prevention. Agency for Health Care Policy and Research and National Heart, Lung, and Blood Institute. *Clin Pract Guidel Quick Ref Guide Clin*. 1995;17:1–23.**

78. **Williams MA, Haskell WL, Ades PA, et al. Resistance exercise in individuals with and without cardiovascular disease: 2007 update: a scientific statement from the American Heart Association Council on Clinical Cardiology and Council on Nutrition, Physical Activity, and Metabolism. *Circulation*. 2007;116(5):572–584.**

79. Williams PT. Physical fitness and activity as separate heart disease risk factors: a meta-analysis. *Med Sci Sports Exerc*. 2001;33(5): 754–761.

80. Wisloff U, Asbjom S, Loennechen JP, et al. Superior cardiovascular effect of aerobic interval training versus moderate continuous training in heart failure patients: a randomized study. *Circulation*. 2007; 115(24):3086–3094.

81. Yu S, Yarnell JW, Sweetnam PM, Murray L. What level of physical activity protects against premature cardiovascular death? The Caerphilly study. *Heart*. 2003;89(5):502–506.

SELECTED REFERENCES FOR FURTHER READING

American Association of Cardiovascular and Pulmonary Rehabilitation. *Guidelines for Pulmonary Rehabilitation and Programs*. 3rd ed. Champaign (IL): Human Kinetics; 2004.

Armstrong LE, Casa DJ, Millard-Stafford M, Moran DS, Pyne SW, Roberts WO. American College of Sports Medicine position stand. Exertional heat illness during training and competition. *Med Sci Sports Exerc*. 2007;39(3):556–572.

Castellani JW, Young AJ, Ducharme MB, Giesbrecht GG, Glickman E, Sallis RE. American College of Sports Medicine Position Stand: Prevention of cold injuries during exercise. *Med Sci Sports Exerc*. 2006;38(11):2012–2029.

Fletcher GF, Balady GJ, Amsterdam EA, et al. Exercise standards for testing and training. American Heart Association Scientific Statement. *Circulation*. 2001;104:1644–1740.

Pescatello LS, Franklin BA, Fagard R, Farquhar WB, Kelley GA, Ray CA. American College of Sports Medicine position stand. Exercise and hypertension. *Med Sci Sports Exerc*. 2004;36(3):533–553.

INTERNET RESOURCES

- American Academy of Orthopaedic Surgeons: www.aaos.org
- American Heart Association: www.americanheart.org
- American Red Cross: www.redcross.org
- National Athletic Trainers' Association: www.nata.org
- National Safety Council: www.nsc.org
- Occupational Safety and Health Administration: www.osha.gov

Exercise Prescription in Patients with Cardiovascular Disease

Current public health recommendations state that all healthy adults aged 18 to 65 years need moderate-intensity activity for a minimum of 30 minutes on 5 days each week or vigorous-intensity aerobic activity for a minimum of 20 minutes on 3 days each week (50,108). In addition, adults should include resistance training involving the major muscle groups at least 2 days per week (112). Exercise is also recommended for the elderly (79), those with chronic disease (79), patients with heart disease, and those at risk for developing heart disease (6,70). Similar to other patients at increased risk who plan to participate in an exercise program, it is recommended that a physician or midlevel provider first evaluate the individual to determine if he or she can exercise safely (42).

DISEASE-SPECIFIC EFFECTS ON PHYSIOLOGIC RESPONSES AND FITNESS

Patients with cardiovascular disease may demonstrate a normal or abnormal cardiovascular response during a single bout of exercise, depending on the severity of disease and other factors (Table 35-1), (60,61). Normal and abnormal cardiovascular responses are discussed below.

HEART RATE

> **1.3.23-CES:** Describe the normal and abnormal chronotropic and inotropic responses to exercise testing and training.

> **1.5.2-CES:** Describe mechanisms and actions of medications that may affect exercise testing and prescription (i.e., β-blockers, nitrates, calcium channel blockers, digitalis, diuretics, vasodilators, antiarrhythmic agents, bronchodilators, antilipemics, psychotropics, nicotine, antihistamines, over-the-counter (OTC) cold medications, thyroid medications, alcohol, hypoglycemic agents, blood modifiers, pentoxifylline, antigout medications, and anorexiants/diet pills).

A normal response to maximal exercise testing involves the patient achieving a heart rate (HR) that is within two standard deviations of an age-predicted maximum value, then decreasing back to baseline fairly quickly during recovery (22,38). Failure to achieve 85% of the predicted maximum HR, in the absence of β-adrenergic blocking agents or other medications that affect the chronotropic response, is termed **chronotropic incompetence**. This finding during exercise, even as an isolated anomaly, is predictive of the presence of coronary artery disease (CAD) and is associated with increased risk of morbidity and

> > > KEY TERMS

Angina: Chest pain, pressure, discomfort, or fullness that occurs as a result of coronary artery stenosis, which prevents an increased blood flow and oxygen delivery to the myocardium during exercise, creating a temporary mismatch between oxygen delivery and oxygen demand. The chest pain resolves with rest.

Chronotropic incompetence: An attenuated heart rate response to exercise; failure to achieve a heart rate that is ≥85% or within two standard deviations of the age-predicted maximum.

Heart failure: Condition created by disease or injury in which myocardial contraction/relaxation function

is abnormal to the extent that the heart is no longer able to pump blood at a rate commensurate with the requirement of metabolizing tissues.

Ischemic cascade: The temporal sequence of cellular, hemodynamic, electrocardiographic, and symptomatic expressions occurring during ischemia.

Rate–pressure product: Surrogate of myocardial oxygen consumption, computed as the product of heart rate and systolic blood pressure.

TABLE 35-1. COMPARISON OF PEAK ARM AND LEG RESPONSES IN HEALTHY SUBJECTS AND THOSE WITH HEART FAILURE AND CARDIAC TRANSPLANT

	PEAK HR ($b \cdot min^{-1}$)	OXYGEN CONSUMPTION ($L \cdot min^{-1}$)	RATE PRESSURE PRODUCT $\times 10^3$ ($b \cdot mm\,Hg \cdot min^{-1}$)
Healthy			
Arm	140 ± 13	1.50 ± 0.38	28.5 ± 3.9
Leg	162 ± 45	2.28 ± 0.150	32.5 ± 4.5
Heart failure			
Arm	128 ± 17	1.08 ± 0.22	20.5 ± 5.2
Leg	144 ± 14	1.48 ± 0.30	24.1 ± 4.0
Transplant			
Arm	135 ± 4	1.15 ± 0.07	24.8 ± 2.0
Leg	145 ± 4	1.60 ± 0.09	27.8 ± 1.9

HR, heart rate.

Rate pressure product = peak HR × peak systolic blood pressure.

Adapted from Keteyian SJ, Marks CRC, Brawner CA, et al. Responses to arm exercise in patients with compensated heart failure. *J Cardiopulm Rehabil.* 1996;16:366–371. Keteyian S, Marks CRC, Levine AB, et al. Cardiovascular responses of cardiac transplant patients to arm and leg exercise. *Eur J Appl Physiol.* 1994;68:441–444.

mortality (22,69). After exercise, increased parasympathetic tone causes the HR to decrease fairly quickly. Measurement of the HR at 1 or 2 minutes into recovery and comparing these rates with peak HR is termed *HR recovery*. Abnormal HR recovery, defined as a decrease in HR of <12 bpm at 1 minute while walking and <22 bpm at 2 minutes if supine, predicts future cardiac mortality (30).

BLOOD PRESSURE

Because of a reduction in systemic vascular resistance in the metabolically more active muscles during exercise, the normal diastolic blood pressure (BP) response is to remain constant or decrease slightly during exercise. Conversely, the normal response of systolic BP during incremental exercise is to increase progressively by about 10 ± 2 mm Hg·MET^{-1} (metabolic equivalent), with a plateau at peak exercise. In patients with CAD, systolic BP during exercise may respond normally or may disproportionately increase or inappropriately decrease. Exertional hypertension during an exercise test is defined as a systolic BP of >250 mm Hg or diastolic BP >115 mm Hg. Exertional hypotension is defined as a decrease of systolic BP below resting BP of ≥10 mm Hg during exercise. In the absence of BP-lowering or after-load–reducing medications such as β-adrenergic blocking agents and angiotensin II–converting enzyme inhibitors, a failure of systolic BP to increase with exercise is considered an abnormal systolic BP response to exercise (42). Exertional systolic hypotension or hypertension are both associated with an increased risk of cardiac events (31,55), and although an increase in diastolic BP of 10 mm Hg or more may also be associated with CAD, it is more often a marker for future hypertension (37,99,113).

CARDIAC OUTPUT AND OXYGEN UPTAKE

Peak $\dot{V}O_2$ in healthy, active individuals typically is between 30 and 45 mL·kg^{-1}·min^{-1}. In patients with CAD,

however, the increase in peak $\dot{V}O_2$ may be reduced (6). In a two-site study involving more than 2,800 patients, Ades et al. showed that mean exercise capacity as measured by peak $\dot{V}O_2$> was 19.3 ± 6.1 mL·kg^{-1}·min^{-1} for men with CAD and 14.5 ± 3.9 mL·kg^{-1}·min^{-1} for women with CAD (1). In general, this reduction in peak $\dot{V}O_2$ in patients with cardiovascular disease often exceeds 20% or more when compared with age-matched, healthy persons. The magnitude of reduction in peak $\dot{V}O_2$ varies in part with the severity of the heart disease in that $\dot{V}O_2$ below the twentieth percentile for age and sex is associated with increased risk of death from all causes.

A patient's reduced ability to transport and use oxygen is primarily caused by a diminished cardiac output, a reduced peak blood flow within the peripheral musculature, and peripheral skeletal muscle cellular abnormalities that effect oxygen utilization and energy production. Cardiac output (HR × stroke volume) during exercise may be reduced because of either chronotropic incompetence or left ventricular dysfunction secondary to prior myocardial infarction (MI), transient coronary ischemia, or a nonischemic cardiomyopathy that results in a reduced ejection fraction and stroke volume (26). With exercise training, $\dot{V}O_2$ can be increased approximately 15% to 30% in sedentary patients, as well as in those with heart disease (45,48,106).

SCIENTIFIC AND PHYSIOLOGIC RATIONALE FOR EXERCISE THERAPY IN PATIENTS WITH HEART DISEASE

 1.2.1-HFS: Knowledge of the physiologic and metabolic responses to exercise associated with chronic disease (heart disease, hypertension, diabetes mellitus, and pulmonary disease).

 1.2.2-CES: Compare and contrast the differences between typical, atypical, and vasospastic angina and how these may differ in specific subgroups (i.e., men, women, diabetes).

> **1.2.11-CES: Describe the cardiorespiratory and metabolic responses in myocardial dysfunction and ischemia at rest and during exercise.**

Typical symptoms associated with heart disease are **angina**, dyspnea on exertion, orthopnea, peripheral edema, palpitations, dizziness, and syncope. These symptoms can be experienced individually or in combination. Symptoms, other than chest pain, that occur with physical activity may be considered as an anginal equivalent. Control of symptoms is of paramount importance in the treatment of patients with heart disease and an important reason for referral to a cardiac rehabilitation program.

The development of angina represents the cumulative impact of a sequence of pathophysiologic events referred to as the **ischemic cascade** (52,80). The ischemic cascade has been studied during percutaneous transluminal coronary angioplasty, atrial pacing, and exercise testing. It begins with the imbalance between myocardial oxygen supply and demand and produces an ischemic event that causes initial cellular abnormalities leading to abnormalities in diastolic function, with subsequent abnormalities in systolic function. Next, electrocardiographic (ECG) changes, such as ST-segment depression, occur, and, finally, the patient may or may not experience angina. After the myocardial oxygen supply and demand imbalance is corrected at the cellular level, the process is reversed: Angina resolves first, then the ECG changes, followed by improvement in systolic function and finally normalization of diastolic dysfunction.

Berger et al. (14) found that although hemodynamic abnormalities were seen in nearly all patients with CAD studied during ischemia, radionuclide evidence of global or regional wall motion abnormalities were only noted in 80% of patients, and ECG and symptomatic evidence of ischemia occurred in only 50% and 30% of patients, respectively. Thus, it is of fundamental importance to understand that although ischemia results in abnormalities of diastolic and systolic function in the majority of patients, ECG changes and angina are seen less frequently. Finally, some patients—such as those with diabetes or who have undergone cardiac transplant—experience ST-segment depression without angina (i.e., silent ischemia), whereas others may experience angina without ST-segment depression.

MYOCARDIAL OXYGEN DEMAND

Physiologic variables that increase myocardial oxygen demand are increasing HR, increasing left ventricular preload, and increasing myocardial contractility. At rest and during exercise, myocardial oxygen consumption can be reliably estimated by the product of HR and systolic BP. This is called the **rate–pressure product** (aka *double prod-*

uct). The normal maximal exercise response results in a rate–pressure product of 25,000 or higher (109).

> **1.1.11-CES: Knowledge of acute and chronic adaptations to exercise for those with cardiovascular, pulmonary, and metabolic diseases.**

> **1.5.2-CES: Describe mechanisms and actions of medications that may affect exercise testing and prescription (i.e., β-blockers, nitrates, calcium channel blockers, digitalis, diuretics, vasodilators, antiarrhythmic agents, bronchodilators, antilipemics, psychotropics, nicotine, antihistamines, OTC cold medications, thyroid medications, alcohol, hypoglycemic agents, blood modifiers, pentoxifylline, antigout medications, and anorexiants/diet pills).**

> **1.5.3-CES: Recognize medications associated in clinical setting, their indications for care, and their effects at rest and during exercise (i.e., β-blockers, nitrates, calcium channel blockers, digitalis, diuretics, vasodilators, antiarrhythmic agents, bronchodilators, antilipemics, psychotropics, nicotine, antihistamines, OTC cold medications, thyroid medications, alcohol, hypoglycemic agents, blood modifiers, pentoxifylline, antigout medications, and anorexiants/diet pills).**

For patients with CAD and angina symptoms, the rate–pressure product is generally a reproducible indicator of the myocardial oxygen demand at which angina initially occurs (i.e., the angina threshold). This is important when treating patients with CAD. For example, consider the patient who undertakes a graded exercise test (GXT), walks for 6 minutes, and stops because of angina at a rate pressure product of 193 (HR of 140 bpm times systolic BP of 138 mm Hg divided by 1,000). After the test, this patient's doctor prescribes a β-adrenergic blocking agent (i.e., β-blocker) as a means to attenuate the increases in both HR and systolic BP during exercise. After 1 month of taking this medication, a repeat test is conducted and reveals a longer total exercise time of 7.2 minutes, a lower peak rate pressure product of 156 (HR of 120 bpm times systolic BP of 130 mm Hg divided by 1,000), an increased MET level, and the test is now stopped because of fatigue rather than angina. This means this patient can now exercise longer and do so symptom-free. And just like a β-blocker, regular exercise training also lowers HR and BP responses during submaximal exercise and also creates a rightward shift in the rate–pressure product (Fig. 35-1). This shift in the rate–pressure product curve demonstrates why a patient can engage in routine and leisure-time activities with fewer symptoms.

MYOCARDIAL OXYGEN SUPPLY

As mentioned, ischemia occurs as a result of an imbalance between myocardial oxygen supply and demand. To better appreciate the pathophysiology leading to angina

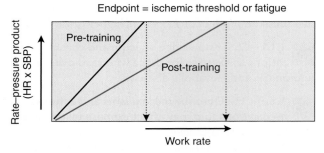

FIGURE 35-1. Regular exercise training attenuates myocardial O_2 demand during exercise, as estimated by the rate–pressure product. HR, heart rate; SBP, systolic blood pressure.

in patients with stable CAD, one must understand the four basic pathogenic factors that affect myocardial O_2 supply: coronary artery stenosis with endothelial dysfunction, microvascular dysfunction, abnormalities of the autonomic nervous system, and abnormalities of coagulation and fibrinolytic systems. This discussion focuses on the effects of how a chronic exercise program might contribute to ameliorating several of these components (Table 35-2).

Coronary artery stenosis influences myocardial oxygen supply and can be further divided into the components of plaque formation, collateral artery formation, and endothelial dysfunction. To date, three trials address the issue of whether a combined intervention of aggressive risk factor modification and exercise training is associated with a slowing of progression or regression of obstructive CAD (49,87). Although the individual effect of exercise, per se, was not isolated, the Stanford Coronary Risk Intervention Project (SCRIP) revealed that the mean rate of plaque progression in the combined risk factor modification and exercise training group was half that of patients in the usual care group (49).

Shuler et al. (100) also randomized patients with heart disease to either a combined risk factor modification plus exercise (n = 56) group or a usual care (n = 55) group. At 1 year, the intervention group demonstrated no change in the luminal diameter, but the usual care group had a significant decrease in luminal diameter of 0.13 ± 0.45 mm. Repeat angiography at 6 years continued to demonstrate significantly less progression in the intervention group. Interestingly, a poststudy subgroup analysis (100) aimed at isolating the direct effects of exercise in just those subjects in the intervention group revealed that those expending <1,000 kcal per week experienced the greatest amount of disease progression, subjects expending >1,400 kcal per week showed improved cardiopulmonary fitness, and subjects expending >1,500 kcal per week demonstrated the slowest rate of disease progression. In fact, partial regression of CAD was observed in patients training at an energy expenditure of 2,200 kcal or more per week.

Currently the evidence that exercise causes collateral blood vessel formation in humans is unclear and involves a limited number of trials that include small sample sizes. Belardinelli et al. (12) randomized 46 patients with chronic coronary artery disease and impaired left ventricular (LV) function into a group that exercised versus a nonexercising control group. The group that trained had significant improvement in contractile response to dobutamine and thallium activity. In a subgroup of trained patients, both improvements were correlated with an improvement in coronary collateral score, suggesting additional coronary collateral formation. However, Hambrecht et al. (46) and Niebauer et al. (81) assessed the combined effects of <3 hours of exercise per week and a low-fat diet on collateral formation in patients with CAD compared with patients receiving usual care. After 1 year, there was no significant difference between the groups with respect to coronary collateral formation.

TABLE 35-2. PATHOPHYSIOLOGIC EFFECTS OF EXERCISE AND EXERCISE TRAINING

PATHOPHYSIOLOGIC VARIABLE	ACUTE EXERCISE	CHRONIC EXERCISE TRAINING
Vascular		
Vascular stenosis	—	Partial regression ($>2,200$ kcal·wk^{-1})
Coronary collaterals	—	—
Endothelial dysfunction	—	↓
Capillary flow	—	↑
Autonomic nervous symptoms		
Parasympathetic	↓	↑
Sympathetic	↑	↓
Hemostatic		
Fibrinogen	↑	↓
Factor VII	—	—
Platelet aggregation	↑	↓
Fibrinolysis	↓	↑
Viscosity	↑	↓

↑, increase; ↓, decrease; —, no effect.

Abnormal endothelial function in patients with CAD was first described in 1986 by Ludmer et al (71). Whereas normal coronary arteries dilate in response to intracoronary acetylcholine, a paradoxical vasoconstriction is observed in patients with CAD or chronic **heart failure**, as well as those with multiple risk factors for CAD. Endothelial dysfunction is thought to result from a decreased production of nitric oxide within vascular smooth muscle cells. Using invasive techniques, Hambrecht et al. showed that regular exercise training partially normalizes endothelial dysfunction and improves myocardial blood flow (47).

ADDITIONAL PHYSIOLOGIC VARIABLES

During rest and exercise, the autonomic nervous system, through a complex interplay of the parasympathetic and sympathetic components, mediates changes in HR, BP, and vascular tone (i.e., systemic blood flow). Patients with previous MI (15,41) and patients with chronic heart failure (82,83) often have abnormalities of autonomic function at rest and during exercise, as manifested by decreased parasympathetic and increased sympathetic activity. This often manifests itself as an elevated resting HR and an attenuated peak exercise HR response.

Another measure of autonomic functions, the beat-to-beat (measured in milliseconds) variation in R-R intervals known as HR variability (HRV), serves as a surrogate assessment for parasympathetic activity. After an MI, mean values of all measures of HRV are attenuated by about one third, when compared with age- and sex-matched healthy control subjects. Mean values of HRV improve with time but never return to normal. The magnitude of the reduction reflects the amount of the myocardial damage. Even after making adjustments for abnormal LV function and ventricular ectopy, patients with attenuated parasympathetic activity manifested as a reduced HRV have a fivefold increase in mortality (63). Although much less precise, plasma norepinephrine represents yet another marker for sympathetic activity. Patients with heart failure often have elevated plasma (and urinary) norepinephrine levels at rest, with such elevations associated with worsening heart failure and representing a strong and independent predictor of future mortality (29).

Chronic exercise training partially reverses autonomic dysfunction in patients with cardiovascular disease. Among patients with chronic heart failure, Roveda et al. (95) showed a 33% decrease in muscle sympathetic nervous system activity with just 4 months of exercise training, returning muscle sympathetic nervous system activity back to levels similar to that in normal controls. Additionally, exercise trials involving patients recovering from an MI demonstrate significant improvement in HRV (75,107). Finally, exercise training results in decreased resting and exercise plasma norepinephrine levels in both MI patients and patients with heart failure (11,28,57,76).

Koenig (65) and Imhof and Koenig (54) describe the relationship between hemostatic components, cardiovascular disease (CVD) risk, and exercise. Abnormalities in the concentrations of hemostatic elements, such as fibrinogen, factor VII, and platelet hyperactivity, as well as fibrinolytic elements, such as tissue plasminogen activator, have been identified as cardiovascular risk factors (54,65,77,105). The viscosity of the blood is also important to coronary blood flow. The major determinants of blood viscosity are hematocrit and fibrinogen levels. Increased fibrinogen levels are associated with a twofold increase in the risk for cardiovascular events. Increased factor VII levels, platelet hyperactivity, and decreased tissue plasminogen activator levels have also been shown to be predictors of coronary events but to a lesser degree (23,51,115). Much, but not all, of the literature describes an inverse relationship for moderate- to high-intensity exercise training and fibrinogen levels. Whereas there is no evidence that factor VII levels are affected by acute exercise, endurance exercise increases activity in the fibrinolytic system. Long-term exercise training trials in patients with a history of an MI report reductions in erythrocyte rigidity, platelet aggregation, and adherence. Carroll et al. (23) and others (39,66) demonstrate an inverse relationship between hematologic parameters, such as plasma viscosity and hematocrit, and physical activity parameters, such as leisure-time physical activity and maximum oxygen consumption in patients with a history of MI. It is important to point out that most of the studies addressing the relationship between exercise and the level of hemostatic components involved individuals without known CAD.

MORBIDITY, MORTALITY, AND SAFETY OF CARDIAC REHABILITATION

The 1995 Agency for Heath Care Policy and Research (AHCPR) Clinical Practice Guidelines for Cardiac Rehabilitation (111) states that "total and cardiovascular mortality are reduced in patients following myocardial infarction who participate in cardiac rehabilitation exercise training, especially as a component of multifactorial rehabilitation." This statement is based primarily on two meta-analyses of randomized controlled trials of cardiac rehabilitation conducted in the late 1980s (85,86) that showed a 25% reduction in mortality at 3 years among patients participating in multifactorial cardiac rehabilitation. A review of the literature by AHCPR found no difference in the rate of nonfatal MIs between the cardiac rehabilitation group and the control population. A recent meta-analysis of trials, including those published during the past decade, confirmed that cardiac rehabilitation reduced all-cause mortality by approximately 25% without a reduction in nonfatal MI (104).

 1.7.19-CES: Describe the indications and methods for ECG monitoring during exercise testing and training.

The initial classification of cardiac rehabilitation into phases I, II, III, and IV is less used today. Instead, cardiac rehabilitation is now often thought of as a continuum of care including inpatient cardiac rehabilitation, early outpatient cardiac rehabilitation, and maintenance and follow-up cardiac rehabilitation (8). The goals of inpatient cardiac rehabilitation are to minimize the deconditioning that occurs as a result of bed rest during hospitalization and begin to educate the patient about risk-factor modification and the lifestyle changes necessary to reduce future mortality and morbidity. Today, inpatient cardiac rehabilitation is limited by the increasingly shortened hospital stays for the uncomplicated cardiac patient. Outpatient cardiac rehabilitation is separated into early outpatient and maintenance cardiac rehabilitation, with each phase differing based on extent of supervision and monitoring, subject independence, and time from the event (4). Outpatient cardiac rehabilitation aims include improving exercise performance and modifying cardiac risk factors meant to reduce future all-cause and cardiac mortality (4).

Nontraditional exercise programs are effective and safe in selected populations (111). DeBusk et al. (34), as well as others, have reported their experience with medically directed at-home rehabilitation after an uncomplicated MI. At 26 weeks, the adherence rate was 72% and 71% for home and group training, respectively. No training complications occurred in either group. When compared with usual care, the patients involved in home training demonstrated a significantly greater functional capacity. These findings support the concept that medically directed at-home rehabilitation has the potential to increase the availability and decrease the cost of exercise for low-risk survivors of acute MI.

The incidence of fatal and nonfatal cardiac events occurring during or shortly after a traditional cardiac rehabilitation exercise session is low. Fatal events occur at a rate of 1 in 900,000 patient hours of participation in supervised exercise training, with most events occurring in patients considered to be at high risk for cardiac events. The rate of nonfatal MI during cardiac rehabilitation is approximately 1 in 250,000 patient hours (104,111).

> **1.11.4-CES: Understand the most recent cardiac and pulmonary rehabilitation Centers for Medicare Services (CMS) rules for patient enrollment and reimbursement (e.g., diagnostic current procedure terminology [CPT] codes, diagnostic related groups [DRG]).**

Insurance reimbursement for cardiac rehabilitation has long been regulated by the Centers for Medicare Services (CMS). Before March 2006, the diagnoses covered for Medicare beneficiaries were stable angina with CAD, MI, and coronary artery bypass graft (CABG) surgery. More recently, CMS has added percutaneous coronary intervention (PCI), valve surgery, and heart transplant. Con-

gestive heart failure (CHF) has yet to be added; however, the results of the HF-Action Trial (Heart Failure—A Controlled Trial Investigating Outcomes of Exercise Training) was released in late 2008 and ultimately will help clarify the efficacy and role of exercise in the treatment of patients with heart failure.

EXERCISE PRESCRIPTION AND PROGRAMMING

> **1.7.4-CES: Design, implement, and supervise individualized exercise prescriptions for people with chronic disease and disabling conditions or who are young or elderly.**

> **1.7.5-CES: Design a supervised exercise program beginning at hospital discharge and continuing for up to 6 months for the following conditions: MI, angina; left ventricular assist device (LVAD); congestive heart failure, percutaneous coronary intervention (PCI); CABGs; medical management of CAD; chronic pulmonary disease; weight management; diabetes; metabolic syndrome; and cardiac transplants.**

> **1.7.40-HFS: Ability to explain and implement exercise prescription guidelines for apparently healthy patients, increased risk patients, and patients with controlled disease.**

> **1.7.41-HFS: Ability to adapt frequency, intensity, duration, mode, progression, level of supervision, and monitoring techniques in exercise programs for patients with controlled chronic disease (e.g., heart disease, diabetes mellitus, obesity, hypertension), musculoskeletal problems (including fatigue), pregnancy and/or postpartum, and exercise-induced asthma.**

Individuals with chronic illnesses such as MI, heart failure, and stroke have rates of sedentary behavior of 30% to 40%, exceeding the general population rate of 24% (24,33) (Table 35-3). The previously cited meta-analyses of secondary prevention in patients having previously suffered an MI (85,86,104), combined with data from primary prevention observational studies (18,88,89), provide strong evidence that exercise, whether measured as physical activity or physical fitness levels, reduces all-cause and cardiovascular mortality. In apparently healthy men at baseline, the Harvard Alumni Study (88,89) demonstrated a dose response curve to exercise, with the benefits of exercise beginning at an expenditure of 500 kcal per week and continuing through 2,500 kcal per week, at which point the reduction of the endpoints of MI and death are maximized. Men with a weekly energy expenditure below 2,000 kcal were at 64% higher risk for MI and death than classmates with a higher energy expenditure per week. Blair et al. (17,18) reported that only a modest level of fitness is necessary to begin achieving

TABLE 35-3. SUMMARY OF EFFECTS OF CARDIORESPIRATORY EXERCISE TRAINING ON SELECTED CARDIOVASCULAR RISK FACTORS

RISK FACTOR	EFFECT
Smoking	By itself: little or no effect
	Exercise should be part of a comprehensive smoking cessation program
Lipid abnormalities	
Cholesterol	Little or no effect
LDL cholesterol	Little or no effect
HDL cholesterol	Mild to moderate increase
Hypertension	Reduces incidence (especially among white men)
Systolic	Reduced: average, 6 mm Hg
Diastolic	Reduced: average, 5 mm Hg
Obesity	Exercise alone: mild effect
	Exercise should be part of a comprehensive weight-management program

HDL, high-density lipoprotein; LDL, low-density lipoprotein.

the benefits of reduced mortality from CVD in persons without CAD. There was again noted a strong and graded association between fitness and mortality because of all causes, cardiovascular disease, and cancer, with the greatest benefit occurring in the most fit. These findings form the basis for the American Association of Cardiovascular and Pulmonary Rehabilitation (AACVPR)'s (4) risk stratification for sedentary lifestyle into three categories, with ≥1,500 kcal per week being low risk, 700 to 1,499 kcal per week being intermediate risk, and <700 kcal per week being high risk for CAD. The information on patients who already have CAD, however, is limited, and there are no significant data to define the necessary caloric expenditure to reduce mortality. The question often asked is: "Do those patients who already have coronary artery disease need exercise prescriptions with an even higher level of physical activity?" Hambrecht et al.'s observation that 2,200 kcals of physical activity are needed each week to cause regression of coronary artery disease suggest that higher levels of physical activity may be needed, perhaps as much as 2,000 to 2,200 kcal per week to reduce mortality in patients who already have CAD (46). Additional studies are needed to determine the ideal caloric expenditure during exercise for patients with CAD.

Two separate groups have evaluated the physical activity levels of patients in cardiac rehabilitation. Patients participating in a maintenance program (e.g., phase 4 cardiac rehabilitation) after an MI or coronary revascularization were found to expend 230 kcal to 270 kcal per 45-minute rehabilitation session (2,97). Another study evaluated total weekly caloric energy expenditure among patients participating in a maintenance cardiac rehabilitation program and confirmed that the average patient, exercising three times per week in the program, expended

~830 kcal per week (96). In this study, patients were also found to be active outside of the program, expending an additional 675 kcal per week. Combining rehabilitation-based and home-based exercise, 72% of these patients exceeded 1,000 kcal, and 43% exceeded 1,500 kcal per week in weekly energy expenditure. Patients 70 years and older; those with a body mass index (BMI) of 30 or higher; and women, regardless of race, were the least likely to achieve the 1,500-kcal goal recommended by AACVPR (4).

When implementing exercise training in patients with heart disease, there are specific issues to be addressed with respect to the specific cardiac issue. The next several subsections review this information. Table 35-4 also provides a brief overview of some of these issues.

CORONARY ARTERY DISEASE

> **1.3.22-CES: Describe the differences in physiologic responses to various modes of ergometry (e.g., treadmill, cycle and arm ergometers) as they relate to exercise testing and training.**

> **1.4.9-CES: Identify potentially hazardous arrhythmias or conduction defects observed on the ECG at rest, during exercise, and during recovery.**

> **1.4.19-CES: Identify and describe the significance of ECG abnormalities in designing the exercise prescription and in making activity recommendations.**

To prevent deconditioning while in the hospital, patients who suffer an MI should be enrolled in inpatient cardiac rehabilitation. The cardiac patient can start with slow ambulation as soon as he or she is stabilized, usually the second or third day. Much of the deterioration in exercise tolerance during an inpatient stay can be countered through simple exposure to orthostatic or gravitational stress (by intermittent sitting or standing) and range-of-motion ROM exercises (32). The patient's activity level is increased from sitting to standing and to ambulation while being monitored for adverse responses. If there are no adverse responses noted, the patient may progress with ambulation as tolerated. Monitoring may include HR, BP, and cardiac telemetry before and during exercise (4).

After discharge from the hospital, the patient should automatically be enrolled in outpatient cardiac rehabilitation: a program of secondary prevention and exercise. The initial step is to risk stratify the patient into low, intermediate, or high risk for cardiac events while exercising (GETP8, Chapter 2). The general principles of prescribing exercise apply to patients enrolled in an outpatient cardiac rehabilitation program (4,93). The duration of each exercise session should gradually be increased until the patient is training at least 20 to 60 minutes most days of the week. Exercising large muscle groups through rhythmic activity such as walking, cycling, rowing, or stair climbing is a

TABLE 35-4. SUMMARY OF UNIQUE EXERCISE PRESCRIPTION ISSUES AMONG PATIENTS WITH CARDIOVASCULAR DISEASE

ILLNESS	INTENSITY	COMMENTS
Coronary artery disease	40/50%–85% of HRR	To affect mortality, frequency, duration, and intensity of training should sum to yield a weekly energy expenditure >1,500 kcal·wk^{-1}.[a,b]
Angina or equivalent	40/50%–85% of HRR with necessary adjustment to keep upper HRR limit to no more than 10 beats below ischemic threshold	Consider a prophylactic nitroglycerin 15 min before anticipated exertion if symptoms limit routine ADLs or ability to exercise.
Myocardial infarction	40/50% –85% of HRR	Achieve 1,500–2,000 kcal of energy expenditure through physical activity each week.[a,b]
PTCA with or without stent	40/50%–85% of HRR	Achieve 1,500–2,000 kcal of energy expenditure through physical activity each week.[a,b]
CABG or valve surgery	40/50%–85% of HRR	Restrict upper-body movement until sternum is healed (6–12 wk).
Heart failure	40/50%–70% of HRR	If needed, initially guide exercise intensity at 60% of HRR and adjust duration to three bouts of 10 min each, progressing to 30–40 min. As patient progresses, maintain upper rate below ventilatory threshold.
Cardiac transplant	RPE 11–14	Restrict upper-body resistance exercises until sternum is healed (6–12 wk).
Pacemaker, ICD, biventricular, RCT	10% below activation threshold	Avoid activities that stretch the arms. After 8 wk, nonballistic activities may be resumed, and ballistic activities may be resumed after 12 wk.

ADLs, activities of daily living; CABG, coronary artery bypass graft; HRR, heart rate reserve; ICD, implantable cardiac defibrillator; PTCA, percutaneous transluminal coronary angioplasty; RCT, cardiac resynchronization therapy; RPE, rating of perceived exertion.

[a]American Association of Cardiovascular and Pulmonary Rehabilitation. *Guidelines for Cardiac Rehabilitation and Secondary Prevention.* 4th ed. Champaign (IL): Human Kinetics; 2004. p. 65–66, 118–120.

[b]Shuler G, Hambrecht R, Schlierf G, et al. Regular exercise and low fat diet—effects on progression of coronary artery disease. *Circulation.* 1992;86:1–11.

cornerstone of outpatient cardiac rehabilitation programs. Because training benefits are specific to the activity performed, both the legs and the arms need to be trained (27). The exercise session should have warm-up and cool-down phases (5–10 min), including stretching, ROM, and low-intensity aerobic activity. Among patients with CAD, a low-intensity warm-up may help them avoid the occurrence of ST-segment depression, threatening arrhythmias, and transient LV dysfunction (9,10). Similar to recovery from a maximal exercise stress test, the cooldown phase after exercise training may help facilitate the gradual return of HR and BP to resting values and therefore reduce the likelihood of either postexercise hypotension/dizziness or a postexercise increase in plasma catecholamine levels (36). The above training parameters may need to be modified based on an individual patient's symptoms and medication use.

> **1.1.10-CES: Discuss the effects of isometric exercise in individuals with cardiovascular, pulmonary, and/or metabolic diseases.**

> **1.3.30-CES: Discuss the appropriate use of static and dynamic resistance exercise for individuals with cardiovascular, pulmonary, and metabolic disease.**

> **1.7.16-CES: Describe the principle of specificity as it relates to the mode of exercise testing and training.**

> **1.7.20-CES: Discuss the appropriate use of static and dynamic resistance exercise for individuals with cardiovascular, pulmonary, and metabolic diseases and conditions.**

In addition to cardiovascular exercise, it is important for patients with CAD to include a resistance-training program. A 2007 scientific statement of the American Heart Association (AHA) (112) endorsed by the American College of Sports Medicine (ACSM) recommended mild to moderate resistance training for improving muscular strength and endurance, preventing and managing a variety of chronic medical conditions, and modifying risk factors. Although dynamic resistance exercise for the upper and lower body is now commonly recommended as part of a structured cardiac rehabilitation program (92), there are still limited data on the effects of resistance training among moderate- to high-risk cardiac patients. Currently, isometric exercises are not recommended among this population because of a potential significant rise in systolic and diastolic blood pressure. Moderate-intensity dynamic resistance exercise (defined as 50%–60% of one repetition maximum [1RM]) results in improved muscle strength and endurance, both of which are important for the safe return to activities of daily living (ADLs), vocational and avocational activities, and maintaining independence. However, it remains unclear to what extent, if any, cardiovascular risk factors such as hyperlipidemia and hypertension are favorably modified by resistance training in patients with CVD (92). Data from current meta-analysis have shown a small reduction of 3 and 4 mm Hg for resting systolic blood pressure and diastolic blood pressure, respectively (25,67,112).

> **1.7.10-CES: Organize graded exercise testing (GXT) and clinical data to counsel patients regarding issues such as activities of daily living (ADLs), return to work, and physical activity.**

> **1.7.17-CES: Design strength and flexibility programs for individuals with cardiovascular, pulmonary, and/or metabolic diseases; the elderly; and children.**

> **1.7.22-CES: Design, describe, and demonstrate specific resistance exercises for major muscle groups for patients with cardiovascular, pulmonary, and metabolic diseases and conditions.**

A commonly recommended resistance-training program involves performing one set of eight to 10 regional exercises, performed 2 to 3 days per week (43,68,112). Typically, these programs involve starting at a low weight and progressing to 10 to 15 repetitions. While resistance training at 50% to 70% of a 1RM, the rate–pressure product should not exceed that prescribed for endurance exercise, and perceived exertion should remain between 11 and 14 on the Borg scale (68,112) (see Table 4.7 in GETP8). Patients undergoing a catheterization with or without PCI and those recovering from an uncomplicated MI may begin a resistance-training program as early as 3 and 5 weeks after the event, respectively (4). Patients undergoing CABG surgery or valve surgery involving a sternotomy should avoid upper-limb resistance training until sternal healing has occurred, generally 6 to 12 weeks after surgery. Patients may benefit by first training the upper limbs with elastic bands and hand weights before progressing to resistance-type exercise machines (4).

ANGINA

Exercise, lifestyle behavior changes, and medical compliance are key for people with stable angina and help reduce overall cardiac risk and prevent or retard progression of atherosclerotic plaques (87). It was initially thought that the threshold at which the myocardium becomes ischemic and angina occurs is reproducible and, as mentioned earlier, can be estimated by the rate–pressure product (RPP). Subsequent work by Garber et al. (43) and others (13,74,94) demonstrated that the angina threshold varies with the type of exercise performed. They found that the RPP at the ischemic threshold varied depending on whether one was performing a maximal stress test or a longer submaximal exercise session. The ischemic threshold occurred at a lower HR during sustained submaximal exercise and

daily activities at home than during a maximal stress test. Circadian rhythm also plays a role (94) in that the ischemic threshold was found to be lower at 1 PM than 8 AM and 9 PM. Forearm vascular resistance was increased at 8 AM and 9 PM compared with 1 PM, suggesting that increased vascular resistance may be one of the causes for the variability in angina threshold.

However, for a given patient performing a specific activity at the same time of the day, there did appear to be reproducibility in the RPP at which angina occurs (94). Therefore, one goal for patients with angina is to perform routine daily activities at a lower RPP, thus reducing the amount of angina and fatigue they experience. Another goal is to increase the amount of work, home activity, or exercise they can perform at a given RPP (4,42) or below their ischemic threshold (Fig. 35-1).

Exercise programming for patients with angina requires that they first recognize and understand their symptoms. They need to identify the nature of their angina (e.g., location, precipitating factors, associated symptoms, and radiation pattern) and understand that there are no clinical benefits derived from exercising with such discomfort or pain. In cardiac rehabilitation there are rating scales (e.g., 1 to 4) to help assess the severity of symptoms. Patients also need to identify which activities precipitate their angina and modify the situation accordingly. For example, if walking in the cold causes chest discomfort, then they should exercise indoors or consider wearing a scarf or other protective wear over their mouth to warm inhaled air. Similarly, if carrying out the garbage, walking the dog, or mild exercise regularly causes chest pain, they should talk with their doctor about taking sublingual nitroglycerin beforehand. Finally, in the cardiac rehabilitation setting, it is not uncommon for the patient who regularly experiences angina at relatively low workloads (e.g., 2 METs) to take one sublingual nitroglycerin about 15 minutes before starting their warm-up. This practice usually allows these patients to exercise in a pain-free manner and at slightly higher workloads. Also, it may be beneficial to include a longer warm-up (≥10 min) to help minimize or avoid ischemia.

> **1.4.9-CES: Identify potentially hazardous arrhythmias or conduction defects observed on the ECG at rest, during exercise, and recovery.**

> **1.4.19-CES: Identify and describe the significance of ECG abnormalities in designing the exercise prescription and in making activity recommendations.**

> **1.7.10-CES: Organize GXT and clinical data to counsel patients regarding issues such as ADLs, return to work, and physical activity.**

> **1.7.13-CES: Describe the importance of warm-up and cool-down sessions with specific reference to angina and ischemic ECG changes, and for overall patient safety.**

For patients with evidence of exercise-induced ischemia (i.e., angina, ECG changes), the upper HR for exercise training should be set 10 or more beats below the HR or RPP at which ischemia was first noticed during a GXT (4,5). Although determining the ischemic threshold during a regular exercise test is usually possible, doing so for a patient who completed a stress imaging study, such as a stress echo or radionuclide, is much more difficult. This is because myocardial ischemia may manifest itself as angina, ST-segment depression, ventricular arrhythmias, or abnormal BP response (53). Finally, if needed, it may be prudent to simply have the patient complete a regular ECG stress test to help identify ischemic threshold.

> **1.5.2-CES: Describe mechanisms and actions of medications that may affect exercise testing and prescription (i.e., β-blockers, nitrates, calcium channel blockers, digitalis, diuretics, vasodilators, antiarrhythmic agents, bronchodilators, antilipemics, psychotropics, nicotine, antihistamines, OTC cold medications, thyroid medications, alcohol, hypoglycemic agents, blood modifiers, pentoxifylline, antigout medications, and anorexiants/diet pills).**

> **1.5.3-CES: Recognize medications associated in clinical setting, their indications for care, and their effects at rest and during exercise (i.e., β-blockers, nitrates, calcium channel blockers, digitalis, diuretics, vasodilators, antiarrhythmic agents, bronchodilators, antilipemics, psychotropics, nicotine, antihistamines, OTC cold medications, thyroid medications, alcohol, hypoglycemic agents, blood modifiers, pentoxifylline, antigout medications, and anorexiants/diet pills).**

Medications such as β-blockers, nitrates, calcium channel blockers, and others may influence the ischemic threshold. As a result, it is prudent to ensure that patients take their medications between 3 and 10 hours of undergoing an exercise test administered for the purpose of establishing the correct exercise training HR range. In fact, a test should be cancelled and rescheduled if a patient "forgets" to take β-blocker medication, because the HR response will not be representative of what the patient will actually experience during exercise training. Finally, another exercise test should be completed if a patient's medication or dose is changed, although this is not always possible because of insurance reimbursement issues.

MYOCARDIAL INFARCTION

> **1.7.10-CES: Organize GXT and clinical data to counsel patients regarding issues such as ADLs, return to work, and physical activity.**

Following inpatient cardiac rehabilitation, it is suggested that patients who have suffered an MI begin an outpatient rehabilitation program. When starting an outpatient cardiac rehabilitation program, it is generally recommended that patients who have suffered an MI first start at the lower end of their training intensity (40%–60% of $\dot{V}O_2$ or HR reserve method or 11–13 on the ratings of perceived exertion scale) (4). Patients should participate in three nonconsecutive days of cardiac rehabilitation per week, with each exercise session consisting of a 5- to 10-minute warm-up and cool-down period (4) and progressively increase exercise intensity and duration up to 85% of HR reserve method and 20 to 60 minutes, respectively. As patients progress, they should be encouraged to adopt an active life style, including exercise and daily activities, so that they expend >1,500 kcal each week (4,46,88,89). These recommendations form the framework of exercise prescription for those with stable CAD; however, they will need to be modified based on the patient's other medical diseases.

REVASCULARIZATION (CORONARY ARTERY BYPASS GRAFT AND PERCUTANEOUS CORONARY INTERVENTION)

The three medical/surgical treatment modalities for coronary heart disease—medications, PCI, and CABG—are discussed in Chapter 6. The effects of anti-ischemic medications are discussed in the previous section on angina. Patients undergoing revascularization by either PCI or CABG surgery are expected to demonstrate an improved exercise response. Signs of ischemia during exercise, such as angina, ST-segment depression, and hemodynamic abnormalities (i.e., chronotropic incompetence, blunted BP response) are often eliminated or occur at higher-intensity activities after revascularization. In short, the benefits and limitations of exercise are the same for patients after revascularization as they are for all patients after an MI.

> **1.7.10-CES: Organize GXT and clinical data to counsel patients regarding issues such as ADLs, return to work, and physical activity.**

Recommendations for exercise programming for patients after PCI are generally the same as for other patients with CAD. However, because patients undergoing PCI frequently do not experience myocardial damage or extensive surgery, they can sometimes begin cardiac rehabilitation, return to work, and resume ADLs much sooner. In fact, cardiac rehabilitation can begin within 48 hours after the procedure (98). Patients undergoing CABG surgery often begin rehabilitation as early as 2 weeks after surgery, with the initial focus on aerobic-type exercises. All upper-body exercise should be limited to ROM and light repetitive activities such as arm ergometry until 4 to 8 weeks after surgery (4). Following the initial wound healing of revascularization, patients should be able to exercise up to 85% of HR reserve method, 3 to 4 days per week, for 20 to 60 minutes. After the sternum is healed at 6 to 12 weeks, patients can then begin a resistance-training program similar to other patients with cardiovascular disease (4).

VALVE DYSFUNCTION/REPAIR/REPLACEMENT

Heart valve abnormalities, such as stenosis and regurgitation, increase the work the heart must perform to meet the body's demands by reducing the effective cardiac output at any given heart rate (19). As a result, myocardial hypertrophy can develop. Over time this may lead to mild diastolic dysfunction or a decrease in ventricular distensibility. Exercise will not improve or change the function of the valves, but it will help to improve the efficiency of oxygen extraction by the skeletal muscles and improve the work capacity of the individual (19). Recommendations for exercise training and participation in competitive sports for patients with cardiovascular disease are contained in the AHA/ACC Guidelines for Valvular Heart Disease (19) and the Bethesda Conference Task Force 3: Valvular Heart Disease (20). In general, patients with mild disease who are asymptomatic, have normal LV function, and have normal pulmonary artery pressures are not restricted from participating in competitive sports (19,20). Patients with aortic regurgitation or mitral regurgitation that have more than a mildly dilated LV or abnormal systolic function should avoid competitive sports (19,20). Because of the danger of sudden death, it is recommended that patients with moderate to severe symptomatic aortic stenosis or asymptomatic patients with severe aortic stenosis not participate in vigorous or competitive exercise (19). Most of the changes in the myocardium that develop because of faulty valve function are partially reversible after surgery, if cardiac function has not been compromised long enough for permanent remodeling to occur. This length of time is variable among individuals (19).

The majority of valve abnormalities can be corrected with surgical procedures. Following surgery patients are encouraged to begin an exercise program to prevent any other heart problems. It is advised that patients follow the same guidelines as CABG patients following surgery. They may begin an exercise program 2 to 4 weeks following surgery, with upper-body exercise limited to ROM and light repetitive activities such as arm ergometry until 12 weeks after surgery (4). Following the initial wound healing, patients should be able to exercise up to 85% of HR reserve, 3 to 4 days per week, for 20 to 60 minutes.

In addition, patients with bioprosthetic or mechanical valves should limit themselves to low- to moderate-intensity exercise training. Patients on warfarin (Coumadin) for mechanical valves or atrial fibrillation should avoid contact sports (19,20).

HEART FAILURE

A hallmark symptom of patients with chronic heart failure is exercise intolerance or dyspnea on exertion. Compared with age-matched healthy normal individuals, peak exercise capacity is reduced by an average of 30% to 40% in patients with heart failure (91).

Several mechanisms have been identified to explain the observed exercise intolerance, including a reduction in peak cardiac output (~40%), chronotropic incompetence, and a reduced stroke volume. In addition, the ability to increase blood flow to the more metabolically active skeletal muscles during exercise is attenuated, mostly because of both an exaggerated increase in plasma norepinephrine level and sympathetic tone and endothelial dysfunction. There are also abnormalities in the skeletal muscle, such as a reduction in myosin heavy chain I isoforms, reduced activity of the enzymes associated aerobic metabolism, and a reduction in fiber size (91).

Current evidence (59,73,91) indicates that moderate exercise is generally safe and results in improvements in quality of life, autonomic balance (i.e., parasympathetic activity), exercise tolerance (peak $\dot{V}O_2$, ~15%–35%), endothelial function, chronotropic responsiveness, and skeletal muscle function. Exercise training provides a mild, favorable antiremodeling effect, including a 2- to 4-percentage-point increase in ejection fraction and a small decrease in LV end-diastolic volume (44). Patients with decompensated heart failure should not be involved in an exercise program. Single center data has been favorable for morbidity & mortality (11). The HF action trial reported at the 2008 AHA meeting that cardiac rehabilitation reduced cardiac specific morbidity & mortality. Also, this study showed that exercise is safe in the heart failure population.

Compared with apparently healthy people and those with ischemic heart disease and normal ventricular function, there are only a few differences relative to prescribing exercise in patients with heart failure. Specifically, duration of activity may initially need to be adjusted to allow these patients more opportunity for rest and to progress at their own pace. In fact, some patients may better tolerate discontinuous training involving short bouts of exercise interspersed with bouts of rest (78,114). Patients should be encouraged to progressively increase exercise duration, as tolerated, until they are able to tolerate one bout of 30 minutes or more. When prescribing exercise for patients with heart failure, one must also consider the etiology. Specifically, the cause of the heart failure may be either ischemic or nonischemic, and if it is the former, then the guidelines for prescribing exercise in patients with angina may also need to be followed.

> **1.7.10-CES: Organize GXT and clinical data to counsel patients regarding issues such as ADLs, return to work, and physical activity.**

Research indicates that different exercise intensities are able to increase exercise tolerance yet still yield generally similar relative gains in cardiorespiratory fitness (91). Based on these data, for the first few exercise sessions, it is appropriate to guide the upper end of exercise intensity at 60% of HR reserve method, titrated based on a patient's subjective feelings of fatigue using the rating of perceived exertion scale of 11 to 14. In view of conflicting reports about whether there is a further decrease in LV function when patients with chronic heart failure train above ventilatory threshold (VT) (84,91,102), it seems prudent to set exercise intensity at 60% to 70% of HR reserve, or, if available, below the identified VT. This type of testing requires the use of a metabolic cart to measure cardiorespiratory variables during a stress test and determination of the VT using the V-slope method (7,103).

Presently, in cardiac rehabilitation programs in the United States, it is left to the clinicians in the program to decide whether to use ECG telemetry monitoring when exercising patients with heart disease, both with and without heart failure, based on a patient's risk for exercise-related events (4). Although ECG telemetry monitoring during cardiac rehabilitation is common in the United States, it is important to point out that such an approach is not used in either Canada or Europe. Albeit limited, analysis of safety data from several clinical trials suggest that ECG monitoring may not be necessary when exercising patients with chronic heart failure (40,62,73).

CARDIAC TRANSPLANT

> **1.7.10-CES: Organize GXT and clinical data to counsel patients regarding issues such as ADLs, return to work, and physical activity.**

Every year, approximately 3,000 cardiac transplants are performed worldwide in patients with end-stage heart failure. For adults undergoing this procedure, the 1- and 3-year survival rates are approximately 86% and 80%, respectively (56). Despite receiving a donor heart with normal systolic function with subsequent improvement in functional capacity, cardiac transplant recipients continue to experience exercise intolerance after surgery that is about 40% to 50% below that of age-matched normal individuals (56). This exercise intolerance is believed to be primarily attributable to the absence of efferent sympathetic innervation of the myocardium, affecting heart rate and contractility responses, residual skeletal muscle abnormalities developed before transplantation because of heart failure, and decreased skeletal muscle strength (56).

After surgery, medical management focuses on preventing rejection of the donor heart by suppressing immune system function, while avoiding complicating side effects such as infections, hyperlipidemia, hypertension, osteoporosis, diabetes, certain cancers, and accelerated graft atherosclerosis of the epicardial and intramural coronary arteries. Except for cyclosporine, which may cause an increase in BP at rest and during submaximal exercise, none of the other medications used to control immune system rejection in cardiac transplant recipients appears to influence the cardiorespiratory response of these patients during acute bout of exercise or prevent the development of a safe exercise prescription for aerobic conditioning (56) or resistance training.

Because of the denervated myocardium, at least during the first year after transplantation, many differences in the cardiorespiratory and neuroendocrine responses are evident at rest, during exercise, and in recovery in cardiac transplant recipients (101). These abnormalities include an elevated resting HR (often >90 bpm); elevated systolic and diastolic BPs at rest, partly attributable to increased plasma norepinephrine and the immunosuppressive medications (i.e., cyclosporine and prednisone); an attenuated increase in HR during submaximal work; a lower peak HR and peak stroke volume; a greater increase in plasma norepinephrine during exercise; and a delayed slowing of HR in recovery (56). Delayed HR in recovery is thought to be attributable to increased levels of plasma norepinephrine, exerting its positive chronotropic effect in the absence of vagal efferent innervation (3).

To prescribe exercise and guide exercise intensity in cardiac transplant recipients in the first year after surgery, it is best to simply disregard all HR-based methods because of the abnormal HR control in these patients (58). For example, it is common to find persons with cardiac transplant within the past year achieving an exercise HR during training that not only exceeds 85% of peak but is often equal to or greater than the peak rate attained during their last symptom-limited exercise test. Ratings of perceived exertion between 11 and 14 should be used to guide exercise training intensity (56,58).

Among cardiac transplant patients who undergo exercise training, exercise capacity increases by about 15% to 40%; resting HR is unchanged or decreases slightly; peak HR increases; there is little change in peak stroke volume or cardiac dimensions; and quality of life is favorably altered (56). In a comprehensive prospective, randomized trial, Kobashigawa et al. (64) showed a 49% increase in peak $\dot{V}O_2$ and a 23 bpm increase in peak HR.

In addition, cardiac transplant patients (and patients with stable heart failure before transplant) can benefit from a systematic program of resistance training because of a leg-strength deficit that contributes to the reduced exercise capacity that persists before and after surgery. Braith and Edwards (21) showed that resistance training improves muscular endurance and also partially restores bone mineral density and addresses the skeletal muscle abnormalities (i.e., strength development, lipid content, fiber size) that commonly occur because of long-term corticosteroid therapy. A progressive resistance training program of seven to 10 exercises that focus on the legs, back, arms, and shoulders, started 6 to 12 weeks after transplant surgery and performed two times per week, is recommended (21).

PACEMAKERS, IMPLANTABLE CARDIAC DEFIBRILLATORS, AND ARRHYTHMIAS

Pacemakers and implantable cardiac defibrillators (ICD) are small devices implanted in the body to monitor and regulate the electrical activity of the heart. In general, the exercise training prescription is unaltered for patients with these devices. Often the devices are implanted because of concurrent cardiovascular disease.

Functional capacity may be improved with pacemakers because of an improved HR response to exercise. Rate-responsive pacemakers respond to exercise by sensing movement or respiration and gradually increase HR until the upper rate of the pacemaker is reached. The type of ramp-up programmed into the pacemaker determines how quickly the HR is increased in response to exercise. Both the ramp and the upper rate limit of the pacemaker are adjustable to maximize a patient's exercise performance. The pacemaker upper rate limit is usually set so it is 10% or more beats below ischemic threshold (90,92). Biventricular pacemakers (i.e., cardiac resynchronization therapy [CRT]) are used for the treatment of heart failure. Indications for a biventricular pacemaker include LV dysfunction with left bundle branch block, poor functional capacity, and evidence of asynchronous ventricular contraction. Unlike traditional pacemakers, these pace both the right and left ventricles. Biventricular pacemakers are designed to act just like other pacemakers and may or may not have internal cardiac defibrillator (ICD) capacity (35). Data demonstrate that functional capacity (i.e., peak $\dot{V}O_2$) and quality of life are improved with the use of a biventricular pacemaker (72,110).

ICDs are devices that detect abnormal heart rhythms and deliver an electrical shock if a dangerous rhythm is detected (90). Exercise intensity in patients with an ICD should be set at least 10 beats below the programmed firing threshold. For many patients, this is not a big concern because they are taking a medication (i.e., β-adrenergic blocking agents) that prevents their HR from increasing to the ICD firing threshold, which is often between 150 and 180 bpm. Exercise tests performed to evaluate ischemia in patients with pacemakers or ICDs require imaging studies during the test because of the abnormal resting ECG. Patients should be restricted from raising the arms above the head for 6 weeks following implantation of a pacemaker or ICD (90).

Often patients with CVD will also have atrial and/or ventricular arrhythmias during exercise. Regular exercise training favorably alters cardiac autonomic regulation which provides a possible means of preventing dangerous arrhythmias (16). Patients with atrial fibrillation have irregular HRs that prevent the use of standard exercise HR prescriptions. These patients should guide their exercise intensity using the Borg rating of perceived exertion scale. Patients presenting with frequent premature ventricular contractions (PVCs) should also be monitored closely and for longer periods. If there is a set HR at which the PVCs become more frequent, the exercise prescription may be set 10 beats below this heart rate, especially if they become symptomatic. Most of these patients will also require further testing to determine the impact on these arrhythmias and to help the physician better control them.

SUMMARY

Exercise programming following the guidelines of the ACSM, AHA, AACVPR, and the Surgeon General as reviewed in this chapter allows patients with a variety of cardiovascular diseases to exercise safely (4,108,112). The inclusion of exercise in the treatment of these patients is beneficial because of its favorable effects on risk factors, symptoms, functional capacity, physiology, and quality of life. Finally, and possibly most important, all patients with cardiovascular disease should be encouraged to participate in exercise because of its real or likely positive impact on mortality and morbidity.

REFERENCES

1. Ades PA, Savage PD, Brawner CA, et al. Aerobic capacity in patients entering cardiac rehabilitation. *Circulation*. 2006;113:2706–2712.
2. Ades H, Savage PD, Brochu M, et al. Low caloric expenditure in cardiac rehabilitation. *Am Heart J*. 2000;140:527–533.
3. Albrecht AE, Lillis D, Pease MD, et al. Heart rate and catecholamine responses during exercise and recovery in cardiac transplant recipients. *J Cardiopulm Rehabil*. 1993;13:182–187.
4. **American Association of Cardiovascular and Pulmonary Rehabilitation. *Guidelines for Cardiac Rehabilitation and Secondary Prevention*. 4th ed. Champaign (IL): Human Kinetics; 2004. p. 65–66, 118–120.**
5. American College of Sports Medicine. *American College of Sports Medicine's Exercise Management for Persons with Chronic Disease and Disabilities*. Champaign (IL): Human Kinetics; 1997.
6. **American College of Sports Medicine. Exercise for patients with coronary artery disease. Position Stand. *Med Sci Sports Exerc*. 1994;26:i–v.**
7. Arena R, Myers J, Williams MA, et al. Assessment of functional capacity in clinical and research settings: a scientific statement from the American Heart Association committee on exercise, rehabilitation, and prevention of the council on clinical cardiology and the council on cardiovascular nursing. *Circulation*. 2007; 116: 329–343.
8. **Balady GJ, Williams MA, Ades PA, et al. Core components of cardiac rehabilitation/secondary prevention programs: 2007 update. *Circulation*. 2007;115:2675–2682.**
9. Barnard RJ, Gardner GW, Diaco NV, et al. Cardiovascular responses to sudden strenuous exercise: heart rate, blood pressure and ECG. *J Appl Phys*. 1973;34:833–837.
10. Barnard RJ, MacAlpin R, Katus AA, et al. Ischemic response to sudden strenuous exercise in healthy men. *Circulation*. 1973; 48: 936–942.
11. Belardinelli R, Georgiou D, Cianci G, et al. Randomized, controlled trial of long-term moderate exercise training in chronic heart failure: effects on functional capacity, quality of life, and clinical outcome. *Circulation*. 1999;99:1173–1182.
12. Belardinelli R, Georgiou D, Ginzton L, et al. Effects of moderate exercise training on thallium uptake and contractile response to low-dose dobutamine of dysfunctional myocardium in patients with ischemic cardiomyopathy. *Circulation*. 1998;97:553–561.
13. Benhorin J, Pinsker G, Moriel M, et al. Ischemic threshold during two exercise testing protocols and during ambulatory electrocardiographic monitoring. *J Am Coll Cardiol*. 1993;22:671–677.
14. Berger HJ, Reduto LA, Johnstone DE, et al. Global and regional left ventricular response to cycle exercise in coronary artery disease: assessment by quantitative radionuclide angiocardiography. *Am J Med*. 1979;66:13–21.
15. Bigger JT, Fleiss JL, Steinman RC, et al. Frequency domain measures of heart period variability and mortality after myocardial infarction. *Circulation*. 1992;85:164–171.

16. Billman GE. Aerobic exercise conditioning: a nonpharmacological antiarrhythmic intervention. *J Appl Phys.* 2001;92:446–454.

17. Blair SN, Kohl HW, Gorgon NF, et al. How much physical activity is good for health? *Annu Rev Public Health.* 1992;13:99–126.

18. Blair SN, Kohl HW, Paffenbarger RS, et al. Physical fitness and all cause mortality. *JAMA.* 1989;262:2395–2401.

19. Bonow RO, Carabello BA, Chatterjee K, et al. ACC/AHA 2006 guidelines for the management of patients with valvular heart disease: a report of the American College of Cardiology/American Heart Association Task Force on Practice Guidelines (Writing Committee to Develop Guidelines for the Management of Patients with Valvular Heart Disease). *Circulation.* 2006;e84–e231. Available at: http://www.american heart.org.

20. Bonow RO, Cheitlin MD, Crawford MH, et al. Bethesda Conference; Task Force 3: valvular heart disease. *J Am Coll Cardiol.* 2005;45:1334–1340.

21. Braith RW, Edwards DG. Exercise following heart transplantation. *Sports Med.* 2000;30:171–192.

22. Brener SJ, Pashkow FJ, Harvey SA, et al. Chronotropic response to exercise predicts angiographic severity in patients with suspected or stable coronary artery disease. *Am J Cardiol.* 1995;76: 1228–1232.

23. Carroll S, Cooke CB, Butterfly RJ. Physical activity, cardiorespiratory fitness, and the primary components of blood viscosity. *Med Sci Sports Exerc.* 2000;32:353–385.

24. Centers for Disease Control and Prevention. Prevalence of sedentary lifestyle: behavioral risk factor surveillance system, United States, 1991. *MMWR Morb Mortal Wkly Rep.* 1991;42:576–579.

25. **Chobanian AV, Bakrisg GL, Black NR, et al. The seventh report of the joint national commission (JNC) VII on detection evaluation and treatment of high blood pressure: the JNC VII report. *JAMA.* 2003;289:2560–2672.**

26. Clausen JP. Circulatory adjustments to dynamic exercise and effects of physical training in normal subjects and in patients with coronary artery disease. In: Sonneblick H, Lesch M, editors. *Exercise and Heart Disease.* New York: Grune and Stratton; 1977. p. 39–75.

27. Clausen JP, Trap-Jensen J, Lassen NA. The effects of training on heart rate during arm and leg exercise. *Scand J Clin Lab Invest.* 1970;26:295–301.

28. Coats AJS, Adamopoulos, S, Rnadaelli A, et al. Controlled trial of physical training in chronic heart failure. *Circulation.* 1992; 85: 2119–2131.

29. Cohn JN, Levine TB, Olivari MT. Plasma norepinephrine as a guide to prognosis in patients with chronic congestive heart failure. *New Engl J Med.* 1984;311:819–823.

30. Cole CR, Blackstone EH, Paskow FJ, et al. Heart-rate recovery immediately after exercise as a predictor of mortality. *New Engl J Med.* 1999;341:1351–1357.

31. Comess KA, Fenster PE. Clinical implications of the blood pressure response to exercise. *Cardiology.* 1981;68:233–244.

32. Convertino VA. Effect of orthostatic stress on exercise performance after bed rest: relation to in-hospital rehabilitation. *J Cardiopulm Rehabil.* 1983;3:660–663.

33. Crespo CJ, Keteyian SJ, Heath GW, et al. Leisure time physical activity among US adults. *Arch Intern Med.* 1996;156:93–98.

34. DeBusk RF, Haskell WL, Miller NH, et al. Medically directed at-home rehabilitation soon after clinically uncomplicated acute myocardial infarction: a new model for patient care. *Am J Cardiol.* 1985;55:251–257.

35. Delnoy PP, Ottervanger JP, Luttikhuis HO, et al. Sustained benefit of cardiac resynchronization therapy. *J Cardiovasc Electrophys.* 2007;18(3):298–302.

36. Dimsdale JE, Hartly H, Guiney T, et al. Postexercise peril: plasma catecholamines and exercise. *JAMA.* 1984;251:630–632.

37. Dlin R, Hanne N, Silverberg DS, et al. Follow-up of normotensive men with exaggerated blood pressure response to exercise. *Am Heart J.* 1983;106:316–320.

38. Ellestad MH, Wan MK. Predictive implications of stress testing: follow-up of 2700 subjects after maximum treadmill stress testing. *Circulation.* 1975;51:363–369.

39. Elwood PC, Yarnell JWG, Pickering J, et al. Exercise, fibrinogen and other risk factors for ischaemic heart disease: Caerphilly prospective heart disease study. *Br Heart J.* 1993;69:183–187.

40. **European Heart Failure Training Group. Experience from controlled trials of physical training in chronic heart failure. *Eur Heart J.* 1998;19:466–475.**

41. Farrell T, Paul V, Cripps T, et al. Baroreflex sensitivity and electrophysiological correlates in patients after acute myocardial infarction. *Circulation.* 1991;83:945–952.

42. **Fletcher GF, Balady GJ, Amsterdam EA, et al. Exercise standards for testing and training: a statement for healthcare professionals from the American Heart Association. *Circulation.* 2001;104: 1694–1740.**

43. Garber CE, Carleton RA, Camaione DN, et al. The threshold for myocardial ischemia varies with coronary artery disease depending on the exercise protocol. *J Am Coll Cardiol.* 1991;17: 1256–1262.

44. Giannuzzi P, Temporelli PL, Corra U, et al. Antiremodeling effect of long-term exercise training in patients with stable chronic heart failure. *Circulation.* 2003;108:554–559.

45. Hambrecht R, Niebauer J, Fiehn E. Physical training in patients with stable chronic heart failure: effects on cardiorespiratory fitness and ultrastructural abnormalities of leg muscles. *J Am Coll Cardiol.* 1995;25:1239–1249.

46. Hambrecht R, Niebauer J, Marburger CH, et al. Various intensities of leisure time physical activity in patients with coronary artery disease: effects of cardiorespiratory fitness and progression of coronary artherosclerotic lesions. *J Am Coll Cardiol.* 1993;22: 468–477.

47. Hambrecht R, Wolf A, Gielen S, et al. Effect of exercise on coronary endothelial function in patients with coronary artery disease. *New Engl J Med.* 2000;342:454–460.

48. Hartung GH, Rangel R. Exercise training in post-myocardial infarction patients: comparison of results with high risk coronary and post-bypass patients. *Arch Phys Med Rehabil.* 1988;62: 147–150.

49. Haskell WL, Alderman EL, Fair JM, et al. Effects of intensive multiple risk factor reduction on coronary atherosclerosis and clinical cardiac events in men and women with coronary artery disease. *Circulation.* 1994;89:975–990.

50. **Haskel WL, Lee I-Min, Pate KE, et al. Physical activity and public health: updated recommendation for adults from the American College of Sports Medicine and the American Heart Association. *Med Sci Sports Exerc.* 2007;39:1423–1439.**

51. Heinrich J, Balleisen L, Schulte H, et al. Fibrinogen and factor VII in the prediction of coronary risk: results of PROCAM study in healthy men. *Arterioscler Thromb.* 1994;14:54–59.

52. Heller GV, Ahmed I, Tilkemeier PL, et al. Comparison of chest pain, electrocardiographic changes and thallium-201 scintigraphy during varying exercise intensities in men with stable angina pectoris. *Am J Cardiol.* 1991;68:569–574.

53. Hoberg E, Schuler G, Kunze B, et al. Silent myocardial ischemia as a potential link between lack of premonitoring symptoms and increased risk of cardiac arrest during physical stress. *Am J Cardiol.* 1990;65:583–589.

54. Imhof A, Koenig W. Exercise and thrombosis. *Cardiol Clin.* 2001;19:389–400.

55. Irving JB, Bruce RA, DeRouen TA. Variations in and significance of systolic pressure during maximal exercise (treadmill) testing: relation to severity of coronary artery disease and cardiac mortality. *Am J Cardiol.* 1977;39:841–848.

56. Keteyian SJ, Brawner C. Cardiac transplant. In: Durstine JL, Moore GE, editors. *ACSM's Exercise Management for Persons with Chronic Disease and Disabilities.* Champaign (IL): Human Kinetics; 2001. p. 70–75.

57. Keteyian SJ, Brawner CA, Schairer JR, et al. Effects of exercise training on chronotropic incompetence in patients with heart failure. *Am Heart J.* 1999;138:2343–2240.

58. Keteyian SJ, Ehrman J, Fedel F, Rhoads K. Heart rate-perceived exertion relationship during exercise in orthotopic heart transplant patients. *J Cardiopulm Rehabil.* 1990;10:287–293.

59. Keteyian SJ, Levine AB, Brawner CA. A randomized controlled trial of exercise training in patients with heart failure. *Ann Intern Med.* 1996;124:1051–1057.

60. Keteyian SJ, Marks CRC, Brawner CA, et al. Responses to arm exercise in patients with compensated heart failure. *J Cardiopulm Rehabil.* 1996;16:366–371.

61. Keteyian S, Marks CRC, Levine AB, et al. Cardiovascular responses of cardiac transplant patients to arm and leg exercise. *Eur J Appl Physiol.* 1994;68:441–444.

62. Keteyian SJ, Mellett PA, Fedel FJ, et al. Electrocardiographic monitoring during cardiac rehabilitation. *Chest.* 1995;107: 1242–1246.

63. Kleiger RE, Miller JP, Bigger JT, et al. Decreased heart rate variability and its association with increased mortality after acute myocardial infarction. *Am J Cardiol.* 1987;59:256–262.

64. Kobashigawa JA, Leaf DA, Lee N, et al. A controlled trial of exercise rehabilitation after heart transplantation. *New Engl J Med.* 1999;34:272–277.

65. Koenig W. Haemostatic risk factors for cardiovascular diseases. *Eur Heart J.* 1998;19(suppl C):C39–C43.

66. Koenig W, Sund M, Döring A, et al. Leisure-time physical activity but not work-related physical activity is associated with decreased plasma viscosity: results from a large population sample. *Circulation.* 1997;95:335–341.

67. Kokkinos P, Narayan P, Colleran J, et al. Effects of regular exercise on blood pressure and left ventricular hypertrophy in African-American men with severe hypertension. *New Engl J Med.* 1995;333:1462–1467.

68. Kraemer WJ, Adams K, Cafarelli E, et al. American College of Sports Medicine position stand. Progression models in resistance training for healthy adults. *Med Sci Sports Exerc.* 2002;34: 364–380.

69. Lauer MS, Okin PM, Larson MG, et al. Impaired heart rate response to graded exercise: prognostic implications of chronotropic incompetence in the Framingham Heart Study. *Circulation.* 1996;93: 1520–1526.

70. Leon AS, Franklin BA, Costa F, et al. Cardiac rehabilitation and secondary prevention of coronary heart disease. *Circulation.* 2005;111:369–376.

71. Ludmer PL, Selwyn AP, Shook TL, et al. Paradoxical vasoconstriction induced by acetylcholine in atherosclerotic coronary arteries. *New Engl J Med.* 1986;315:1046–1051.

72. McCullough PA, Abraham WT. Does quality of life evidence assist in the selection of patients for resynchronization therapy? *Cardiac Electrophysiology Review.* 2003;7(1):71–76.

73. McKelvie RS, Teo KK, Roberts R, et al. Effects of exercise training in patients with heart failure: the exercise prescription trial (EX-ERT). *Am Heart J.* 2002;144:23–30.

74. McLenachan JM, Weidinger FF, Barry J, et al. Relations between heart rate, ischemia and drug therapy during daily life in patients with coronary artery disease. *Circulation.* 1991;83:1263–1270.

75. Malfatto G, Facchini M, Bragato R, et al. Short and long term effects of exercise training on the tonic autonomic modulation of heart rate variability after myocardial infarction. *Eur Heart J.* 1996;17:532–538.

76. Malfatto G, Facchini M, Sala L, et al. Effects of cardiac rehabilitation and beta-blocker therapy on heart rate variability after first acute myocardial infarction. *Am J Cardiol.* 1998;81:834–840.

77. Meade TW, Ruddock V, Stirling Y, et al. Fibrinolytic activity, clotting factors and long term incidence of ischemic heart disease in the Northwick Park Heart Study. *Lancet.* 1993;342:1076–1079.

78. Meyers K, Schwaibold M, Westbrook S, et al. Effects of short-term exercise training and activity restriction on functional capacity in patients with severe chronic heart failure. *Am J Cardiol.* 1996;78:1017–1022.

79. Nelson ME, Rejeski WJ, Blair SN, et al. Physical activity and public health in older adults: recommendation from the American College of Sports Medicine and the American Heart Association. *Circulation.* 2007;116:1094–1105.

80. Nesto RW, Kowalchuk GJ. The ischemic cascade: temporal sequence of hemodynamic, electrocardiographic, and symptomatic expressions of ischemia. *Am J Cardiol.* 1987;57:23C–30C.

81. Niebauer J, Hambrecht R, Marburger C, et al. Impact of intensive physical exercise and low fat diet on collateral vessel formation in stable angina pectoris and angiographically confirmed coronary artery disease. *Am J Cardiol.* 1995;76:771–775.

82. Nolan J, Batin PD, Andrews R, et al. Prospective study of heart rate variability and mortality in chronic heart failure evaluation and assessment of risk trial (UK-heart). *Circulation.* 1998;98:1510–1516.

83. Nolan J, Flapan AD, Capewell S, et al. Decreased cardiac parasympathetic activity in chronic heart failure. *Br Heart J.* 1992;67: 482–485.

84. Normandin EA, Camaione DN, Clark BA III, et al. A comparison of conventional vs anaerobic threshold exercise prescription methods in subjects with left ventricular dysfunction. *J Cardiopulm Rehabil.* 1993;13:110–116.

85. O'Conner GT, Burning JE, Yusuf S, et al. An overview of randomized trials of rehabilitation with exercise after myocardial infarction. *Circulation.* 1989;80:234–244.

86. Oldridge NB, Guyatt GH, Fischer ME, et al. Cardiac rehabilitation after myocardial infarction: combined experience of randomized trials. *JAMA.* 1988;260:945–950.

87. Ornish D, Brown SE, Scherwitz LW, et al. Can lifestyle changes reverse coronary heart disease? *Lancet.* 1990;336:129–133.

88. Paffenbarger RS, Hyde RT, Wing AL, et al. Physical activity, all-cause mortality, and longevity of college alumni. *New Engl J Med.* 1986;314:605–613.

89. Paffenbarger RS, Wing AL, Hyde RT. Physical activity as an index of heart attack risk in college alumni. *Am J Epidemiol.* 1978; 108:161–175.

90. Pashkow FJ. Patients with implanted pacemakers or implanted cardioverter defibrillators. In: Wenger N, Hellerstein H, editors. *Rehabilitation of the Coronary Patient.* 3rd ed. New York: Churchill Livingstone; 1992. p. 431–438.

91. Pina IL, Apstein CS, Balady GJ. Exercise and heart failure: a statement from the American Heart Association Committee on exercise, rehabilitation and prevention. *Circulation.* 2003; 107: 1210–1225.

92. Pollock ML, Franklin BA, Balady GJ, et al. Resistance exercise individuals with and without cardiovascular disease: benefits, rationale, safety, and prescription. An advisory from the Committee on Exercise, Rehabilitation, and Prevention, Council on Clinical Cardiology, American Heart Association. *Circulation.* 2000;101: 828–833.

93. Pollock ML, Gasser GA, Butcher JD, et al. The recommended quantity and quality of exercise for developing and maintaining cardiorespiratory and muscular fitness, and flexibility in healthy adults. Position Stand. *Med Sci Sports Exerc.* 1998;30:972–991.

94. Quyyumi AA, Panza JA, Diodati JG, et al. Circadian variation in ischemic threshold. *Circulation.* 1992;86:22–28.

95. Roveda F, Middlekauff HR, Rondon MUPB, et al. The effects of exercise training on sympathetic neural activation in advanced heart failure. *J Am Coll Cardiol.* 2003;42:854–860.

96. Schairer JR, Keteyian SJ, Ehrman JK, et al. Leisure-time physical activity in patients in maintenance cardiac rehabilitation. *J Cardiopulm Rehabil.* 2003;23:260–265.

97. Schairer JR, Kostelnik T, Proffett SM, et al. Caloric expenditure during cardiac rehabilitation. *J Cardiopulm Rehabil.* 1998;18: 290–294.

98. Schelkum PH. Exercise after angioplasty: How much? How soon? *Phys Sportsmed.* 1992;20:199–212.

99. Sheps DS, Ernst JC, Briese FW, et al. Exercise-induced increase in diastolic pressure: indicator of severe coronary artery disease. *Am J Cardiol.* 1979;43:708–712.

100. Shuler G, Hambrecht R, Schlierf G, et al. Regular exercise and low fat diet—effects on progression of coronary artery disease. *Circulation.* 1992;86:1–11.

101. Squires RW, Leung TC, Cyr NS, et al. Partial normalization of heart rate response to exercise after transplantation: frequency and relationship to exercise capacity. *Mayo Clin Proc.* 2002;77: 1295–1300.

102. Strzelczk TA, Quigg RJ, Pfeifer PB. Accuracy of estimating exercise prescription intensity in patients with left ventricular systolic dysfunction. *J Cardiopulm Rehabil.* 2001;21:158–163.

103. **Task Force of the Italian Working Group on Cardiac Rehabilitation and Prevention. Statement on cardiopulmonary exercise testing in chronic heart failure due to left ventricular dysfunction: recommendations for performance and interpretation. Part III: Interpretation of cardiopulmonary exercise testing in chronic heart failure and future applications. *Eur J Cardiovasc Prev Rehabil.* 2006;13:485–494.**

104. Taylor RS, Brown A, Ebrahim S, et al. Exercise-based rehabilitation for patients with coronary heart disease: systematic review and meta-analysis of randomized controlled trials. *Am J Med.* 2004;116:682–692.

105. Thallow E, Eriksen J, Sandvik L, et al. Blood platelet count and function are related to total and cardiovascular death in apparently healthy men. *Circulation.* 1991;84:613–616.

106. Thompson PD. The benefits and risks of exercise training in patients with chronic coronary artery disease. *JAMA.* 1988;259: 1537–1540.

107. Tiukinhoy S, Beohar N, Hsie M. Improvement in heart rate recovery after cardiac rehabilitation. *J Cardiopulm Rehabil.* 2003;23:84–87.

108. **U.S. Department of Health and Human Services. *Physical Activity and Health: A Report of the Surgeon General.* Atlanta: U.S. Department of Health and Human Services, Centers for Disease Control and Prevention, National Center for Chronic Disease Prevention and Health Promotion; 1996. Publication no: S/N 017-023-00196-5.**

109. Wasserman K, Hansen JE, Sue DY, et al. *Principles of Exercise Testing and Interpretation.* 3rd ed. Baltimore: Lippincott, Williams & Wilkins; 1999.

110. Wasserman K, Sun XG, Hansen JE. Effect of biventricular pacing on the exercise pathophysiology of heart failure. *Chest.* 2007; 132(1):250–261.

111. **Wenger NK, Froelicher ES, Smith LK, et al. *Cardiac Rehabilitation.* Clinical Practice Guideline No. 17. Rockville (MD): U.S. Department of Health and Human Services, Public Health Ser-**vice, Agency for Heath Care Policy and Research, and the National Heart, Lung, and Blood Institute; October 1995. ACHPR Publication No. 96-0672.

112. **Williams MA, Haskell WL, Ades PA, et al. Resistance exercise in individuals with and without cardiovascular disease: 2007 update. *Circulation.* 2007;116:572–584.**

113. Wilson N, Meyer E. Early prediction of hypertension using exercise blood pressure. *Prev Med.* 1981;10:62–68.

114. Wisloff U, Stoylen, A, Loennechen JP, et. al. Superior cardiovascular effect of aerobic interval training versus moderate continuous training in heart failure patients. *Circulation.* 2007;115: 3086–3094.

115. Womack CJ, Nagelkirk PR, Coughlin AM. Exercise-induced changes in coagulation and fibrinolysis in healthy populations and patients with cardiovascular disease [Review]. *Sports Med.* 2003; 33(11):795–807.

SELECTED REFERENCES FOR FURTHER READING

American Association of Cardiovascular and Pulmonary Rehabilitation. *Guidelines for Cardiac Rehabilitation and Secondary Prevention Programs.* 4th ed. Champaign (IL): Human Kinetics; 2004.

American College of Sports Medicine. *ACSM's Exercise Management for Persons with Chronic Diseases and Disabilities.* 2nd ed. Champaign (IL): Human Kinetics; 2003.

Brubaker P, Kaminsky LA, Whaley, MH. *Coronary Artery Disease: Essentials of Prevention and Rehabilitation Programs.* Champaign (IL): Human Kinetics; 2002.

Fardy PS, Franklin BA, Pocari JP, Verrill DE. *Guidelines for Cardiac Rehabilitation and Secondary Prevention Programs.* Champaign (IL): Human Kinetics; 1999.

Graves JE, Franklin BA. *Resistance Training for Health and Rehabilitation.* Champaign (IL): Human Kinetics; 2001.

Pashkow FJ, Dafoe WA. *Clinical Cardiac Rehabilitation: A Cardiologist's Guide.* 2nd ed. Philadelphia: Lippincott, Williams & Wilkins; 1999.

INTERNET RESOURCES

- AACVPR: American Association of Cardiovascular and pulmonary Rehabilitation: www.aacvpr.org
- American College of Sports Medicine (position stands): www.acsm.org/publications/positionStands.htm
- American Heart Association (scientific statements and practice guidelines list): www.americanheart.org/presenter.jhtml?identifier ≥2158
- National Clinical Guideline Clearinghouse: www.guideline.gov
- National Heart Lung and Blood Institute Clinical Guidelines: www.nhlbi.nih.gov/guidelines

Exercise Prescription in Patients with Pulmonary Disease

36

CHAPTER

EPIDEMIOLOGY

Acute and chronic diseases of the upper and lower respiratory tract account for one third of all physician consultations. Also, it is estimated that one third of hospitalized patients have a problem with their respiratory system regardless of the immediate cause of admission. By definition, pulmonary diseases affect the lungs, including their airways, blood vessels and parenchyma. The common symptoms of pulmonary disease are shortness of breath, wheezing, cough, expectoration of sputum, and chest pain or discomfort. The most common pulmonary diseases in order of importance are chronic obstructive pulmonary disease (COPD), asthma, sleep apnea, and pulmonary vascular disease. Sleep apnea will not be discussed further in this chapter, but one of its symptoms, daytime hypersomnolence, can affect physical activity with predictable limitations. Other conditions, such as bronchiectasis, cystic fibrosis, pleural effusion, ventilatory muscle weakness, and disorders of ventilatory control will be discussed briefly where they have distinguishing features that differ from the common diseases.

CHRONIC OBSTRUCTIVE PULMONARY DISEASE

Chronic obstructive pulmonary disease (COPD) is a major cause of mortality, morbidity, and disability worldwide and certainly within the United States (97). The National Health and Nutritional Examination Survey (NHANES III) estimated the prevalence of COPD to be at 24.0 million adults (67). COPD is ranked as the fourth

> > > KEY TERMS

Asthma: A disease of the lung characterized by airflow obstruction that is usually completely reversible and is usually associated with airway hyperreactivity.

Atelectasis: Collapse of part or all of a lung caused by a blockage of an airway (bronchus) or by external pressure on the lung.

Bronchiectasis: A relatively uncommon destructive lung disease characterized by irreversible dilatation of the distal bronchi, impaired clearance of sputum, and chronic infection.

Chronic bronchitis: Chronic inflammation of the conducting airways associated with the inhalation of noxious particles or gases (usually tobacco smoke).

Chronic obstructive pulmonary disease (COPD): Chronic bronchitis and emphysema.

Emphysema: Considered an element of COPD that primarily destroys the connective tissue structure of the lung, resulting in enlargement of distal air spaces.

Interstitial lung disease (ILD): A group of restrictive pulmonary diseases involving pathology primarily confined to the lung parenchyma.

Obstructive pulmonary disease: A category of diseases of the pulmonary system characterized by increased airway resistance, which is a major physiologic limitation.

Pulmonary arterial hypertension (PAH): Elevation of pulmonary arterial pressure usually associated with pulmonary vascular disease.

Pulmonary vascular disease: A category of lung diseases that affect the pulmonary vasculature by destruction or remodeling.

Restrictive pulmonary disease: A category of lung diseases in which the underlying pathologic process involved with each disease interferes with ability for normal lung expansion.

Ventilatory control: Mechanism that adjusts pulmonary ventilation to match metabolic requirements or to control acid-base state.

leading cause of death worldwide and is projected to rise to the third leading cause by 2015, just behind cardiovascular disease and cancer. The socioeconomic implications are enormous. A recent report by the Centers for Disease Control and Prevention showed that COPD is responsible for 8 million outpatient medical visits and 1.5 million emergency department visits. During the same year, COPD was responsible for 1.9%, or 726,000, of all hospitalizations, and this diagnosis was listed as a major contributing illness for 25 million additional hospitalizations (67). Dollars spent on this diagnosis are estimated to be in the billions, with $20 billion linked to direct and $11 billion linked to indirect medical costs (53). COPD accounts for approximately 120,000 deaths per year in the United States; since 2000, more women than men have succumbed to this disease (50).

ASTHMA

Asthma is also a common disease and is estimated to affect approximately 16 million Americans, one third of whom are children, making it the most common chronic childhood disease (10). Asthma has attracted public attention because it affects children and young adults. This disease claims more than 4,000 lives per year in the United States, and many of the victims are relatively young, dying of acute severe asthma, which in many cases might have been preventable (7). Asthma is characterized by chronic airway inflammation and reversible airflow obstruction, at least in its earlier stages (5). Asthma is linked to 100 million days missed from work or school and 470,000 hospitalizations annually in the U.S. (7). The monetary costs are substantial (128) and reflect both direct medical costs (hospital admissions and cost of medications) and indirect nonmedical costs (time lost from work, premature death) (118).

INTERSTITIAL LUNG DISEASE

Interstitial lung disease (ILD) encompasses several distinct disease entities, each of which tends to result in pulmonary fibrosis or scarring of the lung parenchyma. The most significant of these diseases is called idiopathic pulmonary fibrosis (IPF) and, although a misnomer, this label is meant to mean that the cause of the disease is unknown. About 50,000 individuals in the United States are thought to have IPF. Other conditions that are associated with pulmonary fibrosis include connective tissue disease, such as rheumatoid arthritis and systemic lupus erythematosus; pneumoconioses, such as coal-workers lung and asbestosis; and extrinsic allergic alveolitis in response to inhaled organic materials like fungi. Although much less common than the obstructive diseases (COPD and asthma), pulmonary fibrosis can result in markedly deranged physiology and serious impact on exercise performance.

PULMONARY VASCULAR DISEASE

In recent years, pulmonary vascular diseases have been gaining attention. Although less common, like interstitial lung diseases, the pulmonary vascular diseases can have marked effect on exercise performance and require special precautions in exercise testing and prescription. As pulmonary vascular disease progresses, vascular remodeling tends to increase pulmonary vascular resistance, resulting in pulmonary hypertension. The World Heath Organization has recently proposed a new categorization of pulmonary hypertension (109). This classification divides pulmonary hypertension into (a) pulmonary arterial hypertension (PAH); (b) pulmonary venous hypertension; (c) pulmonary hypertension associated with pulmonary diseases; including chronic hypoxemia; (d) pulmonary hypertension as a result of thromboembolic disease; and (e) miscellaneous disorders directly affecting the pulmonary vasculature. There are several causes associated with PAH, the most devastating of which is called primary pulmonary hypertension. Other causes include connective tissue diseases, such as progressive systemic sclerosis (scleroderma), human immunodeficiency virus (HIV), and exposure to anorexigenic drugs. The estimated incidence of primary pulmonary hypertension is 1 to 2 cases per million persons in the general population, and it is seen more commonly in women than in men (1.7 women per man) (101). Other causes of pulmonary hypertension may be relatively common but underdiagnosed. Reliable estimates of the prevalence of this condition are difficult to obtain because of the diversity of identifiable causes.

PATHOPHYSIOLOGY

A basic understanding of the pathophysiology of the different pulmonary diseases, particularly in the context of exercise performance, improves the efficacy and success of any exercise program for these patients. The design of the exercise program can be enhanced by recognizing disease features that can be used to individualize the program and optimize the individual exercise response. Through this knowledge base, elements key to the evaluation or assessment of the exercise response become more apparent, providing further direction to modifications that will enhance program design. Acquiring this knowledge base can be a large and complicated task, particularly if the diseases are approached in an individual manner. This task can be simplified by grouping diseases based on physiologic similarities. Four groups of diseases can be defined and named for their primary limitation: obstructive pulmonary disease, restrictive pulmonary disease, pulmonary vascular disease, and disturbances in ventilatory control. The physiologic pattern associated with each category can be generally applied to all the diseases within the respective category.

CHRONIC OBSTRUCTIVE PULMONARY DISEASE

Chronic obstructive pulmonary disease is a preventable and treatable disease in which the characteristic abnormality is chronic airway inflammation in response to exposure to noxious particles and gases (16,97). The most common etiology by far is tobacco smoking, although exposure to environmental tobacco smoke (passive smoking) is also recognized to be important, as well as occupational or environmental exposures, which are now thought to be responsible for about 20% of the cases of COPD. The term COPD encompasses chronic bronchitis and emphysema. Disease severity is staged according to guidelines set by the Global Initiative for Chronic Obstructive Lung Disease (GOLD) (97) (Table 36-1). Chronic bronchitis is defined by its histopathology, which is predominantly neutrophilic airway inflammation; but the clinical syndrome is still defined by symptoms such as sputum production on most days of the week for more than 3 months for at least 2 consecutive years (1). By contrast, the primary abnormality in emphysema involves destruction of alveolar septae and enlargement of the air spaces distal to the terminal bronchioles (57). COPD is recognized as an inflammatory disease of the airways with increased numbers of alveolar macrophages, neutrophils, and cytotoxic T lymphocytes, accompanied by release of multiple inflammatory mediators (e.g., oxygen free radicals, chemokines, cytokines, and growth factors) (16). An imbalance between neutrophil-derived proteases (e.g., neutrophil elastase and matrix metalloproteinases) and antiprotease defense mechanisms are characteristic of emphysema (16). One example of the genetic predisposition to developing emphysema is alpha-1 protease inhibitor deficiency, an inherited condition that accounts for 1% to 2% of cases of emphysema (2). From a practical standpoint, it is usually difficult to separate chronic bronchitis from emphysema, and the majority of individuals manifest a combination of both conditions.

The chronic inflammation common to COPD leads to progressive narrowing of small airways in the lung, thus increasing airway resistance. The destruction of lung connective tissue and loss of alveolar attachments in emphysema reduces lung elastic recoil. Both mechanisms hinder exhalation and tend to cause air trapping in regions of the lung with increased time constants for lung emptying. This process results in static hyperinflation that can be measured at rest. However, of particular importance during exercise as a result of increased respiratory rate and increased minute ventilation is dynamic hyperinflation. With dynamic hyperinflation, lung volumes increase even further.

Hyperinflation is central to understanding the pathophysiology of lung mechanics in COPD (Fig. 36-1)(33). Of all the spirometric measures in obstructive pulmonary disease, inspiratory capacity, a measure of hyperinflation, correlates best with patient-reported outcomes such as dyspnea, exercise capacity, and quality of life (84,87). At higher operational lung volumes, the increased elastic and threshold work of breathing contributes to dyspnea. Also, the configuration of the diaphragm tends to be low and flat, which diminishes its mechanical efficiency during inspiration. Factors that increase ventilatory work also affect energy expenditure and oxygen requirement. When ventilatory muscle work exceeds oxygen supply, ventilatory muscle fatigue and exercise termination can result (34). The negative effects of dynamic hyperinflation during exercise include increased elasticity; increased threshold work of breathing, which contributes to dyspnea and early exercise termination; and the potential for reduced venous return and cardiac output as a result of the increased intrathoracic pressure (86).

A recent article by Celli et al. (28) proposed the use of a new index, the BODE index, to more accurately rate the severity of COPD and predict the risk of death attributable to respiratory and nonrespiratory causes. The BODE index is a 10-point multidimensional scale that assigns points based on the results of four measures: body mass index (B), airflow obstruction (O), dyspnea (D), and exercise capacity (E). Airflow obstruction is measured by the FEV_1 (forced expiratory volume in 1 second) (75,92); dyspnea with the Medical Research Council (MRC)

TABLE 36-1. GLOBAL INITIATIVE FOR CHRONIC OBSTRUCTIVE LUNG DISEASE: GUIDELINES FOR CHRONIC OBSTRUCTIVE PULMONARY DISEASE STAGING

SEVERITY	STAGE	FEV_1[a]	SYMPTOMS[b]
Mild	I	>80%	Intermittent symptoms
Moderate	II	50%–80%	Persistent symptoms
Severe	III	30%–50%	Exacerbations
Very severe	IV	<30% or <50% with chronic respiratory failure	Respiratory failure

FEV_1, forced expiratory volume in 1 second.

[a]FEV_1 values are based on postbronchodilator measurements.

[b]Symptom categories are useful in clinical management but might not correlate with FEV_1.

Adapted from Global Initiative for Chronic Obstructive Lung Disease. Available at: www.goldcopd.com. See also Cooper CB, Tashkin DP. Recent developments in inhaled therapy in stable chronic obstructive pulmonary disease. *BMJ.* 2005;330(7492):640–644.

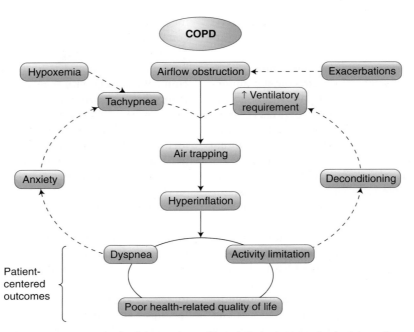

FIGURE 36-1. Central role of air trapping and hyperinflation in the pathophysiology of chronic obstructive pulmonary disease (COPD). Although related to increased airwal resistance, hyperinflation correlates more directly with patient centered outcomes. Activity limitation leads to deconditioning, which in turn, increases ventilatory requirements establishing a cycle of decline leading to worsening hyperinflation. Anxiety and hypoxemia cause tachypnea, which worsens hyperinflation by allowing less time for exhalation. From reference 30.

dyspnea scale (22) ; and exercise capacity, measured by the best of two trials on the 6-minute walking test (114) (Table 36-2).

> **1.5.3-CES: Recognize medications associated in the clinical setting, their indications for care, and their effects at rest and during exercise (i.e., β-blockers, nitrates, calcium channel blockers, digitalis, diuretics, vasodilators, antiarrhythmic agents, bronchodilators, antilipemics, psychotropics, nicotine, antihistamines, over-the-counter (OTC) cold medications, thyroid medications, alcohol, hypoglycemic agents, blood modifiers, pentoxifylline, antigout medications, and anorexiants/diet pills).**

> **1.5.1-HFS: Knowledge of common drugs from each of the following classes of medications and describe the principal action and the effects on exercise testing and prescription: antianginals, antihypertensives, antiarrhythmics, anticoagulants, bronchodilators, hypoglycemics; psychotropics, and vasodilators.**

Optimizing respiratory system mechanics before implementing an exercise program is essential for patients with COPD. Many COPD patients demonstrate a degree of reversibility with bronchodilator therapy, particularly assessed in terms of inspiratory capacity and hyperinflation. The GOLD guidelines have outlined the list of pharmacologic interventions advocated for COPD but do not provide a clear selection sequence for these agents. A recent review of inhaled therapies in COPD has proposed a three-step approach for mild, moderate, and severe disease (43,90). A combination of an inhaled short-acting anticholinergic agent (ipatropium) plus a short-acting β-agonist agent (e.g., albuterol) is beneficial before exercise and useful to relieve dyspnea (3). More recently, the long-acting anticholinergic bronchodilator tiotropium has become available, along with the long-acting β-adrenoreceptor agonists salmeterol and formoterol. These long-acting drugs will gain acceptance because of their sustained bronchodilator efficacy and convenience (e.g., tiotropium is a once-daily medication). Evidence suggests that inhaled corticosteroids should be prescribed for patients with severe COPD (FEV_1 <50%) to reduce the frequency of acute exacerbations. They are most efficacious in those patients who have frequent

TABLE 36-2. BODE INDEX

POINTS ON BODE INDEX

Variable	0	1	2	3
FEV_1 (% predicted)	≥56	50–64	36–49	≤35
Distance walked in 6 minutes (m)	≥350	250–349	150–249	≤149
MMRC dyspnea scale	0–1	2	3	4
BMI	>21	≤21		

BODE, body mass index (B), airflow obstruction (O), dyspnea (D), and exercise capacity (E); BMI, body mass index; FEV_1, forced expiratory volume in 1 second; MMRC, Modified Medical Research Council dyspnea scale.

Adapted from Celli BR, Cote CG, Marin JM, et al. The body-mass index, airflow obstruction, dyspnea, and exercise capacity index in chronic obstructive pulmonary disease. *N Engl J Med.* 2004;350:1005–1012.

exacerbations (e.g., two or more per year) (36,110). Inhaled agents are usually preferred over oral agents because of their rapid onset and low side-effect profile.

After lung mechanics are optimized by bronchodilator therapy, the need for oxygen supplementation should be assessed. The underlying mechanism for hypoxia in COPD involves regional mismatching between ventilation and perfusion (27). Ventilation is wasted within regions of the lung where emphysema is the dominant pathology and the capillary bed is destroyed. This type of gas exchange abnormality is known as dead-space ventilation. However, COPD is a heterogeneous disease, and there are other regions of the lungs where perfusion is relatively preserved but ventilation is impaired because of airway narrowing. This results in lung units with low ventilation-perfusion ratios, causing venous admixture of deoxygenated blood with oxygenated blood from other regions of the lung. The net result is a reduction in the oxygen content of systemic arterial blood. Thus, dead-space ventilation and venous admixture can be viewed at opposite ends of the spectrum of gas exchange abnormality or ventilation/perfusion mismatching (V/Q mismatch).

Increased dead-space ventilation affects exercise performance by increasing ventilatory requirement at a given metabolic rate. In circumstances in which ventilatory capacity is limited, dead-space ventilation can result in ventilatory limitation and directly contribute to exercise limitations. Venous admixture lowers arterial oxy-hemoglobin saturation and can result in desaturation during exercise, particularly when blood flow though V/Q mismatch areas increases with increased cardiac output. Desaturation, or failure of adequate gas exchange, is a serious cause of exercise limitation but can be overcome to some extent by providing supplemental oxygen.

ASTHMA

The relationship between COPD and asthma has undergone much debate throughout the years (16,41,106). The classic definition for asthma is airflow obstruction that is completely reversible and usually associated with airway hyperreactivity (41). One perspective considers chronic bronchitis, emphysema, and asthma as distinct diseases, sometimes with overlapping features (9). An alternative perspective, the so-called Dutch hypothesis (41,95,106), claims that asthma, chronic bronchitis, and emphysema are components of a single disease. The reality of varying degrees of disease overlap adds to the difficulty in differentiating these diseases clinically. For now, the general consensus is that COPD refers to chronic bronchitis and emphysema alone. Certainly it is erroneous these days to think of asthma as being reversible or responsive to bronchodilator therapy and COPD as being irreversible. The reality is that COPD is, by definition, partially reversible, and often the bronchodilator response is impressive, particularly after combined classes of bronchodilators (3). Asthma, on the other hand, becomes less responsive to bronchodilator therapy with poor control and over time (60,119).

The pathology of asthma consists of chronic airway inflammation, smooth muscle hyperplasia and hypertrophy, mucous hypersecretion, distal airway plugging, and atelectasis. The disruption of ventilation-perfusion matching in the lungs causes hypoxemia (116).

Triggers that induce the inflammatory cascade are important to recognize and avoid if possible (5,116). Triggers can include allergens and inhaled irritants. Common aeroallergen triggers are dust mites, animal dander, pollen, mold spores, and inhaled irritants (e.g., smoke, airborne particulates). Occupational or nonallergic triggers include invisible particulate matter (e.g., PM-10, fumes, diesel exhaust) and gases (oxides of nitrogen, oxides of sulphur and ozone). Some individuals exhibit aspirin sensitivity, frequently in association with nasal polyps. The effect of these triggers is dose dependent and often immediate. However, symptoms that occur after allergen exposure can sometimes manifest a delayed onset that occurs 6 to 8 hours after exposure. Seasonal variations are not uncommon. In sensitive individuals, cool air and humidity can also serve as triggers because of the affect on airway tone. Some patients have exercise-induced asthma. in which the stimulus to bronchoconstriction is thought to be respiratory heat exchange at higher levels of ventilation. Trigger avoidance, suppression of inflammation, and prophylaxis (i.e., before exercise) are essential elements in asthma management (5).

Asthma is a clinical diagnosis, although bronchial provocation studies are used by some to confirm or refute the diagnosis (5,116). The traditional test for exercise-induced asthma recommends an exercise stimulus of >80% of maximum heart rate for 6 minutes. A maximal cardiopulmonary exercise test (CPX) can be also used as a provocation study to identify exercise-induced asthma (35,38). A 10% fall in FEV_1 is considered abnormal; a fall of 15% appears to be more diagnostic of exercise-induced bronchoconstriction (EIB) (38). This usually occurs about 10 minutes after exercise, with recovery by 30 minutes after the exercise stimulus.

Asthma severity can be divided into four levels of severity: mild intermittent, mild persistent, moderate, and severe (4,10). See Box 36-1 for classifications of asthma severity (10). The frequency and severity of both basal symptoms and exacerbations determine the level of severity. The most recent guidelines, however, emphasize the importance of including the level of asthma control in the evaluation of disease severity (Table 36-3). Each severity level corresponds to a specific step approach, which defines general treatment options.

Short-acting β-agonist drugs, such as albuterol, with effectiveness lasting 4 to 6 hours, are the drugs of choice for rapid relief of symptoms related to acute

BOX 36-1 CLASSIFICATION OF ASTHMA SEVERITY BY CLINICAL FEATURES BEFORE TREATMENT

INTERMITTENT

Symptoms less than once a week

Brief exacerbations

Nocturnal symptoms not more than twice a month

- FEV_1 or PEF ≥80% predicted
- PEF or FEV_1 variability <20%

MILD PERSISTENT

Symptoms more than once a week but less than once a day

Exacerbations may affect activity and sleep

Nocturnal symptoms more than twice a month

- FEV_1 or PEF ≥80% predicted
- PEF or FEV_1 variability <20%–30%

MODERATE PERSISTENT

Symptoms daily

Exacerbations may affect activity and sleep

Nocturnal symptoms more than once a week

Daily use of inhaled short-acting β_2-agonist

- FEV_1 or PEF 60%–80% predicted
- PEF or FEV_1 variability >30%

SEVERE PERSISTENT

Symptoms daily

Frequent exacerbations

Frequent nocturnal asthma symptoms

Limitation of physical activities

- FEV_1 or PEF ≤60% predicted
- PEF or FEV_1 variability >30%

FEV_1, forced expiratory volume in 1 second; PEF, peak expiratory flow. From: Global Initiative on Asthma: www.ginasthma.org.

bronchoconstriction (5,15,81). Long-acting β-agonist bronchodilators, such as salmeterol and formoterol, result in improvement of airflow for up to 12 hours (5,15,81). Because of their delayed onset of action, long-acting β-agonist inhalers are not recommended for "rescue" relief of bronchoconstriction. Side effects of β-agonists—such as tachycardia, palpitations, dysrhythmias, and tremor—

require consideration in the context of exercise and could potentially compromise the exercise response (5,15,81).

In summary, successful asthma management requires trigger awareness, environmental controls, peak flow monitoring, and pharmacotherapy based on illness severity. Important considerations in the management of exercise-induced asthma include recognition of symptoms

TABLE 36-3. LEVELS OF ASTHMA CONTROL

CHARACTERISTIC	CONTROLLED (ALL OF THE FOLLOWING)	PARTLY CONTROLLED (ANY MEASURE PRESENT IN ANY WEEK)	UNCONTROLLED
Daytime symptoms	None (twice or less/week)	More than twice/week	
Limitations of activities	None	Any	
Nocturnal symptoms/ awakening	None	Any	Three or more features of partly controlled asthma present in any week
Need for reliever/rescue treatment	None (twice or less/week)	More than twice/week	
Lung function (PEF or FEV_1)[a]	Normal	<80% predicted or personal best (if known)	
Exacerbations	None	One or more/year[b]	One in any week[c]

PEF, peak expiratory flow; FEV_1, forced expiratory volume in 1 second.

[a]Lung function is not a reliable test for children 5 years and younger.

[b]Any exacerbation should prompt review of maintenance treatment to ensure that it is adequate.

[c]By definition, an exacerbation in any week makes that an uncontrolled asthma week.

From Global Strategy for Asthma Management and Prevention. Available at: www.ginasthma.org, p. 23.

and pretreatment with bronchodilator therapy. Management of exercise-induced asthma is much more attainable when chronic bronchial inflammation is kept under control.

BRONCHIECTASIS

Bronchiectasis is an inflammatory condition characterized by irreversible damage and dilatation of the bronchi (102,108). Regions of bronchiectasis in the lung commonly become chronically infected. Acute exacerbations of this disease influence the amount, color, and tenacity of mucus produced. Mucociliary clearance is altered in bronchiectasis, with retained secretions imposing a significant clinical problem.

Cystic fibrosis (CF) is an important cause of bronchiectasis in the United States and Europe, and this disorder has a genetic basis. The age at onset for CF is characteristically childhood, but genetic testing has enabled the identification of adult-onset disease linked to variable gene penetrance. Recurrent and chronic lung infection with resistant bacterial pathogens, particularly gram-negative organisms such as *Pseudomonas* species and nontuberculous mycobacteria, is common in CF.

Airflow obstruction occurs in up to 50% of individuals with bronchiectasis (76). In some patients, the airflow obstruction is associated with bronchial hyperresponsiveness, as demonstrated by bronchial provocation with methacholine. This observation may represent coexisting asthma (17). Administration of an inhaled bronchodilator should be considered but should be determined on an individual basis. One study (76) demonstrated improved airflow after inhaled ipratropium bromide ion, suggesting that bronchoconstriction in bronchiectasis is mediated by reflex vagal mechanism related to airway irritation (60,119).

Bronchopulmonary hygiene is fundamental to the management of bronchiectasis (102,108). The treatment involves a combination of adequate hydration to reduce mucous tenacity and chest physiotherapy implemented either manually or with the aid of mechanical devices (24,102,108). Theoretically, exercise performance could be improved in bronchiectasis by implementing bronchopulmonary hygiene and clearing mucous plugging, thereby improving gas exchange.

INTERSTITIAL LUNG DISEASE

Interstitial lung disease implies that the primary site of pathophysiologic abnormality is the lung parenchyma (76). Multiple classifications are proposed for the ILDs. The classification scheme used in this chapter includes infiltrating (e.g. edema, amyloid, or tumor), inflammatory (idiopathic interstitial pneumonias and acute respiratory distress syndrome), and infectious processes. As a result of inflammation of fibrosis of the interstitial space, the lungs become stiff and noncompliant, causing restric-

tive physiology and diffusion impairment. Reduced compliance limits the increase in tidal volume during exercise and results in a disproportionate rise in the breathing frequency. Respiratory rates will often exceed 50 breaths per minute, and the breathing pattern is both rapid and shallow. As with obstructive disease, when the ventilatory requirement of exercise reaches the limited ventilatory capacity, there will be exercise impairment. Some lung diseases are classically characterized by a combination of both restriction and obstruction (76). The diseases typically associated with both processes include sarcoidosis, hypersensitivity pneumonitis, and pulmonary (Langerhans) histiocytosis (76). Different natural histories are encountered for each ILD, and fluctuations in disease severity are likely to influence the exercise potential.

Compared with COPD, there has been relatively little investigation of the exercise physiology of the ILDs (51,68–70). Recently, some authors have argued for the usefulness of exercise testing in the evaluation of at least some restrictive pulmonary diseases (71). Abnormalities of gas exchange are particularly evident with the ILDs. Loss of pulmonary capillary bed and ventilation-perfusion mismatching cause increased dead-space ventilation and exercise-induced hypoxemia (51,68–71). The diffusing capacity is usually low, with restrictive disease reflecting impaired gas diffusion through the alveolar-capillary membrane (76). This abnormality might not translate into clinically significant hypoxemia at rest because there is adequate pulmonary capillary transit time to allow complete diffusion equilibrium of the oxygen molecules. However, during exercise, the reduced pulmonary capillary transit time in conjunction with slowed diffusion can result in significant hypoxemia (51,68–70,72).

OTHER RESTRICTIVE PULMONARY DISEASES

Whereas interstitial lung diseases can be viewed as causing restriction by reducing lung compliance, there are other extrapulmonary diseases that cause restriction (76). The most important to consider are pleural effusion, chest wall deformity, and ventilatory muscle weakness. There are many causes of pleural effusions, including pneumonia, heart failure, renal disease, liver disease, and malignancy. Chest wall deformities can be related to kyphoscoliosis, or they may accompany chronic neuromuscular diseases, such as muscular dystrophy, myopathy, or postpolio syndrome. The same neuromuscular diseases, plus others such as acute postinfectious polyneuropathy (Guillain-Barre syndrome) and myasthenia gravis, can cause ventilatory muscle weakness.

The extrapulmonary causes of restriction have common pathophysiologic features that pertain to exercise. Both reduced chest wall compliance and ventilatory muscle weakness compromise ventilatory capacity by limiting the ability to increase in tidal volume. As a result, increases in minute ventilation tend to rely more on

BOX 36-2	WORLD HEALTH ORGANIZATION DISEASE CLASSIFICATION OF THE CAUSE OF PULMONARY HYPERTENSION

1. Pulmonary arterial hypertension
2. Pulmonary venous hypertension
3. Pulmonary hypertension associated with pulmonary disease or chronic hypoxemia

4. Pulmonary hypertension because of chronic thromboembolic disease
5. Pulmonary hypertension because of disorders directly affecting pulmonary vasculature

Adapted from Simonneau G, Galie N, Rubin LJ, et al. Clinical classification of pulmonary hypertension. *J Am Coll Cardiol.* 2004;43(suppl S):5S–12S.

increased breathing frequency. During maximal incremental exercise, it is not unusual to see a breathing frequency $>50 \cdot min^{-1}$ in this type of patient. In those circumstances in which the ventilatory requirement for exercise approaches or equals the reduced ventilatory capacity, ventilatory limitation will be the cause of exercise limitation.

PULMONARY VASCULAR DISEASES

Under normal conditions, the pulmonary vascular system is a low-pressure circuit with a low vascular resistance (76). Vascular resistance can be altered by disease. The mechanism depends on whether the vessel is a primary disease target. Box 36-2 shows the World Health Organization (WHO) disease classifications based on the cause of pulmonary hypertension. The distinction of etiology has both prognostic and therapeutic value. Primary pulmonary hypertension (PPH) exemplifies the vessel wall as the primary disease target (76). This disease is rare and mostly sporadic in occurrence, with only 10% of the cases demonstrating genetic linkage (76). Risk factors predisposing to PPH include connective tissue diseases, chronic liver disease, HIV infection, cocaine or amphetamine use, and dietary agents such as fenfluramine and tryptophan. Diagnosis of PPH is complex, and readers are referred to McGoon et al. (72) for a detailed overview. The determination of disease severity of pulmonary hypertension follows the criteria used by the American

Heart Association outlined for congestive heart failure (Box 36-3) (59).

Secondary pulmonary hypertension demonstrates an indirect effect of disease on pulmonary vascular resistance. Diseases that can lead to the development of secondary pulmonary hypertension include pulmonary fibrosis, COPD, and left-sided heart disease (76). Prognostic and therapeutic implications underscore the importance of making the distinction between primary and secondary pulmonary hypertension (59,76).

DISORDERS OF VENTILATORY CONTROL

Ventilatory control is mediated either through metabolic or behavioral pathways (76). Metabolic pathways are triggered by changes in carbon dioxide or oxygen tension or changes in acid–base balance (pH) detected by chemoreceptors. Chemoreceptors are located either centrally, such as in the brain, or peripherally, such as in the carotid bodies. Ventilatory control through behavioral pathway originates from the brain cortex and supramedullary region. Disorders in breathing control are classified as hyperventilation or hypoventilation syndromes.

Hyperventilation Syndromes

Acute hyperventilation syndromes are characterized by episodes of hypocapnia and respiratory alkalosis. This occurs in relation to anxiety disorders or acute panic

BOX 36-3	WORLD HEALTH ORGANIZATION CLASSIFICATION OF THE SEVERITY OF ILLNESS FOR PULMONARY HYPERTENSION

Class I	Asymptomatic, no physical limitations
Class II	Mild limitation of physical activity. Comfortable at rest.
	Breathless on exertion.
Class III	Marked limitation of physical activity. Comfortable at rest.
	Unduly breathless on exertion.
Class IV	Unable to perform any physical activity. Symptomatic at rest.
	Right heart failure

Adapted from Simonneau G, Galie N, Rubin LJ, et al. Clinical classification of pulmonary hypertension. *J Am Coll Cardiol.* 2004;43(suppl S):5S–12S.

attacks. In the context of exercise, the minute ventilation is inappropriately high for the metabolic rate because of factors other than lactic acid accumulation. Excess carbon dioxide excretion leads to an increase in the respiratory exchange ratio (R). The associated hypocapnia can cause lightheadedness and paraesthesia, which can themselves contribute to exercise intolerance. Ventilatory reserve is reduced and in certain circumstances (e.g., patients with chronic obstructive or restrictive lung disease), this could precipitate ventilatory limitation and exercise termination.

Hypoventilation Syndromes

Hypoventilation syndromes can be the result of reduced ventilatory drive from the central nervous system or, alternatively, the inability to maintain alveolar ventilation because of severe mechanical abnormalities of the respiratory system or disturbances in gas exchange. With hypoventilation, the minute ventilation is inappropriately low for the metabolic rate, and arterial carbon dioxide tension increases, creating a respiratory acidosis. Hypoventilation is rarely seen in the context of incremental exercise, usually in association with severe obstructive or restrictive lung diseases.

Two hypoventilation syndromes—obstructive sleep apnea and obesity hypoventilation syndrome—deserve brief consideration (76). These syndromes are more often encountered within the obese population. Obstructive sleep apnea syndrome is characterized by failure to maintain upper-airway patency during sleep either because of anatomic deformities of the upper airway or because of loss of supportive muscle tone (49). In obese individuals, the accumulation of fat around the upper airway is a significant contributory factor. Episodes of nocturnal apnea lead to classic manifestations of sleep fragmentation, day-

time hypersomnolence, and cognitive impairment. Systemic arterial hypertension is frequently associated with this disorder. Obesity hypoventilation syndrome, historically known as Pickwickian syndrome, is seen in morbidly obese individuals (62). These individuals have diminished ventilatory drive with hypoxemia and hypercapnia reflective of chronic respiratory failure. They develop insensitivity to hypercapnia. In the longer term, the chronic hypoxemia associated with hypoventilation syndromes predisposes patients to cor pulmonale and right-sided heart failure.

Hypoventilation syndromes can be treated with assisted ventilation using noninvasive apparatus. Obstructive sleep apnea is treated with continuous positive airway pressure (CPAP) during sleep to prevent upper-airway collapse, whereas obesity hypoventilation syndrome requires bilevel intermittent positive pressure (BiPAP) to augment alveolar ventilation.

EXERCISE RESPONSES IN PULMONARY DISEASE

Exercise intolerance is the hallmark of chronic lung disease. Foremost among the symptoms that limit exercise is dyspnea and/or fatigue because of some combination of the pathologic changes in lung function noted above. These may be exacerbated by physical deconditioning, anxiety secondary to exertional shortness of breath, and declining motivation. As shown in Figure 36-2 (32), this is a vicious cycle leading to further exercise intolerance and increased ventilatory requirements at a given workload. Exercise tolerance is reduced in chronic lung diseases because of ventilatory and gas exchange limitations, cardiac and respiratory muscle dysfunction, and skeletal muscle disuse and/or dysfunction. Specific limitations to exercise

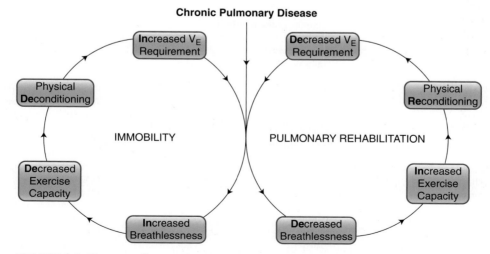

FIGURE 36-2. Diagram to illustrate the vicious cycle (on left) of disabling breathlessness physical inactivity, and deconditioning in chronic pulmonary disease. Pulmonary rehabilitation that includes exercise training offers a favorable cycle (on right) of reconditioning, restoration of functional capacity, and improved quality of life. From reference 33.

in chronic pulmonary disease and their influence on exercise prescription are shown in Table 36-4.

ACUTE RESPONSES TO EXERCISE

The acute responses to exercise resulting from those factors that limit tolerance because of the specific limitations imposed by chronic lung diseases are listed in Box 36-4. The goals surrounding the exercise component of pulmonary rehabilitation are to alleviate these functional limitations (Box 36-5).

CHRONIC EXERCISE RESPONSES: EVIDENCE-BASED OUTCOMES

The chronic responses to exercise training in patients with lung disease are dependent on several factors, including disease severity, initial level of fitness, supplemental oxygen, and optimal management of bronchodilator therapy in patients with airflow limitation (99). A patient's ability to tolerate endurance exercise at intensities above the metabolic (lactate) threshold may also influence the extent to which endurance performance is improved (26). Typical adaptations to exercise training are shown in Box 36-6. Supporting evidence for these adaptations will be noted throughout this chapter. Evidence is based on a recent American College of Chest Physicians (ACCP)/American Association of Cardiovascular and Pulmonary Rehabilitation (AACVPR) report on evidence-based clinical practice guidelines for pulmonary rehabilitation (PR), along with grading for their strength of evidence and balance of benefits to risks/burdens (99). Table 36-5 contains a key for the ACCP grading of these benefits.

THE EXERCISE PRESCRIPTION

Recently published, the Joint ACCP/AACVPR Evidence-Based Clinical Practice Guidelines for Pulmonary Rehabilitation (99) provide strong recommendations for exercise training as a mandatory component of pulmonary rehabilitation. The 2006 American Thoracic Society

---

TABLE 36-4. SPECIFIC LIMITATIONS TO EXERCISE IN CHRONIC PULMONARY DISEASE AND HOW THEY INFLUENCE EXERCISE PRESCRIPTION

SPECIFIC EXERCISE LIMITATION	THRESHOLDS INFLUENCING INTENSITY PRESCRIPTION	GOALS AND TARGETS FOR EXERCISE PRESCRIPTION
Physical deconditioning (i.e., premature lactic acidosis)	Lactic acidosis (metabolic threshold)	Reconditioning exercise Target intensity should be above metabolic threshold
Ventilatory limitation (e.g., $\dot{V}Emax$, MVV)	Dyspnea	Increase ventilatory capacity
	Dyspnea	Improve respiratory system mechanics (PFTs)
	Lactic acidosis (metabolic acidosis)	Mitigate lactic acidosis through reconditioning Reduce ventilatory requirement
	Hypoventilation	Increase respiratory muscle strength Offer ventilatory assistance Improve breathing efficiency (reduce VD/VT)
	Hypoxemia (desaturation)	Prevent desaturation with supplemental oxygen
Ventilatory inefficiency (e.g., dynamic hyperinflation in COPD or high VD/VT)	Bronchoconstriction or airway collapse	Relieve expiratory airflow obstruction Optimize bronchodilator therapy
	Tachypnea Hypoventilation	Reduce respiratory rate Teach breathing techniques Teach panic control
Gas exchange failure (i.e., hypoxemia or hypercapnia)	Desaturation Respiratory acidosis	Prevent hypoxemia and hypoventilation Use supplemental oxygen Offer assisted ventilation
Cardiovascular limitations (e.g., myocardial ischemia, hypertension, pulmonary vascular disease)	Angina Hypertension Dysrhythmia	Cardiovascular monitoring ECG telemetry BP during exercise Adjust intensity range for safety Adjust cardiovascular medications
Symptomatic limitations	Dyspnea Anxiety Fear	Psychotherapy Desensitization Mastery Panic control

BP, blood pressure; COPD, chronic obstructive pulmonary disease; ECG, electrocardiogram; MVV, maximum voluntary ventilation; PFT, pulmonary function test.

Adapted from: Cooper CB. Exercise in chronic pulmonary disease: aerobic exercise prescription. *Med Sci Sports Exerc.* 2001;33(7):S671–S679.

BOX 36-4 ACUTE RESPONSES TO EXERCISE IN CHRONIC LUNG DISEASES

Obstructive diseases

Reduced $\dot{V}O_2$ max

Reduced metabolic (lactate) threshold

Reduced muscular strength

Reduced ventilatory reserve

Increased VD/VT

Increased ventilatory equivalents for O_2 [$\dot{V}E/\dot{V}O_2$) and CO_2 ($\dot{V}E/\dot{V}CO_2$)

Increased difference between arterial and end-tidal partial pressures for CO_2 ($PaCO_2 - P_{ET}CO_2$)

Increased difference between alveolar and end-tidal partial pressures for O_2 ($PAO_2 - PaO_2$)

No increase in ventilatory equivalent for CO_2 at maximum exercise

Respiratory acidosis

Hypoxemia depending on the presence of low VA/Q lung units

High heart rate reserve (HRmax predicted − HRmax measured)

Low O_2 pulse

Early-onset lactic acidosis

Restrictive diseases

Reduced $\dot{V}O_2$max

Reduced metabolic (lactate) threshold

Reduced $\Delta\dot{V}O_2/\Delta WR$ slope

Increased VD/VT

Increased ventilatory equivalents for O_2 ($VE/\dot{V}O_2$) and CO_2 ($\dot{V}E/\dot{V}CO_2$)

Increased difference between arterial and end-tidal partial pressures for CO_2 ($PaCO_2 - P_{ET}CO_2$)

No increase in ventilatory equivalent for CO_2 at maximum exercise

Respiratory acidosis

Hypoxemia that is usually progressive

Ratio of tidal volume to inspiratory capacity (VT/IC) that ≈ 1 at low levels of work

Muscular weakness

Adapted from Wasserman K. Exercise tolerance in the pulmonary patient. In: Casaburi R, Petty TL, editors. *Principles and Practice of Pulmonary Rehabilitation*. Philadelphia: W.B. Saunders; 1993. p. 119–121.

BOX 36-5 GOALS OF PULMONARY REHABILITATION

Improve exercise performance and activities of daily living

Alleviate dyspnea

Restore a positive outlook

Reduce the work of breathing

Normalize arterial blood gases

Increase mechanical efficiency

Improve nutrition

Improve emotional state

Decrease health-related costs

Lengthen survival

Adapted from Celli BR. Pulmonary rehabilitation for COPD: a practical approach for improving ventilatory conditioning. *Postgrad Med*. 1998;103: 159–160, 167–158, 173–156.

(ATS)/European Respiratory Society (ERS) Statement on Pulmonary Rehabilitation (82) has updated the scientific evidence for the physiologic effects of chronic lung disease and the role of pulmonary rehabilitation in affecting change in the ensuing functional limitations. Practice guidelines summarizing these recommendations were included.

Exercise training improves exercise tolerance and may also improve motivation to exercise as well as psychological and cognitive outcomes (48,91,124). The exercise training component of PR programs should be comprehensive, providing cardiopulmonary endurance (aerobic) exercise, muscle strengthening, and joint range-of-motion exercise. The addition of inspiratory muscle training may be of value for some patients, particularly those with low inspiratory muscle strength (6,99). After medical evaluation and optimization of bronchodilator and oxygen therapy, a maximal cardiopulmonary exercise test can be valuable in defining the specific physiologic limitations to exercise, assessing the safety of exercise, and helping formulate the exercise prescription. When this is not possible or is inappropriate, functional exercise assessments, such the 6-minute walk test (114) or the shuttle walk test (112), can provide helpful information for setting the

BOX 36-6 CHRONIC ADAPTATIONS TO EXERCISE IN PEOPLE WITH CHRONIC LUNG DISEASE

1. Maximal endurance exercise
   Improved aerobic capacity ($\dot{V}O_{2max}$)
   Increased maximal work rate
   Improved 6-minute walking distance

2. Submaximal endurance exercise
   Higher metabolic (lactate) threshold
   Increased endurance (longer duration at same work rate)
   Reduced heart rate[a]
   Reduced $\dot{V}O_2$[a]
   Reduced perception of effort[a]
   Reduced blood lactate[a]
   Reduced $\dot{V}CO_2$[a]
   Reduced minute ventilation[a]

3. Peripheral muscle performance
   Increased upper- and lower-body peripheral muscle strength and endurance
   Improved rate of force development
   Improved mechanical efficiency

4. Symptoms
   Decreased dyspnea
   Less fear and anxiety because of sensations of breathlessness
   Improved quality of life

[a]Compared with the same absolute pretraining work rates.

exercise prescription and for progress monitoring. In physiologic terms, this type of test is similar to a maximum test.

The majority of research studying the effects of exercise training in chronic lung diseases has been completed in patients with COPD. To date, there are no evidence-based guidelines for exercise training in other forms of lung disease. It is reasonable to believe, however, that the general principles of training recommended by expert groups and evidence-based practice guidelines for the COPD population can also be applied to other forms of chronic lung disease when appropriate, disease-specific

modifications are employed. The following sections summarize recommendations for endurance training, resistance training, flexibility exercise, and inspiratory muscle training in patients with COPD. Subsequent sections will describe concerns and modifications that should be considered in disease-specific applications for exercise training in patients with chronic lung diseases other than COPD.

The use of exercise assessments on the patient with chronic respiratory diseases will quantify exercise tolerance, aid in developing training recommendations, and

TABLE 36-5. AMERICAN COLLEGE OF CHEST PHYSICIANS RELATIONSHIP OF STRENGTH OF THE SUPPORTING EVIDENCE TO THE BALANCE OF BENEFITS TO RISKS AND BURDENS

Strength of Evidence	BALANCE OF BENEFITS TO RISKS AND BURDENS[a]			
	Benefits Outweigh Risks/Burdens	Risks/Burdens Outweigh Benefits	Evenly Balanced	Uncertain
High	1A	1A	2A	
Moderate	1B	1B	2B	
Low or very low	1C	1C	2C	2C

[a]1A, 1B, 1C, strong recommendation.

2A, 2B, weak recommendation.

2C, weak recommendation.

DESCRIPTION OF BALANCE OF BENEFITS TO RISKS/BURDENS SCALE

Benefits clearly outweigh the risks and burdens	Certainty of imbalance
Risks and burdens clearly outweigh the benefits	Certainty of imbalance
The risks/burdens and benefits are closely balanced	Less certainty
The balance of benefits to risks and burdens is uncertain	Uncertainty

Adapted from Pulmonary Rehabilitation: Joint ACCP/AACVPR Evidence-Based Clinical Practice Guidelines. *Chest.* 2007;131:4S–42S.

provide a baseline for progress monitoring and program efficacy. These assessments may also be used to identify relationships between exercise intensity and symptoms such as hypoxemia, exercise-induced bronchospasm, cardiac abnormalities, or musculoskeletal limitations. Assessment instruments for endurance performance include laboratory methods such as incremental and constant work-rate cardiopulmonary exercise testing (11,35) performed on treadmills or cycle ergometers, and functional exercise tests such as 6-minute walk distance tests (114) and shuttle tests (111,112). For resistance training, the one-repetition maximum procedure (14) may be useful and is safely applied in patients with chronic pulmonary diseases (61). Tests are also available for assessing flexibility and range of motion (11).

Endurance (Aerobic) Exercise Training

Individualized exercise prescriptions for people with chronic lung disease include application of the familiar FITT (Frequency, Intensity, Time, and Type) framework (73) adjusted to patient capabilities, disease specific limitations, therapeutic objectives, and goals. It is important to note that the intensity and duration guidelines should be considered together, as they dictate the total energy expenditure of an exercise session. Warm-up and cool-down periods should be integrated into the training session as described below. A summary of current evidence-based guidelines for endurance exercise training in patients with COPD and, for comparison, in older healthy adults is presented in Table 36-6.

Warm-up

A 5- to 10-minute warm-up, including whole-body low- to moderate-intensity cardiovascular (aerobic) and local muscle endurance exercise, provides a gradual transition to higher-intensity exercise performed during the conditioning phase. The warm-up period is valuable for increasing muscle temperature, improving oxygen exchange, and speeding nerve impulse transmission (13). Warm-up activities should be similar to those to be performed in the subsequent training period and not induce shortness of breath. Joint readiness, the gradually increasing movement of the joints to be used during the conditioning period, should be included. Stretching exercise is often incorporated into the warm-up period but should be considered as a distinct segment and performed after warm-up exercise or cool-down. See **flexibility** section below.

Cool-down

The purpose of the cool-down period is to return the body to pre-exercise conditions by gradually decreasing the exercise intensity. Avoiding an abrupt stop in the activity maintains blood pressure through the action of the peripheral muscle pump and thus helps prevent blood pooling leading to dizziness, syncope, and cardiac arrhythmias. Cool-down also reduces the risk of postexercise bronchospasm (9). The duration of the cool-down is dependent on the intensity of the previous exercise and is normally 3 to 10 minutes. Stretching can be added at the end of the cool-down but should not be considered as the primary cool-down activity.

TABLE 36-6. SUMMARY OF EVIDENCE-BASED GUIDELINES FOR CARDIOVASCULAR ENDURANCE (AEROBIC) EXERCISE TRAINING

REFERENCE	GROUP	FREQUENCY	INTENSITY	TIME	TYPE	STRENGTH OF EVIDENCE
(5)	Patients with COPD	≥3 d·week⁻¹	Low intensity		Walking Cycling	IB[a]
			High intensity High and low	>30 min	Swimming Upper-body ergometer	IA[a]
(3)	Older, healthy adults	5 d·week⁻¹ 3 d·week⁻¹	Moderate[b] Vigorous[b]	≥30 min ≥20 min	Walking Other aerobic activity	I (A)[c]
			Combinations			IIa (B)[c]

COPD, chronic obstructive pulmonary disease.

[a] See Table 36-5.

[b] Rating exercise at 5 to 6 on a 10-point scale (the Borg 10-point scale was not specified) for "moderate" exercise (5 d·week⁻¹) and 7 to 8 on the 10-point scale for vigorous exercise (3 d·week⁻¹) or a combination of these.

[c] Based on the American College of Cardiology/American Heart Association approach to assigning the classification of recommendations and level of evidence.

Classification of Recommendations

I: Conditions for which there is evidence and/or general agreement that a given procedure or treatment is useful and effective (should; is recommended; is indicated; is useful/effective, beneficial)

IIa: Weight of evidence/opinion is in favor of usefulness/efficacy (is reasonable; can be useful, effective, or beneficial; is probably recommended or indicated)

Levels of Evidence

A: Data derived from multiple randomized clinical trials

B: Data derived from a single randomized trial or from nonrandomized studies

Frequency

Three to five days per week of endurance exercise training is recommended (9,82,99), with supervised sessions, directed by at least one clinical exercise professional, required to achieve optimal health-related and physiologic benefits. This guideline is consistent with recommendations for frequency of endurance exercise training in healthy older adults (78). Two supervised sessions plus one or more home sessions may be an acceptable alternative to three supervised sessions, but whether home exercise is effective in promoting health benefits or a physiologic training effect is equivocal.

Intensity

Defining appropriate or optimal intensity targets for patients with chronic lung disease is difficult. In some cases, general exercise intensity recommendations for healthy individuals may be used (11). However, ventilatory limitations, dyspnea, skeletal muscle dysfunction, exercise tolerance, motivation, oxygen transport, cardiac function, and patient safety contribute variable limitations on tolerable levels of exertion in these patients (Table 36-4).

When possible, high-intensity training produces greater benefit in patients with COPD than lower-intensity training (26) and as a practice guideline should be encouraged when appropriate (82). Alternatively, lower-intensity prescriptions may be more appropriate at the onset of rehabilitation for those with poor exercise tolerance, for long-term adherence, and for "metabolic fitness" (42) that may lead to health benefits other than improved physical function. For patients with mild to moderate COPD or controlled asthma, use of intensity guidelines set for older adults (78) may be appropriate (Table 36-6). Current evidence-based clinical practice guidelines grade the recommendation of higher versus lower training intensity as moderately strong or 1B (Table 36-5), whereas both high- and low-intensity exercise training are given a grade of strong, or1A, for their ability to produce clinical benefits in patients with COPD (99).

Cardiopulmonary exercise testing can provide valuable information regarding safety and patient limitations as well as anchor points for setting training intensity and for progress monitoring. Empirical evidence suggests that intensities exceeding 60% of maximum work rate or maximum $\dot{V}O_2$ are adequate to elicit a training effect (82), and training intensities representing 80% to 95% of maximum work rate have been used successfully in patients with COPD (21,85,100). In one study, higher-intensity but not moderate-intensity exercise resulted in reduced dyspnea at rest and submaximal exercise and increased 12-minute walk distance (45). *High intensity* and *moderate intensity* are relative terms and do not indicate high absolute workloads because these are significantly reduced in patients with COPD (99). Intensity targets based on percentage of estimated maximal heart rate or

heart rate reserve may be difficult in patients with chronic lung disease (31). Resting heart rate is often elevated in individuals with chronic lung disease, particularly if their severity is advanced (107). The exercise limitations seen in these patients, as well as the effects of some medication, prohibit attainment of the predicted value of peak heart rate and thus its use in intensity calculations. Maximal cardiopulmonary exercise testing obviates this problem because a symptom-limited maximum heart rate can be measured along with maximum work rate. The $\dot{V}O_2$ and work rate at the metabolic or gas exchange threshold may also be determined. These data may then be used with symptom scores (rating of perceived exertion, dyspnea scales) collected during the maximal cardiopulmonary exercise test to generate appropriate training intensities (23,29,58,122).

There may be a reluctance to use higher-intensity exercise in individuals with moderate to severe lung disease. Estimating the maximum sustainable exercise intensity may be determined by: (a) recognizing the difference between "perceived level of exertion" and "dyspnea" ; (b) avoiding sustained ventilatory loads close to ventilatory capacity, which would correlate to a "moderate" dyspnea index; and (c) aiming for an exercise intensity level that is 60% to 80% of the maximum capability for that individual. Sustained exercise intensity levels higher than these recommendations predispose to muscle fatigue and exhaustion. If the respiratory muscle fatigue is sustained, respiratory failure can ensue. Although skeletal muscle fatigue is better tolerated, it still influences the frequency at which exercise can be performed (32,66,104). Distinguishing between perceived exertion and dyspnea is essential but difficult because they are not mutually exclusive (66). The former represents the degree of peripheral muscle fatigue and weakness, and the latter represents the degree of breathlessness.

When maximal cardiopulmonary exercise testing is unavailable or inappropriate, submaximal testing may prove useful. Although there are no specific intensity guidelines that use heart rate indices, heart rates that are correlated with symptom scores, such Borg rating of perceived exertion (RPE) (23) or dyspnea scales (58,66), determined during submaximal exercise, such as a 6-minute walk test, can provide an objective measure of training intensity and progress monitoring. In clinical practice, RPE and dyspnea scores provide self-adjusting anchors for intensity prescriptions. That is, as fitness improves, work rates will increase at the same symptom score. Periodic assessment of this relationship provides a mechanism for progress monitoring. Intensity targets of 4 to 6 on the 0 to 10 category/ratio Borg perceived exertion scale (23) are reasonable (82). Regardless of the intensity utilized, monitoring oxygen saturation in patients with more severe disease should be part of the exercise regimen, at least during the initial few weeks of training. Values for oxygen saturation during exercise should be maintained at ≥90% (9).

Time

No specific guidelines for training-session duration have been set for patients with chronic lung disease. However, an initial goal of 30 (range 20–60) minutes has been suggested, with a goal of progressing to 60 to 90 minutes as tolerated (9,30). Because training intensity in part dictates achievable training duration, attempting to achieve an intensity target that is set too high may preclude attainment of target duration. Patients with chronic lung disease often do not achieve 30 minutes of continuous endurance training until several weeks into their rehabilitation program, even at lower intensities. Training frequencies of 3 to 5 days per week have been recommended for healthy older adults, depending on the intensity with which the exercise is performed (78) (Table 36-6). These general guidelines for healthy individuals may be successfully adapted to patients with chronic lung disease as well.

One approach to achieving target duration is to decrease the exercise intensity. Although this might be a desirable solution, another option is to apply the aerobic exercise prescription in intervals for several weeks with the goal of achieving 30 minutes or more of cumulative aerobic exercise with each session. Interval training with bouts of higher-intensity exercise interspersed with periods of lower intensity has proven to be equally (12,96,123) or more (45,122) effective at eliciting significant physiologic training effects than lower-intensity exercise. One study in patients with severe COPD has shown differing physiologic responses to interval versus continuous training (37).

Type

Patients with chronic lung disease typically use lower-extremity modalities, such as treadmills and cycle ergometers. This has practical value in improving performance of the muscles of ambulation. Treadmill exercise is usually preferred by patients and exercise professionals because of its similarity to everyday walking and greater relevance to many activities of daily living. Cycle ergometry can be used as a means of varying the exercise mode and may be preferred in patients with arthritis, joint deformities, or morbid obesity because of its low impact on the musculoskeletal system. Cycle ergometry might also be chosen if the clinical exercise professional finds difficulty with monitoring, such as pulse oximetry, sphygmomanometry, or electrocardiography during treadmill exercise.

Other modes of endurance exercise training may be used successfully, including track walking, rowing, arm ergometry, stepping, swimming, water aerobics, modified aerobic dance, and seated aerobics (9). Patient participation in selecting one or more appropriate (e.g., large muscle group, rhythmic exercise) exercise training modes will likely add enjoyment and contribute to long-term compliance, and is recommended.

Previous ACCP/AACVPR evidence-based guidelines for pulmonary rehabilitation emphasized the scientific evidence in favor of aerobic exercise training using the large muscle groups of the legs (6). Current evidence-based (82) and practice guidelines (99) provide new support for the use of upper-extremity exercise specifically for developing upper-limb exercise capacity and reduced ventilation and oxygen cost during unsupported arm activity.

On the Use of Supplemental Oxygen During Exercise

Maintenance of oxyhemoglobin saturation (SaO_2) during exercise at levels $\geq 88\%$ is generally recommended (9). Assessments of exercise performance will aid in identifying exercise intensities at which patients become hypoxemic, and periodic monitoring of SaO_2 by pulse oximetry will help guide administration of supplemental oxygen therapy. At least from a safety perspective, supplemental oxygen administered during exercise training is recommended for patients with severe resting or exercise-induced hypoxemia (99). Although inconclusive, supplemental oxygen administered to patients who do not experience significant exercise-induced desaturation has been shown to allow higher training intensities and improved constant work rate performance (99). Thus, in this case, supplemental oxygen is not routinely recommended.

Resistance Exercise Training

Disuse deconditioning is common in patients with COPD because of the vicious cycle of increasing ventilatory limitations, shortness of breath, and consequent decreases in physical activity. This contributes to skeletal muscle disuse atrophy and loss of muscle strength, power, and endurance. In addition, myopathies in skeletal muscle attributable to systemic inflammation, oxidative stress, blood gas abnormalities, and use of corticosteroids are proposed as mechanisms of skeletal muscle dysfunction (8). Evidence is available suggesting that loss of muscle strength is proportional to the loss of muscle mass in patients with COPD and that there is preferential loss of muscle size and strength in the lower limbs (20). That peripheral muscle dysfunction contributes to the exercise intolerance seen in chronic respiratory diseases has received considerable attention (8,89) and is shown to be significantly and independently related to increased use of healthcare resources (40). Recent evidence-based and scientific guidelines for pulmonary rehabilitation (82,99) clearly emphasize the value of resistance exercise training for increasing muscle strength and muscle mass for both upper and lower extremities. Strength of evidence is graded at 1A (i.e., highest recommendation).

There is no consensus regarding the characteristics of an optimal resistance training program for patients with pulmonary disease. However, templates for program

TABLE 36-7. SUMMARY OF RECOMMENDATIONS AND SUGGESTIONS FOR RESISTANCE EXERCISE TRAINING IN PATIENTS WITH COPD AND IN OLDER ADULTS

REFERENCE	GROUP	FREQUENCY	INTENSITY	SETS	REPETITIONS	REST	EXERCISES
Storer (115)	COPD	2–3 d·week^{-1}	50%–60% 1RM initially Progress to 85% 1RM	1–3	10–12 initially Progress to 6–10	1–3 min	8–10
O'Shea et al. (88)	COPD	2–3 d·week^{-1}	50%–85% 1RM	2–4	6–12		3–9
Nelson et al. (78)	Healthy, older adults	≥2 d·week^{-1}	Moderate to high^a	1 or more	10–15		8–10

COPD, chronic obstructive pulmonary disease; 1RM, 1 repetitive maximum.

^{a}Moderate intensity is defined as 5 to 6 on a 0 to 10 scale; high intensity is 7 to 8 on a 0 to 10 scale.

design have emerged from reviews of research in resistance training for individuals with COPD that have resulted in successful outcomes (88,115) and current guidelines for healthy older adults (78) (Table 36-7).

As with endurance (aerobic) exercise training, resistance training utilizes a warm-up, exercise period, and cool-down. The purposes of the warm-up and cool-down are similar but executed in slightly different ways in resistance training. The same FITT framework used with endurance training is applicable for resistance training as well. Progression should follow as tolerated, followed by maintenance of gains as outlined in Chapter 7 of the GETP8.

Warm-up

Warm-up sets using very light resistance before the exercise to be performed will provide specific local muscle temperature increase. Gradually increasing the range of motion through this warm-up set will also help provide joint readiness. Movements should be done slowly, starting with shorter range of motion and progressing to full range of motion by the end of the warm-up set. If desired, a light stretch for the muscles used in that specific exercise could also be performed.

Cool-down

Cool-down following strength training exercise requires only easy walking or cycling and perhaps light stretching and joint mobility exercises. This is primarily to give the patient a sense of comfort and gradual return to resting conditions.

Frequency

Two to three nonconsecutive days per week of resistance training is recommended for patients with COPD (9,88,99,115) and is consistent with recently published recommendations for strength training in older adults (78). On each of these days, participants perform sets of resistance training for at least the large muscle groups of the upper and lower extremity.

Intensity

In resistance training, the load imposed is usually considered to represent the intensity of a given training segment, i.e., a repetition or a set. Current recommendations for intensity range between 70% and 85% of the one repetition maximum (1RM). This will result typically in 8 to 10 repetitions performed. Older individuals may reduce this to 60% to 70% 1RM (~10–15 repetitions). However, there are some considerations in using percent 1RM loads. First, the training stimulus at a fixed percentage of 1RM varies with the muscle mass used and the training state of the subject (54,55). Thus, 70% of 1RM for the leg press exercise may result in a different number of repetitions completed per set than for triceps extensions at the same 70% 1RM load. Second, the number of repetitions that can be performed at 50% 1RM versus 85% 1RM varies considerably. At least in healthy individuals, 50% 1RM loads correspond to greater than 15 repetitions; similarly, 85% of 1RM corresponds to about six repetitions (14). These different combinations of load and repetitions predict different training effects (14). Third, assigning loads on the basis of percent 1RM requires frequent reassessment of the 1RM so that load may be increased proportionally with strength increases over time. This can be tedious and time-consuming as readjustments in load become necessary for progression. The 1RM is a highly effort-dependent measure requiring maximal force production, thus increasing the risk of injury. However, when testing is carefully conducted by experienced personnel, the 1RM procedure appears to be safe in patients with COPD (61). An alternative approach proposed by Nelson et al. for older, healthy adults makes use of perceptual ratings in which moderate exercise is rated at 5 to 6 on a zero- to 10-point scale (0 = no movement) and high-intensity exercise at 7 to 8 on the zero to 10 scale (78).

Recently, Hoff et al. demonstrated the effectiveness of high-intensity resistance training in which the rate of force production was emphasized (56). Twelve patients with COPD (FEV_1 <60% of predicted) were randomized to either 8 weeks of three times weekly leg press exercise training (four sets of five repetitions at 85%–90% 1RM) or to a nonexercising control group. Compared with controls, the exercising subjects showed significant improvements in 1RM strength, dynamic rate of force development, static peak force, mechanical efficiency of leg cycling (31%), and FEV_1 (21%). Although these data are encouraging, studies confirming these observations will be important. Until then, practitioners might consider this approach with select patients. Caution is recommended with regard to injury prevention through technique instruction, warm-up, and progression toward these higher-intensity levels with a base conditioning period.

Time

Strength training should be a component of a comprehensive exercise rehabilitation program for patients with COPD that includes endurance training and flexibility exercise as well as resistance training. Total training session time for endurance and strength exercise, when reported, has ranged between 40 and 90 minutes. Using reasonable assumptions for time per repetition, the strength-training portion of a comprehensive pulmonary rehabilitation program could be completed within 20 to 40 minutes, assuming one set of 8 to 12 repetitions performed for 8 to 10 exercises interspersed with 2 to 3 minutes rest between sets (115). This estimate may be modified based on disease severity and program design. The number and choice of exercises may be dictated by patient goals and needs assessment (e.g., improving ability to climb stairs in the patient's domicile) or by contraindications such as arthritic joints or osteoporosis (a potential problem in patients undergoing long-term corticosteroid therapy). A free-weight squat, for example, would typically not be appropriate in the COPD population. However, a seated leg press exercise or repetitions of standing up from a bench or chair while holding progressively heavier weights may be acceptable alternatives. If patients cannot stand up from the chair or bench with their body weight alone, the seat height may be elevated or direct supervision may be necessary.

The rest interval between sets should also be considered. An ideal rest period between sets is difficult to establish for the patient with COPD primarily because of varying degrees of dyspnea and/or oxyhemoglobin desaturation. Although a 1-minute rest interval between sets might be attempted in selected patients who are performing a higher-intensity training bout, in practice, most patients will require a 2- to 3-minute period of rest.

Type

Many types of resistance training are available, including machine weights, free weights, elastic resistance, weighted balls, and body weight. Choice of equipment is often dictated by what is available. However, almost any form of resistance will suffice as long as it can be graded in its application, is safe to use, and has some motivational appeal to the participant. Consideration should be given to the minimal weight that can be set for any given exercise. Some types of weight machines have minimal resistances that are too high or weights that are in increments that are too large for some patients who exhibit significant atrophy and weakness. For some, the use of free weights may be contraindicated because of balance/safety issues. Elastic resistance can provide low force requirements and may be ideal for some very debilitated patients.

Flexibility

Flexibility is recognized as a component of a comprehensive exercise training regimen and should be performed with the objective of "maintaining the flexibility necessary for regular physical activity and daily life" (78). The health-related benefits of good flexibility are not established, and no specific guidelines for patients with chronic respiratory diseases are available. However, recent recommendations for flexibility exercise training in healthy older adults (78) are relevant, as are general guidelines for healthy individuals (11). These include performing flexibility exercises at least 2 days/week for at least 10 minutes each day (classification IIb and level of evidence B for older healthy adults) (78). Table 36-8 summarizes the recommendations for healthy older adults and general American College of Sports Medicine (ACSM) guidelines for prescriptions to improve flexibility. Although systematic reviews of the literature (52,117) cannot confirm the value of stretching for either injury prevention or delayed onset muscle soreness, neither is there evidence to discontinue its practice. Additional research is needed to demonstrate the extent to which flexibility is lost with aging, whether regular stretching reduces or reverses this loss, and whether improved flexibility confers health benefits not obtained from other forms of exercise.

Warm-up

It is generally acknowledged that flexibility exercises are best performed after a warm-up or cool-down to make use of the increased muscle temperature and pliability of the warm muscle. Stretching exercises should not be considered as the sole activity of the warm-up phase of an exercise training session.

Cool-down

As with stretching during warm-up, utilizing the cool-down period for range-of-motion activities makes use of

TABLE 36-8. SUMMARY OF RECOMMENDATIONS AND SUGGESTIONS FOR FLEXIBILITY TRAINING IN HEALTHY OLDER ADULTS

REFERENCE	FREQUENCY	INTENSITY[a]	TIME	TYPE	BODY PARTS	STRENGTH OF EVIDENCE
(3)	≥ 2 d·week^{-1}		• >10 min·d^{-1}			IIb (B)
(2)	≥ 2 d·week^{-1}		• >10 min·d^{-1} • 4 or more repetitions per muscle group • 15–60 s (static stretches) • 6-s contraction → 15–30-s assisted stretch (PNF)	Ballistic Static Dynamic PNF	Major muscle tendon groups of the body	

PNF, proprioceptive neuromuscular facilitation.

[a]Intensity was not specified by either expert group; pain-free range of motion or mild discomfort are common recommendations. Care should be taken to emphasize good breathing techniques and to avoid the Valsalva maneuver.

warmer muscles that facilitate improved stretching responses. It is not likely that risk of muscle injury will occur as is seen in some athletic groups when stretching is performed too soon during the cool-down period.

Frequency

At a minimum, stretching exercises are recommended whenever endurance exercise or resistance exercise training is performed. If flexibility exercises are pain free in their intensity, they can be performed as often as the individual wishes.

Intensity

The general recommendation for stretching intensity suggests mild to moderate discomfort or pain-free stretching.

Time

Current recommendations for healthy older adults recommend at least 10 minutes of flexibility activities. These are reasonable to apply to the patient with chronic pulmonary disease. This is based on the time required to complete three to four repetitions of a 15- to 20-second static stretch for the major muscle-tendon groups (e.g., neck, shoulders, upper and lower back, pelvis, hips, and legs). Holding stretches for up to 60 seconds may enhance benefits.

Type

Methods of stretching include ballistic, dynamic, proprioceptive neuromuscular facilitation, and static. There are no specific data on the efficacy of different modes of stretching in the population of patients with chronic lung diseases. However, it is reasonable to assume that all but the ballistic stretching method may be used in supervised programs with practitioners knowledgeable in the different stretching methods.

Respiratory (Inspiratory) Muscle Training

Many patients with COPD experience inspiratory muscle weakness that leads to increased breathlessness and de-

creased exercise tolerance. As reported in the 2007 Joint ACCP/AACVPR Practice Guidelines, several recent randomized controlled trials (63,65,103,126,127) have demonstrated positive physiologic and patient-centered effects from inspiratory muscle training. However, the results of these studies, as well as their single-center design with relatively few patients, have not convinced the ACCP/AACVPR to change their previous evidence-based practice guidelines (6), which now state that (a) inspiratory muscle training should be considered in selected patients who have decreased inspiratory muscle strength and breathlessness, despite receiving optimal medical therapy; and (b) overall, the scientific evidence does not support the routine use of inspiratory muscle training as an essential component of pulmonary rehabilitation (grade 1B) (99). The ATS/ERS practice guidelines (82) provide similar recommendations that "although the data are inconclusive, inspiratory muscle training could be considered as adjunctive therapy in pulmonary rehabilitation, primarily in patients with suspected or proven respiratory (i.e. inspiratory) muscle weakness."

Guidelines for inspiratory muscle training have been provided by the AACVPR (9) and include the following.

Frequency

The goal for frequency is 4 to 5 days per week.

Intensity

The goal for intensity is 30% to 35% maximal inspiratory pressure measured at the mouth (Pimax).

Time

The goal for time is two 15-minute sessions per day or one 30-minute session per day.

Type

Three types of inspiratory muscle training are used: inspiratory resistance training (19), threshold loading (46), and isocapneic hyperventilation (105). There is no demonstrated superiority of one method over another to suggest its preferred use (82).

DISEASE-SPECIFIC PRECAUTIONS AND ACTIONS/ASSESSMENTS THAT MAY BE REQUIRED BEFORE, DURING, OR AFTER EXERCISE

General Safety Concerns for Exercise Training in People with Chronic Lung Disease

Exercise training in patients with chronic lung disease is generally considered safe, even with high relative intensities, when training guidelines are correctly applied with due consideration of individual patients' exercise tolerance and thresholds limiting exercise intensity (Table 36-4).

Cardiopulmonary exercise testing is valuable in assessing overall safety of exercise training, and the availability of supplemental oxygen during training helps maintain appropriate levels of oxygen saturation, thus reducing hypoxemia and dyspnea. Periodic monitoring by pulse oximetry and visual analog scales for dyspnea are helpful in this regard (22, 29). Optimal bronchodilator therapy improves lung function by reducing airflow obstruction and thereby reduces breathlessness and wheeze. Pursed-lip breathing should be taught, practiced, and performed as needed to lower end-expiratory lung volume and improve the subsequent inhalation (83,120,121). In resistance training, proper biomechanics for lifting technique reduces the risk of musculoskeletal injury; avoidance of the Valsalva maneuver during lifting reduces the risk of developing high intrathoracic pressures, thereby decreasing venous return and cardiac output. Periodic blood pressure measurements may be necessary in some hypertensive patients to monitor the pressor response to exercise.

Asthma

Recently reviewed by Ram et al., research investigating the effects of exercise training in patients with asthma is limited by small numbers of randomized controlled trials and subjects, different outcome measures, missing data, and by different study durations (98). Bearing this in mind, the authors concluded from their review that exercise training generally resulted in statistically significant improvements in maximum work rate, peak $\dot{V}O_2$, maximum heart rate, and maximum exercise ventilation. However, the absolute changes were small. There was no evidence of improved lung function or evidence that the improved measures of cardiopulmonary performance translate into improved physical function.

Unlike COPD, the airflow obstruction in asthma is considered reversible. Recommendations for exercise training include avoidance of triggers resulting in bronchoconstriction, adequate warm-up, and use of bronchodilators before exercise (9). Exercise can be a significant stimulus

for bronchoconstriction (i.e., EIB) and is common in untreated asthma (64) but can be well controlled with optimal therapy (25,94). EIB may also occur in some who do not otherwise have asthma (125). Tests to determine the presence of EIB are described in detail elsewhere (35,38). Briefly, the test requires a two-step process: First, an exercise stimulus of >80% of maximum heart rate is applied for 6 to 8 minutes of exercise on a motor-driven treadmill or cycle ergometer to increase the minute ventilation to 40% to 60% of the expected value. Second, serial FEV_1 measurements are obtained by spirometry at 5, 10, 15, 20, and 30 minutes postexercise; occasionally measurements at 1 and 3 minutes are also obtained. An abnormal response is defined by a fall of >10% below the baseline FEV_1 at each interval, although a fall of >15% has also been recommended, particularly if challenge tests are performed in the field (38). Blood pressure and oxygen saturation should be measured throughout the test and recovery periods. Although unusual, upper-airway abnormalities other than asthma may also exhibit positive challenge tests and may be distinguished from EIB through examination of the flow-volume loop (38). A diagnostic cardiopulmonary exercise test may also be used as a provocation study to identify exercise-induced asthma (35,93). Severe bronchoconstriction is a potential hazard following challenge testing. Immediate administration of nebulized bronchodilators and oxygen usually provide successful treatment (38). Tests should be appropriately supervised by trained technicians and, in the case of higher-risk individuals, by a physician.

The comprehensive exercise training program described for patients with COPD is directly applicable to individuals with asthma when airway obstruction is adequately managed with bronchodilator therapy and triggers to bronchoconstriction (such as cold, dry, dusty air and inhaled pollutants) are removed. Warm-up and bronchodilator therapy before exercise will often reduce the occurrence of EIB (9).

Interstitial Lung Disease

Unlike the chronic obstructive lung diseases, ILD is seen as a restrictive spirometric abnormality with low lung volumes, reduced diffusing capacity leading to gas exchange abnormalities, and increased respiratory frequency. Whatever the underlying cause, ILD is usually characterized by interstitial or alveolar inflammation and/or fibrosis. As with COPD, the primary limitation to exercise is dyspnea. However, whereas exertional dyspnea seen in COPD is the result of ventilatory impairment, hyperinflation, and skeletal muscle disuse atrophy or dysfunction, dyspnea occurring in patients with ILD is more often because of gas exchange abnormality (77). Oxygen desaturation is a hallmark of ILD (9) even when supplemental oxygen is provided at high flow rates. Use of pulse oximetry to periodically verify that oxygen saturation remains above 88% during exercise is important.

Relatively few studies have been conducted in patients with ILD. However, it appears that the functional improvements from pulmonary rehabilitation seen in patients with ILD are similar (39,77) or just slightly less (44) than in patients with COPD. A recent study (77) demonstrated improvements in exercise endurance, quality of life, and dyspnea symptoms in 26 patients completing an 8-week training program. Fifteen subjects were reassessed after 1 year. They showed maintenance of treadmill test performance, but improvements in quality of life and dyspnea were not maintained. Hospital admissions were reduced in these patients in comparison with the previous year.

In general, the exercise training recommendations used in patients with COPD apply to those with the ILDs when modifications are adapted to the individual's exercise tolerance. During exercise training, careful application of intensity and duration guidelines is recommended in these patients. Despite the functional improvements that might result from exercise training, higher-intensity exercise may still result in deranged gas exchange, desaturation, and incapacitating dyspnea.

Bronchiectasis

Bronchiectasis is a chronic destructive lung disease characterized by airflow obstruction and chronic infection leading to shortness of breath and exercise intolerance. Symptoms include cough, sputum production, and wheeze (79). Very few studies have investigated the role of pulmonary rehabilitation in this condition. Smidt et al. (113) identified only one systematic review of exercise training in bronchiectasis that qualified for inclusion in their best-evidence summary of exercise training in chronic diseases (24). Based on this single review, it was concluded that there is insufficient evidence to support or refute the effectiveness of exercise therapy for patients with bronchiectasis. Published contemporaneously with the Smidt et al. report, Newall et al. (79) found that a small number of patients with bronchiectasis who were randomized to 8 weeks of three-times-weekly sessions of 45 minutes of high-intensity exercise training improved exercise tolerance, but the addition of inspiratory muscle training provided no added benefit. Neither exercise training nor inspiratory muscle training affected 24-hour sputum clearance. Based on the limited data available, application of exercise training guidelines suggested for patients with COPD should be appropriate for patients with bronchiectasis.

Pulmonary Arterial Hypertension

Exercise training in PAH is a serious undertaking with the necessity for precautions that exceed those employed in other chronic lung diseases. In patients with PAH, pulmonary pressures can increase suddenly and dramatically during exercise, predisposing them to right ventricular decompensation and cardiovascular collapse (18). Sudden death has been reported during exercise in individuals with PAH; the underlying mechanism is postulated as acute right ventricular pressure overload or cardiac arrhythmia. This suggests that some patients with PAH may require electrocardiogram monitoring. Hypoxemia reflects the severity of PAH, and when significant during exercise, it often requires supplemental oxygen (76). Fatigue and weakness are important manifestations of PAH and reflect the inability to meet metabolic demands of exercise. This is accentuated by early-onset lactic acidosis. Other symptoms include resting tachycardia, substernal chest pain, presyncope (dizziness), and syncope (loss of consciousness). These, along with oxygen saturation, should be carefully monitored (9).

Before exercise training, patients' medical treatment should be optimized and exercise training sessions closely supervised by experienced personnel (9). Recommendations for exercise training in patients with PAH include lower-intensity exercise training, avoidance of arm ergometry or resistance exercise training that may result in a Valsalva maneuver, and avoidance of floor exercise (9). Recently, however, Mereles et al. demonstrated that stable, medically optimized patients with severe, chronic PAH could undergo rather rigorous exercise training (74). In this 15-week randomized controlled trial with crossover design, patients completed a closely supervised inpatient training phase (7 d · week^{-1} for 3 weeks) that was immediately followed by 12 weeks of home training. The inpatient training consisted of 10- to 25-minute progressive interval training (up to 60%–80% peak heart rate) and 5 d · week^{-1} of walking for 60 minutes. Additionally, patients performed light (0.5–1.0 kg) dumbbell resistance training for 30 min 5 d · week^{-1}. Home training consisted of 5 d · week^{-1} of leg cycling for 15 to 30 minutes at target heart rate, 3 d · week^{-1} dumbbell training, and 2 d · week^{-1} of walking. Home training was monitored by twice-weekly telephone calls. Significant improvements in 6-minute walk distance of 85 m and 75 m were seen after 3 weeks of training in the primary training group and in the control group that crossed over to training, respectively. Further, slight improvement or maintenance of change was noted at 15 weeks. In addition, significant improvements were observed in quality of life (SF-36), maximum work rate, maximum heart rate, peak $\dot{V}O_2$, as well as $\dot{V}O_2$ and work rate at the anaerobic (measured by gas exchange) threshold. The training was well tolerated, with no adverse events reported. The authors caution, however, that exercise training in patients with PAH can have serious adverse effects. It is important to note that the Mereles et al. study began in the hospital and was carefully supervised and monitored by personnel experienced with these patients. As noted in an accompanying editorial, carefully designed exercise is safe and beneficial, at

BOX 36-7 COMPONENTS OF PULMONARY REHABILITATION PROGRAM

Patient education

Pulmonary anatomy, physiology, and disease pathophysiology

Diagnostic testing

Treatment (including oxygen, medications, surgery)

Bronchial hygiene techniques

Exercise training

Breathing retraining

Endurance, strength, and flexibility training, including of the upper and lower extremities

Ventilatory muscle training

Energy conservation techniques

Self-management

Self-assessment and symptom management

Infection control (avoidance, early intervention, and immunization)

Environmental control

Indications for seeking medical advice and resources

Sleep disturbances

Sexuality and intimacy

Nutrition

Smoking cessation

Psychosocial intervention and support

Community services, including patient and family support groups

Advance care planning

Recreation and leisure activities and travel

Stress management

Adapted from Haynes JM. AARC clinical practice guideline: pulmonary rehabilitation. *Respir Care.* 2002;47:617–625.

least in the short term, for patients with pulmonary arterial hypertension (80). These data are encouraging, but remain to be confirmed by larger groups of patients with PAH in which there is more random selection and perhaps greater diversity in patient characteristics. Although the results are impressive, considerable training time was invested, which begs the question whether other patients with PAH can tolerate and/or complete such a program and whether a less rigorous regimen would produce similar results.

IMPLEMENTATION OF PULMONARY REHABILITATION PROGRAMS

Pulmonary rehabilitation is a structured, "evidence-based, multidisciplinary, and comprehensive intervention for patients with chronic lung diseases who are symptomatic and often have decreased daily life activities" (82). The comprehensive nature of PR addresses both physical and psychological needs and facilitates a holistic approach to lung disease management with well-defined objectives (Box 36-5) and evidence-based practice guidelines and outcomes (82,99). The components of a comprehensive pulmonary rehabilitation are outlined in Box 36-7. Recommended guidelines for implementing the exercise training component of PR are summarized in Tables 36-6 through 36-8. The building blocks for these guidelines are discussed throughout this chapter, along with the observed responses to the exercise.

The optimal length of time over which to implement the initial PR program is not clear (99). In general, although

the evidence is weak, programs that are of longer duration (e.g., >12 weeks) result in greater sustained benefits than shorter programs (ACCP/AACVRP grade 2C; Table 36-5). The available research suggests that many variables, including the variations in types of PR programs, program participants, and program content, affect benefits that may be derived. Somewhat surprisingly, even 6 to 12 weeks of PR have yielded durable benefits that have persisted for 12 to 18 months following completion of the program. However, despite the apparent sustainability of benefit from relatively short-term PR, these benefits eventually disappear when exercise training ceases (47,100). This, as well as the unquestioned value of exercise training in patients with chronic lung disease, clearly suggests the need for long-term maintenance strategies. Possible approaches include repeat PR courses, participation in maintenance cardiac/pulmonary rehabilitation programs, guided and monitored home exercise, self-management, participation in exercise programs available in community settings, or combinations of these. Research is needed to identify successful options for long-term maintenance PR programs that address problems such as sustainable motivation, adherence, cost, and accessibility.

SUMMARY

By adapting basic exercise training guidelines to patient capabilities and disease-specific concerns, exercise in chronic lung disease can be performed successfully regardless of the illness severity level. Disease-specific concerns can be easily identified with a basic understanding of lung pathophysiology as it relates to pattern recognition for each of the disease categories. These principles also facilitate identification of the proper therapeutic interventions. Incorporating modifications based on the individual's response to exercise can further augment individualization of the exercise program. The response to exercise is best judged by understanding basic pathophysiology and recognizing the meaning and measurement of certain signs and symptoms.

REFERENCES

1. Committee on the Aetiology of Chronic Bronchitis, Medical Research Council. Definition and classification of chronic bronchitis for clinical and epidemiological purposes: a report to the Medical Research Council by their Committee on the Aetiology of Chronic Bronchitis. *Lancet.* 1965;1:775–779.
2. **American Thoracic Society. Guidelines for the approach to the patient with severe hereditary alpha-1-antitrypsin deficiency. *Am Rev Respir Dis.* 1989;140:1494–1497.**
3. COMBIVENT Inhalation Aerosol Study Group. In chronic obstructive pulmonary disease, a combination of ipratropium and albuterol is more effective than either agent alone: an 85-day multicenter trial. *Chest.* 1994;105:1411–1419.
4. **Expert Panel Report 3: Guidelines for the diagnosis and management of asthma. NIH Publication No. 07-4051, 2007.**
5. **Expert Panel Report 2: Guidelines for the diagnosis and management of asthma. NIH Publication No. 97-4051141. 1997.**
6. **ACCP/AACVPR Pulmonary Rehabilitation Guidelines Panel. American College of Chest Physicians. American Association of Cardiovascular and Pulmonary Rehabilitation. Pulmonary rehabilitation: joint ACCP/AACVPR evidence-based guidelines. *Chest.* 1997;112:1363–1396.**
7. National Institutes of Health Data Fact Sheet: Asthma, Statistics. NIH Publication No. 55-798140. 1999.
8. **American Thoracic Society and European Respiratory Society. Skeletal muscle dysfunction in chronic obstructive pulmonary disease: a statement of the American Thoracic Society and European Respiratory Society. *Am J Respir Crit Care Med.* 1999;159:S1–40.**
9. **American Association of Cardiovascular and Pulmonary Rehabilitation. *AACVPR Guidelines for Pulmonary Rehabilitation Programs.* Champaign (IL): Human Kinetics; 2004.**
10. **Global Strategy for Asthma Management and Prevention, Global Initiative for Asthma (GINA) 289. 2006. Available at: www.ginasthama.org. Last accessed 11/19/08.**
11. **American College of Sports Medicine. *Guidelines for Exercise Testing and Prescription.* Philadelphia: Lippincott Williams and Wilkins; 2008.**
12. Arnardottir RH, Boman G, Larsson K, Hedenstrom H, Emtner M. Interval training compared with continuous training in patients with COPD. *Respir Med.* 2007;101:1196–1204.
13. Astrand P-O, Rodahl K. *Textbook of Work Physiology.* New York: McGraw-Hill, Inc.; 1986. p. 627–628.
14. Baechle TR, Earle RW, Wathen D. Resistance training. In: Baechle TR, Earle RW, editors. *Essentials of Strength Training and Conditioning.* Champaign (IL): Human Kinetics; 2000. p. 406–417.
15. Barnes PJ. Asthma management: can we further improve compliance and outcomes? *Respir Med.* 2004;98(Suppl A):S8–9.
16. Barnes PJ, Shapiro SD, Pauwels RA. Chronic obstructive pulmonary disease: molecular and cellular mechanisms. *Eur Respir J.* 2003;22: 672–688.
17. Barnes PT, Drazen JM, Rennard S, Thompson NC. *Asthma and COPD Basic Mechanisms and Clinical Management.* Boston: Elsevier; 2000.
18. Barst RJ, McGoon M, Torbicki A, et al. Diagnosis and differential assessment of pulmonary arterial hypertension. *J Am Coll Cardiol.* 2004;43:40S–47S.
19. Belman MJ, Shadmehr R. Targeted resistive ventilatory muscle training in chronic obstructive pulmonary disease. *J Appl Physiol.* 1988;65:2726–2735.
20. Bernard S, LeBlanc P, Whittom F, et al. Peripheral muscle weakness in patients with chronic obstructive pulmonary disease. *Am J Respir Crit Care Med.* 1998;158:629–634.
21. Bernard S, Whittom F, Leblanc P, et al. Aerobic and strength training in patients with chronic obstructive pulmonary disease. *Am J Respir Crit Care Med.* 1999;159:896–901.
22. Bestall JC, Paul EA, Garrod R, Garnham R, Jones PW, Wedzicha JA. Usefulness of the Medical Research Council (MRC) dyspnoea scale as a measure of disability in patients with chronic obstructive pulmonary disease. *Thorax.* 1999;54:581–586.
23. Borg G. *Borg's Perceived Exertion and Pain Scales.* Champaign (IL): Human Kinetics; 1998.
24. Bradley J, Moran F, Greenstone M. Physical training for bronchiectasis. *Cochrane Database Syst Rev.* 2002;3:CD002166.
25. Carlsen KH, Carlsen KC. Exercise-induced asthma. *Paediatr Respir Rev.* 2002;3:154–160.
26. Casaburi R, Patessio A, Ioli F, Zanaboni S, Donner CF, Wasserman K. Reductions in exercise lactic acidosis and ventilation as a result of exercise training in patients with obstructive lung disease. *Am Rev Respir Dis.* 1991;143:9–18.
27. Celli BR. Pathophysiology of chronic obstructive pulmonary disease. In: Hodgkin JE, Celli BR, Connors GL, editors. *Pulmonary Rehabilitation: Guidelines to Success.* Philadelphia: Lippincott, Williams & Wilkins; 2000. p. 41–55.
28. Celli BR, Cote CG, Marin JM, et al. The body-mass index, airflow obstruction, dyspnea, and exercise capacity index in chronic obstructive pulmonary disease. *N Engl J Med.* 2004;350:1005–1012.
29. Chida M, Inase N, Ichioka M, Miyazato I, Marumo F. Ratings of perceived exertion in chronic obstructive pulmonary disease—a possible indicator for exercise training in patients with this disease. *Eur J Appl Physiol Occup Physiol.* 1991;62:390–393.
30. Cooper CB. Exercise in chronic pulmonary disease: aerobic exercise prescription. *Med Sci Sports Exerc.* 2001;33:S671–679. Review. Erratum in: *Med Sci Sports Exerc.* 2001;33:2009, following table of contents.
31. Cooper CB. Exercise in chronic pulmonary disease: aerobic exercise prescription. *Med Sci Sports Exerc.* 33:S671-679. Review. Erratum in: Med Sci Sports Exerc 2001 Sep;2033(2009):following table of contents., 2001
32. Cooper CB. Exercise in chronic pulmonary disease: limitations and rehabilitation. *Med Sci Sports Exerc.* 2001;33:S643–646.
33. Cooper CB. The connection between chronic obstructive pulmonary disease symptoms and hyperinflation and its impact on exercise and function. *Am J Med.* 2006;119:21–31.
34. Cooper CB. The connection between chronic obstructive pulmonary disease symptoms and hyperinflation and its impact on exercise and function. *Am J Med.* 2006;119:21–31.
35. Cooper CB, Storer TW. *Exercise Testing and Interpretation: A Practical Approach.* New York: Cambridge University Press; 2001.
36. Cooper CB, Tashkin DP. Recent developments in inhaled therapy in stable chronic obstructive pulmonary disease. *BMJ.* 2005;330: 640–644.
37. Coppoolse R, Schols AM, Baarends EM, et al. Interval versus continuous training in patients with severe COPD: a randomized clinical trial. *Eur Respir J.* 1999;14:258–263.
38. **Crapo RO, Casaburi R, Coates AL, et al. Guidelines for methacholine and exercise challenge testing—1999. This official statement of the American Thoracic Society was adopted by the ATS Board of Directors, July 1999. *Am J Respir Crit Care Med.* 2000;161:309–329.**
39. Crouch R, MacIntyre NR. Pulmonary rehabilitation of the patient with nonobstructive lung disease. *Respir Care Clin N Am.* 1998; 4:59–70.

40. Decramer M, Gosselink R, Troosters T, Verschueren M, Evers G. Muscle weakness is related to utilization of health care resources in COPD patients. *Eur Respir J.* 1997;10:417–423.

41. Desai TJ, Karlinsky JB. OPD: Clinical manifestations, diagnosis, and treatment. In: Crapo JD, Glassroth J, Karlinsky J, King TE, editors. *Baum's Textbook of Pulmonary Diseases*. Philadelphia: Lippincott, Williams & Wilkins; 2004. p. 204–246.

42. Despres JP, Lamarche B. Low-intensity endurance exercise training, plasma lipoproteins and the risk of coronary heart disease. *J Intern Med.* 1994;236:7–22.

43. Ferguson GT, Cherniack RM. Management of chronic obstructive pulmonary disease. *N Engl J Med.* 1993;328:1017–1022.

44. Foster S, Thomas HM 3rd. Pulmonary rehabilitation in lung disease other than chronic obstructive pulmonary disease. *Am Rev Respir Dis.* 1990;141:601–604.

45. Gimenez M, Servera E, Vergara P, Bach JR, Polu JM. Endurance training in patients with chronic obstructive pulmonary disease: a comparison of high versus moderate intensity. *Arch Phys Med Rehabil.* 2000;81:102–109.

46. Gosselink R, Wagenaar RC, Decramer M. Reliability of a commercially available threshold loading device in healthy subjects and in patients with chronic obstructive pulmonary disease. *Thorax.* 1996; 51:601–605.

47. Griffiths TL, Burr ML, Campbell IA, et al. Results at 1 year of outpatient multidisciplinary pulmonary rehabilitation: a randomised controlled trial. *Lancet.* 2000;355:362–368.

48. Guell R, Resqueti V, Sangenis M, et al. Impact of pulmonary rehabilitation on psychosocial morbidity in patients with severe COPD. *Chest.* 2006;129:899–904.

49. Guilleminault C, Abad VC. Obstructive sleep apnea syndromes. *Med Clin North Am.* 2004;88:611–630, viii.

50. Han MK, Postma D, Mannino D, et al. Gender and chronic obstructive pulmonary disease: why it matters. *Am J Respir Crit Care Med.* 2007;176:1179–1184.

51. Harris-Eze AO, Sridhar G, Clemens RE, Zintel TA, Gallagher CG, Marciniuk DD. Role of hypoxemia and pulmonary mechanics in exercise limitation in interstitial lung disease. *Am J Respir Crit Care Med.* 1996;154:994–1001.

52. Herbert R, de Noronha M. Stretching to prevent or reduce muscle soreness after exercise. *Cochrane Database Syst Rev.* 2007;CD 004577.

53. Hilleman DE, Dewan N, Malesker M, Friedman M. Pharmacoeconomic evaluation of COPD. *Chest.* 2000;118:1278–1285.

54. Hoeger WWK, Barette SL, Hale DF, Hopkins DR. Relationship between repetitions and selected percentages of one repetition maximum. *J Appl Sports Sci Res.* 1987;1:11–13.

55. Hoeger WWK, Hopkins DR, Barette SL, Hale DF. Relationship between repetitions and selected percentages of one repetition maximum: a comparison between untrained and trained males and females. *J Appl Sports Sci Res.* 1990;4:47–54.

56. Hoff J, Tjonna AE, Steinshamn S, Hoydal M, Richardson RS, Helgerud J. Maximal strength training of the legs in COPD: a therapy for mechanical inefficiency. *Med Sci Sports Exerc.* 2007;39:220–226.

57. Hogg JC, aSenior RM. Chronic obstructive pulmonary disease. Part 2: Pathology and biochemistry of emphysema. *Thorax.* 2002;57:830–834.

58. Horowitz MB, Littenberg B, Mahler DA. Dyspnea ratings for prescribing exercise intensity in patients with COPD. *Chest.* 1996;109: 1169–1175.

59. **Hunt SA, Baker DW, Chin MH, et al. ACC/AHA Guidelines for the Evaluation and Management of Chronic Heart Failure in the Adult: Executive Summary A Report of the American College of Cardiology/American Heart Association Task Force on Practice Guidelines (Committee to Revise the 1995 Guidelines for the Evaluation and Management of Heart Failure): Developed in Collaboration with the International Society for Heart and Lung Transplantation; endorsed by the Heart Failure Society of America. *Circulation.* 2001; 104:2996–3007.**

60. Jeffery PK, Godfrey RW, Adelroth E, Nelson F, Rogers A, Johansson SA. Effects of treatment on airway inflammation and thickening of basement membrane reticular collagen in asthma: a quantitative light and electron microscopic study. *Am Rev Respir Dis.* 1992;145:890–899.

61. Kaelin ME, Swank AM, Adams KJ, Barnard KL, Berning JM, Green A. Cardiopulmonary responses, muscle soreness, and injury during the one repetition maximum assessment in pulmonary rehabilitation patients. *J Cardiopulm Rehabil.* 1999;19:366–372.

62. Koenig SM. Pulmonary complications of obesity. *Am J Med Sci.* 2001;321:249–279.

63. Larson JL, Covey MK, Wirtz SE, et al. Cycle ergometer and inspiratory muscle training in chronic obstructive pulmonary disease. *Am J Respir Crit Care Med.* 1999;160:500–507.

64. Lee TH, Anderson SD. Heterogeneity of mechanisms in exercise induced asthma. *Thorax.* 1985;40:481–487.

65. Lisboa C, Villafranca C, Leiva A, Cruz E, Pertuze J, Borzone G. Inspiratory muscle training in chronic airflow limitation: effect on exercise performance. *Eur Respir J.* 1997;10:537–542.

66. Mahler DA, Horowitz MB. Perception of breathlessness during exercise in patients with respiratory disease. *Med Sci Sports Exerc.* 1994;26:1078–1081.

67. Mannino DM, Buist AS. Global burden of COPD: risk factors, prevalence, and future trends. *Lancet.* 2007;370:765–773.

68. Marciniuk DD, Sridhar G, Clemens RE, Zintel TA, Gallagher CC. Lung volumes and expiratory flow limitation during exercise in interstitial lung disease. *J Appl Physiol.* 1994;77:963–973.

69. Marciniuk DD, Watts RE, Gallagher CG. Dead space loading and exercise limitation in patients with interstitial lung disease. *Chest.* 1994;105:183–189.

70. Markovitz GH, Cooper CB. Exercise and interstitial lung disease. *Curr Opin Pulm Med.* 1998;4:272–280.

71. Mascolo MC, Truwit JD. Role of exercise evaluation in restrictive lung disease: new insights between March 2001 and February 2003. *Curr Opin Pulm Med.* 2003;9:408–410.

72. McGoon M, Gutterman D, Steen V, et al. Screening, early detection, and diagnosis of pulmonary arterial hypertension: ACCP evidence-based clinical practice guidelines. *Chest.* 2004;126:14S–34S.

73. **American College of Sports Medicine. *Guidelines for Exercise Testing and Prescription*. Philadelphia: Lippincott Williams and Wilkins; 2008.**

74. Mereles D, Ehlken N, Kreuscher S, et al. Exercise and respiratory training improve exercise capacity and quality of life in patients with severe chronic pulmonary hypertension. *Circulation.* 2006;114:1482–1489.

75. Miller MR, Hankinson J, Brusasco V, et al. Standardisation of spirometry. *Eur Respir J.* 2005;26:319–338.

76. Murray JF, Nadel JA. Part 2: Manifestations and diagnosis of respiratory disease. In: *Textbook of Respiratory Medicine*. 3rd edition JF Murray and Sanodal editors Philadelphia: WB Saunders, 2000.

77. Naji NA, Connor MC, Donnelly SC, McDonnell TJ. Effectiveness of pulmonary rehabilitation in restrictive lung disease. *J Cardiopulm Rehabil.* 2006;26:237–243,

78. **Nelson ME, Rejeski WJ, Blair SN, et al. Physical activity and public health in older adults: recommendation from the American College of Sports Medicine and the American Heart Association. *Med Sci Sports Exerc.* 2007;39:1435–1445.**

79. Newall C, Stockley RA, Hill SL. Exercise training and inspiratory muscle training in patients with bronchiectasis. *Thorax.* 2005;60: 943–948.

80. Newman JH, Robbins IM. Exercise training in pulmonary hypertension: implications for the evaluation of drug trials. *Circulation.* 2006;114:1448–1449.

81. Newman KB, Mason UG 3rd, Schmaling KB. Clinical features of vocal cord dysfunction. *Am J Respir Crit Care Med.* 1995;152:1382–1386.

82. **Nici L, Donner C, Wouters E, et al. American Thoracic Society/European Respiratory Society statement on pulmonary rehabilitation. *Am J Respir Crit Care Med.* 2006;173:1390–1413.**

83. Nield MA, Soo Hoo GW, Roper JM, Santiago S. Efficacy of pursed-lips breathing: a breathing pattern retraining strategy for dyspnea reduction. *J Cardiopulm Rehabil Prev.* 2007;27:237–244.

84. O'Donnell DE, Fluge T, Gerken F, et al. Effects of tiotropium on lung hyperinflation, dyspnoea and exercise tolerance in COPD. *Eur Respir J.* 2004;23:832–840.

85. O'Donnell DE, McGuire M, Samis L, Webb KA. General exercise training improves ventilatory and peripheral muscle strength and endurance in chronic airflow limitation. *Am J Respir Crit Care Med.* 1998;157:1489–1497.

86. O'Donnell DE, Revill SM, Webb KA. Dynamic hyperinflation and exercise intolerance in chronic obstructive pulmonary disease. *Am J Respir Crit Care Med.* 2001;164:770–777.

87. O'Donnell DE, Voduc N, Fitzpatrick M, Webb KA. Effect of salmeterol on the ventilatory response to exercise in chronic obstructive pulmonary disease. *Eur Respir J.* 2004;24:86–94.

88. O'Shea SD, Taylor NF, Paratz J. Peripheral muscle strength training in COPD: a systematic review. *Chest.* 2004 ;126:903–914.

89. Palange P, Wagner PD. The skeletal muscle in chronic respiratory diseases: summary of the ERS research seminar in Rome, Italy, February 11–12, 1999. *Eur Respir J.* 2000;15:807–815.

90. **Pauwels RA, Buist AS, Ma P, Jenkins CR, aHurd SS. Global strategy for the diagnosis, management, and prevention of chronic obstructive pulmonary disease: National Heart, Lung, and Blood Institute and World Health Organization Global Initiative for Chronic Obstructive Lung Disease (GOLD): executive summary. *Respir Care.* 2001;46:798–825.**

91. Paz-Diaz H, Montes de Oca M, Lopez JM, Celli BR. Pulmonary rehabilitation improves depression, anxiety, dyspnea and health status in patients with COPD. *Am J Phys Med Rehabil.* 2007;86:30–36.

92. Pellegrino R, Viegi G, Brusasco V, et al. Interpretative strategies for lung function tests. *Eur Respir J.* 2005;26:948–968.

93. **American Thoracic Society/American College of Chest Physicians. ATS/ACCP Statement on cardiopulmonary exercise testing. *Am J Respir Crit Care Med.* 2003;167:211–277.**

94. Pierson WE, Voy RO. Exercise-induced bronchospasm in the XXIII summer Olympic games. *N Engl Reg Allergy Proc.* 1988;9:209–213.

95. Postma DS Boezen HM. Rationale for the Dutch hypothesis: allergy and airway hyperresponsiveness as genetic factors and their interaction with environment in the development of asthma and COPD. *Chest.* 2004;126:96S–104S; discussion 159S–161S.

96. Puhan MA, Busching G, Schunemann HJ, VanOort E, Zaugg C, Frey M. Interval versus continuous high-intensity exercise in chronic obstructive pulmonary disease: a randomized trial. *Ann Intern Med.* 2006;145:816–825.

97. **Rabe KF, Hurd S, Anzueto A, et al. Global strategy for the diagnosis, management, and prevention of chronic obstructive pulmonary disease: GOLD executive summary. *Am J Respir Crit Care Med.* 2007;176:532–555.**

98. Ram FS, Robinson SM, Black PN, Picot J. Physical training for asthma. *Cochrane Database Syst Rev.* 2005;CD001116,

99. **Ries AL, Bauldoff GS, Carlin BW, et al. Pulmonary Rehabilitation: Joint ACCP/AACVPR Evidence-Based Clinical Practice Guidelines. *Chest.* 2007;131:4S–42S.**

100. Ries AL, Kaplan RM, Limberg TM, Prewitt LM. Effects of pulmonary rehabilitation on physiologic and psychosocial outcomes in patients with chronic obstructive pulmonary disease. *Ann Intern Med.* 1995;122:823–832.

101. Rubin LJ. Primary pulmonary hypertension. *N Engl J Med.* 1997; 336:111–117.

102. Ryu JH, Myers JL, Swensen SJ. Bronchiolar disorders. *Am J Respir Crit Care Med.* 2003;168:1277–1292.

103. Sanchez Riera H, Montemayor Rubio T, Ortega Ruiz F, et al. Inspiratory muscle training in patients with COPD: effect on dyspnea, exercise performance, and quality of life. *Chest.* 2001;120:748–756.

104. Sassi-Dambron DE, Eakin EG, Ries AL, Kaplan RM. Treatment of dyspnea in COPD: a controlled clinical trial of dyspnea management strategies. *Chest.* 1995;107:724–729.

105. Scherer TA, Spengler CM, Owassapian D, Imhof E, Boutellier U. Respiratory muscle endurance training in chronic obstructive pulmonary disease: impact on exercise capacity, dyspnea, and quality of life. *Am J Respir Crit Care Med.* 2000;162:1709–1714.

106. Sciurba FC. Physiologic similarities and differences between COPD and asthma. *Chest.* 2004;126:117S–124S; discussion 159S–161S.

107. Sietsema K. Cardiovascular limitations in chronic pulmonary disease. *Med Sci Sports Exerc.* 2001;33:S656–661.

108. Silverman E, Ebright L, Kwiatkowski M, Cullina J. Current management of bronchiectasis: review and 3 case studies. *Heart Lung.* 2003;32:59–64.

109. Simonneau G, Galie N, Rubin LJ, et al. Clinical classification of pulmonary hypertension. *J Am Coll Cardiol.* 2004;43:5S–12S.

110. Sin DD, McAlister FA, Man SF, Anthonisen NR. Contemporary management of chronic obstructive pulmonary disease: scientific review. *JAMA.* 2003;290:2301–2312.

111. Singh SJ, Morgan MD, Hardman AE, Rowe C, Bardsley PA. Comparison of oxygen uptake during a conventional treadmill test and the shuttle walking test in chronic airflow limitation. *Eur Respir J.* 1994;7:2016–2020.

112. Singh SJ, Morgan MD, Scott S, Walters D, Hardman AE. Development of a shuttle walking test of disability in patients with chronic airways obstruction. *Thorax.* 1992;47:1019–1024.

113. Smidt N, de Vet HC, Bouter LM, et al. Effectiveness of exercise therapy: a best-evidence summary of systematic reviews. *Aust J Physiother.* 2005;51:71–85.

114. **American Thoracic Society. ATS statement: guidelines for the six-minute walk test. *Am J Respir Crit Care Med.* 2002;166(1): 111–117.**

115. Storer TW. Exercise in chronic pulmonary disease: resistance exercise prescription. *Med Sci Sports Exerc.* 2001;33:S680–692.

116. Sutherland ER, Kraft M, Crapo JD. Diagnosis and treatment of asthma. In: Crapo JD, Glassroth J, Karlinsky JJ, King TE, editors. *Baum's Textbook of Pulmonary Diseases.* Philadelphia: Lippincott, Williams & Wilkins; 2004. p. 179–198.

117. Thacker SB, Gilchrist J, Stroup DF, Kimsey CD Jr. The impact of stretching on sports injury risk: a systematic review of the literature. *Med Sci Sports Exerc.* 2004;36:371–378.

118. Thompson S. On the social cost of asthma. *Eur J Respir Dis Suppl.* 1984;136:185–191.

119. Tiddens H, Silverman M, Bush A. The role of inflammation in airway disease: remodeling. *Am J Respir Crit Care Med.* 2000;162: S7–S10.

120. Tiep BL. Pursed lips breathing—easing does it. *J Cardiopulm Rehabil Prev.* 2007;27:245–246.

121. Tiep BL, Burns M, Kao D, Madison R, Herrera J. Pursed lips breathing training using ear oximetry. *Chest.* 1986;90:218–221.

122. Vallet G, Ahmaidi S, Serres I, et al. Comparison of two training programmes in chronic airway limitation patients: standardized versus individualized protocols. *Eur Respir J.* 1997;10:114–122.

123. Varga J, Porszasz J, Boda K, Casaburi R, Somfay A. Supervised high intensity continuous and interval training vs. self-paced training in COPD. *Respir Med.* 2007;101:2297–2304.

124. Verrill D, Barton C, Beasley W, Lippard WM. The effects of short-term and long-term pulmonary rehabilitation on functional capacity, perceived dyspnea, and quality of life. *Chest.* 2005;128: 673–683.

125. Weiler JM. Exercise-induced asthma: a practical guide to definitions, diagnosis, prevalence, and treatment. *Allergy Asthma Proc.* 1996;17:315–325.

126. Weiner P, Magadle R, Beckerman M, Weiner M, Berar-Yanay N. Comparison of specific expiratory, inspiratory, and combined muscle training programs in COPD. *Chest.* 2003;124:1357–1364.

127. Weiner P, Magadle R, Beckerman M, Weiner M, Berar-Yanay N. Maintenance of inspiratory muscle training in COPD patients: one year follow-up. *Eur Respir J.* 2004;23:61–65.

128. Weiss KB, Sullivan SD. The economic costs of asthma: a review and conceptual model. *Pharmacoeconomics.* 1993;4:14–30.

SELECTED REFERENCES FOR FURTHER READING

American Association of Cardiovascular Pulmonary Rehabilitation. *AACVPR Guidelines for Pulmonary Rehabilitation Programs.* 2nd ed. Champaign (IL): Human Kinetics; 1998.

Cooper CB, Storer TW. *Exercise Testing and Interpretation: A Practical Approach.* New York: Cambridge University Press; 2001.

Crapo JD, Glassroth J, Karlinsky J, King TE, editors. *Baum's Textbook of Pulmonary Diseases.* 7th ed. Philadelphia: Lippincott, Williams & Wilkins; 2004.

Durstine JL, Moore GE, editors. *ACSM's Exercise Management for Persons with Chronic Diseases and Disabilities.* 2nd ed. Champaign (IL): Human Kinetics; 2002.

INTERNET RESOURCES

- American Thoracic Society (statements): www.thoracic.org/statements
- Global Initiative for Asthma (GINA) Workshop Reports: www.ginasthma.com/
- Global Initiative for Chronic Lung Disease: www.goldcopd.com
- National Asthma Education and Prevention Program (Expert Panel report 2: Guidelines for the diagnosis and management of asthma): www.nhlbi.nih.gov/guidelines/asthma/asthgdln.htm
- National Clinical Guideline Clearinghouse (Pulmonary Rehabilitation): www.guideline.gov/summary/summary.aspx?doc_id=3211&nbr=2437&string=lung+and+exercise

Diabetes mellitus is characterized by abnormal glucose metabolism resulting from defects in insulin release, action, or both (6,30). This complex disease requires rigorous self-management combined with an appropriate balance of nutritional intake, medication(s), and regular physical activity (PA)/exercise for blood glucose control.

This chapter focuses on the most common forms of diabetes, including type 1 diabetes mellitus (T1DM), type 2 diabetes mellitus (T2DM), and gestational diabetes mellitus (GDM). Each type of diabetes is distinct in etiology and subsequent exercise programming. Safe and effective exercise recommendations are presented to assist in diabetes management and any accompanying complications.

EPIDEMIOLOGY AND PATHOPHYSIOLOGY OF DIABETES

Diabetes mellitus is a heterogeneous disease that is composed of three major categories: T1DM, T2DM, and GDM (30). Diagnostic and classification criteria of diabetes focus on cause and pathogenesis (30) (see Chapter 8). Although T1DM is one of the most common chronic diagnosed diseases in children, diagnosis of T2DM in youth has risen dramatically over the past decade (13). The burden of diabetes disproportionately affects minorities: the prevalence rates are about twofold greater in Hispanic Americans, African Americans, Native Americans, Asians, and Pacific Islanders compared with non-Hispanic whites (21).

> > > KEY TERMS

Autonomic neuropathy: Disease affecting the nerves innervating the heart, gastrointestinal, and genitourinary tract; cardiovascular autonomic neuropathy is most common, studied, and clinically important of this neuropathy.

Glycosylated hemoglobin (A_{1c}): Test to assess glycemic control that reflects a time-averaged blood glucose concentration over the previous 2 to 3 months.

Hyperglycemia: High blood glucose level (e.g., blood glucose ≥ 126 mg$\cdot$dL^{-1}).

Hypoglycemia: Low blood glucose level (e.g., blood glucose <70 mg$\cdot$dL^{-1}).

Insulin resistance: A condition in which there is a relative lack of insulin action in insulin-sensitive tissues to maintain normal glucose levels.

Ketoacidosis: High level of blood ketones (β-hydroxybutyrate, acetoacetate).

Metabolic syndrome (MetS): A syndrome characterized by a constellation of disorders, including insulin resistance/diabetes, obesity, central adiposity, glucose intolerance, dyslipidemia, and hypertension.

Nephropathy: A disease affecting the kidneys resulting in excessive urinary protein.

Peripheral neuropathy: Disease affecting the nerves in the extremities, especially the lower legs and feet, resulting in loss of sensation.

Retinopathy: A disease affecting the retina of the eye.

Type 1 diabetes mellitus: Immune-mediated disease that selectively destroys the pancreatic β-cells, leading to a "central defect" in insulin release upon stimulation.

Type 2 diabetes mellitus: Disease usually afflicting persons older than the age of 40 years that is directly related to insulin resistance; there is a current increasing prevalence in younger children/adolescents.

Diabetes increases the onset of diabetes-related complications (DRCs), which exacerbate morbidity and increase the likelihood of physical limitation or disability (8,12). Hyperglycemia for an extended period is linked with chronic DRCs that worsen macrovascular, microvascular, and neural processes. Because of daily fluctuations in blood glucose occurring in diabetes, therapeutic interventions purposefully address effective blood glucose control, heart disease risk factors, and prevention of DRCs (12,25). Further information regarding DRCs and metabolic syndrome (MetS) are presented in Chapter 8.

CLINICAL FEATURES OF DIABETES MELLITUS

The diagnosis of diabetes mellitus is based on established criteria (6,30) (see Chapter 8). After diagnosis, clinical emphasis is placed on frequent blood glucose monitoring (i.e., three to six glucose checks per day) in conjunction with diet and PA to control glucose levels and reduce risk of complications (7,12). Glycemic control is assessed using glycosylated hemoglobin (A_{1c}), which reflects a time-averaged blood glucose concentration over the previous 2 to 3 months. The recommended A_{1c} goal is set at <7.0%, which is approximately1% above the nondiabetic range (A_{1c} = 4.0%–6.0%). The A_{1c} is recommended to be assessed every 3 to 4 months (6,12).

Assessment of overall health, especially identification of coexisting cardiovascular disease (CVD) risk factors and DRCs, are essential components of effective diabetes care (6,12). Current recommendations focus on aggressive management of CVD risk factors (12,19,25). Glucose-lowering agents are the primary medications used in diabetes management, supplemented by indicated drugs to prevent CVD, such as antihypertensive drugs, lipid-lowering agents, and antiplatelet medications (12,21).

Whereas body weight is usually normal or reduced in T1DM, obesity is highly prevalent in T2DM and GDM. Body mass index (BMI) often exceeds 30 $kg \cdot m^{-2}$, and abdominal girth is large (men ≤102 cm or 40 in; women ≥88 cm or 35 in) in those with T2DM and GDM, placing many patients at high risk for CVD and cancer (12,21). Therefore, weight loss is a primary treatment goal to improve insulin action in persons with T2DM (12). Table 37-1 provides the major characteristics of T1DM and T2DM diabetes.

GLUCOSE REGULATION

Precise hormonal and metabolic events that normally regulate glucose homeostasis are disrupted in diabetes because of defects in insulin release, action, or both, and result in an excess release of counterregulatory hormones. Glucose control requires near-normal balance between hepatic glucose production and peripheral glucose uptake, combined with effective insulin responses. With diabetes, a reduced ability to precisely match glucose production and use results in daily glucose fluctuations. This requires adjustments in the dosage of exogenous insulin or oral agent(s). Ideally, a patient will learn how to make these adjustments on his or her own. These adjustments should be combined with necessary changes in dietary intake, particularly when anticipating exercise or PA. Information about the use of insulin and oral agents to treat diabetes is provided in Chapter 8.

> **1.5.3-CES: Recognize medications associated in the clinical setting, their indications for care, and their effects at rest and during exercise.**

TABLE 37-1. MAJOR CHARACTERISTICS OF TYPE 1 AND TYPE 2 DIABETES

FACTOR	TYPE 1	TYPE 2
Age at onset	Usually early but may occur at any age	Usually older than age 30 years but may occur at any age
Type of onset	Usually abrupt	Slow progression
Genetic susceptibility	HLA-related DR3 and DR4, ICAs, IAAs	Frequent genetic background; not HLA related
Environmental factors	Virus, toxins, autoimmune stimulation	Obesity, poor nutrition, physical inactivity
Islet cell antibody	Present at onset	Not observed
Endogenous insulin	Minimal or absent	Stimulated response either adequate but delayed secretion or reduced but not absent; insulin resistance present
Nutritional status	Thin, catabolic state	Obese or normal
Symptoms	Thirst, polyuria, polyphagia, fatigue	Mild or frequently none
Ketosis	Common at onset or during insulin deficiency	Resistant to ketosis except during infection or stress
Control of diabetes	Often difficult, with wide glucose fluctuation	Variable; helped by dietary adherence, weight loss, exercise
Dietary management	Essential	Essential; may suffice for glycemic control
Insulin	Required for all	Required for ~40%
Oral hypoglycemics	Not effective	Effective
Vascular or neurologic	Seen in most after 5 or more years of diabetes	Frequent

HLA, human leukocyte antigen; DR, D-related antigen; ICA, islet cell antibodies; IAA, insulin autoantibodies.

Adapted from Shulman CR. Diabetes mellitus: definition, classification, and diagnosis. In: Galloway JA, Potvin JH, Shulman CR, editors. *Diabetes Mellitus.* 9th ed. Indianapolis: Lilly Research Laboratories; 1988.

Insulin Injections or Continuous Subcutaneous Insulin Infusion

Type 1 diabetes mellitus requires multiple daily insulin injections or continuous subcutaneous insulin infusion (CSII) to facilitate glucose uptake and control glucose levels (12). Exercise can accelerate mobilization of insulin if the injection site is in close proximity to an exercising muscle. Recommendations for pre-exercise injections typically suggest injection into the abdominal fat tissue. Insulin dosage (pump or injection) may be need to be reduced before exercise to avoid hypoglycemia. Insulin adjustments involve a trial-and-error process that requires understanding of insulin action and the impact of exercise, food intake, and medication on glucose variability, combined with frequent routine self–blood glucose monitoring (SBGM) (15). Regular PA combined with frequent SBGM is the cornerstone for safe and effective glucose control.

Oral Hypoglycemic Agents

Oral agents are widely prescribed for T2DM when onset is recent and little (e.g., units <20) or no insulin is taken (12). As with insulin injections, oral agents are prescribed individually or in combination to optimize glucose control in T2DM. Three major groups of oral agents are used to control glucose, and their mechanisms of action and effects of exercise are discussed below.

β-Cell Stimulants for Insulin Release

Drugs that stimulate insulin release are taken at mealtime to stimulate insulin release and manage postprandial glycemia. Because of insulin stimulation, these oral agents can lead to hypoglycemia with or without exercise. The prolonged length of action in these oral agents increases risk for low blood glucose and requires more frequent monitoring when a patient is regularly exercising.

Drugs to Improve Insulin Sensitivity

Some of the drugs in this class improve insulin sensitivity in muscle tissue, adipose tissue, and the liver, and others promote muscle glucose uptake and inhibit hepatic glucose output. The effect mainly improves the action of insulin at rest, not during exercise, so their risk of causing exercise-associated hypoglycemia is unlikely (15).

Drugs That Abate Intestinal Absorption of Carbohydrates

Drugs that decrease carbohydrate absorption rate and slow the increase in postprandial blood glucose level don't directly affect exercise. However, they can delay effective treatment of hypoglycemia during activities by slowing the absorption of carbohydrates ingested to treat this condition (15).

TREATMENT

Exercise intervention for persons with diabetes involves a multidisciplinary team of specialists that includes the diabetes physician, diabetes nurse educator, registered dietician, and exercise physiologist to facilitate patient education and lifestyle changes to manage this disease (12). Intensive SBGM, combined with balancing diet, oral drugs or exogenous insulin (or both), and regular PA/exercise are established cornerstones of therapy to facilitate near-normal to normal metabolic function (12). Self-management skills are essential to the successful management of diabetes, and use of diabetes self-management education (DSME) is an important tool to improve control (12).

The primary goal of therapy for all persons with diabetes focuses on SBGM to achieve acceptable blood glucose control (A_{1c} <7.0%), thereby limiting the development and progression of DRCs (12). Both T1DM (9) and T2DM (10) show reduced risk for retinopathy, nephropathy, and neuropathy with intensive therapy and the potential for a reduction of CVD and related risk factors with improved glycemic control.

> **1.2.5-CES: Examine the role of lifestyle on cardiovascular risk factors, such as hypertension, blood lipids, glucose tolerance, and body weight.**

Cardiovascular risk factors, along with symptomatic and asymptomatic CVD, are common in diabetes (6,19,25). Identification of macrovascular disease and comorbidities of diabetes and aggressive intervention are crucial in minimizing their progression, particularly factors linked with the MetS (19,25,29). CVD morbidity and mortality in diabetes can be favorably affected through lifestyle interventions. Prudent lifestyle interventions in diabetes care focus on minimizing progression of CVD through management of CVD risk factors. Lifestyle strategies lower CVD risk factors by favorably affecting blood pressure (BP), blood lipids, glucose tolerance, and body weight. Lifestyle strategies for managing CVD risk in diabetes include (a) dietary intervention in which calories and fat intake are limited, (b) weight management and/or weight loss, (c) regular PA/exercise, (d) smoking cessation, and (e) DSME (12). The coexistence of multiple CVD risk factors (e.g., MetS), along with hyperglycemia, requires a vigilant lifestyle intervention to reduce risk and prevent CVD (19,25).

> **1.7.14-CES: Identify and explain the mechanisms by which exercise may contribute to reducing disease risk or rehabilitating individuals with cardiovascular, pulmonary, and metabolic diseases.**

> **1.2.8-CES: Describe the influence of exercise on cardiovascular, pulmonary, and metabolic risk factors.**

Engaging in regular PA/exercise is an important therapeutic intervention to assist in managing diabetes (31). When combined with lifestyle measures, regular aerobic exercise in persons with diabetes reduces CVD risk factors (14,19,25). Regular PA/exercise facilitates improved blood glucose control in T2DM and may offer a similar benefit in GDM (3,7). Although regular exercise fails to favorably control glucose in those with T1DM (4), exercise can be a safe and effective adjunct therapy for diabetes management (11). Improved glucose control attenuates progression of CVD disease processes (3,4,11,35). Exercise, in combination with medical nutrition therapy and weight loss, has been demonstrated to favorably modify lipids and lipoproteins, thereby lowering CVD risk in persons with diabetes (4,11,14). Also, reductions in BP have been demonstrated through exercise and weight loss, and may be partially explained by improved insulin sensitivity and loss of abdominal fat (35). A 7% to 10% reduction in body weight is recommended (12,36), and this has important outcomes related to BP, glucose control, and CVD risk. Glucose control is favorably affected through exercise in T2DM and in some GDM by an increased insulin sensitivity of skeletal muscle. Lowering A_{1c} for those with diabetes reduces risk for DRCs (12) and CVD (19,36). In those with diabetes, regular PA/exercise has many benefits, including improvement of cardiovascular, metabolic, and psychological health; primary and secondary prevention of CVD; and prevention of diabetes-specific complications (19,25,35).

ACUTE AND CHRONIC EXERCISE-RELATED PHYSIOLOGIC RESPONSES IN DIABETES

> **1.1.11-CES: Knowledge of acute and chronic adaptations to exercise for those with cardiovascular, pulmonary, and/or metabolic diseases.**

The acute effect of exercise on diabetes improves insulin sensitivity, facilitates glucose uptake, and aids in glucose homeostasis (11,31). Usually, an acute bout of exercise lowers blood glucose for 24 hours to 72 hours postexercise (27,31). Thus, acute effects of exercise are transient and short-lived.

The favorable effects of chronic exercise have been reported for T1DM (4,11,39) and T2DM (4,11,34,37) (Table 37-2). Regular aerobic and resistance training combined with medical nutrition therapy promotes improved cardiovascular function, along with favorable changes in lipids and lipoproteins, BP, body mass, fat-free mass (maintain or increase), fat mass, body fat distribution, insulin sensitivity, glucose control (T2DM only) and metabolism, and postprandial thermogenesis (3,4,11,39). These physiologic changes usually result in a lowering of the daily medication dose (e.g., insulin or oral agent) needed to manage glucose levels for T1DM and T2DM, and in some GDM.

TABLE 37-2. EFFECTS OF EXERCISE IN DIABETES MELLITUS

PARAMETER	TYPE 1	TYPE 2
Cardiovascular		
Aerobic capacity or fitness level	⇑	⇑/⇔
Resting pulse rate and rate–pressure product	⇓	⇓
Resting BP in mild-moderate hypertensives	⇓	⇓
HR at submaximal loads	⇓	⇓
Lipid and Lipoprotein Alterations		
HDL	⇑	⇑
LDL	⇓/⇔	⇓/⇔
VLDL	⇓	⇓
Total cholesterol	⇔	⇔
Risk ratio (total cholesterol/HDL)	⇓	⇓
Anthropometric Measures		
Body mass	⇓/⇔	⇓
Fat mass, especially in obese persons	⇓	⇓
Fat-free mass	⇑	⇑/⇔
Metabolic Parameters		
Insulin sensitivity and glucose metabolic machinery	⇑	⇑
A_{1c}	⇔	⇓
Postprandial thermogenesis or thermic effect of food	⇑	⇑
Presumed Psychological Outcomes		
Self-concept and self-esteem	⇑	⇑
Depression and anxiety	⇓	⇓
Stress response to psychological stimuli	⇓	⇓

BP, blood pressure; HDL, high-density lipoprotein; HR, heart rate; LDL, low-density lipoprotein; VLDL, very low-density lipoprotein; ↑, increase; ↓, decrease; ⇔, no change.

American College of Sports Medicine and American Diabetes Association. Diabetes mellitus and exercise: a joint position statement of the American College of Sports Medicine and the American Diabetes Association. *Med Sci Sport Exerc*. 1997;29:i–vi. American Diabetes Association. Physical activity/exercise and diabetes: position statement. *Diabetes Care*. 2004;27(suppl 1):S58–S64.

Regular exercise training improves glucose control only in T2DM, primarily through increased insulin sensitivity (3,4,17,18,27,37). Additionally, improved glucose uptake through increased insulin sensitivity has been demonstrated in GDM (7,11). Although exercise improves insulin sensitivity, little or no improvement in glucose control has been demonstrated in T1DM after regular exercise training (4,39).

Regular exercise may also favorably alter stress-related psychological factors and cognitive function in diabetes (27,37). Depression is common in diabetes (12), and regular PA/exercise may assist in countering this debilitating psychoemotional state. Overall, regular PA/exercise may offer quality-of-life improvements for individuals with diabetes that other therapies fail to achieve.

EXERCISE PRESCRIPTION IN DIABETES

 1.3.28-CES: Describe the aerobic and anaerobic metabolic demands of exercise testing and training in individuals with cardiovascular, pulmonary, and/or metabolic diseases undergoing exercise testing or training.

Comprehensive diabetes therapy includes participation in regular PA and intentional exercise (24). Given the benefits of a physically active lifestyle, an exercise physiologist must also recognize the associated risks as previously mentioned. Identifiable limitations (e.g., presence of disease complications) and precautions (e.g., degree of glucose control) must be addressed before an exercise program can be developed.

SCREENING

 1.7.11-CES: Describe relative and absolute contraindications to exercise training.

Uncontrolled diabetes is a relative contraindication to exercise training. Before exercise sessions, SBGM is essential to make any adjustments in insulin or caloric intake for glucose management. In the presence of low insulin levels, insulin-stimulated glucose uptake in skeletal muscle is reduced, and exercise-induced hepatic glucose output is excessive, resulting in hyperglycemia or elevated blood glucose (e.g., >126 mg·dL^{-1}). After glucose levels exceed 250 to 300 mg·dL^{-1}, urinary ketones appear and represent excessive fat metabolism, and they contribute to diabetic ketoacidosis (DKA) if glycemia remains uncontrolled. This scenario requires insulin to be administered to lower the glucose level and re-establish euglycemia. In the presence of excess insulin, hepatic glucose production is blunted, and glucose uptake into exercising muscle is heightened by exercise when insulin is high. This scenario can result in hypoglycemia, or low blood glucose (e.g., blood glucose <80 mg·dL^{-1}), and requires that insulin be reduced and rapidly absorbed carbohydrates (10–20 g) be ingested before beginning an exercise session to increase blood glucose to an acceptable level (11,15).

 4.2.1-HFS: Knowledge of metabolic risk factors or conditions that may require consultation with medical personnel before testing or training, including obesity, MetS, thyroid disease, kidney disease, diabetes or glucose intolerance, and hypoglycemia.

A thorough preactivity screening of the patient's clinical status is recommended to ensure safe and effective participation (24,27,34). Coexisting morbidities in the diabetes health profile are important to determine whether the clinical status is acceptable for safely engaging in exercise and to determine the need for monitoring of each session.

Before commencing exercise, prudent screening for vascular and neurologic complications, including silent ischemia, are warranted, along with identification of the presence of CVD risk factors and MetS. Persons with diabetes are stratified in the high-risk category, according to recommended guidelines (5), and a stress test is strongly recommended before initiating moderate to vigorous exercise irrespective of the patient's cardiac risk profile (4,25,27,34). Specific indications for a stress test to be administered include the presence of one or more of the criteria shown in Box 37-1 (12,34). Procedures for general exercise testing and testing in persons with diabetes are discussed in Chapters 21 and 24.

 1.7.16-CES: Describe the principle of specificity as it relates to the mode of exercise testing and training.

For those with diabetes, glucose response to exercise can vary with each exercise session. Through the use of daily glucose logs, the patient can better understand his/her glucose response to an exercise bout. Just as exercise adaptations are specific to the type of training, so too is the glucose response. Caution should be exercised when changing from one mode of exercise to another or modifying intensity/duration of a session because of unpredictable glycemic fluctuations (24).

BOX 37-1	**INDICATIONS FOR STRESS TESTING WITH DIABETES**

- Known or suspected cardiovascular disease (e.g., coronary artery disease, peripheral arterial disease)
- Age >35 years
- Age >25 years if duration of diabetes >10 years for type 1 or >15 years for type 2
- Presence of any additional risk factors for cardiovascular disease
- Microvascular disease
- Autonomic neuropathy

> **1.1.10-CES: Discuss the effects of isometric exercise in individuals with cardiovascular, pulmonary, and/or metabolic diseases.**

Although aerobic exercise and dynamic resistance training are favorably recommended, the possible use of isometric exercise in diabetes is viewed with extreme caution. Exposure to isometric exercise causes marked elevations in systolic and diastolic BP, and a postexercise increase in blood glucose in those with diabetes (24,31). Because of the significant pressor response and rise in BP and its potential to worsen DRCs, isometric exercise is contraindicated and may compromise safety of exercise for persons with diabetes who have poor left ventricular function (40). If normal ventricular function is assured through appropriate diagnostic testing (e.g., echocardiography, catheterization), then isometric exercise may be permitted.

AEROBIC EXERCISE PRESCRIPTION

In general, aerobic exercise programming for diabetes without complications follows the frequency, intensity, duration, and types of activities presented in Table 37-3. Each exercise session is composed of a warm-up, aerobic-based exercise, and a cool-down phase. Supervised exercise for nondiseased diabetes is recommended and encouraged during initial phases of an exercise program to aid in monitoring signs/symptoms, response to exercise, and glucose levels, whereas supervision of exercise in postevent or surgical diabetes patients is necessary.

> **1.7.13-CES: Describe the importance of warm-up and cool-down sessions with specific reference to angina and ischemic electrocardiogram (ECG) changes, and for overall patient safety.**

At least a 5- to 10-minute period of warm-up is warranted for those with diabetes before progressing to moderate intensity exercise. Warm-up before the conditioning phase (a) facilitates transition from rest to exercise via increasing blood flow, body temperature, oxygen disassociation, and metabolism; (b) reduces susceptibility to muscular injury, improves joint range of motion, and improves muscular performance; and (c) decreases occurrence of

electrocardiogram (ECG) changes consistent with myocardial ischemia, angina onset, ventricular arrhythmias, and transient left ventricular dysfunction (5). Thus, warm-up improves physiologic function, reduces untoward outcomes of sudden strenuous exercise, and enhances overall patient safety.

Cool-down after exercise should be an active, low-level recovery period that progressively reduces exercise intensity to allow gradual redistribution of blood from the extremities to other tissue and to prevent sudden reduction in venous return, thereby reducing the possibility of postexercise hypotension or even syncopal events. Heart rate monitoring can be effective in determining recovery from an exercise bout. Medication for hypertension, or other vasodilators, may require individuals to participate in a longer period of active cool-down (5).

> **1.7.18-CES: Determine appropriate testing and training modalities according to the age, functional capacity, physical ability, and health status of the individual.**

Training modalities selected for the exercise prescription are commonly predicated on patient goals, preferences, and abilities, along with fitness level and orthopedic limitations. Nearly 80% of adults with diabetes are obese (12), and most with T2DM have low aerobic capacity (18). The selection of equipment for exercise training is important to ensure appropriate intensity level is achieved without discomfort and the activity is preferred by the patient. Careful selection of the exercise modality, not only for those with diabetes but for everyone, can improve the likelihood of sustaining the exercise habit.

> **1.7.40-HFS: Ability to explain and implement exercise prescription guidelines for apparently healthy patients, increased-risk patients, and patients with controlled disease.**

In T1DM without complications, exercise recommendations are closely aligned with apparently healthy persons (39), whereas recommendations for T2DM are more closely aligned with obesity and hypertension guidelines (27,34) because of the prevalence of these comorbidities

TABLE 37-3. RECOMMENDED FITT PROGRAM FOR AEROBIC TRAINING IN DIABETES

VARIABLE	T1DM	T2DM
Frequency	3–7 d·wk^{-1}	3–7 d·wk^{-1}
Intensity	50%–80% HRR	50%–80% HRR^a
	RPE = 12–16 (6–20 scale)	RPE = 12–16 (6–20 scale)
Time	20–60 min·session^{-1} moderate intensity	20–60 min·session^{-1}
	(e.g., 600 METs·min·wk^{-1})	At least 150 min·wk^{-1} at moderate intensity (e.g., 600 METs·min·wk^{-1} or 90 min·wk^{-1} at vigorous intensity (540 METs·min·wk^{-1})
Type^a	Walk; bicycle; jogging; water aerobic activities	walk; bicycle; water aerobic activities

FITT, fitness, intensity, time, type; T1DM, type 1 diabetes mellitus; T2DM, type 2 diabetes mellitus; HRR, heart rate reserve; RPE, rating of perceived exertion; MET, metabolic equivalent.

^{a}Persons may require non–weight-bearing activity or alternating with weight-bearing activities because of orthopedic limitations and/or peripheral vascular disease.

in T2DM. Also, T2DM patients are recommended to engage in at least 150 minutes of moderate-intensity exercise (e.g., 600 metabolic equivalents [METs] $\cdot$ min $\cdot$ wk^{-1}) each week or 90 minutes of vigorous exercise (e.g., 540 METs $\cdot$ min $\cdot$ wk^{-1}) each week, primarily focusing on caloric expenditure and weight management issues (11). For long-term weight loss maintenance, larger volumes of exercise (7 h/wk of moderate or vigorous activity) for T2DM are recommended (11). In GDM, moderate physical exercise is warranted in women with medical approval because of its glucose-lowering effects (7). Consideration of personal interests, past and/or present activity habits, and goals and needs of a PA program are critical for successful participation, especially in T2DM (3,14,27). Those who use insulin may prefer to engage in daily PA to improve the balance between insulin dose and caloric needs (3,11,15).

> **1.7.41-HFS: Ability to adapt frequency, intensity, duration, mode, progression, level of supervision, and monitoring techniques in exercise programs for patients with controlled chronic disease (e.g., heart disease, diabetes mellitus, obesity, hypertension), musculoskeletal problems (including fatigue), pregnancy and/or postpartum, and exercise-induced asthma.**

Initial exercise program sessions may require modifications in intensity and duration for persons with diabetes. Each acute bout of exercise can have a variable effect on blood glucose, so to prevent untoward glycemic outcomes, lower intensity and duration are initially recommended for persons with diabetes, particularly T2DM (3,34) and GDM (7), because of fitness level, clinical status, and coexisting CVD risk factors (obesity, hypertension). Given the coexistence of risk factors (e.g., hypertension, obesity) observed in T2DM and GDM, walking is a preferred low-impact mode of exercise to lessen joint loading, whereas general activity mode recommendations for those with T1DM are similar to those without diabetes. Excess body weight may limit weight-bearing exercise, whereas lower impact activities, such as recumbent cycle ergometer and aquatic activities (aquacise or swimming), are prudent activities to reduce joint stress. Although bench stepping is lower impact, care should be used in its implementation, particularly in those with arthritis or orthopedic limitations of the lower extremities. In developing an exercise prescription for someone with diabetes, there may be a need to adapt a mode of exercise that will improve the likelihood of meeting the goals and needs of the patient.

> **1.7.8-CES: Demonstrate exercise equipment adaptations necessary for different age groups, physical abilities, and other potential contributing factors.**

To ensure adherence of an exercise program, the mode of exercise and potential equipment modification(s) may be necessary in patients with diabetes, particularly those who are physically disabled or those with weight management/obesity issues, low-back concerns, peripheral neuropathy, or low fitness level. Common exercise equipment adaptations primarily center on use of lower-impact machines, and when bicycle or rowing ergometer activity is recommended, a wide-seated platform is more appropriate and comfortable. Exercise equipment adaptations for those with physical disabilities should follow universal design and use of facilities to maximize opportunities of access and adaptation.

Precautions of Aerobic Training

> **1.7.7-CES: Prescribe exercise using nontraditional modalities (e.g., bench stepping, elastic bands, isodynamic exercise, water aerobics, yoga, tai chi, etc.) for individuals with cardiovascular, pulmonary, or metabolic disease.**

Moderate-intensity exercise is strongly recommended for persons with diabetes (3,4,11,24,27,39). It may be necessary to obtain physician approval for previously sedentary patients to perform vigorous exercise (>60% $\dot{V}O_{2max}$). Non–weight-bearing or low-impact activities (e.g., recumbent cycle ergometer, aquacise, elastic bands, yoga, tai chi) may be useful alternatives for T2DM and GDM to lessen joint stress, yet provide functional fitness programming for selected patients. Activities performed lying on the back or belly are contraindicated for GDM (see Chapter 41) before giving birth (7). Usually, activity other than walking requires physician approval for GDM to limit complicating outcomes.

RESISTANCE-TRAINING EXERCISE PRESCRIPTION

> **1.7.17-CES: Design strength and flexibility programs for individuals with cardiovascular, pulmonary, and/or metabolic diseases; the elderly; and children.**

Resistance training is recommended for persons with diabetes who have no complications (3,4,11,34) and follow apparently healthy guidelines, with age and experience as prime considerations in program development (Table 37-4). Appropriate attention to modifying the intensity of the lifting session may reduce the risk for elevations in BP, glucose, and onset of musculoskeletal injury (3,11). Research suggests that higher-intensity resistance exercise is safe and effective in lowering A$_{1c}$ (20,22). Recommending higher-intensity resistance-training exercises for those with diabetes should be done with caution. For safe and effective exercise participation, it is imperative that glucose levels be carefully managed.

Traditional resistance training may be supplemented with the use of nontraditional activities. For improved muscular strength, endurance, and balance exercises, tai

TABLE 37-4. RECOMMENDED FITT PROGRAM FOR RESISTANCE TRAINING IN DIABETES

VARIABLE	T1DM	T2DM
Frequency	2–3 d·wk^{-1}	2–3^a d·wk^{-1}
Intensity	60%–80% 1RM low to moderate	60%–80% 1RM lower intensity
	RPE ~14–16 (6–20 scale)	RPE ~11–15 (6–20 scale)
Time	8–12/exercise	8–12 (up to 20)/exercise
	2–3 sets/exercise	2–3 sets/exercise
Type of exercise	All major muscle groups	All major muscle groups
	Upper body: 4–5 exercises	Upper body: 4–5 exercises
	Lower body: 4–5 exercises	Lower body: 4–5 exercises

FITT, fitness, intensity, time, type; T1DM, type 1 diabetes mellitus; T2DM, type 2 diabetes mellitus; 1RM, 1 repetitive maximum; RPE, rating of perceived exertion.
^{a}3 d/wk is strongly encouraged (11,34).

chi has been safely performed by and can provide functional outcomes for those with diabetes.

Precautions of Resistance Training

> **1.3.30 and 1.7.20-CES: Discuss the appropriate use of static and dynamic resistance exercise for individuals with cardiovascular, pulmonary, and metabolic disease.**

Although studies have found that moderate- to high-intensity resistance training provoked no ECG evidence of ischemia, it is recommended that lifts be dynamic and at a moderate intensity to ensure a safe and effective program. Patients should be apprised of the Valsalva maneuver and encouraged to breathe on effort to avoid untoward outcomes of resistance training, particularly with respect to increased BP that may contribute to retinal damage (1,16). Therefore, prescribing resistance training exercises for those with diabetic retinopathy may be contraindicated.

FLEXIBILITY EXERCISE PRESCRIPTION

Static flexibility exercises are recommended in persons with diabetes who have no complications and follow apparently healthy guidelines, with age and experience as prime considerations in program development (Table 37-5). Traditional stretches are recommended to be performed after an active warm-up and should not require considerable skill or flexibility; however, appropriate modification(s) of

TABLE 37-5. RECOMMENDED FITT PROGRAM FOR FLEXIBILITY TRAINING IN TYPE 1 AND 2 DIABETES

Variable	T1DM
Frequency	2–3 d·wk^{-1}
Intensity	Stretch to ROM tightness
Time	15–30 s/stretch
	2–4 reps/stretch
Type of stretching exercise	Upper body: 4–5 exercises
	Lower body: 4–5 exercises

FITT, fitness, intensity, time, type; T1DM, type 1 diabetes mellitus; ROM, range of motion.

stretches because of joint limitations, obesity, or pregnancy restrictions may be necessary.

> **1.3.9-CES: Instruct the test participant in the use of the ratings of perceived exertion (RPE) scale and other appropriate subjective rating scales, such as the dyspnea, pain, claudication, and angina scales.**

Exercise intensity can be objectively derived from heart rate, as well as subjectively determined through proper use of the ratings of perceived exertion (RPE) scale. Informing the patient to accurately identify their level of effort during exercise is useful and important feedback. In reflecting exercise effort, patients must be familiarized with the Borg rating scale used for RPE determination. Perceived effort of the patient must be aligned with the numeric rating scale. Routinely during an exercise bout, the patient will be asked to identify his/her subjective estimate of effort by stating a numeric equivalent of the verb that best describes one's perceived effort. Ensuring appropriate interpretation of the response requires that the exercise practitioner "restate" the number out loud to confirm a correct rating.

Other subjective rating scales used during exercise bouts (e.g., dyspnea, claudication, and angina scales) follow similar procedures of administration and aid the exercise practitioner in providing a safe exercise environment for patients with diabetes (5).

> **1.7.3-CES: Design an appropriate exercise prescription in environmental extremes for those with cardiovascular, pulmonary, and metabolic diseases.**

Patients with diabetes should be encouraged by their exercise professional (e.g. exercise physiologist) to engage in other types of PA outside of scheduled exercise sessions. In some instances, patients may anticipate exercising in an environment that modifies the normal exercise prescription. For instance, exercising at altitude (a) lowers aerobic capacity and requires that intensity/duration be reduced because of hypoxia; (b) increases work, sympathetic response, and sweating, which can cause hypoglycemia and requires reduced insulin/medications with frequent glucose monitoring and feeding; and (c) fosters onset of dehydration and requires increased water consumption (31). Additionally, diabetes increases likelihood of dehydration. Ensuring proper hydration in any environmental condition is important for the exercise professional to convey. Exercising in a thermally challenging environment (e.g., hot and/or humid) can pose difficulties for those with diabetes because of hydration issues and heightened glucose metabolism. Exercise professionals (e.g., exercise physiologists) should offer precautionary measures and prevention strategies to avoid dehydration and/or hypoglycemia in those with diabetes. In some instances, outdoor exercise should be postponed to ensure a safe environment in which to participate. Exercise professionals should apprise patients of risks and educate them on the management of expected environmental challenges.

Throughout the exercise session, the exercise physiologist must ensure the safety of the patient. One important aspect of safety when supervising an exercise session is to ensure the patient checks his/her blood glucose and take appropriate steps whenever hypoglycemia occurs, as recommended (4,12,34).

> **1.7.23-CES: Identify procedures for pre-exercise assessment of blood glucose, determining safety for exercise and avoidance of exercise-induced hypoglycemia in patients with diabetes; also the management of postexercise hypoglycemia when it occurs.**

Glucose control must be maintained in order for exercise to be safe and effective. Self–blood glucose monitoring is recommended so that adjustments in medications, caloric intake, or both can be made to preserve euglycemia (12). Self–blood glucose monitoring is recommended before and after each exercise session in persons with diabetes, and a blood glucose value ranging between 100 and 250 mg·dL^{-1} is recommended to participate safely in exercise (11,14,24). If blood glucose is elevated (e.g., >250–300 mg·dL^{-1}) before exercise, an acute bout tends to cause further elevation in blood glucose (hyperglycemia). Exercise in this scenario can still occur, provided there is no evidence of urinary ketones. Conversely, if blood glucose is within the low-normal range (e.g., <100 mg·dL^{-1}) before exercising, an acute bout tends to accelerate blood glucose lowering and increase risk for hypoglycemia. To avoid hypoglycemia, consumption of 20 to 30 g of carbohydrates is recommended before exercising (12,13). Also, extra carbohydrates may need to be ingested during and after exercise predicated on intensity and duration of the exercise bout.

If postexercise hypoglycemia occurs, the exercise physiologist should encourage the patient with diabetes to consume 20 to 30 g of carbohydrate and monitor blood glucose after 5 minutes. This sequence of carbohydrate consumption and blood glucose monitoring should proceed until the patient's blood glucose has reached a normal level (e.g., ≥80 mg·dL^{-1}) (12). Acute exercise has a postexercise influence on diabetes for 24 to 72 hours (4,11). Thus, vigilant SBGM before, after, and several hours after the exercise bout is critical to prevent severe glucose excursions causing hypoglycemia.

EXERCISE PRESCRIPTION FOR PATIENT WITH DIABETES AND CARDIAC DISEASE

> **1.7.6-CES: Knowledge of the concept of activities of daily living (ADLs) and its importance in the overall rehabilitation of the individual.**

Patients with diabetes who suffer a myocardial event or undergo surgery are strongly encouraged to participate in exercise and aggressive lifestyle modification to prevent future CVD complications (14,19,25). The inpatient cardiac rehabilitation setting (i.e., phase I) provides awareness of and education about the role of regular PA/exercise. Moreover, an ability to perform activities of daily living (ADLs), from bedside activities to functional performance, increases the likelihood of independent living and improves psychoemotional status (5,14).

For patients with diabetes, participation in cardiac rehabilitation is warranted to aid in secondary prevention of CVD by aggressive risk-factor modification and disease management (14,19). Cardiac rehabilitation staff should follow and enforce all the previous stated guidelines regarding pre– and post–blood glucose assessment and treatment for the patient with diabetes.

> **1.7.9-CES: Identify patients who require a symptom-limited exercise test before exercise training.**

In patients with diabetes who will be performing a vigorous exercise program (i.e., >60% peak V̇O$_2$), it is recommended to administer a symptom-limited exercise test before supervised exercise training because of the increased risk of silent ischemia, hypertension, dyslipidemia, poor metabolic control, and advanced CVD (14,19). From the symptom-limited exercise test, stratification of risk and level of supervision and monitoring should be determined and utilized to develop the exercise training routine. Supervised exercise programming for outpatient settings is strongly recommended (14). Because of diabetes, these patients are likely to be stratified as moderate-to-higher risk for exercise participation.

> **1.7.5-CES: Design a supervised exercise program beginning at hospital discharge and continuing for up to 6 months for the following conditions: myocardial infarction; angina; left ventricular assist device; congestive heart failure; percutaneous coronary intervention; coronary artery bypass graft(s); medical management of coronary artery disease (CAD); chronic pulmonary disease; weight management; diabetes; metabolic syndrome; and cardiac transplants.**

Exercise prescription for those with diabetes from hospital discharge to 6 months postdischarge follows an equivalent protocol established for those without diabetes (see Chapter 28). Initial exercise programs for diabetes focuses on lowering intensity/duration, monitoring of clinical responses, and ensuring assessment of blood glucose to ensure safe and effective exercise participation (14). Precautions in exercise programs for diabetes address potential risks and DRCs. Hypoglycemia awareness may be blunted in those taking β-blocker medication (15). In diabetes, autonomic neuropathy may limit work capacity and result in a higher resting and lower peak heart rate than age-matched normals (38). Under this circumstance, a symptom-limited graded exercise test is recommended to set safe upper heart rate limits (14).

Exercise sessions may begin with low-to-moderate intensity for 10-minute bouts performed two to three times per day. Modest increases in frequency, intensity, and duration require careful consideration because of diabetes, CVD, and possible DRCs and obesity (14). Monitoring of signs/symptoms aid in determining progression of the exercise performed. Because of peripheral neuropathy, palpation-type heart rate monitoring may need to be complemented with either a heart rate (HR) monitor (e.g., Polar-type HR monitor) or RPE to monitor intensity of activities performed at home. Ensuring accurate use of RPE in the clinical setting can help ensure safe participation. Because volume of PA/exercise is important in recovery, it is recommended that patients with diabetes accumulate additional energy expenditure outside the center-based program. Overall, a 6-month target for diabetes patients is to achieve a frequency of at least 3 to 5 $d \cdot wk^{-1}$ (up to 7 $d \cdot wk^{-1}$) at a low to moderate intensity (50%–85% of heart rate reserve) for at least 30 to 40 minutes (e.g. ~600 $METs \cdot min \cdot wk^{-1}$) and a maximum of 60 minutes (1,200 $METs \cdot min \cdot wk^{-1}$) (14). The importance of increasing daily PA is an important part of the rehabilitation plan and should be emphasized.

> **1.5.5-CES: Practice disease/case management responsibilities, including daily follow-up concerning patient needs, signs and symptoms, physician appointments, and medication changes for patients with chronic diseases, including cardiovascular, pulmonary, metabolic diseases, comorbid conditions, arthritis, osteoporosis, and renal dysfunction/transplant/dialysis.**

Throughout the cardiac rehabilitation timeline (phases I–IV), it is recommended that the cardiac rehabilitation staff oversee patient progress. Responsibilities for cardiac rehabilitation staff in patients with diabetes involves follow-up with regards to (a) satisfactory glucose levels before, during, and postexercise, especially early in rehabilitation; (b) management of medications that are taken for diabetes control and coexisting CVD risk factors (e.g., weight, hypertension, dyslipidemia) to reduce untoward risks of exercise (e.g., hypoglycemia and hypotension); (c) exercise being performed without change of sign/symptoms, and exercise prescription updates routinely provided when warranted; (d) PA counseling to improve recreational, occupational, or domestic function and limit dysfunction or disability onset; and (e) ensuring follow-up with diabetes specialist(s) for routine care and assessment of diabetes management, particularly A_{1c} (14). These management aspects constitute important aspects in cardiac rehabilitation for those who have diabetes. A structured exercise program patterned after a cardiac rehabilitation model for diabetes is feasible and effective in improving fitness, glycemic control, and CVD risk factors.

The clinical exercise program must consider personal interests as well as past and present activity habits. The goals and needs of an exercise prescription for patients with diabetes are critical in determining whether the exercise habit will be sustained, especially in persons with T2DM (4,23). Additionally, past exercise habits can provide important information regarding present exercise preferences and behaviors.

Diabetes increases risk for cardiac events (14,25). When an event occurs, cardiac rehabilitation is strongly recommended (14). Counseling the patient with diabetes about postevent ability to return to regular domestic, recreational, and occupational physical activities is important for the patient to comprehend.

> **1.7.10-CES: Organize graded exercise test and clinical data to counsel patients regarding issues such as ADLs, return to work, and physical activity.**

Exercise professionals must review clinical data to counsel patients. Medical history, physical examination, and testing outcomes are central to data acquisition (14). Review medical history for current cardiovascular medical and surgical diagnoses, and procedures performed; comorbidities; signs/symptoms of CVD; diagnosed history of DRCs (eye, kidney, feet, or nervous systems); medications (dose, frequency and compliance); and cardiovascular risk profile, along with A_{1c}. Review physical examination for assessment of cardiac function (HR, BP), pulmonary function, findings from inspection of lower extremities and presence of arterial pulses, postcardiac procedure wound site, orthopedic and neuromuscular status, and cognitive function. Review testing outcomes to obtain 12-lead ECG and perceived health-related quality of life or health status (e.g. SF-36). From these data, patient counseling can address a variety of issues, including ADLs, PA, and return to work.

Initial interaction with a patient should evaluate any signs/symptoms of DRCs and episodes of hypoglycemia. Presence of DRCs may limit certain activities. Assessment of the current level of ability to be self-sufficient by performing ADLs independently should be performed. It is important to emphasize that ADLs that the patient is capable of performing independently should be done as a start to regular independent PA. Evaluation of PA through the use of a questionnaire or other objective measure of PA (e.g., pedometer) and assessment of occupational PA requirements may be useful. If appropriate, determine current level of PA relative to age, sex, and daily life (gardening, yard work, household tasks, driving, sports, sexual activity). Most importantly, evaluate personal qualities of the patient, including self-confidence, readiness to change behavior, barriers to increasing PA, and social support structure to make beneficial changes. Recovery emphasis for the person with diabetes is similar to that for nondiabetics and is placed on the goal of returning to work and the necessary steps to undertake to achieve this goal (14).

The exercise professional must continually provide advice, professional support, and counseling of sustaining ADLs and PA for the patient with diabetes from initial evaluation to follow-up (14). Following a cardiac event, maintaining an active lifestyle is an important goal. Educational materials should be provided to support advice given to the patient. Aggressive risk-factor-reduction education and awareness is prudent, along with intensive SBGM, for patients with diabetes (14,19,25). Through regular participation in PA/exercise and making appropriate lifestyle changes, fitness is improved, CVD risk is lowered, body weight/fat is decreased, and participation in recreational, occupational, and domestic activities is more easily accommodated. Regular PA participation also facilitates psychoemotional health, reduces stress, promotes functional independence, and enhances self-care independence (14). These outcomes are of primary importance for people with diabetes.

> ### 1.11.4-CES: Understand the most recent cardiac and pulmonary rehabilitation Centers for Medical Care Services (CMS) rules for patient enrollment and reimbursement (e.g., diagnostic current procedure terminology [CPT] codes, diagnostic related groups [DRG]).

Cardiac rehabilitation is recommended, but third party coverage is critical for the patient with diabetes to participate. Staff must understand enrollment and reimbursement issues for cardiac rehabilitation in patients with diabetes. CMS rules for enrolling patients with diabetes in cardiac rehabilitation are equivalent to those without diabetes (20). Although diabetes alone is not covered, traditional CVD codes are covered for the patient with diabetes who has suffered a recent cardiac event or undergone surgery. CVD codes linked with cardiac rehabilitation are presented in Chapter 49.

Risks and Precautions of Exercise in Diabetes

> ### 1.7.2-CES: Compare and contrast benefits and risks of exercise for individuals with risk factors for or established cardiovascular, pulmonary, and metabolic diseases.

Exercise provides definitive benefits and certain risks for persons with diabetes. When performed properly, the benefits will far outweigh the risks for an individual patient.

Although favorable changes occur in cardiovascular and hemodynamic function, insulin action and sensitivity, glucose metabolism, weight management, and CVD risk reduction, these benefits must be weighed against risks of exercise for patients with diabetes. A safe and effective exercise program for diabetes minimizes the acute risks and long-term complications while maximizing the benefits. Two common risks associated with exercise in diabetic patients are hypoglycemia and hyperglycemia; however, practical precautions can be taken to reduce the risk or avoid their onset (Table 37-6). Essential to preventing risk onset is SBGM (3,4,11,14). Exercise-induced hypoglycemia is most common for those who require exogenous insulin, has been observed in those taking oral sulfonylureas, and may exist for meglitinide (15). To prevent hypoglycemia, glucose monitoring before and after exercise is required, as well as reducing insulin dosage (e.g., 50% to 90% of daily dosage) based on duration and intensity (15), along with personal experience. For those taking oral sulfonylureas, preventing exercise-induced hypoglycemia requires pre-exercise SBGM with adjustments that may require increased carbohydrate ingestion or reduced dosage of exogenous insulin. In some cases, physician-recommended reduction of oral drug is necessary (15).

Hyperglycemia is a common outcome in insulin-requiring and poorly managed diabetes and is a common outcome in the presence of low insulin levels (15). If pre-exercise glucose is >250 mg · dL^{-1}, the acute effect of exercise is to augment release of counterregulatory hormones (e.g., catecholamines, glucagon), causing excessive hepatic glucose production, which exceeds blood glucose uptake in skeletal muscle because of a lack of adequate insulin. Hence, those who require exogenous insulin may need to postpone any exercise until their glucose level is better controlled because exercise worsens glucose levels and may contribute to excessive urinary ketones (e.g., metabolic by-products of fatty acids) that can be dangerous and potentially fatal if very high levels of ketosis is achieved (12).

COMPLICATIONS OF DIABETES

> ### 1.5.8-CES: Recognize patient clinical need for referral to other (non–Clinical Exercise Specialist®) allied health professionals (e.g., behavioralist, physical therapist, diabetes educator).

Diabetes poses challenges for exercise professionals because of increased morbidity and mortality from vascular and neurologic disease processes. Macrovascular (e.g., coronary, cerebrovascular, and peripheral), microvascular (e.g., retinal, kidney), and neural (e.g., peripheral and

TABLE 37-6. PRACTICAL RECOMMENDATIONS FOR EXERCISES FOR PERSONS WITH DIABETES MELLITUS

Perform SBGM	Check before and after each exercise session. Allows the patient to understand glucose response to PA. It is important to ensure that glucose is in relatively good control before beginning exercise. If blood glucose is:
	>250 mg·dL^{-1} to 300 mg·dL^{-1}+ ketones, exercise should be postponed. > 250–300 mg·dL^{-1} without ketones exercise ok, but no vigorous exercise.
	<100 mg·dL^{-1}, eat a snack consisting of easily absorbed carbohydrates ($\sim$20–30 g)
	100–240 mg·dL^{-1}, exercise is recommended.
Keep a daily log	Record the time of day the SBGM values are obtained and the amount of any pharmacologic agent (e.g., oral drugs, insulin). Also, approximate the time (min), intensity (HR), and distance (miles or meters) of exercise session. Over time, this aids the patient in understanding the type of glucose response to anticipate from an exercise bout.
Plan for exercise sessions	How much (e.g., time and intensity) exercise is anticipated allows adjusting insulin or oral drugs.
	If needed, carry extra carbohydrate feedings ($\sim$10–15 g·30 min^{-1}) to limit hypoglycemia.
	Hydrate before and rehydrate after each exercise session to prevent dehydration.
Modify caloric intake accordingly	Through frequent SBGM, caloric intake can be regulated more carefully on days of and after exercise.
Adjust insulin accordingly	If using insulin, reduce rapid- or short-acting insulin dosage by 50% to limit hypoglycemia episodes.
Exercise with a partner	This affords a support system for the exercise habit. Initially, diabetic patients should exercise with a partner until their glucose response is known.
Wear a diabetes identification tag	A diabetes necklace or shoe tag with relevant medical information should always be worn. Hypoglycemia and other problems can arise that require immediate attention.
Wear good shoes	Always wear proper-fitting and comfortable footwear with socks to minimize foot irritations and limit orthopedic injury to the feet and lower legs.
Practice good hygiene	Always take extra care to inspect feet for any irritation spots to prevent possible infection. Tend to all sores immediately, and limit any irritations.

HR, heart rate; PA, physical activity; SBGM, self–blood glucose monitoring.

autonomic nerves) diseases are common and constitute the DRCs that develop and worsen with poor glucose control and diabetes management (12). The onset and progression of vascular and neural complications of diabetes often cause physical limitation and varying levels of disability and are linked with depression and cognitive deficits (12). Thus, the quality of life in those with diabetes can be adversely affected without aggressive management and intervention. For those who have difficulty managing his/her diabetes, in whom glucose levels are chronically elevated, it is prudent to refer to allied health professionals (e.g., diabetes educator, diabetes nurse, registered dietician) to aid in improved diabetes management and care (12).

EXERCISE RECOMMENDATIONS FOR SPECIFIC DIABETES-RELATED COMPLICATIONS

DRCs are linked with diabetes and require careful screening. The presence of DRCs is not a contraindication for exercise, and the benefits of low- to moderate-intensity exercise generally outweigh the risks presented in diabetes. Although precautions and limitations must be recognized, with prudent modifications, a safe exercise plan can be achieved when the clinical status and existing complications are thoroughly assessed in the screening process. Discussion of exercise considerations for individuals with complicated diabetes follows, and a summary of considerations is shown in Table 37-7.

AUTONOMIC NEUROPATHY

This complication broadly affects the involuntary functions of the body, including the cardiac, vascular, gastrointestinal, and genitourinary systems. When autonomic neuropathy affects the innervation of the heart, it is referred to as cardiovascular autonomic neuropathy (CAN), and its presence is linked with poor prognosis and premature mortality (38).

> **1.4.11-CES: Identify resting and exercise ECG changes associated with cardiovascular disease, hypertensive heart disease, cardiac chamber enlargement, pericarditis, pulmonary disease, and metabolic disease.**

Clinical features of CAN include silent ischemia (ST depression) and infarction (Q waves), tachycardia at rest and early in exercise, reduced maximal HR and exercise intolerance, exercise-induced hypotension after strenuous activity, thermoregulatory dysfunction, a tendency to dehydrate, and hypoglycemia unawareness (38). If postural hypotension is present, inadequate HR and BP responses are observed with incremental work. Consequently, PA for these persons should focus on lower-intensity activities in which mild changes in HR and BP are more easily tolerated and lessen ventricular ectopy (38). Any exercise program for persons with CAN should be viewed with caution and requires physician approval, supervised exercise, and careful monitoring; it may require a clinical setting for safe exercise (38).

TABLE 37-7. SPECIAL PRECAUTIONS: RECOMMENDING EXERCISE FOR PATIENTS WITH DIABETES COMPLICATIONS

COMPLICATION	PRECAUTION
Autonomic neuropathy[a]	Likelihood of hypoglycemia, abnormal BP ($\Uparrow/\Downarrow$), and impaired thermoregulation. Abnormal resting HR ($\Uparrow$) and maximal HR ($\Downarrow$). Impaired SNS or PNS nerves yield abnormal exercise HR, BP, and SV. Use of RPE is suggested. Prone to dehydration and hyper/hypothermia.
Peripheral neuropathy	Avoid exercise that may cause trauma to the feet (e.g., prolonged hiking, jogging, or walking on uneven surfaces). Non–weight-bearing exercises (e.g., cycling, chair exercises, swimming) are most appropriate. Aquatics are not recommended if active ulcers are present. Regular assessment of the feet recommended. Keep feet clean and dry. Choose shoes carefully for proper fit. Avoid activities requiring a great deal of balance.
Nephropathy	Avoid exercise that increases BP (e.g., weight lifting, high-intensity aerobic exercise) and refrain from breath holding. High BP is common. Lower intensity is recommended.
Retinopathy[a,b]	With proliferative and severe stages of retinopathy, avoid vigorous, high-intensity activities that involve breath holding (e.g., weight lifting and isometrics) or overhead lifting. Avoid activities that lower the head (e.g., yoga, gymnastics) or that risk jarring the head. Consult an ophthalmologist for specific restrictions and limitations. In the absence of stress test HR, use of RPE is recommended (10–12 on 20 scale).
Hypertension	Avoid heavy weight lifting or breath holding. Perform dynamic exercises using large muscle groups, such as walking and cycling at a low to moderate intensity. Follow BP guidelines. In the absence of stress test HR, use of RPE is recommended (10–12 on 6–20 scale).
All patients	Carry identification with diabetes information. Maintain hydration (drink fluids before, during, and after exercise). Avoid exercise in the heat of the day and in direct sunlight (wear hat and sunscreen when in the sun).

BP, blood pressure; HR, heart rate; RPE, rating of perceived exertion; PNS, parasympathetic nervous system; SNS, sympathetic nervous system; SV, stroke volume; ↑, increase; ↓, decrease.

[a]Submaximal exercise testing is recommended for patients with proliferative retinopathy and autonomic neuropathy.

[b]If patient has proliferative retinopathy and has recently undergone photocoagulation or surgical treatment or is not properly treated, exercise is contraindicated.

Reprinted with permission from Campaigne BN, Lampman RL. *Exercise in the Clinical Management of Diabetes Mellitus.* Champaign (IL): Human Kinetics; 1994.

PERIPHERAL NEUROPATHY

Peripheral neuropathy (PN) affects the extremities, especially the lower legs and feet, and results in loss of sensation, or desensate feet (38). Poor wound healing and ulcerations leading to amputation are common. Proper daily hygiene is essential to limit sores from progressing from a poorly healing wound to ulceration. Exercise combined with loss of sensation can lead to musculoskeletal injury through overstretching, loss of balance, or falling, in addition to infection with minor irritations from footwear (38). Thus, persons with desensate feet require non–weight-bearing activities to lessen onset of foot ulcerations, bunions, and foot deformity (38).

Exercise for persons with PN should focus on low-intensity activities, as gauged by RPE, and range-of-motion activities for major joints to prevent or minimize contractures and maintain function. Non–weight-bearing activities that improve balance and awareness of the lower extremities are encouraged for persons with PN (38). Properly fitted and comfortable footwear and socks for walking are important to minimize the likelihood for undetectable sores in persons with PN, which can evolve into infections if unnoticed. Frequent visual inspection of the feet is also recommended.

NEPHROPATHY

This DRC affects the kidneys and is present when excessive urinary protein is present (microalbuminuria >30 and <300 mg · dL^{-1}) and accompanied by hypertension (30). Hypertension is a precursor to progression of nephropathy and must be controlled. Controlled hypertension limits BP excursions with exercise as well as any resulting albuminuria. Glucose control is central to reducing presence of albuminuria and delaying the onset or progression of this complication to end-stage renal disease (30). Exercise recommendations for persons with nephropathy focus on low- to moderate-intensity aerobic and resistance exercise, proper hydration strategies used for apparently healthy persons, and avoidance of activities that cause excessive elevation in BP (e.g., Valsalva maneuver, high-intensity aerobic or strength exercises) (4,11,12). Specific exercise testing and training recommendations may be found in Chapter 28.

RETINOPATHY

Diabetic retinopathy occurs in varying degrees of severity in the form of either nonproliferative diabetic retinopathy or proliferative diabetic retinopathy (PDR) (1). BP and glucose control are essential in limiting progression of retinopathy. Although PA/exercise increases systemic and retinal BP, few studies have shown a worsening of retinopathy related to exercise (1,16). There are some recommended limitations to PA/exercise, as shown in Table 37-8. Research has shown that low-intensity training in a mixed group of persons with types 1 and 2 diabetes with PDR improved cardiovascular function by 15% without adverse retinal outcomes (16). Recommended precautions for exercise in patients with retinopathy are shown in Box 37-2 (16).

TABLE 37-8. DIABETIC RETINOPATHY: CONSIDERATIONS FOR ACTIVITY LIMITATION

LEVEL OF DR	ACCEPTABLE ACTIVITIES	DISCOURAGED ACTIVITIES	OCULAR AND ACTIVITY RE-EVALUATION
No DR	Dictated by medical status	Dictated by medical status	12 months
Mild NPDR	Dictated by medical status	Dictated by medical status	6–12 months
Moderate NPDR	Dictated by medical status	Activities that dramatically increase BP, such as power lifting, heavy Valsalva maneuver	
Severe NPDR		Limit systolic BP, Valsalva maneuvers, active jarring, boxing, heavy competitive sports	2–4 months (may require laser surgery)
PDR	Low-impact cardiovascular conditioning: swimming (not diving); walking; low-impact aerobics; stationary cycling; endurance exercises	Low-impact cardiovascular jarring: weight lifting, jogging, high-impact aerobics, racquet sports, strenuous trumpet playing	1–2 months (may require laser surgery)

BP, blood pressure; DR, diabetic retinopathy; NPDR, nonproliferative diabetic retinopathy; PDR, proliferative diabetic retinopathy.

Reprinted with permission from Aeillo LP, Wong J, Cavallerano JD, Bursell S-E, Aiello LM. Retinopathy. In: Ruderman N, Devlin J, Schneider S, Kriska A, editors. *Handbook of Exercise in Diabetes.* 2nd ed. Alexandria (VA): American Diabetes Association; 2002. p. 401–413.

LIMITATIONS AND CONTRAINDICATIONS

Because of the increased risk for vascular and neural diseases related to diabetes, it is imperative that safe limits of exercise are established and that onset and progression of DRCs are reduced. To this end, there are potential contraindications to exercise for those with diabetes that follow previously established guidelines (3). Depending on the patient's clinical status, those with heart disease, in combination with advanced CAN, PN, nephropathy, or retinopathy, may be limited to lower-intensity exercise, and more vigorous exercise is contraindicated (12). Also, poor glucose control above 250 mg $\cdot$ dL^{-1} with or without ketones is a relative contraindication for persons with diabetes to safely participate in exercise (3,27).

BOX 37-2 — RECOMMENDED PRECAUTIONS FOR EXERCISE IN DIABETES WITH RETINOPATHY

- Limit systolic BP to <170 mm Hg.
- Use HR and RPE from BP increase during exercise to establish safe intensity.
- Avoid heavy or effortful exercise, which causes dramatic BP increases, as in strength training (use of Valsalva maneuver) or when using performing activities with the arms overhead.
- Advise annual eye examinations, which are needed to establish the level of retinopathy and its progression for exercise modification.

BP, blood pressure; HR, heart rate; RPE, rating of perceived exertion.

From Aeillo LP, Wong J, Cavallerano JD, Bursell S-E, Aiello LM. Retinopathy. In: Ruderman N, Devlin J, Schneider S, Kriska A, editors. *Handbook of Exercise in Diabetes.* 2nd ed. Alexandria (VA): American Diabetes Association; 2002. p. 401–413.

EFFICACY AND IMPLEMENTATION OF SUPERVISED EXERCISE PROGRAMS FOR PATIENTS WITH DIABETES

Diabetes is now considered a vascular equivalent to CVD (19,25,26). Regular PA/exercise is an important cornerstone in diabetes care and therapy. Current recommendations suggest that both aerobic and resistance training can improve cardiac and skeletal muscle functions, physiologic capabilities, and glucose and fat mobilization and utilization (4,11). Commensurate with these favorable exercise adaptations and lifestyle interventions is the CVD risk reduction to reduce the risk of a myocardial infarction and/or improve mortality rates in people with diabetes (12,19,25). Therefore, patients with diabetes can derive significant health outcomes through participation in supervised exercise programs.

> **1.7.4-CES: Design, implement, and supervise individualized exercise prescriptions for people with chronic disease and disabling conditions, or who are young or elderly.**

Before initiating an exercise program, the exercise professional must review and evaluate the current health status of a patient with diabetes, especially noting the presence of hypertension, obesity, dyslipidemia, tobacco use, glucose control (A$_{1c}$ %), PA habits, physical or orthopedic issues, and all medications. Patient education regarding the benefits and risks of exercise and long-term outcomes is essential, and attention to ensuring proper footwear is important. One must provide patient awareness regarding the need to check blood glucose before and after exercise, so that the patient remembers to always bring his/her glucometer. Design of the exercise prescription should include aerobic and resistance training, along with being based on current health status, existing comorbid conditions, assessment findings (if available), and patient goals. Any concerns of the healthcare professional regarding the exercise prescription for the patient with diabetes may require consultation with his/her physician.

The exercise prescription should specifically identify the FITT (frequency, intensity, time, type) for aerobic, resistance training, and flexibility exercise. For aerobic exercise, the FITT is F = 3–7 d·wk^{-1}; I = 50%–80% heart rate reserve (HRR) and/or RPE ~12–16; T = 20–60 min·d^{-1}, accumulating ~150 min·wk^{-1}; T = treadmill walking, recumbent cycling, or other appropriate modes of exercise. For resistance exercise, the FITT is F = 2–3 d·wk^{-1}; I = 8–12 reps/set to moderate fatigue; T = 1–3 sets of 8–12 upper-/lower- body exercises; T = handheld weight, machine weights, elastic bands, and free weights. In order to develop a more "precise" exercise prescription, the Compendium of Physical Activities should be utilized (2). The compendium assigns a specific MET level to an activity, which allows the exercise professional to estimate both MET·min·wk^{-1} and total energy expenditure. For flexibility exercise, the FITT is F = each exercise session; I = moderate tension to tightness; T = repeat each stretch 2–4 times for 15–30 s·stretch^{-1} of 8–12 upper- and lower- body muscle groups; T-static stretches. For each aerobic exercise session, a warm-up of 5 to 10 minutes and an active cool-down of at least 5 to 10 minutes will be performed (14).

Implementation of the exercise prescription entails recording of exercise performed each session and glucose levels before and after exercise. Initial exercise sessions will focus on ensuring proper form while exercising, as well as comfort level. Education and awareness of RPE, signs/symptoms of muscular fatigue, dyspnea, chest pain, and monitoring of intensity either by heart rate or RPE should be reviewed and implemented (14).

Glucose monitoring should be performed before warm-up and after cool-down sessions, especially when beginning or modifying an exercise program (4,11). On days when resistance training is performed with aerobic exercise, it may be prudent to check blood glucose after the resistance-training session. Also, glucose monitoring may be necessary early in the program during the aerobic phase to avoid hypoglycemia (24). To assure safe and effective exercise sessions, the exercise professional should be prepared to handle potential hypoglycemia with 20 to 30 g of simple carbohydrates (12).

The warm-up session for the patient should be at a low-level intensity for accommodation. Heart rate, RPE, and signs/symptoms of exertion must be monitored to ensure appropriate level of warm-up. Communication is important to ensure that the patient understands and is able to communicate clearly while exercising. Hypoglycemia awareness is important for the exercise professional to understand and be able to identify in individual patients. After a period of about 5 to 10 minutes, the exercise intensity will be gradually increased, and monitoring by the exercise professional should continue every 2 to 3 minutes throughout the aerobic session. Initially,

the duration of the aerobic phase may not reach 30 minutes; however, the long-term goal is to achieve at least 150 minutes (~600 METs·min·wk^{-1}) each week, with a goal of expending at least 1,000 kcals per week (12,34). Workload may be increased to 2,000 + kcals per week when weight loss or control is warranted. The cool-down will proceed at a low exercise intensity with continued monitoring. Blood glucose monitoring will take place, and nutrient consumption will be performed as appropriate.

> **1.7.22-CES:** Design, describe, and demonstrate specific resistance exercises for major muscle groups for patients with cardiovascular, pulmonary, and metabolic diseases and conditions.

Resistance training should commence at low-level intensities, and in the absence of 1-repetition max (1RM) data, RPE should be used to determine intensity of lifting. The patient must be individually instructed in the use of all resistance-training equipment. Program development should balance upper- and lower-body exercises, and progression of resistance exercise should alternate between the upper and lower body. Initially, one set of each exercise should be performed; the long-term goal is to achieve 2 to 3 sets of each exercise. After the resistance-training session is completed, a blood glucose check should be performed, which is especially important during the initial several sessions of the exercise program.

Flexibility exercises should focus on low-back flexibility and other major muscle groups of the upper and lower extremities. The patient should be instructed on each movement, and proper form should be emphasized to optimize the stretch, while breathing cues are continually provided.

SUMMARY

Regular PA/exercise is an essential part of the therapeutic regimen in diabetes management and care. Diabetes presents challenges for the exercise professional (e.g., exercise physiologist) that require comprehensive evaluation of patient status, assessment of patient ability, and individualizing the exercise prescription to meet the needs and goals of those with diabetes. Careful attention to the patient and their diabetes-related comorbidities is a must for safe and effective exercise training.

REFERENCES

1. Aeillo LP, Wong J, Cavallerano JD, Bursell S-E, Aiello LM. Retinopathy. In: Ruderman N, Devlin J, Schneider S, Kriska A, editors. *Handbook of Exercise in Diabetes*. 2nd ed. Alexandria (VA): American Diabetes Association; 2002. p. 401–413.
2. Ainsworth BE, Haskell WL, Whitt MC, et al. Compendium of physical activities: an update of activity codes and MET intensities. *Med Sci Sports Exerc*. 2000;32:S498–516.
3. Albright A, Franz M, Hornsby G, et al. Exercise and type 2 diabetes. Position Stand. *Med Sci Sport Exerc*. 2000;32:1345–1360.

4. American College of Sports Medicine and American Diabetes Association. Diabetes mellitus and exercise: a joint position statement of the American College of Sports Medicine and the American Diabetes Association. *Med Sci Sport Exerc.* 1997;29:i–vi.

5. American College of Sports Medicine. *ACSM's Guidelines for Exercise Testing and Prescription.* 8th ed. Philadelphia:Lippincott, Williams & Wilkins; 2009. p. 232–237.

6. American Diabetes Association. Diagnosis and classification of diabetes mellitus. *Diabetes Care.* 2007;30(suppl 1):S42–S47.

7. American Diabetes Association. Gestational diabetes mellitus: position statement. *Diabetes Care.* 2004;27(suppl 1):S88–S93.

8. American Diabetes Association. Hyperglycemic crises in patients with diabetes mellitus. *Diabetes Care.* 2004;27(suppl 1):S94–S102.

9. American Diabetes Association. Implications of the Diabetes Control and Complications Trial: position statement. *Diabetes Care.* 2003;26(suppl 1):S25–S27.

10. American Diabetes Association. Implications of the United Kingdom Prospective Diabetes Study: position statement. *Diabetes Care.* 2003;26(suppl 1):S28–S32.

11. American Diabetes Association. Physical activity/exercise and diabetes: position statement. *Diabetes Care.* 2004;27(suppl 1):S58–S64.

12. American Diabetes Association. Standards of medical care in diabetes—2007: position statement. *Diabetes Care.* 2007;30(suppl 1): S4–S41.

13. American Diabetes Association. Type 2 Diabetes in children and adolescents: position statement. *Diabetes Care.* 2000;23(3):381–389.

14. Balady, GJ, Williams MA, Ades PA, et al. Core components of cardiac rehabilitation/secondary prevention programs: 2007 update. A scientific statement from the American Heart Association Exercise, Cardiac Rehabilitation, and Prevention Committee, the Council on Clinical Cardiology; the Councils on Cardiovascular Nursing, Epidemiology and Prevention, and Nutrition, Physical Activity, and Metabolism; and the American Association of Cardiovascular and Pulmonary Rehabilitation. *Circulation.* 2007;115:2675–2682.

15. Berger M. Adjustment of insulin and oral agent therapy. In: Ruderman N, Devlin J, Schneider S, Kriska A, editors. *Handbook of Exercise in Diabetes.* 2nd ed. Alexandria (VA): American Diabetes Association; 2002. p. 365–381.

16. Bernbaum M, Alber SG, Cohen JD, Drimmer A. Cardiovascular conditioning in individuals with diabetic retinopathy. *Diabetes Care.* 1989;12:740–742.

17. Boulé NG, Haddad E, Kenny GP, Wells GA, Sigal RJ. Effects of exercise on glycemic control and body mass in type 2 diabetes mellitus: a meta-analysis of controlled clinical trials. *JAMA.* 2001;286: 1218–1227.

18. Boulé NG, Kenny GP, Haddad E, Wells GA, Sigal RJ. Meta-analysis of the effect of structures exercise training on cardiorespiratory fitness in type 2 diabetes. *Diabetologia.* 2003;46:1071–1081.

19. Buse JB, Ginsberg HN, Bakris GL, et al. Primary prevention of cardiovascular diseases in people with diabetes mellitus: a scientific statement from the American Heart Association and the American Diabetes Association. *Circulation.* 2007;115:114–126.

20. Castenada C, Layne JE, Munoz-Orians L, et al. A randomized controlled trial of resistance exercise training to improve glycemic control in older adults with type 2 diabetes. *Diabetes Care.* 2002;25: 2335–2341.

21. Centers for Disease Control and Prevention. National Diabetes Fact Sheet: National estimates and general information on diabetes in the United States—2005. Atlanta: U.S. Department of Health and Human Services, Centers for Disease Control and Prevention; 2005.

22. Dunstan DW, Daly RM, Wen N, et al. High intensity resistance training improves glycemic control in older patients with type 2 diabetes. *Diabetes Care.* 2002;25:1729–1736.

23. Durak E, Hill E. Medical reimbursement issues. In: Ruderman N, Devlin J, Schneider S, Kriska A, editors. *Handbook of Exercise in Diabetes.* 2nd ed. Alexandria (VA): American Diabetes Association; 2002. p.673–678.

24. Gordon N. The exercise prescription . In: Ruderman N, Devlin J, Schneider S, Kriska A, editors. *Handbook of Exercise in Diabetes.* 2nd ed. Alexandria (VA): American Diabetes Association; 2002. p. 269–288.

25. Grundy SM, Benjamin IJ, Burke GL, et al. Diabetes and cardiovascular disease: a statement for healthcare professionals from the American Heart Association. *Circulation.* 1999;100:1134–1146.

26. Haffner SM, Lehto S, Ronnemaa T, Pyorala K, Laakso M. Mortality from coronary heart disease in subjects with type 2 diabetes and in nondiabetic subjects with and without prior myocardial infarction. *N Engl J Med.* 1998;339:229–234.

27. Hornsby WG, Albright AL. Diabetes. In: Durstine L, Moore G, editors. *ACSM's Exercise Management for Persons with Chronic Disease and Disabilities.* 2nd ed. Champaign (IL): Human Kinetics; 2003. p. 133–141.

28. Joint National Committee on Prevention, Detection, Evaluation, and Treatment of High Blood Pressure. The seventh report of the Joint National Committee on Prevention, Detection, Evaluation, and Treatment of High Blood Pressure (JNC-VII). *JAMA.* 2003; 289:2560–2572.

29. National Institutes of Health and National Heart, Lung, and Blood Institute. Clinical guidelines on the identification, evaluation, and treatment of overweight and obesity in adults: evidence report. Bethesda (MD): NIH Publication No. 98-4083; 1998.

30. Expert Committee on the Diagnosis and Classification of Diabetes Mellitus. Report of the Expert Committee on the Diagnos is and Classification of Diabetes Mellitus. *Diabetes Care.* 2004;27 (suppl 1): S5–S35.

31. Riddell MC, Ruderman N, Berger M, Vranic M. Exercise physiology and diabetes: from antiquity to the age of the exercise sciences. In: Ruderman N, Devlin J, Schneider S, Kriska A, editors. *Handbook of Exercise in Diabetes.* 2nd ed. Alexandria (VA): American Diabetes Association; 2002. p. 3–15.

32. Ruderman N. A target population for diabetes prevention: the metabolically obese, normal-weight individual. In: Ruderman N, Devlin J, Schneider S, Kriska A, editors. *Handbook of Exercise in Diabetes.* 2nd ed. Alexandria (VA): American Diabetes Association; 2002. p. 235–249.

33. Shulman CR. Diabetes mellitus: definition, classification, and diagnosis. In: Galloway JA, Potvin JH, Shulman CR, editors. *Diabetes Mellitus.* 9th ed. Indianapolis: Lilly Research Laboratories; 1988.

34. Sigal RJ, Kenny GP, Wasserman DH, Castaneda-Sceppa C. Physical activity/exercise and type 2 diabetes: technical review. *Diabetes Care.* 2004;27(10):2518–2539.

35. Stewart KJ. Exercise training and the cardiovascular consequences of type 2 diabetes and hypertension: plausible mechanisms for improving cardiovascular health. *JAMA.* 2002;288(13):1622–1631.

36. The Diabetes Prevention Program Research Group. Impact of intensive lifestyle and metformin therapy on cardiovascular disease risk factors in the diabetes prevention program. *Diabetes Care.* 2005;28(4):888–894.

37. U.S. Department of Health and Human Services. Physical activity and health: a report of the Surgeon General. Atlanta: U.S. Department of Health and Human Services, Centers for Disease Control and Prevention, National Center for Chronic Disease Prevention and Health Promotion; 1996.

38. Vinik AI, Erbas T. Neuropathy. In: Ruderman N, Devlin J, Schneider S, Kriska A, editors. *Handbook of Exercise in Diabetes.* 2nd ed. Alexandria (VA): American Diabetes Association; 2002. p. 463–496.

39. Wasserman D, Zinman B. Exercise in individuals with IDDM. *Diabetes Care.* 1994;17:924–937.

40. Waxman S, Nesto RW. Cardiovascular complications. In: Ruderman N, Devlin J, Schneider S, Kriska A, editors. *Handbook of Exercise in Diabetes.* 2nd ed. Alexandria (VA): American Diabetes Association; 2002. p. 415–432.

SELECTED REFERENCES FOR FURTHER READING

American College of Sports Medicine. *ACSM's Exercise Management for Persons with Chronic Disease and Disabilities*. 2nd ed. Champaign (IL): Human Kinetics; 2003.

American Diabetes Association. Clinical practice recommendations: 2007. *Diabetes Care*. 2007;30(suppl 1):S1–103.

American Diabetes Association. Physical activity/exercise and diabetes mellitus: position statement. *Diabetes Care*. 2003;26(suppl 1): S73–S77.

Ruderman N, Devlin J, Schneider S, Kriska A, editors. *Handbook of Exercise in Diabetes*. 2nd ed. Alexandria (VA): American Diabetes Association; 2002.

INTERNET RESOURCES

- American College of Sports Medicine (position stands): www.acsm.org/publications/positionstands.htm
- American Diabetes Association (diabetes and cardiovascular disease): www.s2mw.com/heartofdiabetes/cardio.html
- American Diabetes Association: www.diabetes.org/for-health-professionals-and-scientists/professionals.jsp
- American Society of Diabetes Educators: www.aadenet.org
- Centers for Disease Control and Prevention. National Center for Chronic Disease Prevention and Health Promotion (diabetes public health resource): www.cdc.gov/diabetes/index.htm

Exercise Prescription for Patients with Comorbidities and Other Chronic Diseases

Current trends show that Americans are living longer while the number of U.S. citizens with chronic diseases continues to increase. In the past 100 years, life expectancy at birth in the United States increased from less than 50 years to more than 76 years (1,4). The U.S. Census Bureau projects that by 2030, the number of adults 65 years of age and older will be approximately 70 million, and by 2050, persons 85 years of age and older are expected to compose 5% of the population, or nearly 20 million people (4,5,10,19,28,74,75,106). Concerned healthcare providers, including exercise professionals, are faced with maintaining quality of life, limiting chronic diseases, and reducing the number of disabilities in this aging population (67).

Chronic diseases and disabilities associated with a sedentary lifestyle are important because maintaining a physically active lifestyle does affect health. Approximately 80% of individuals aged 65 years or older are living with at least one chronic health problem, and another 50% are living with two (9,11,87). Currently, the American Heart Association (AHA) and the American College of Sports Medicine (ACSM) list sedentary lifestyle as a controllable risk factor for many chronic health problems. Notably lifestyle, not just aging, is a leading cause for many chronic diseases and disabilities. As the aging process occurs, many bodily physiologic and function changes take place. For example, less ability to maintain one's balance, slower reaction time, loss of flexibility or joint motion, decreased lean body mass, increased interstitial fat, reduced blood levels of estrogen and androgen, and decreased muscle strength and endurance are all experienced with aging (6,11).

Discouraging as these aging processes sound, the deterioration of physiologic and functional changes are delayed by a lifestyle that emphasizes increased daily physical activity and/or planned regular exercise. Regular physical activity and/or planned exercise programming helps reduce body fat, body weight, resting blood pressure, and resting heart rate while improving cognitive and cardiopulmonary function and sleep quality (116). Physical activity aides in maintaining muscle mass, joint flexibility, and bone mineralization despite advancing age. An active lifestyle increases neuromuscular coordination, balance, and agility, all of which can be important in the prevention of falls, possibly reducing the likelihood of a disability while increasing the ability of independence as aging occurs. Thus, a lifestyle that incorporates a lifetime of increased daily physical activity and planned exercise results in reduced chronic disease risk for coronary heart disease (CHD), diabetes, and other debilitating conditions, such as arthritis and osteoporosis (5,6,11,52,67,74, 75,87,104,105,113).

In this chapter, we discuss strategies for managing, preventing, and improving the functional deterioration brought on by hyperlipidemia, hypertension, obesity, peripheral arterial disease (PAD), and stroke, all diseases of

> > > KEY TERMS

Apraxia: Inability to make purposeful bodily motions or movements.

Claudication: Cramping, painful sensation in skeletal muscles of the lower extremity, most commonly related to Atherosclerosis in the lower extremities.

Dyslipidemia: Abnormal blood levels of triglyceride and/or cholesterol-carrying lipoproteins affecting one or all of the subfractions of blood lipids; characteris-

tically, these levels are abnormally high, though some forms of dyslipidemia can include low values (typically of high-density lipoprotein cholesterol).

Hypertonia: Abnormally increased amount of tension in resting skeletal muscle.

Vertebrobasilar: Pertaining to the part of cerebral circulation that is supplied by the vertebral and basilar arteries in the neck and head.

aging that increase the risk for developing heart disease and cardiovascular complications. These can lead to a difficult downward spiral and deterioration in functional capacity. Exercise management in these populations serves to reduce risk for chronic diseases and secondary conditions or disorders while optimizing functional capacity, ability to perform basic and instrumental activities of daily living, and improve overall quality of life.

EPIDEMIOLOGY AND PATHOPHYSIOLOGY

> **4.2.1-HFS: Knowledge of metabolic risk factors or conditions that may require consultation with medical personnel before testing or training, including obesity, metabolic syndrome, thyroid disease, kidney disease, diabetes or glucose intolerance, and hypoglycemia.**

HYPERLIPIDEMIA

Hyperlipidemia or **dyslipidemia** is primary in determining CHD risk and is formally defined as the consequence of a variety of genetic, environmental, and pathologic factors resulting in elevated blood cholesterol and triglyceride levels. Factors associated with dyslipidemia include sex, age, body fat distribution, cigarette smoking, some medications, genetic background, dietary habits, and whether physically activity or regular participation in exercise is built into daily activities.

An estimated 107 million Americans have blood cholesterol levels that exceed 200 $mg \cdot dL^{-1}$ (13). Current guidelines from the National Cholesterol Education Program Adult Treatment Panel III (NCEP ATP III) state that CHD risk increases dramatically when blood cholesterol level is $\geq$240 $mg \cdot dL^{-1}$ (32), and this accounts for about 38 million Americans. The remaining 69 million individuals with blood cholesterol levels between 200 $mg \cdot dL^{-1}$ and 239 $mg \cdot dL^{-1}$ are considered to have borderline-high CHD risk (32).

Lipids are not soluble in water (i.e., are hydrophobic) and do not mix well with body fluids. In order for these lipids to move around the body, they must combine with proteins (apolipoproteins) to form lipoproteins, or micelle particles. Four principal lipoprotein classes exist and are classified by density (which is dictated by both lipid and protein content). Chylomicrons are derived from intestinal absorption of *exogenous dietary fat*. Very-low-density lipoproteins (VLDL) are smaller and more dense than chylomicrons and are synthesized primarily by the liver; some VLDL particles are also derived from chylomicron breakdown. Liver VLDL is mostly responsible for movement of endogenous triglyceride. Low-density lipoprotein (LDL) particles represent the final stage of catabolism of VLDL and are the primary carrier of cholesterol (LDL-C). Intermediate-density lipoprotein (IDL) and lipoprotein(a) [Lp(a)], are intermediate steps in this pathway and are LDL subfractions. In addition, other LDL subfractions include small and large particles (the small and more dense particles are more atherogenic than the larger and less dense). High-density lipoprotein (HDL) particles transport cholesterol (HDL-C) from all areas in the body back to the liver for degradation and disposal. This process, known as reverse cholesterol transport, is a major cardioprotective function of HDL as it counters the atherogenic effects of LDL within the arterial wall. HDL particles include the subfractions of the larger and less dense HDL_2 (cardioprotection is associated with HDL_2) and the smaller, more dense HDL_3 particles. The characteristics of HDL and other lipids and lipoproteins are listed in Table 38-1.

Several key enzymes regulate intravascular lipoprotein metabolism: lipoprotein lipase (LPL), hepatic lipase (HL), lecithin-cholesterol acyltransferase (LCAT), and cholesterol ester transfer protein (CETP). Together with plasma lipoproteins, these enzymes foster the movement and exchange of triglyceride and cholesterol between lipoproteins, the intestine, liver, and extrahepatic tissues. Several lipoprotein metabolic pathways exist, but the LDL receptor pathway and reverse cholesterol transport account for most of the cholesterol and triglyceride movement in the blood. When either genetic or unfavorable environmental influences affect the function of these pathways, dyslipidemia results, and CHD risk is increased.

Elevated blood cholesterol, triglycerides, LDL-C, and HDL-C are linked with clinical manifestations of CHD, but through scientific investigations, the initiation and progression of atherosclerotic CHD depends greatly on the presence of elevated LDL-C. Therefore, LDL-C is the primary lipoprotein target in the NCEP ATP III intervention algorithm (32). The evidence in support of elevated triglyceride or hypertriglyceridemia as an independent risk factor for CHD is less clear and appears more strongly associated with CHD risk in women than in men (32,51). Regardless, large amounts of triglyceride are found in all coronary atherosclerotic plaques, and blood triglyceride levels need be determined when assessing an individual's CHD risk (32,35,51). Recommendations for classifying levels of blood cholesterol, triglyceride, and LDL-C in regard to CHD risk are summarized in Table 38-2. The recommended LDL-C goal for high-risk persons is 100 $mg \cdot dL^{-1}$, but when disease is present, an LDL-C goal of 70 $mg \cdot dL^{-1}$ is desired (47).

Another lipid condition associated with increased CHD risk is exaggerated postprandial lipemia, which is a prolonged amount of time required for the removal of chylomicrons or their movement into extrahepatic tissue. Exaggerated postprandial lipemia adversely affects endothelial function and contributes to atherosclerotic plaque formation. In healthy persons, postprandial

TABLE 38-1. CHARACTERISTICS OF PLASMA LIPIDS AND LIPOPROTEINS

Lipid/Lipoprotein	Source	Protein %	Total Lipid %	TG	Chol	Phosp	Free Chol	Apolipoprotein
							COMPOSITION	
					Percentage of Total Lipid			
Chylomicron	Intestine	1–2	98–99	88	8	3	1	Major: A-IV, B-48, B-100, H Minor: A-I, A-II, C-I, C-II, C-III, E
VLDL	Major: Liver Minor: Intestine	7–10	90–93	56	20	15	8	Major: B-100, C-III, E, G Minor: A-I, A-II, B-48, C-II, D
IDL	Major: VLDL Minor: Chylomicron	11	89	29	26	34	9	Major: B-100 Minor: B-48
LDL	Major: VLDL Minor: Chylomicron	21	79	13	28	48	10	Major: B-100 Minor: C-I, C-II, (a)
HDL$_2$	Major: HDL$_3$	33	67	16	43	31	10	Major: A-1, A-II, D, E, F Minor: A-IV, C-I, C-II, C-III
HDL$_3$	Major: Liver and intestine Minor: VLDL and Chylomicron Remnants	57	43	13	46	29	6	Major: A-1, A-II, D, E, F Minor: A-IV, C-I, C-II, C-III
Chol	Liver and diet			70–75	25–30			
TG	Diet and liver			100	100			

VLDL, very-low-density lipoprotein; IDL, intermediate-density lipoprotein; LDL, low-density lipoprotein; HDL, high-density lipoprotein; Chol, cholesterol; TG, triglycerides; Phosp, phospholipid.

TABLE 38-2. LOW-DENSITY LIPOPROTEIN CHOLESTEROL GOALS AND CUTPOINTS FOR THERAPEUTIC LIFESTYLE CHANGES AND DRUG THERAPY IN DIFFERENT RISK CATEGORIES

RISK CATEGORY	LDL GOAL	LDL LEVEL AT WHICH TO INITIATE THERAPEUTIC LIFESTYLE CHANGES	LDL LEVEL AT WHICH TO CONSIDER DRUG THERAPY
CHD or CHD risk Equivalents (10-year risk >20%)	<100 mg·dL^{-1}	≥100 mg·dL^{-1}	≥130 mg·dL^{-1} (100–129 mg·dL^{-1}:drug optional)[a]
2 + risk factors (10-year risk ≥20%)	<130 mg·dL^{-1}	≥130 mg·dL^{-1}	10-year risk 10%–20%: ≥130 mg·dL^{-1} 10-year risk <10%: ≥160 mg·dL^{-1}
0–1 risk factor[b]	<160 mg·dL^{-1}	≥160 mg·dL^{-1}	≥190 mg·dL^{-1} (160–189 mg·dL^{-1}: LDL-lowering drug optional)

CHD, coronary heart disease; LDL, low-density lipoprotein.

[a] Some authorities recommend use of LDL-lowering drugs in this category if an LDL cholesterol <100 mg·dL^{-1} cannot be achieved by therapeutic lifestyle changes. Others prefer use of drugs that primarily modify triglycerides and high-density lipoprotein (HDL) (e.g., nicotinic acid or fibrate). Clinical judgment also may call for deferring drug therapy in this subcategory.

[b] Almost all people with 0 to 1 risk factor have a 10-year risk <10%, thus 10-year risk assessment in people with 0 to 1 risk factor is not necessary.

From National Cholesterol Education Program. Executive Summary of the Third Report of the National Cholesterol Education Program (NCEP) Expert Panel on Detection, Evaluation, and Treatment of High Blood Cholesterol in Adults (Adult Treatment Panel III). *JAMA*. 2001;285(19):2486–2497.

triglyceride levels return to baseline levels within 8 to 10 hours after consumption of dietary fat (84).

HYPERTENSION

High blood pressure, or hypertension, is a major health concern. In the United States, an estimated 65 million Americans older than the age of 18 have systolic blood pressure >140 mm Hg with a diastolic blood pressure >90 mm Hg (33). Hypertension prevalence trends unfortunately indicate a continued growth rate, whereas control of the condition is inadequate (25,33,57). A person with normal systolic blood pressure of 120 mm Hg and diastolic pressure of 80 mm Hg at age 55 years has a 90% lifetime risk of developing hypertension (25). Because of the likelihood for developing this condition is high, the Joint National Commission VII (JNC VII) developed a classification scheme containing the designation prehypertension, which is defined as a systolic between 120 and 139 and a diastolic of 80 to 89 mm Hg (Table 38-3) (25). High blood pressure is a disorder with multiple factors contributing to elevated systolic and diastolic pressures. Mean arterial pressure is the product of cardiac output and total peripheral resistance; MAP = CO × TPR. Many factors can contribute to high blood pressure

by altering cardiac output and/or total peripheral resistance. Factors influencing blood pressure include genetics, susceptibility to renal retention of excess sodium, sympathetic nervous system hyperactivity, renin-angiotensin system, hyperinsulinemia or insulin resistance, and endothelial cell dysfunction (92,117).

Despite the fact that numerous factors contributing to hypertension are known, the underlying cause(s) of high blood pressure is poorly understood for most people with hypertension. In such cases, this is termed *essential hypertension*. In contrast, *secondary hypertension* refers to high blood pressure that is secondary to other disorders of the renal, endocrine, and nervous systems. Diagnosis of these disorders is beyond the scope of this chapter, other than to note that these disorders are reversible and this is the desired course of treatment for secondary hypertension.

Hypertension presents differently in younger than in older individuals. In adults, isolated systolic hypertension (systolic pressure >140 mm Hg and diastolic pressure <90 mmHg) is rare before 50 years of age. Among older adults, however, isolated systolic hypertension is the most common form of hypertension. Another form of high blood pressure is pulmonary hypertension, an elevation of pulmonary artery pressure that often presents with symptoms of dyspnea and fatigue, and may be accompanied by syncope and substernal chest pain. Pulmonary hypertension can accompany other forms of pulmonary disease, as well as heart disease (66,81).

The reason that blood pressure is a serious health problem is that it leads to many serious and debilitating diseases, including CHD, congestive heart failure, atrial fibrillation, cerebrovascular disease, end-stage renal disease, PAD, aortic aneurysm, and retinal disease. Hypertension is one of the three major contributing factors (along with obesity and hyperlipidemia) to the metabolic syndrome that predisposes people for cardiovascular disease and diabetes mellitus (31).

TABLE 38-3. CLASSIFICATION OF BLOOD PRESSURE FOR ADULTS

BP CLASSIFICATION	SBP (mm Hg)	DBP (mm Hg)
Normal	<120	and <80
Prehypertension	120–139	or 80–89
Stage 1 hypertension	140–159	or 90–99
Stage 2 hypertension	≥160	or ≥100

BP, blood pressure; SPB, systolic blood pressure; DBP, diastolic blood pressure; mm Hg, millimeters of mercury.

From Chobanian AV, Bakris GL, Black HR, et al. Seventh Blood Pressure Report of the Joint National Committee on Detection, Evaluation, and Treatment of High Blood Pressure. JNC 7—complete version. *Hypertension*. 2003;42:1206–1252.

OVERWEIGHT AND OBESITY

Overweight and obesity are major public health concerns for many developed countries throughout the world. In the United States, obesity prevalence rates doubled in adults between 1980 and 2002 (34), and by 2004, almost one third of U.S. adults were classified as obese (77). The most recent estimates indicate that 66% of all U.S. adults are classified as overweight, as indicated by a body mass index (BMI) ≥ 25 kg·m^{-2}; 32% are classified as obese, with a BMI ≥ 30 kg·m^{-2}; and 5% are classified as extremely obese, with a BMI ≥ 40 kg·m^{-2} (49). Overweight and obesity are also linked to numerous chronic diseases, including coronary artery disease (CAD), diabetes mellitus, many forms of cancer, and numerous musculoskeletal problems (73).

Fat is the body's major form of energy storage and is found throughout all body regions. When energy intake exceeds expenditure, the excess energy mounts up in these fat storage sites, and weight gain occurs. Several medical conditions exist, however, that promote weight gain. These include endocrine disorders, such as Cushing syndrome or newly discovered hypothyroidism; side effects of some medications; and smoking cessation. However, treatable medical causes for obesity are uncommon, and in most individuals, overweight and obesity are the result of sedentary lifestyle and/or increased calorie consumption (73).

Obesity is associated with an increased rate of death from cardiovascular disease as well as all causes, such as cancer, gallbladder disease, arthritis, poor quality of life (QOL), and risk of falling (29). Excess fat deposition in the abdominal region, commonly referred to as *central obesity* or *abdominal obesity,* is often associated with a condition referred to as *metabolic syndrome,* which is a group of risk factors that correlate with increased risk for cardiovascular disease. Comorbidities common with obesity, such as hypertension, type 2 diabetes, dyslipidemia, and obstructive sleep apnea, also increase CAD risk. Additionally, unhealthy lifestyle habits found among many obese individuals—such as diets high in sugar, simple carbohydrates, or starch and saturated fat, in combination with sedentary activity levels—promote CAD disease risk through various mechanisms.

PERIPHERAL ARTERIAL DISEASE

Peripheral arterial disease is the manifestation of atherosclerosis in systemic arteries outside of the heart. Technically, this therefore includes the carotid or renal arteries, but these vessels are usually referred to by name, and PAD refers to atherosclerosis in the lower limbs. Approximately 10 million Americans have PAD, with an occurrence of more than 10% in people aged 60 years and older (26). Diabetes mellitus, hypertension, and smoking are major PAD risk factors (72). Patients with PAD have a six-times-greater risk of dying from CHD compared with individuals without PAD (101).

Common signs and symptoms of PAD are calf pain (usually the primary symptom), leg numbness or weakness, cold legs or feet, sores on lower extremities that won't heal, color change in legs, hair loss on legs, and toenail color change. Whether a patient has some or all of these signs or symptoms depend on the disease severity. As the severity of PAD worsens, the individual typically develops exertional leg pain, known as **claudication**, which is much like a muscle cramp. As PAD worsens, the symptoms can become so severe to limit the person's ability to perform activities of daily living (39). Claudication does not go away if the person continues to walk; it is only relieved by rest. The pain, as with ischemia of the heart, is the result of a mismatch between oxygen delivery and metabolic oxygen demand. This occurs in the working tissue, secondary to flow-limiting stenosis upstream in the arterial trunks. Although ischemia of the heart is potentially dangerous, intermittent ischemia of the skeletal muscles, as with PAD, is uncomfortable, but not dangerous. However, if the pain progresses to resting pain, there is a possibility of gangrene and subsequent tissue loss.

Estimates vary, but claudication is found in less than half of persons afflicted with PAD (14). Reasons for not having claudication in all persons with PAD are not completely clear. Some reasons why PAD patients do not experience claudication are that they may not walk far or fast enough to induce muscle ischemic symptoms because of comorbidities such as pulmonary disease or arthritis, have neuropathies that deaden nerve endings in the legs as with diabetes, have atypical symptoms unrecognized as intermittent claudication, fail to mention their symptoms to their physician, or have sufficient collateral arterial channels to tolerate their arterial obstruction (14).

CEREBROVASCULAR STROKE/TRANSIENT ISCHEMIC ATTACK

Stroke ranks third among all causes of U.S. deaths, only behind CHD and cancer. An estimate of 700,000 Americans suffer new or recurrent strokes each year, resulting in 273,000 deaths (12). As a result, stroke accounts for about 1 of every 15 U.S. deaths. Stroke incidence rate is 1.25 times greater in men than women. However, women account for approximately 61% of stroke deaths in the United States each year (12). Stroke death rates are higher in blacks than in whites. Fortunately, the good news is that from 1993 to 2003, the U.S. stroke death rate fell 19%, and the actual number of stroke deaths declined by 0.7% (12).

Ischemic and hemorrhagic strokes are the two major stroke types, with ischemic-type stroke accounting for approximately 88% of all strokes. Ischemic strokes can be classified into three major groups by the nature of the risk factors:

- Nonmodifiable: age, race/ethnicity, sex, and family history

- Modifiable: atrial fibrillation, CAD, other types of cardiac disease (e.g., asymptomatic carotid stenosis), hypertension, cigarette smoking, hyperlipidemia, diabetes mellitus, hyperinsulinemia, insulin resistance, and sickle cell disease
- Potentially modifiable: physical inactivity, obesity, alcohol abuse, hyperhomocysteinemia, drug abuse, hypercoagulability, hormone replacement therapy, oral contraceptive use, and inflammatory processes (42)

Additionally, a previous transient ischemic attack (TIA) should be considered a strong indicator to intervene for any modifiable or potentially modifiable risk factors for stroke. Atherosclerosis is the most common underlying cause of ischemic stroke, and all of the major modifiable CHD risk factors are included in the above listing.

Hemorrhagic strokes account for the remaining 12% of all strokes. Two major hemorrhagic stroke categories are defined; intracerebral hemorrhage and subarachnoid hemorrhage. Most intracerebral hemorrhages are related to hypertension, whereas a subarachnoid hemorrhage is most likely a result of a ruptured aneurysm, also often precipitated by hypertension. Hemorrhagic strokes although less common than ischemic strokes, are more likely to be fatal within 30 days. On the other hand, hemorrhagic stroke survivors are less likely to be severely disabled when compared with survivors of ischemic strokes (43).

MEDICAL MANAGEMENT

> **1.5.2-CES: Describe mechanisms and actions of medications that may affect exercise testing and prescription (i.e., β-blockers, nitrates, calcium channel blockers, digitalis, diuretics, vasodilators, antiarrhythmic agents, bronchodilators, antilipemics, psychotropics, nicotine, antihistamines, over-the-counter (OTC) cold medications, thyroid medications, alcohol, hypoglycemic agents, blood modifiers, pentoxifylline, antigout medications, and anorexiants/diet pills).**

> **1.5.3-CES: Recognize medications associated in the clinical setting, their indications for care, and their effects at rest and during exercise (i.e., β-blockers, nitrates, calcium channel blockers, digitalis, diuretics, vasodilators, antiarrhythmic agents, bronchodilators, antilipemics, psychotropics, nicotine, antihistamines, OTC cold medications, thyroid medications, alcohol, hypoglycemic agents, blood modifiers, pentoxifylline, antigout medications, and anorexiants/diet pills).**

Because the diseases presented in this chapter very often occur together, they are presented as such here as opposed to separate chapters for each. As comorbidities, medical management is sometimes interconnected, and the lifestyle modification and exercise planning and programming for these conditions is highly interconnected. Provided here is a cursory discussion of the medical management of these conditions followed by discussion of exercise management and programming.

HYPERLIPIDEMIA

The evidence-based medical management of hyperlipidemia is well described in the National Cholesterol Education Program (NCEP) Adult Treatment Panel (ATP) III recommendations (71). Refer to these materials for complete guidance. In brief, lipid management is triaged into three risk classes: low risk, moderate risk, and high risk. People who are low risk have at most one risk factor; those at moderate risk have two or more risk factors, but do not have known cardiovascular disease (or equivalent). High-risk individuals have a history of CAD or have atherosclerosis in peripheral arteries (most typically carotid, aorta, iliac, femoral, or popliteal) or diabetes.

The degree of recommended lipid lowering is determined by the level of risk. The primary target of lipid lowering recommended in NCEP ATP III is the LDL cholesterol. Secondary targets include the HDL cholesterol and triglycerides. The LDL goals of therapy are shown in Table 38-2.

Triglycerides are a secondary risk factor under NCEP ATP III. A normal fasting triglyceride is <150 mg·dL^{-1}, borderline high is 150 to 199 mg·dL^{-1}, high is 200 to 499 mg·dL^{-1}, and very high would be ≥500 mg·dL^{-1}. In the current epidemic of obesity, high triglycerides are commonly seen in people with type 2 diabetes or with metabolic syndrome, though high triglycerides can be an isolated finding (e.g., type V hyperlipidemia, or *familial hypertriglyceridemia*). Evidence is mounting that high triglycerides are an independent risk factor for atherosclerosis (17,76).

HDL cholesterol levels are considered low when they are <40 mg·dL^{-1}. NCEP ATP III does not make recommendations about raising the HDL cholesterol, but many experts feel that HDL should also be treated if the value is low, particularly if it is <30 mg·dL^{-1} and/or if the ratio of total cholesterol to HDL is higher than about 5.0.

Lifestyle factors are very important in managing hyperlipidemia, in particular diet and exercise. In the past, expert opinion held that it was possible to "eat your way through any lipid-lowering therapy" (107), and although that remains possible, it is more difficult to do now because of modern potent statin class medications that were not available a few years ago. The core of lifestyle recommendations in NCEP ATP III is the TLC diet (Therapeutic Lifestyle Change) (71). This recommended nutritional composition is shown in Table 38-4 (71).

These nutritional recommendations are reasonably similar in all chronic conditions requiring lifestyle intervention as part of medical management. In addition, physical activity recommendations that are in line with the ACSM/Centers for Disease Control (CDC) guidelines on exercise are recommended (35).

TABLE 38-4. NUTRIENT COMPOSITION OF THE THERAPEUTIC LIFESTYLE CHANGES DIET

NUTRIENT	RECOMMENDED INTAKE
Saturated fat[a]	<7% of total calories
Polyunsaturated fat	Up to 10% of total calories
Monounsaturated fat	Up to 20% of total calories
Total fat	25%–35% of total calories
Carbohydrate[b]	50%–60% of total calories
Fiber	20–30 $g \cdot day^{-1}$
Protein	Approximately 15% of total calories
Cholesterol	<200 $mg \cdot day^{-1}$
Total calories (energy)[c]	Balance energy intake and expenditure to maintain desirable body weight/prevent weight gain

[a]Trans fatty acids are another low-density-lipoprotein–raising fat that should be kept at a low intake.

[b]Carbohydrate should be derived predominantly from foods rich in complex carbohydrates, including grains, especially whole grains, fruits, and vegetables.

[c]Daily energy expenditure should include at least moderate physical activity (contributing approximately 200 Kcal per day).

From: National Cholesterol Education Program Expert Panel. Detection, evaluation, and treatment of high blood cholesterol in adults (adult treatment panel III): executive summary. Washington (DC): National Heart, Lung, and Blood Institute, National Institutes of Health; 2001.

When people do not achieve the recommended lipid levels within 12 weeks of diet and exercise, drug therapy is recommended. There are now multiple randomized controlled trials showing that HMG CoA reductase inhibitors (statins) prevent cardiovascular events and death from myocardial infarctions. Accordingly, statins are first line therapy for LDL lowering. Many patients are given single-drug statin therapy at a high dose, although it is known that combination therapy at a lower dose is typically more effective at lowering the LDL and also has fewer side effects. The main rationale to use combination therapy is that the interrelated metabolic pathways involved in cholesterol metabolism often adjust by up-regulating gene expression and thereby reducing the impact of monotherapy.

Additional classes of lipid-lowering drugs include bile acid sequestrants, fibric acids, nicotinic acid, and cholesterol absorption blocking agents. All of these drugs by themselves have good safety profiles, but some combinations are known to increase risk of serious side effects (36). Statins and fibric acid derivatives can cause myopathy and severe rhabdomyolysis, with the potential complications of kidney failure and death. Nonetheless, some patients who have extremely high cardiovascular risk sometimes end up on both classes of drugs (36).

Caution is given with the use of statins and exercise intervention. These drugs are rarely associated with exertional rhabdomyolysis, as reflected by muscle symptoms and blood levels of creatine kinase (CK) (107). This is often medically managed by the physician, but the clinical exercise specialist working with patients on this also should be aware of this possibility. Numerous patients have normal blood levels of creatine kinase (CK) but report muscle symptoms that resolve when the statin was stopped (85,97,98,110). In such individuals, it is difficult to discriminate between delayed-onset muscle soreness and statin side effects.

HYPERTENSION

The diagnosis of hypertension requires three separate occasions when the systolic blood pressure is ≥140 or the diastolic blood pressure is ≥90 (Table 38-3). Measurement of blood pressure should be obtained after the subject has been seated quietly for at least 5 minutes, because the exertion of walking is likely to mildly elevate blood pressure.

Once the diagnosis is made, recommendations are to use a trial of lifestyle intervention before the prescription of antihypertensive medications (73). Typically, a low-sodium diet or a diet such as DASH (Dietary Approaches to Stop Hypertension) is prescribed (58). Alcohol can also exacerbate high blood pressure. Although one to two alcoholic beverages a day can reduce cardiovascular mortality, beyond this increases the risk of poor blood pressure control (115). Thus, people with high blood pressure should be counseled on a low-sodium-, vegetable-, and fruit-oriented diet, with only modest alcohol consumption. Such changes in diet can be expected to reduce systolic blood pressure by 2 to 14 mm Hg. Also, weight loss can yield a 5 to 20 mm Hg reduction in systolic blood pressure.

In addition to dietary changes, exercise can achieve another 5 to 7 mm Hg reductions in systolic and diastolic blood pressure (82). Also, in many people, elevated blood pressure is a consequence of inadequate coping skills to life stressors. For such individuals, stress management training is an appropriate intervention before, or perhaps concurrent with, antihypertensive medications.

Many patients are not able to achieve sufficient reductions in blood pressure with lifestyle modification and end up taking medications. The goal of hypertension medical management is to achieve a blood pressure of <120/80 mm Hg. Many patients can achieve this on only one medication, but most patients achieve better control on two medications. Some require three or more medications to achieve the target range of blood pressure. The most common initial medication is a diuretic. In the United States, this is most often hydrochlorothiazide because it is available as an inexpensive generic drug and is well tolerated. Another common drug class used as a first- or second-line agent is β-receptor antagonists (i.e., β-blockers). Many β-blockers are also available in generic formulations in the United States.

Many physicians prefer to prescribe antihypertensive drugs that reduce afterload as a mechanism of action, especially angiotensin-converting enzyme inhibitors (ACEIs) and angiotensin receptor blockers (ARBs). These classes of medications have an **ergomimetic** profile in that they decrease peripheral vascular resistance, much as occurs with exercise. However, except in persons with diabetes, there is no current research to support that afterload reducers are better than other approaches to hypertensive therapy; in fact, diuretics and β-blockers reduce cardiovascular mortality. Although there is reason to believe that reduction in cardiovascular mortality is a pressure-related phenomenon, this is not known for certain; thus, there is good rationale for using diuretics and β-blockers initially, then moving to other classes of medications. One must also consider the potential side effects of diuretics and β-blockers in those who are active and athletic (e.g., fatigue-reduced physical performance, decreased libido).

PERIPHERAL ARTERIAL DISEASE

Medical management of PAD is similar to management of CAD. The mainstay of treatment is lifestyle modification to reduce the primary risk factors of PAD, which are hypertension, smoking, and diabetes. The recommended approach to lifestyle modification in this population is similar to that outlined above for hypertension and hyperlipidemia, and will not be reiterated here.

Surgical management of PAD depends on the severity of circulatory inadequacy. In the most severe cases, in which tissue becomes nonviable, the vascular anatomy cannot be repaired, and amputation is the only choice. In less severe cases, the magnitude of circulatory impairment is often estimated in a vascular lab, where an ankle-brachial index (ABI) is obtained (Table 38-5). An ABI is the ratio of pressures in the posterior tibial or dorsalis pedis artery and brachial artery, taken while the patient is supine. The lower the ratio, particularly when it is below 0.9, the more severe of a blood flow limitation exists. Also, one can obtain other images of the vascular anatomy, such as arteriograms or magnetic resonance angiograms (MRAs). The main purpose of such imaging is to determine whether the arteries can be repaired with bypass grafts or angioplasty with stent placement.

Medical management of PAD is quite similar to that of CAD. Goals are to normalize blood pressure and cholesterol, promote smoking cessation, and provide antithrombosis therapy for patients who have had a stent implanted, as well as therapy to relieve the symptoms of intermittent claudication.

TABLE 38-5. ANKLE BRACHIAL INDEX

≥1.30	Noncompressible vessel
1.00–1.29	Normal
0.91–0.99	Borderline (equivocal)
0.41–0.90	Mild to Moderate PAD
0.00–0.40	Severe PAD

PAD, peripheral arterial disease.

From: Hirsch AT, Haskal ZJ, Hertzer NR, et al. ACC/AHA 2005 guidelines for the management of patients with peripheral arterial disease (lower extremity, renal, mesenteric, and abdominal aortic): executive summary. *J Am Coll Cardiol.* 2006;47:1239–1312.

Smoking cessation success rates improve about twofold or more when counseling is coupled with nicotine replacement, nicotine receptor blockade, and/or antidepressant therapy. Nicotine replacement is best achieved with transdermal patches, but also can be delivered with chewing gum. Nicotine replacement in combination with antidepressant therapy, best documented for bupropion, improves successful smoking cessation. Bupropion alone is also helpful. More recently, the nicotine receptor partial agonist varenicline has come under Food and Drug Administration (FDA) approval in the United States. Varenicline appears to be superior to bupropion, and compared with placebo, varenicline appears to triple the probability of being smoke-free at 12 months (99). Medical management to support smoking cessation should not be overlooked in patients with PAD.

In patients who have had a stent placed, the antiplatelet agent clopidogrel is used to prevent thrombosis. Clopidogrel is also used in patients with intermittent claudication but who do not receive a stent. In addition, cilostazol, from a different class of antiplatelet agents, is indicated specifically for intermittent claudication. These drugs, despite being approved for similar mechanisms of action, have different clinical benefits. Clopidogrel is primarily beneficial in preventing restenosis and/or thrombosis. Cilostazol is indicated for the symptom of intermittent claudication and is used specifically to reduce pain and increase walking distance. These medications can also be combined, but this seems to be an uncommon practice.

OVERWEIGHT AND OBESITY

Chapter 33 reviews the techniques of weight management in detail. The cornerstone of management for overweight and obesity is lifestyle modification emphasizing diet and exercise. In some patients for whom lifestyle modification is insufficient, FDA-approved weight loss medications or bariatric surgery (for morbidly obese patients with a BMI ≥40 or ≥35 with comorbid conditions) may be considered. Recent evidence demonstrated a beneficial mortality effect following bariatric surgery (99).

CEREBROVASCULAR STROKE/TRANSIENT ISCHEMIC ATTACK

Medical management of carotid and **vertebrobasilar** atherosclerosis is almost identical to PAD; the main difference is that cilostazol has not been approved for use in cerebrovascular disease.

Medical management of patients who have had a stroke is an extensive and highly complex problem that would require several chapters to address the many kinds of disabilities that result from strokes. In this chapter, we will confine our comments to a few major points. First, patients who have had a stroke often die from cardiovascular disease. It is therefore important that people who are disabled by stroke receive adequate and intensive cardiovascular risk-reduction interventions. Second, some strokes resolve and have minimal residual impact, and others may leave the patient in a permanent hemiplegic state and with ataxia. The medical needs will be dramatically different, depending on the severity of the disability, and exercise programming will need to be appropriately individualized. Third, all lifestyle modification intervention programming rely on cognitive therapy, and the cognitive decline associated with cerebrovascular disease needs to be factored into the design of the lifestyle/exercise program. Unfortunately, this remains an uncommon skill, and more knowledge is needed to better understand how to work with cognitively impaired individuals (21).

EXERCISE RESPONSES AND ADAPTATIONS

 1.1.11-CES: Knowledge of acute and chronic adaptations to exercise for those with cardiovascular, pulmonary, and metabolic diseases.

 1.2.8-CES: Describe the influence of exercise on cardiovascular, pulmonary, and metabolic diseases.

 1.7.2-CES: Compare and contrast benefits and risks of exercise for individuals with risk factors for or established cardiovascular, pulmonary, and/or metabolic diseases.

In this section, we will consider the acute exercise response and the adaptations to chronic exercise training.

HYPERLIPIDEMIA

Generally, unless the dyslipidemia is long-standing and has led to CHD or secondary illness, the exercise response to a single exercise session will not be altered as a result. After a single exercise session, blood triglycerides and postprandial lipemia are reduced, and HDL-C is usually, but not always, increased (27,46). Typically, these effects have no discernable symptoms. However, dyslipidemia can lead to secondary illness, such as angina or claudication, and these secondary problems often alter the exercise response in accordance with that problem. In these cases, attention is given to the exercise response in view of these other secondary conditions.

Exceptions to this rule include individuals with genetic disorders. For example, individuals who have an extremely high triglyceride or cholesterol level can have inadequate oxygen supply to vital tissues, such as the heart or brain, and are at greater risk for stroke and/or myocardial infarctions. It is best to gain control of the dyslipidemia with medical management before the patient begins exercising, and supervised exercise is recommended. Because familial (or genetic) dyslipidemic patients are usually prescribed various medications for other conditions, the type and dosage of their medications should be noted before undergoing exercise testing or training.

Regular participation in physical activity is shown to cause beneficial changes in people with normal lipid and lipoprotein concentrations, as well as in most persons with dyslipidemia. Beneficial changes include the following: decreased triglyceride (60), increased HDL-C (but not always) (64,65), and increased lipoprotein enzyme activity (LPL, LCAT, and CETP) (64,65). These exercise training changes enhance reverse cholesterol transport and are augmented further by a low-fat diet, weight loss, and reduction in adiposity. Thus, exercise training can directly (e.g., by increased LPL activity) and indirectly (e.g., by reductions in body weight and body fat) improve blood lipid and lipoprotein profiles. Work by Kraus et al. (61) demonstrates that the volume of exercise completed on a weekly basis is more important than the exercise intensity for affecting favorable blood lipid and lipoprotein changes. They showed that regular aerobic exercise can induce favorable changes in LDL subfractions (e.g., converting smaller, denser LDLs to larger, less dense LDLs), thus reducing cardiovascular risk.

Abnormal blood lipid and lipoprotein profiles can result from congenital deficiencies, and patients having these deficiencies have substantially different lipid and lipoprotein responses to routine physical activity from that seen in healthy individuals. For example, LPL activity is not increased by exercise training in those with LPL deficiency; nor does HDL-C concentration increase in individuals with low HDL (hypoalphalipoprotein syndrome). The mechanisms responsible for changes in dyslipidemic conditions as a consequence of exercise training are unclear and in many cases are likely to be different from those reported for healthy subjects.

HYPERTENSION

A single dynamic exercise session usually induces a normal rise in systolic blood pressure from baseline in hypertensive persons who are not on medications. Often, the slope of the pressor response is either exaggerated or diminished. On the other hand, when the baseline blood pressure level is elevated, the absolute level of systolic blood pressure attained during dynamic exercise is usually higher in hypertensive persons than in normal persons. Furthermore, diastolic blood pressure typically stays constant or is slightly higher during dynamic exercise. Rarely does the diastolic blood pressure decrease. A rise in diastolic blood pressure during dynamic exercise is likely the result of an impaired vasodilatory response (79).

Aerobic or endurance exercise usually produces immediate decreases in blood pressure of similar magnitude to exercise training programs and may persist up to 22 hours after the exercise (82,83). After 30 to 45 minutes of moderate-intensity dynamic exercise in persons with hypertension, there can be reductions of 10 to 20 mm Hg in systolic blood pressure during the initial 1 to 3 hours postexercise (6).

Mechanisms for the decrease in blood pressure after exercise training are not well understood. Decreased plasma norepinephrine levels, increases in circulating vasodilator substances, improvements in hyperinsulinemia, and altered renal function are all possible explanations. Hypertension that goes untreated is often accompanied by limitations in exercise tolerance. Also, some antihypertensive drugs impair exercise performance (see Appendix A in GETP8) (48). Nevertheless, when hypertension is controlled with lifestyle modification and well-tolerated antihypertensive medications, exercise tolerance typically improves over the long term.

Resistance training is commonly advised today, but the cardiovascular responses to a single resistance exercise session are quite different from a session of endurance exercise. Heavy-resistance exercise in particular elicits a pressor response causing only moderate heart rate and cardiac output increases, relative to those seen with dynamic endurance exercise, though systolic and diastolic blood pressure can increase dramatically more than that seen in endurance exercise. The 2004 ACSM position stand on exercise and blood pressure recommends aerobic exercise as an indicated intervention in hypertension, with resistive training as an *adjunct* (82). Logically, this must be dynamic resistive exercise training, because there are no data to suggest that static exercise has any benefit. Thus, strength/resistive training are suggested for overall fitness, but in a person with hypertension, the clinical exercise specialist must be concerned about an exaggerated pressor response.

PERIPHERAL ARTERIAL DISEASE

The primary effect of PAD on a single exercise session is the development of claudication pain. Prospective exercise training studies demonstrate beneficial improvement in exercise tolerance in patients with claudication (38,63,88,111). Exercise-induced improvements in walking ability are well established, but the degree of exercise training is varied across studies. Clinical benefits are reported after 4 weeks of exercise training and continue to accrue for 6 months of regular exercise participation (38,41). Thus, exercise training is important, but the dose-response relationship is not fully clear.

Symptoms of intermittent claudication are improved by exercise training. Possible mechanisms for this increased exercise tolerance include increased leg blood flow, better redistribution of blood flow, improved hemorheologic and fibrinolytic properties of blood (e.g., reduced viscosity), greater reliance on aerobic metabolism because of a higher concentration of oxidative enzymes, less reliance on anaerobic metabolism, an improvement in the efficiency of walking economy and oxygen uptake kinetics, and an increased free-living daily energy expenditure (6,102).

OVERWEIGHT AND OBESITY

A single exercise session has little impact on being overweight or obese, but exercise can have deleterious effects on the obese person who overdoes a single exercise routine. Obesity increases the load on weight-bearing joints and spine and can impair thermoregulation in hot environmental conditions. Exercise is often a very uncomfortable experience for persons with obesity. Thus, exercise training for the obese must be undertaken with care. Nonetheless, exercise training is a key component for success in long-term lifestyle management of obesity. Although exercise training is modestly effective in reducing body weight 5% to 10% in moderate obesity, there is some question as to its effectiveness in morbid obesity.

The exact exercise training dose necessary to control weight is not yet defined. Emerging evidence suggests that exercise time ranging from 45 to 60 minutes per day on most days of the week is most effective for preventing weight regain in overweight and obese adults (29,53,59,94). For weight control, ACSM recommends approximately 60 minutes per day on most days of the week (54), whereas the International Association for the Study of Obesity recommends 60 to 90 minutes per day on most days of the week (93). Recent research concerning exercise intensity supports that moderate- (40%–60% of $\dot{V}O_2max$) intensity exercise has a positive impact on health parameters (112) and is likely as effective for weight control as vigorous-intensity exercise (53). Consequently, a sensible recommendation is for obese patients to work toward weight loss and continue long-term exercise training for weight maintenance. A logical approach to this goal is a moderate-intensity exercise regimen for 60 minutes or more on most days of the week for a total of 240 minutes/week or more (68).

Physical activity is believed to affect body fat distribution by promoting visceral fat loss in the abdomen. This reduction of abdominal fat decreases the risk of the diseases associated with visceral body fat distribution. The effects of exercise training on metabolism are not well established. Metabolic rate, including the caloric cost of physical activity, is shown to decline with weight reduction via caloric restriction (16,50). In the starvation state, however, the maintenance of metabolic rate through exercise may not always counteract the reduction mediated by food restriction. Despite this, exercise training has positive effects on glucose metabolism in both the moderately obese and the morbidly obese. These benefits of exercise include decreasing fasting glucose, decreasing fasting insulin, increasing glucose tolerance, and decreasing insulin resistance/increasing insulin sensitivity. These changes are achieved, in some instances, without changes in body weight or body fat. Other reports show that the more dramatic changes in glucose metabolism occurred in those who exhibited the greatest reduction in deep abdominal fat (18,40,56,69,78,89,90,91).

CEREBROVASCULAR STROKE/TRANSIENT ISCHEMIC ATTACK

The severity of neurologic involvement and existing comorbidities that occur in those with stroke greatly affects one's ability to perform bodily movements, including exercise. The following items are examples of potential effects of neurologic deficits on exercise.

- Muscle weakness, limited range of motion, and impaired sensation may limit independent ambulation or ability to exercise in the standing position.
- Lack of adequate balance may interfere with the ability to perform stationary cycle exercise.
- Weakness and/or limited range of motion of the arm or leg may also interfere with a person's ability to maintain desired speed during ergometry.
- Receptive aphasia, mental confusion, and/or **apraxia** may interfere with the ability to understand and follow directions during exercise testing or training sessions.

Cognitive and behavioral sequelae may influence compliance with and retention of an exercise program. Involvement of the frontal lobe can result in lack of initiation, apathy, easy frustration, loss of inhibition, and impaired cognitive and executive functions. Lesions in the temporal lobe may cause difficulties with new learning, memory deficits, and possible outbursts of aggression. Involvement of the areas of the brain mediating perception and arousal may lead to difficulty screening irrelevant sensory input in the environment and focusing on important cues.

Because the majority of strokes occur in elderly individuals, participation in aerobic exercise may be further complicated by the arthritic, orthopedic, and cardiovascular problems common in this population. Although most individuals with traumatic brain injuries are young, their general physical capacities and endurance may be severely limited secondary to orthopedic and other injuries incurred at the time of the accident. Also, seizures, another comorbidity associated with brain injury, may pose a safety concern during exercise.

Motor function deficits may interfere with exercise performance. In previous studies, only 20% to 34% of individuals with stroke were able to achieve 85% of age-predicted maximal heart rate (6). People with a traumatic brain injury typically exhibit aerobic capacities about 67% to 74% below predicted ability level (6). These individuals typically have much higher submaximal heart rates during cycle ergometry when compared with age-matched controls without physical impairments.

Exercise training may have differential impacts on people who have experienced a stroke and those who have sustained a brain injury. Most individuals with a recent history of stroke are highly deconditioned, exhibiting a peak oxygen consumption ($\dot{V}O_2$ peak) that is about half that achieved by age-matched individuals without a previous cerebral vascular accident (CVA) (55). This deconditioned state, however, leaves tremendous room for improvement. If a person with CVA recovers enough motor function to take part in a leg cycle exercise program, aerobic training studies suggest that 60% increases in $\dot{V}O_2$ peak might be expected (45). Endurance training not only has the potential to increase aerobic capacity but may also increase self-selected walking speed, decrease reliance on assistive devices during ambulation, and increase functional mobility scores.

Resistance training also has positive effects in those who suffered from a CVA. In particular, several studies have shown strong associations between paretic knee-extension torque and locomotion ability and between both hip flexor and ankle plantar flexor strength of the paretic limb and walking speed after stroke (44). These data suggest that a carefully planned resistance-training regimen might be beneficial for some selected individuals who have suffered a CVA.

EXERCISE PRESCRIPTION FOR CHRONIC CONDITIONS

> **1.3.30-CES: Discuss the appropriate use of static and dynamic resistance exercise for individuals with cardiovascular, pulmonary, and metabolic diseases.**

> **1.7.4-CES: Design, implement, and supervise individualized exercise prescriptions for people with chronic disease and disabling conditions, or who are young or elderly.**

> **1.7.40-HFS: Ability to explain and implement exercise prescription guidelines for apparently healthy patients, increased-risk patients, and patients with controlled disease.**

> **1.7.41-HFS: Ability to adapt frequency, intensity, duration, mode, progression, level of supervision, and monitoring techniques in exercise programs for patients with controlled chronic disease (e.g., heart disease, diabetes mellitus, obesity, hypertension), musculoskeletal problems (including fatigue), pregnancy and/or postpartum, and exercise-induced asthma.**

> **1.7.20-CES: Discuss the appropriate use of static and dynamic resistance exercise for individuals with cardiovascular, pulmonary, and metabolic diseases.**

In adapting an exercise program to meet the needs of a specific population, one must know that group well. The exercise prescription for an apparently healthy individual is described in Chapters 28 and 29. This prescription can and should be modified for the individual for the specific needs related to their diagnosis. Remember that each person has individual signs and symptoms, needs, and goals related to his or her diagnosis. The exercise prescription should focus on these specific needs and be updated continuously as the individual progresses.

HYPERLIPIDEMIA

Exercise for the hyperlipidemic patient is considered adjuvant therapy used in conjunction with reduced energy intake and dietary fat consumption. If after 12 weeks of this treatment blood lipids and lipoproteins are not controlled, lipid-lowering medications, the primary method for controlling hyperlipidemia, are initiated. This will have no effect on the exercise prescription for these patients.

Assuming no other chronic conditions, the same exercise prescription that is used for a healthy adult is commonly used for the hyperlipidemic patient with several additional considerations. In order for the hyperlipidemic patient to affect lipid and lipoprotein levels, they must expend a large quantity of calories (30). Not only are large quantities of energy expenditure required for lipid and lipoprotein change, but also different energy expenditure thresholds for different lipids and lipoproteins exist. For example, triglyceride concentrations are lower in hypertriglyceridemic men after 2 weeks of aerobic exercise when at least 45 minutes of exercise per day is performed on consecutive days, whereas total plasma cholesterol concentration usually remains unchanged even after 1 year of exercise training unless body weight is concomitantly reduced (30). On the other hand, HDL-C concentrations are frequently increased by exercise regimens requiring 1,000 to 1,200 kcal of energy expenditure per week for a minimal training period of 12 weeks (30). Inactive subjects may also have a lower exercise threshold than physically active persons for HDL-C change. In any case, inactive persons can expect a favorable change in blood lipids within several months when an exercise threshold is met.

HYPERTENSION

If an individual has uncontrolled hypertension (i.e., blood pressure >200/110 mm Hg), exercising is not recommended until after initiating drug, although some individuals with occasional blood pressure elevations to this level may initiate exercise training (48). This latter point should be evaluated on a case-by-case basis. However, when blood pressure is controlled, endurance training can safely be added to the treatment regimen. The exercise program for a hypertensive individual is similar as that for healthy adults. Exercise should utilize large muscle groups doing aerobic activities that are usually completed on most, but preferably all, days per week. The exercise duration ranges from 30 to 60 minutes at an exercise-intensity 40% to 60% of $\dot{V}O_2 R$. Interestingly, exercise training at somewhat lower intensities appears to lower blood pressure as much as, if not more than, exercise at higher intensities (82). The latter is especially important in certain specific populations of persons with hypertension, such as those who are elderly or who have chronic diseases in addition to hypertension.

Strength or resistive training is recommended for hypertensive persons, but endurance exercise training must be included because resistance training, with the exception of circuit weight training, has not consistently been shown to lower blood pressure. A resistance training regimen of 8 to 10 different exercises at 60% to 80% of the 1 repitition maximum (1RM) and targeting major muscle groups is recommended (48).

Several special considerations deserve mention. One should not allow a hypertensive individual to exercise when resting systolic pressure is >200 mm Hg or diastolic pressure is >110 mm. Also, exercise should not be attempted until the excessive exercise pressor response is well controlled by medications. An initial goal of 700 kcal expenditure per week is recommended, with a long-term energy expenditure goal of 2,000 kcal per week. Note that this weekly dose of energy expenditure for hypertension may be higher than the dose recommended for hyperlipidemia.

PERIPHERAL ARTERIAL DISEASE

Exercise programs for patients with PAD are designed with a goal of improving claudication pain symptoms and reducing cardiovascular risk factors (114). Most patients with PAD should perform interval walking or stair climbing (i.e., weight-bearing activities) three to five times a week at an intensity that causes pain to reach a 3 score on a 4-point scale (see GETP8, Fig. 5.4) (39,48). The onset of claudication will usually occur in approximately 5 minutes, and exercise is stopped when the pain reaches the 3 on the 4-point intensity scale. Full pain-free recovery is encouraged between intervals. This type of program may start with 10 to 20 minutes of exercise (not exercise plus rest) per session at 40% of $\dot{V}O_2 R$ or heart rate reserve (HRR), and gradually progress to 30 to 60 $min \cdot d^{-1}$ at 60% of $\dot{V}O_2 R$ or HRR, over a period of about 6 months. Non–weight-bearing tasks (e.g., cycling) are recommended for warm-up and cool-down. Medical clearance should include a physical exam, blood screening, and assessment and treatment of any potentially hazardous or exercise-limiting comorbid medical condition. A graded exercise test before beginning and after several weeks of exercise training is completed is useful to detect potential cardiac ischemia and to quantify symptom-limited exercise tolerance. One should understand that the presence of PAD increases the risk that other vascular abnormalities exist.

Special considerations exist for individuals with PAD, including the need for an aggressive lifestyle and lipid management. With an exercise training program, repeated submaximal treadmill tests to evaluate time to pain and maximum walking distance or 6-minute walk tests are helpful to properly gauge progress. Unfortunately, these are typically not available because of insufficient third-party reimbursement, and many patients are not willing to pay for the cost of these tests. Remember that improvements in walking ability may unmask signs and symptoms of angina pectoris and the presence of CHD. Also, cold weather may exacerbate symptoms, requiring the need for longer warm-ups (8). These patients often do better in a controlled environment. Finally, a quality of life questionnaire (e.g., Short Form 36) and watching for changes in comorbid conditions can be extremely useful in both designing and measuring individual progress.

OVERWEIGHT AND OBESITY

Although the primary objective of exercise in the treatment of obesity is to expend more calories, the optimal approach to increase energy expenditure is debatable. The exercise prescription must optimize energy expenditure yet minimize potential for injury. On the other hand, exercise should be enjoyable and practical and fit into the lifestyle of the individual.

The energy expenditure of the actual exercise, as well as that of the recovery period, otherwise known as excess postexercise oxygen consumption (EPOC), is considered in the total energy expenditure for a single exercise session. There is considerable debate on whether two or more short sessions a day will produce a higher total energy expenditure (exercise + EPOC) than one longer session of the same intensity. The use of two or more shorter sessions is recommended because the elevated energy expenditure of recovery is sustained for a longer period of time than after a single exercise session. On the other hand, a single longer exercise session provides an advantage in substrate utilization and for ease of incorporation into some individuals' lifestyles.

Whether substrate utilization is important for weight reduction is not clear. Total calories expended are the primary goal for body fat reduction. In this regard, certain considerations and recommendations for the exercise prescription include non–weight-bearing exercise and activities; increases in daily living activities like walking; the incorporation of resistance training as part of the exercise regiment; daily exercise or at least 5 or more days per week, with a goal of maximizing the amount of daily/weekly caloric expenditure; sessions of 30 to 60 minutes per day performed continuously or in bouts no

shorter than 10 minutes; and exercise intensity at 40% to 60% of $\dot{V}O_2 R$ or HRR. Providing that risk of injury is minimal, exercise intensities of 50% to 75% of $\dot{V}O_2 R$ or HRR may be prescribed once a regular exercise routine is established (7,48,49,112).

Exercise programs that include high-resistance activities (e.g., free weights, resistance machines) can lead to preferential retention of lean body weight. However, aerobic activity has more potential to decrease fat weight than does resistance training because the aerobic exercises can be sustained for a longer time, allowing more energy to be expended.

Exercise is not effective if the patient is not motivated or ready to make the necessary changes. Motivational strategies are often required to help patients move into readiness for change. These strategies include using goal setting and decision/balance sheets.

Injury prevention is an important consideration in exercise for obese adults. Physical injury is a principle reason for discontinuation of exercise. Excess body weight can accelerate deterioration of osteoarthritis. Another important concern in obese individuals is thermoregulation.

In sum, the following considerations are important for exercise programming in obese populations: the prevention of overuse injury; history of injury; adequate flexibility, warm-up, and cool-down sessions; a gradual progression of intensity and duration; the use of low-impact or non–weight-bearing exercises; thermoregulation; neutral temperature and humidity; times of day, cool times being the best; adequate hydration; and clothing (should be loose fitting). Other considerations may be dependent on associated diseases that coexist with obesity. Further information about exercise training for the overweight and obese individual can be found in Chapter 33.

CEREBROVASCULAR STROKE/ TRANSIENT ISCHEMIC ATTACK

Overall medical management and exercise program design for the patient following a stroke is highly individualized and is in accordance with the severity of the stroke. Before exercise training is started, all other conditions resulting from the stroke and the factors associated with stroke must be taken into consideration. Hypertension is one of the primary risk factors for stroke, and uncontrolled hypertension must be controlled before exercise training begins. Exercise training programs for individuals with stroke should focus at increasing the level of physical fitness and at reducing CHD risk factors. Aerobic conditioning can positively alter many of the risk factors associated with stroke, including hypertension, glucose regulation, blood lipid profile, and body fat.

Patients that survive traumatic brain injury are at risk for sustaining permanent cognitive and behavioral sequelae that might interfere with their ability to follow directions for exercise testing and training. Cognitive deficits include memory loss and decreased rate of information processing, whereas behavioral problems include loss of impulse control, increased agitation, and impaired mood control. Many of these deficits can be addressed using cognitive retraining, behavioral management, and medication. Ideally, these should take place before beginning an exercise training program.

Aerobic exercise training mode depends on the individual's ability and choice, but the various modes used for exercise testing are also used for exercise training. Suggested exercise frequency is three to five sessions per week, with the exercise intensity based on the subject's initial fitness level. A very unfit individual, or one who is limited because of consequences of the stroke, will likely have to begin at exercise intensities equivalent to 40% to 50% $\dot{V}O_2$ peak (79). Exercise duration also depends on the subject's initial fitness level. Intermittent (interval training) protocols are often employed during the initial weeks of training because of the extremely deconditioned level of many patients after a stroke or a traumatic brain injury. Exercise professionals should aim for at least a 20-minute exercise duration (or two 10-minute exertion periods). Once an individual comfortably completes a 20-minute aerobic exercise period, the exercise duration should be gradually increased until the individual completes an exercise session equivalent to a caloric expenditure of 300 kcal. Depending on individual preference and ability, this may be achieved with shorter exercise sessions at a higher intensity or a longer exercise session at lower exercise intensities.

Previously, resistance exercise was thought to cause further increases in muscle tone in those individuals demonstrating **hypertonia and/or spasticity**. Therefore, resistance exercise training programs were often not included in the rehabilitation programs of many individuals following traumatic brain injury (TBI) or stroke. These fears have proven unfounded, and resistance exercises are often prescribed to address muscle weakness identified during the fitness assessment (3,80,103). Use of resistance exercise in persons with stroke has not, however, been demonstrated to be universally effective in improving functional capacity. In large part, this is related to complexity of studying such individuals and in designing a representative control group. Some data suggest that progressive resistance exercise training does not improve clinical outcomes (70). Clarification of the role of resistance exercise training will likely involve timing of the program relative to the brain injury/stroke, nature/severity of the neurologic deficits, and careful study design that examines the role of resistance exercise not as specific therapy, but as additional therapy to a standard rehabilitation regimen.

Individuals with neurologic impairments may have difficulty with preparatory postural adjustments and recruiting strength quickly enough to combat a loss of balance. Thus, some of the positions typically used for resistance training may need modification. For example, many healthy individuals perform dumbbell exercises while standing to increase upper-body strength. A person who has difficulty maintaining standing balance should perform these exercises unilaterally while holding onto a bar or other stationary object. They could also perform these exercises from a seated position.

Behavioral factors (e.g., impulsivity, a tendency to display outward aggression, lack of judgment, misunderstanding directions) exhibited by a patient following TBI must be considered when selecting the most appropriate environment for exercise. A patient who lacks complete judgment will need closer exercise supervision, whereas the individual who displays outward aggression may not succeed in certain group exercise settings. Patients who are easily agitated/frustrated or highly distractible should be scheduled for exercise during a quieter time of the day or work out in an area with fewer distractions. The patient who lacks initiative is likely to be more successful in a group setting.

EXERCISE TRAINING SUPERVISION

Individuals with chronic diseases benefit from some type of supervised exercise program. This supervision can be in various forms. One may take part in a medically supervised program, such as cardiovascular and pulmonary rehabilitation programs. Others may choose to take part in a program offered by a local gym. Finally, individuals may choose to exercise at home. Any of these choices are good; however, some type of supervision is believed to improve long-term outcomes and adherence to a more active lifestyle (15,20,22,24,37,95,96).

For those taking part in a medically supervised program, the highest level of supervision is usually offered. However, for most chronic diseases, a third-party reimbursement is not available, and medically supervised exercise can become quite expensive over time. The next choice is a public gym. In this setting, the supervision level varies based on the level of expertise of those operating the facility. Here again, no reimbursement is readily available, except possibly from work as a health incentive. This too can be quite expensive, but is usually less than that of the medical model. The final choice of home exercise is the least expensive. However, it is also the one with the least supervision. In this situation, it is important to have communication between the individual and his/her physician in developing the correct exercise program. All choices can provide equal benefits. The main difference is the level and expertise of supervision. This choice is best made by the individual after discussing all options with the exercise professional.

ECONOMIC BURDEN OF CHRONIC DISEASES

The diseases discussed in this chapter place heavy economic burdens on the world. Hypertension is a prime example of this burden. The current direct and indirect costs of hypertension are $59.7 billion, underscoring the social and economic burden of the problem. Hypertension is the most common primary diagnosis in America and is a major contributor to the metabolic syndrome (31). Hyperlipidemia is estimated to affect approximately 107 million Americans, who have blood cholesterol levels exceeding 200 mg·dL^{-1} (13). PAD affects approximately 5 million to 10 million American adults (101). Obesity-related conditions account for approximately 7% of total healthcare costs in the United States, and the direct and indirect costs of obesity are in excess of $117 billion annually (100). This is because an estimated 66% of adults are labeled as overweight, 32% obese, and 5% extremely obese (77). In the United States, more than 700,000 strokes are estimated this year, but at least 500,000 are preventable (108).

CONSEQUENCES OF PHYSICAL INACTIVITY

Considerable data are available on the detrimental physiologic effects of bed rest and restricted physical activity on health. Most individuals with a chronic disease become less active. This, in turn, leads to a cycle of deconditioning that results in the impairment of multiple physiologic systems. Some specific consequences of inactivity for individuals with a chronic disease include reduced cardiorespiratory fitness, osteoporosis, impaired circulation to the lower extremities, diminished self-concept, greater dependence on others for normal activities of daily living, and reduced ability for normal social interactions. As with any disease, the physical abilities and response to exercise, or lack thereof, varies tremendously among individuals. These variations are largely determined by one or more of the following: the severity and/or progression of the disease, response to treatments, and presence of concomitant illnesses. Large variations between individuals make expected health benefits from increased physical activity less predictable. However, the majority of the diseases discussed in this chapter do have generalized benefits from increased physical activity.

BENEFITS OF EXERCISE REVIEW

Benefits from exercise training are usually related to functional capacity and quality of life, although some populations also benefit from decreased morbidity and mortality. Furthermore, it is sometimes possible to decrease the doses of medications and reap a direct financial return on investment. There has been some success in predicting outcome for cardiac rehabilitation patients, and this technique may be useful for other populations. Until then, exercise training is probably worthwhile in any person with a chronic disease or disability. In contrast, a person who has several diseases and/or disabilities may gain little or may even be adversely affected by exercise training. Thus, it is difficult to know who is too sick to benefit from an exercise program. In people who are too sick to improve, it usually soon becomes apparent that exercise is of little benefit. Unfortunately, it is not currently possible to know how much someone will benefit from a given exercise program, and in many cases, it is impossible to compare the benefits with costs in monetary terms. Better methods of predicting adaptation would improve goal setting and improve risk-benefit as well as cost-benefit analyses.

Research shows that programs designed for the chronic diseases mentioned in this chapter are often quite successful in either managing or decreasing the signs and symptoms associated with those diseases. Also, physically active persons with hypertension and those with higher levels of cardiorespiratory fitness have markedly lower mortality rates than sedentary and less-fit persons. Programs consisting of moderate-intensity exercise are effective for weight control and weight loss, especially when coupled with dietary modifications. In general, most diseases respond favorably to exercise and physical activity. The exact intensity, duration, and frequency are still not known for many (or most) diseases. This is because of the highly individualized nature of each of these chronic diseases.

REFERENCES

1. Accreditation Counsel for Graduate Medical Education. Available from: www.seniorjournal.com/NEWS/Eldercare/5-02-27Medical-Training.htm. Accessed August 20, 2006.

2. **National Institute on Aging, Department of Health and Human Services. Action Plan for Aging Research: Strategic Plan for Fiscal Years 2001–2005. National Institute on Aging, Department of Health and Human Services. NIH publication No. 01-4951. Bethesda, MD May 2001.**

3. Ada L, Dorsch S, Canning CG. Strengthening interventions increase strength and improve activity after stroke: a systematic review. *Aust J Physiother.* 2006;52(4):241–248.

4. **Agency for Healthcare Research and Quality. Centers for Disease Control and Prevention. Physical activity and older Americans: benefits and strategies. June 2002. Available from: www.ahrq. gov /ppip/activity.htm. Accessed August 20, 2006.**

5. **American College of Sports Medicine. Position stand: Recommended quantity and quality of exercise for developing and maintaining cardiorespiratory and muscular fitness in health adults. *Med Sci Sports Exerc.* 1990;22(2):265–274.**

6. Durstine JL, Moore GE, editors, *ACSM's Exercise Management for Persons with Chronic Diseases and Disabilities.* 2nd ed. Champaign (IL): Human Kinetics; 2003.

7. **American College of Sports Medicine. Position stand: The recommended quantity and quality of exercise for developing and maintaining cardiorespiratory and muscular fitness, and flexibility in adults. *Med Sci Sports Exerc.* 1998;30:975–991.**

8. **American College of Sports Medicine. Position stand: Prevention of cold injuries during exercise. *Med Sci Sports Exerc.* 2006;38: 2012–2029.**

9. **American College of Sports Medicine. *ACSM's Guidelines for Exercise Testing and Prescription.* 4th ed. Philadelphia: Lippincott Williams & Wilkins; 2000.**

10. American College of Sports Medicine. The recommended quantity and quality of exercise for developing and maintaining fitness in healthy adults. *Med Sci Sports Exerc.* 1978;10(3):vii–x.

11. American Heart Association. Web site [Internet]. Available from: www.americanheart.org. Accessed August 20, 2006.

12. American Heart Association. Heart disease and stroke statistics — 2006 update. A report from the American Heart Association Statistics Committee and Stroke Statistics Subcommittee. *Circulation.* 2006;113:e85–e151.

13. American Heart Association. Cholesterol Statistics. Available from: http://216.185.112.5/presenter.jhtml?identifier=4506. Accessed November 2, 2006.

14. Aronow WS. Management of peripheral arterial disease. *Cardiol Rev.* 2005;13(2):61–68.

15. Ashworth NL, Chad KE, Harrison EL, Reeder BA, Marshall SC. Home versus center based physical activity programs in older adults. *Cochrane Database Syst Rev.* 2005;(1):CD004017.

16. Atkinson RL, Walberg-Rankin J. Physical activity, fitness, and severe obesity. In: Bouchard C, Shephard RJ, Stephens T, editors. Physical Activity, Fitness, and Health. Champaign (IL): Human Kinetics; 1994. p. 696–711.

17. Bansal S, Buring JE, Rifai N, Mora S, Sacks FM, Ridker PM. Fasting compared with non-fasting triglycerides and risk of cardiovascular events in women. *JAMA.* 2007;298(3):309–316.

18. Bell LM, Watts K, Siafarikas A, et al. Exercise alone reduces insulin resistance in obese children independently of changes in body composition. *J Clin Endocrinol Metab.* 2007;92(11):4230–4235.

19. Blair SN, Kampert JB, Kohl HW III. Influences of cardiorespiratory fitness and other precursors on cardiovascular disease and all-cause mortality in men and women. *JAMA.* 1996;276(3):205–210.

20. Bock BC, Albrecht AE, Traficante RM, et al. Predictors of exercise adherence following participation in a cardiac rehabilitation program. *Int J Behav Med.* 1997;4(1):60–75.

21. Bowen A, Lincoln NB. Cognitive rehabilitation for spatial neglect following stroke. *Cochrane Database Syst Rev.* 2007;(2):CD003586.

22. Burke LE, Dunbar-Jacob JM, Hill MN. Compliance with cardiovascular disease prevention strategies: a review of the research. *Ann Behav Med.* 1997;19(3):239–263.

23. Cahill K, Stead LF, Lancaster T. Nicotine receptor partial agonists for smoking cessation. *Cochrane Database Syst Rev.* 2007;(1): CD006103.

24. Carlson JJ, Norman GJ, Feltz DL, et al. Self-efficacy, psychosocial factors, and exercise behavior in traditional versus modified cardiac rehabilitation. *J Cardiopulm Rehabil.* 2001;21(6):363–373.

25. **Chobanian AV, Bakris GL, Black HR, et al. Seventh Blood Pressure Report of the Joint National Committee on detection, evaluation, and treatment of high blood pressure. JNC 7—complete version. *Hypertension.* 2003;42:1206–1252.**

26. Criqui MH. Peripheral arterial disease—epidemiological aspects. *Vasc Med.* 2001;6(3 Suppl):3–7.

27. Crouse S, O'Brien B, Grandjean P, et al. Effects of exercise training and a single session of exercise on lipids and apolipoproteins in hypercholesterolemic men. *J Appl Physiol.* 1997;83:2019–2028.

28. Duffy FD, Schnirring L. How to counsel patients about exercise: an office friendly approach. *Phys Sportsmed.* 2000;28(10):53–58.

29. Duncan JJ, Gordon NF, Scott CB. Women walking for health and fitness: how much is enough? *JAMA.* 1991;266(23):3295–3299.

30. Durstine JL, Peel JB. Dyslipidemia. In: Durstine JL, Moore GE, LaMonte MJ, Franklin BA. Pollock's Textbook of Cardiovascular Disease Rehabilitation. 1st ed. Champaign (IL): Human Kinetics; 2008. (In preparation for 2008 release).

31. Ehrman JK, Gordon PM, Visich PS, Keteyian SJ, editors. *Clinical Exercise Physiology* 2nd ed. Champaign (IL): Human Kinetics; 2008.

32. **National Cholesterol Education Program Expert Panel on Detection, Evaluation, and Treatment of High Blood Cholesterol in Adults. Executive Summary of the Third Report of the National Cholesterol Education Program (NCEP) Expert Panel on Detec-**

tion, Evaluation, and Treatment of High Blood Cholesterol in Adults (Adult Treatment Panel III) *JAMA.* 2001;285: 2486–2497.

33. Fields LE, Burt VL, Cutler JA, et al. The burden of adult hypertension in the United States 1999 to 2000 a rising tide. *Hypertension.* 2004;44:398–404.

34. Flegal KM, Carroll MD, Ogden CL, Johnson CL. Prevalence and trends in obesity among US adults, 1999–2000. *JAMA.* 2002;288: 1723–1727.

35. Fletcher B, Berra K, Ades P, et al. Managing abnormal blood lipids: a collaborative approach. *Circulation.* 2005;112:3184–3209.

36. Fletcher G, Bufalina V, Costa F, et al. Efficacy of drug therapy in the secondary prevention of cardiovascular disease and stroke. 2007; 99(6):S1–S35.

37. Forkan R, Pumper B, Smyth N, et al. Exercise adherence following physical therapy intervention in older adults with impaired balance. *Phys Ther.* 2006;86(3):401–410.

38. Gardner AW, Poehlman ET. Exercise rehabilitation programs for the treatment of claudication pain: a meta-analysis. *JAMA.* 1995;274 (12):975–980.

39. Gardner AW, Montgomery PS, Flinn WR, Katzel LI. The effect of exercise intensity on the response to exercise rehabilitation in patients with intermittent claudication. *J Vasc Surg.* 2005;42:702–709.

40. Giannopoulou I, Fernhall B, Carhart R, et al. Effects of diet and/or exercise on the adipocytokine and inflammatory cytokine levels of postmenopausal women with type 2 diabetes. *Metabolism.* 2005; 54(7):866–875.

41. Gibellini R, Fanello M, Bardile AF, et al. Exercise training in intermittent claudication. *Int Angiol.* 2000;19(1):8–13.

42. **Goldstein LB, Adams R, Becker K, et al. AHA scientific statement: Primary prevention of ischemic stroke. *Circulation.* 2001; 103:163–182.**

43. Gordon NF, Contractor A, Leighton RF. Resistance training for hypertension and stroke patients. In: Graves JE, Franklin BA, editors. Resistance Training for Health and Rehabilitation. Champaign (IL): Human Kinetics; 2001.

44. **Gordon NF, Gulanik M, Costa F, et al. AHA scientific statement: Physical activity and exercise recommendations for stroke survivors. *Circulation.* 2004;109:2031–2041.**

45. Gordon WA, Sliwinski M, Echo J, et al. The benefits of exercise in individuals with traumatic brain injury: a retrospective study. *J Head Trauma Rehabil.* 1998;134:58–67.

46. Grandjean PW, Crouse SF, Rohack JJ. Influence of cholesterol status on blood lipid and lipoprotein enzyme responses to aerobic exercise. *J Appl Physiol.* 2000;89(2):472–480.

47. Grundy SM, Cleeman JI, Merz CNB, et al. Implications of recent clinical trial for National Cholesterol Education Program Adult Treatment Panel III Guidelines. *Circulation.* 2004;110:227–239.

48. American College of Sports Medicine. *ACSM's Guidelines for Exercise Testing and Training.* 8th ed. Balitmore: Lippincott Williams and Wilkins; 2009.

49. **Haskell WL, Lee IM, Pate RR, et al. Physical activity and public health: updated recommendations from the American College of Sports Medicine and the American Heart Association. *Med Sci Sports Exerc.* 2007;39(8):1423–1434.**

50. Hill JO, Drougas HJ, Peters JC. Physical activity, fitness, and moderate obesity. In: Bouchard C, Shephard RJ, Stephens T, editors. Physical Activity, Fitness, and Health. Champaign (IL): Human Kinetics; 1994. p. 684–695.

51. Hokanson JE, Austin MA. Plasma triglyceride is a risk factor for cardiovascular disease independent of high-density lipoprotein cholesterol: a meta-analysis of population-based prospective studies. *J Cardiovasc Risk.* 1996;3:213–219.

52. Hui EK, Rubenstein LZ. Promoting physical activity and exercise in older adults. *JAMA.* 2006;7(5):310–314.

53. Jakicic JM, Winters C, Lang W, Wing RR. Effects of intermittent exercise and use of home exercise equipment on adherence,

weight loss, and fitness in overweight women: a randomized trial. *JAMA.* 1999;282(16):1554–1560.

54. Jakicic JM, Clark K, Coleman E, et al. American College of Sports Medicine position stand: appropriate intervention strategies for weight loss and prevention of weight regain for adults. *Med Sci Sports Exerc.* 2001;33(12):2145–2156.

55. Jankowski LW, Sullivan SJ. Aerobic and neuromuscular training: effect on the capacity, efficiency, and fatigability of patients with traumatic brain injury. *Arch Phys Med Rehabil.* 1990;71:500–504.

56. Janssen I, Fortier A, Hudson R, Ross R. Effects of an energy-restrictive diet with or without exercise on abdominal fat, intermuscular fat, and metabolic risk factors in obese women. *Diabetes Care.* 2002;25(3):431–438.

57. Joint National Committee on Detection, Evaluation, and Treatment of High Blood Pressure. The 6th Report of the Joint National Committee on detection, evaluation, and treatment of high blood pressure (JNC VI). *Arch Intern Med.* 1997;157:2413–2446.

58. Karanja N, Lancaster KJ, Vollmer WM, et al. Acceptability of sodium-reduced research diets, including the Dietary Approaches to Stop Hypertension diet, among adults with prehypertension and stage 1 hypertension. *J Am Diet Assoc.* 2007;107(9):1530–1538.

59. Klem WL, Wing RR, McGuire MT, et al. A descriptive study of individuals successful at long-term maintenance of substantial weight loss. *Am J Clin Nutr.* 1997;66:239–246.

60. Kokkinos PF, Holland JC, Narayan P., et al. Miles run per week and high-density lipoprotein cholesterol levels in healthy, middle-aged men. *Arch Intern Med.* 1995;155:415–420.

61. Kraus WE, Houmard JA, Duscha BD, et al. Effects of the amount and intensity of exercise on plasma lipoproteins. *N Engl J Med.* 2002;347(19):1483–1492.

62. Laurie N. Healthy People 2010: setting the nation's public health agenda. *Acad Med.* 2000;75:12–13.

63. Leng GC, Fowler B, Ernst E. Exercise for intermittent claudication. *Cochrane Database Syst Rev.* 2000;(2):CD000990.

64. Leon AS, Gaskill SE, Rice T, et al. Variability in the response of HDL cholesterol to exercise training in the Heritage Family Study. *Int J Sports Med.* 2002;23:1–9.

65. Leon AS, Rice T, Mandel S, et al. Blood lipid response to 20 weeks of supervised exercise in a large biracial population. The Heritage Family Study. *Metabolism.* 2000;49:513–520.

66. Mason RJ, Broaddus VC, Murray JF, Nadel JA. eds. *Murray and Nadel's Textbook of Respiratory Medicine.* 4th ed. Philadelphia,: W.B. Saunders Company; 2005.

67. McDermott AY, Mernitz H. Exercise and older patients: prescribing guidelines. *Am Fam Physician.* 2006;74(3):437–444.

68. Miller WM, McCullough PA. Obesity. In: Durstine JL, Moore GE, LaMonte MJ, Franklin BA. *Pollock's Textbook of Cardiovascular Disease Rehabilitation.* 1st ed. Champaign (IL): Human Kinetics; 2008. (In preparation for 2008 release).

69. Miyatake N, Nishikawa H, Morishita A, et al. Daily walking reduces visceral adipose tissue areas and improves insulin resistance in Japanese obese subjects. *Diabetes Res Clin Pract.* 2002;58(2):101–107.

70. Moreland JD, Goldsmith CH, Huijbregts MP, et al. Progressive resistance strengthening exercises after stroke: a single-blind randomized controlled trial. *Arch Phys Med Rehabil.* 2003;84(10):1433–1440.

71. National Cholesterol Education Program Expert Panel. Detection, evaluation, and treatment of high blood cholesterol in adults (adult treatment panel III): executive summary. Washington (DC): National Heart, Lung, and Blood Institute, National Institutes of Health; 2001.

72. National Heart, Lung, and Blood Institute. Seventh Report of the Joint National Committee on Prevention, Detection, Evaluation and Treatment of High Blood Pressure—JNC VII Bethesda (MD): U.S. Department of Health and Human Services; 2004. 04-52302003.

73. National Institutes of Health and National Heart, Lung, and Blood Institute. Clinical guidelines on the identification, evalua-tion, and treatment of overweight and obesity in adults—the evidence report. *Obes Res.*1998;6(suppl 2):51S–209S.

74. Nied RJ, Franklin B. Promoting and prescribing exercise for the elderly. *Am Fam Physician.* 2002;65(3):419–428.

75. Nimalasuriya K, Frank E. A new key to improving the health of patients and of the whole population: physicians preach what they practice. American College of Preventive Medicine 2006. Available from: http://medscape.com/viewarticle/522907. Accessed August 21, 2006.

76. Nordestgaard BG, Benn M, Schnohr P, Tybjaerg-Hansen A. Nonfasting triglycerides and risk of myocardial infarction, ischemic heart disease, and death in men and women. *JAMA.* 2007; 298(3):299–308.

77. Ogden CL, Carroll MD, Curtin LR, et al. Prevalence of overweight and obesity in the United States, 1999–2004. *JAMA.* 2006;295:1549–1555.

78. O'Leary VB, Marchetti CM, Krishnan RK, et al. Exercise-induced reversal of insulin resistance in obese elderly is associated with reduced visceral fat. *J Appl Physiol.* 2006;100(5):1584–1589.

79. Palmer-McLean K, Harbst KB. Stroke and brain injury. In: Durstine JL, editor. *ACSM's Exercise Management for Persons with Chronic Diseases and Disabilities.* 2nd ed. Champaign (IL): Human Kinetics; 2003. p. 238–246.

80. Patten C, Lexell J, Brown HE. Weakness and strength training in persons with poststroke hemiplegia: rationale, method, and efficacy. *J Rehabil Res Dev.* 2004;41(3A):293–312.

81. Pescatello LS. Hypertension. In: Durstine JL, Moore GE, LaMonte MJ, Franklin BA. *Pollock's Textbook of Cardiovascular Disease Rehabilitation.* 1st ed. Champaign (IL): Human Kinetics; 2008. (In preparation for 2008 release).

82. Pescatello LS, Franklin D, Fagard R, et al. American College of Sports Medicine. Position stand: Exercise and hypertension. *Med Sci Sports Exerc.* 2004;36:533–553.

83. Pescatello LS, Guidry MA, Blanchard BE, et al. Exercise intensity alters postexercise hypotension. *J Hypertens.* 2004;22: 1881–1888.

84. Petitt DS, Cureton KJ. Effects of prior exercise on postprandial lipemia: a quantitative review. *Metabolism.* 2003;52:418–424.

85. Phillips PS, Haas RH, Bannykh S, et al. Statin-associated myopathy with normal creatine kinase levels. *Ann Intern Med.* 2002;137: 581–585.

86. Centers for Disease Control and Prevention. *Physical Activity and Health: A Report from the Surgeon General.* December 17, 1999. 48(SS08):1–6.

87. Pratt M, Macera CA, Wang G. Higher direct medical costs associated with physical inactivity. *Phys Sportsmed.* 2000;28:63–70.

88. Regensteiner JG. Exercise in the treatment of claudication: assessment and treatment of functional impairment. *Vasc Med.* 1997;2(3): 238–242.

89. Ross R, Dagnone D, Jones PJ, et al. Reduction in obesity and related comorbid conditions after diet-induced weight loss or exercise-induced weight loss in men: a randomized, controlled trial. *Ann Intern Med.* 2000;133(2):92–103.

90. Ross R, Janssen I, Dawson J, et al. Exercise-induced reduction in obesity and insulin resistance in women: a randomized controlled trial. *Obes Res.* 2004;12(5):789–798.

91. Ryan AS, Nicklas BJ, Berman DM. Aerobic exercise is necessary to improve glucose utilization with moderate weight loss in women. *Obesity (Silver Spring).* 2006;14(6):1064–1072.

92. Saltin B, Boushel R, Secher N, Mitchell J, editors. *Exercise and Circulation in Health and Disease.* Champaign (IL): Human Kinetics; 2000.

93. Saris WHM, Blair SN, van Baak MA, et al. How much physical activity is enough to prevent unhealthy weight gain? Outcome of the IASO 1st stock conference and consensus statement. *Obes Rev.* 2003;4:101–114.

94. Schoeller DA, Shay K, Kushner RF. How much physical activity is needed to minimize weight gain in previously obese women? *Am J Clin Nutr.* 1997;66:551–556.

95. Shaughnessy M, Resnick BM, Macko RF. Testing a model of poststroke exercise behavior. *Rehabil Nurs.* 2006;31(1):15–21.

96. Shepich J, Slowiak JM, Keniston A. Do subsidization and monitoring enhance adherence to prescribed exercise? *Am J Health Promot.* 2007;22(1):2–5.

97. Sinzinger H, Schmid P, O'Grady J. Two different types of exercise-induced muscle pain without myopathy and CK-elevation during HMG-Co-enzyme-A-reductase inhibitor treatment. *Atherosclerosis.* 1999;143(2):459–460.

98. Sinzinger H. Statin-induced myositis migrans. *Wien Klin Wochenschr.* 2002;114(21–22):943–944.

99. Sjöström L, Narbro K, Sjöström CD, et al. Effects of bariatric surgery on mortality in Swedish obese subjects. *N Engl J Med.* 2007;357(8):818–820.

100. Stein CJ, Colditz GA. The epidemic of obesity. *J Clin Endocrinol Metab.* 2004;89:2522–2525.

101. Stein R, Hriljac I, Halperin JL, et al. Limitation of the resting ankle-brachial index in symptomatic patients with peripheral arterial disease. *Vasc. Med.* 2006;11:29–33.

102. Stewart KJ, Hiatt WR, Regensteiner JG, Hirsch AT. Exercise training for claudication. *N Engl J Med.* 2002;347(24):1941–1951.

103. Taylor NF, Dodd KJ, Damiano DL. Progressive resistance exercise in physical therapy: a summary of systematic reviews. *Phys Ther.* 2005;85(11):1208–1223.

104. The Active for Life Program Office. Conference Report: The Role of Midlife and Older Consumers in Promoting Physical Activity through Healthcare, 2002.

105. The American Heart Association Web site [Internet]. Available from www.aha.org. Accessed on August 20, 2006.

106. The Centers for Disease Control and Prevention Web site [Internet]. Available from: www.cdc.org. Accessed June 20, 2007.

107. The National Heart Lung Blood Institute Web site [Internet]. Available from: www.nhlbi.nih.gov/chd/Tipsheets/daily.htm. Accessed June 23, 2007.

108. The National Stroke Association Web site [Internet]. Available from: www.stroke.org/site/DocServer/STROKE_101_Fact_Sheet.pdf?docID=4541.

109. Thompson PD, Zmuda JM, Domalik LJ, et al. Lovastatin increases exercise-induced skeletal muscle injury. *Metabolism.* 1997;46(10):1206–1210.

110. Torgovnick J, Arsura E. Statin-associated myopathy with normal creatine kinase levels. *Ann Intern Med.* 2003;138(12):1007; author reply 1008–1009.

111. Tsai JC, Chan P, Wang CH, et al. The effects of exercise training on walking function and perception of health status in elderly patients with peripheral arterial occlusive disease. *J Intern Med.* 2002;252(5):448–455.

112. U.S. Department of Health and Human Services. **Physical activity and health: a report of the Surgeon General. Atlanta: U.S. Department of Health and Human Services, Centers for Disease Control and Prevention, and National Center for Chronic Disease Prevention and Health Promotion; 1996.**

113. Wenger NK, Scheidt S, Weber MA. Exercise and elderly persons. *Am J Geriatr Cardiol.* 2001;10(5):241–242.

114. Womack CJ, Gardner AW. Peripheral arterial disease. In: Durstine JL, editor. *ACSM's Exercise Management for Persons with Chronic Diseases and Disabilities.* 2nd ed. Champaign (IL): Human Kinetics; 2003. p. 81–85.

115. Xin X, He J, Frontini J, et al. Effects of alcohol reduction on blood pressure: a meta-analysis of randomized controlled trials. *Hypertension.* 2001;38:1112–1117.

116. Youngstedt SD. Effects of exercise on sleep. *Clin Sports Med.* 2005;24(2):355–365.

117. Zipes DP, Libby P, Bonow RO, Braunwald E, editors. *Braunwald's Heart Disease: A Textbook of Cardiovascular Medicine.* 7th ed. Philadelphia: W.B. Saunders Company; 2005.

SELECTED REFERENCES FOR FURTHER READING

Ad Hoc Committee on Reporting Standards. Suggested standards for reports dealing with lower extremity ischemia. *J Vas Surg.* 1986;4:80–94.

Blair SN, Kohl HW, Barlow CE, Gibbons LW. Physical fitness and all-cause mortality in hypertensive men. *Ann Med.* 1991;23:307–312.

Durstine JL, Grandjean PW, Davis PG, Ferguson MA, Alderson NL, DuBose KD. The effects of exercise training on serum lipids and lipoproteins: a quantitative analysis. *Sports Med.* 2001;31(15):1033–1062.

Gordon NF. *Stroke: Your Complete Exercise Guide.* Champaign (IL): Human Kinetics; 1993.

Verrill D, Shoup E, Boyce L, Fox B, Moore A, Forkner T. Recommended guidelines for body composition assessment in cardiac rehabilitation: a position paper by the North Carolina Cardiopulmonary Rehabilitation Association. *J Cardiopulm Rehabil.* 1994;14:104–121.

INTERNET RESOURCES

- National Heart, Lung and Blood Institute: www.nhlbi.nih.gov
- National Hypertension Association: www.nathypertension.org
- National Lipid Association: www.lipid.org
- National Stroke Association: www.stroke.org
- North American Association for the Study of Obesity (NAASO): www.naaso.org

Exercise Prescription for People with Osteoporosis

EPIDEMIOLOGY

Osteoporosis is a skeletal disorder characterized by compromised bone strength that results in an increased susceptibility to fracture (35,85). It is estimated that more than 200 million people worldwide currently have osteoporosis (20), and the prevalence is expected to increase with the increasing lifespan and aging population (21). In the United States alone, an estimated 44 million individuals (55% of the population older than 50 years) have low bone mass or osteoporosis. This number is predicted to increase to 61.4 million by the year 2020 (82). Because osteoporosis is seen mainly as a disease that affects women, men often go undiagnosed and untreated, yet men are increasingly at risk for osteoporotic fractures.

The clinical relevance of osteoporosis is the dramatic increase in risk of fracture. More than 1.5 million fractures are associated with osteoporosis each year. **Osteoporotic fractures** are low-trauma fractures that occur with forces generated by a fall from a standing height or lower and are most common at the spine, hip, and wrist. Regardless of fracture site, adults who fracture are at much greater risk of fracturing again at any location (25). It is estimated that one in two women and one in four men older than 50 years of age will suffer from an osteoporotic-related fracture in their lifetime. To put this in perspective, a woman's risk of hip fracture is equal to her combined risk of breast, uterine, and ovarian cancers (82), and men have a greater risk of developing osteoporosis than prostate cancer. Hip fractures are considered to be the most devastating consequences of osteoporosis because they are associated with severe disability and increased mortality (77). Furthermore, the economic burden of hip fractures is substantial, with an estimated worldwide annual cost of $131.5 billion (42). The combination of all osteoporotic fractures cost the U.S. healthcare system approximately $17 billion per year, and these annual costs are projected to reach $50 billion by the year 2040 (59).

Osteoporosis is a silent disease: if not detected early, fractures may occur without warning because of reduced bone strength and increased load on the bone at a given time. Therefore, much attention is focused on early prevention, detection, and treatment of osteoporosis. The purpose of this chapter is to provide a brief overview of the pathogenesis, diagnosis, risk assessment, prevention, and treatment of osteoporosis—with special emphasis placed on the role of exercise in building and maintaining a strong skeleton and thereby offsetting skeletal fragility.

BONE PHYSIOLOGY

Bone is a biphasic material with crystals of hydroxyapatite (calcium-phosphate mineral) incorporated in a collagen matrix. The collagen gives bone flexible properties, and the mineral adds stiffness. This material is fashioned into two types of bone. **Cortical bone** (also referred to as compact bone) is dense and stiff and comprises the shaft of long bones as well as provides a shell of protection around **trabecular bone** (Fig. 39-1). Trabecular bone (also referred to as *cancellous* or *spongy bone*) is more porous and flexible and is found in flat bones, the ends of long bones, and in cuboidal bones (e.g., vertebrae). In trabecular bone, the bone material is in the form of plates and struts called *trabeculae*.

The characteristics of bone that determine its strength include the *quantity* of bone material present (the "mass" component), the *quality* of the material (i.e., material properties), and the distribution of the material in space (*structure* or *geometry*). These factors are determined by the dynamic cellular activities known as bone **modeling** and **remodeling**, which are regulated by bone's hormonal and mechanical environments. Modeling is the *independent* action of **osteoclasts** (bone-resorbing cells) and **osteoblasts** (bone-forming cells) on the surfaces of bone, whereby new bone is added along some surfaces and removed from others. Modeling affects the size and shape of bones and is especially important for reshaping long bones as they grow in length during adolescence or in response to changing mechanical load throughout life. Remodeling (Fig. 39-2) is a localized process that in-

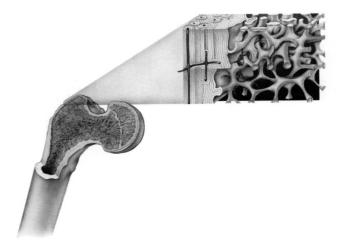

FIGURE 39-1. Bone is a dynamic tissue that is vascularized and innervated. *Cortical* bone is dense and stiff and makes up the shaft of long bones. Cortical bone also provides a shell of protection around *trabecular* bone, which is more porous and flexible and is found at the ends of long bones and in vertebrae. The external surface of bone is called the *periosteal* surface. The inner surface of long bones lining the medullary canal (containing bone marrow) is called the *endocortical* surface. The distance between the endocortical and periosteal surfaces in any given cross section is referred to as the *cortical thickness*. (Adapted from DAMS.)

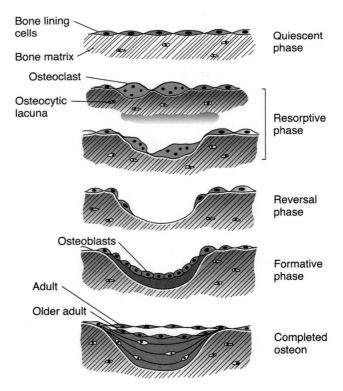

FIGURE 39-2. Bone remodeling is the *coupled* actions of osteoclasts and osteoblasts whereby a portion of older bone is resorbed by osteoclasts and replaced with newly formed bone by osteoblasts. The new bone begins as unmineralized matrix (osteoid). Eventually, the osteoid incorporates mineral. (From DAMS.)

volves the *coupled* action of osteoclasts and osteoblasts, in which osteoclasts first resorb a pit of older bone and osteoblasts are subsequently recruited to the site to form and mineralize new bone. This process happens throughout the lifespan and occurs diffusely throughout the skeleton. Like any material subjected to repetitive loading, fatigue damage is incurred. However, unlike inert materials, bone is able to replace damaged bone with new bone through the process of remodeling (87).

PATHOPHYSIOLOGY

Although osteoporosis denotes skeletal fragility, osteoporotic fractures are the result of *both* skeletal fragility and increased rate of falls. Osteoporotic fractures are a function of the reduced strength of a bone and the load on the bone at any given time, where the load must exceed bone strength for the fracture to occur. A majority of hip and wrist fractures occur as a consequence of falling. Thus, factors influencing both bone strength *and* risk of falling are important for fracture prevention.

SKELETAL FRAGILITY

Many skeletal characteristics contribute to bone strength, and consequently, bone fragility, including the quantity of bone material present, the quality of the material, and the distribution of the material within the bone structure.

Bone Quantity

Bone "quantity" refers to the amount of bone material present (i.e., the bone mass). The average pattern of change in bone mass across the lifespan is displayed graphically in Figure 39-3. The actual pattern of bone change is more dynamic than shown, both during growth

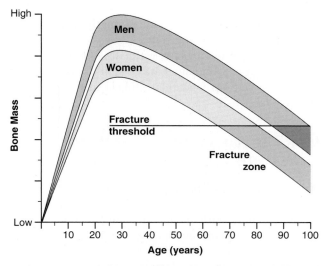

FIGURE 39-3. Normal pattern of bone mineral accretion and loss throughout the lifespan in men and women. (Permission requested.)

and in later life. For example, approximately 26% of total adult bone mass is accrued in a 2-year period during adolescence (9). This is approximately equivalent to the amount lost in later life (26). Overall, global bone formation continues at a faster pace than bone resorption until peak bone mineral accretion is attained sometime in the second or third decade (depending on site, region, and gender). In later life, the process of bone formation in each remodeling site no longer equals the bone that was resorbed, and thus, a small amount of bone is lost with each new remodeling cycle. This is referred to as a negative **bone balance**.

In later life, gonadal hormones (testosterone, estrogen) decrease in both men and women. Estrogen suppresses activation of new remodeling cycles, and thus, low estrogen levels partially contribute to an increased rate of remodeling (108). As resorption precedes formation in the process of remodeling, and formation and subsequent mineralization are time-intensive processes, an increase in the rate of remodeling results in temporary decreases in bone mass. Although temporary losses in bone mass lead to a transient increase in bone fragility, increased rates of remodeling with a negative bone balance lead to sustained bone loss of approximately 9% to 13% (91) during the first 5 years after menopause. Bone turnover eventually slows to a rate similar to premenopausal years. Men also experience age-related bone loss but without the rapid period of loss (16).

Bone Material Quality

Although the amount of bone in the human skeleton decreases with menopause and advancing age, there is evidence that properties of the remaining bone material may change with age in a way that increases susceptibility to fracture. Bone material from older individuals is less able to absorb energy before failure, likely because of increased mean tissue mineralization and changes in collagen properties that are associated with advancing age (22). Bone, like all loaded structural materials, is subject to fatigue damage in the form of microcracks that increase in number and length with advancing age (113). Microdamage accumulation is associated with reduced bone strength (81).

Bone Structure

Another important component of bone strength is the structure and geometry of bone—that is, how the material is distributed in space. Subtle changes in cross-sectional geometry can markedly increase bone strength with little or no changes in bone mass or density. Structural differences in cortical bone geometry may partially explain some of the differences in fracture rates between men and women. During growth, boys have greater gains in periosteal (outer) diameter, while girls have a narrowing of the endocortical (inner) surface, resulting in a greater overall bone size in boys that remains throughout life (33,99). In later life, bone is lost primarily from the endosteal surfaces (inner surface of long bones and intracortical surfaces within the cortex). Thus, the cortex becomes more porous and the cortices become thinner and more fragile. To offset these losses, bone may be added to the periosteum (outside surface of bone), thereby increasing the diameter of bone and maintaining the strength of the structure in bending (13,100,101). However, as more bone is resorbed from the endocortical surface than is formed on the periosteal surface, the cortices continue to thin, becoming fragile and more likely to fracture.

Microarchitecture of trabecular bone is also an important contributor to skeletal fragility (50). For example, if the resorption phase of remodeling is too aggressive, as is seen at menopause and thereafter, trabeculae may be penetrated and entire trabecular elements lost (Fig. 39-4). In these cases, the loss in structural strength is exaggerated far out of proportion to the amount of bone lost (92). Furthermore, trabeculae that remain intact may be thinned by excessive remodeling, creating a weakness in the ability to bear loads.

FALLS

Although skeletal fragility increases susceptibility to fracture, it would be of little concern if damaging loads, such as those generated in a fall, were prevented. A majority of hip fractures occur after a sideways fall and landing on the hip (36,110). The incidence of falls increases with age because several sensory systems that control posture (vestibular, visual, and somasensory) become compromised with advancing age. Furthermore, muscle mass

and strength, which prevent instability and correct imbalance, decline 30%–50% between the ages of 30 and 80 (51).

DIAGNOSIS OF OSTEOPOROSIS

There is currently no direct method to measure bone strength noninvasively. Therefore, identification of individuals with osteoporosis relies on the use of noninvasive technology to measure surrogates of bone strength. A measurement of **bone mineral density** (BMD) by dual energy x-ray absorptiometry (DXA) is the primary factor involved in the diagnosis of osteoporosis (1). BMD represents the amount of bone per unit *area* and is currently the most commonly used surrogate of bone strength in clinical settings. The World Health Organization (WHO) has defined **osteopenia** (low bone mass) as a site-specific bone density between 1.0 and 2.5 standard deviations less than the mean for young white adult women, and **osteoporosis** as a bone density that is 2.5 standard deviations less than the mean for young white adult women (85,112). Expressing an individual's BMD relative to the young adult mean is referred to as a T-score (i.e., T ≤2.5 = osteoporosis). These criteria were developed based on population data of primarily white women. Controversy exists among experts as to how this criterion applies to men, children, and various ethnic groups (5,85). Furthermore, as these categories were derived from BMD data at the hip, the application of these criteria to other skeletal sites is questionable (44,45). Despite these issues, BMD measurements have been shown to predict 60%–70% of a patient's risk for fracture (80), therefore making them better predictors of fracture than the measurement of lipids in predicting heart disease (44,80,112).

New software such as the Hip Structure Analysis Program and new technology such as quantitative computed tomography (QCT), peripheral QCT (pQCT), and magnetic resonance imaging (MRI) are used to better assess important components of bone strength such as bone geometry and cortical and trabecular volumetric density and, therefore, provide better estimates of bone strength. However, these technologies are currently used primarily in research settings, and their clinical utility is not yet clearly established.

RISK FACTORS FOR OSTEOPOROTIC FRACTURE

Despite the appreciable capabilities of BMD measurements in predicting fracture, combining multiple risk factor assessment with a measure of BMD may more accurately determine overall fracture risk (44,80,112). This notion is strengthened by the observation that the presence of multiple risk factors is a better predictor of hip fracture than low bone density alone (44). Many risk

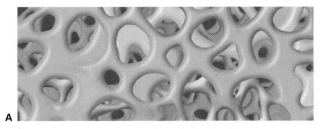

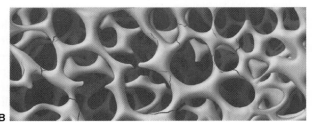

FIGURE 39-4. Slice of trabecular bone in normal **(A)** and osteoporotic **(B)** individual showing loss of trabecular connectivity and increased microcracks with ageing. (From DAMS.)

BOX 39.1	OSTEOFIT: A COMMUNITY-BASED PHYSICAL ACTIVITY PROGRAM FOR WOMEN WITH OSTEOPOROSIS

> **1.7.7-CES:** Prescribe exercise using nontraditional modalities (e.g., bench stepping, elastic bands, isodynamic exercise, water aerobics, yoga, tai chi, etc.) for individuals with cardiovascular, pulmonary, or metabolic diseases.

> **1.7.17-CES:** Design strength and flexibility programs for individuals with cardiovascular, pulmonary, and metabolic diseases, the elderly, and children.

AN EFFECTIVE EXERCISE PROGRAM IN OSTEOPOROTIC WOMEN: OSTEOFIT

Osteofit is an exercise-based program designed by the staff of the British Columbia Women's Hospital Centre Osteoporosis Program in Vancouver, Canada (http://www.osteofit.org/) (51). In a study of the efficacy of Osteofit in women aged 65–85 with osteoporosis, the women who completed the Osteofit program had (a) increased ability to undertake ADLs, (b) decreased back pain, (c) increased general health, (d) decreased fear of falling, and (e) improved falls risk profiles (18, 61). Importantly, the benefits of this program have been shown to persist even 1 year postintervention (62). This community-based program for women and men with osteoporosis aims to reduce participant's risk of falling and improve their functional ability, thereby enhancing quality of life. It differs from typical senior exercise classes by specifically targeting posture, balance, gait, coordination, and hip and trunk stabilization rather than general aerobic fitness. A typical class consists of a warm-up, a workout, and a relaxation component, all of which are outlined here (Fig. 39-5).

Warm-up: The general 10- to 15-minute warm-up is done to music and commences with gentle range of motion exercises for the major joints, which are performed either seated or standing. Static stretching exercises are usually not included. The warm-up ends with walking and simple dance routines with tempos of between 110 and 126 beats per minute so that participants can remain in control.

Workout: The workout consists of strengthening and stretching exercises intended to improve posture by combating medially rotated shoulders, chin protrusion (excessive cervical extension), thoracic kyphosis, and loss of lumbar lordosis. Exercises to improve balance and coordination may progress from heel raises and toe pulls to the mildly challenging two-legged heel-toe rock and the more challenging tandem walks and obstacle courses. Hip stabilization is trained using leg exercises (e.g., hip abduction and extension) or balance exercises. Trunk stabilization is addressed when the participant is cued and positioned to do all standing exercises with resistance for the arms (e.g., biceps curls) and shoulders (e.g., lateral arm raises). The abdominal muscles strengthened in their function as stabilizers rather than as prime movers. Exercises to improve functional ability include chair squats and getting up and down from the floor. Exercises are arranged so that upper and lower body activities are alternated to reduce the risk of tendon pain. If the class includes more than one set of an exercise, the sets are separated by a short rest period. Repetitions are kept to between 8 and 16, and weights are relatively light so that participants do not work to fatigue with each set. The exercises are arranged so that the less strenuous exercises, such as hamstring stretching, are at the end of the workout.

Relaxation: The last few minutes of the class are devoted to relaxation techniques such as deep breathing, progressive muscle tensing and relaxing, and visualizations to a background of soft music and/or nature sounds.

---

factors for osteoporosis and fracture have been identified, including age, family history of fracture, previous fracture, physical inactivity, and medication use, among others (Table 39-1). Advancing age is perhaps one of the best predictors of fracture because the risk of a hip fracture increases three to six times from 50 to 80 years, independent of BMD status (21,46).

Because of estrogen's effect on suppression of remodeling, hypogonadism is an important risk factor in both men and women. In men, hypogonadism can be caused by several conditions including hypopituitarism, hyperprolactinemia, overtraining, and inadequate energy intake. In young women, hypogonadism secondary to amenorrhea may be associated with inadequate energy intake (67). When taken to the extreme, the so-called female athlete triad syndrome (amenorrhea, disordered eating, and osteoporosis) is thought to be associated with increased risk for osteoporosis (2), although the prevalence of all three components of the triad is low (52). Menopause, whether spontaneous or due to surgery, chemotherapy, or radiotherapy, is also associated with increased risk of osteoporosis and fracture.

History of fracture is another important risk factor for subsequent fragility fractures, with a twofold increase in

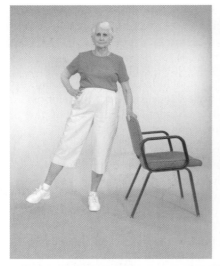
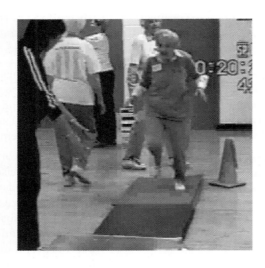
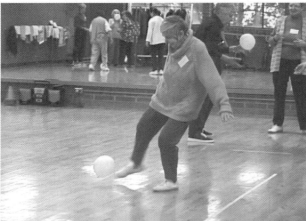
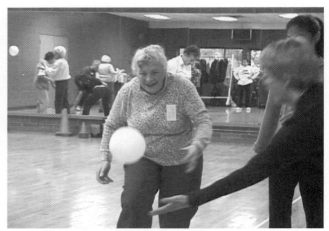

FIGURE 39-5. Women participating in the Osteofit class community-based program for falls prevention that includes strength and agility training. (Photos courtesy of K. Khan.)

risk of hip fracture following a previous hip or spinal fracture (53). Several medications can increase risk of osteoporosis, including glucocorticoids, which result in greater losses in spine bone mass. However, bone loss can be reduced by use of inhaled glucocorticoid therapy (109). Use of medications such as anticonvulsants, glucocorticosteroids and adrenocorticotropin, gonadotropin-releasing hormone agonists, immunosup- pressants, and heparin (long term) have also been associated with osteoporosis and fracture risk (83). Furthermore, several conditions

are associated with secondary osteoporosis, including hyperthyroidism and gastric surgery (44).

As discussed previously, factors related to risk of falls have important considerations. Exercise professionals should pay close attention to neuromuscular deficits, balance, and coordination in older individuals, particularly those with osteopenia or osteoporosis, who would be at increased risk of fracture in the case of a fall. Improving these deficits is equally (if not more) important in older individuals than attempting to increase bone integrity.

TABLE 39-1. RISK FACTORS FOR OSTEOPOROTIC FRACTURES

Age	**Neuromuscular disorders**	Excessive alcohol consumption
Previous fragility fracture	**Cigarette smoking**	Long-term immobilization
Glucocorticoid therapy	**Low body weight**	Low dietary calcium intake
High bone turnover	Premature menopause	Vitamin D deficiency
Family history of hip fracture	Primary or secondary amenorrhoea	Female sex
Poor visual acuity	Primary or secondary hypogonadism in men	Asian or white ethnic origin

Bold text indicates characteristics that capture aspects of fracture risk over and above that provided by bone mineral density. Adapted from Kanis, 2002 (14).

Falls are correlated with physiological impairments associated with aging such as slow reaction time, loss of balance, and muscular weakness (17,65). Psychological factors, such as fear of falling, are also associated with falls (17). Other risk factors associated with fall risk include orthostatic hypotension, Parkinson disease, stroke, depression, epilepsy, eye diseases, osteoarthritis, peripheral neuropathy, delirium, anemia, diabetes mellitus, depression, cognitive impairment, vitamin D deficiency, syncope, and many medications. Therefore, these factors should all be considered when determining risk, treatment, and preventative strategies regarding osteoporotic fracture (51).

CLINICAL MANAGEMENT

Although prevention of osteoporosis is important, once an individual is diagnosed with the disease, attention is turned to treatment to offset initial and subsequent fractures. Management strategies involve both pharmacological therapy and lifestyle modifications.

PHARMACOLOGICAL THERAPY

 1.5.3-CES: Recognize medications associated in the clinical setting, their indications for care, and

their effects at rest and during exercise (i.e., beta-blockers, nitrates, calcium channel blockers, *Digitalis*, diuretics, vasodilators, antiarrhythmic agents, brochodialators, antilipemics, psychotrophics, nicotine, antihistimes, over-the-counter cold medications, thyroid medications, alcohol, hypoglycemic agents, blood modifiers, pentoxifylline, antigout medications, and anorexiants/diet pills).

Several pharmacological agents (listed in Table 39-2) have been approved by the U.S. Food and Drug Administration (FDA) for the treatment of osteoporosis. These agents can be categorized by whether they act on remodeling (antiremodeling drugs) or directly on formation (anabolic drugs). Antiremodeling agents include bisphosphonates, salmon calcitonin, hormone replacement therapy (HRT), and selective estrogen receptor modulators (SERMs, raloxifene). These drugs act by suppressing the resorption phase of the remodeling cycle and thus allow existing cavities to fill, resulting in an increase in bone density. Also, by suppressing resorption, these agents can reduce loss of connectivity and trabecular thinning associated with menopause and aging. One of the major hormones regulating calcium homeostasis is parathyroid hormone (PTH), which is secreted in response to falling serum calcium levels. PTH helps to regulate serum calcium levels by (a) stimulating bone resorption in

TABLE 39-2. MEDICAL THERAPIES AVAILABLE FOR THE TREATMENT OR PREVENTION OF OSTEOPOROSIS

DRUG CLASS	NAME OF DRUG	BRAND NAME
Estrogens[a]	Estrone sulfate	Ogen
	Conjugated estrogen	Premarin
	Transdermal estrogen	Estraderm
	Estropipate	Ortho-Est
	Esterified estrogen	Estratab
	Conjugated estrogen + medroxyprogestrone acetate[b]	Premphase
		PremPro
		Activella
Calcitonin[c]	Synthetic salmon calcitonin	MiaCalcin
		Calcimar
Bisphosphonates	Alendronate[d]	Fosamax
	Risedronate[d]	Actonel
	Etidronate[e]	Didronel
SERMs	Raloxifene[f]	Evista
	Tamoxifene	Nolvadex
Others	Isoflavones (natural flavonoids)	
	Tibolone or ipriflavone (synthetic flavonoids)	
	Calcitriol or other vitamin d metabolites	
	Teriparatide[f] or other parathyroid hormones[g]	
	Sodium fluoride[g]	

SERM, selective estrogen receptor modulator.

[a]All estrogens have FDA approval for prevention of osteoporosis, but only Premarin is approved for treatment.

[b]Premphase, PremPro, and Activella are estrogen and progesterone taken in combination. Premphase and PremPro are FDA approved for the treatment of osteoporosis; Activella is approved for prevention of osteoporosis.

[c]Both calcitonins are approved for prevention, but only MiaCalcin is approved for treatment of osteoporosis.

[d]Alendronate and risedronate have FDA approval for both prevention and treatment of osteoporosis. Alendronate is also approved for treatment of osteoporosis in men.

[e]Etidronate has FDA approval but not with an osteoporosis indication in the United States.

[f]FDA-approved treatment of osteoporosis.

[g]Approval pending for an osteoporosis indication.

the presence of adequate vitamin D, (b) increasing intestinal calcium absorption, and (c) enhancing resorption of calcium in the kidney (51). Although PTH can stimulate both bone formation and bone resorption, when administered intermittently it results in net bone formation, and it is thus classified as an anabolic agent (83). Recombinant PTH is an anabolic drug that works by stimulating an increase in osteoblastic bone formation.

Because of the role of estrogen in suppression of osteoclast function and progestins in stimulating osteoblast activity, HRT has been shown to increase BMD at the spine and hip in women during the postmenopausal years when substantial losses are typically observed. However, approximately 40% of women who begin HRT treatment choose to stop taking the medication because of its many side effects (29). Furthermore, HRT is associated with an increased risk of coronary disease, stroke, and breast and ovarian cancer (34). For women unable to take HRT because they are at high risk of ovarian and breast cancer, the SERM raloxifene is a treatment option because it does not stimulate breast or endometrial tissues (58).

LIFESTYLE MODIFICATIONS

Because of difficulty implementing long-term lifestyle changes, the exercise professional can play a large role in facilitating adherence to these changes in the patient with osteoporosis. All postmenopausal women and older men, regardless of fracture risk, should be encouraged to engage in behavior modifications, including adequate calcium (1000–1500 mg $\cdot$ d^{-1}) and vitamin D (400–800 IU $\cdot$ d^{-1}) intake, regular exercise, smoking cessation, avoidance of excessive alcohol intake, and visual correction to decrease fall risk. Of these lifestyle modifications, exercise is the only one that can simultaneously ameliorate low BMD, augment muscle mass, promote strength gain, and improve dynamic balance—all of which are independent risk factors for fracture (47,84). However, there is currently no direct evidence that exercise reduces the risk of osteoporotic fracture, and there likely will not be until large, well-funded trials are conducted. Nevertheless, clinicians and exercise professionals should embrace the theoretical basis behind exercise prescription in osteoporosis prevention and treatment (51). Exercise prescription for individuals diagnosed with osteoporosis is outlined at the end of the chapter.

EXERCISE AND OSTEOPOROSIS

PHYSIOLOGICAL RESPONSE TO EXERCISE

This section reviews both the acute and chronic physiologic responses to exercise in those with osteoporosis.

Acute Physiological Response

Bone is a dynamic tissue capable of continually adapt to its changing mechanical environment. When a bone is loaded in compression, tension, or torsion, bone tissue is deformed. Deformation of bone tissue, or the relative change in bone length, is referred to as **strain**. Bone tissue strain causes fluid within the bone to move past the cell membrane of **osteocytes**—the bone cells that are embedded throughout bone tissue and are connected with one another, to other bone cells, and with the bone marrow through slender dendritic processes. The current prevailing theory in the bone field is that this fluid flow along the osteocyte and its cell processes causes a release of molecular signals that lead to osteoclast and osteoblast recruitment to (re)model bone to better suit its new mechanical environment. This process of turning a mechanical signal into a biochemical one is called **mechanotransduction**.

Chronic Physiological Response

It has been suggested by Harold Frost that the response of bone to its mechanical environment is controlled by a "mechanostat" that aims to keep bone tissue strain at an optimal level by homeostatically altering bone structure (31). Indeed, when bone is subjected to lower than customary loads (as in space flight and immobilization), bone will adapt by ridding itself of excess mass. Alternately, when bone is subjected to higher loads such as uncustomary exercise, bone will become stronger by altering its structure and increasing in mass. Although mechanotransduction is an acute response to exercise, the adaptation of bone structure through modeling and remodeling takes up to several months to complete. Bone does not respond to exercise by solely adding mass randomly to the skeleton. Rather, from animal studies, it is clear that bone is added where strains are the highest—typically on the periosteal surface in long bones (95). This has the effect of increasing the diameter of long bones, making them stronger in bending, because small increases in bone mass applied to appropriate locations can increase bending strength dramatically.

Remodeling is a process that not only performs the task of removing excess bone or adding bone on trabecular surfaces in youth but also repairs fatigue-damaged bone. With the increase in bone tissue strain that occurs with exercise, damage in the form of microcracks results. This damage is targeted for removal by osteoclasts, and new bone is formed in its place (87). Thus, one of the chronic effects of exercise on the skeleton involves the maintenance of bone strength through targeted remodeling.

Traditional imaging techniques such as DXA are unable to capture fine structural changes in bone and therefore may underestimate the benefits of exercise on the skeleton (41). Furthermore, mineralization of newly formed bone is an ongoing process on the order of months to years. Recall that resorption precedes formation in remodeling; therefore, the effects of exercise on the skeleton may take up to several months to be fully realized.

OSTEOGENIC ACTIVITIES

> **1.7.16-CES: Describe the principal of specificity as it relates to the mode of exercise testing and training.**

Bone responds to loading in a site-specific manner. That is, bone will be added in locations where adequate strain is generated. Thus, to optimize bone health at the hip, for example, physical activity should load the hip region through muscle force or ground reaction forces. Evidence from animal studies suggests that effective exercise programs for bone health should result in high strain rates and unusual strain distributions (i.e., loading in directions the bone is unaccustomed to). In practical terms, an osteogenic (bone-forming) exercise regimen should require high mechanical forces at high rates of force application produced in versatile movements (95,106). New evidence also suggests inserting rest between loading cycles can optimize the bone response to loading (94,105). That is, bone cells seem to saturate after a short loading period. In animal studies, bone loses more than 95% of its mechanosensitivity after only 20 loading cycles (95,106). For example, doing 10 jumps three times per day with 2–4 hours of rest between sets should be more effective for bone health than doing 30 jumps all at one time.

Although generally high magnitude and high strain rate lead to an optimal bone response, strain patterns can be altered to stimulate bone adaptation. For example, low magnitude strains that were otherwise ineffective stimulated an osteogenic response in mature animals if 10 seconds of rest were inserted between loading bouts (105) or if they were generated at a very high frequency (>20 Hz or cycles$\cdot$s^{-1}) (43,96,97). These novel strain applications have important implications for interventions in individuals with low bone mass such as osteoporotic adults (discussed later).

PHYSICAL ACTIVITY DURING ADOLESCENCE: PREVENTION OF OSTEOPOROSIS

Although osteoporosis is a disease associated with advancing age, there is almost universal consensus that early-life experiences are important in reducing the risk of osteoporosis in later life (26). The amount of bone mineral accrued during growth is recognized as an important predictor of bone mineral status in older adults (26,66). The observation that more than 25% of adult bone mineral is laid down during the 2 years surrounding the age of peak linear growth emphasizes the importance of the adolescent years in optimizing bone mineral ac-

crual (8). It is estimated that as much bone mineral is laid down during this period as an adult will lose from 50 to 80 years of age (4,8). Thus, optimizing bone mineral accrual during the growing years would seem to be an essential ingredient for the prevention of osteoporosis later in life (24).

A number of excellent reviews have all concluded that appropriate physical activity augments bone development (7,10,11,68,74). Retrospective human studies clearly indicate that bone responds more favorably to physical activity undertaken during childhood and adolescence than during adulthood (6,7,28,88). Mechanical loading studies using animal models lend strong support to these human studies (9,23,27,28,37,40,49,56,63,90, 95,106).

Numerous randomized controlled intervention studies aimed to investigate the change in bone mass or strength in children secondary to an exercise intervention. In general, these demonstrate a positive effect for physical activity during growth and development. Interventions were diverse, and activities ranged from moderate (running) to high (jumping) impact performed for 10–40 minutes, two to three times per week. In all studies of pre- and early-pubertal children, BMD increased more in the intervention group than in controls at various regions of the proximal femur and/or lumbar spine (15,32,39,70,71,76,79). Generally, the magnitude of the augmented response over 7–10 months varied from 1% at the trochanteric region of the proximal femur (76) to ~3% at the femoral neck for a high-impact jumping intervention (32,79). When moderate activity was increased through daily physical education, a positive effect on bone accretion in prepubertal girls was also noted (107). In a school-based intervention with a 10-minute moderate-impact circuit training three times per week, the benefit doubled if the intervention continued for a second school year. Bone mass benefits increased from 2% to approximately 4% at the femoral neck and lumbar spine in both boys and girls (69,72). These and other studies suggest that the bone response to loading is optimized in pre- and early-puberty (premenarche in girls) (14,39,48, 111,94).

Exercise Prescription for Optimizing Bone Development in Youth

> **1.7.4-CES: Design, implement, and supervise individualized exercise prescriptions for people with chronic disease and disabling conditions and people who are young or elderly.**

The ACSM position stand on physical activity and bone health (54) states that exercise to optimize bone health in children and adolescents should involve 10–20 minutes, three days per week, of impact activities such as plyometrics, jumping, moderate-intensity resistance training, and participation in sports that involve running and jumping (soccer, basketball). Since the publication of this position stand, a new trial of exercise in youth has further elucidated the appropriate anabolic dose of exercise to strengthen the growing skeleton. A pilot study of a simple jumping intervention, "Bounce at the Bell," showed that 10 jumps, three times per day, over 8 months was associated with a significant increase in proximal femur (+2.3%) and intertrochanteric region (+3.2%) BMD (75). To perform their jumps, children simply stood next to their desk and jumped for <1 minute, three times per day when the bell rang. The intervention took <3 minutes per day and required no equipment or special training from teachers. Although more work is needed to confirm these results, these data suggest that interventions can be very simple and short and still be effective at improving bone development; they may be excellent adjunctive exercises to those recommended in the ACSM position stand.

EXERCISE AND BONE HEALTH IN ADULTHOOD

The goal of exercise in adulthood should be to offset bone loss that is observed during this time in life, rather than adding bone mass to the skeleton as in youth. Trials of exercise lasting 8–12 months in premenopausal women generally show increased BMD by 1%–3% at the loaded sites (spine and hip) compared to controls (30,38,64, 102–104). Differences between exercisers and controls in the premenopausal cohorts are attributed to gains in bone mineral of exercisers (12,38), attenuation of bone loss in exercisers, or a combination of bone gain in exercisers and bone loss in controls (30). Trials of exercise in premenopausal women (ages 22–49) with favorable outcomes involved jogging, strength training, aerobics, and jumping exercises (51).

Traditionally, there is far less research attention regarding the effects of exercise on bone health in men versus women (86). This paucity of research is not justified by the observations of the exponential increase in incidence of hip fracture in men as they age (although this happens 5–10 years later than for women) (86). Of the few studies performed in older men, most found positive effects of resistance training on BMD at loaded sites. Menkes et al. report that 16 weeks of resistance training in 59-year-old men resulted in a 3.8% increase in femoral neck BMD compared with controls (78). Similarly, Ryan et al. found that 16 weeks of resistance training in 61-year-old men resulted in a 2.8% increase in femoral neck BMD compared with controls (98). Overall, studies in adults indicate that exercise, if done with adequate load such as resistance (weight training) and impact (i.e., jump) training, are effective at attenuating bone loss observed with advancing age (51).

Exercise Prescription to Preserve Bone Health during Adulthood

 1.7.9-CES: Identify patients who require a symptom-limited exercise test prior to exercise training.

> **1.7.40-CES: Ability to explain and implement exercise prescription guidelines for apparently healthy clients, increased risk clients, and clients with controlled disease.**

Prior to beginning a new exercise program, all individuals with osteoporosis or who are at risk should be encouraged to consult with their physician. No special recommendations for performing an exercise evaluation exist for this population, and the recommendation is to consider the need for an exercise evaluation as one would for any individual.

The ACSM position stand on physical activity and bone health states that exercise to preserve bone health during adulthood should involve 30–60 minutes per day of a combination of moderate-to-high intensity weight-bearing endurance activities (three to five times per week), resistance exercise (two to three times per week), and jumping activities (54). Weight-bearing endurance activities include tennis, stair climbing, and jogging at least intermittently during walking. Activities should involve jumping, including volleyball and basketball, and resistance exercises, such as weightlifting, and these should target all major muscle groups (54).

EXERCISE IN ELDERLY AND OSTEOPOROTIC INDIVIDUALS

Exercise Testing in Osteoporosis

> **5.2.1-HFS: Knowledge of musculoskeletal risk factors or conditions that may require consultation with medical personnel before testing or training, including acute or chronic back pain, osteoarthritis, rheumatoid arthritis, osteoporosis, inflammation/pain, and low back pain.**

> **1.3.9-CES: Instruct the test participant in the use of the RPE [rate of perceived exertion] scale and other appropriate subjective rating scales, such as the dypsnea, pain, claudication, and angina scales.**

> **1.3.22-CES: Describe the differences in the physiological responses to various modes of ergometry (e.g., treadmill, cycle and arm ergometers) as they relate to exercise testing and training.**

> **1.7.18-CES: Determine appropriate testing and training modalities according to the age, functional capacity, and health status of the individual.**

Exercise testing is not contraindicated for those with osteoporosis. However, because of the nature of the disease, if an exercise test is indicated, certain measures must be taken into consideration to ensure maximal safety. As with any exercise test, instruct the test participant in the use of the RPE and pain scales. Because the majority of individuals with osteoporosis are older in age and sedentary, they should be considered as moderate risk for atherosclerotic disease (see GETP8 Table 2.1). Based on this, it is recommended that a physician be present if a maximal exercise test is performed (see GETP8 Fig. 2.4). When exercise tests are performed in individuals with osteoporosis, the following should be considered:

- Use of cycle ergometry as an alternative to treadmill exercise testing to assess cardiovascular function may be indicated in patients with severe vertebral osteoporosis for whom walking is painful.
- Vertebral compression fractures leading to a loss of height and spinal deformation can compromise ventilatory capacity and result in a forward shift in the center of gravity. The latter may affect balance during treadmill walking.
- Maximal muscle strength testing may be contraindicated in patients with severe osteoporosis, although there are no established guidelines for contraindications for maximal muscle strength testing.

> **1.7.10-CES: Organize GXT [graded exercise test] and clinical data to counsel patients regarding issues such as ADL [activities of daily living], return to work, and physical activity.**

As with all patient populations, the trained exercise professional should work in consultation with the physician or other referring licensed healthcare provider to counsel patients regarding activities of daily living (ADL), return to work, and physical activity. The results of an exercise test are useful in determining the safety of performing these activities and the maximal metabolic equivalent (MET) threshold for activities that a person should be allowed to perform.

> **1.5.2-CES: Describe the mechanisms and actions of medications that may affect exercise testing and prescription, i.e., beta-blockers, nitrates, calcium channel blockers, *Digitalis*, diuretics, vasodilators, antiarrhythmic agents, brochodialators, antilipemics, psychotrophics, nicotine, antihistimes, over-the-counter cold medications, thyroid medications, alcohol, hypoglycemic agents, blood modifiers, pentoxifylline, antigout medications, and anorexiants/diet pills.**

The effects of any of the FDA-approved medications for the specific prevention and treatment of osteoporosis (e.g., calcium, vitamin D, calcitonin, bisphosphonates, fluoride, estrogens, and androgens) on acute or chronic exercise responses have not been extensively studied. However, there is no evidence that any of these agents would affect exercise response during testing with the possible exception of estrogen, which has an acute vasodilator effect and may alter electrocardiographic responses to exercise during an exercise test. This effect has been seen in studies using large doses of estrogen but has not been demonstrated in doses used with estrogen or HRT (3,55).

> **1.7.15-CES: Describe common gait, movement, and coordination abnormalities as they relate to exercise testing and programming.**

Osteoporosis can preclude detection of abnormal responses associated with heart diseases during an exercise test because performance may be limited by the symptoms of osteoporosis, thus preventing the individual from achieving an adequate heart rate and blood pressure response necessary for an accurate diagnosis. Severe kyphosis (rounding of the upper spine) is one such example unique to osteoporosis that may limit an exercise test because of an imposed mechanical limitation on respiratory muscle function. Ideally, a maximum effort test should be used, assuming no contraindications exist and the appropriate supervision is provided. A maximal capacity test is preferred so that more accurate exercise heart rates can be prescribed based off of the heart rate reserve method. If a maximal test is contraindicated or cannot be performed, the rating of perceived exertion (RPE) to guide exercise intensity is appropriate for this population. However, if the population is at moderate or high risk for cardiovascular disease, it would be prudent to closely assess the patient for indications of ischemia (e.g., angina equivalents) or excessive exercise intensity (e.g., excessive heart rate or blood pressure responses).

Exercise Prescription in Patients with Osteoporosis

> **1.7.41-HFS: Ability to adapt frequency, intensity, duration, mode, progression, level of supervision, and monitoring technique in exercise programs for patients with controlled chronic disease (e.g., heart disease, diabetes mellitus, obesity, hypertension), with musculoskeletal problems (including fatigue), during pregnancy and/or postpartum, and with exercise-induced asthma.**

> **1.7.4-CES: Design, implement, and supervise individualized exercise prescriptions for people with chronic disease and disabling conditions and people who are young or elderly.**

> **1.5.8-CES: Recognize patient clinical need for referral to other (non-ES) allied health professionals (e.g., behavioralist, physical therapist, diabetes educator, nurse, etc.).**

> **1.5.9-CES: Recognize patients with chronic pain who may be in a chronic pain management treatment program and who may require special adaptations during exercise testing and training.**

> **1.7.8-CES: Demonstrate exercise equipment adaptations necessary for different age groups, different**

physical abilities, and other potential contributing factors.

> **1.5.10-CES: Recognize exercise testing and training needs of patients with joint replacements or prostheses.**

Prior to prescribing exercise for the patient with osteoporosis, especially those who have recently experienced a fracture, an exercise professional should consult with the clients' physician. For patients with debilitating osteoporosis and severe pain or recent joint replacement, exercise program options will be limited. These patients should typically work with a physical therapist or rehabilitation specialist until mobile. There is a high prevalence of back pain in patients with osteoporosis, which is related to limited functional ability (60). Thus, pain management may be an important part of the care for osteoporotic individuals. It may be necessary to begin exercise prescription with a warm-pool-based program (e.g., hydrotherapy), which, although non-weight-bearing, can improve flexibility and muscle strength. In light of the rapid and profound effects of immobilization and bed rest on bone loss, and the poor prognosis for recovery of bone mineral content after remobilization, even the frailest elderly people should remain as physically active as their health permits to preserve skeletal integrity. If a person cannot tolerate active exercises, functional electrical stimulation may improve vital muscle strength in preparation for active strengthening as pain diminishes (51).

> **1.3.30-CES: Discuss the appropriate use of static and dynamic resistance exercise for individuals with cardiovascular, pulmonary, and metabolic disease.**

> **1.2.3-HFS: Knowledge of risk factors that may be favorably modified by physical activity habits.**

As stated in the ACSM position stand on physical activity and bone health (54), "exercise programs for elderly women and men should include not only weight-bearing endurance and resistance activities aimed at preserving bone mass, but also activities designed to improve balance and prevent falls." However, few well-designed trials have tested the efficacy of such programs. A 20-week strength, posture, and balance program, Osteofit, improved dynamic balance in females with osteoporosis. In a study of females with a history of spinal fracture, a 10-week balance, strengthening, stretching, and relaxation program resulted in a significant reduction in pain and use of analgesia and increased quality of life (73). In both men and women with osteoporosis, 12 months of balance and strength training resulted in improved BMD, balance, and aerobic capacity (57). Although these trials indicate that exercise has beneficial effects on *surrogates* of osteoporotic fracture, well-designed studies with fracture endpoints are needed to fur-

ther guide exercise prescription in men and women with osteoporosis.

> **1.7.11-CES: Describe relative and absolute contraindications to exercise training.**

> **1.7.6-CES: Knowledge of the concept of "activities of daily living" (ADLs) and its importance in the overall rehabilitation of the individual.**

Contraindicated Exercises for Individuals with Osteoporosis

Several general types of exercise are contraindicated for people with osteoporosis because they can generate large forces on relatively weak bone. Twisting movements (e.g., golf swing), dynamic abdominal exercises (e.g., sit-ups), and excessive trunk flexion should all be avoided because they can all result in vertebral fracture. Osteoporotic individuals should be taught correct form for ADLs such as bending to pick up objects to avoid vertebral fractures. Furthermore, exercises that involve abrupt or explosive loading, or high-impact loading, are contraindicated in persons with osteoporosis.

Flexibility Training for Individuals with Osteoporosis

A program to increase flexibility can also benefit osteoporotic patients because decreased flexibility can cause problems with posture. However, many of the commonly prescribed exercises for increasing flexibility, especially of the hamstring muscles, involve spinal flexion and must be avoided. There is little consensus on the optimal training program for increasing flexibility in individuals with osteoporosis, but good suggestions are available from many sources including Chapter 7 of the ACSM's eighth edition of the *Guidelines for Exercise Testing and Prescription* and Pearlmutter et al. (89). As with resistance training, slow and controlled movements should be the rule with stretching; ballistic-type stretching should be avoided.

Aerobic Training for Individuals with Osteoporosis

The primary reasons for prescribing aerobic exercise for those with osteoporosis are to increase aerobic fitness and work capacity, decrease cardiovascular disease risk factors, help maintain bone strength, and improve balance. Aerobic exercise for those with osteoporosis should primarily involve weight-bearing modes of exercise such as walking. For those with more significant osteoporosis-induced pain who cannot tolerate weight-bearing activities, cycling, swimming, or water aerobics are possible alternatives. Aerobic exercise should be performed according to the ACSM's eighth edition of the *Guidelines for Exercise Testing*, approximately 3–5 days per week at an intensity of 40% to 70% of $\dot{V}O_2$ reserve or heart rate reserve (HRR). An initial goal of 20–30 minutes per session is reasonable but may be shorter at the beginning in cases of extreme deconditioning. Orthopedic limitations may slow progress or mandate the use of additional supports, such as handrails for walking. Once 20–30 minutes becomes well tolerated, the duration can slowly be increased in much the same fashion as with healthy populations. If the individual is severely limited by pain, the physician should be consulted prior to exercise participation. Aerobic exercises that involve forward flexion of the spine such as rowing should be avoided.

> **1.7.20-CES: Discuss the appropriate use of static and dynamic resistance exercise for individuals with cardiovascular, pulmonary, and cardiovascular disease.**

Resistance Training in Patients with Osteoporosis

Resistance training offers a good option to meet both the bone health and falls prevention criteria on an individual basis. Resistance training requires little skill and has the added advantage of being highly adaptable to changes in both magnitude and strain distribution. In addition, increases in strength and muscle size have been demonstrated after resistance training, even in elderly individuals, which has the added benefit of reducing these patients' risk of falls (17,19,93).

Improving muscle strength helps to conserve bone and muscle mass and enhance dynamic balance. Resistance training with free weights, machines, calisthenics, and elastic bands are recommended for osteoporotic populations with the loads ideally being directed over the long axis of the bone (axial loading). A resistance exercise prescription, for individuals at risk for osteoporosis, should follow the FITT principal outlined in the ACSM's *Guidelines for Exercise Testing* that recommends 2 to 3 days per week, of 8–12 repetitions, at a moderate (60%–80%) intensity of one time the repetition maximum (1-RM). For those with established osteoporosis, the only limitation in this exercise prescription should be to limit the resistance training intensity to the moderate level because of the risk of fracture. Additionally, those with osteoporosis should avoid any ballistic or jumping activities that are recommended for those who are at risk. The overall goal for both groups is to perform weight-bearing and resistance exercise for 30–60 minutes each exercise session.

REFERENCES

1. U.S. Preventive Services Task Force. Clinical guidelines: screening for osteoporosis in postmenopausal women: recommendations and rationale. *Ann Intern Med.* 2002;137:526–8.
2. American College of Sports Medicine. ACSM position stand on the female athlete triad. *Med Sci Sports Exerc.* 1997;29:i–ix.
3. American College of Sports Medicine. ACSM position stand on osteoporosis and exercise. *Med Sci Sports Exerc.* 1995;27:i–vii.
4. Arlot ME, Sornay-Rendu E, Garnero P, Vey-Marty B, Delmas PD. Apparent pre- and postmenopausal bone loss evaluated by DXA at different skeletal sites in women: the OFELY cohort. *J Bone Miner Res.* 1997;12:683–90.
5. Bachrach LK. Assessing bone health in children: who to test and what does it mean? *Pediatr Endocrinol Rev.* 2005;2(Suppl 3):332–6.
6. Bailey D, McCulloch R. Osteoporosis: are there childhood antecedents for an adult health problem? *Canadian J Ped.* 1992;4:130–4.
7. Bailey DA, Faulkner RA, McKay HA. Growth, physical activity, and bone mineral acquisiton. In: Holloszy JO, editor. *Exerc Sport Sci Rev.* Williams & Wilkins; 1996. p. 233–66.
8. Bailey DA, Maring AD, McKay HA, et al. Calcium accretion in girls and boys during puberty: a longitudinal analysis. *J Bone Miner Res.* 2000;15:2245–50.
9. Bailey DA, McKay HA, Mirwald RL, et al. A six year longitudinal study of the relationship of physical activity to bone mineral accrual in growing children: the University of Saskatchewan Bone Mineral Accrual Study. *J Bone Miner Res.* 1999;14:1672–9.
10. Barr SI, McKay HA. Nutrition, exercise and bone status in youth. *Int J Sport Nutr.* 1998;8:124–42.
11. Bass SL, Eser P, Daly R. The effect of exercise and nutrition on the mechanostat. *J Musculoskelet Neuronal Interact.* 2005;5:239–254.
12. Bassey EJ, Ramsdale SJ. Increase in femoral bone mineral density in young women following high impact exercise. *Osteoporosis Int.* 1994;4:72–5.
13. Beck TJ, Orekovic TL, Stone KL, et al. Structural adaptation to changing skeletal load in the progression toward hip fragility: the study of osteoporotic fractures. *J Bone Miner Res.* 2001;16:1108–19.
14. Blimkie C, Rice S, Webber C. Effects of resistance training on bone mineral content and density in adolescent females. *Can J Physiol Pharmacol.* 1996;74:1025–33.
15. Bradney M, Pearce G, Naughton G, et al. Moderate exercise during growth in prepubertal boys: changes in bone mass, size, volumetric density, and bone strength: a controlled prospective study. *J Bone Miner Res.* 1998;13:1814–21.
16. Burger H, de Lact C, vanDaele PL, et al. Risk factors for increased bone loss in an elderly population: the Rotterdam Study. *Am J Epidemiol.* 1998;147:871–79.
17. Carter ND, Kannus P, Khan KM. Exercise in the prevention of falls in older people: a systematic literature review examining the rational and the evidence. *Sports Med.* 2001;31:427–38.
18. Carter ND, Khan KM, Petit MA, et al. Results of a 10 week community based strength and balance training in 65–75 year old women with osteoporosis. *Br J Sports Med.* 2001;35:348–51.
19. Chilibeck PD, Sale DG, Webber CE. Exercise and bone mineral density. *Sports Med.* 1995;19:103–22.
20. Cooper C. Epidemiology of osteoporosis. *Osteoporos Int.* 1999;9:S2–S8.
21. Cummings SR, Melton L. Epidemiology and outcomes of osteoporotic fractures. *Lancet.* 2002;359:1761–7.
22. Currey JD. *Bones.* 2nd ed. Princeton (NJ): Princeton University Press; 2002.
23. Daly R, Saxon L, Turner C, et al. The relationship between muscle size and bone geometry during growth and in response to exercise. *Bone.* 2004;34:281–7.
24. Daly RM, Petit MA. *Optimizing Bone Mass and Strength: The Role of Physical Activity and Nutrition.* Basel: Karger, 2007.
25. Delmas PD, Genant HK, Crans CG, et al. Severity of prevalent vertebral fractures and the risk of subsequent vertebral and nonvertebral fractures: results from the MORE trial. *Bone.* 2003;33:522–32.
26. Faulkner RA, Bailey DA. Osteoporosis: a pediatric concern? *Med Sport Sci.* 2007;51:1–12.
27. Forwood MR, Baxter-Jones AD, Beck TJ, et al. Physical activity and strength of the femoral neck during the adolescent growth spurt: a longitudinal analysis. *Bone.* 2006;38:576–83.
28. Forwood MR, Burr DB. Physical activity and bone mass: exercises in futility? *Bone Miner.* 1993;21:89–112.
29. Friedlander AH, Jones LJ. The biology, medical management, and podiatric implications of menopause. *J Am Podiatr Med Assoc.* 2002;92:437–43.

30. Friedlander AL, Genant HK, Sadowsky S, et al. A two-year program of aerobics and weight training enhances bone mineral density of young women. *J Bone Miner Res*. 1995;10:574–85.

31. Frost HM. Bone's mechanostat: a 2003 update. *Anat Rec Part A*. 2003;275A:1081–101.

32. Fuchs RK, Bauer JJ, Snow CM. Jumping improves hip and lumbar spine bone mass in prepubescent children: a randomized controlled trial. *J Bone Miner Res*. 2001;16:148–56.

33. Garn SM. *The Earlier Gain and Later Loss of Cortical Bone*. Springfield (IL): CC Thomas; 1970.

34. Gass M, Dawson-Hughes B. Preventing osteoporosis-related fractures: an overview. *Am J Med*. 2006;119:3S–11S.

35. **Genant HK, Cooper C, Poor G, et al. Interim report and recommendations of the World Health Organization Task-Force for Osteoporosis. *Osteoporos Int*. 1999;10:259–64.**

36. Guesens P, Autier P, Boonen S, et al. The relationship among history of falls, osteoporosis, and fractures in postmenopausal women. *Arch Phys Med Rehabil*. 2002;83:903–6.

37. Haapasalo H, Kannus P, Sievanen H, et al. Development of mass, density, and estimated mechanical characteristics of bones in Caucasian females. *J Bone Miner Res*. 1996;11:1751–60.

38. Heinonen, A., Kannus P, Sievanen H, et al. Randomized controlled trial of effect of high-impact exercise on selected risk factors for osteoporotic fractures. *Lancet*. 1996;348:1343–7.

39. Heinonen A, Sievanen H, Kannus P, et al. High-impact exercise and bones of growing girls: a 9-month controlled trial. *Osteoporosis Int*. 2000;11:1010–7.

40. Janz K, Burns T, Levy S, et al. Everyday activity predicts bone geometry in children: the Iowa bone development study. *Med Sci Sports Exerc*. 2004;36:1124–31.

41. Jarvinen T, Kannus P. Sievanen H. Have the DXA-based exercise studies seriously underestimated the effects of mechanical loading on bone? *J Bone Miner Res*. 1999;14:1634–5.

42. Johnell O. The socioeconomic burden of fractures: today and in the 21st century. *Am J Med*. 1997;103:20S–26S.

43. Judex S, Boyd S, Qin Y-X, et al. Adaptations of trabecular bone to low magnitude vibrations result in more uniform stress and strain under load. *Annal Biomed Engin*. 2003;31:12–20.

44. Kanis JA. Diagnosis of osteoporosis and assessment of fracture risk. *Lancet*. 2002;359:1929–1936.

45. **Kanis JA, Gluer CC. An update on the diagnosis and assessment of osteoporosis with densitometry: Committee of Scientific Advisors, International Osteoporosis Foundation. *Osteoporos Int*. 2000;11:192–202.**

46. Kanis JA, Johnell O, Oden A, et al. Ten year probabilities of osteoporotic fractures according to BMD and diagnostic thresholds. *Osteoporos Int*. 2001;12:989–95.

47. Kannus P. Preventing osteoporosis, falls, and fractures among elderly people. *Br Med J*. 1999;318:205–6.

48. Kannus P, Haapasalo H, Sankelo M, et al. Effect of starting age of physical activity on bone mass in the dominant arm of tennis and squash players. *Ann Intern Med*. 1995;123:27–31.

49. Kannus P, Haapasalo H, Sievanen H, et al. The site-specific effects of long-term unilateral activity on bone mineral density and content. *Bone*. 1994;15:279–84.

50. Kazakia GJ, Majumdar S. New imaging technologies in the diagnosis of osteoporosis. *Rev Endocr Metab Disord*. 2006;7:67–74.

51. Khan K, Mckay H, Kannus P, et al. *Physical Activity and Bone Health*. Champaign (IL): Human Kinetics; 2001.

52. Khan KM, Liu-Ambrose T, Sran MM, et al. New criteria for female athlete triad syndrome? As osteoporosis is rare, should osteopenia be among the criteria for defining the female athlete triad syndrome? *Br J Sports Med*. 2002;36:10–13.

53. Klotzbuecher CM, Ross PD, Landsman PB, et al. Patients with prior fractures have increased risk of future fractures: a summary of the literature and statistical synthesis. *J Bone Miner Res*. 2000; 15:721–7.

54. **Kohrt WM, Bloomfield SA, Little KD, et al. American College of Sports Medicine position stand: physical activity and bone health. *Med Sci Sports Exerc*. 2004;36:1985–96.**

55. Kohrt WM, Ehsani AA, Birge SJ. HRT preserves increases in bone mineral density and reductions in body fat after a supervised exercise program. *J Appl Physiol*. 1998;S4:1506–12.

56. Kontulainen S, Kannus P, Haapasalo H, et al. Good maintenance of exercise-induced bone gain with decreased training of female tennis and squash players: a prospective 5-year follow-up study of young and old starters and controls. *J Bone Miner Res*. 2001; 16:195–201.

57. Kronhed AC, Moller M. Effects of physical exercise on bone mass, balance skill and aerobic capacity in women and men with low bone mineral density, after one year of training—a prospective study. *Scand J Med Sci Sports*. 1998;8:290–8.

58. Labovitz JM, Revill K. Osteoporosis: pathogenesis, new therapies and surgical implications. *Clin Podiatr Med Surg*. 2007;24:311–32.

59. Lane NE. Epidemiology, etiology, and diagnosis of osteoporosis. *Am J Obstet Gynecol*. 2006;194:S3–S11.

60. Liu-Ambrose T, Eng JJ, Khan KM, et al. The influence of back pain on balance and functional mobility in 65- to 75-year-old women with osteoporosis. *Osteoporos Int*. 2002;13:868–73.

61. Liu-Ambrose T, Khan KM, Eng JJ, et al. Resistance and agility training reduce fall risk in women aged 75 to 85. *J Am Geriatr Soc*. 2004;52:657–65.

62. Liu-Ambrose TY, Khan KM, Eng JJ, et al. The beneficial effects of group-based exercises on fall risk profile and physical activity persist 1 year postintervention in older women with low bone mass: follow-up after withdrawal of exercise. *J Am Geriatr Soc*. 2005;53:1767–73.

63. Lloyd T, Petit MA, Lin HM, Beck TJ. Lifestyle factors and the development of bone mass and bone strength in young women. *J Pediatr*. 2004;144:776–82.

64. Lohman T, Going S, Pamenter R, et al. Effects of resistance training on regional and total bone mineral density in premenopausal women: a randomized prospective study. *J Bone Miner Res*. 1995; 10:1015–24.

65. Lord SR, Sambrook PN, Gilbert C, et al. Postural stability, falls and fractures in the elderly: results from the Dubbo Osteoporosis Epidemiology Study. *Med J Aust*. 1994;6:684–91.

66. Loro ML, Sayre J, Roe TF, et al. Early identification of children predisposed to low peak bone mass and osteoporosis later in life. *J Clin Endocrinol Metab*. 2000;85:3908–18.

67. Loucks AB, Verdun M, Heath EM. Low energy availability, not stress of exercise, alters LH pulsatility in exercising women. *J Appl Physiol*. 1998;84:37–46.

68. MacKelvie KJ, Khan KM, McKay HA. Is there a critical period for bone response to weight-bearing exercise in children and adolescents? A systematic review. *Br J Sports Med*. 2002;36:250–7.

69. MacKelvie KJ, Khan KM, Petit MA, et al. A school-based exercise intervention elicits substantial bone health benefits: a 2-year randomized controlled trial in girls. *Pediatrics*. 2003;112:e447–e452.

70. MacKelvie KJ, McKay HA, Khan KM, Crocker PRE. Defining the window of opportunity: a school-based loading intervention augments bone mineral accrual in early, but not pre-, pubertal girls. *J Pediatr*. 2001;139:501–8.

71. MacKelvie KJ, McKay HA, Petit MA, et al. Bone mineral response to a 7-month randomized controlled, school-based jumping intervention in 121 prepubertal boys: associations with ethnicity and body mass index. *J Bone Miner Res*. 2002;17:834–44.

72. MacKelvie KJ, Petit MA, Khan KM, et al. Bone mass and structure are enhanced following a 2-year randomized controlled trial of exercise in prepubertal boys. *Bone*. 2004;34:755–64.

73. Malmros B, Mortenson L, Jensen MB, et al. Positive effects of physiotherapy on chronic pain and performance in osteoporosis. *Osteoporos Int*. 1998;8:215–21.

74. McKay HA, Khan KM. Bone mineral acquisition during childhood and adolescence: physical activity as a preventative measure. In: Henderson JE, Goltzman D, editors. *The Osteoporosis Primer*. Cambridge: Cambridge University Press; 2000. p. 170–84.

75. McKay HA, MacLean L, Petit MA, et al. "Bounce at the Bell": a novel program of short bouts of exercise improves proximal femur bone mass in early pubertal children. *Br J Sports Med*. 2005;39:521–6.

76. McKay HA, Petit MA, Schutz RW, et al. Augmented trochanteric bone mineral density after modified physical education classes: a randomized school-based exercise intervention study in prepubescent and early pubescent children. *J Pediatr*. 2000;136:156–62.

77. Melton LJ, Cooper C. Magnitude and impact of osteoporosis and fractures. In: Marcus R, Feldman D, Kelsey J, editors. *Osteoporosis*. San Diego: Academic Press; 2001. p. 557–67.

78. Menkes A, Mazel S, Redmond R, et al. Strength training increases regional bone mineral density and bone remodeling in middle-aged and older men. *J Appl Physiol*. 1993;74:2478–84.

79. Morris FL, Naughton GA, Gibbs JL, et al. Prospective 10-month exercise intervention in pre-menarcheal girls: positive effects on bone and lean mass. *J Bone Miner Res*. 1997;12:1453–62.

80. Moyad MA. Osteoporosis, part I: risk factors and screening. *Urol Nurs*. 2002;22:276–9.

81. Nagaraja S, Couse TL, Guldberg RE. Trabecular bone microdamage and microstructural stresses under uniaxial compression. *J Biomech*. 2005;38:707–16.

82. National Osteoporosis Foundation. *American's Bone Health: The State of Osteoporosis and Low Bone Mass*. Washington (DC): National Osteoporosis Foundation; 2002.

83. National Osteoporosis Foundation. *Physician's Guide to Prevention and Treatment of Osteoporosis*. Washington (DC): National Osteoporosis Foundation; 2003.

84. Nelson ME, Fiatore MA, Morganti CM, et al. Effects of high-intensity strength training on multiple risk factors for osteoporotic fractures: a randomized controlled trial. *JAMA*. 1994;272:1909–14.

85. **National Institute of Health. *NIH Consensus: Osteoporosis, Prevention, Diagnosis, and Therapy*. NIH Consensus Statement 17; March 27–29, 2000.**

86. Orwoll ES. Osteoporosis in men: epidemiology, pathophysiology and clinical characterization. In: Marcus R, Feldman D, Kelsey J, editors. *Osteoporosis*. San Diego: Academic Press; 1996.

87. Parfitt AM. Targeted and nontargeted bone remodeling: relationship to basic multicellular unit origination and progression. *Bone*. 2002;30:5–7.

88. Parfitt AM. The two faces of growth: benefits and risks to bone integrity. *Osteoporosis Int*. 1994;4:382–98.

89. Pearlmutter LL, Bode BY, Wildinson WE, Maricic MH. Shoulder range of motion in patients with osteoporosis. *Arthritis Care Res*. 1995;8:194–8.

90. Petit MA, Beck TJ, Lin HM, et al. Femoral bone structural geometry adapts to mechanical loading and is influenced by sex steroids: the Penn State Young Women's Health Study. *Bone*. 2004;35:750–9.

91. Ravn P, Hetland ML, Overgaard K, Christiansen C. Premenopausal and postmenopausal changes in bone mineral density of the proximal femur measured by dual-energy X-ray absorptiometry. *J Bone Miner Res*. 1994;9:1975–80.

92. Recker RR. Skeletal fragility and bone quality. *J Musculoskelet Neuronal Interact*. 2007;7:54–5.

93. Robertson MC, Campbell AJ, Gardner MM, Devlin N. Preventing injuries in older people by preventing falls: a meta-analysis of individual-level data. *J Am Geriatr Soc*. 2002;50:905–11.

94. Robling AG, Burr DB, Turner CH. Recovery periods restore mechanosensitivity to dynamically loaded bone. *J Exp Biol*. 2001;204:3389–99.

95. Robling AG, Castillo AB, Turner CH. Biomechanical and molecular regulation of bone remodeling. *Annu Rev Biomed Eng*. 2006; Apr. 3.

96. Rubin C, Turner AS, Bain S, et al. Low mechanical signals strengthen long bones. *Nature (London)*. 2001;412:603–4.

97. Rubin CT, Sommerfeldt DW, Judex S, Qin Y. Inhibition of osteopenia by low magnitude, high-frequency mechanical stimuli. *Drug Discov Today*. 2001;15:848–58.

98. Ryan AS, Treuth MS, Rubin MA, et al. Effects of strength training on bone mineral density: hormonal and bone turnover relationships. *J Appl Physiol*. 1994;77:1678–84.

99. Seeman E. From density to structure: growing up and old on the surfaces of bone. *J Bone Miner Res*. 1997;12:509–21.

100. Seeman E. Pathogenesis of bone fragility in women and men. *Lancet*. 2002;359:1841–50.

101. Seeman E, Delmas PD. Bone quality—the material and structural basis of bone strength and fragility. *N Engl J Med*. 2006;25:2250–61.

102. Sinaki M, Wahner HW, Bergstralh EJ, et al. Three-year controlled, randomized trial of the effect of dose-specified loading and strengthening exercises on bone mineral density of spine and femur in nonathletic, physically active women. *Bone*. 1996;19:233–44.

103. Snow-Harter C, Bouxsein M, Lewis B, et al. Effects of resistance and endurance exercise on bone mineral status of young women: a randomized exercise intervention trial. *J Bone Miner Res*. 1992;7:761–9.

104. Snow-Harter C, Marcus R. Exercise, bone mineral density, and osteoporosis. *Exerc Sport Sci Rev*. 1991;19:351–88.

105. Srinivasan S, Agans SC, King KA, et al. Enabling bone formation in the aged skeleton via rest-inserted mechanical loading. *Bone*. 2003;33:946–55.

106. Turner CH, Robling AG. Designing exercise regimens to increase bone strength. *Exerc Sport Sci Rev*. 2003;31:45–50.

107. Valdimarsson O, Linden C, Johnell O, et al. Daily physical education in the school curriculum in prepubertal girls during 1 year is followed by an increase in bone mineral accrual and bone width—data from the prospective controlled Malmo Pediatric Osteoporosis Prevention Study. *Calcif Tissue Int*. 2006;78:65–71.

108. Vanderschueren D, Venken K, Ophoff J, et al. Clinical review: sex steroids and the periosteum—reconsidering the roles of androgens and estrogens in periosteal expansion. *J Clin Endocrinol Metab*. 2006;91:378–82.

109. VanStaa TP, Leufkens HGM, Abenhaim L, et al. Use of oral corticosteroids and risk of fractures. *J Bone Miner Res*. 2001;16:581–8.

110. Wei TS, Hu CH, Wang SH, Hwang KL. Fall characteristics, functional mobility and bone mineral density as risk factors of hip fracture in the community-dwelling ambulatory elderly. *Osteoporos Int*. 2001;12:1050–5.

111. Witzke KA, Snow CM. Effects of plyometric jump training on bone mass in adolescent girls. *Med Sci Sport Exerc*. 2000;32:1051–7.

112. **World Health Organization. *Assessment of Fracture Risk and Its Application to Screening for Postmenopausal Osteoporosis*. Geneva: World Health Organization; 1994. p. 1–129.**

113. Zioupos P. Accumulation of in-vivo fatigue microdamage and its relation to biomechanical properties in ageing human cortical bone. *J Microsc*. 2001;201:270–8.

SELECTED REFERENCES FOR FURTHER READING

Daly RM, Petit MA, editors. *Optimizing Bone Mass and Strength: The Role of Physical Activity and Nutrition*. Karger Pubs. Med Sci Sports Exerc vol. 51; 2007.

Lord S, Sherrington C, Menz HB. *Falls in Older People: Risk Factors and Strategies for Prevention*. Cambridge: Cambridge University Press; 2000.

Khan K, McKay HA, Kannus P et al. *Physical Activity and Bone Health*. Champaign (IL): Human Kinetics; 2001.

Kohrt WM et al. Amercian College of Sports Medicine position stand: physical activity and bone health. *Med Sci Sports Exerc*. 2004;36:1985–96.

INTERNET RESOURCES

- Action Schools BC: http://www.actionschoolsbc.ca/Content/Home.asp
- American Academy of Physical Medicine and Rehabilitation: How PM&R Physicians Use Exercise to Prevent and Treat Osteoporosis: http://www.aapmr.org/condtreat/other/osteotreat.htm
- American Society of Bone and Mineral Research: Webcast on Bone Quality: What Is It and Can We Measure It?" http://aap2capital-reach.com/esp1204/servlet/tc?cn=asbmr&c=10169&s=20292&e=4 521&& American Society of Bone and Mineral Research: Bone Curriculum: http://depts.washington.edu/bonebio/ASBMRed/ASBMRed.html
- Mayo Clinic: Exercise and Osteoporosis: http://www.mayoclinic.com/ health/osteoporosis/HQ00643
- National Institutes of Health: Osteoporosis and Related Bone Diseases National Resource Center: http://www.niams.nih.gov/bone/
- National Osteoporosis Foundation: http://www.nof.org/
- Osteofit: http://www.osteofit.org/
- Prevention of Falls Network Europe (ProFaNE): http://www.profane.eu.org/
- U.S. Bone and Joint Decade: http://www.usbjd.org/

Exercise Prescription in Those with Arthritis

> **1.7.4-CES:** Design, implement, and supervise individualized exercise prescriptions for people with chronic disease and disabling conditions, or who are young or elderly.

> **5.2.1-HFS:** Knowledge of musculoskeletal risk factors or conditions that may require consultation with medical personnel before testing or training, including acute or chronic back pain, osteoarthritis, rheumatoid arthritis, osteoporosis, inflammation/pain, and low-back pain.

More than 100 arthritic diseases and conditions have been identified, with muscle and/or joint involvement being the commonality. The most common types include **osteoarthritis (OA)**, **fibromyalgia**, and **rheumatoid arthritis (RA)**. An additional group of arthritic diseases that have special exercise needs fall into a category called **spondyloarthropathies**, of which the most common is **ankylosing spondylitis (AS)** (3). Between 2003 and 2005, more than 46 million Americans reported having physician-diagnosed arthritis. This represents more than 21% of the adult population (one in every five adults); past the age of 65, the percentage increases to approximately 50% (17).

The economic, social, and psychological costs of arthritis are significant. Arthritis is currently the leading cause of disability in the United States, with 18.9 million (8.3% of the population) reporting limitations in activity because of their arthritis (Fig. 40-1). Within the next few decades, the total number with arthritis is projected to increase to 67 million, with an even larger percentage in the 65-and-older age group than in the current population (55). The estimated total cost attributable to arthritis, both direct and indirect, was $128 billion in 2003 (18).

There are no current estimates of the frequency of each type of arthritis, but earlier studies give some idea of the potential distribution. Osteoarthritis is the most prevalent form of arthritis, with almost 85% of all those affected having this joint-specific problem. Although the other arthritis forms have lower prevalence, their pathologies are systemic. Thus, the resultant impact on the individual is often significant. Fibromyalgia has an estimated prevalence of 2% of the U.S. population (3.7 million) (63), whereas rheumatoid arthritis is approximately 1% (>2.1 million persons) (17). Ankylosing spondylitis affects roughly 1% to 2% of the population (130 out of 100,000 individuals). Its distribution is atypical of the rheumatic diseases, as it is more prevalent

> > > KEY TERMS

COX-1: An enzyme that is necessary for normal physiologic function of the stomach, kidney, and platelets.

COX-2: An enzyme involved in the production of prostaglandin, which produces inflammation and contributes to acute pain.

Cytokines: Small proteins that can either step up or step down the immune response.

Cyclo-oxygenase (COX): An enzyme found in two main forms, COX-1 and COX-2.

Fibromyalgia: A rheumatologic syndrome characterized by chronic widespread pain in the muscles, ligaments, and joints.

Osteoarthritis: A degenerative disease that affects the articular cartilage and the underlying subchondral bone.

Rheumatoid arthritis: An inflammatory disease with the major symptoms of pain, swelling, stiffness, and reduced joint mobility.

Spondyloarthropathy: A rheumatic disease that causes inflammation and calcification of joints, especially present in the spine.

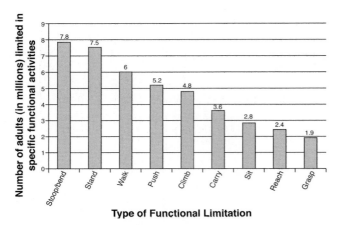

FIGURE 40-1. Specific functional activity limitations for adults with arthritis. (From: 2002 National Health Interview Survey Arthritis Surveillance Fact Sheet: www.cdc.gov/arthritis/data_statistics/ national_data_nhis.htm#impact.)

in men than women (3). Other forms of arthritis, such as gout, compose the rest of the arthritic population.

OSTEOARTHRITIS

Osteoarthritis (OA), also known as degenerative joint disease, is joint specific. The joints in the hands have the greatest prevalence of arthritis. The most common weight-bearing joints that are affected are the knees, followed by the hips (26,33,63).

CLINICAL FEATURES AND DIAGNOSIS

The primary symptom with OA is joint pain and stiffness, usually associated with degeneration of the joint cartilage (Fig. 40-2). However, the relationship between radiographic diagnosis of OA and the presence of symptoms is not predictable. Only 25% to 50% of people with radiographic evidence of OA have symptoms, whereas others

with severe symptoms sometimes have limited medical evidence of OA (2,33,63). Thus, diagnosis is based on several different features and can include both laboratory and clinical tests, radiographic and clinical results, or purely clinical features. For the knee, the criteria for a clinical diagnosis include age older than 50 years, stiffness lasting less than 30 minutes, crepitus (crackling sound), bony tenderness, bony enlargement, and no palpable warmth of the joint (2).

As the joint structure alters, motion becomes limited, and the muscles adjacent to the joint atrophy. Several studies have identified significant weakness in the quadriceps muscles, although it is not known whether this weakness happens before or results from the joint disease (38,56).

Because of the loss of motion of the joint and muscle atrophy, physical mobility is decreased. Functional assessment usually reflects difficulties with activities of daily living that require the involved joints. Thus, individuals with arthritis in the upper extremities report problems with lifting, carrying, and dressing, whereas those with lower-extremity arthritis have problems with climbing stairs, ambulation, and getting in and out of a chair. As mobility declines and pain and stiffness increase, loss of independence and quality of life occur (26,33).

ETIOLOGY

The etiology of primary OA has not yet been identified, although numerous factors have been shown to increase the risk of developing OA. Aging used to be considered the cause of OA, however, although it is a risk factor, evidence suggests that aging alone does not cause the changes associated with OA. An examination of other risk factors reveals some of the rationale for proposed etiologies of OA. The most common risk factors include previous injury to the joint, malalignment of the joint, and obesity. Any of these can result in abnormal load distributions in the joint, which alters the accompanying biomechanics. These risk factors have not only been correlated to the development of arthritis, but also to the progression of the disease.

Burr and Radin hypothesize that initial failure to absorb the altered loads results in microcracks in the subchondral tissue and reactivation of the secondary center of ossification (14). These primary changes lead to a cascading cycle: thinning of the articular cartilage, leading to increased joint stresses and loads. On radiographs, the progression of arthritis is observed as joint-space narrowing, followed by changes in the subchondral bone and osteophyte (bone spur) formation along the joint line (69). As the cartilage degrades, more stress is transmitted to the underlying bone, resulting in further deformation and decreased shock-absorbing capability (57). Although this proposed etiology of arthritis has yet to be confirmed,

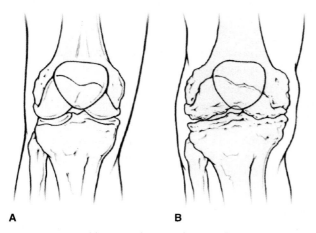

A   **B**

FIGURE 40-2. Healthy (**A**) and osteoarthritic (**B**) knees.

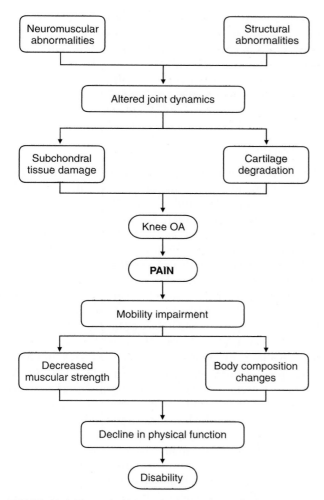

FIGURE 40-3. Theoretical biomechanical pathways for knee osteoarthritis (OA) and subsequent disability.

others have similarly proposed that an increase of abnormal loads may result in OA (see Fig. 40-3). Several studies have found either abnormal external knee adduction or extension moments in individuals with OA (1,73). Furthermore, some have noted an association between altered biomechanics and the severity and progression of OA (8,73,74,94,104,105). One potential cause of a change in biomechanics and load absorption is injury. A phenomenon that has been identified following injury to the knee is quadriceps activation failure (QAF). Additionally, individuals with knee OA have been shown to have more QAF than those without OA, regardless of age of sex (56). Fitzgerald et al. suggested that the activation failure moderates the interaction between quadriceps strength and function (38).

Although not necessarily the cause of OA, inflammation is present and appears to be related to progression of the disease. Inflammatory cytokines (interleukin-1 beta [IL-1beta]) have been found in the joint fluids of patients with OA. Others have found increased serum concentrations of cytokines (interleukin-6 [IL-6], tumor necrosis

factor alpha [TNF-alpha]) and another inflammatory marker, acute phase reactant C-reactive protein (CRP), in individuals with OA (87,103,107). Several longitudinal studies have shown that elevated serum levels of specific cytokines predicts the progression of knee OA, as determined by radiographic changes in the joint (42,61,88, 103,117). Importantly, some of these studies have shown that the level of inflammatory marker in the blood was related to the individual's functional status and severity (both pain and radiographic evidence) of joint disease (88,117). It has been suggested that the cytokines may be one factor affecting cartilage loss observed in OA, as the cytokines may stimulate catabolism of the articular cartilage and inhibit chondrocyte formation (90).

Although it has been noted that obesity is a risk factor for the development and progression of OA, this relationship has usually been attributed to the increased loads that are transmitted to the lower-extremity joints. However, Nicklas et al. note that individuals who are obese have higher concentrations of inflammatory markers than individuals who are not overweight (86). Furthermore, they showed that those who lost weight also had decreases in CRP, IL-6, and TNF-alpha receptor 1 levels as compared with controls. Thus, inflammation may be an important mediator related to the progression of the disease and function for individuals who are obese (86).

TREATMENTS

Although exercise was initially used to maintain or improve function, many studies have found that it can reduce pain. The use of supplements has been investigated, initially for proposed effects on cartilage and later for potential pain mediation. Medical treatment is focused on pain relief, usually through the use of anti-inflammatory medications. When medications are not enough to control pain, orthopedic procedures directed at the joint are utilized.

Exercise Response

Early studies on individuals with arthritis showed deficits in strength, flexibility, and aerobic capacity as compared with age-matched individuals without arthritis. These deficits are associated with the decreased ability to perform activities of daily living. Much of the difference appears because of a more sedentary lifestyle. As the joint becomes painful and stiff, the tendency is to decrease activity in an effort not to exacerbate the problem. However, numerous studies have shown that most exercise does not aggravate the symptoms nor increase the progression of the arthritis (31).

The most common aerobic activity that has been used for training is walking. Walking programs ranged from 8 weeks to 3 months, and many of the earlier studies used low- to moderate-intensity levels for the program.

Although the assessment of aerobic capacity varies from study to study, most studies showed improved aerobic capacity and walking time in conjunction with decreases in pain and disability (11,31,61,79). A few studies have looked at jogging from the perspective of impact on the prevalence and progression of arthritis. These studies have shown that jogging neither increases the chances of developing arthritis nor the progression of the disease (12). In fact, longitudinal work has shown that runners with arthritis reported less pain and better function than sedentary individuals with arthritis (12). The use of jogging as a training method for research has been limited to jogging in the water. Although the group that jogged in the water showed improvements in aerobic capacity, endurance, and pain as compared with a control group, the results were mixed when compared with a walking program (79). Cycling has also been used successfully as a training technique in one of the few studies that compared the effect of two different training intensities (68). Patients training for 10 weeks at either 40% or 70% of heart rate reserve (HRR) reported decreased pain, which was similar in both groups despite the higher-intensity group performing nearly twice as much total work.

Water-based activities have often been promoted for those with arthritis, emphasizing the decreased load on the joints and increased comfort. However, the few studies that have used water-based activities have not focused on aerobic capacity as a measure. In a larger yearlong study, Cochrane et al. found significant improvement in quality-of-life measures and physical function for the group that exercised in the water (23).

Resistance training has been examined both as an independent exercise program and in conjunction with aerobic activities. Most programs have focused on lower-extremity resistance training and have demonstrated gains in strength and decreased pain. Improvements in strength translate to better function and balance in patients with OA (36,37). Another study found that strength training resulted in better stair-climbing ability, but the aerobic group reported better quality of life. Importantly, when resistance training was combined with aerobic training, significant improvements in balance, strength, and aerobic capacity—and decreases in disability and pain, as well as body weight—were found (32,75).

A popular alternative form of exercise, particularly with older individuals, is tai chi. Currently, there is only one published study on tai chi and OA. Although Hartman et al. found no significant changes in mobility, they did find that those who participated in the tai chi program had improved self-efficacy scores for arthritis symptoms (51).

Exercise has also been studied for its role in weight control for overweight or obese individuals with arthritis because of the relationship of body weight and arthritis. The combination of diet and exercise resulted in greater improvements in self-reported function, mobility, and pain than either of those interventions alone or a health education intervention (75,76). The authors noted that subjects who lost between 7.5% and 11.0% of their body weight had significantly better self-reported function than subjects who lost less weight or no weight at all, with an apparent dose-related response.

Exercise Prescription

Although management guidelines for OA of the knee and hip recommend exercise therapy, the specifics—such as frequency, intensity, and mode—have not been addressed. Unfortunately, there is a wide variety in the programs that have been studied. The most common frequency is 3 days/week with 1-hour sessions. However, there is no evidence to suggest that individuals with arthritis cannot follow the recommendations for 5 days/week of moderate-intensity aerobic activity. Until recently, the emphasis was on mild intensity, as many feared that higher intensities would exacerbate symptoms. However, several studies have used standard American College of Sports Medicine (ACSM) intensity guidelines without detrimental effects (11,32,77,79). As with any patient, the exercise prescription must consider the individual's current level of activity. Initial aerobic exercise should be at the lower levels of moderate intensity (~40% HRR) for individuals who have been sedentary. Additionally, some researchers have noted that the use of initial durations of 10 minutes, with several sessions per day, has been shown to improve initial adherence for patients with lower-extremity arthritis (79). Progression of intensity and duration should follow ACSM guidelines, with the goal of 30 or more minutes of continuous exercise of moderate intensity.

Resistance training has been shown to be an important component of a training program for those with arthritis (31,77). Resistance-training regimens that have been used range from body-weight activities, such as partial squats, to the use of specialized equipment (32,77). Resistance training should meet the ACSM guidelines of 2 to 3 days/week, training multiple muscle groups. Initial intensity may need to be low (10% of 1 repetitive maximum [1RM]) for individuals with severe arthritis, but loads of 40%–60% of 1RM, or the 10–15RM, are otherwise appropriate. It may be necessary to modify the activity to accommodate reductions in range of motion (ROM) because of the arthritis. Finally, individuals with arthritis often note times of increased joint pain and stiffness, sometimes accompanied by swelling. During these flare-ups, it may be wisest to decrease the intensity of the exercise program.

The third traditional component of an exercise program, flexibility, is a vital part of arthritis treatment. Flexibility and ROM activities address the stiffness and loss of motion that is a primary result of arthritis. Although there is no research on the optimal number of days per week, clinical reports suggest that daily ROM activities are best. Movement through the normal, available range, repeated 5 to 10 times, appears to decrease symptoms of stiffness and may be repeated throughout the day as needed.

Pharmacologic Treatment

The American College of Rheumatology recommends acetaminophen for patients with mild to moderate pain (54). Side effects of acetaminophen include the potential for upper gastrointestinal (GI) bleeding and liver damage. Anti-inflammatory medications have also become increasing popular as an initial therapy for OA. The most common of these medications are the nonsteroidal anti-inflammatory drugs (NSAIDs). NSAIDs include aspirin, ibuprofen, and naproxen. They exert anti-inflammatory and usually analgesic actions through their inhibition of the enzyme **cyclo-oxygenase (COX)** (see Key Terms). Side effects include an increased chance of GI bleeding. COX-2 selective inhibitors (Celebrex) decrease the risk of GI side effects; however, some have been associated with increased risk of cardiovascular disease events (e.g., myocardial infarction) (91). Because of some of the rarer but serious side effects, it has been suggested that individuals should be continually monitored for signs of renal toxicity, hypertension, and limb edema (15,101). Interestingly, although acetaminophen and selective and nonselective NSAIDs are commonly considered the first line of defense for mild to moderate OA, Fraenkel et al. (39) reported that many patients with symptomatic knee OA preferred a topical pain medication (Capsaicin) because of its negligible side effects. Hence, patients were willing to accept a less effective treatment in exchange for a much lower risk of side effects.

The dietary supplements glucosamine and chondroitin, separately and in combination, have gained widespread use for the treatment of OA. Glucosamine is thought to promote proteoglycan and glycosaminoglycan synthesis, important components of cartilage. Chondroitin is responsible, with collagen and noncollagenous glycoproteins, for giving cartilage its resiliency and inhibiting synovial degradative enzymes (24,65).

Previous clinical trials that compared glucosamine with a placebo suggest that it is moderately effective in reducing pain or improving function for those with hip or knee OA (52,70,71). McAlindon et al. (71) noted in their meta-analysis that many of these studies suffer from methodological problems, but overall, it seems probable that glucosamine and chondroitin have some efficacy in treating the symptoms of OA with few reported side effects (52,71).

Studies of combination therapy of glucosamine and chondroitin have shown reductions in pain in adults with OA, although each study has used supplements in addition to glucosamine and chondroitin (24,92,97,102). Two studies of patients with knee OA found combination therapy along with manganese ascorbate was effective in reducing pain after 4 and 6 months, respectively (39,64). As with many nonsurgical treatments of OA, the best results occur in patients with mild to moderate disease (71).

Surgical Treatment

When noninvasive treatments of knee OA fail to relieve pain and improve function, several surgical treatment options may be considered. Several of the surgical methods involve arthroscopic surgery that usually involves a method to "clean out" the joint. Débridement is a method to trim torn and damaged cartilage and may be combined with joint lavage, or "washing" of the joint. Joint lavage may also be performed alone. Lavage and débridement are the most common surgical procedures for mild to moderate knee OA, accounting for approximately 650,000 procedures (89). The success of these procedures varies, but approximately 50% of the patients report pain relief from either procedure (82). A randomized, controlled trial comparing arthroscopic débridement with lavage found no difference in clinical, functional, patient overall well-being, and blinded physician global outcomes between the groups. After 1 year, 44% of the patients who underwent surgery reported improvements in their global assessment versus 58% for the lavage group (19). A randomized, placebo-controlled trial to determine the efficacy of arthroscopic lavage and débridement using a simulated arthroscopic débridement procedure as a placebo surgery found no difference in pain or function between the lavage, débridement, and placebo surgery groups (82).

The second category of surgical procedures commonly used in patients with OA is total knee replacement (TKR) or arthroplasty. Total knee replacement is most commonly performed in knees with severe OA. The most common age range for TKR is 60 to 75 years. Patients younger than 55 years will increase the stress placed on a TKR, increasing the likelihood of a second procedure. Hence, younger patients are usually considered for alternative procedures, such as unicompartmental knee replacement (partial knee replacement) or osteotomy to improve alignment. TKR is a safe and effective treatment for end-stage knee OA. The mortality rate is 0.5%, and improvements in pain, function, and health-related quality of life appear rapid and substantial in 90% of the patients (85).

FIBROMYALGIA

Similar to other rheumatologic conditions, fibromyalgia afflicts women more often than men; roughly 80% to 90% of individuals with fibromyalgia are women. Fibromyalgia affects about 3.4% of women and 0.5% of men (118).

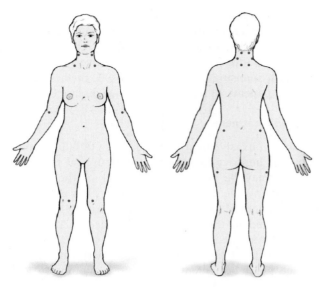

FIGURE 40-4. Tender points for the diagnosis of fibromyalgia. •, tender points.

CLINICAL FEATURES AND DIAGNOSIS

Fibromyalgia is a rheumatologic syndrome characterized by chronic widespread pain in muscles, ligaments, and joints, as well as a heightened tenderness at discrete anatomic locations called *tender points* (Fig. 40-4) (22,119). Historically, fibromyalgia has been diagnosed by the process of elimination. Specifically, fibromyalgia is diagnosed when the subject experiences widespread chronic pain in the absence of other identifiable pathology. Individuals with fibromyalgia have a decreased pain threshold (allodynia) during digital palpation or dolorimetry at these tender points. Besides chronic pain and tender points, individuals with fibromyalgia frequently have additional symptoms, including sleep disturbance, chronic fatigue, psychological distress, morning stiffness, and irritable bowel syndrome (118).

The American College of Rheumatology (ACR) 1990 Criteria for the Classification of Fibromyalgia (Table 40-1) continues to serve as the primary guidelines for the diagnosis of fibromyalgia (119). The main criteria are widespread pain for at least 3 months, bilateral pain, and pain on palpation with a force of 39 N (i.e., equivalent to 4 kg) at 11 or more of 18 tender-point sites (93,119).

Although the ACR criteria serve as the main diagnostic guidelines, they have received numerous criticisms. Criticisms include heterogeneity of pain attributes, problems with consistency of diagnosis, and the actual validity of tender-points assessment (22). The current definition of fibromyalgia is thought to capture only 20% of individuals with chronic widespread pain.

ETIOLOGY

No definite causal mechanism for fibromyalgia has been identified, but many have been hypothesized. Most of

---

TABLE 40-1. AMERICAN COLLEGE OF RHEUMATOLOGY 1990 CRITERIA FOR FIBROMYALGIA

CRITERION	DEFINITION
1. History of widespread pain	Pain is considered widespread when all of the following are present: pain in the left side of the body, pain in the right side of the body, pain above the waist, and pain below the waist. In addition, axial skeletal pain (cervical spine or anterior chest or thoracic spine or low back) must be present. In this definition, shoulder and buttock pain is considered as pain for each involved side. "Low back" pain is considered lower segment pain.
2. Pain in 11 of 18 tender-point sites on digital palpation (Fig. 40-4)	Pain on digital palpation must be present in at least 11 of the following 18 tender-point sites:

* Occiput: Bilateral, at the suboccipital muscle insertions
* Low cervical: Bilateral, at the anterior aspects of the intertransverse spaces at C5–C7
* Trapezius: Bilateral, at the midpoint of the upper border
* Supraspinatus: Bilateral, at origins above the scapula spine near the medial border
* Second rib: Bilateral, at the second costochondral junctions, just lateral to the junctions on upper surfaces
* Lateral epicondyle: Bilateral, 2 cm distal to the epicondyles
* Gluteal: Bilateral, in upper outer quadrants of the buttocks in the anterior folds of muscle
* Greater trochanter: Bilateral, posterior to the trochanteric prominence
* Knee: Bilateral, at the medial fat pad proximal to the joint line

Digital palpation should be performed with an approximate "force" of 4 kg. For a tender point to be considered "positive," the subject must state that palpation was painful. "Tender" is not to be considered "painful."

From Wolfe F, Smythe HA, Yunus MB, et al. The American College of Rheumatology 1990 criteria for the classification of fibromyalgia. *Arthritis Rheum.* 1990;33:160–172.

these hypotheses focus on the abnormal levels of nociceptive hormones and neurotransmitters in subjects with fibromyalgia. Particular attention has been paid to the function of the hypothalamic-pituitary-adrenal (HPA) axis and its associated chemical pain mediators, which include (among others) cortisol, growth hormone, insulinlike growth factor-1, substance P, and serotonin (27). Additionally, genetics and environmental factors (e.g., muscle trauma; certain infections, such as hepatitis C, Lyme disease, Epstein-Barr virus) are possible mechanisms in the development of fibromyalgia (22).

Glucocorticoid deficiency may result in pain, and individuals with fibromyalgia exhibit moderate basal hypocortisolism (13,27). It remains unclear, however, whether low cortisol levels represent a cause or effect of chronic pain. Moreover, low levels of growth hormone in fibromyalgia subjects could be related to sleep disturbances. Growth hormone is secreted primarily during stages 3 and 4 of non-REM sleep (9), and fibromyalgia patients exhibit an abnormal sleep pattern, particularly for stages 3 and 4 (80).

Substance P is a peptide that may be important in the neurotransmission of pain. Numerous studies have shown two- to threefold average increases in substance P in the cerebrospinal fluid of subjects with fibromyalgia (10,66,99,112,115). Moreover, a prospective study showed that increases in medication-free substance P concentration were directly related to increased levels of pain and tenderness in fibromyalgia patients (99). Finally, recent studies have shown a probable reason for the efficacy of antidepressants in the treatment of fibromyalgia. A study of the effects of tricyclic antidepressants (TCAs) on rats showed a down-regulation of substance P in the limbic system (106), and a human study of the antidepressant St. John's wort showed a dose-dependent decrease in substance P (35).

Patients with fibromyalgia have abnormalities in collagen metabolism that are related to increased inflammation. More specifically, Salemi et al. (100) found that abnormalities in collagen metabolism were correlated with increased levels of IL-1beta, IL-6, and TNF-alpha in roughly one third of fibromyalgia subjects. These data suggest that there is a connection between collagen abnormalities and pain-inducing inflammation in a subset of the fibromyalgia population, which may help explain why some fibromyalgia sufferers experience pain relief from NSAIDs.

TREATMENTS

There is currently no cure for fibromyalgia. Treatment is focused on the management of pain and associated symptoms using nonpharmacologic and pharmacologic therapies separately or in combination (96).

Exercise Response

Exercise therapy is the most common treatment, although much debate still exists regarding the optimal frequency, duration, and intensity of exercise therapy in individuals with fibromyalgia (21). The most effective treatment is a combination exercise along with cognitive behavioral therapy and education carried out by an interdisciplinary team that includes physicians, nurses, clinical exercise specialists, occupational therapists, psychologists, and others.

Short-term aerobic exercise interventions are generally successful in improving function and pain in patients with fibromyalgia. Richards and Scott (98) examined the effects of a 3-month, $2 \, d \cdot wk^{-1}$ aerobic exercise intervention in 136 patients and found significant improvements in self-reported global assessment of well-being compared with a flexibility and relaxation attention control group. Tender-point count was not significantly different at the end of the intervention period; however, a 1-year follow-up revealed improved pain levels in the aerobic group. Compliance for both groups was low, with only 53% of the participants attending at least one third of the sessions. Fatigue, pain, and Medical Outcomes Study Questionnaire Short Form (SF-36) scores did not differ between the groups. Gowans et al. (43,44) randomized 51 fibromyalgia patients into either a 23-week aerobic exercise program or a control group and found the exercise group significantly improved mood, 6-minute walk distance, and self-efficacy relative to the control group. A meta-analysis of 16 randomized clinical trials that compared various forms of aerobic exercise with control groups found a significant treatment effect with improvements in aerobic performance, tender-point pain threshold, and pain (16). It has been speculated that exercise in the water may reduce pain, thus promoting better adherence to a program. Assis et al. (7) compared deep-water running with land-based exercise and found similar improvements in aerobic measures and depression scores, with fewer reports of pain during the activity.

Strength training may attenuate the accelerated decline in physical function common in patients with fibromyalgia. Jones et al. (59) enrolled 68 women with fibromyalgia into either a 12-week strength-training or a flexibility program. Following training, there were no significant differences between the groups in isokinetic strength, number of tender points, pain, fatigue, sleep, depression, anxiety, or quality of life. In contrast, Hakkinen et al. (47) found significant increases in leg strength in fibromyalgia patients randomized to a progressive strength-training group versus a control group. The trained patients also reported significant decreases in fatigue and depression. The authors concluded that strength training is a safe and effective intervention for patients with fibromyalgia.

Taken together, it appears that aerobic—and to a lesser extent, resistance training—results in short-term improvements in function, mood, self-efficacy, and pain in fibromyalgia patients. Future investigations need to examine the long-term benefits of aerobic and resistance training in fibromyalgia patients.

Exercise Prescription

The most fundamental rule for recommending exercise for patients with fibromyalgia is to individualize the prescription. Exercise prescription should ideally begin with a detailed assessment that includes both the individual's fitness level and pain and then follows a progression so that severe pain from overexertion is avoided at all times. Many of the exercise clinical trials that reported low adherence indicated that the intervention exacerbated patients' pain. Dawson and Tiidus (25) suggest beginning at one to two times/week, with a goal of 3 to 4 days/week. They note that a training heart rate of <75% of maximum seems to be tolerated more readily, along with shorter durations (10–30 minutes). Walking and running have been successfully used in several studies, although some have suggested that exercise in the water might not only provide the appropriate cardiovascular stimulus, but also have better compliance (7). Similar to recommendations for other systemic arthropathies, exercise duration may need to be decreased during flare-ups.

Although there are currently no research-based recommendations for resistance training for those with fibromyalgia, studies that have used resistance training have used up to 50% to 70% of 1RM with a frequency of 2 days/week (59).

Pharmacologic Treatment

Antidepressants are a common pharmacologic treatment for fibromyalgia. The most popular include TCAs, selective serotonin reuptake inhibitors (SSRIs), and dual reuptake inhibitors. This class of antidepressants increases neurotransmission and has a positive analgesic effect. TCAs improve sleep, pain, and fatigue, but their effect on mood is less definitive (96). SSRIs have proven effective for major depressive disorders, but their effectiveness for fibromyalgia patients has been inconsistent and appears less than TCAs (6,78,120). Dual reuptake inhibitors are similar pharmacologically to TCAs but have a better analgesic effect and diminished side effects (30).

NSAIDs have also been used to treat fibromyalgia. Goldenberg et al. (41) compared naproxen, amitriptyline (a TCA), and the combination of naproxen and amitriptyline with a placebo in patients with fibromyalgia. The authors found no significant effect of naproxen; however, amitriptyline was significantly better than the placebo on all outcomes, including pain, sleep difficulties, fatigue, and tender-point scores. Several other trials have also failed to find significant improvements in pain using NSAIDs in the treatment of fibromyalgia (62,78). Hence, it appears that NSAIDs are of limited use in the treatment of fibromyalgia.

RHEUMATOID ARTHRITIS

There is two to three times greater mortality among rheumatoid arthritis (RA) patients than in the general population. Especially significant is the increased risk of coronary artery disease as compared with age-matched controls (20). The number of new cases of RA that occur in a population each year has decreased during the past few decades, with a reduction in the prevalence from 61.2 per 100,000 persons (1955–1964) to 32.7 per 100,000 persons (1985–1994) (29,111).

CLINICAL FEATURES AND DIAGNOSIS

Rheumatoid arthritis is an inflammatory disease, associated with autoimmune dysfunction, which attacks the joint capsule. The resultant major symptoms are pain, swelling, stiffness, and reduced joint mobility. Inflammatory periods are characterized by an abnormal increase in the cells of the synovial membrane, a thickening of this membrane, and a further increase in joint swelling. As the disease progresses, cartilage and bone that participate in joint articulations are degraded. In severe cases, the bones fuse together, resulting in a further loss of function and increased pain and deformity (Fig. 40-5).

Diagnosis is based on a combination of at least four signs and symptoms (Table 40-2) (5). The rheumatoid factor (RF) is a blood test used to diagnosis RA, although a positive RF test result can also indicate the presence of other diseases, such as Sjögren syndrome, systemic

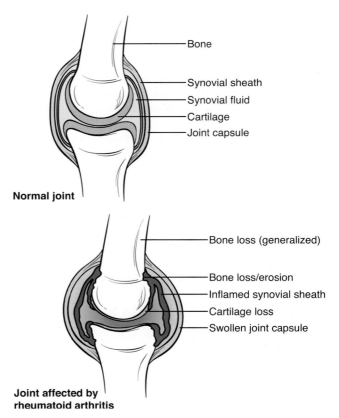

FIGURE 40-5. Normal and rheumatoid arthritic joints. (From the National Institutes of Health: Handout on Health: Rheumatoid arthritis: www.niams.nih.gov/Health_Info/Rheumatic_Disease/default.asp.)

TABLE 40-2. REVISED 1987 AMERICAN RHEUMATISM ASSOCIATION CRITERIA FOR RHEUMATOID ARTHRITIS

CRITERION[a]	DEFINITION
1. Morning stiffness	Morning stiffness in and around the joints, lasting at least 1 hour before maximal improvement
2. Arthritis of three or more joint areas	Swelling of at least three joint areas for at least 6 weeks. The 14 possible areas are right or left PIP, MCP, wrist, elbow, knee, ankle, and MTP joints.
3. Arthritis of hand joints	Swelling of the wrist, MCP, or PIP joint for at least 6 weeks
4. Symmetrical arthritis	Simultaneous involvement of the same joint areas (as defined in #2) on both sides of the body (bilateral involvement of PIPs, MCPs, or MTPs is acceptable without absolute symmetry)
5. Rheumatoid nodules	Subcutaneous nodules over bony prominences or extensor surfaces or in juxta-articular regions
6. Serum rheumatoid factor	Abnormal level of serum rheumatoid factor as detected by a method that is positive in <5% of normal control subjects
7. Radiographic changes	Radiographic changes typical of rheumatoid arthritis on posteroanterior hand and wrist radiographs, which must include erosions or unequivocal bony decalcification localized in or most marked adjacent to the involved joints

MCP, metacarpophalangeal; MTP, metatarsophalangeal; PIP, proximal interphalangeal.

[a]At least four criteria must be fulfilled for classification as rheumatoid arthritis.

From Arnett FC, Edworthy SM, Bloch DA, et al. The American Rheumatism Association 1987 revised criteria for the classification of rheumatoid arthritis. *Arthritis Rheum.* 1988;31:315–324.

lupus, and systemic sclerosis (53). Approximately 80% of patients with RA have a positive RF test result.

Chronic inflammatory diseases such as RA cause premature aging (110). Diseases that take decades to advance during normal aging—such as atherosclerosis, osteoporosis, muscle wasting, and sleep disorders—change dramatically within a few months in those with RA. Women are affected two to three times more often than men, with the peak incidence occurring between the sixth and seventh decades of life (29).

ETIOLOGY

The development of RA has both genetic and environmental (i.e., nongenetic) determinants. The genetic contribution is estimated at 60% (50,67). Studies that have advanced our understanding of RA genetics include a 1978 study by Stastny (108), who found a link between the human leukocyte antigen system (specifically HLA-DR4) and RA and Gregersen et al. (45) in 1987, who advanced the case for a genetic link by finding a one-in-six chance of developing a higher risk in individuals who are homozygous for a polymorphism of the HLA gene (*HLA-DRB*0408*).

Environmental, or nongenetic, factors linked to the occurrence of RA include age, hormonal factors, infection, smoking, and obesity (60). More specifically, the incidence of RA increases with age, is rare in women before menarche, has declined in women with the increased use of oral contraception, is widely believed to be linked to some type of infection, and is higher in smokers and in individuals with a body mass index of 30 kg/m² or above. After the onset of RA, the severity of the disease is related to the DR4 alleles, which are alternative forms of the HLA gene; onset after the age of 60 years; being female; and smoking, which initially decreases pain but ultimately increases the risk for lung and blood vessel involvement (111).

TREATMENTS

A variety of treatment options for RA, including exercise, medications, and surgery, will be described.

Exercise Response

Patients with RA have reduced muscle strength and compromised joint ROM that decreases mobility and increases pain (46). Initially, the primary concern regarding exercise with RA patients was that it would exacerbate the chronic inflammation associated with the disease (95). However, numerous studies have demonstrated that exercise does not increase symptoms or physiologic indicators of the disease (58). Furthermore, some of the more recent studies have shown that vigorous, high-intensity workloads result in better fitness gains while still not exacerbating symptoms (84).

Long-term dynamic strength training has a positive effect on muscle strength, self-reported physical function, and physical performance in women with RA (48,95). As little as 1.4 exercise sessions per week for 24 months provided these positive effects without exacerbating disease activity, as evidenced by inflammatory biomarkers or joint degradation. Importantly, these more recent studies have used workloads that are within ACSM guidelines (50%–70% of 1RM, 10–15 reps, 3–4 sets) (48). Long-term follow-up in a similar study of those who participated in a strength-training program showed continued benefits after 5 years (49).

Aerobic exercise also appears to have a positive effect. A 12-month aerobic weight-bearing exercise program significantly improved self-reported function and activity level, and bone mineral density and disease activity remained unchanged (116). One of the few studies to examine the question of intensity used both biking and resistance training. Although the conservative exercise program used isometric exercises with no resistance, the other group did both isometric and isokinetic training using 70% maximal voluntary contractions and biked at 60% of maximal heart rate. The authors found that those participating in the more intense program had fewer swollen joints, less pain, and lower biomarkers with better joint mobility at both 12 and 24 weeks (113). In a study that focused on exercise adherence to an intensive program, ACSM guidelines were followed for aerobic bicycle exercise. The authors not only found an adherence rate of 81% after 2 years, but also showed that high adherence was associated with lower disease activity and pain scores (83).

Exercise Prescription

Although exercise—including joint ROM, resistance exercise, and aerobic conditioning—is recommended for management of RA, specific guidelines regarding type, frequency, and intensity of exercise have not been addressed (4). However, an analysis of 15 randomized clinical trials suggests that aerobic exercises (e.g., walking, aquatics, bicycling) performed three times per week for 30 to 60 minutes per session at an intensity of 60% to 85% of maximum heart rate successfully improve aerobic capacity and muscle strength. Furthermore, resistance training (e.g., use of weight machines, dumbbells, elastic bands) performed two to three times weekly at 50% to 80% of maximal voluntary contraction improves strength and does not have a detrimental effect on pain (109).

Similar to the recommendations for exercise prescription for those with OA, initial intensities should be modified based on previous activity and current joint pain. Joint ROM may be limited and should be considered in activity selection. Flare-ups are more common with RA, thus necessitating the ability to modify the program based on changes in the disease activity.

Pharmacologic Treatment

A mainstay of the treatment of RA is pharmacologic therapy (4,114). Pharmacologic therapy for the treatment of RA includes NSAIDs, disease-modifying antirheumatic drugs (DMARDs), glucocorticoids (steroids), and biologic therapies. NSAIDs reduce swelling, pain, and inflammation but have some serious side effects, including stomach bleeding and ulcers (management guidelines note a twofold risk for complications as compared with an individual with OA). DMARDs include injectible or oral gold, hydroxychloroquine, penicillamine, sulfasalazine, methotrexate, azathioprine, cyclosporine, and lefluomide. This classification of drugs also works to suppress the immune system and is thought to slow the progression of the disease and reduce cartilage degradation. Possible side effects include liver and kidney damage. Glucocorticoids (steroids), such as prednisone, methylpredinsone, cortisone, and hydrocortisone, reduce

TABLE 40-3. MEDICATIONS USED IN THE TREATMENT OF RHEUMATOID ARTHRITIS

CATEGORY	EXAMPLES (TRADE NAMES)
NSAIDs	Aspirin
	Ibuprofen (Advil, Motrin IB)
	Ketoprofen (Orudis)
	Naproxen (Naprosyn)
	Celecoxib (Celebrex)
DMARDs	Gold, injectable or oral
	Antimalarials (Plaquenil)
	Penicillamine (Cuprimine, Depen)
	Sulfasalazine (Azulfidine)
	Methotrexate (Rheumatrex)
	Azathioprine (Imuran)
	Cyclosporine (Sandimmune, Neoral)
	Lefluomide (Arava)
Glucocorticoids (steroids)	Prednisone (Deltasone, Orasone)
	Methylprednisolone (Medrol)
Biologic therapy	Etanercept (Enbrel)

DMARDs, disease-modifying antirheumatic drugs; NSAIDs, nonsteroidal antiinflammatory drugs.

inflammation and suppress the immune response. The most serious side effect is the increased risk of infection. Biologic therapies work to suppress joint inflammation that is thought to play a role in cartilage degradation by blocking the action of certain cytokines, specifically, TNF (81). Table 40-3 lists the general categories of drugs used in the treatment of RA.

Surgical Treatment

Age, disease severity, degree of disability, and the combination of involved joints are important considerations in the timing of orthopedic interventions. Less definitive orthopedic procedures include synovectomy (excision of inflamed synovial tissue), tendon realignment, and arthroscopic débridement. These procedures can improve alignment, reduce synovial tissue, control pain, provide stability, and improve function in some RA patients. These techniques can also prolong periods of good function and delay the need for replacement procedures (40). After all other options have been exhausted, joint replacement results in vastly improved function and reduced pain (72).

ADDITIONAL FACTORS

It is important to recognize that there are some other factors that should be considered when prescribing exercise for an individual with arthritis. As OA or RA progresses, joint stability is often compromised. Modifications may be necessary to the activity, such as using a machine versus free weights or modifying a position. For example, increasing seat height and decreasing pedal load reduces joint pain with cycling. With severe joint instability, a brace may be necessary. Improper joint alignment (e.g., excessive knee varus) has been shown to negatively affect progression of the disease and may also warrant activity modification or joint protection. Balance and proprioception have also been shown to be compromised with lower-extremity arthritis, and incorporation of balance and kinesthetic activities into a training program has resulted in even greater improvements in some activities, such as stair climbing (28). Knowledge of the type and severity of the arthritis is essential. For example, ankylosing spondylitis results in a loss of joint mobility, especially in the spine. Flexibility exercises are needed on a regular basis to slow the progression of the loss of motion and maintain function (34).

SUMMARY

Arthritis and chronic joint symptoms, both physician diagnosed and undiagnosed, affect more than 70 million Americans and are the leading cause of disability (17). Arthritis increases pain, reduces strength, restricts mobility, and lowers health-related quality of life. Furthermore, it has been shown that individuals with some of the systemic arthropathies have a higher risk for chronic heart disease and hypertension. There are no known cures for arthritis; however, exercise appears to improve the clinical symptoms of a variety of rheumatic diseases, including OA, fibromyalgia, and RA.

REFERENCES

1. Al-Zahrani KS, Bakheit AM. A study of the gait characteristics of patients with chronic osteoarthritis of the knee. *Disabil Rehabil.* 2002; 24:275–280.
2. Altman R, Asch E, Bloch D, et al. The American College of Rheumatology criteria for the classification and reporting of osteoarthritis of the knee. *Arthritis Rheum.* 1986;29:1039–1049.
3. American College of Rheumatology. Ankylosing spondylitis. Available from: www.rheumatology.org/public/factsheets/as.asp. Accessed May 22, 2007.
4. American College of Rheumatology. Guidelines for the management of rheumatoid arthritis: 2002 update. *Arthritis Rheum.* 2002;46:328–346.
5. Arnett FC, Edworthy SM, Bloch DA, et al. The American Rheumatism Association 1987 revised criteria for the classification of rheumatoid arthritis. *Arthritis Rheum.* 1988;31:315–324.
6. Arnold LM, Hess EV, Hudson JI, et al. A randomized, placebo-controlled, double-blind, flexible-dose study of fluoxetine in the treatment of women with fibromyalgia. *Am J Med.* 2002;112:191–197.
7. Assis MR, Silva LE, Alves AMB, et al. A randomized controlled trial of deep water running: clinical effectiveness of aquatic exercise to treat fibromyalgia. *Arthritis Rheum.* 2006;55:57–65.
8. Baliunas AJ, Hurwitz DE, Ryals AB, et al. Increased knee joint loads during walking are present in subjects with knee osteoarthritis. *Osteoarthritis Cartilage.* 2002;10:573–579.
9. Bennett RM. Beyond fibromyalgia: ideas on etiology and treatment. *J Rheumatol.* 1989;19(suppl):185–191.
10. Bradley LA, Alarcon GS. Is Chiari malformation associated with increased levels of substance P and clinical symptoms in persons with fibromyalgia? *Arthritis Rheum.* 1999;42:2731–2732.
11. Brousseau L, Pelland L, Wells G, et al. Efficacy of aerobic exercises for osteoarthritis (Part II): a meta-analysis. *Phys Ther Rev.* 2004;9: 125–145.
12. Bruce B, Fries J, Lubeck DP. Aerobic exercise and its impact on musculoskeletal pain in older adults: a 14 year prospective, longitudinal study. *Arthritis Res Ther.* 2005;7:R1263–R1270.
13. Buchwald D. Fibromyalgia and chronic fatigue syndrome: similarities and differences. *Rheum Dis Clin North Am.* 1996;22:219–243.
14. Burr DB, Radin EL. Microfractures and microcracks in subchondral bone: are they relevant to osteoarthrosis? *Rheum Dis Clin North Am.* 2003;29:675–685.
15. Burris JE. Pharmacologic approaches to geriatric pain management. *Arch Phys Med Rehabil.* 2004;85:S45–S49.
16. Busch A, Schachter CL, Peloso PM, Bombardier C. Exercise for treating fibromyalgia syndrome. *Cochrane Database Syst Rev.* 2002; CD003786,
17. Centers for Disease Control and Prevention. Prevalence of doctor-diagnosed arthritis and arthritis-attributable activity limitation—United States, 2003–2005. *MMWR Morb Mortal Wkly Rep.* 2006;55 (40):1089–1092.
18. Centers for Disease Control and Prevention. National and state medical expenditures and lost earnings attributable to arthritis and other rheumatic conditions—United States, 2003. *MMWR Morb Mortal Wkly Rep.* 2007;56(01):4–7.
19. Chang RW, Falconer J, Stulberg SD, et al. A randomized, controlled trial of arthroscopic surgery versus closed-needle joint lavage for patients with osteoarthritis of the knee. *Arthritis Rheum.* 1993;36:289–296.
20. Chung CP, Oeser A, Avalos I, et al. Utility of the Framingham risk score to predict the presence of coronary atherosclerosis in patients with rheumatoid arthritis. *Arthritis Res Ther.* 2006;8:R186.
21. Clarke SR, Jones KD, Burckhardt CS, Bennett RM. Exercise for patients with fibromyalgia: risk versus benefits. *Curr Rheumatol Rep.* 2001;3:135–146.
22. Clauw DJ, Crofford LJ. Chronic widespread pain and fibromyalgia: what we know, and what we need to know. *Best Pract Res Clin Rheumatol.* 2003;17:685–701.
23. Cochrane T, Davey RC, Matthes Edwards SM. Randomised controlled trial of the cost-effectiveness of water-based therapy for lower limb osteoarthritis. *Health Technology Assessment.* 2005;9:iii–76.
24. Das A Jr, Hammad TA. Efficacy of a combination of FCHG49 glucosamine hydrochloride, TRH122 low molecular weight sodium chondroitin sulfate and manganese ascorbate in the management of knee osteoarthritis. *Osteoarthritis Cartilage.* 2000;8:343–350.
25. Dawson KA, Tiidus PM. Physical activity in the treatment and management of fibromyalgia. *Crit Rev Phys Rehab Med.* 2005;17:53–64.
26. Davis MA, Ettinger WH, Neuhaus JM. The role of metabolic factors and blood pressure in the association of obesity with osteoarthritis of the knee. *J Rheumatol.* 1988;15:1827–1832.
27. Demitrack MA, Crofford LJ. Evidence for and pathophysiologic implications of hypothalamic-pituitary-adrenal axis dysregulation in fibromyalgia and chronic fatigue syndrome. *Ann N Y Acad Sci.* 1998;840:684–697.
28. Diracoglu D, Aydin R, Baskent A, Celik A. Effects of kinesthesia and balance exercise in knee osteoarthritis. *J Clin Rheumatol.* 2005;11:303–310.
29. Doran MF, Pond GR, Crowson CS, et al. Trends in incidence and mortality in rheumatoid arthritis in Rochester, Minnesota, over a forty-year period. *Arthritis Rheum.* 2002;46:625–631.
30. Dwight MM, Arnold LM, O'Brien H, et al. An open clinical trial of venlafaxine treatment of fibromyalgia. *Psychosomatics.* 1998;39:14–17.
31. Ettinger WH Jr, Afable RF. Physical disability from knee osteoarthritis: the role of exercise as an intervention. *Med Sci Sports Exerc.* 1994;26:1435–1440.
32. Ettinger WH Jr, Burns R, Messier SP, et al. A randomized trial comparing aerobic exercise and resistance exercise with a health education program in older adults with knee osteoarthritis. The Fitness Arthritis and Seniors Trial (FAST). *JAMA.* 1997;277:25–31.
33. Felson DT, Naimark A, Anderson J, et al. The prevalence of knee osteoarthritis in the elderly. The Framingham Osteoarthritis Study. *Arthritis Rheum.* 1987; 30:914–918.
34. Fernández-de-las-Peñas C, Alonso-Blanco C, Alguacil-Diego IM, Miangolarra-Page JC. One-year follow-up of two exercise inter-

ventions for the management of patients with ankylosing spondylitis. *Am J Phys Med Rehabil.* 2006;85:559–567.

35. Fiebich BL, Hollig A, Lieb K. Inhibition of substance P-induced cytokine synthesis by St. John's wort extracts. *Pharmacopsychiatry.* 2001;34 (Suppl 1):S26–S28.

36. Fisher NM, Gresham G, Pendergast DR. Effects of a quantitative progressive rehabilitation program applied unilaterally to the osteoarthritic knee. *Arch Phys Med Rehabil.* 1993;74:1319–1326.

37. Fisher NM, Pendergast DR. Effects of a muscle exercise program on exercise capacity in subjects with osteoarthritis. *Arch Phys Med Rehabil.* 1994;75:792–797.

38. Fitzgerald GK, Piva SR, Irrgang JJ, Bouzubar F, Starz TW. Quadriceps activation failure as a moderator of the relationship between quadriceps strength and physical function in individuals with knee osteoarthritis. *Arthritis Rheum.* 2004;51:40–48.

39. Fraenkel L, Bogardus ST Jr, Concato J, Wittink DR. Treatment options in knee osteoarthritis: the patient's perspective. *Arch Intern Med.* 2004;164:1299–1304.

40. Gerber LH, Hicks JE. Surgical and rehabilitation options in the treatment of the rheumatoid arthritis patient resistant to pharmacologic agents. *Rheum Dis Clin North Am.* 1995;21:19–39.

41. Goldenberg DL, Felson DT, Dinerman H. A randomized, controlled trial of amitriptyline and naproxen in the treatment of patients with fibromyalgia. *Arthritis Rheum.* 1986;29:1371–1377.

42. Goldring MB. Osteoarthritis and cartilage: the role of cytokines. *Curr Rheumatol Rep.* 2000;2:459–465.

43. Gowans SE, DeHueck A, Voss S, et al. Effect of a randomized, controlled trial of exercise on mood and physical function in individuals with fibromyalgia. *Arthritis Rheum.* 2001;45:519–529.

44. Gowans SE, DeHueck A, Voss S, Silaj A, Abbey SE. Six-month and one-year followup of 23 weeks of aerobic exercise for individuals with fibromyalgia. *Arthritis Rheum.* 2004;51:890–898.

45. Gregersen PK, Silver J, Winchester RJ. The shared epitope hypothesis: an approach to understanding the molecular genetics of susceptibility to rheumatoid arthritis. *Arthritis Rheum.* 1987;30:1205–1213.

46. Hakkinen A, Haanonan P, Nyman K, Hakkinen K. Aerobic and neuromuscular performance capacity of physically active females with early or long-term rheumatoid arthritis compared to matched healthy women. *Scand J Rheumatol.* 2002;31:345–350.

47. Hakkinen A, Hakkinen K, Hannonen P, Alen M. Strength training induced adaptations in neuromuscular function of premenopausal women with fibromyalgia: comparison with healthy women. *Ann Rheum Di.s* 2001;60:21–26.

48. Häkkinen A, Pakarinen A, Hannonen P, et al. Effects of prolonged combined strength and endurance training on physical fitness, body composition and serum hormones in women with rheumatoid arthritis and healthy controls. *Clin Exp Rheum.* 2005;23:505–512.

49. Häkkinen A, Sokka T, Hannonen P. A home-based two-year strength training period in early rheumatoid arthritis led to good long-term compliance: a five year followup. *Arthritis Rheum.* 2004;51:56–62.

50. Harney S, Wordsworth BP. Genetic epidemiology of rheumatoid arthritis. *Tissue Antigens.* 2002;60:465–473.

51. Hartman CA, Manos TM, Winter C, et al. Effects of tai chi training on function and quality of life indicators in older adults with osteoarthritis. *J Am Geriatr Soc.* 2000;48:1553–1559.

52. Hauselmann HJ. Nutripharmaceuticals for osteoarthritis. *Best Pract Res Clin Rheumatol.* 2001;15:595–607.

53. Hess EV. In: Schumacher HR, editor. *Rheumatoid Arthritis.* Atlanta: Arthritis Foundation; 1988. p. 83–96.

54. Hochberg MC, Dougados M. Pharmacological therapy of osteoarthritis. *Best Pract Res Clin Rheumatol.* 2001;15:583–593.

55. Hootman JM, Helmick CG. Projections of US prevalence of arthritis and associated activity limitations. *Arthritis Rheum.* 2006;54:226–229.

56. Hurley MV. The effects of joint damage on muscle function, proprioception and rehabilitation. *Man Ther.* 2001;2:11–17.

57. Hurwitz DE, Sumner DR, Andriacchi TP, Sugar DA. Dynamic knee loads during gait predict proximal tibial bone distribution. *J Biomech.* 1998;31:423–430.

58. Jones G, Halberti J, Crotty M, et al. The effect of treatment on radiological progression in rheumatoid arthritis: a systematic review of randomized placebo-controlled trials. *Rheumatology.* 2003;42:6–13.

59. Jones KD, Burckhardt CS, Clark SR, et al. A randomized controlled trial of muscle strengthening versus flexibility training in fibromyalgia. *J Rheumatol.* 2002;29:1041–1048.

60. Kaipiainen-Seppanen O, Aho K, Isomaki H, Laakso M. Shift in the incidence of rheumatoid arthritis toward elderly patients in Finland during 1975–1990. *Clin Exp Rheumatol.* 1996;14:537–542.

61. Kovar PA, Allegrante JP, MacKenzie CR, et al. Supervised fitness walking in patients with osteoarthritis of the knee: a randomized, controlled trial. *Ann Intern Med.* 1992;116:529–534.

62. Lautenschlager J. Present state of medication therapy in fibromyalgia syndrome. *Scand J Rheumatol.* 2000;113(suppl):32–36.

63. Lawrence RC, Helmick CG, Arnett FC, et al. Estimates of the prevalence of arthritis and selected musculoskeletal disorders in the United States. *Arthritis Rheum.* 1998;41:778–799.

64. Leffler CT, Philippi AF, Leffler SG, et al. Glucosamine, chondroitin, and manganese ascorbate for degenerative joint disease of the knee or low back: a randomized, double-blind, placebo-controlled pilot study. *Mil Med.* 1999;164:85–91.

65. Lippiello L, Woodward J, Karpman R, Hammad TA. In vivo chondroprotection and metabolic synergy of glucosamine and chondroitin sulfate. *Clin Orthop.* 2000;381:229–240.

66. Liu Z, Welin M, Bragee B, Nyberg F. A high-recovery extraction procedure for quantitative analysis of substance P and opioid peptides in human cerebrospinal fluid. *Peptides.* 2000;21:853–860.

67. MacGregor AJ, Snieder H, Rigby AS, et al. Characterizing the quantitative genetic contribution to rheumatoid arthritis using data from twins. *Arthritis Rheum.* 2000;43:30–37.

68. Mangione KK, McCully K, Gloviak A, Lefebvre I, Hofmann M, Craik R. The effects of high-intensity and low-intensity cycle ergometry in older adults with knee osteoarthritis. *J Gerontol.* 1999;54(A):M184–M190.

69. Martin DF. Pathomechanics of knee osteoarthritis. *Med Sci Sports Exerc.* 1994;26:1429–1434.

70. Mazieres B, Loyau G, Menkes CJ, et al. Chondroitin sulfate in the treatment of gonarthrosis and coxarthrosis: 5-months result of a multicenter double-blind controlled prospective study using placebo. *Rev Rhum Mal Osteoartic.* 1992;59:466–472.

71. McAlindon TE, LaValley MP, Gulin JP, Felson DT. Glucosamine and chondroitin for treatment of osteoarthritis: a systematic quality assessment and meta-analysis. *JAMA.* 2000;283:1469–1475.

72. McCoy TH, Salvati EA, Ranawat CS, Wilson PD Jr. A fifteen-year follow-up study of one hundred Charnley low-friction arthroplasties. *Orthop Clin North Am.* 1988;19:467–476.

73. Messier SP, Devita P, Cowan RE, et al. Do older adults with knee osteoarthritis place greater loads on the knee during gait? A preliminary study. *Arch Phys Med Rehabil.* 2005;86:703–705.

74. Messier SP, Loeser RF, Hoover JL, et al. Osteoarthritis of the knee: effects on gait, strength, and flexibility. *Arch Phys Med Rehabil.* 1992;73:29–36.

75. Messier SP, Loeser RF, Miller GD, et al. Exercise and dietary weight loss in overweight and obese older adults with knee osteoarthritis: the Arthritis, Diet, and Activity Promotion Trial. *Arthritis Rheum.* 2004;50:1501–1510.

76. Messier SP, Loeser RF, Mitchell MN, et al. Exercise and weight loss in obese older adults with knee osteoarthritis: a preliminary study. *J Am Geriatr Soc.* 2000;48:1062–1072.

77. Messier SP, Thompson CD, Ettinger WH. Effects of long-term aerobic or weight training regimens on gait in an older, osteoarthritic population. *J Appl Biomech.* 1997;13:205–225.

78. Miller LJ, Kubes KL. Serotonergic agents in the treatment of fibromyalgia syndrome. *Ann Pharmacother.* 2002;36:707–712.

79. Minor MA, Hewett JE, Webel RR, et al. Efficacy of physical conditioning exercise in patients with rheumatoid arthritis and osteoarthritis. *Arthritis Rheum.* 1989;32:1396–1405.

80. Moldofsky H, Scarisbrick P, England R, Smythe H. Musculoskeletal symptoms and non-REM sleep disturbance in patients with "fibrositis syndrome" and healthy subjects. *Psychosom Med.* 1975; 37:341–351.

81. Moreland LW, Baumgartner SW, Schiff MH, et al. Treatment of rheumatoid arthritis with a recombinant human tumor necrosis factor receptor (p75)-Fc fusion protein. *N Engl J Med.* 1997;337: 141–147.

82. Moseley JB, O'Malley K, Petersen NJ, et al. A controlled trial of arthroscopic surgery for osteoarthritis of the knee. *N Engl J Med.* 2002;347:81–88.

83. Munneke M, DeJong A, Zwinderman AH, et al. Adherence and satisfaction of rheumatoid arthritis patients with a long-term intensive dynamic exercise program (RAPIT Program). *Arthritis Rheum.* 2003;49:665–672.

84. Munneke M, deJong Z, Zwinderman AH, et al. Effect of a high-intensity weight-bearing exercise program on radiologic damage progression of the large joints in subgroups of patients with rheumatoid arthritis. *Arthritis Rheum.* 2005;53:410–417.

85. **National Institutes of Health. NIH consensus statement on total knee replacement.** *NIH Consens Stat Sci Statements.* **2003;Dec 8–10, 20:1–32.**

86. Nicklas BJ, Ambrosius W, Messier SP, et al. Diet-induced weight loss, exercise, and chronic inflammation in older, obese adults: a randomized controlled clinical trial. *Am J Clin Nutr.* 2004;79: 544–551.

87. Otterness IG, Swindell AC, Zimmerer RO, et al. An analysis of 14 molecular markers for monitoring osteoarthritis: segregation of the markers into clusters and distinguishing osteoarthritis at baseline. *Osteoarthritis Cartilage.* 2000;8:180–185.

88. Otterness IG, Weiner E, Swindell AC, et al. An analysis of 14 molecular markers for monitoring osteoarthritis: relationship of the markers to clinical end-points. *Osteoarthritis Cartilage.* 2001;9: 224–231.

89. Owings MF, Kozak LJ. Ambulatory and inpatient procedures in the United States, 1996. *Vital Health Stat.* 1998;13:1–119.

90. Pelletier JP, Martel-Pelletier J, Abramson SB. Osteoarthritis, an inflammatory disease: potential implication for the selection of new therapeutic targets. *Arthritis Rheum.* 2001;44:1237–1247.

91. Psaty BM, Furberg CD. COX-2 inhibitors-lessons in drug safety. *N Engl J Med.* 2005;352:1133–1135.

92. Pujalte JM, Llavore EP, Ylescupidez FR. Double-blind clinical evaluation of oral glucosamine sulphate in the basic treatment of osteoarthrosis. *Curr Med Res Opin.* 1980;7:110–114.

93. Quintner JL, Cohen ML. Fibromyalgia falls foul of a fallacy. *Lancet.* 1999;353:1092–1094.

94. Radin EL, Yang KH, Riegger C, et al. Relationship between lower limb dynamics and knee joint pain. *J Orthop Res.* 1991;9:398–405.

95. Rall LC, Roubenoff R, Cannon JG, et al. Effects of progressive resistance training on immune response in aging and chronic inflammation. *Med Sci Sports Exerc.* 1996;28:1356–1365.

96. Rao SG, Bennett RM. Pharmacological therapies in fibromyalgia. *Best Pract Res Clin Rheumatol.* 2003;17:611–627.

97. Reginster JY, Deroisy R, Rovati LC, et al. Long-term effects of glucosamine sulphate on osteoarthritis progression: a randomised, placebo-controlled clinical trial. *Lancet.* 2001;357:251–256.

98. Richards SC, Scott DL. Prescribed exercise in people with fibromyalgia: parallel group randomised controlled trial. *BMJ.* 2002;325:185.

99. Russell IJ, Fletcher EM, Vipraio GA, et al. Cerebrospinal fluid (CSF) substance P (SP) in fibromyalgia; changes in CSF SP over time parallel changes in clinical activity. *J Musculoskeletal Pain* [Internet]. 1998. Available from: www.haworthpress.com.

100. Salemi S, Rethage J, Wollina U, et al. Detection of interleukin 1beta (IL-1beta), IL-6, and tumor necrosis factor-alpha in skin of patients with fibromyalgia. *J Rheumatol.* 2003;30:146–150.

101. Schnitzer TJ. Osteoarthritis management: the role of cyclooxygenase-2-selective inhibitors. *Clin Ther.* 2001; 23:313–326.

102. Shankland WE. The effects of glucosamine and chondroitin sulfate on osteoarthritis of the TMJ: a preliminary report of 50 patients. *Cranio.* 1998;16:230–235.

103. Sharif M, Shepstone L, Elson CJ, et al. Increased serum C reactive protein may reflect events that precede radiographic progression in osteoarthritis of the knee. *Ann Rheum Dis.* 2000;59:71–74.

104. Sharma L, Hurwitz DE, Thonar EJ, et al. Knee adduction moment, serum hyaluronan level, and disease severity in medial tibiofemoral osteoarthritis. *Arthritis Rheum.* 1998;41:1233–1240.

105. Sharma L, Song J, Felson DT, et al. The role of knee alignment in disease progression and functional decline in knee osteoarthritis. *JAMA.* 2001;286:188–195.

106. Shirayama Y, Mitsushio H, Takashima M, et al. Reduction of substance P after chronic antidepressants treatment in the striatum, substantia nigra and amygdala of the rat. *Brain Res.* 1996;739:70–78.

107. Spector TD, Hart DJ, Nandra D, et al. Low-level increases in serum C-reactive protein are present in early osteoarthritis of the knee and predict progressive disease. *Arthritis Rheum.* 1997;40:723–727.

108. Stastny P. Association of the B-cell alloantigen DRw4 with rheumatoid arthritis. *N Engl J Med.* 1978;298:869–871.

109. Stenstrom CH, Minor MA. Evidence for the benefit of aerobic and strengthening exercise in rheumatoid arthritis. *Arthritis Rheum.* 2003;49:428–434.

110. Straub RH, Scholmerich J, Cutolo M. The multiple facets of premature aging in rheumatoid arthritis. *Arthritis Rheum.* 2003;48:2713–2721.

111. Symmons DP. Epidemiology of rheumatoid arthritis: determinants of onset, persistence and outcome. *Best Pract Res Clin Rheumatol.* 2002;16:707–722.

112. Vaeroy H, Helle R, Forre O, et al. Elevated CSF levels of substance P and high incidence of Raynaud phenomenon in patients with fibromyalgia: new features for diagnosis. *Pain.* 1988;32:21–26.

113. van den Ende CHM, Breedveld FC, le Cessie S, Bijkmans BAC, de Mug AW, Hazes JMW. Effect of intensive exercise on patients with active rheumatoid arthritis: a randomized clinical trial. *Ann Rheum Dis.* 2000;59:615–621.

114. van Schaardenburg D. Rheumatoid arthritis in the elderly: prevalence and optimal management. *Drugs Aging.* 1995;7:30–37.

115. Welin M, Bragee B, Nyberg F, Kristiansson M. Elevated substance levels are contrasted by a decrease in met-enkephalin-arg-phe-levels in CSF from fibromyalgia patients. *J Musculoskelet Pain.* 1995; 3(suppl 1):4.

116. Westby MD, Wade JP, Rangno KK, Berkowitz J. A randomized controlled trial to evaluate the effectiveness of an exercise program in women with rheumatoid arthritis taking low dose prednisone. *J Rheumatol.* 2000;27:1674–1680.

117. Wolfe F. The C-reactive protein but not erythrocyte sedimentation rate is associated with clinical severity in patients with osteoarthritis of the knee or hip. *J Rheumatol.* 1997;24:1486–1488.

118. Wolfe F, Ross K, Anderson J, et al. The prevalence and characteristics of fibromyalgia in the general population. *Arthritis Rheum.* 1995;38:19–28.

119. **Wolfe F, Smythe HA, Yunus MB, et al. The American College of Rheumatology 1990 criteria for the classification of fibromyalgia.** *Arthritis Rheum.* **1990;33:160–172.**

120. Zijlstra TR, van de Laar MA. The lack of a placebo effect in a trial of fluoxetine in the treatment of fibromyalgia. *Am J Med.* 2002; 113:614–615.

SELECTED REFERENCES FOR FURTHER READING

Brandt KD. *Osteoarthritis* (Rheumatic Disease Clinics of North America). Philadelphia: Elsevier Science Health Science; 2003.

Brent S, Wilk KE. *Clinical Orthopaedic Rehabilitation.* 2nd ed. Philadelphia: Mosby; 2003.

Centers for Disease Control and Prevention. Prevalence of doctor-diagnosed arthritis and possible arthritis—30 states, 2002. *MMWR Morbid Mortal Wkly Rep.* 2004;53:383–388.

Fransen M, McConnell S, Bell M. Exercise for osteoarthritis of the hip or knee. *Cochrane Database Syst Rev.* 2003;(3):CD004286.

Green WB, Snider RK. *Essentials of Musculoskeletal Care.* 2nd ed. Rosemont (IL): American Academy of Orthopaedic Surgeons; 2001.

Hakkinen A. Effectiveness and safety of strength training in rheumatoid arthritis. *Curr Opin Rheumatol.* 2004;16:132–137.

Haq I, Murphy E, Dacre J. Osteoarthritis. *Postgrad Med J.* 2003;79: 377–383.

Jette AM, Keysor JJ. Disability models: implications for arthritis exercise and physical activity interventions. *Arthritis Rheum.* 2003;49: 114–120.

Jordan KM, Arden NK, Doherty M, et al. Standing Committee for International Clinical Studies Including Therapeutic Trials ESCISIT. EULAR Recommendations 2003: An evidence based approach to the management of knee osteoarthritis: Report of a Task Force of the Standing Committee for International Clinical Studies Including Therapeutic Trials (ESCISIT). *Ann Rheum Dis.* 2003;62: 1145–1155.

Krebs D, Herzog W, McGibbon CA, Sharma L. Work group recommendations: 2002 Exercise and Physical Activity Conference. St. Louis. *Arthritis Rheum.* 2003;49:261–262.

O'Dell JR. Therapeutic strategies for rheumatoid arthritis. *N Engl J Med.* 2004; 350:2591–2602.

Roubenoff R. Exercise and inflammatory disease. *Arthritis Rheum.* 2003; 49:263–266.

Sahrmann S. *Diagnosis and Treatment of Movement Impairment Syndromes.* Philadelphia: Mosby; 2001.

van Gool CH, Penninx BWJH, Kempen GIJM, et al. Effects of exercise adherence on osteoarthritis-related performance and disability. *Arthritis Care Res.* 2005;53:24–32.

INTERNET RESOURCES

- American College of Rheumatology Practice Guidelines: www.rheumatology.org/publications/guidelines/index.asp?aud=prs
- Arthritis Foundation (Bulletin on the Rheumatic Diseases): www.arthritis.org/research/bulletin/archives.asp
- Arthritis Foundation (Research Update): www.arthritis.org/research/ResearchUpdate/archives.asp
- HealthTalk Rheumatoid Arthritis: www.healthtalk.com/rheumatoidarthritis/index.cfm
- National Guideline Clearinghouse (Exercise Prescription for Older Adults with Osteoarthritis Pain: Consensus Practice Recommendations): www.guideline.gov/summary/summary.aspx?doc_id=3188&nbr=2414&string=arthritis
- National Guideline Clearinghouse (Osteoarthritis: AAOS Clinical Guideline on Osteoarthritis of the Knee): www.guideline.gov/summary/summary.aspx?doc_id=3856&nbr=3069&string=arthritis
- National Guideline Clearinghouse (Osteoarthritis: AAOS Clinical Guideline on Osteoarthritis of the Knee [Phase II]): www.guideline.gov/summary/summary.aspx?doc_id=4584&nbr=3374&string=arthritis; www.rheumatology.org/public/factsheets/as.asp; www.cdc.gov/arthritis/data_statistics/national_data_nhis.htm#impact

Exercise Prescription in Special Populations: Women, Pregnancy, Children, and the Elderly

This chapter describes exercise testing and exercise prescription for several special populations, specifically women, especially women during pregnancy; children and adolescents; and older adults.

WOMEN

Women have become increasingly more interested in physical activity and sport as a result of the passing of Title IX legislation. The recent obesity epidemic has also provided an impetus for many women to begin taking part in physically active lifestyles. This interest in improving activity and fitness levels has led to more focus on women and exercise. Physiologic differences between men and women may necessitate special considerations when developing exercise prescriptions.

EXERCISE RESPONSE

Compared with men, women have lower absolute and relative $\dot{V}O_{2max}$ values. This difference in $\dot{V}O_{2max}$ is because men have a greater amount of muscle mass as well as increased hemoglobin levels. Women also have a lower blood volume compared with men and, consequently, lower stroke volumes, which lead to increased heart rates to maintain cardiac output (109). In terms of strength, women are able to generate nearly the same force as men when the weight lifted is compared with lean body mass (108).

EXERCISE TESTING

Generally, the adult guidelines for standard exercise testing apply to both men and women (see Chapters 19 and 20).

EXERCISE PRESCRIPTION

Generally, the adult guidelines for standard exercise prescription apply to both men and women (see Chapters 28 and 29).

SPECIAL CONSIDERATIONS

> **1.8.15-HFS: Knowledge of nutritional factors related to the female athlete triad syndrome (i.e., eating disorders, menstrual cycle abnormalities, and osteoporosis).**

Women have an increased level of body fat, which necessary to maintain a healthy menstrual cycle and support pregnancy. Lean body mass is lower compared with men because of the higher levels of body fat. Lower lean body mass is related to lower $\dot{V}O_{2max}$ and decreased overall strength in women compared with men (34). Because of monthly hormonal flux, women experience regular menstrual cycles. The menstrual cycle typically does not affect the ability to continue regular exercise. Estrogen has a protective effect against heart disease in women, hence the later development of cardiovascular disease in women (73). Female athletes may experience amenorrhea, a cessation of the menstrual cycle, as a result of reduced energy availability or energy deficiency. Energy deficiency is defined in the literature as an energy imbalance that may emerge if excessive expenditure demands are not compensated for by an increase in dietary intake (67–69).

Oftentimes in athletes, amenorrhea is accompanied by eating disorders and osteoporosis, contributing to the female athlete triad. Middle-aged women experience

---

Adolescent: A person between the onset of puberty and maturation, 13 to 18 years old.

Child: A person between birth and puberty, defined as younger than 13 years old.

Growth: Increase in size of a body part or body as a whole.

Maturation: The process and progress toward reaching the adult state.

menopause, which is the cessation of the menstrual cycle, because of age-related lower levels of estrogen and progesterone. Symptoms of menopause may be attenuated by regular exercise in these women (28). As a result of menopause, women lose the protective effect of estrogen against heart disease (73). Cardiovascular disease risk then approaches that of men; therefore, regular exercise should be continued.

PREGNANCY

Pregnancy is a time when a woman's body undergoes significant anatomic and physiologic changes. These changes are caused by the release of gestational hormones that allow for appropriate changes to occur in the body to create the optimal environment for the fetus. Healthy pregnant women without exercise contraindications (see Box 8.1 in *ACSM's Guidelines for Exercise Testing and Prescription*, 8th edition) are encouraged to exercise throughout the pregnancy. Regular exercise during pregnancy provides benefits to the mother and child (31,32). Benefits include reduced risk of excessive weight gain and a decreased risk of development of conditions associated with pregnancy, such as gestational diabetes mellitus and pregnancy-induced hypertension (86).

The American College of Sports Medicine (ACSM) endorses guidelines (74) regarding exercise in pregnancy and the postpartum period set forth by the American College of Obstetricians and Gynecologists (2,3) and the Joint Committee of the Society of Obstetricians and Gynecologists of Canada and the Canadian Society for Exercise Physiology (CSEP) (31). These guidelines outline the importance of exercise during pregnancy and also provide guidance on exercise prescription and contraindications to beginning and continuing exercise during pregnancy.

EXERCISE RESPONSE

Pregnancy has a major effect on the physiologic responses women have to exercise. Table 8.1 in *ACSM's Guidelines for Exercise Testing and Prescription*, 8th edition, provides an overview of these responses that are detailed in this chapter.

Metabolic Response

Changes in the anatomy and physiology of pregnant women lead to differing exercise responses compared with a nonpregnant woman. Oxygen uptake during weight-dependent exercise is increased, whereas oxygen uptake during weight-independent exercise is unchanged during pregnancy (25).

Cardiovascular Response

During exercise, pregnant women have increased heart rates primarily caused by increased levels of gestational hormones in the first trimester (24). During subsequent trimesters, heart rate is elevated to maintain blood pressure. Blood volume increases by approximately 50% during pregnancy to accommodate the needs of both the mother and fetus (35). This increase in blood volume increases stroke volume and cardiac output. Systolic and diastolic blood pressures remain unchanged during pregnancy. A decrease in total peripheral resistance attenuates the increase in blood volume that typically would cause blood pressure to increase (111).

Ventilatory Response

Minute ventilation ($\dot{V}E$) increases during pregnancy because of increased ventilatory sensitivity. A lower ventilatory threshold and an increase in the sensitivity to CO_2 cause tidal volume and breathing frequency to increase (111). Because of the increased $\dot{V}E$, both ventilatory equivalent for oxygen ($\dot{V}E/\dot{V}O_2$) and ventilatory equivalent for carbon dioxide ($\dot{V}E/\dot{V}CO_2$) increase.

Fetal Response

Factors that can elicit a fetal response to exercise include blood flow and oxygen delivery, heat dissipation, and glucose availability. A decrease in any of these factors can adversely affect the fetus. The degree of the effect depends on the intensity of the exercise. Higher-intensity exercise will cause a greater decrease in any of the factors compared with moderate-intensity exercise. Women who exercise regularly before and during pregnancy have increased blood flow, oxygen, and nutrient delivery to the uterus, reducing the risk of adversely affecting the fetus during exercise. Also, women who exercise tend to divert more blood flow to the skin and begin to sweat sooner, allowing heat to dissipate more quickly without causing a dangerously increased fetal temperature (23). These adaptations allow women to comfortably exercise during pregnancy without risk to fetal health.

EXERCISE TESTING

Maximal exercise testing should not be performed in pregnant women unless medically necessary. If a maximal exercise test is warranted, the test should be performed with physician supervision. An equation for predicting peak oxygen uptake ($\dot{V}O_{2peak}$) from peak heart rate and peak speed and grade achieved during incremental, submaximal treadmill exercise has been validated for women during pregnancy (74). Women who have been sedentary before pregnancy or who have a medical condition (see Box 8.1 in the *ACSM's Guidelines for Exercise Testing and Prescription*, 8th edition) should receive clearance from their physician before beginning an exercise program.

EXERCISE PRESCRIPTION

> **1.7.22-HFS: Skill to teach and demonstrate appropriate modifications in specific exercises for groups such as older adults, pregnant and postnatal women, obese persons, and persons with low-back pain.**

The CSEP Physical Activity Readiness Medical Examination for Pregnancy (PARmed-X for Pregnancy) is used for screening pregnant women before participating in exercise programs (see Figure 8.1 in the *ACSM's Guidelines for Exercise Testing and Prescription*, 8th edition) (112). The recommended exercise prescription for pregnant women is generally consistent with recommendations for the general adult population. However, it is important to monitor and adjust exercise prescriptions according to the woman's symptoms, discomforts, and abilities during pregnancy.

Physical activity should be performed on at least 3 days, preferably every day of the week. Physical activity should be of moderate intensity (40%–60% $\dot{V}O_2$ reserve [$\dot{V}O_2R$]). If peak VO_2 is known, then workloads associated with 40% to 60% of $\dot{V}O_2R$ may be calculated. In nonpregnant women, $\dot{V}O_2R$ is typically translated into a target heart rate (HR) using equivalent percentages of heart rate reserve (HRR). However, because pregnancy raises resting HR and lowers maximal HR, the HRR method is ineffective unless true resting and maximal HRs are known. Given the rarity of maximal testing during pregnancy, neither the $\dot{V}O_2R$ nor HRR method of prescribing exercise intensity is commonly used. Alternatives include using rating of perceived exertion (RPE) (12–14 on a scale of 6–20) or the "talk test" (being able to maintain a conversation during activity) to monitor exercise intensity. General guidelines for physical activity during pregnancy are summarized in Table 41-1. If HR is to be used to establish intensity, ranges that correspond to moderate-intensity exercise have been developed for pregnant women based on age (Table 41-2) (31).

The duration of physical activity should be at least 15 $min \cdot d^{-1}$, gradually increasing to at least 30 $min \cdot d^{-1}$ of accumulated physical activity. The type of physical activity should be dynamic and rhythmic in nature and use large muscle groups. Aerobic activities include walking,

TABLE 41-1. PHYSICAL ACTIVITY RECOMMENDATIONS FOR PREGNANT WOMEN

Frequency	3 $d \cdot wk^{-1}$, preferably daily
Intensity	Moderate (40%–60%) RPE 12–14 (6–20 scale) Talk test
Duration	15–30 minutes
Mode	Aerobic activity

RPE, rating of perceived exertion.

TABLE 41-2. MODIFIED HEART RATE TARGET ZONES FOR MODERATE-INTENSITY AEROBIC EXERCISE IN PREGNANCY

MATERNAL AGE (yr)	HEART RATE TARGET ZONE (beats $\cdot min^{-1}$)
<20	140–155
20–29	135–150
30–39	130–145
≥40	125–140

From Davies GA, Wolfe LA, Mottola MF, MacKinnon C. Joint SOGC/CSEP clinical practice guideline: exercise in pregnancy and the postpartum period. *Can J Appl Physiol*. 2003;28:330–41.

cycling, and swimming. Pregnant women should avoid contact sports and sports/activities that may cause loss of balance or trauma to the mother or fetus. Examples of sports/activities to avoid include soccer, basketball, ice hockey, horseback riding, and vigorous-intensity racquet sports.

SPECIAL CONSIDERATIONS

Pregnant women who have been sedentary or who have a condition that inhibits them from engaging in recommended levels of physical activity should gradually increase activity with the goal of meeting guidelines previously mentioned. Morbidly obese women and women with medical conditions related to pregnancy, gestational diabetes mellitus, or pregnancy-induced hypertension should receive clearance from their physician before beginning an exercise program. Exercise prescriptions should be adjusted according to the medical condition, symptoms, and functional capacity of the women.

Exercise should be terminated should any of the following occur: vaginal bleeding, dyspnea before exertion, dizziness, headache, chest pain, muscle weakness, calf pain or swelling, preterm labor, decreased fetal movement, and amniotic fluid leakage. In the case of calf pain and swelling, thrombophlebitis should be ruled out (2).

Pregnant women should avoid exercising in the supine position after the first trimester to ensure that venous obstruction to the fetus does not occur. Pregnant women should also avoid performing the Valsalva maneuver during exercise. For the safety of the woman and the fetus, exercise should take place in a thermoneutral environment, and the woman should be adequately hydrated to avoid heat stress.

During pregnancy, the metabolic demand increases by approximately 300 $kcal \cdot d^{-1}$. Regular exercise also increases the metabolic demand, which depends on the intensity and duration of the workouts. Women should increase caloric intake to meet the caloric costs of both pregnancy and exercise. This will ensure that the mother and fetus are receiving proper nutrients to sustain the pregnancy.

Pregnant women may participate in a strength-training program. The program should incorporate low resistance lifts (40%–60% of estimated one repetition maximum [1RM]) and high repetition sets (12–15 repetitions). During strength training, women should avoid the supine position and the Valsalva maneuver.

Generally, exercise in the postpartum period may begin approximately 4 to 6 weeks after delivery and with permission from a physician. Women who deliver via cesarean section may require more than 6 weeks after delivery to begin exercise. Deconditioning typically occurs during the initial postpartum period, so women should gradually increase exercise until prepregnancy physical fitness levels are achieved.

CHILDREN AND ADOLESCENTS

> **1.7.3-HFS: Knowledge of the benefits and precautions associated with exercise training across the lifespan (from youth to elderly).**

> **1.7.7-HFS: Knowledge of and the ability to describe the unique adaptations to exercise training in children, adolescents, and older participants with regard to strength, functional capacity, and motor skills.**

In 2003–2004, 33.6% of U.S. children and adolescents were classified as overweight or obese (79). Current trends indicate that this number will increase over the next few years. Most children participate in adequate amounts of physical activity (30). However, physical activity levels decrease through adolescence such that the majority of adolescents are not participating in sufficient amounts of physical activity to meet recommended guidelines (19). Decreased levels of physical activity during childhood and adolescence tend to track as lower levels of physical activity in adulthood (70). These findings provide evidence that children who adopt a physically active lifestyle may have a better chance of continuing this behavior later in life.

Cardiovascular disease (CVD) risk factors that are present in youth also have a tendency to track into adulthood. Youth who are overweight are more likely to have a higher prevalence of CVD risk factors than their normal-weight peers. In children and adolescents, the presence of CVD risk factors may indicate the future development of disease, which manifests much later in life. Risk factors that track into adulthood include dyslipidemia, hypertension, obesity, impaired glucose tolerance, and sedentary behavior (102). Each of these risk factors can be modified positively through physical activity. Therefore, it is important that children become physically active during childhood and continue this behavior through adolescence into adulthood, so that their risk of CVD and all-cause mortality is reduced.

In addition to benefits that physical activity has on physical health and fitness, physical activity also has a positive influence on academic performance (26) and self-esteem. Because of the protective and health benefits of habitual physical activity, it is important that children are physically active and that they continue this behavior through adolescence into adulthood (102).

EXERCISE RESPONSE

As a result of growth and maturation processes, children's physiologic responses to exercise differ from those of adults (see Table 8.2 in the ACSM's *Guidelines for Exercise Testing and Prescription*, 8th edition). Children's smaller stature and body weight, in addition to the immaturity of their physiologic regulatory systems, requires special consideration when exercising.

Children have lower absolute oxygen uptake ($\dot{V}O_2$ [$L \cdot min^{-1}$]) values compared with adults. However, because of the immaturity of the metabolic system and scaling, children's relative oxygen uptake ($\dot{V}O_2$ [$mL \cdot kg^{-1} \cdot min^{-1}$]) is higher than in adults. Children are also less economical than adults, resulting in a higher relative oxygen consumption, especially during locomotor activities. According to the geometric principles of scaling, smaller organisms are expected to have higher metabolic rates (relative to body mass) than are larger organisms.

Cardiovascular Response

Children's stroke volumes at submaximal and maximal exercise are lower than adult values. Children's submaximal and maximal HRs are generally higher than adult HRs at corresponding workloads. Cardiac output is slightly lower in children. Because of lower cardiac outputs, the systolic and diastolic blood pressures are lower in children (50,90).

Ventilatory Response

Minute ventilation ($\dot{V}E$) is lower in children than in adults. Children have a higher breathing frequency than adults, however, children tend to not breathe as deeply. Children use less oxygen per breath, which may be because of a shorter ventilatory cycle, a result of a higher breathing frequency. The oxygen cost of ventilation is also higher in children because of their more frequent, shallow breaths (50,90).

Thermoregulatory Response

Children also have immature thermoregulatory systems. Children have a higher threshold for sweating and have a lower perspiration rate than adults. These thermoregulatory responses require that youth exercise in thermoneutral environments and be properly hydrated so as not to overheat. Special care must be taken to avoid ambient temperatures that are greater than body temperature, as children will gain heat more quickly than adults because of their greater surface area to body mass ratio (50,90).

EXERCISE TESTING

 1.5.11-CES: Address exercise testing and training needs of elderly and young patients.

Generally, the adult guidelines for standard exercise testing apply to children and adolescents (see Chapters 19 and 20). The exercise testing protocol and mode of testing (treadmill versus cycle) should be based on the reason the test is being performed and the functional capacity of the child or adolescent. Typically, treadmills elicit a higher peak oxygen uptake ($\dot{V}O_{2\,peak}$) and maximum heart rate (HR_{max}). Cycle ergometers provide less risk for injury but need to have the ability to adjust to the size of the child or adolescent. Before testing, children and adolescents should be familiarized with the test protocol and procedure. This familiarization with the procedure serves to minimize stress and maximize the potential for a successful test. Compared with adults, children and adolescents are mentally and psychologically immature and may require extra motivation and support during the exercise test (83).

In addition to traditional clinical fitness testing, health/fitness testing may be performed outside of the clinical setting. Fitness testing may occur in places such as schools or community centers. In these types of settings, the FITNESSGRAM test battery may be used to assess the components of health-related fitness in youth (54). The components of health-related fitness covered in this battery include cardiorespiratory capacity, muscular strength, muscular endurance, flexibility, and body composition. Criterion-referenced standards are available for this test.

EXERCISE PRESCRIPTION

1.7.4-CES: Design, implement, and supervise individualized exercise prescriptions for people with chronic disease and disabling conditions, or who are young or elderly.

1.7.5-HFS: Knowledge of how to select and/or modify appropriate exercise programs according to age, functional capacity, and limitations of the individual.

1.7.6-HFS: Knowledge of the differences in the development of an exercise prescription for children, adolescents, and older participants.

Aerobic Activity

The exercise prescription guidelines outlined below for children and adolescents establish the minimal amount of physical activity needed to achieve the various components of health-related fitness. These recommendations are based on a combination of evidence-based guidelines developed by an expert panel and from the National Association for Sport and Physical Education (NASPE), the governing body for physical education (75,98).

Physical activity should be performed at least 3 to 4 $d \cdot wk^{-1}$, preferably daily. Physical activity should be of moderate (physical activity that noticeably increases breathing, sweating, and HR) to vigorous (physical activity that substantially increases breathing, sweating, and HR) intensity. These intensities are intended to approximate 40% to 59% and 60–85% of $\dot{V}O_2$ reserve, respectively. RPE scales, such as the OMNI Scale, may also be used to set the intensity of activity (see Fig. 26.2). Youth should participate in 30 $min \cdot d^{-1}$ of moderate and 30 $min \cdot d^{-1}$ of vigorous intensity to total 60 $min \cdot d^{-1}$ of accumulated physical activity. To achieve recommended levels of physical activity, youth should participate in a variety of activities that are enjoyable and developmentally appropriate, which may include locomotor activities, active games, dance, and sports. Table 41-3 presents a summary of physical activity guidelines for children and adolescents.

Strength Training

1.7.8-CES: Demonstrate exercise equipment adaptations necessary for different age groups, physical abilities, and other potential contributing factors.

1.7.17-CES: Design strength and flexibility programs for individuals with cardiovascular, pulmonary and/or metabolic diseases, the elderly, and children.

Previous research indicates that children and adolescents may safely participate in strength-training activities (8). Strength gains achieved by prepubescent youth typically occur as a result of neuromuscular adaptations; postpubescent youth can achieve hypertrophic adaptations because of the presence of anabolic hormones. Recommendations for resistance training include a moderate intensity (60%–80% of estimated 1RM), 8 to 15 repetitions for one to three sets, no more than 2 $d \cdot wk^{-1}$. It is of primary importance that youth receive proper instruction and supervision (8). Also, youth should be able to properly fit the equipment being used for training. Equipment that is too large for children and adolescents impedes them from using proper form while training, which may increase their risk of injury.

TABLE 41-3. PHYSICAL ACTIVITY RECOMMENDATIONS FOR CHILDREN AND ADOLESCENTS

Frequency	3–4 $d \cdot wk^{-1}$, preferably daily
Intensity	Moderate to vigorous
Duration	60 minutes (accumulated)
Mode	Activities that are enjoyable and developmentally appropriate

Flexibility

Youth should regularly participate in activities that promote increased levels of flexibility. Increased flexibility translates into an increased range of motion, which is advantageous in certain sporting activities. Children and adolescents should participate in flexibility activities at least 3 $d \cdot wk^{-1}$, preferably every day. Intensity of the stretch should be at the point of mild discomfort, and then have the individual back off slightly. The stretch should be held between 10 and 30 seconds. Static stretching should be emphasized in youth, with each major muscle group targeted during stretching sessions.

Special Considerations

Because of the increasing prevalence of childhood obesity and decreasing levels of daily physical activity in youth, children and adolescents who are overweight or physically inactive may not be able to achieve 60 $min \cdot d^{-1}$ of physical activity. It is important to gradually increase the duration and frequency of physical activity to achieve this goal. Gradual progression will aid in the avoidance of exercise program dropout and lower the risk of injury. In this population, every effort should be made to decrease sedentary activities, such as television watching, surfing the Internet, and playing stationary video games. It is also important that youth are exposed to a variety of activities that promote lifelong activity and fitness (i.e., walking and cycling).

Children and adolescents with diseases or disabilities such as asthma, diabetes mellitus, obesity, cystic fibrosis, and cerebral palsy should have their exercise prescriptions tailored to their condition, symptoms, and functional capacity. With most of these disease states, youth have a lower level of cardiorespiratory fitness compared with their healthy counterparts. This low level of fitness may be the result of the children with these disease states being sedentary, either because of the inability to exercise or physicians and/or parents who encourage inactivity (5). In most cases, youth with these disease states are able to exercise, usually with the result of increased fitness and decreased symptoms of the disease.

OLDER ADULTS

> **1.7.4-CES: Design, implement, and supervise individualized exercise prescriptions for people with chronic disease and disabling conditions, or who are young or elderly.**

> **1.7.6-CES: Knowledge of the concept of activities of daily living (ADLs) and its importance in the overall rehabilitation of the individual.**

> **1.7.20-HFS: Knowledge of the concept of activities of daily living (ADLs) and its importance in the overall health of the individual.**

Currently, disparities exist among population groups in levels of physical activity that exaggerate the negative health consequences of a sedentary lifestyle. According to the 1996 Surgeon General's Report on Physical Activity and Health, demographic groups at highest risk for inactivity are the elderly, women, minorities, those with low income or educational background, and those with disabilities or chronic health conditions (102). As might be expected, these are the same demographic groups that both bear a large burden of the diseases amenable to prevention and treatment with exercise (40) and yet often have the least access and opportunity for health-promotion efforts related to physical activity. Therefore, exercise and fitness specialists should identify and understand barriers to physical activity faced by particular population groups and be prepared to develop programs and tools that address these barriers.

Previous objectives for the nation have primarily focused on physical activities designed to improve cardiorespiratory fitness and prolong life. However, it is now recognized that older adults can benefit from physical activities designed to ensure functional independence throughout life as well. The specific physical fitness components that provide continued physical function as individuals age include muscle strength, cardiovascular and muscular endurance, balance, and flexibility. The problems of mobility impairment, falls, arthritis, osteoporotic fractures, and functional status are clearly related to muscle strength and mass (33,58,94,96,104), and thus strengthening activities, although important for all age groups, are particularly important for older adults. Age-related loss of strength, muscle mass, and bone density, which are most dramatic in women, may be attenuated by strengthening exercises and regained even afterward with appropriate resistance training (1,9,48,93,99). Unfortunately, national survey data indicate that women in general report lower-than-average adult participation levels for strength training (11% vs. 16%) (20). Additionally, despite the evidence on safety and efficacy in even frail elders, the prevalence rate for resistive exercise is even lower among the old (6% at ages 65–74) or the very old (4% older than age 75) (20). Individuals in this latter age group, particularly older than the age of 85, are primarily women, making an understanding of the risks and benefits of exercise in this population a priority.

RATIONALE FOR EXERCISE IN OLDER ADULTS

The rationale for the integration of a physical activity prescription into geriatric healthcare is based on four essential concepts (84,85). First, there is a great similarity between the physiologic changes that are attributable to disuse and those that have been typically observed in aging populations, leading to the speculation that the way in which we age may in fact be greatly modulated with attention to activity levels. Second, chronic diseases increase with age, and exercise has now been shown to be an independent risk factor and/or potential treatment for most of the major causes of morbidity and mortality in western societies, a potential which is currently vastly underutilized (13,41,55,85). Third, traditional medical interventions don't typically address disuse syndromes accompanying chronic disease, which may be responsible for much of their associated disability. Exercise is particularly good at targeting syndromes of disuse (103). Finally, many pathophysiologic aberrations that are central to a disease or its treatment are specifically addressed only by exercise, which therefore deserves a place in the mainstream of medical care, not as an optional adjunct.

It is clear that the optimum approach to "successful aging" or to healthcare in the older population cannot ignore the overlap of these areas. In some cases, exercise can be used to avert "age-related" decrements in physiologic function and thereby maximize function and quality of life in the elderly. On the other hand, the combination of exercise and sound nutrition, particularly in relation to favorable alterations in body composition, will have numerous important effects on risk factors for chronic disease as well as the disability that accompanies such conditions. Therefore, understanding the effects of aging on exercise capacity and how habitual physical activity can modify this relationship in the older adult, including its specific utility in treating medical diseases, is critical for healthcare practitioners of all disciplines.

EXERCISE TESTING

 1.5.11-CES: Address exercise testing and training needs of elderly and young patients.

When exercise is prescribed for healthcare goals, its use by the individual should be systematically reviewed and adjusted over time, like any other medical intervention, via exercise testing. Such assessments and tracking should be built into any exercise prescription for older adults. Periodically performing exercise-capacity assessments and reviewing activity logs will form the primary means of assessing compliance and adaptation over time, and it is recommended that such discussions be included in counseling sessions/group meetings at regular intervals. Often errors in training technique (particularly lack of regularity, progression, and appropriate intensity) will be uncovered in this way. The primary goal of the exercise prescription is to change exercise behavior and fitness itself. Additionally, secondary goals may be improvements in specific symptoms or conditions, such as arthritis pain, depression, sleep disturbance, angina, time to claudication, glucose control, or blood pressure, and appropriate measurements may be made to gauge progress in these areas as well. However, as some things are slow to change—i.e., the effects not dramatic in the short term—it is best not to overly emphasize goals such as weight loss or the need for antihypertensive medicines as

the participant may be discouraged rather than encouraged by the results.

Most health outcomes appear to be related to the accumulated volume and intensity of exercise, and so monitoring compliance will theoretically provide evidence that the benefits are occurring (14,15,22,80,84,85,94,96). However, there may be benefit also in monitoring the improvements in cardiovascular fitness from training, as aerobic capacity itself has an even stronger relationship to mortality than level of physical activity. Documenting improvements in fitness may have a reinforcing effect on long-term behavioral adaptations as well. Improved fitness across domains of exercise capacity may be shown by:

- Improved measurements of maximal aerobic capacity
- Decreased HR and blood pressure response to a fixed submaximal workload
- Decreased RPE for a fixed submaximal workload
- Improved strength
- Ability to lift a submaximal load more times
- Ability to withstand postural stress or negotiate obstacles
- Improved joint range of motion

EXERCISE TESTING FOR THE OLDEST SEGMENT OF THE POPULATION

Aerobic Capacity Testing

Because treadmill testing and indirect calorimetry are not always available or feasible, particularly in frail older adults older than 75 years, field estimates of aerobic capacity and cardiovascular responses are usually substituted. A simple way to do this in clinical practice that requires minimal equipment is the 6-minute walk test (46). This test has been used as an index of rehabilitation in cardiac and pulmonary patients, and is known to improve with effective interventions. With training, pulse and blood pressure at 6 minutes should decrease, and distance covered should increase. In young or very fit individuals, a running test is usually needed, as they do not have room for much improvement on a walking test. Alternatives to the 6-minute walk are walking a fixed distance (e.g., 400 m), climbing multiple flights of stairs as rapidly as possible, or stepping up and down a single step for several minutes, followed by the measurements above. Availability of stairs and the potential for musculoskeletal injury because of balance, hip and knee arthritis, or vision problems make rapid-stepping tests less desirable in the older adult, however.

In evaluating the responses to aerobic exercise, the reduced fatigue and/or breathlessness during submaximal exercise will be of greater magnitude than the increase in maximal aerobic capacity, if this is measured. Because most ADLs take place at submaximal workloads, this benefit should be readily appreciable to the older adult as well. Large improvements in maximal aerobic capacity are not seen in "lifestyle" approaches to aerobic exercise and are likely to occur only after structured, high-intensity progressive aerobic training (22). Therefore, to avoid discouraging a compliant exerciser who is doing an appropriate *volume* of exercise to achieve health benefits, but perhaps not at an *intensity* required for improvements in maximal aerobic capacity, it is best to concentrate on the improved tolerance for submaximal workloads that is likely to have accrued instead. In addition to clinical testing for such improved tolerance, as above, it is a good idea to ask older adults their current RPE for series of tasks performed at home at regular intervals. Providing this as written or visual "proof of progress" over the course of several months will reinforce the positive change in behavior that has occurred and emphasize the relevance of the exercise prescription to daily life.

Strength Testing

If maximal strength itself cannot be measured or is not considered safe or feasible in an elderly individual, there is an option that is commonly used to rate effort during a lift, using a scale of perceived exertion, such as the Borg scale (11). On this scale from 6 to 20, a rating of 15 to 18 (hard to very hard) is equivalent to 80% of maximum lifting capacity in studies conducted in young and older adults, and is therefore an appropriate training goal (43,66). The technique is as follows: As soon as the person performs the lift with the first weight selected, he or she should be asked to rate how difficult it was to lift. If it was given a score less than 15, than the next higher weight available can be used, until the appropriate range is reached. If a weight that is too heavy is selected, as long as proper form and breathing and speed of lifting are adhered to, the only thing that can happen is that the person will be unable to cover the full range of motion or complete a full set of repetitions. Older adults, particularly older men and women, rarely if ever voluntarily choose weights that are too heavy. On the other hand, there is a great tendency to choose weights that are far too light to be optimally therapeutic. The negative effects of exercising at a subtherapeutic intensity are many: discouragement at lack of progress; delayed recovery from atrophy and illness; and limited improvements in arthritis, mobility, balance, and other outcomes. In the end, this approach is quite counterproductive. There is, in fact, no evidence that the often presumed positive benefits of using lighter-than-recommended weights (e.g., prevention of injury, minimizing dropout, addressing fears of lifting heavy objects, avoiding cardiovascular events) actually occur.

PRE-EXERCISE ASSESSMENT IN OLDER ADULTS

Most older adults, despite the presence of chronic diseases and disabilities, are able to undertake and benefit from an exercise prescription that is tailored to their physiologic capacities, comorbidities, and neuropsychological and behavioral needs. The relative few permanent exclusions to any structured exercise are generally severe irreversible conditions that are obvious exclusions because of the nature of the specific exercise prescription under consideration or the risk the exercise would impose on the health status of the individual (49,107). There may be some forms of exercise that even permanently bed-bound patients or those with severe behavioral problems may engage in, but they are not able to participate in the usual aerobic, resistive, or balance exercises described below. For some older adults, such as those with critical aortic stenosis, cardiac or peripheral vascular ischemia at rest, or an enlarging aortic aneurysm or known cerebral aneurysm (when surgery is not an option because of other medical considerations or very advanced age), any exercise that significantly elevates cardiac workload or blood pressure is considered high risk and therefore not recommended. It is anticipated that relatively few older adults (even those in long-term care) would be excluded from all exercise programs based on items in this category (Table 41-4), outside of those with severe forms of dementia.

The majority of questions about exercise prescription eligibility will be because of items in the "temporary exclusion" category, so judgments must be made based on the severity of the diagnosis, timing of the event in question, and re-evaluation after a diagnostic workup or adjustment of medications is made. It is anticipated that most older adults in this category will be able to be reclassified as appropriate for exercise once their condition has been treated or stabilized. Each of the items listed in Table 41-4 in this category are discussed briefly below, with a rationale for the approach to management that maximizes safety of the exercise prescription and is consistent with ACSM current guidelines.

For older adults with no items in these exclusions columns, a clinical exercise specialist may initiate an exercise program without further review. However, should a change in health status occur after exercise has begun (such as one of the items from the temporary exclusion category), physician review should be requested at that time.

Acute Change in Mental Status or Delirium

Because these symptoms may be indicative of an emerging disease process such as metabolic disorder, fluid imbalance, drug toxicity, systemic infection, or transient ischemic attack, exercise must be delayed until appropriate diagnostic tests have determined the cause of the altered mental status. It is sometimes difficult to recognize delirium when it is superimposed on a chronic dementia, but the characteristic features of fluctuation throughout the day and decreased attention span should differentiate

TABLE 41-4. EVALUATION OF APPROPRIATENESS OF EXERCISE PRESCRIPTION IN OLDER ADULTS

I. STOP! PERMANENT EXCLUSION	II. WAIT! TEMPORARY EXCLUSION	III. GO! EXERCISE RECOMMENDED
If any boxes in this column are checked, individual is ineligible for any exercise prescription at this time.	If any boxes in this column are checked, follow protocols for further evaluation of these concerns with medical personnel before reevaluating for appropriateness/modification of exercise prescription.	If only boxes in this column are checked, individual is suitable for exercise prescription without additional evaluation by medical personnel at this time.
a. ☐ End-stage congestive heart failure	**a.** ☐ Acute change in mental status or delirium, psychosis	**a.** ☐ Arthritis, stable
b. ☐ Permanent bed-bound status	**b.** ☐ Cerebral hemorrhage within the past 3 months	**b.** ☐ Chronic obstructive pulmonary disease, asthma
c. ☐ Severe cognitive impairment or behavioral disturbance	**c.** ☐ Exacerbation of chronic inflammatory joint disease or osteoarthritis	**c.** ☐ Congestive heart failure, stable
d. ☐ Unstable abdominal, thoracic, or cerebral aneurysm	**d.** ☐ Eye surgery within the past 6 weeks	**d.** ☐ Coronary artery disease, stable
e. ☐ Untreated severe aortic stenosis	**e.** ☐ Fracture in healing stage	**e.** ☐ Chronic renal failure
f. ☐ Other _____	**f.** ☐ Hernia, symptomatic (abdominal or inguinal) or bleeding hemorrhoids	**f.** ☐ Cancer (history or current)
	g. ☐ Myocardial infarction or cardiac surgery within past 3 months	**g.** ☐ Chronic liver disease
	h. ☐ Other acute illness or change in symptoms	**h.** ☐ Chronic venous stasis
ASSESSMENT OF ADL FUNCTIONAL PERFORMANCE Check the appropriate boxes below for the individual's actual performance over the last 7 days in each activity	**i.** ☐ Proliferative diabetic retinopathy or severe nonproliferative retinopathy	**i.** ☐ Dementia, cognitive impairment
	j. ☐ Pulmonary embolism or deep venous thrombosis within 3 months	**j.** ☐ Depression, anxiety, low morale
1. INDEPENDENT: received hands-on assistance or supervision/cueing ≤ 2 times in last 7 days;	**k.** ☐ Soft-tissue injury, healing	**k.** ☐ Diabetes
	l. ☐ Active suicidality or suicidal ideation	**l.** ☐ Drugs causing muscle wasting (steroids)
2. INDEPENDENT WITH SUPERVISION: used setup help (e.g., cutting food, laying out clothing, locking wheelchair)	**m.** ☐ Systemic infection	**m.** ☐ Frailty
	n. ☐ Uncontrolled blood pressure (>160/100)	**n.** ☐ Falls, history of hip fracture
3. DEPENDENT	**o.** ☐ Uncontrolled diabetes mellitus (FBS>200 mg/dL)	**o.** ☐ Gait and balance disorders, mobility impairment

	1	2	3	**p.** ☐ Uncontrolled malignant cardiac arrhythmia (ventricular tachycardia, complete heart block, atrial flutter, symptomatic bradycardia)	**p.** ☐ Hypertension
g. Walking in room	☐	☐	☐	**q.** ☐ Unstable angina (at rest or crescendo pattern, ECG changes)	**q.** ☐ HIV infection
h. Transfers	☐	☐	☐	**r.** ☐ Other	**r.** ☐ Hyperlipidemia
i. Dressing	☐	☐	☐		**s.** ☐ Malnutrition, poor appetite
j. Eating	☐	☐	☐		**t.** ☐ Neuromuscular disease
k. Is wheelchair his/her primary mode of locomotion?	☐ Yes	☐ No			**u.** ☐ Obesity
					v. ☐ Osteoporosis
					w. ☐ Parkinson disease
					x. ☐ Peripheral vascular disease
					y. ☐ Stroke, stable

ADL, activities of daily living; ECG, electrocardiogram; FBS, fasting blood sugar; HIV, human immunodeficiency virus.

it from stable cognitive impairment. Once delirium has cleared, or the cause of the cognitive impairment or psychosis is identified and stable, exercise participation is no longer restricted. Residual underlying mental impairment will require lower exercise leader–to–older adults ratios than can be used with cognitively intact older adults. Some individuals with dementia may have an exacerbation of symptoms of disorientation, paranoia, or behavioral disturbance toward the late afternoon or evening hours ("sundowning"). If this syndrome is present, it is important to plan exercise sessions for such older adults to coincide with a more favorable time of the day that facilitates their optimal participation.

Cerebral Hemorrhage within the Past 3 Months

Hemorrhagic stroke because of intracerebral or subarachnoid bleeding is far less common than ischemic stroke because of thrombosis or embolism, accounting for about 30% of all strokes. In its acute phase, it is a contraindication to any activity that has the potential to significantly raise intracerebral or systemic arterial pressure for fear of extending the area of bleeding. There is no clear evidence to indicate when progressive resistance or aerobic exercise may begin, but general physical therapy is initiated as soon as the patient is able, and it is likely that low- to moderate-intensity exercise (both aerobic and resistive) is not detrimental in this phase. However, current guidelines suggest waiting for 3 months posthemorrhagic stroke before initiating progressive resistance training or other kinds of strenuous exercise. Therefore, in the absence of more definitive data, waiting until the subacute stage of recovery, approximately 8 to 12 weeks postintracerebral bleed, is recommended. If other features of cardiovascular status and blood pressure are stable at that time, the program can be initiated without modification.

By contrast, thrombotic or embolic stroke is not a contraindication to exercise training as prescribed in this program. If hemodynamic status is stable, progressive resistance and aerobic and balance training may be added to other elements of physical therapy during the recovery from ischemic stroke. Alternatively, it may be initiated once formal physical therapy has ended as a means to continue and extend the benefits of acute rehabilitation to the subacute and chronic phases of recovery.

In all forms of stroke, particular attention should be paid to proper breathing technique to avoid excessive rises in mean arterial pressure that may occur during the Valsalva maneuver (straining against a closed glottis). Although the cerebral and ocular circulations are protected to some extent against acute rises in blood pressure via autoregulatory pathways governing vasoconstriction of the cerebral vessels, this pathway can be overridden by extreme rises in pressure. Such rises are associated with very heavy loads, sustained contractions, breath holding, and the Valsalva maneuver, which is why such techniques

are not indicated, whether or not stroke is present. Again, more data are needed on the use of resistance or aerobic training during the early recovery period of ischemic stroke, but both appear to be well-tolerated and efficacious in this setting.

Exacerbation of Chronic Inflammatory Joint Disease or Osteoarthritis

Although both resistance and aerobic exercise have been shown to be beneficial for function and pain in chronic arthritis, there are times during a flare-up of the disease that such exercise needs to be avoided or modified. Usually this is a temporary condition affecting one or more joints that will resolve with appropriate diagnosis, treatment, and time, thus allowing exercise prescription to be initiated in standard or modified form. Appropriate steps may include:

- Evaluation of other possible causes of joint pain, including fracture, dislocation, rotator cuff, cartilage or ligament tear, septic or gout-related inflammation in the joint, referred neurologic pain, spinal stenosis, and carpal tunnel syndrome, which require specific therapeutic interventions
- Modification of pain or anti-inflammatory medications to provide better coverage of symptoms
- Prescription of a period of isometric strength training of the muscles around the affected joint(s), with a transition to dynamic strength training as soon as symptoms have stabilized
- Modification of positions or ranges of motion of the standard exercises to accommodate particular musculoskeletal restrictions in individual older adults

It should be emphasized that if the affected joint (such as a hip or knee) is unable to be improved because of very severe disease/deformity/pain, this should not be used as a rationale to avoid all resistance training. By contrast, such individuals, whose independence and mobility are threatened by progressive joint disease and surrounding muscle atrophy from disuse, are in *great need* of strengthening exercises for their upper body. This is because they will rely increasingly on shoulder and triceps strength to assist with transfers when lower-extremity pain and reduced range of motion are present and progressive. Such prophylactic use of progressive resistance training to offset impending disability by improving the capacity of uninvolved muscle groups and joints to assist with the activity is preferable to the simple use of assistive devices such as higher chair seats, or "adaptive maneuvers" such as rocking back and forth to rise from a chair. Assistive devices or alternative strategies such as rocking do not improve the underlying physiologic capacity of the person to perform the task and should therefore be used as adjuncts when needed, but not considered appropriate as an isolated approach to such impairments.

Eye Surgery within the Past 6 Weeks

Recent ophthalmologic procedures, such as cataract extraction, laser treatments, or other surgery, require a period of healing during which elevations of intraocular pressure are contraindicated. The exact duration of this recovery period is not known with precision, and ophthalmologists may impose restrictions for periods ranging from a few days to 6 weeks. Therefore, it is recommended that any older adult who has had such procedures should have clearance by his or her ophthalmologist before engaging in the exercises. In general, the risk is low; however, it is prudent to seek specific clearance in individual cases, given the lack of a consensus among practitioners or any clinical trial evidence on which to base guidelines.

The kinds of activities that should be specifically avoided in older adults with healing eye surgery include:

- Lowering the head below the heart
- Direct impact to eye or surrounding tissues
- High impact, jolting activities (jumping, jogging)
- Any activity or situation that causes very high elevations in blood pressure

Thus, walking, stepping, or cycling at low-to-moderate intensities, or typical resistance training as outlined in these guidelines, are not in this category and can be resumed as soon as clearance is obtained.

Fracture in Healing Stage

Specific timing of resistance training after a fracture will depend on the type and stability of fracture, surgical treatment, casting or immobilization, and pain control. Therefore, clearance should be sought from the orthopedic surgeon, physiatrist, or physical therapist directing the care during acute rehabilitation. For fractures involving a cast, isometric resistance exercises can and *should* be initiated immediately after fixation in most cases, and will prevent the rapid muscle atrophy associated with periods of immobilization in this situation. Once immobilization is no longer needed, isometric training can be replaced with dynamic training to regain the maximum range of motion and strength across the affected joints.

Hip fractures will be followed by a period of partial weight bearing and restrictions in hip motions in some cases, depending on the type of surgical fixation used, stability of the fracture site, and underlying degree of osteopenia around the prosthesis. Hip adduction, flexion, and internal rotation are often prohibited for a period after prosthetic joint implantation, for example. Communication with the therapist or surgeon will be required to establish the nature and time course of such restrictions in individual cases. In general, by 6 weeks postoperatively, the majority of patients with fractured hips who have regained ambulatory status will be full weight bearing and no longer require hip movement restrictions. At this time, or whenever the surgeon approves, standard exercises may be initiated, and these will complement and extend other aspects of rehabilitation. Lower-extremity resistance exercises (hip abduction, extension, flexion, knee extension and flexion, and plantar flexion) and balance training are particularly important to the recovery of gait, balance, and function in this cohort and do not place the person at risk of prosthetic dislocation once surgically stable. For those patients who do not regain ambulatory status, arm strengthening will be critical for the optimization of independence in transfer activities, and leg exercises in seated or modified standing postures should be included as possible.

Symptomatic Hernia (Abdominal or Inguinal) or Bleeding Hemorrhoids

The elevation in intra-abdominal pressure during weightlifting exercise may increase symptoms in an unrepaired hernia or bleeding hemorrhoid. This will need to be evaluated on an individual basis. In some cases, avoiding breath holding, straining, and the Valsalva maneuver will be sufficient to prevent symptoms, and training can be initiated. In others, any elevation in pressure is intolerable, and it may be necessary to treat the hernia surgically or with mechanical supports. In general, umbilical hernias that are small and reducible are not associated with pain, bowel obstruction, or strangulation, and do not preclude training with moderate loads, although they may enlarge with higher loads. More worrisome are large or painful inguinal hernias, which may require surgical evaluation and delay of exercise initiation. Previously repaired hernias are not a contraindication to resistance training; however, careful instruction on breathing techniques and monitoring for hernia pain or protrusion during exercise should be carried out, as these individuals are at risk for recurrence.

Myocardial Infarction or Cardiac Surgery within Past 3 Months

Exercise has been shown to be an effective strategy after myocardial infarction or cardiac surgery to improve mortality, reduce secondary events, and improve quality of life. Cardiac rehabilitation programs include both aerobic and resistive training after medical stabilization, and therefore exercise is appropriate for such patients as part of their overall rehabilitation. However, older adults with a recent cardiac event should be cleared by a physician and monitored for physical signs or symptoms of heart disease, as they are at higher risk for recurrent events than other older adults are. Precautions that apply to the cardiac patient in particular include:

- Avoiding the Valsalva maneuver at all times
- Avoiding sustained, isometric contractions
- Observing rest periods between repetitions and sets as prescribed

- Exercising in supervised setting with emergency plan in place for facility
- Stopping exercise immediately if there is any suspicion of angina, arrhythmias, or ischemia during exercise
- Warming up and cooling down with slow walking before and after more vigorous exercise

Proliferative Diabetic Retinopathy or Severe Nonproliferative Retinopathy

There are case reports of retinal bleeding or detachment occurring in response to extreme elevations in blood pressure associated with very heavy power lifting or sustained isometric contractions with Valsalva maneuver. Individuals with severe retinopathy are at higher risk for retinal detachment and bleeding under normal conditions, and therefore significant elevations in arterial and intraocular pressure (such as those associated with strenuous exercise or head-down positioning) should be avoided in such conditions. Milder degrees of retinopathy and nonproliferative retinopathy (such as is usually seen with hypertensive disease or type 2 diabetes in older adults) do not preclude resistive or aerobic exercises as normally prescribed. Therefore, it is recommended that older adults with retinopathy of moderate to severe degree be evaluated by an ophthalmologist before beginning an exercise regimen. Because retinal hemorrhage or detachment is in many cases preventable with prophylactic laser treatment, such exams are indicated in all adults with hypertension and diabetes on an annual basis, regardless of exercise participation. Most adults with mild or moderate retinopathy are appropriate for the moderate- to high-intensity aerobic and resistive exercises. Avoiding sustained contractions, breath holding, isometric contractions, the Valsalva maneuver, and holding the head below the level of the heart minimizes risk.

Pulmonary Embolism or Deep Venous Thrombosis within 3 Months

In the acute phase, it is possible that the mechanical and hemodynamic factors associated with exercise of any kind could cause a clot to break off or move in the circulation, causing further symptoms or pulmonary infarction. It is not known precisely what the risk of exercise is in this situation, but prudence suggests avoiding strenuous activity until full anticoagulation has been achieved and the clot has organized and is unlikely to expand or embolize further. Although the precise timing of such a period of waiting is unknown, a conservative approach is to review all older adults with a pulmonary or deep venous thrombosis in the past 3 months before initiating exercise. It is likely that the majority of such individuals may begin exercise earlier than 3 months after the event, as long as anticoagulant status is stable and hemodynamic or respiratory status is not compromised. Falling while on anticoagulants will increase the risk for soft-tissue bleeding and bruising,

so particular care should be taken during transfer activities before and after exercises, when postural blood pressure changes may be prevalent, as well as in the handling of heavy weights that could be dropped onto legs or feet. Padding the front of the shin with a woolen leg warmer or thick sock may be necessary to prevent bruising from the placement of ankle weights, if used.

Soft-Tissue Injury (Healing)

Depending on the nature of the injury, various periods of rest may be needed in the face of acute soft-tissue trauma or surgery. If sutures have been placed, once they are removed and skin closure has been achieved, exercise may in general be resumed. Sprains, strains, bruises, skin lacerations, dislocations, and other injuries should be evaluated on a case-by-case basis for the timing of exercise. In general, it is best to continue exercising the nonaffected body parts to avoid disuse and behavioral disruption. In addition, isometric exercises of the affected body part may be continued to prevent muscle atrophy without causing additional injury to joints, tendons, ligaments, or other affected tissues.

Suicidal Ideation

Although depression may be treated with moderate- to high-intensity exercise, an older adult who currently expresses passive ("I wish I was dead") or active ("I have a plan to take my life") suicidal ideation must be immediately referred to a qualified psychiatric/medical professional. Older men who live alone are the cohort at the highest risk of suicide out of all depressed individuals, and such sentiments should never be dismissed. Once antidepressant treatment has been initiated, exercise may be a strong adjunctive or alternative form of therapy prescribed for clinical depression.

Systemic Infection

During acute systemic infections, there is an increased risk of dehydration, arrhythmias, pericarditis, myocarditis, ischemia, delirium, and fatigue, all of which affect both the safety and feasibility of exercise training. Therefore, it is recommended that while a febrile condition or systemic infection exists, exercise be temporarily put on hold. For nonsystemic minor infections, such as a small skin infection or minor upper-respiratory symptoms, clinical judgment may be used to direct the nature and intensity of the physical activities that are undertaken.

Uncontrolled Blood Pressure (>160/100 mm Hg)

Although all kinds of exercise elevate blood pressure acutely during the phase of muscle contraction, the chronic effect of training in nonhypertensives and hypertensives is to lower blood pressure slightly. Weightlifting exercises cause moderate elevations in systolic and diastolic blood pressure for several beats while the muscle is contracted, and then a rapid return to baseline values or below baseline values in the recovery period between lifts. Therefore, if blood pressure is currently out of control, exercise should not be initiated until better levels are achieved (e.g., approximately 150/95 mm Hg or lower on most readings). There are no definitive data on exactly what cutoff should be used, but in general, hypertension needs to be controlled whether exercise is planned or not, so general recommendations for monitoring and treating hypertension in the elderly should be followed. This is particularly true for type 2 diabetic patients, who are at much higher risk for vascular complications of their disease if hypertension is uncontrolled. For individuals with mild to moderate elevations in pressure (140–170/90–100 mm Hg), review by a physician with a plan for dietary, pharmacologic, and physical activity management of the hypertension is appropriate, and resistive or aerobic exercises are both appropriate in this setting. Until blood pressure is under better control, it may be prudent in some individuals to monitor blood pressure and pulse responses to exercise. In addition, in all individuals with hypertension, one should avoid very strenuous aerobic exercise, very heavy loads, sustained contractions, isometric handgrip, and Valsalva maneuver during lifting to minimize blood pressure excursions.

Uncontrolled Diabetes Mellitus (Fasting Blood Glucose >200 mg · dL^{-1})

As with hypertension, diabetes is in general an indication *for* exercise; however, in the acute stage when metabolic control is very poor, exercise may cause blood glucose levels to deteriorate further. In the insulin-resistant type 2 diabetic patient, there is usually no danger of severe ketosis or acidosis, but the rise in blood glucose may produce symptoms of fatigue or altered mental state, as well as infections, diuresis, and dehydration. Therefore, it is recommended that glucose control be improved to some extent before initiating a new exercise regimen. Fasting glucose values between 140 and 200 mg · dL^{-1} are not a contraindication to exercise prescription but require physician review of the overall management plan. Both aerobic and resistance training exert marked beneficial effects on insulin resistance and glucose tolerance, even in the absence of weight loss or dietary change, and should therefore be a central part of the management of type 2 diabetes, whereas other forms of exercise or low-intensity exercise have generally not been shown to have metabolic benefit. Optimally, exercise sessions should coincide with peak elevations in blood glucose 1 to 2 hours after meals (particularly after breakfast) and thus minimize swings in glucose levels throughout the day. Those who require insulin injections as well should not exercise directly after taking insulin unless they have had a meal in between. In some cases, doses of medications may

need to be lowered if sustained, regular exercise regimens are incorporated into the lifestyle of the patient. Monitoring HgA$_{1c}$ levels every 3 months during exercise training will help to define the exercise effect and any needed adjustments in dietary or pharmacologic management.

Uncontrolled Malignant Cardiac Arrhythmia (Ventricular Tachycardia, Complete Heart Block, Atrial Flutter, Symptomatic Bradycardia)

These conditions require obvious attention by the physician regardless of the intent to prescribe exercise. In some cases, control cannot be achieved with drugs or pacemakers, and the patient may be unsuitable for exercise at all because of the potential danger of inducing sustained ventricular tachycardia, hypotension, complete heart block, or ischemia. The majority of older adults with arrhythmias will not fall into this category, however. Nonmalignant arrhythmias—such as isolated premature atrial or ventricular contractions, couplets, atrial fibrillation at a controlled rate, or totally paced rhythms—do not preclude aerobic or resistive training. They may indicate the need to search for underlying etiologies, such as dehydration, thyroid disease, electrolyte disturbance, ischemia, or pulmonary disease, however, and such conditions should be evaluated and treated before the introduction of significant changes in physical activity levels.

Unstable Angina (at Rest or Crescendo Pattern, Electrocardiogram Changes)

Although chronic stable angina and ischemic heart disease are indications for exercise, unstable angina and undiagnosed chest pains must be evaluated fully before commencing exercise. The exact nature of the investigations will depend on the clinical presentation and the level of medical intervention agreed on by the patient and the caregivers. Once the cardiac diagnosis is made and symptoms are controlled surgically or pharmacologically, exercise may begin as in other kinds of cardiac rehabilitation situations. Resistive and aerobic exercise are both safe and effective in such patients when prescribed with attention to standard principles. Resistance training is sometimes more tolerable than aerobic training in patients with a low threshold for ischemia. This occurs because of the more modest HR response and nonsustained blood pressure response to resistive exercise, resulting in a lower average double product during exercise (heart rate–pressure product). The double product is a noninvasive index of myocardial oxygen demand and therefore can be used as a marker of the ischemic threshold. In addition, diastolic pressure (and therefore coronary perfusion) tends to rise rather than fall (as in aerobic exercise), again minimizing ischemic potential. The same precautions listed above that reduce the risk of blood pressure and intraocular pressure elevations are relevant here to minimize the likelihood of ischemia in this setting. A very small proportion of patients will have uncontrolled ischemia at rest despite treatment, and exercise is contraindicated in such individuals.

Management of Older Adults with No Exclusions to Exercise

All of the listed conditions (Table 41-4) are in fact *indications* to exercise, rather than reasons to limit exercise participation (47). This assumes, of course, that the condition is currently well managed with medical or other treatment modalities, and no recent changes in symptoms or level of disease have occurred. Reintroduction of exercise after prolonged periods of injury or convalescence is crucial to prevent the vicious spiral of declining function otherwise seen in recurrent exacerbations of chronic illness.

EXERCISE PRESCRIPTION IN OLDER ADULTS

> **1.7.7-HFS: Knowledge of and ability to describe the unique adaptations to exercise training in children, adolescents, and older participants with regard to strength, functional capacity, and motor skills.**

> **1.7.8-CES: Demonstrate exercise equipment adaptations necessary for different age groups, physical abilities, and other potential contributing factors.**

> **1.7.15-CES: Describe common gait, movement, and coordination abnormalities as they relate to exercise testing and programming.**

> **1.7.8-HFS: Knowledge of common orthopedic and cardiovascular considerations for older participants and the ability to describe modifications in exercise prescription that are indicated.**

Exercise Prescription Implementation: Prioritize Physical Activity Needs in Relation to Risks

It is quite likely that after initial screening, many problems and needs will be identified in the typically sedentary older individual. Therefore, it becomes important to know how to deliver the prescription in logical stages that are palatable and feasible, and have some likelihood of successful implementation. In most cases, it is recommended to start with only one mode of exercise (balance, strength, endurance, flexibility) and let the older adult get used to the new routine of exercise before adding other components. This approach obviously requires attention to risk factors, medical history, physical exam findings, and personal preferences, and will be different for each individual. However, there are a few generalizations that can be made.

If significant deficits in muscle strength or balance are identified, than these should be addressed before the initiation of aerobic training. Prescribing progressive aerobic training in the absence of sufficient balance or strength is likely to result in knee pain, fear of falling, falls, and limited ability to progress aerobically, and is not recommended. Attempting to ambulate those who cannot lift their body weight out of a chair or maintain standing balance is a suboptimal approach. Paying attention to the physiologic determinants of transfer ability and ambulation, and targeting these specifically with the appropriate exercise prescription when reversible deficits are uncovered, is more likely to succeed.

In some cases, the older adults may benefit equally from resistance or aerobic training (e.g., for the treatment of depression) but the decision is made based on ability to tolerate one form of exercise over another (10,96). Severe osteoarthritis of the knee, recurrent falls, and a low threshold for ischemia may make resistance training safer than aerobic training as an antidepressant treatment in this case. Prioritization requires careful consideration of the risks and benefits of each mode of activity, as well as the current health status and physical fitness level.

Aerobic Activity

Cardiovascular endurance training refers to exercise in which large muscle groups contract many times (thousands of times at a single session) against little or no resistance other than that imposed by gravity. The purpose of this type of training is to increase the maximal amount of aerobic work that can be carried out, as well as to decrease the physiologic response and perceived difficulty of submaximal aerobic workloads. Extensive adaptations in the cardiopulmonary system, peripheral skeletal muscle, circulation, and metabolism are responsible for these changes in exercise capacity and tolerance. Many different kinds of exercise fall into this category, including walking and its derivatives (hiking, running, dancing, stair climbing, biking, swimming, ball sports, etc.). The key distinguishing feature between activities that are primarily aerobic versus resistive in nature is the much larger degree of overload to the muscle in resistance training. Obviously, there may be some overlap if aerobic activities are altered to increase the loading to muscle, as in resisted stationary cycling or stair-climbing machines. However, such activities are still primarily aerobic in nature, as they do not cause fatigue within a very few contractions as resistance training does, and they therefore do not cause the kinds of adaptations in the nervous system and muscle that lead to marked strength gain and hypertrophy.

Modes of Aerobic Exercise

There are many more kinds of cardiovascular exercise available than is the case for strengthening exercise. The decision about how to train aerobically depends on factors such as preference, access, likelihood of injury, and health-related restrictions or desired benefits. In general, although there are differences in oxygen consumption among various kinds of aerobic exercise, unless one is training for a particular sport, personal preference can provide much of the direction in this regard, as long-term compliance will require that an enjoyable pursuit has been selected. Given attention to the intensity and volume requirements below, most activities can contribute to improvements in cardiovascular efficiency, reduction of metabolic risk factors, and reduced risk of many chronic diseases. Two other factors assume importance in older adults, and older women in particular. The first is the beneficial effects of weight-bearing aerobic activities on bone density. The loading of bone is critical to this outcome, so that non–weight-bearing aerobic activities (such as swimming and biking) have not been shown to maintain or increase bone density, whereas walking, jogging, and stepping have positive effects in cross-sectional and longitudinal studies (100). Second, high-impact activities, such as jogging, jumping, and running, although beneficial for bone formation in children and premenopausal women (51,57), have been associated with high rates of knee and ankle injuries, even in healthy older adults, and have not yet been shown to increase bone density by themselves (6). In older adults with preexisting arthritis, such high-impact activities are neither feasible nor recommended, as they are even more likely to result in injuries and exacerbations of arthritis in this cohort. Balancing the skeletal need for weight-bearing or high-impact loading and the safety requirements of the joints and connective tissues for low-impact loading, one would therefore favor exercises such as walking, dancing, hiking, or stair climbing over running, step aerobics, or jumping rope in most older adults. Men and women without underlying arthritis may generally perform high-impact activities safely as long as muscle and ligament strength and joint structure is normal. It has been suggested anecdotally that concurrent resistance training may prevent much of the joint problems and injuries incurred during typical high-impact aerobic pursuits, but this remains to be shown experimentally.

Overall, walking and its derivations surface as the most widely studied, feasible, safe, accessible, and economical mode of aerobic training for men and women of most ages and states of health. This does not require special equipment or locations and does not need to be taught or supervised (except in the cognitively impaired, very frail, or medically unstable individual). Walking bears a natural relationship to ordinary ADLs, making it easier to integrate into lifestyle and functional tasks than any other mode of exercise. Therefore, it is theoretically more likely to translate into improved functional independence and mobility than other types of aerobic exercise.

Intensity of Aerobic Exercise

The intensity of aerobic exercise refers to the amount of oxygen consumed ($\dot{V}O_2$), or energy expended, per minute while performing the activity, which will vary from about 5 kcal·min^{-1} for light activities, to 7.5 kcal·min^{-1} for moderate activities, to 10 to 12 kcal·min^{-1} for very heavy activities. Energy expenditure increases with increasing body weight for weight-bearing aerobic activities, as well as with inclusion of larger muscle mass and increased work (force × distance) and power output (work/time) demands of the activity. Therefore, the most intensive activities are those that involve the muscles of the arms, legs, and trunk simultaneously, necessitate moving the full body weight through space, and are done at a rapid pace (e.g., cross-country skiing). Adding extra loading to the body weight (backpack, weight belt, wrist weights) increases the force needed to move the body part through space and therefore increases the aerobic intensity of the work performed.

The intensity of aerobic work can be calculated by measuring the actual consumption of oxygen using measurements of inspired and expired gases, which are analyzed for their oxygen and carbon dioxide content. Because this method is normally only available in research facilities or clinical laboratories, estimations are usually made by assessing cardiovascular responses or subjective rating of effort by the participant. The rise in HR is directly proportional in normal individuals in sinus rhythm to the increasing oxygen consumption or aerobic workload. Thus, monitoring HR has traditionally been a primary means of both prescribing appropriate intensity levels as well as following training adaptations when direct measurements of oxygen consumption are not available. The HRR method is the most useful estimate of intensity based on HR, and training intensity is normally recommended at a moderate (40%–59%) to vigorous (60%–84%) level (53). Calculation of target HRs using HRR is described in Chapter 28.

Difficulties with an intensity prescription based on HR in the older adult include the presence of arrhythmias, pacemakers, or β-blockers (systemic or ophthalmologic) that will alter the HR response to exercise. Therefore, a more easily obtainable and reliable estimate of aerobic intensity is to prescribe a moderate level as 12 to 14, or a vigorous level as 15 to 17, on the RPE scale, which runs from 6 to 20 (11). At a moderate level, the exerciser should note increased pulse and respiratory rate, but still be able to talk. This scale has been validated for use in men and women, young and old, those with coronary disease and healthy adults, and is therefore of widespread applicability (59). It is easy to teach and is a means to "supervise" training intensity from afar, by means of written diaries or telephone calls, making it cost-effective in community programs and healthcare settings. Usually a visual representation of the RPE scale is used to increase accuracy, but assessment can even be done without this prop in patients who are blind or cannot read.

As is the case with all other forms of exercise, to maintain the same relative training intensity over time, the

TABLE 41-5. INCREASING THE INTENSITY OF AEROBIC EXERCISE FOR OLDER ADULTS

MODE OF EXERCISE	WAYS TO INCREASE INTENSITY
Walking	Add small weights around wrists
	Swing arms
	Use "race walking" style
	Add inclines, hills, stairs
	Carry weighted backpack or waist belt[a]
	Push a wheelchair or stroller (with someone in it)
Cycling	Increase pedaling speed
	Increase resistance to pedals
	Add hills
	Add backpack[a]
	Add child carrier to back of bike
Water activities	Use arms and legs in strokes
	Add resistive equipment for water
	Increase pace
Tennis	Convert from doubles to singles game
Golf	Carry clubs[a]
	Eliminate golf cart
Dance	Increase pace of movements
	Add more arm and leg movements

[a]Avoid flexing the spine when doing this to prevent excessive compressive forces on the thoracic spine.

absolute training load must be increased as fitness improves. In younger individuals, typically walking may be changed to jogging and then running to increase intensity as needed. More appropriate in older or frail adults are progressive alterations in workload that increase energy expenditure without converting to a high-impact form of activity. Examples of how to prescribe such progression for various modes of aerobic exercise are given in Table 41-5. The workloads should be progressed based on ratings of effort at each training session. Once the perceived exertion slips below 12 on the RPE scale, the workload should be increased to maintain the physiologic stimulus for continued cardiovascular adaptation. As with resistance training, the most common error in aerobic training is *failure to progress*, which results in an early suboptimal plateau in cardiovascular and metabolic improvement.

Volume of Aerobic Exercise

In most very old, frail adults, aerobic exercise is not being used for the *prevention* of premature mortality, cardiovascular disease, diabetes, or hypertension, or for the treatment of obesity. Therefore, it is likely that 60 to 120 minutes of exercise each week will be sufficient to provide benefits in the domains of improved maximal and submaximal cardiovascular efficiency, psychological well-being, and control of chronic diseases such as arthritis, diabetes, peripheral vascular disease, chronic lung disease, coronary artery disease, and congestive heart failure, for example (84). It should be noted, however, that very little research on aerobic training in very old or

frail adults has actually been conducted, and most recommendations are simply extrapolated from studies in younger individuals.

It has been shown that aerobic exercise does not need to be carried out at a single session to provide training effects and may be broken up into bouts of 10 minutes at a time to reach the desired volume of training (84). Shorter-duration sessions than this have not been evaluated for efficacy, although public health recommendations for integrating short bouts of even 5 minutes into the daily routine have been made recently. Very frail adults may only tolerate 2 to 5 minutes of walking or other aerobic activities initially, and a reasonable goal is to increase tolerance for longer workloads until 10 to 20 minutes of exercise can be sustained without resting. This would provide substantial functional benefit in the nursing home, as walking for 20 minutes would likely enable the older adults to get to almost any location in the home without having to stop and rest.

Overall, a session or sessions of aerobic exercise carried out at least once every 3 days adding up to about 60 minutes a week appears to be the minimal prescription justifiable based on the currently available literature. Higher volumes of exercise than this (such as 30 minutes per day, most days per week) are frequently recommended by public health authorities (47), although the evidence for such recommendations is not clear-cut. It is not recommended to exercise in very long bouts once or twice a week as an alternative to several shorter sessions, as this is likely to result in overuse muscle soreness and injuries. The risk of sudden death during physical activity appears to be limited to those who do not exercise on a regular basis (at least 1 hour per week), which is another reason for advocating regular, moderate doses of exercise rather than periodic high-volume training.

Supervision and Setting

Most people will be familiar with the basic principles of most common forms of aerobic exercise (e.g., walking, biking, swimming), so that this modality of exercise is frequently carried out in unsupervised settings. Exceptions to this general rule may be made in special circumstances, such as in cardiac rehabilitation settings or with frail adults, when safety may be a concern. In addition, when new techniques are introduced (e.g., aerobic dance, aqua aerobics) or when compliance needs to be more intensively monitored for efficacy (as in the treatment of obesity or diabetes), supervision may be required. It is often possible to graduate to a partially monitored program after a new routine has been established to increase flexibility and yet maintain reinforcing contact and supervision. It should be remembered that a group setting or supervised program does not automatically ensure higher exercise compliance in older adults. King et al. have shown that *choice* is the most important determinant of compliance, and if barriers to supervised participation away from home (such as dislike of group exercise, need to care for a family member, lack of transportation, financial costs, inclement weather, inconvenient scheduling or work commitments) outweigh the benefits (perceived safety, access to trainers, support of group members, socialization), then there is no advantage to prescribing center-based, supervised exercise (61,62). Assessing an older adult's preferences in this regard is most important early in the prescriptive process to avoid failure and behavioral relapse.

Monitoring Progress

The best way to monitor progress in an aerobic training program is to review an activity log kept by the participant, including frequency, duration, and HR or RPE of exercise sessions. This can be simply recorded on an ordinary calendar posted on the refrigerator in the spaces for each day of the month, as follows:

Walking, 20 minutes, RPE 14

If such monthly calendars are reviewed periodically by an appropriate member of the healthcare team, advice can be given on a timely basis about patterns, volume, and intensity of exercise so as to enhance compliance and optimize efficacy. For example, if a diabetic patient is noted to be exercising in long bouts at intervals 5 days apart on average, advice may be given to change to shorter bouts every 3 days. Events that typically trigger long bouts of noncompliance (e.g., illness, injury, depression, work commitments, vacation, babysitting responsibilities) can be identified and relapse prevention strategies put into place to avert such patterns.

Benefits of Aerobic Exercise

The benefits of aerobic exercise have been extensively studied over the past 40 years, and the most important of these for older adults are listed in Table 41-6. They include a broad range of physiologic adaptations that are in general opposite to the effects of aging on most body systems, as well as major health-related clinical outcomes. The health conditions that are responsive to aerobic exercise include most of those of concern to older adults: osteoporosis, heart disease, stroke, breast cancer, diabetes, obesity, hypertension, arthritis, depression, and insomnia (85). These physiologic and clinical benefits form the basis for the inclusion of aerobic exercise as an essential component of the overall physical activity prescription for healthy aging.

Risks of Aerobic Exercise

The major potential risks of aerobic exercise are listed in Table 41-7. Most of these adverse events are preventable with attention to the underlying medical conditions

TABLE 41-6. BENEFITS OF AEROBIC EXERCISE IN OLDER ADULTS

PHYSIOLOGIC ADAPTATION	PREVENTION OR TREATMENT OF DISEASE
Increased bone density	Arthritis
Decreased total body and visceral adipose tissue	Breast cancer
Decreased fibrinogen levels	Chronic insomnia
Decreased sympathetic and hormonal response to exercise	Colon cancer
Decreased LDL, increased HDL levels	Coronary artery disease
Decreased postural blood pressure response to stressors	Depression
Increased heart rate variability	Hyperlipidemia
Increased neural reaction time	Hypertension
Increased blood volume and hematocrit	Impotence
Increased energy expenditure	Obesity
Increased glycogen storage in skeletal muscle	Osteoporosis
Increased oxidative enzyme capacity in skeletal muscle	Overall and cardiovascular mortality
Increased glucose disposal rate	Peripheral vascular disease
Increased mitochondrial volume density in skeletal muscle	Prostate cancer
Decreased resting heart rate and blood pressure	Stroke
Increased GLUT-4 receptors in skeletal muscle	Type 2 diabetes mellitus
Decreased arterial stiffness	
Increased maximal aerobic capacity	
Increased stroke volume during exercise[a]	
Increased capillary density in skeletal muscle	
Increased insulin sensitivity	
Improved glucose toleranc	
Increased cardiac contractility during exercise[a]	
Decreased heart rate/BP response to submaximal exercise	
Increased oxygen extraction by skeletal muscle	

BP, blood pressure; HDL, high-density lipoprotein; LDL, low-density lipoprotein.
[a]Observed only in older endurance-trained men thus far.

present, appropriate choices as regards the modality of exercise used, avoiding exercise during extreme environmental conditions, wearing proper footwear and clothing, and minimizing or avoiding exercise during acute illness or in the presence of new, undefined symptoms. All older adults should have yearly ophthalmologic exams for glaucoma and retinal changes, and therefore exercise programming should be delayed until this routine health screen has been completed to avoid complications. If someone has had recent ophthalmologic surgery, exercise is contraindicated for several weeks to avoid raising intraocular pressure, and the exact recommendations should be obtained from the ophthalmologist in these cases. Metabolic complications are rare unless diabetes is out of control at the time exercise is initiated or dehydration or acute illness are present. Most fluid balance problems can be handled by exercising in reasonable

TABLE 41-7. THE RISKS OF AEROBIC EXERCISE IN OLDER ADULTS

MUSCULOSKELETAL	CARDIOVASCULAR	METABOLIC
Falls	Arrhythmia	Dehydration
Foot ulceration or laceration	Cardiac failure	Electrolyte imbalance
Fracture, osteoporotic or traumatic	Hypertension	Energy imbalance
Hemorrhoids[a]	Hypotension	Heat stroke
Hernia[a]	Ischemia	Hyperglycemia
Joint or bursa inflammation, exacerbation of arthritis	Pulmonary embolism	Hypoglycemia
Ligament or tendon strain or rupture	Retinal hemorrhage or detachment, lens detachment	Hypothermia
Muscle soreness or tear	Ruptured cerebral or other aneurysm	Seizures
Stress incontinence	Syncope or postural symptoms	

[a]Primarily associated with increased intra-abdominal pressure during resistive exercise, but may occur if Valsalva maneuver occurs during aerobic activities.

temperature and humidity only and drinking extra fluid on exercise days.

Cardiovascular complications are most likely if ischemic heart disease is not well controlled medically or surgically before exercise initiation, if warning signs are ignored, or if sudden vigorous exercise is tried in a previously completely sedentary individual. When done properly, both aerobic and resistance training have been shown to reduce the incidence of angina and medication use in cardiac rehabilitation settings, and are indicated as part of standard medical management of coronary artery disease. Although claudication is mentioned as a possible adverse side effect of exercise in those with peripheral vascular disease, there is an important treatment caveat here. It has been shown that aerobic exercise significantly increases exercise tolerance in patients with peripheral vascular disease (i.e., time to claudication) (42). However, it may work optimally if continued for about 30 to 90 seconds if possible after the onset of claudication, and then a rest period taken. This is different from angina or any of the other symptoms listed in Table 41-7, for which exercise should be stopped immediately if they occur.

Musculoskeletal problems are more common than any other risk of aerobic exercise, particularly in the novice or very frail woman. Often if significant weakness or balance impairment is present, it is best to avoid aerobic exercise altogether until strength and balance have been improved sufficiently with specific training, so as to allow safe weight-bearing exercise such as walking. If this is not done, falls, arthritis pain, fear of falling, and muscle fatigue will be so limiting that effective aerobic training is precluded. Warming up muscles gently with slow movements before aerobic routines is important to avoid soft-tissue injury. The most important point is to avoid high-impact activities (such as jumping, step aerobics, jogging) in those with pre-existing arthritis or weak muscles and ligaments, as this is a principle cause of sports-related injury.

Muscle-Strengthening Activity

> **1.7.17-CES: Design strength and flexibility programs for individuals with cardiovascular,**

pulmonary, and/or metabolic diseases, the elderly, and children.

> **1.7.22-HFS: Skill to teach and demonstrate appropriate modifications in specific exercises for groups such as older adults, pregnant and postnatal women, obese persons, and persons with low-back pain.**

Progressive resistance training (PRT) is one of the four basic modalities of exercise that is recommended for older adults as part of a balanced physical activity program, whether this is formalized as an exercise prescription or integrated into lifestyle changes. Progressive resistance training is the process of challenging the skeletal muscle with an unaccustomed stimulus, or load, such that neural and muscle tissue adaptations take place, leading ultimately to increased muscle force producing capacity (strength) and muscle mass. In this kind of exercise, the muscle is contracted slowly just a few times in each session against a relatively heavy load. Any muscle may be trained in this way, although usually 8 to 10 major muscle groups with clinical relevance are trained for a balanced and functional outcome (101,107).

Equipment

There are many ways to carry out PRT (106). Equipment may range from only body weight to technologically sophisticated pneumatic or hydraulic resistance-training machines. A listing of the general types of equipment available and considerations for their use is presented in Chapter 29. In general, in the older adult, machine-based training allows the most robust adaptations to be achieved, offers maximum safety, and requires less technique to be learned. Free weights, on the other hand, offer significant advantages in terms of cost and flexibility in programming, may provide a better stimulus for motor coordination and balance, and are the only option in most home and limited-space settings.

Intensity

Several authors have recommended that elderly or frail adults should use a lower intensity (approximately 60% of the 1RM, or a weight that can be lifted 12–15 times before fatiguing). Although these suggestions are made as though they resulted from experimental trials or clinical experience, in fact virtually all of the randomized controlled trials of resistance training in the elderly that have resulted in large gains in strength have used an intensity of approximately 80% of the 1RM. There is no evidence that this intensity is unsafe or poorly tolerated in men or women, healthy or frail, up to 100 years of age (39,40), or even those in early outpatient cardiac rehabilitation, for example (101). By contrast, low-intensity training results in negligible or modest gains in strength and associated clinical benefits (33,94) and cannot therefore be recommended if the primary intent of training is to increase muscle size and strength.

Volume

The volume of resistance training refers to the frequency of sessions and the number of sets and repetitions (lifts) performed during each session for each muscle group. This subject has generated a great deal of debate among scientists, trainers, and athletes. But a review of the existing scientific data does allow some useful conclusions to be drawn.

Frequency

Depending on the access to training, motivation of the individual, and other circumstances, training frequency should therefore be tailored to maximize adherence without compromising physiologic and clinical benefits. It is most effective to recommend training frequencies of 3 days per week in the older adult. Because compliance generally does not exceed 60% to 70% of recommended sessions long term unless entirely supervised, this level of compliance will still result in two sessions per week on average. Thus, a reasonable physiologic response is achievable. If there is only one session a week planned, and it is missed because of illness, vacation, or other activities, then 2 full weeks will elapse between training, which may result in lost strength, disruption of progress, soreness, or loss of commitment to the new behavior in the interval. In addition, with only one session a week (with the possible exception of trunk muscle training) (87), it will take longer for a level of competence and clinical benefit to be reached that will lead to sustained adherence.

Some individuals like to train every day, particularly if they notice psychological benefits from participation. This can be accomplished by exercising different muscle groups on different days: for example, arm exercises on Monday, Wednesday, and Friday, and leg exercises on Tuesday, Thursday, and Saturday. This still allows individual muscle groups to recover between training sessions, but provides an activity for the person 6 days per week. Such shorter sessions (15 minutes or so) may fit better into some schedules than a few long sessions each week and may thus enhance overall compliance. A similar approach has been advocated with cardiovascular training,

as intermittent short bouts of exercise appear to be as beneficial in most ways as longer sessions. In all cases, a balance must be achieved between preferences, convenience, barriers such as time or transportation, access to trainers or equipment, and known physiologic requirements before a rational prescription can be formulated that maximizes compliance and adaptation.

Setting and Supervision

Resistance training is a novel activity for most older men and women, and supervision is recommended in some form initially to ensure proper technique, provide confidence, and, most importantly, ensure progression to appropriate levels of intensity. This supervision may take the form of hands-on training or a combination of visits, videos, telephone calls, mail, or feedback on activity logs. Most unsupervised weightlifting programs in the elderly suffer more from low intensity than from low compliance. This will markedly limit the adaptation that accrues and therefore needs to be addressed in any program implementation or exercise prescription. Success in getting older adults to progress to higher weights requires continuous supervision, although this may gradually shift from direct supervision to more remote means of providing feedback. Given adherence to the principles of intensity, form, and volume, the setting is quite flexible and will primarily depend on issues such as cost, transportation, availability of trainers, spouse or other dependent needs at home, living situation, health status, cognition, and functional or mobility impairments. Cognitive impairment does not preclude training, but it does mandate long-term supervision. It has been demonstrated that compliance is highest when older adults are allowed to choose the setting in which they wish to exercise and that not all older adults want to exercise in a group, as has sometimes been wrongly assumed (62). One of the major factors that predicts lack of involvement in a nursing home exercise program is the patient characteristic of not participating in groups of any kind as assessed by the nursing staff. So determination of such barriers to adoption and preferences for setting is crucial to successful behavior change in relation to all modes of exercise.

Benefits

Increases in muscle size and strength following appropriate PRT are not seen with other forms of exercise and are also not obtainable with low-intensity PRT. Therefore, if a primary goal of exercise is to prevent or treat sarcopenia, then there is no effective substitute for this modality of exercise. The hypertrophic response to training does appear to be affected by health status, anabolic hormonal milieu, nutritional substrate availability, changes in protein synthesis with age, and other factors yet to be identified (17,64,71,77,105,106). Previous suggestions that women do not undergo hypertrophy as effectively as men appear to be related to differences in training intensity and age of the subjects in these trials rather than reflecting a true sex difference in training adaptation. It is clear that exogenous anabolic steroids can augment the hypertrophic response to resistive exercise in young men (63); they appear to have the same effect in older men as well (12). However, trials with growth hormone or its secretagogues, or estrogen, have thus far largely failed to show benefit in terms of muscle mass or strength in older adults when given alone or in combination with resistance training.

Risks

Progressive resistance training has been thought of as a relatively risky form of exercise in the past and has therefore been sometimes avoided by healthcare professionals in their counseling of older adults. However, a wealth of literature over the past 10 years indicates that this modality of exercise is in fact quite safe and is more feasible in many groups of patients and frail elders than is cardiovascular exercise, as illustrated in Box 41-1. There are relatively few medical contraindications to PRT, as outlined in Box 41-2. Apart from these specific circumstances, resistance training is a realistic option even in very frail elderly individuals. Frailty is not a contraindication to strength training, but conversely one of the most important reasons to prescribe it.

The potential risks of resistance training are primarily musculoskeletal injury and cardiovascular events. Musculoskeletal injury is largely preventable with attention to the following points:

- Adherence to proper form
- Isolation of the targeted muscle group
- Slow velocity of lifting
- Limitation of range of motion to the pain-free arc of movement
- Avoidance of use of momentum and ballistic movements to complete a lift

---

BOX 41-1   INDICATIONS FOR CHOOSING RESISTANCE TRAINING OVER AEROBIC TRAINING

- Severe arthritis preventing weight-bearing activity
- Lower-extremity fracture with casting
- Inability to support body weight
- Foot ulceration or ankle injury
- Severe balance disorder or recurrent falls precluding safe standing or walking
- Amputation of lower extremities without prostheses
- Chronic lung disease and hypoxia with aerobic exercise
- Low threshold for ischemia with aerobic exercise

BOX 41-2   MEDICAL CONTRAINDICATIONS TO RESISTANCE TRAINING

- Unstable angina, untreated severe left main coronary artery disease
- Angina, hypotension, or arrhythmias provoked by resistance training
- Significant exacerbation of musculoskeletal pain with resistance training
- End-stage congestive heart failure
- Failure to thrive, terminal illness
- Severe valvular heart disease

- Use of machines or chairs with good back support
- Observation of rest periods between sets and rest days between sessions

A distinction should be made between delayed onset muscle soreness (DOMS), a normal response to the initiation or increase in intensity of PRT, and an acute musculoskeletal injury because of training, such as a ligament tear, sprain, hernia, or muscle rupture. DOMS presents as a dull, diffuse aching sensation over the trained muscle group that starts the day following exercise and peaks about 48 hours after the session, but may take several days to completely resolve. This symptom complex gradually diminishes and disappears in the first few weeks of continuous training, but will resurface after interruptions to the training schedule.

Delayed onset muscle soreness is related to the damage caused to the muscle by mechanical stretch and loading, which in turn stimulates a reactive inflammatory response, characterized by damage to muscle cell membranes, cytokine elevations, intracellular edema, and leukocyte infiltrates (27). Ultimately, this process is not harmful and does not need to be suppressed or treated, as the attempt to repair this damage results in a desirable adaptation of increased protein synthesis and fiber hypertrophy. It is thought that the eccentric (lowering, lengthening) contraction is what produces most of the damage. However, because the damage ultimately leads to hypertrophy, eccentric contractions should not be avoided but in fact emphasized in training programs for older adults with low muscle mass.

An acute injury, by contrast, will be felt during or just after the exercise session itself and is more likely to be perceived as sudden in onset, sharp, easily localizable, often allowing identification of the exact site of injury. Such events should always provoke a response known as RICE:

- Rest
- Ice
- Compression
- Elevation

Ice can be applied via use of a cold pack for 15 to 20 minutes every hour in the acute phase. Compression with an elastic bandage so as to limit fluid accumulation will minimize pain, as does elevating the arm or leg if possible. Such a protocol serves to immobilize the affected joint and lessen the edema and inflammatory infiltrate that will otherwise occur. Additionally, if there is a dislocation, fracture, or other serious injury, stabilization of the bones and ligaments is crucial before definitive diagnosis and treatment. Weight-bearing and all other activity should be restricted until appropriate medical care is available.

In patients with pre-existing arthritis, there may be intermittent exacerbation of joint symptoms or inflammation with the initiation of PRT. However, the overall effect of training is to decrease chronic arthritis pain over time (38,52,88,92). During periods of disease flare-up, it may be necessary to switch to isometric contractions, lower the weight lifted, limit the range of motion through which the load is lifted, or insert additional days of rest between training sessions. It is advisable to continue isometric contractions if nothing else, as this will prevent loss of strength and will not further increase pain. Once the symptoms have lessened, normal exercise sessions may resume.

The circulatory response to PRT has been a matter of fear and controversy, and there is much misperception about the actual changes that occur. The blood pressure changes are difficult to measure during PRT because of the transient nature of the rises and the fact that blood pressure falls almost immediately after a repetition is completed. This makes monitoring of intra-arterial pressure the only accurate way to gather such information. The best study of these factors has been completed in older men by Benn et al. (7) and additional reviews of the literature provided by McCartney (72). The HR response to PRT is in general lower than that which is due to aerobic exercise such as walking up an incline or stair climbing, whereas the increase in systolic blood pressure tends to be intermediate between walking and stair climbing. Diastolic pressure elevations are greater with PRT than aerobic exercise, thus increasing mean arterial pressure to a greater degree. The rate pressure product (the product of systolic blood pressure and HR), which is felt to be representative of myocardial oxygen demand, is greatest for stair climbing, followed by weightlifting and walking. The authors concluded from these studies that older adults engaged in high-intensity weightlifting exercise are exposed to no greater peak circulatory stress than that created by a few minutes of inclined walking and much less than that elicited by climbing three to four flights of stairs. In addition, it has been pointed out that although the double product during weightlifting and some forms of aerobic work are similar, the contribution of HR is much higher in aerobic work, whereas the mean pressure is higher in weightlifting. The slower HR and increased diastolic pressure during PRT compared with aerobic work would facilitate diastolic filling and coronary artery perfusion, both desirable outcomes in an older individual, particularly someone with diastolic dysfunction (impaired relaxation and filling) or coronary artery disease (13). Consistent with these observations are the reports of patients who exhibit ischemia or angina during treadmill work but not during weightlifting exercises at a similar elevation of the double product. In the largest series of maximum strength tests yet reported, in 26,000 individuals undergoing testing, not a single cardiovascular event occurred (44). Additionally, the literature suggests a reduction in ischemic signs and symptoms after PRT in cardiac patients, attesting to the safety of this form of exercise even in individuals with heart disease.

In contrast to typical weightlifting regimens, the response to a sustained isometric contraction of a small muscle mass is a more substantial increase in arterial pressure; therefore, this mode of training is not recommended unless joint pain temporarily precludes dynamic training. Circulatory responses increase with the intensity of the relative load and the number of repetitions in a set. The augmentation in blood pressure is also contributed to by increased intrathoracic pressure during a Valsalva maneuver, which is transmitted directly to the arterial vasculature, causing a rise in pressure. The Valsalva maneuver is difficult to avoid when lifting loads >85% of the 1RM and is invoked with lower loads when muscles are fatigued. Thus, keeping lifting intensity at about 80% of the 1RM and limiting sets to eight repetitions (rather than "to fatigue" as has sometimes been suggested) should minimize the contribution to circulatory stress of the Valsalva. The circulatory response is least during the eccentric (lowering) phase of the repetition and highest during the static and early part of the concentric phase. Thus, emphasizing the duration of the eccentric contraction will both moderate cardiovascular stress and maximize adaptations that lead to hypertrophy and is thus highly recommended for older adults in particular. A summary of the major factors related to circulatory responses in weightlifting exercise is presented in Box 41-3.

BOX 41-3	FACTORS RELATED TO INCREASED CIRCULATORY STRESS DURING RESISTANCE TRAINING

- Higher relative intensity of load lifted
- Static contractions
- Early phase of concentric contraction
- Greater muscle mass used
- Performance of a Valsalva maneuver
- Increasing number of repetitions
- Fatigue of muscles

Circulatory stress = increase of heart rate and blood pressure in response to resistive exercise.

Patients with unstable cardiovascular signs and symptoms, as noted in Box 41-2, should not begin any exercise regimen, including weightlifting, without medical evaluation.

Special Considerations in Older Men and Women

There is no need to change the specifics of the exercise prescription given above to be more suitable for older men and women. They will lift lower absolute loads than younger adults because of their generally smaller muscle mass, but the relative load recommended is exactly the same. Their adaptations should be similar if this principle is observed.

Special consideration should be given to erector spinae and upper-back muscles, which contribute to back extension (89). Stimulation of these muscle groups will strengthen the bones of the thoracic and lumbar spine and counteract the forces promoting osteopenic vertebral compression fractures in high-risk men and women.

Disorders of gait and balance and falls are prevalent in older men and women and therefore training programs should always include the ankle dorsiflexors and plantar flexors, hip abductors, hip extensors, and knee extensors and flexors if possible. Those who are already wheelchair bound or nearly so will benefit from triceps and shoulder exercises to increase independence in transfers and wheelchair mobility.

Abdominal muscle strengthening is of interest to many older men and women for perceived aesthetic reasons (even in 90-year-old nursing home older adults) and to therapists for its contribution to good posture, balance, and control of low-back pain symptoms because of degenerative changes in the spine and surrounding tissues.

Monitoring Progress

It is imperative to monitor progress in PRT, as adaptation depends on maintenance of the training stimulus, which means continuous increases in absolute load. Many techniques suitable for enhancing compliance are discussed in Chapter 42, but in regards to this modality of training in particular, the need for documentation of the training load (by the individual or the trainer) is paramount (113). Providing this feedback in graphic form is particularly useful for reinforcing the presence or absence of appropriate progression, as training loads should increase steadily and continuously if appropriate technique is being followed. For some individuals, it may also be important to monitor target symptoms or functions that may change during the course of training, such as angina, shortness of breath, falls, insomnia, depressive symptoms, ability to climb stairs, use of assistive devices, fear of falling, blood glucose levels, waist, and arm or calf circumference. Deciding what goals are important and realistic in the beginning and monitoring progress in domains that are meaningful to the older adult will provide the most effective motivation. Because strength increases are the most dramatic outcome usually, periodically testing maximum strength is a good idea if equipment is available. If it isn't, a simple test, such as recording the amount of time it takes the adult to stand up and sit down 5 or 10 times in a row, will provide a proxy index of lower-extremity muscle power. In addition, the perceived exertion in response to lifting the weights that were used in the first week of training can be remeasured over time to demonstrate how much easier tasks that once seemed difficult are after training. Any adverse events attributable to the exercise should also be tracked on logs so that appropriate investigation and/or adjustments in training regimens can be made.

Enhancing Balance with Resistance Training

Standard high-intensity PRT has been shown to improve mobility and balance (81). The feasibility and efficacy of a specific balance-enhancing technique incorporated directly into the PRT routine in a group of older adults of average age 84 with a history of falling or gait and balance problems has been recently tested. As outlined in Box 41-4, they were instructed to gradually reduce the hand support during their standing weightlifting exercises, but otherwise follow the general principles outlined above. They exercised 3 days per week over a 12-week period. The exercises in which these balance-enhancing postures were included were the hip extensors, hip flexors, hip abductors, knee flexors, and plantar flexors. This training regimen resulted in large improvements in static and dynamic balance, as follows:

Usual gait speed:	6% increase
Maximal gait speed:	10% increase
Tandem stand time:	162% increase
One-legged stand time:	126% increase
Tandem walk time:	6% increase
Errors made during tandem walk:	55% decrease

BOX 41-4 **ADDING BALANCE TRAINING TO RESISTIVE EXERCISES**

Step 1: Hold onto chair or table with two hands during standing resistive exercises (hip flexion, hip abduction, hip extension, knee flexion, and plantar flexion).

Step 2: Hold on with one hand only.

Step 3: Hold on with one fingertip only.

Step 4: Keep both hands 2 inches above chair or table.

The ability to incorporate such balance-enhancing postures into PRT is a distinct advantage of free-weight modes of training, including standing postures. Even if an adult does not have balance impairments at the time of initial prescription, it is prudent to instruct him/her in this adaptation of standard technique for standing exercises, as it does not take any extra time to complete the session and may prevent decrements in balance from occurring in the future. Studies are continuing on the long-term adaptations to this enhanced form of resistance training.

Integration of Strength Training into Daily Activities

Although PRT is usually conceptualized as a discreet "exercise" activity, there are in fact ways to incorporate elements of PRT into daily life in the same way that aerobic activities are. The guiding principles underlying such incorporation are listed in Table 41-8.

Balance Exercises for Frequent Fallers or Individuals with Mobility Problems

Balance training is probably the least well defined of the various exercise modalities. Despite the use of balance-enhancing modalities for decades by physical therapists and others working with adults and children with developmental or degenerative neurologic diseases affecting balance, only recently have there been well-controlled formalized studies of techniques and outcomes (18,65,84). The recognition that balance impairment is a risk factor for falls and hip fracture even in adults without identifiable neurologic disease has expanded the potential target population for balance training to the general aging cohort. The pressing need for definitive outcome data on feasibility and efficacy of various intervention techniques has stimulated quantitative research that will assist in the development of clinical protocols. In the meantime, the balance prescription must be formulated from a variety of evidence collected in epidemiologic studies, experimental trials, and clinical practice. It should be noted that in many cases, it is difficult to compare the results across trials, as investigators have used unique training interventions and different outcome measures as well (18,21,56,91,95).

Any activity that increases one's ability to maintain balance in the face of a threat to stability may be considered a balance-enhancing activity. Common stressors include:

- Narrowing of the base of support
- Perturbation of the ground support
- Decrease in proprioceptive sensation
- Diminished or misleading visual inputs
- Disturbed vestibular system input
- Increased compliance of the support surface
- Movement of the center of mass of the body away from the vertical

On a day-to-day basis, stressors may also include things such as environmental hazards to traverse, postural hypotension, and drugs that affect central nervous system function. The plethora of conditions that contribute to gait and balance abnormalities in older adults requires a multifactorial approach to balance enhancement and falls prevention. What is presented below is a summary of exercise techniques that have favorable effects on this physiologic capacity and therefore form an important part of the exercise prescription for older adults.

Balance-enhancing activities affect the central nervous system control of balance and coordination of movement

TABLE 41-8. INCORPORATING STRENGTHENING INTO DAILY ACTIVITIES

PRINCIPLE	EXAMPLES
Use smallest possible muscle mass to accomplish task.	Rise from a chair without using arms to assist. Lift heavy objects with one arm instead of two. Stand on one leg. Climb stairs using hands only lightly for balance on rails.
Resist gravity.	Sit down slowly. Lower body weight slowly up and down stairs. Lower packages slowly. Lift slowly rather than swinging objects into position.
Do not use momentum to assist with tasks.	Don't rock body to rise from a low chair or sofa.
Perform isometric contractions when resting.	Push down on floor with toes when sitting. Hook toes under sofa and pull up while sitting. Stand on one leg whenever waiting in line. Push out against chair arms with forearms and upper arm while sitting. Extend spine against back of chair while sitting. Press legs together when sitting or lying. Do abdominal crunches while riding in cars or buses. Place hands palms up under desk and pull up while sitting. Push head back against high-backed seat. Perform Kegel (pelvic floor) exercises any time.

or augment the peripheral neuromuscular system response to signals that balance is threatened. Resistance training likely improves balance by specifically enhancing the strength of postural control muscles of the trunk and lower extremities, particularly ankles, hips, and knees, so that the person is able to mount a more robust response to a given stressor (81). It is not known whether resistance training also changes the neural recruitment of these muscles in response to perturbations in balance so that they are activated more quickly or in better sequence, but this may be an additional beneficial adaptation. Even when only seated resistance training is performed, improvements in static and dynamic balance can be demonstrated in the elderly. Inclusion of standing postures, particularly if hand support is gradually withdrawn, has an even more potent effect on balance.

General Technique

The general approach to the enhancement of balance should rely on theoretical principles that are designed to elicit adaptations in the central neurologic control of posture and equilibrium. The basic idea is to progressively challenge the system with stressors of increasing difficulty in three different domains:

1. Narrowing the base of support for the body
2. Displacing the center of mass to the limits of tolerance
3. Removing or minimizing contributions of visual, vestibular, and proprioceptive pathways to balance

Each of these will be considered in turn.

Narrowing the Base of Support   This is one of the most commonly used techniques and is quite effective. The person is instructed to stand in postures of increasing difficulty, as follows:

- Feet apart with assistive device
- Feet apart without assistive device
- Feet together (tandem; touching along entire length)
- Semitandem stand (feet touching but the toe of one foot is at the instep of the other foot)
- Heel-to-toe stand (toe of one foot is touching the heel of the foot in front)
- One-legged stand (one foot only is on the ground)
- Toe stand (standing on tip-toe with both or only one foot)
- Heel stand (standing on both heels)

These postures have been presented in order of increasing difficulty, with the possible exception of the final two postures (toe stand and heel stand), which may present variable challenges to an individual depending not only on balance capacity, but also on muscle strength, presence of arthritis, peripheral edema, range of motion in the ankle, and other podiatric problems. To prescribe such exercise, each of the above postures should be tried under direct supervision to see where in this hierarchy he or she begins to have difficulties maintaining balance. A useful technique is to ask the person to hold the desired posture for 15 seconds. If this is done successfully (without moving feet, grabbing for support, or falling), then the next more difficult posture is tried. Obviously it is essential that the examiner be close to the person at all times to prevent a fall. Wherever difficulty is first noted (defined as inability to hold the stance for the full 15 seconds), this is the level that is prescribed as the initial "training" posture. Training involves practicing this posture (see below for volume) until it is mastered and then progressing to the next higher level of difficulty. We have seen, for example, that community-dwelling men and women of average age 80 begin to have difficulty at the level of the heel-to-toe stand (37,45,81,82). By contrast, frailer individuals in a nursing home may find the feet-together position initially difficult or impossible.

In addition to the static postures noted above, the principle of narrowing the base of support can be applied to dynamic movements as well, such as during heel-to-toe walking. This can be taken to a higher level of difficulty by tandem walking backward or with the eyes closed, or on a flat board 3 to 4 inches wide that serves as a balance beam.

As long as the basic principle is followed, it does not matter whether the stances are done by themselves as a discreet training session; are incorporated into strength-training sessions; are practiced while carrying out daily activities, such as standing in line, cooking, doing housework, or talking on the phone; or form part of a more extensive routine of yoga, tai chi, or dance. The essential feature is progression driven by challenging the person with tasks that are slightly beyond their reach to induce favorable adaptations.

Displacing the Center of Mass   The goal of this mode of training is to move the body weight through space toward the limits of sway, just short of where balance is lost. All movement involves some displacement of the center of mass, even simple walking, but as a person's resources improve, more difficult and challenging displacement tasks can be mastered. In its simplest form, the person can be asked to stand still with his or her feet slightly apart, and keeping the body rigid, lean forward, backward, and to each side as far as possible without having to move one's feet to maintain balance. Other ways of displacing the center of mass include:

- Turning in a circle
- Shifting weight from side to side
- Stepping over obstacles, such as a step or book
- Turning or leaning while holding a heavy object, such as a book or dumbbell, out in front of the chest
- Crossover walking, sideways walking, heel walking
- Moving weighted arms or legs out to the front or side (as in standing resistive exercises with free weights)
- Balancing on a large ball or rocker platform (available in many physical therapy settings)

Practicing tai chi and yoga involves many postures that similarly perturb the center of mass as well as diminishing the base of support within simple or more complex movements; thus, these exercises fall into the above theoretical constructs as well (65,114). If complicated forms of these exercises cannot be mastered, there are simpler versions that have been distilled and tested and found to be feasible and effective in older adults, resulting in reduced fall rates, as well as decreased fear of falling. By contrast, training using sophisticated balance platforms has not yet been shown to necessarily improve these clinical outcomes, although improvements in balance capacity tested on the same machine may be seen (110). Exercise classes including tai chi are now available in many senior centers and local gyms and are thus economical and highly accessible to many older adults. Compared with the high cost and lack of access to computerized balance training systems, as well as perhaps greater efficacy in falls prevention (115), tai chi or other kinds of functional balance-stressing movements are therefore recommended in preference to balance platform training at this point for most older adults. However, it is recognized that there are many groups of clinical patients, such as those with Parkinson disease, stroke, brain injury, or other neurologic conditions, who may benefit from balance platform training in an acute rehabilitation setting. There is a need for research into appropriate transition protocols for such clinical populations, which may involve use of the low-tech methods outlined above for more chronic rehabilitation or home settings.

Minimizing Contributions of Visual and Proprioceptive Pathways The ability to tolerate a narrowed base of support or shift in the center of mass will be markedly impaired if sensory inputs to balance control are reduced. This is most simply accomplished by closing the eyes during any of the movements mentioned in the preceding two sections. This should only be done after the posture in question has already been completely mastered with eyes open. It is also best to try this under direct supervision of a trainer or another exerciser, particularly in high-risk adults. In addition, positioning in between a wall and a chair or other object is recommended for maximal safety.

Decreased proprioceptive input can be accomplished by practicing standing postures on a highly compliant surface, such as a pillow, piece of foam, mattress, or quilt. Using a mattress has the added advantage of providing a "safety net" should balance be lost during the attempt. This should allow safer progression to higher levels of difficulty without fear of injury. It is a good idea to teach adults strategies on how to get up from a fall before undertaking any balance training so that the fear of this outcome is reduced. Again, no progression to reduced proprioceptive input should be made until the standard movements on a hard surface can be completed competently (without loss of balance). Obviously, the combination of decreased

vision and proprioception will be even more difficult than either adaptation alone. Proprioceptive input can be lessened in stages by inserting foam or mattresses of increasing thickness under the feet during training. A simple log sheet can be made to track the postures and these additional modifications on a weekly basis to monitor progress.

All balance movements should be done slowly and with deliberation, as this stresses the control systems more and produces better physiologic adaptation. As with resistance training, increased speed serves to substitute momentum for the appropriate physiologic domain (strength, balance) and therefore undercuts desired stress on the system. It can be seen, for example, that an exercise such as heel walking is actually easier when done rapidly rather than slowly, so the challenge and adaptation will be greater when the slow speed is practiced. One of the outcomes of the tai chi intervention reported above was that the older participants walked and moved more slowly after training, and their deliberation in movement was felt to be related to their reduced fear of falling and subsequent fall rates (110).

Intensity

Intensity in balance training refers to the degree of difficulty of the postures, movements, or routines practiced. The appropriate level of difficulty or "intensity" for any balance-enhancing exercise is the highest level that can be tolerated without inducing a fall or near-fall. In a supervised session, the individual can be pushed to the limits of such tolerance, as safety is assured by the physical presence of the trainer. In an unsupervised setting, the person should be told to try movements only up to the level that they fail to master completely. For example, if the goal is to hold the heel-to-toe stand for 15 seconds, then if someone can only hold the posture for 10 seconds before grabbing the wall for support, this is the appropriate initial training intensity. Progression in intensity is the key to improvement, as in other exercise domains, but this concept of mastery of the previous level before progression must be adhered to for safety. This is particularly important in frail elders, who are at highest risk of falls, osteoporotic fractures, and other injuries.

Volume and Frequency

No definite statement can be made at this time about the minimum effective dose of balance training techniques described above. Regimens have ranged from 1 to 7 days per week, and from once a day to several times per day (4,95). A reasonable recommendation would appear to be 2 to 3 days per week, but it is noted that this is more a matter of convention rather than an evidence-based recommendation. It is likely that as with other forms of training, a dose-response relationship exists, although thresholds have not been defined. There is no evidence that any negative effects are seen with high-volume training. Therefore, for adults with significant balance impairments that require intervention, training 3 to 7 days per week may be advantageous. On the other hand, healthy, normal adults may require only preventive practice 1 day a week or so for maintenance of mobility and function. Many more studies are needed in this area to define the recommendation further.

Choose several different exercises within the basic types of exercises (narrowed base of support, displacement of center of mass), and repeat each exercise two to three times at the most difficult level that falls short of being "mastered." It is unlikely that increasing the number of repetitions of a task that can be easily accomplished (e.g., the semitandem stand) will lead to improvements in balance, but just a few repetitions of a difficult task (such as standing on one leg) will lead to favorable adaptations. As with PRT, the emphasis should be on progressing to higher degrees of difficulty rather than high volumes of training. Tai chi and similar forms of exercise have been successfully prescribed for 45 minutes to 1 hour 2 to 3 days per week, but again, minimum effective doses are unknown.

Supervision and Setting

Balance training can generally be accomplished without the need for specialized equipment, which means that it can be done anywhere. The only supervision requirement relates to safety considerations and the level of risk of the individual for a fall during training. In the case of tai chi or yoga, an instructor may be needed for a length of time to teach the discipline and assure correct form. Practicing balance on a carpeted or other soft surface (such as a lawn) is desirable if available. If balance is impaired to begin with, supervision is highly recommended until capacity improves. Progression to each higher level of intensity should only be attempted after verification by a trainer or other individual that mastery has been achieved. A group setting is convenient, as exercisers can learn from each other's form, provide supervision and encouragement, and thereby challenge each other to progress with more confidence. Many trainers have used such group settings not only to teach balance exercises, but to deliver psychological interventions designed to reduce fear of falling and increase self-efficacy, talk about the safety enhancements of the home environment, practice techniques for getting up from a fall, discuss ways to get help in an emergency, and uncover other fall and fracture risks (e.g., postural hypotension, impaired vision, nutritional habits) that may benefit from treatment. Thus, the multifactorial nature of falls makes the use of a group setting for balance exercise delivery perhaps more important than it is in other modalities of exercise.

Benefits

Balance training has been shown to result in improved balance performance, decreased fear of falling, decreased incidence of falls, and increased ability to participate in other activities that may have been limited by gait and balance difficulties (84,95). It is expected, although not proven, that such changes would ultimately lead to improvements in functional independence, reduce hip fractures and other serious injuries, and improve overall quality of life. Such long-term outcomes will require larger studies of longer duration than those that have been reported to date. In particular, there is a need for data on the feasibility and efficacy of balance training in the very old and frail, in whom deficits are larger, fall risk is usually multifactorial, and cognitive impairments or degenerative neurologic diseases exist. All of these factors may alter the robustness of the physiologic adaptation achieved with training.

Balance training does not generally result in increased strength or aerobic capacity by itself. However, there may be some maintenance of muscle strength from the isometric contractions that occur during many of the balance-enhancing and one-legged postures and the bent-knee stance during tai chi. In addition, to the extent that balance training results in increased overall physical activity and mobility, these other activities may lead to improvements in strength and endurance.

Risks

The only real risk of balance training is loss of balance, resulting in a fall or injury or increased fear of falling. This is preventable with attention to the factors governing progression, intensity, setting, and supervision. There is little or no elevation in pulse or blood pressure during these kinds of exercises, so that cardiovascular events are not an expected or reported consequence. Musculoskeletal injury, other than that resulting from a fall, would also be unlikely.

It should be noted that there might be exacerbation of pre-existing arthritic pain or inflammation of the knee during prolonged one-legged standing or tai chi postures requiring a semicrouched stance. These positions may have to be adapted or avoided in those with significant weight-bearing pain in the joint. However, once quadriceps muscle strength improves with appropriate resistive exercises (see above), these kinds of movements may be tolerable. Impaired flexibility may also limit some tai chi or yoga postures initially and may lead to injury if range of motion is forced in the beginning. Gradual progression over time in the complexity of postures should prevent most injuries to soft tissues.

Integrating the Balance Prescription into Daily Life

Many activities in daily life can be turned into a balance-enhancing movement or position with a little creativity, making balance training one of the easiest modalities of exercise to integrate. Some examples of how this can be accomplished are listed below:

- Every time you are standing in line, cooking, combing your hair, or doing dishes, move your feet closer together, or stand on one leg if possible during the task; alternate legs every 15 to 30 seconds.

- When crossing a room or other short distance, tandem, heel, toe, crossover, or sideways walk for 10 to 20 feet instead of normal walking.
- Carry small items (books, cartons of milk) by holding them out at arm's length while you walk (without bending the spine).
- Close your eyes or stand on one leg while riding a moving bus or train (hold onto a bar for support lightly if needed).
- Attempt to rise from a chair without use of the arms. Next, advance to rising, using only one leg for support. The same may be practiced when sitting back down.

As with balance training sessions, none of these "integrated exercises" should be tried if they are beyond the current capacity of the individual. With time, these habits will become reinforced, and more and more opportunities to improve balance will appear throughout the normal daily routine. Challenge groups who are training together to think of creative ways to modify tasks and activities that are relevant to them in this way. Such group participation in exercise recommendations will serve as a motivational tool to increase overall training volume and optimally enhance the functional benefits of this modality of exercise. By turning "waiting in line" into an opportunity to exercise, you will never look at standing in line quite the same way again.

SPECIAL CONSIDERATIONS

Special Considerations in the Older Woman

Women respond as well as men to aerobic training, given the same level of training. Less robust responses in terms of aerobic capacity or weight loss appear to be because of reduced volume and/or intensity of training in many studies involving women. There does appear to be a difference in the way in which men and women adapt to cardiovascular training, however. Endurance-trained older men have been shown to increase exercise-related cardiac contractility and stroke volume during aerobic work (36), whereas this central adaptation has not yet been observed in older women (76,78,97). Older women adapt to aerobic training with peripheral changes, such as increased oxidative enzyme capacity, mitochondrial volume density, and capillary density in skeletal muscle, and these peripheral changes are responsible for the overall increase in maximal oxygen consumption achieved.

Another consideration in older women that may escape detection is exercise-induced or exacerbated urinary incontinence (29). This symptom may be so limiting that it precludes exercise participation entirely in some women and should be considered when compliance is low despite delivery of appropriate training and behav-

ioral methods. The incontinence in this case is usually stress incontinence related to weakened pelvic floor muscles and collagen resulting from the low estrogenic state of postmenopausal women not on hormone replacement therapy, as well as aging of muscle and connective tissue, and birth trauma. Although a complete discussion of urinary incontinence is beyond the scope of this chapter, a few points are worth emphasizing. Losses of urine when standing, coughing, sneezing, or initiating exercise are often because of stress incontinence secondary to the rise in intra-abdominal pressure caused by these activities. The presence of such symptoms should be part of the pre-exercise assessment of the older woman. If there are any other urinary symptoms, such as dysuria, frequency, urge incontinence, or hematuria, referral for medical evaluation is necessary. If not, then the simple measures outlined in Box 41-5 can be instituted to minimize the occurrence of incontinent episodes. Pelvic floor muscle exercises are essentially isometric resistance training for the levator ani muscles, which prevent the urethra from descending in response to increases in intra-abdominal pressure as noted above (16,60). An effective regimen is as follows:

- Hold a maximal contraction of levator ani muscles (without Valsalva) for 5 seconds; these muscles can be identified during pelvic exam or as the muscles that are used voluntarily to stop the stream of urine.
- Rest for 10 seconds.
- Repeat above steps for a total of 10 minutes.
- Complete this 10-minute session four times per day every day.

Success rates for pelvic muscle exercises vary widely (30%–60%), most likely because compliance with such a 40-minute regimen every day is quite low and contrac-

BOX 41-5	STEPS TO MINIMIZE URINARY INCONTINENCE RELATED TO EXERCISE

- Void before activity.
- Drink extra fluid after exercise rather than before or during sessions.
- Avoid all caffeine- and alcohol-containing foods and beverages for at least 3 hours before exercise.
- Minimize breath holding and use of Valsalva maneuver during exercise.
- Practice pelvic muscle-strengthening exercises.
- Minimize high-impact activities.
- Use intravaginal support or external pad during exercise.
- Review medications and dosing schedule with physician.

tions are submaximal. Biofeedback has been used as a way to show women when they are effectively producing contractile force with these muscles (16). An approach to compliance that may be behaviorally attractive is to tell women with stress incontinence to perform the pelvic muscle contractions whenever they are sitting at rest or riding in a car, or during rest periods between sets of a weightlifting regimen. In this way, the pelvic training does not actually take any "extra" time during the day and will become automatic once the habit is established. If the problem is not resolved with these simple measures, referral to a specialist is indicated for more specific treatment or medication management.

Finally, the generally lower muscle mass and tendency for gait disorders and falls seen in older women compared with men means that aerobic training is rarely indicated as an isolated exercise prescription in this population. The older and more frail the individual, the more this is true. It is reasonable, therefore, to start with strength and balance training, and add aerobic training only when there has been some improvement in these other areas. It should be remembered that there is little or no evidence that aerobic training significantly improves strength, muscle mass, or balance, although such statements are often made in general exercise guidelines for the older adult or healthcare provider.

Integration of Exercise into Daily Activities

Among all the modalities of exercise, cardiovascular exercise is perhaps the easiest to integrate into daily activities. It simply requires a few behavioral decisions to be made that can be adhered to with reasonable success. For example, decisions could be made to:

- Never use an escalator or elevator when stairs are available.
- Never take the car for errands that can be accomplished via a 10-minute walk or less.
- Do not use remote-control devices.
- Substitute manual devices (lawn mowers, egg beaters, brooms) for mechanical devices whenever possible.
- Park in the most remote corner of the parking lot whenever shopping.

If some of these things appear too difficult initially (such as climbing five flights of stairs while carrying home the groceries), they can be gradually added. For example, a person might start by taking the elevator four flights, walking the final flight, and advance to walking the entire way. This approach is very effective because it adheres to both the behavioral principle of "shaping"—taking small steps at a time—as well as the physiologic principle of incremental progression of volume and intensity of training. Immediate feedback on fitness is available as well, as the person notices the ability to climb all five flights of stairs with minimal effort after a few short

weeks. Although it may seem that all of these alterations in routine are time-consuming, the advantage is that no additional time is required for a discrete endurance training session of 20 to 30 minutes during the course of the day. Often, waiting for a busy elevator actually takes longer than climbing the flight of stairs, and the time taken circling the parking lot looking for a close space could have been better spent walking the extra distance.

Older adults of long-term-care facilities present a special problem in terms of "lifestyle" exercise prescription. In a nursing home patient, it is difficult to find stairs to climb or lawns to mow, so walking groups initiated around regularly scheduled activities when staff are available already (such as going to the dining room for meals or other activities) may have the best chance of success. As older adults improve in fitness, instead of walking directly to the dining room, extra laps around the ward can be added to extend the walk to at least 10 minutes for those who are able. Three such walks a day will complete a 30-minute aerobic regimen 7 days a week with minimal time commitment or extra resources needed. The most fit older adults should be encouraged to push wheelchair-bound older adults on these walks, as this will free staff to help less-able older adults ambulate and will also increase the aerobic intensity of the walk for the fitter older adults. Additionally, the psychological benefits of increased self-esteem and morale may be substantial when older adults are encouraged to do this, as they are given back an essential care-giving role that may have been lost on entry to the long-term-care facility.

REFERENCES

1. Ades PA, Savage PD, Cress ME, et al. Resistance training on physical performance in disabled older female cardiac patients. *Med Sci Sports Exerc.* 2003;35(8):1265–70.
2. American College of Obstetricians and Gynecologists. Exercise during pregnancy and the postpartum period. ACOG Committee Opinion (No. 267, January 2002). *Int J Gynaecol Obstet.* 2002;77:79–81.
3. Artal R, O'Toole M. Guidelines of the American College of Obstetricians and Gynecologists for exercise during pregnancy and the postpartum period. *Br J Sports Med.* 2003;37:6–12; discussion 12.
4. Baker MK, Atlantis E, Fiatarone Singh MA. Multi-modal exercise programs for older adults. *Age Ageing.* 2007;36(4):375–81.
5. Bar-Or O. Pathophysiological factors which limit the exercise capacity of the sick child. *Med Sci Sports Exerc.* 1986;18:276–82.
6. Bassey E, Rothwell M, Littlewood J, Pye D. Pre- and postmenopausal women have different bone density responses to the same high-impact exercise. *J Bone Miner Res.* 1998;13:1805–13.
7. Benn S, McCartney N, McKelvie R. Circulatory responses to weight lifting, walking and stair climbing in older males. *J Am Geriatr Soc.* 1996;44:121–5.
8. Bernhardt DT, Gomez J, Johnson MD, et al. Strength training by children and adolescents. *Pediatrics.* 2001;107:1470–2.
9. Binder EF, Yarasheski KE, Steger-May K, et al. Effects of progressive resistance training on body composition in frail older adults: results of a randomized, controlled trial. *J Gerontol A Biol Sci Med Sci.* 2005;60(11):1425–31.
10. Blumenthal JA, Babyak MA, Moore KA, et al. Effects of exercise training on older patients with major depression. *Arch Intern Med.* 1999;159(19):2349–56.

11. Borg G, Linderholm H. Perceived exertion and pulse rate during graded exercise in various age group. *Acta Med Scand.* 1970; 472(Suppl):194–206.

12. Borst SE. Interventions for sarcopenia and muscle weakness in older people. *Age Ageing.* 2004;33(6):548–55.

13. Braith RW, Stewart KJ. Resistance exercise training: its role in the prevention of cardiovascular disease. *Circulation.* 2006;113(22): 2642–50.

14. Brown DW, Brown DR, Heath GW, et al. Associations between physical activity dose and health-related quality of life. *Med Sci Sports Exerc.* 2004;36(5):890–6.

15. Bucksch J. Physical activity of moderate intensity in leisure time and the risk of all cause mortality. *Br J Sports Med.* 2005;39(9): 632–8.

16. Burns PA, Pranikoff K, Nochajski TH, et al. A comparison of effectiveness of biofeedback and pelvic muscle exercise treatment of stress incontinence in older community-dwelling women. *J Gerontol.* 1993;48(4):M167–74.

17. Campbell WW, Leidy HJ. Dietary protein and resistance training effects on muscle and body composition in older persons. *J Am Coll Nutr.* 2007;26(6):696S–703S.

18. Carter ND, Kannus P, Khan M. Exercise in the prevention of falls in older people: a systematic literature review examining the rationale and the evidence. *Sports Med.* 2001;31(6):427–38.

19. Centers for Disease Control and Prevention. Surveillance Summaries. *MMWR Morb Mortal Wkly Rep.* 2003;52:785–8.

20. Centers for Disease Control and Prevention. Strength training among adults aged ≥65 years: United States, 2001. *MMWR Morb Mortal Wkly Rep.* 2004;53(2):25–8.

21. Chang JT, Morton SC, Rubenstein LZ, et al. Interventions for the prevention of falls in older adults: systematic review and meta-analysis of randomised clinical trials. *BMJ.* 2004;328(7441):680.

22. Church TS, Earnest CP, Skinner JS, Blair SN. Effects of different doses of physical activity on cardiorespiratory fitness among sedentary, overweight or obese postmenopausal women with elevated blood pressure: a randomized controlled trial. *JAMA.* 2007;297(19):2081–91.

23. Clapp JF. *Exercising through Your Pregnancy.* Omaha, Nebr.: Addicus Books; 2002.

24. Clapp JF. Maternal heart rate in pregnancy. *Am J Obstet Gynecol.* 1985;152:659–60.

25. Clapp JF. Oxygen consumption during treadmill exercise before, during, and after pregnancy. *Am J Obstet Gynecol.* 1989;161: 1458–64.

26. Coe DP, Pivarnik JM, Womack CJ, Reeves MJ, Malina RM. Effect of physical education and activity levels on academic achievement in children. *Med Sci Sports Exerc.* 2006;38:1515–9.

27. Connolly DA, Sayers SP, McHugh MP. Treatment and prevention of delayed onset muscle soreness. *J Strength Cond Res.* 2003;17(1): 197–208.

28. Daley A, Macarthur C, Stokes-Lampard H, McManus R, Wilson S, Mutrie N. Exercise participation, body mass index, and health-related quality of life in women of menopausal age. *Br J Gen Pract.* 2007;57:130–5.

29. Danforth KN, Shah AD, Townsend MK, et al. Physical activity and urinary incontinence among healthy, older women. *Obstet Gynecol.* 2007;109(3):721–7.

30. Danice KE, Kann L, Kinchen S, et al. Youth risk behavior surveillance—United States, 2005. *MMWR Morb Mortal Wkly Rep.* 2006;55:1–108.

31. Davies GA, Wolfe LA, Mottola MF, MacKinnon C. Joint SOGC/CSEP clinical practice guideline: exercise in pregnancy and the postpartum period. *Can J Appl Physiol.* 2003;28:330–41.

32. Dempsey JC, Butler CL, Williams MA. No need for a pregnant pause: physical activity may reduce the occurrence of gestational diabetes mellitus and preeclampsia. *Exerc Sport Sci Rev.* 2005; 33:141–9.

33. de Vos NJ, Singh NA, Ross DA, Stavrinos TM, Orr R, Fiatarone Singh MA. Optimal load for increasing muscle power during explosive resistance training in older adults. *J Gerontol A Biol Sci Med Sci.* 2005;60(5):638–47.

34. Drinkwater BL. Women and exercise: physiological aspects. *Exerc Sport Sci Rev.* 1984;12:21–51.

35. Duvekot JJ, Cheriex EC, Pieters FA, Menheere PP, Peeters LH. Early pregnancy changes in hemodynamics and volume homeostasis are consecutive adjustments triggered by a primary fall in systemic vascular tone. *Am J Obstet Gynecol.* 1993;169:1382–92.

36. Ehsani AA, Ogawa T, Miller TR, Spina RJ, Jilka SM. Exercise training improved left ventricular systolic function in older men. *Circulation.* 1991;83(1):96–103.

37. Era P, Sainio P, Koskinen S, Haavisto P, Vaara M, Aromaa A. Postural balance in a random sample of 7,979 subjects aged 30 years and over. *Gerontology.* 2006;52(4):204–13.

38. Ettinger WH, Burns Jr R, Messier SP, et al. A randomized trial comparing aerobic exercise and resistance exercise with a health education program in older adults with knee osteoarthritis. The Fitness Arthritis and Seniors Trial (FAST). *JAMA.* 1997;277(1):25–31.

39. Fiatarone MA, O'Neill EF, Ryan ND, et al. Exercise training and nutritional supplementation for physical frailty in very elderly people. *New Engl J Med.* 1994;330:1769–75.

40. Fiatarone MA, Singh M. Exercise comes of age: rationale and recommendations for a geriatric exercise prescription. *J Gerontol A Biol Sci Med Sci.* 2002;57(A):M262–82.

41. Galper DI, Trivedi MH, Barlow CE, Dunn AL, Kampert JB. Inverse association between physical inactivity and mental health in men and women. *Med Sci Sports Exerc.* 2006;38(1):173–8.

42. Gardner A, Katzel L, Sorkin JD, et al. Exercise rehabilitation improves functional outcomes and peripheral circulation in patients with intermittent claudication: a randomized controlled trial. *J Am Geriatr Soc.* 2001;49:755–62.

43. Gearhart RE, Goss FL, Lagally KM, et al. Standardized scaling procedures for rating perceived exertion during resistance exercise. *J Strength Cond Res.* 2001;15(3):320–5.

44. Gordon N, Kohl H, Pollock M, et al. Cardiovascular safety of maximal strength testing in healthy adults. *Am J Cardiol.* 1995;76:851–3.

45. Guralnik JM, Simonsick EM, Ferrucci L, et al. A short physical performance battery assessing lower extremity function: association with self-reported disability and prediction of mortality and nursing home admission. *J Gerontol.* 1994;49(2):M85–94.

46. Guyatt GH, Sullivan MJ, Thompson PJ, et al. The 6-minute walk: a new measure of exercise capacity in patients with chronic heart failure. *Can Med Assoc J.* 1985;132:919–23.

47. **Haskell WL, Lee IM, Pate RR, et al. Physical activity and public health: updated recommendation for adults from the American College of Sports Medicine and the American Heart Association. *Med Sci Sports Exerc.* 2007;39(8):1423–34.**

48. Hauer K, Specht N, Schuler M, et al. Intensive physical training in geriatric patients after severe falls and hip surgery. *Age Ageing.* 2002;31(1):49–57.

49. Heath JM, Stuart MR. Prescribing exercise for frail elders. *J Am Board Fam Pract.* 2002;15(3):218–28.

50. Hebestreit HU, Bar-Or O. Differences between children and adults for exercise testing and prescription. In: Skinner JS, editor. *Exercise Testing and Exercise Prescription for Special Cases.* Philadelphia: Lippincott Williams & Wilkins; 2005. p. 68–84.

51. Heinonen A, Kannus P, Sievanen H, et al. Randomised controlled trial of effect of high-impact exercise on selected risk factors for osteoporotic fractures. *Lancet.* 1996;348(9038):1343–7.

52. Hughes SL, Seymour RB, Campbell RT, et al. Long-term impact of Fit and Strong! on older adults with osteoarthritis. *Gerontologist.* 2006;46(6):801–14.

53. Ingle L. Theoretical rationale and practical recommendations for cardiopulmonary exercise testing in patients with chronic heart failure. *Heart Fail Rev.* 2007;12(1):12–22.

54. Institute for Aerobics Research. *The Prudential FITNESSGRAM Test Administration Manual*. Dallas: Institute for Aerobics Research; 1994.

55. Janssen I, Jolliffe CJ. Influence of physical activity on mortality in elderly with coronary artery disease. *Med Sci Sports Exerc*. 2006; 38(3):418–43.

56. Kannus P, Sievanen H, Palvanen M, et al. Prevention of falls and consequent injuries in elderly people. *Lancet*. 2005;366(9500): 1885–93.

57. Kato T, Terashima T, Yamashita T, et al. Effect of low-repetition jump training on bone mineral density in young women. *J Appl Physiol*. 2006;100(3):839–43.

58. Katsiaras A, Newman AB, Kriska A, et al. Skeletal muscle fatigue, strength, and quality in the elderly: the Health ABC Study. *J Appl Physiol*. 2005;99(1):210–6.

59. Kaufman C, Berg K, Noble J, et al. Ratings of perceived exertion of ACSM exercise guidelines in individuals varying in aerobic fitness. *Res Q Exerc Sport*. 2006;77(1):122–30.

60. Kim H, Suzuki T, Yoshida Y, et al. Effectiveness of multidimensional exercises for the treatment of stress urinary incontinence in elderly community-dwelling Japanese women: a randomized, controlled, crossover trial. *J Am Geriatr Soc*. 2007;55(12):1932–9.

61. King AC, Taylor CB, Haskell WL. Effects of differing intensities and formats of 12 months of exercise training on psychological outcomes in older adults. *Health Psychol*. 1993;12(4):292–300.

62. King AC, Taylor CB, Haskell WL. Effects of differing intensities and formats of 12 months of exercise training on psychological outcomes in older adults; erratum. *Health Psychol*. 1993;2(5):405.

63. King DS, Sharp RL, Vukovich MD, et al. Effect of oral androstenedione on serum testosterone and adaptations to resistance training in young men: a randomized controlled trial. *JAMA*. 1999;281(21): 2020–8.

64. Kryger AI, Andersen JL. Resistance training in the oldest old: consequences for muscle strength, fiber types, fiber size, and MHC isoforms. *Scand J Med Sci Sports*. 2007;17(4):422–30.

65. Kuramoto AM. Therapeutic benefits of tai chi exercise: research review. *WMJ*. 2006;105(7):42–6.

66. Lagally KM, Amorose AJ. The validity of using prior ratings of perceive exertion to regulate resistance exercise intensity. *Percept Mot Skills*. 2007;104(2):534–42.

67. Loucks AB, Laughlin GA, Mortola JF, Girton L, Nelson JC, Yen SS. Hypothalamic-pituitary-thyroidal function in eumenorrheic and amenorrheic athletes. *J Clin Endocrinol Metab*. 1992;75(2):514–8.

68. Loucks AB, Callister R. Induction and prevention of low-T3 syndrome in exercising women. *Am J Physiol*. 1993;264(5 Pt 2): R924–30.

69. Loucks AB, Heath EM. Induction of low-T3 syndrome in exercising women occurs at a threshold of energy availability. *Am J Physiol*. 1994;266(3 Pt 2):R817–23.

70. Malina RM. Tracking of physical activity and physical fitness across the lifespan. *Res Q Exerc Sport*. 1996;67:S48–57.

71. Martel GF, Roth SM, Ivey FM, et al. Age and sex affect human muscle fibre adaptations to heavy-resistance strength training. *Exp Physiol*. 2006;91(2):457–64.

72. McCartney N. Acute responses to resistance training and safety. *Med Sci Sports Exerc*. 1999;31(1):31–37.

73. Mendelsohn ME, Karas RH. The protective effects of estrogen on the cardiovascular system. *N Engl J Med*. 1999;340:1801–11.

74. Mottola MF, Davenport MH, Brun CR, Inglis SD, Charlesworth S, Sopper MM. VO$_2$peak prediction and exercise prescription for pregnant women. *Med Sci Sports Exerc*. 2006;38:1389–95.

75. National Association for Sport and Physical Education. *Physical Activity for Children: A Statement Of Guidelines*. 2nd ed. Reston (VA): NASPE; 1994.

76. Neilan TG, Ton-Nu TT, Jassal DS, et al. Myocardial adaptation to short-term high-intensity exercise in highly trained athletes. *J Am Soc Echocardiogr*. 2006;19(10):1280–5.

77. Norrbrand L, Fluckey JD, Pozzo M, Tesch PA. Resistance training using eccentric overload induces early adaptations in skeletal muscle size. *Eur J Appl Physiol*. 2008;102(3):271–81.

78. Ogawa T, Spina RJ, Martin WH 3rd, et al. Effects of aging, sex, and physical training on cardiovascular responses to exercise. *Circulation*. 1992;86(2):494–503.

79. Ogden CL, Carroll MD, Curtin LR, McDowell MA, Tabak CJ, Flegal KM. Prevalence of overweight and obesity in the United States, 1999–2004. *JAMA*. 2006;295:1549–55.

80. Okazaki K, Iwasaki K, Prasad A, et al. Dose-response relationship of endurance training for autonomic circulatory control in healthy seniors. *J Appl Physiol*. 2005;99(3):1041–9.

81. Orr R, Raymond J, Fiatarone Singh M. Efficacy of progressive resistance training on balance performance in older adults: a systematic review of randomized controlled trials. *Sports Med*. 2008;38(3): 1–51.

82. Ostchega Y, Harris TB, Hirsch R, et al. Reliability and prevalence of physical performance examination assessing mobility and balance in older persons in the US: data from the Third National Health and Nutrition Examination Survey. *J Am Geriatr Soc*. 2000;48(9): 1136–41.

83. Paridon SM, Alpert BS, Boas SR, et al. Clinical stress testing in the pediatric age group: a statement from the American Heart Association Council on Cardiovascular Disease in the Young, Committee on Atherosclerosis, Hypertension, and Obesity in Youth. *Circulation*. 2006;113:1905–20.

84. Paterson DH, Jones GR, Rice CL. Ageing and physical activity: evidence to develop exercise recommendations for older adults. *Can J Public Health*. 2007;98 Suppl 2:S69–108.

85. Pedersen BK, Saltin B. Evidence for prescribing exercise as therapy in chronic disease. *Scand J Med Sci Sports*. 2006;16(s1):3–63.

86. Pivarnik JM, Chambliss HO, Clapp JF, et al. Impact of physical activity during pregnancy and postpartum on chronic disease risk. *Med Sci Sports Exerc*. 2006;38:989–1006.

87. Pollock ML, Graves JE, Bamman MM, et al. Frequency and volume of resistance training: effect on cervical extension strength. *Arch Phys Med Rehabil*. 1993;74(10):1080–6.

88. Rejeski WJ, Ettinger Jr WH, Martin K, et al. Treating disability in knee osteoarthritis with exercise therapy: a central role for self-efficacy and pain. *Arthritis Care Res*. 1998;11(2):94–101.

89. Risch SV, Norvell NK, Pollock ML, et al. Lumbar strengthening in chronic low back pain patients: physiologic and psychological benefits. *Spine*. 1993;18(2):232–8.

90. Rowland TW. *Developmental Exercise Physiology*. Champaign (IL): Human Kinetics; 1996.

91. Rubenstein LZ. Falls in older people: epidemiology, risk factors and strategies for prevention. *Age Ageing*. 2006;35(Suppl 2):ii37–41.

92. Sevick MA, Bradham DD, Muender M, et al. Cost-effectiveness of aerobic and resistance exercise in seniors with knee osteoarthritis. *Med Sci Sports Exerc*. 2000;32(9):1534–40.

93. Seynnes O, Fiatarone Singh MA. Relationship between resistance training intensity and physiological and functional adaptation in frail elders. *J Gerontol A Biol Sci Med Sci*. 2004;59A(4):33–9.

94. Seynnes O, Fiatarone Singh MA, Hue O, et al. Physiological and functional responses to low-moderate versus high-intensity progressive resistance training in frail elders. *J Gerontol A Biol Sci Med Sci*. 2004;59(5):503–9.

95. Sherrington C, Lord SR, Finch CF. Physical activity interventions to prevent falls among older people: update of the evidence. *J Sci Med Sport*. 2004;7(1 Suppl):43–51.

96. Singh NA, Stavrinos TM, Scarbek Y, Galambos G, Liber C, Fiatarone-Singh MA. A randomized controlled trial of high versus low intensity weight training versus general practitioner care for clinical depression in older adults. *J Gerontol A Biol Sci Med Sci*. 2005;60(6):768–6.

97. Spina RJ, Miller TR, Bogenhagen WH, et al. Gender-related differences in left ventricular filling dynamics in older subjects after

endurance exercise training. *J Gerontol A Biol Sci Med Sci.* 1996; 51(3):B232–7.

98. Strong WB, Malina RM, Blimkie CJ, et al. Evidence based physical activity for school-age youth. *J Pediatr.* 2005;146:732–7.

99. Suetta C, Magnusson SP, Rosted A, et al. Resistance training in the early postoperative phase reduces hospitalization and leads to muscle hypertrophy in elderly hip surgery patients—a controlled, randomized study. *J Am Geriat Soc.* 2004;52(12):2016–22.

100. Suominen H. Muscle training for bone strength. *Aging Clin Exp Res.* 2006;18(2):85–93.

101. Taaffe DR. Sarcopenia—exercise as a treatment strategy. *Aust Fam Physician.* 2006;35(3):130–4.

102. **U.S. Department of Health and Human Services. Physical Activity and Health: A Report of the Surgeon General. Washington (DC): U.S. Department of Health and Human Services, Centers for Disease Control and Prevention, National Center for Chronic Disease Prevention and Health Promotion; 1996.**

103. Verhaeghe J, Thomsen JS, van Bree R, et al. Effects of exercise and disuse on bone remodeling, bone mass, and biomechanical competence in spontaneously diabetic female rats. *Bone.* 2000;27(2): 249–56.

104. Visser M, Simonsick EM, Colbert LH, et al. Type and intensity of activity and risk of mobility limitation: the mediating role of muscle parameters. *J Am Geriatr Soc.* 2005;53(5):762–70.

105. Welle S, Totterman S, Thornton C. Effect of age on muscle hypertrophy induced by resistance training. *J Gerontol.* 1996;51A(6):M270–5.

106. Wernbom M, Augustsson J, Thomeé R. The influence of frequency, intensity, volume and mode of strength training on whole muscle cross-sectional area in humans. *Sports Med.* 2007;37(3):225–64.

107. **Williams MA, Haskell WL, Ades PA, et al. Resistance exercise in individuals with and without cardiovascular disease: 2007 update. A scientific statement from the American Heart Association Council on Clinical Cardiology and Council on Nutrition, Physical Activity, and Metabolism. *Circulation.* 2007;116(5):572–84.**

108. Wilmore JH. Alterations in strength, body composition, and anthropometric measurements consequent to a 10-week weight training program. *Med Sci Sports.* 1974;6:133–8.

109. Wilmore JH, Stanforth PR, Gagnon J, et al. Cardiac output and stroke volume changes with endurance training: the HERITAGE Family Study. *Med Sci Sports Exerc.* 2001;33:99–106.

110. Wolf SL, Barnhart HX, Kutner NG, et al. Reducing frailty and falls in older persons: an investigation of tai chi and computerized balance training. *J Am Geriatr Soc.* 1996;44(5):489–96.

111. Wolfe LA. Pregnancy. In: Skinner JS, editor. *Exercise Testing and Exercise Prescription for Special Cases.* Philadelphia: Lippincott Williams & Wilkins; 2005. p. 377–91.

112. Wolfe LA, Mottola MF. *PARmed-X for Pregnancy.* Ottawa: Canadian Society for Exercise Physiology; 2002. p. 1–4.

113. Woodard CM, Berry MJ. Enhancing adherence to prescribed exercise: structured behavioral interventions in clinical exercise programs. *J Cardiopulm Rehabil.* 2001;21(4):201–9.

114. Wu G. Evaluation of the effectiveness of tai chi for improving balance and preventing falls in the older population—a review. *J Am Geriatr Soc.* 2002;50(4):746–54.

115. Zijlstra GA, Van Haastregt JC, van Eijk JT, et al. Interventions to reduce fear of falling in community-living older people: a systematic review. *J Am Geriatr Soc.* 2007;55(4):603–15.

SELECTED REFERENCES FOR FURTHER READING

American College of Obstetricians and Gynecologists. ACOG Committee Opinion (No. 267, January 2002). Exercise during pregnancy and the postpartum period. *Int J Gynaecol Obstet.* 2002;77: 79–81.

Artal R, O'Toole M. Guidelines of the American College of Obstetricians and Gynecologists for exercise during pregnancy and the postpartum period. *Br J Sports Med.* 2003;37:6–12; discussion 12.

Fiatarone Singh M. Exercise comes of age: rationale and recommendations for a geriatric exercise prescription. *J Gerontol Med Sci.* 2002;57(A):M262–82.

Haskell WL, Lee IM, Pate RR, et al. Physical activity and public health: updated recommendation for adults from the American College of Sports Medicine and the American Heart Association. *Med Sci Sports Exerc.* 2007;39(8):1423–34.

Hebestreit HU, Bar-Or O. Differences between children and adults for exercise testing and prescription. In: Skinner JS, editor. *Exercise Testing and Exercise Prescription for Special Cases.* Philadelphia: Lippincott Williams & Wilkins; 2005. p. 68–84.

INTERNET RESOURCES

- American College of Obstetricians and Gynecologists: www.acog.org
- American College of Sports Medicine: www.acsm.org

An explosion of interest, by both the public and health professionals, has emerged with respect to **physical activity** as a means for achieving positive benefits related to health, functioning, and quality of life. Despite this increased interest, available evidence indicates that close to half of Americans do not exercise regularly (i.e., on 4 or more days per week), and one fourth or more do not exercise at all (36,37). Of the 10% (or less) of initially sedentary adults who begin regular physical activity in a year, as many as 50% may drop out within 3 to 6 months, and the recidivism rates are similar among those who were already active. Assisting individuals to stay physically active is a challenge that requires creativity and patience. In addition, finding ways to encourage extremely sedentary individuals to adopt a more active lifestyle represents an increasingly important public health goal. Exercise professionals can take advantage of the current public enthusiasm for becoming more active, as well as the growing literature suggesting strategies that can be effective for enhancing participation in physical activity.

Several health behavior change theories and models have been applied in systematic attempts to change physical activity behavior, with varying results (38). Among the most heuristic of these approaches is the application of social learning/social cognitive theories (2). This approach views such behavior as being initiated and maintained through a complex interaction of personal, behavioral, and environmental factors and conditions

> > > KEY TERMS

Correlate: A variable or factor that is significantly associated with the outcome of interest (e.g., physical activity) and that may be targeted in intervention efforts. Such variables may or may not be part of the causal chain with respect to physical activity participation and may require examination to specifically determine their causal impact.

Intervention strategies: Any technique or approach that aims at enhancing physical activity participation; these strategies can span a range of domains, from individual to policy level.

Physical activity: Any form of repetitive movement, typically involving large muscle groups, that results in energy expenditure.

Physical activity adherence: The percent of physical activity participation, derived by comparing the amount of physical activity engaged in (numerator) with the amount of physical activity recommended or prescribed (denominator).

Physical activity adoption: The initiation or initial increases in physical activity that often accompany an

intervention or that can occur naturally by an individual. Often, the adoption period is considered the initial 3 to 6 months of an intervention or program, although there are no definitive or agreed-upon definitions of the length of this period. In fact, the length of the adoption period is likely to differ depending on the experiences and characteristics of the populations under study. Behavioral indicators of successful physical activity adoption are recommended over often arbitrarily set time periods.

Physical activity maintenance: Sustained physical activity participation that occurs over extended periods of time (i.e., 1 year or longer).

Physical activity participation: The amount of physical activity engaged in more generally, including structured and unstructured (e.g., routine) forms of physical activity.

Predictor: A variable or factor that is associated prospectively with physical activity levels or changes in physical activity over time.

(24). Factors that may play a role in influencing physical activity participation include personal experiences with physical activity; attitudes and perceptions of physical activity; activity-related knowledge, skills, and beliefs; and surrounding physical and social environments or perceptions of those environments. The social learning/social cognitive theoretical approach also emphasizes the individual's ability to self-regulate behavior through setting goals, monitoring progress toward these goals, and modifying resources in the physical and social environment (as well as one's own thoughts or beliefs, as appropriate) to support the goals. Observational learning and modeling by others are important influences. Self-efficacy (i.e., the level of confidence in one's ability to successfully perform a specific behavior or activity) and outcome expectancies (i.e., one's belief that the behavior leads to a desired outcome) are identified to be critical factors that influence which behaviors are attempted and the persistence of the behaviors (2).

Social cognitive theory and related approaches to understanding physical activity behavior have been supplemented in recent years with an increased appreciation for the role of motivational readiness in changing and maintaining physical activity patterns (17). The demand for regularity in performing physical activity to obtain benefits throughout life calls for innovative methods to encourage habitual physical activity. Additionally, factors or correlates that influence initial adoption and early participation in physical activity may differ from those that affect subsequent long-term maintenance. Stage-of-change models that take into account motivational readiness for change (e.g., the transtheoretical model [1]) may better identify strategies that work for individuals in different stages and at different levels of physical activity participation (e.g., sedentary persons contemplating joining a physical activity program, those in the early stage of physical activity adoption, those committed to maintaining a program across the long term).

 1.9.5-HFS: Knowledge of the stages of motivational readiness.

The transtheoretical model proposes that individuals move through five stages of readiness for changing health behaviors (1,28): *precontemplation* (not thinking about changing physical activity), *contemplation* (thinking about changing physical activity), *preparation* (making small changes in physical activity but not to a sufficient level), *action* (meeting physical activity goals but for fewer than 6 months), and *maintenance* (being physically active at the desired level for at least 6 months). However, movement through the stages may not progress in a linear fashion, and individuals often move back and forth through the stages. By understanding and assessing readiness for change, professionals can tailor physical activity interventions and programs to meet a participant's current needs and level of motivation. Questionnaires are

available to assist exercise professionals in evaluating a participant's motivational readiness to change physical activity behavior (see GETP8 Figure 7-4).

Thus, behavior change theories focus on the dynamic relationship between personal attributes and resources, the behavior targeted for change, and influences of the physical and social environment in shaping the **adoption** and **maintenance** of the targeted behavior. Along with similar conceptual approaches, these theories provide a framework for development of physical activity **intervention strategies**. However, theoretical approaches have not often been applied in a comprehensive fashion in physical activity intervention research. In addition, the majority of physical activity intervention studies focus on endurance exercise, often ignoring other forms of activity, such as strength and flexibility training, which are important components of fitness.

In recent years, behavioral theories have been broadened to include ecologic frameworks of physical activity participation, which make more explicit the important interplay between personal-behavioral, social-cultural, and environmental-policy levels of impact and influence (33). Such frameworks underscore the point that physical activity participation is influenced by a complex set of variables that likely change over time.

Although the understanding of the behavior change and maintenance processes continues to develop, several potentially important cognitive, behavioral, social, and environmental variables influencing both initial adoption and longer-term maintenance of physical activity patterns have been identified (16,38) (see GETP8 Box 7-5).

INCREASING ADOPTION AND EARLY ADHERENCE

Adoption of increased physical activity patterns can be enhanced by considering factors in the personal, behavioral, environmental, and program-related spheres.

PERSONAL FACTORS

In the United States as well as in several other industrialized nations, several subgroups remain underactive (36), most notably individuals who are older (particularly women), from ethnic minority groups, less educated, smokers, and overweight. *Health* factors have been shown to have consistent relationships with physical activity level. People with medical problems or disabilities are more likely to be inactive. Health-related barriers and concerns have been found to be particularly important in older age groups, in whom fears of physical activity–related injury often increase (14). Individuals in groups at risk for physical inactivity may benefit from an emphasis on moderate-intensity activities that can be readily adapted for a variety of fitness levels and abilities and incorporated into their daily routines.

In addition, *cognitive and experiential* variables may negatively influence initial participation in regular physical activity, including negative experiences with physical activity; negative perceptions of health status or physical activity ability and skills; lower self-efficacy beliefs (i.e., confidence in the ability to successfully perform a specific physical activity regimen or program); limited outcome efficacy beliefs (i.e., belief that physical activity has value for health, fitness, or related desired outcomes); low levels of perceived physical activity enjoyment and satisfaction; negative perceptions of access to exercise facilities, convenience of the physical activity, or lack of time; limited understanding of personal benefits of physical activity, particularly relative to the "costs" or burden required to undertake a physical activity program (14,16).

Self-efficacy expectations appear to be particularly potent predictors of physical activity participation early on (24). Thus, it is important to focus on individuals' initial feelings of self-efficacy and to help to increase their outcome expectations through shaping early successes. This can be accomplished by helping participants set realistic, personally tailored physical activity goals, providing regular positive feedback and support, and teaching patients to monitor their own physical activity levels as a way of measuring progress and helping them take charge of their programs. Helping patients to plan ahead for inevitable lapses in physical activity participation (i.e., relapse prevention) is another means of encouraging patients to take charge of their own programs and enhance their self-efficacy levels in the face of barriers to their physical activity programs (16,18).

 1.9.4-HFS: Knowledge of extrinsic and intrinsic reinforcement and give examples of each.

In addition, level of self- or *intrinsic motivation* (i.e., internal desires for achievement), as described in self-determination theory and similar perspectives (6,21), may be positively related to continued participation in physical activity. Importantly, intrinsic motivation may be learned when an individual finds personal, self-identified rewards for behavior (e.g., personal achievement, the satisfaction obtained in reaching one's physical activity goals) independent of extrinsic or external reinforcements available for that behavior (12). Such approaches typically involve the acknowledgment of the individual's feelings about the proposed change; providing a personal rationale for the change; providing a choice of alternative behaviors to reduce conflicts regarding making the change; and affirming the importance of individual preferences and experiences (7).

With respect to personal factors, previous experience with physical activity should be explored, along with unreasonable beliefs and misconceptions about physical activity (e.g., the "no pain, no gain" fallacy or myths that older individuals need to "conserve their energy"). For example, many inactive individuals believe that exercise is inherently painful or aversive, and sedentary individuals are often unaware of the benefit of moderate activities (e.g., brisk walking) that may be more appealing and comfortable than more vigorous activity regimens (e.g., high-impact aerobics, running). Professionals can provide specific instruction, accompanied by actual rehearsal and feedback, on appropriate ways of performing specific activities at a safe, beneficial intensity to obtain health-related benefits while avoiding injury.

In addition, a physical activity program should be personally relevant, both in terms of type of activity and goals. For example, if stress reduction is a motivating factor, activities that can be helpful in reducing stress (i.e., not overly competitive, noisy, or demanding) should be targeted. Examples of such activities may include brisk walking, jogging, or bicycling conducted outdoors in pleasant surroundings that allow time to "get away." Alternatively, certain activities that are performed in a noncompetitive manner or that incorporate relaxation techniques, such as yoga, would be appropriate. Targeting an individual's specific interests and goals increases the likelihood for enjoyment and sustained motivation for physical activity.

Additional useful strategies include structuring appropriate expectations concerning physical activity (what can and cannot be accomplished and when results should be expected) as early as possible, stressing the many benefits of making physical activity changes, as well as exploring perceived barriers to increasing physical activity (e.g., unreasonable expectations concerning time or program intensity, fear of embarrassment, failure, boredom). A simple questionnaire or checklist regarding expectations can provide exercise professionals with early clues to such expectations and areas for important problem solving and planning (22).

1.9.1-CES: List and apply behavioral strategies that apply to lifestyle modifications, such as exercise, diet, stress, and medication management.

1.9.1-HFS: Knowledge of behavioral strategies to enhance exercise and health behavior change (e.g., reinforcement, goal setting, social support).

BEHAVIORAL FACTORS

Numerous behavioral and environmental variables enhance initial adoption and early **adherence** to physical activity.

Behavioral factors include the skills to carry out physical activity to facilitate health and quality-of-life benefits while minimizing injury and boredom. Such skills include knowledge and use of behavioral and psychological strategies that assist in the negotiation of barriers and pitfalls that inevitably interfere with regular activity. A useful behavioral skill may be as simple as problem solving specific barriers that the individual is likely to face. A related strategy is relapse prevention, whereby individuals learn how to plan ahead by identifying and preparing for periods when disruption of physical activity is likely (e.g., during holidays). Studies applying relapse-prevention strategies, either alone or in combination with other behavioral strategies, suggest their utility in the promotion, adoption, and maintenance of physical activity (11,13). Another potentially effective strategy is implementation of a decision balance sheet, whereby careful evaluation of expected or experienced benefits and costs of participating are compared. Other self-regulatory skills that appear to promote physical activity participation if used regularly are self-monitoring of progress coupled with ongoing feedback related to success, which may be readily accomplished through the use of written or computerized activity logs. Also, stimulus control or structuring the immediate environment to remind or encourage one to be active (e.g., through the use of visual or auditory reminders or prompts) can be helpful. A summary of behavioral skills and strategies to promote physical activity is given in Box 42-1.

Behavioral Shaping

For sedentary persons, the major objective is to establish a successful physical activity habit that targets the individual's goals while decreasing likelihood for failure. The initial activity prescription should be well within the capabilities of the individual and should be easily accomplished. The activity should also consider preferences, motivation, skills, and life circumstances. For some individuals, shaping may translate into a simple initial increase in activities of daily living (ADLs), for example, walking more at work and at home or taking stairs. For others, the initial prescription may involve some less frequent, structured endurance activity with a concomitant increase in routine activity until more vigorous activity is indicated.

A key consideration in all physical activity program planning should be gradual shaping of the physical activity behavior toward the ultimate goal set forth by the patient and physical activity professional. When physical activity progresses too quickly, adherence is almost always negatively affected. The rate of injury and dropout increases significantly when beginning exercisers are exposed to physical activities of too high an intensity relative to their fitness level, or exposed to very high initial frequency (e.g., 5 or more days per week) or duration (e.g., 45 or more minutes per session). In contrast, after an individual is beyond the initial stages of his or her program, higher intensity, frequency, and duration are often appropriate.

Thus, the physical activity regimen should be initially easy to undertake and gradually incremented, ensuring success at each stage (see GETP8 Table 7-1). As noted earlier, exercise professionals (and beginning exercisers)

BOX 42-1 — BEHAVIORAL SKILLS AND STRATEGIES TO PROMOTE PHYSICAL ACTIVITY

- *Decisional balance:* Identify personal benefits of physical activity and evaluate barriers for change; use benefits for motivation and teach problem-solving skills for overcoming barriers.
- *Self-monitoring:* Record type of activity, intensity, minutes, and calories expended as well as sedentary behaviors, such as time spent sitting, watching television, or computer use; use step counters, particularly for individuals who have not begun structured exercise or find it difficult to keep written logs.
- *Goal setting:* Set realistic short-term and long-term goals for physical activity behaviors; goals should target specific behaviors, be measurable to monitor progress, be realistic, and occur in a reasonable time frame.
- *Commitment:* Make a commitment to healthy behaviors; use behavioral contracts and incentives to enhance motivation.
- *Social support:* Identify and enlist social support to allow participants to share concerns, gain knowledge, receive encouragement, and practice new behaviors; also identify potential saboteurs who could hinder physical activity efforts and then develop strategies and assertiveness skills to deal with them.
- *Stimulus control:* Recognize and control physical, psychological, environmental, and social cues for physical activity behaviors.
- *Relapse prevention:* Identify high-risk situations and plan for potential lapses in physical activity; practice cognitive restructuring to overcome unhelpful or negative thought patterns (e.g., all-or-none thinking).

---

should focus primarily on shaping and maintaining the initial physical activity habit for approximately 6 to 12 weeks rather than rapidly establishing what may eventually be the optimal regimen for desired benefits. This approach emphasizes first establishing behavioral control of the physical activity habit so that beginners are encouraged to simply show up (e.g., "No matter how little you may feel like doing or are able to do, we are working on reinforcing the habit of regular physical activity; the benefits will come, if you can first form the habit"). Of course, finding immediate or short-term benefits of value to the individual in question will serve to increase the likelihood of that person sticking with his/her physical activity regimen long enough to attain other longer-term benefits.

Goal Setting

 1.9.9-HFS: Ability to coach patients to set achievable goals and overcome obstacles through a variety of methods (e.g., in person, phone, and Internet).

The success of behavioral shaping is based on the determination of realistic goals that provide the individual with some motivational challenge but that are likely to be successfully achieved, thus leading to increases in self-efficacy. Key goal-setting principles include that the behavior be:

- Specific: The physical activity behavior should be clearly and precisely established.
- Measurable: The behavior should be something that can be readily monitored.
- Realistic: The behavior should be somewhat challenging but within the individual's capabilities and readily achievable.
- Time-frame specific: The behavior should be accomplished within a specified period.

Enjoyment

For most individuals, it is critically important for adherence that the activity be enjoyable. The physical discomfort that often accompanies early stages of increased activity should be minimized or at least moderated by positive factors and normalized with respect to the individual's expectations. Methods for enhancing enjoyment include tailoring of the types of activities and the format (group or individual, facility or home based). One method of assessing enjoyment is to ask participants to note their level of enjoyment on a range of values from "very unenjoyable" to "very enjoyable" (e.g., scale of 1 to 5). If two or more sessions are "unenjoyable," the exercise regimen should be modified and accompanied, if appropriate for the individual, by additional rewards or incentives.

External Rewards and Incentives

 1.9.4-HFS: Knowledge of extrinsic and intrinsic reinforcement and give examples of each.

As noted previously, the initial steps involved in becoming more physically active are found by many persons to be anything but rewarding. Often it is not until several months into a regular physical activity program that participants begin to report experiencing positive benefits from physical activity on a regular basis. In fact, the longer the period of inactivity and the more unfit the individual, the longer the period may be before any physical activity becomes intrinsically reinforcing (i.e., feels good). Therefore, beginners may need external rewards early in the program for encouragement and motivation.

Use of such rewards is consistent with the process of behavioral shaping in which early approximations of target behaviors require ample reinforcement or rewards for optimal acquisition (i.e., adoption). For highly unfit or inactive individuals, beginner status might extend to 6 months or 1 year, and special external incentives may need to be programmed throughout that time. For other, more fit persons, the beginner phase may occur for only a short time, perhaps as little as 2 to 3 weeks. Generally, the choice of rewards or incentives should reside with the participant, as the incentives people find motivating varies from person to person. However, it is important to help participants identify rewards that will not be counterproductive to desired health goals (e.g., discourage use of high-fat snacks or days off from exercise as rewards). It is also important to recognize that for some individuals, using external rewards or incentives will be unfamiliar, unpalatable, and/or counterproductive and should not be used in such cases.

Social Support

One valuable and reinforcing form of reward is *social support*. Social support is a powerful motivator for many people. It can be delivered in a variety of forms, including through an instructor, exercise partners, family members, coworkers, or neighbors who encourage increased activity, as well as through telephone contacts or letter or e-mail prompts from a health professional. Praise is a critical component of social support, especially for inexperienced, beginning exercisers and completely relapsed former exercisers. To be most effective, encouragement should be both immediate (during or very shortly after the physical activity episode, if possible) and specific. Friends and family members can also be encouraged to participate in physical activity to enhance support. However, others' physical activity pace must be appropriate for the beginner. When support from significant others is active and ongoing, individuals are more likely than those with little or no social support to persist in a physical activity program (33).

Professionals, family members, and helpers should all be cautioned against even well-intentioned nagging or use of other aversive procedures (e.g., using guilt) to induce a person to become more physically active. These counterproductive actions almost inevitably increase the punishing characteristics of physical activity as well as potentially impairing the partnership between the individual and the supportive agent, thus further upsetting the often delicate balance between the motivation to become physically active and remaining inactive.

The use of social support can also be extended and formalized using *written contracts* between the individual and a significant person. Contracts are written, signed agreements that specify the physical activity-related goals in a public format and for which there is value exchange, much like a legal contract. They typically specify short-term, concrete goals and the types of positive consequences that occur upon reaching the goals. The contract should be flexible and avoid rigid daily goals that may be difficult or impossible to meet. In the earlier stages of a program, an appropriate goal might be related to attendance or participation rather than performance. These contracts often work best if developed in tandem with an interested person or helper. Such contracts can help to increase personal responsibility and commitment. Those managing physical activity programs should also consider using contingency management, in which more highly rewarding or preferred activities are made contingent on achieving a particular goal (e.g., watching a favorite television program only after a physical activity session is completed). Another alternative is a written agreement through which the participant agrees in writing to perform or complete certain behaviors or activities that can be useful for persons who are reluctant to sign a behavioral contract. Figure 42-1 presents a sample behavioral contract for physical activity.

The use of appropriate and consistent physical activity role models in the environment can also motivate people to begin and continue exercise. These models should be as similar as possible to the targeted individuals (e.g., some programs use successful graduates as future participant assistants for maximal effectiveness) (16,19). Further-

more, when possible, the physical activity professional should set an appropriate example by exercising with participants and displaying other behaviors that are consistent with an active lifestyle (e.g., taking stairs; walking to accomplish errands; adhering to appropriate exercise safeguards, such as stretching and hydration).

Behavioral Success

Continued adherence usually results from behavioral success rather than education or changes in knowledge; that is, engaging in physical activity on a regular basis subsequently shapes beliefs and attitudes about continuing the activity, rather than vice versa. This may help explain why many individuals, despite being knowledgeable about exercise, are not active. Physical activity professionals can help by pointing out the positive changes and gains being made, no matter how modest. Participants should be shaped such that they engage in some form of regular physical activity regardless of the presence of negative subjective feelings (barring illness or injury) or attitudes. Such regular, successful participation often produces appropriate feelings of mastery and perhaps enjoyment, as well as positive attitudes toward physical activity, a process that enhances the probability of maintaining physical activity.

Date: _____

Client Responsibilities:

1. Over the next 4 weeks, I will walk at least 4 days per week, for a total of at least 30 minutes per day. (I understand that I can break the 30 minutes up into two 15-minute episodes or walk continuously for 30 minutes).

2. For each week that I attain the above set of goals, I will reward myself by putting aside $5 to be used to treat myself to an article of clothing, a movie, or a similar reward.

3. For each week that I don't meet the above set of goals, I will forego watching a favorite TV show (and I will use that time to walk, if possible).

4. I will record my data on my physical activity calendar at the end of each day, and I will evaluate the success of this set of goals (and revise if necessary) on _____ (date) _____ .

My helper in supporting and reminding me about my goals is:

_____

My signature: _____ Date: _____

Helper signature: _____ Date: _____

FIGURE 42-1. Sample behavioral contract.

Self-Monitoring

An important form of establishing behavioral success is *feedback* regarding progress through self-monitoring, or recording physical activity patterns. Feedback stimulates a positive, reactive effect on a wide variety of behaviors. For example, short-term reduction of caloric intake usually results when it is monitored. Similarly, the physical activity habit is frequently enhanced when attendance, general physical activity adherence or performance, or the results of the physical activity program are systematically monitored. Self-monitoring can be used to identify unhelpful patterns or sedentary activities, set goals, monitor progress, and identify barriers as well as prompt physical activity choices. One simple method, especially in those having difficulty engaging in a systematic physical activity, is to provide an inexpensive pedometer or step-counter to track walking and related physical activities. Pedometers have been found to be a cost-efficient, valid, and reliable means for providing motivational feedback across a variety of populations (3).

Feedback can also be delivered by another person or generated through use of self-recorded monitoring sheets, an activity diary, or a graph showing progress in one or more variables, plotted heart rates, and attendance and adherence across time. Computer-generated feedback letters that summarize progress made in the program over time show promise as an efficient, systematic method for providing personalized feedback on a regular basis. When used in conjunction with goals that are reasonable, personally relevant, and short term, feedback can be a powerful motivating factor.

Self-Management

Successful behavior change often correlates with early training in self-management strategies and an understanding of the importance of taking personal responsibility and accountability for physical activity. Individuals must recognize the importance of taking charge of physical activity as a lifelong goal rather than as something that ends when a 12-week class or program is over. Such programs should be thought of as a vehicle for establishing a lifelong habit rather than the means by which physical activity should be defined. Early in all programs, methods to prompt and successfully engage participants in alternate forms of physical activity in a variety of settings and under a variety of circumstances should be outlined, along with relevant relapse prevention tips (Box 42-2). In addition, forming a partnership with each individual that fosters the individual's feelings of autonomy and control with respect to the physical activity program has been increasingly recognized as a potentially important means for facilitating long-term participation (12). Thus, participants should be encouraged to take a self-directed approach to all aspects of physical activity (e.g., goal setting, planning) rather than relying on the professional.

BOX 42-2	METHODS FOR ENGAGING PARTICIPANTS IN PHYSICAL ACTIVITY

SUGGESTIONS FOR PLANNING PHYSICAL ACTIVITY

- Carry exercise clothes or walking shoes in the car; place a pair of walking shoes at work; pack a bag with a set of exercise clothes and shoes so it will be ready when needed.
- Leave exercise clothes or shoes by the bed or the front door.
- Formally schedule physical activity into a weekly planner or calendar.
- Spend time with other physically active people.
- Park the car and walk; take stairs whenever possible.
- Only make decisions concerning whether or not to be physically active or how much to exercise *after* arriving at the designated physical activity site or locale.
- Develop a plan or program for high-risk situations (e.g., travel, holidays) to assist with maintaining physical activity.

SUGGESTIONS FOR A MISSED SESSION (RELAPSE PREVENTION)

- Admit responsibility for the slip.
- Develop a restart plan, including appropriate goals.
- Call physical activity "buddy" for support and motivation.
- Arrange reinforcements or rewards to help restart the activity.
- Simplify or change the routine to accommodate temporary changes in availability or time.
- Begin by simply visiting the usual physical activity place or locale.

ENVIRONMENTAL FACTORS

Several environmental factors can influence initial participation as well as longer-term **adherence** (32,34). These include proximity, access to, and affordability of facilities (for those who prefer facility-based activities); weather; regimen flexibility (type of activity, intensity, location, timing, frequency); convenience and ease of scheduling of the activity (real or perceived); immediate visual or auditory cues and prompts in the environment promoting physical activity (e.g., reminders to exercise); immediate consequences of physical activity for the individual (e.g., discomfort); and social influences and support (e.g., individuals reporting spouses to be neutral or unsupportive of physical activity are more likely to drop out).

Convenience

Three factors related to convenience are important to successful initiation and maintenance of an exercise program. First, it is clear that the greater the effort required to prepare for physical activity (i.e., a long drive to and from an exercise facility and other location issues, having to change clothes for activity), the greater the potential for dropping out (16). Encouraging methods of being physically active in or around the home (the place where many people prefer to exercise) or workplace can make convenience less of a deterrent to adherence. Second, time is often the primary factor leading to perceptions of inconvenience. If a physical activity program is offered within a class structure, having several time options may be helpful. For some people with extreme time constraints, alternatives to a class format are often necessary. A practical alternative is to emphasize ways that individuals can build regular physical activity into their daily routines, such as through using transportation alternatives that facilitate more walking or bicycling, taking stairs, and walking to do errands. It is becoming increasingly recognized that participating in both structured as well as lifestyle physical activity is important for many people to optimize benefits. Although time constraints are typically noted as major reasons for inactivity, regular exercisers complain as much as persons who are not regularly active about such constraints. Thus, perceived available time may reflect, in large part, one's current priorities related to being active or time-management skills rather than actual time limitations. Third, modes of physical activity that require special, costly, or time-consuming preparation (e.g., skiing, swimming) may adversely affect adoption and adherence. Thus, location, time, and mode can be critical factors during early stages of acquisition. Choices should be carefully evaluated by both the participant and the physical activity professional before initiating a physical activity program to help mitigate the negative impact of such factors.

Social Environment

The *social environment* can have a major impact on both physical activity adoption and maintenance. As earlier discussed, family support as well as parental or family level of physical activity are associated with increased physical activity in some population groups (20,23,35). Social support from friends or coworkers may also have a positive effect. In addition, physicians and other health professionals can positively influence physical activity behavior. Individuals should be encouraged to identify and establish appropriate support from others in their social environment as part of behavioral skills training.

Physical Environment

There has been an increasing appreciation of how tangible aspects of the *physical environment* can affect people's physical activity levels throughout the day. For example, research has begun to establish an association of physical activity patterns and preferences with environmental characteristics such as the layout and design of neighborhood streets as well as the presence or absence of such environmental components as sidewalks, streetlights, stray dogs, and neighborhood crime (10,32). As physical activity researchers increasingly collaborate with experts in urban planning, transportation, and environmental development to better understand the influence of the physical environment, the ability to harness such factors to facilitate physical activity participation will increase.

PROGRAM-RELATED FACTORS

With respect to *program-related* factors, the type of physical activity (e.g., swimming, brisk walking, aerobic dance), as well as intensity, duration, and frequency can influence subsequent participation levels.

Format

The format in which the activity is offered (e.g., class, home-based, individual, or group) may also have an important effect on both initial participation and longer-term adherence. Although the majority of community-based physical activity programs are offered in a class or group format, evidence indicates that the public generally prefers programs offered outside of a formal group or facility (10). There are important benefits to long-term adherence with adequately structured home-based regimens (5). The mode, format, and location of physical activity must meet the needs of differing groups of individuals. For example, women generally report a stronger preference for videotaped exercise and aerobic dance than men. Similarly, the workplace has been shown to be a preferred location for undertaking physical activity in some groups, though not in others (9,15).

Intensity

Immediate consequences, including physical activity–related benefits and enjoyment of activity, are other program-related factors likely to have a strong impact on participation levels (22). Conversely, sedentary people persist in inactive patterns principally because sedentary activities are immediately reinforcing and attempts to become physically active are likely to result in immediate aversive sensory or physiologic consequences. Thus, the task of health professionals is to ensure that initial attempts to become more physically active are perceived as generally pain free, enjoyable, and reinforcing by encouraging gradual, progressive increases in physical activity duration, frequency, and intensity, while keeping in mind the individual's physical and psychological readiness to progress (see GETP8 Table 7.4).

Several methods might be considered in properly shaping the behavior to avoid excessive physical activity during the early stages of a program. The talk-sing test (i.e., maintaining an intensity during which talking, but not singing, is possible) is a practical method for monitoring and regulating intensity. In contrast, simply telling participants to "take it easy" in group-based physical activity programs, when the instructor and most of the class are working at a higher level of intensity, is often ineffective. A more effective strategy is to provide an additional role model who demonstrates a lower-intensity alternative. Individuals can also be taught distraction techniques (e.g., music, reading, or TV watching when using indoor equipment) to help refocus their attention from aversive aspects of activity (e.g., increased exertion and sweating).

Heart rate (HR) is a good index of physiologic intensity. Pulse rates can be monitored manually or with portable HR monitors. Rating of perceived exertion (RPE) tracks perception of intensity, which may be as important as physical work (4) (GETP8 Table 4-7). In practice, these measures can be used together. For example, an initial HR of 30% to 45% heart rate reserve (~57%–67% of maximum HR) is recommended in underactive participants for optimal enjoyment and establishment of a habit. This is a light to moderate intensity, which could alternatively be established using an RPE of 10 to 12 on the 6 to 20 scale. It has been shown that even relatively low levels of exercise intensity can be associated with significant health improvements and disease risk reduction (see GETP8 Chapter 7). This is particularly true in special populations, such as older individuals and those with hypertension (26).

Program Incentives

> **1.9.3-HFS: Knowledge of specific techniques to enhance motivation (e.g., posters, recognition, bulletin boards, games, competitions).**

In addition to the behavioral skill of rewarding oneself for meeting physical activity goals, physical activity professionals should consider program-based incentives as a form of extrinsic motivation. Ideas include the use of point systems, competitions, and recognition, which should be based on readily achievable physical activity goals (e.g., attendance or participation) during the early stages of physical activity adoption.

ENHANCING MAINTENANCE

> **1.9.1-CES: List and apply behavioral strategies that apply to lifestyle modifications, such as exercise, diet, stress, and medication management.**

> **1.9.1-HFS: Knowledge of behavioral strategies to enhance exercise and health behavior change (e.g., reinforcement, goal setting, social support).**

In addition to sedentary individuals who may have difficulty initiating physical activity, some individuals spend significant time *restarting* physical activity. Thus, strategies for maintenance should be an integral component of physical activity programming.

RELAPSE PREVENTION

Often individuals stop exercising completely after an inevitable break because of illness or injury, travel, holidays, inclement weather, or increased work demands. One useful step is to prepare in advance (both psychologically and behaviorally) for breaks or lapses in activity that may lead to a full-blown relapse (and a return to the previous sedentary lifestyle) (11,16,18). It should be emphasized that such breaks are inevitable and do not indicate laziness or failure. Early identification of high-risk situations that might lead to inactivity as well as devising strategies to prepare for lapses and for restarting the physical activity program can be effective. Useful relapse preparation plans include identification of alternate activities that can be done in place of the usual activity, planning to exercise as soon as possible after a break, arranging to exercise with someone else, and modifying goals to avoid discouragement (Box 42-2).

REMINDERS OF BENEFITS

It is important to provide continued evidence of relevant personal benefits (physical, social, and psychological) from being regularly active. Physical activity professionals should regularly inquire about benefits and positive outcomes experienced from the current physical activity program. For persons at particular risk for dropping out, these questions should be posed frequently (e.g., one or more times per month). If an individual cannot define the positive aspects of physical activity or, alternatively, provides several negatives, there is serious risk of dropout. Such participants should be targeted for increased attention and support. Having participants regularly revisit their cost–benefits or decisional balance sheet can be useful for reinforcing their personal commitments to be active, as well as revising the physical activity plan to increase the benefits portion of the equation. In addition, training individuals in simple field methods for evaluating changes in their own fitness or physical functioning levels can serve as a powerful motivator for continued physical activity participation (29).

GENERALIZATION TRAINING

From an instructional standpoint, it is wise to avoid discontinuing physical activity programs suddenly, especially if no generalization training has been provided. Generalization training involves expanding the behavior to a different setting to link the behavior with cues or stimuli in the second setting that may help to facilitate ongoing participation. To ensure adherence, the physical activity habit must be generalized or re-established in new environments (e.g., self-initiated, home-based) before discontinuing supervised or programmed, facility-based sessions (30). Generalization may be accomplished in several ways, including requiring off-site, home exercise sessions at an early stage of the program (stimulus generalization); involving family or significant others in physical activity sessions; and adding additional exercises before graduation (response generalization) that are easily maintained in the new environment. Ideally, the responsibility for session supervision, reinforcement, and feedback should be gradually transferred from the instructor to the participant, as well as to helpers in the new environment as the change date approaches. This more closely approximates the conditions likely to be experienced in the maintenance setting.

REASSESSMENT OF GOALS

Regular reassessment of physical activity goals provides an opportunity to verify that they are relevant, realistic, and motivating. Goals that are too long term (e.g., months) or vague (e.g., "I will exercise more") do not provide sufficient motivation to maintain behavior through difficult periods. During the early stages of a physical activity program (i.e., 1–6 months), goals should be adjusted as frequently as necessary (i.e., once every 2 weeks) to maintain physical activity behavior. For maintenance of physical activity, participants should be taught proper goal-setting techniques and convinced of the importance of continuing to set goals to enhance motivation over the long term.

SOCIAL SUPPORT

Continued use of a variety of social support mechanisms is valuable for continued physical activity maintenance. For instance, if the format is a class or group situation, the leader can call participants who miss two classes in a row (one class in high-risk participants). The purpose of such calls is to let individuals know that they are missed and that others notice and care. Other individuals in the class can assume this type of responsibility as well (i.e., a "buddy system"). If physical activity is conducted outside of a formal setting, the physical activity professional may continue support in the form of periodic telephone calls, letters, e-mails, or newsletters. Family members, coworkers, neighbors, and friends should continue to encourage and support the physical activity program, and it may be helpful to include support persons in education efforts to train them in providing continuing support through prompting, modeling, and reinforcing physical activity. Most importantly, individuals should be encouraged to be proactive about seeking out and identifying their own meaningful sources of support; this increases their feel-

ing of ownership and their role in sustaining their physical activity regimen and resources.

RELEVANT REWARDS

 1.9.4-HFS: Knowledge of extrinsic and intrinsic reinforcement and give examples of each.

If use of external rewards are appropriate for the person in question, rewards for meeting physical activity goals should change periodically to maintain motivating impact. Reward systems may include such things as points accumulated as exercise continues to be maintained. Material rewards (e.g., a new exercise outfit or equipment, dinner out, spa treatment) or small rewards such as free time (to read or engage in other enjoyable activities) may ensue from the accumulation of points. Other examples are requiring a monetary deposit that is returned contingent upon achievement of goals (especially behavioral goals such as attendance and participation) or reducing program fees based on program adherence. Preparation for maintenance should also focus on maximizing the rewarding aspects of the physical activity (enjoyment, increased energy, opportunities to socialize or get away) so less dependence is needed on external rewards and there is increased reliance on intrinsic motivation.

FEEDBACK

Self-monitoring and other forms of feedback are useful for noting progress and enhancing motivation. Research in the field continues to support the usefulness of regular self-monitoring of physical activity for long-term maintenance. However, few behavioral strategies evoke more resistance from participants than the prospect of long-term self-monitoring. Individuals should fully participate in designing the self-monitoring strategies that will be the easiest and most convenient for them to maintain. Such strategies can be as simple as noting the number of minutes of moderate-intensity physical activity done throughout the week on a calendar or personal scheduler. As noted earlier, feedback may take the additional form of self-administered fitness tests (e.g., field tests) or professional fitness assessments. Such assessments can be used as a yardstick to measure current compared with past levels of fitness or function and are helpful in setting future goals.

CONTRACTS

Personal contracts should be updated and changed frequently, if necessary, and should include specific goals, rewards, and helpers. Contracts that are too easy do not provide the challenge needed to motivate many individuals. In contrast, contracts that are too difficult lead to frustration, discouragement, and, potentially, injury.

AVOIDING BOREDOM AND ONGOING MONITORING AND MAXIMIZATION OF ENJOYMENT

Individuals should be encouraged to monitor enjoyment and to make activity more enjoyable, especially if it is not meeting their needs or expectations. Physical activity professionals can collaborate to help individuals achieve this goal (e.g., through helping identify new activities, environments, goals, or partners). With a wide variety of physical activities and a diversity of settings in which to conduct activities, the "I'm bored" response should not be allowed to persist and extinguish behavior. Individuals who have achieved improvements in their aerobic conditioning may renew their motivation by trying activities or intensities with a higher level of physical challenge. For some individuals, boredom may be resolved through a regimen involving a variety of activities. For others, one activity conducted in varied settings and formats may be more appropriate. Pairing physical activity with another enjoyable activity (e.g., music, reading or watching TV while on stationary equipment, talking with a friend) can serve as a distraction and increase enjoyment of the exercise session. Often, enjoyable competition (e.g., walkathons) can help to stimulate maintenance and reinvigorate a stale program or regimen.

GENERAL COUNSELING STRATEGIES TO INCREASE PHYSICAL ACTIVITY

> **1.9.10-CES: Facilitation of effective and contemporary motivational and behavior modification techniques to promote behavioral change.**

> **1.9.6-HFS: Knowledge of approaches that may assist less motivated patients to increase their physical activity.**

It is helpful for physical activity professionals to consider the application of specific behavioral skills and exercise prescription within the context of an overall lifestyle approach to physical activity. Applying basic counseling strategies can promote an atmosphere that increases the likelihood of success by facilitating self-directed planning for physical activity.

EMPHASIZE THE IMPORTANCE OF ROUTINE ACTIVITIES

Activities of daily living can help individuals maintain as well as initiate physical activity, especially during times when more structured or vigorous activity is not performed. Current public health guidelines recommend that adults engage in 30 minutes or more of moderate-intensity activities on most days of the week (25). An important aspect to these recommendations is the idea of accumulated activity, which can be accomplished through a variety of

structured and lifestyle physical activities. It is important for individuals to understand that health benefits can be more effectively realized by being active in a variety of ways, both within and outside of formal exercise programs. One method of doing this is to help individuals become aware of times in their daily routines when sedentary activities are performed with little thought or planning (e.g., indiscriminate television viewing). After such time periods are identified, more physically active alternatives can be devised (e.g., going for a walk with family members or dog). Behavior-based interventions have demonstrated that decreasing sedentary activities and increasing lifestyle physical activity can help individuals increase physical activity and fitness (8).

MOTIVATIONAL AND CLIENT-CENTERED COUNSELING TECHNIQUES

In recent years, attention has been given to the application of brief motivational interviewing approaches for health behaviors such as physical activity (31). Motivational interviewing was initially developed as a brief and effective method of helping those with addictive behaviors (primarily alcohol abuse and smoking) increase their motivational readiness to make positive behavior changes. Key components of this approach include acknowledging, normalizing, and gently working through the person's ambivalence concerning physical activity participation; stressing the individual's freedom to choose not to be physically active while at the same time encouraging personal responsibility for change and the consequences of not changing; developing an internal discrepancy for remaining inactive through strategic reflections, feedback, and questions from the counselor; and encouraging the participant to evaluate the pros and cons (i.e., decisional balance) of remaining inactive versus becoming more active (31). Such motivational strategies can be applied via telephone as well as through face-to-face encounters (also see Chapter 44).

> **1.9.2-HFS: Knowledge of the important elements that should be included in each behavior modification session.**

The Five-A's Model has also been used in client-centered counseling for physical activity (27). This model outlines five elements for professionals to use to engage participants in developing a plan for physical activity:

1. Address the agenda or why the participant is there.
2. Assess relevant aspects of current health and activity level, including readiness for change, physical activity history, and expectations.
3. Advise participants of the importance of behavior change, including risks and benefits.
4. Assist individuals in developing a plan for physical activity and overcoming barriers to change.
5. Arrange for follow-up after the plan is implemented.

This model is useful to structure the physical activity counseling session, assess motivational readiness to be active, and tailor recommendations based on the individual's current physical activity level, goals, and stage of change (see GETP8 Box 7.6).

SUMMARY

The variety of factors that influence physical activity demonstrate the importance of developing programs and strategies that fit the needs and preferences of different population groups. By tailoring physical activity programs, professionals may positively influence initial dropout rate (during the critical period, which is the first 3 to 6 months) as well as promote maintenance. Further research evaluating specific methods of tailoring programs to enhance both adoption and maintenance of physical activity is indicated, particularly among subgroups at risk for physical inactivity. In addition, knowledge in this area obtained from studies of endurance exercise should be systematically applied to other dimensions of physical activity, including strength and flexibility training.

Current evidence supports the following recommendations for changing and maintaining physical activity behavior. Behavior (including physical activity) is strongly influenced by its immediate consequences rather than distal, long-term consequences. Increasing the immediately rewarding aspects of physical activity and decreasing the negative aspects increases the likelihood that the behavior will occur. Expectations concerning physical activity–related benefits and outcomes should be addressed during the initial stage of a program. Exploring beliefs, misconceptions, and barriers early in the program sets the stage for realistic goal setting and minimizes disappointment and frustration. To facilitate sustained participation over time, self-management strategies should be encouraged, including ongoing use of self-monitoring, goal setting, problem solving, decisional balance, behavioral commitment, self-assessment, reward systems, stimulus control, relapse prevention, social support, and other strategies. When appropriate, motivational interviewing strategies and other patient-centered approaches can be used when counseling more resistant, inactive individuals and those struggling with ambivalence concerning being more active. Finally, it is advisable to offer choices and encourage self-directed planning as a means of tailoring physical activity programs to fit the changing needs and preferences of participants and to promote a sense of personal control and autonomy.

REFERENCES

1. Bandura A. The anatomy of stages of change. *Am J Health Promot.* 1997;12:8–10.
2. Bandura A. Social cognitive theory: an agentic perspective. *Ann Rev Psychol.* 2001;52:1–26.
3. Bassett DR Jr, Ainsworth BE, Leggett SR, et al. Accuracy of five electronic pedometers for measuring distance walked. *Med Sci Sports Exerc.* 1996;28:1071–7.
4. Borg GAV. Borg's perceived exertion and pain scales. Champaign (IL): Human Kinetics; 1998.
5. Castro CM, King AC. Telephone-assisted counseling for physical activity. *Exerc Sport Sci Rev.* 2002;30:64–8.
6. Deci EL, Ryan RM. *Intrinsic Motivation and Self-Determination in Human Behavior.* New York: Plenum; 1985.
7. Deci EL, Ryan RM. The support of autonomy and the control of behavior. *J Pers Soc Psychol.* 1987;53:1024–37.
8. Dunn AL, Marcus BH, Kampert JB, et al. Comparison of lifestyle and structured interventions to increase physical activity and cardiorespiratory fitness: a randomized trial. *JAMA.* 1999;281:327–34.
9. King AC, Carl F, Birkel L, Haskell WL. Increasing exercise among blue-collar employees: the tailoring of worksite programs to meet specific needs. *Prev Med.* 1988;17:357–65.
10. King AC, Castro C, Wilcox S, et al. Personal and environmental factors associated with physical inactivity among different racial/ethnic groups of U.S. middle- and older-aged women. *Health Psychol.* 2000;19:354–64.
11. King AC, Frederiksen L. Low-cost strategies for increasing exercise behavior: relapse preparation training and social support. *Behav Modif.* 1984;8:3–21.
12. King AC, Friedman R, Marcus B, et al. Harnessing motivational forces in the promotion of physical activity: the Community Health Advice by Telephone (CHAT) Project. *Health Educ Res.* 2002;17:627–36.
13. King AC, Haskell WL, Taylor CB, et al. Group- versus home-based exercise training in healthy older men and women: a community-based clinical trial. *JAMA.* 1991;266:1535–42.
14. King AC, Rejeski WJ, Buchner DM. Physical activity interventions targeting older adults: a critical review and recommendations. *Am J Prev Med.* 1998;15:316–33.
15. King AC, Taylor CB, Haskell WL, DeBusk RF. Identifying strategies for increasing employee physical activity levels: findings from the Stanford/Lockheed exercise survey. *Health Educ Q.* 1990;17:269–85.
16. Marcus BH, Dubbert PM, Forsyth LH, et al. Physical activity behavior change: issues in adoption and maintenance. *Health Psychol.* 2000;19:32–41.
17. Marcus BH, Simkin LR. The transtheoretical model: applications to exercise behavior. *Med Sci Sports Exerc.* 1994;26:1400–4.
18. Marcus BH, Stanton AL. Evaluation of relapse prevention and reinforcement interventions to promote exercise adherence in sedentary females. *Res Q Exerc Sport.* 1993;64:447–52.
19. Martin JE, Dubbert PM, Katell AD, et al. Behavioral control of exercise in sedentary adults: studies 1 through 6. *J Consult Clin Psychol.* 1984;52:795–811.
20. McAuley E, Blissmer B, Marquez DX, et al. Social relations, physical activity, and well-being in older adults. *Prev Med.* 2000;31:608–17.
21. Mullan E, Markland D, Ingledew D. A graded conceptualisation of self-determination in the regulation of exercise behavior: development of a measure using confirmatory factor analytic procedures. *Pers Individ Dif.* 1997;23:745–52.
22. Neff KL, King AC. Exercise program adherence in older adults: the importance of achieving one's expected benefits. *Med Exerc Nutr Health.* 1995;4:355–62.
23. Oka RK, King AC, Young DR. Sources of social support as predictors of exercise adherence in women and men ages 50 to 65 years. *Women's Health: Research on Gender, Behavior, and Policy.* 1995;1:161–75.
24. Oman RF, King AC. Predicting the adoption and maintenance of exercise participation using self-efficacy and previous exercise participation rates. *Am J Health Promot.* 1998;12:154–61.
25. **Pate RR, Pratt M, Blair SN, et al. Physical activity and public health: a recommendation from the Centers for Disease Control**

and Prevention and the American College of Sports Medicine. *JAMA.* 1995;273:402–7.

26. Patten CA, Martin JE. Exercise interventions for older adults with high blood pressure: from efficacy to adherence. *J Prevent Intervent Commun.* 1996;13:111–142.

27. Pinto BM, Goldstein MG, Marcus, BH. Activity counseling by primary care physicians. *Prev Med.* 1998;27:506–13.

28. Prochaska JO, DiClemente CC. Transtheoretical therapy, toward a more integrative model of change. *Psychother Theory Res Prac.* 1982;19:276–87.

29. Rikli RE, Jones CJ. Development and validation of a functional fitness test for community-residing older adults. *J Aging Phys Act.* 1999;7:129–61.

30. Rejeski WJ, Brawley LR. Shaping active lifestyles in older adults: a group-facilitated behavior change intervention. *Ann Behav Med.* 1997;19(suppl):S106.

31. Rollnick S, Mason P, Butler C. *Health Behavior Change: A Guide for Practitioners.* London/New York: Churchill Livingstone; 1999.

32. Sallis JF, Bauman A, Pratt M. Environmental and policy interventions to promote physical activity. *Am J Prev Med.* 1998;15: 379–97.

33. Sallis JF, Owen N. Ecological models of health behavior. In Glanz K, Rimer BK, Lewis FM, editors. *Health Behavior and Health Education: Theory, Research, and Practice.* 3rd ed. San Francisco: Jossey-Bass; 2002. p. 462–84.

34. Sallis JF, Owen N. *Physical Activity and Behavioral Medicine.* Thousand Oaks (CA): Sage Publications; 1999.

35. Treiber FA, Baranowski T, Braden DS, et al. Social support for exercise: relationship to physical activity in young adults. *Prev Med.* 1991;20:737–50.

36. U.S. Department of Health and Human Services. *Physical Activity and Health: A Report of the Surgeon General.* Atlanta: U.S. Department of Health and Human Services, Centers for Disease Control and Prevention, National Center for Chronic Disease Prevention and Health Promotion; 1996.

37. U.S. Department of Health and Human Services. *Healthy People 2010: Understanding and Improving Health.* Washington (DC): U.S. Department of Health and Human Services; 2000.

38. Young DR, King AC. Exercise adherence: determinants of physical activity and applications of health behavior change theories. *Med Exerc Nutr Health.* 1995;4:335–48.

SELECTED REFERENCES FOR FURTHER READING

Blair SN, Morrow JR Jr, eds. Physical activity interventions [theme issue]. *Am J Prev Med.* 1998;15:255–440.

Carron AV, Hausenblas HA, Estabrooks PA. *The Psychology of Physical Activity.* St. Louis: McGraw-Hill; 2002.

Giles-Corti B, Donovan RJ. The relative influence of individual, social and physical environment determinants of physical activity. *Soc Sci Med.* 2002;54:1793–812.

King AC. Interventions to promote physical activity in older adults. *J Gerontol A Biol Sci Med Sci.* 2001;56A(special issue II):36–46.

King AC, Bauman A, Calfas K, eds. Innovative approaches to understanding and influencing physical activity. *Am J Prev Med.* 2002;23 (suppl):1–108.

King AC, Kiernan M, Oman RF, et al. Can we identify who will adhere to long-term physical activity? Application of signal detection methodology as a potential aid to clinical decision-making. *Health Psychol.* 1997;16:380–9.

Marcus BH, Dubbert PM, Forsyth LH, et al. Physical activity behavior change: issues in adoption and maintenance. *Health Psychol.* 2000; 19:32–41.

Sallis JF, Owen N. *Physical Activity and Behavioral Medicine.* Thousand Oaks (CA): Sage Publications; 1999.

Taylor WC, Baranowski T, Young DR. Physical activity interventions in low-income, ethnic minority, and populations with disability. *Am J Prev Med.* 1998;15:334–43.

INTERNET RESOURCES

- Active Living by Design: www.activelivingbydesign.org
- Health Canada, Physical Activity Unit: www.phac-aspc.gc.ca/pau-uap/paguide/
- National Center for Bicycling & Walking: www.bikewalk.org
- National Coalition for Promoting Physical Activity: www.ncppa.org

Supplemental Section: Programmatic and Professional Materials

BONNIE SANDERSON, PhD, FACSM, *Section Editor*

This chapter introduces behavior change theories, gives examples of research applications of each theory, and provides examples of how to apply the theoretical principles to your work with your patients. More in-depth discussion of practical application strategies of behavioral change theories are provided in Chapter 44 (85).

THE IMPORTANCE OF THEORIES

Physical activity is a complex behavior that involves many steps and a series of skills to adopt and maintain. It is impossible to consider all possible influences on physical activity; therefore, psychological theories and models of behavior change can be important to help guide both research and clinical practice (76). Theories provide a framework for understanding the process through which a complex behavior, such as physical activity, changes and is sustained over time. Theories can also provide guidance to practitioners in helping people make behavior changes by understanding the connection between theories and results, how to translate theory into practice, and which specific strategies to recommend (39,76). Theories can help provide techniques and shed light on potential pitfalls in becoming more physically active.

This chapter provides an overview of the theories that have been applied to help understand and guide changes in physical activity behavior in healthy and clinical adult populations (76,83). The theories covered in this chapter include the stages of change for motivational readiness (or the transtheoretical model), decision-making theory, social-cognitive theory, health belief model (HBM), social ecology theory, theories of reasoned action and planned behavior, and relapse-prevention model. The theories were selected for this chapter based on their clinical and research applications. Each of these theories has been applied to studies of physical activity determinants, as well as in studying other health behavior changes (76). Some of the theories (e.g., social cognitive theory [SCT]) have more predictive utility than other theories (e.g., theory of reasoned action [TRA]) (82). Although there may be some theories that are not included in this review (e.g., health action process approach) (77), the theories addressed in this chapter are ones that have been applied most often in relation to physical activity (12,76,83).

INCORPORATING THEORY-BASED TECHNIQUES AND PRINCIPLES INTO WORK WITH PATIENTS

A large body of research addresses the importance of using theory to help guide individuals through behavior changes. Although not all theories or aspects of theories

> > > KEY TERMS

Decisional balance: The comparison of the benefits of making a behavior change versus the costs.

Outcome expectations: The potential results that one would anticipate after performing physical activity (e.g., having more energy, sleeping better).

Processes of change: The strategies that individuals use as they are adopting and maintaining behavior changes.

Relapse prevention: The process by which one maintains long-term behavior change by anticipating

potentially high-risk situations and devising strategies to cope with these situations.

Self-efficacy: An individual's belief and confidence about his or her ability to make specific behavior changes.

Stages of change: A model, also known as the transtheoretical model, that postulates that individuals move through a series of stages that represent increased motivation to be physically active and face common barriers when making a behavior change.

can be applied to all individuals at a given time, theories can be helpful in designing an intervention and in selecting evaluation measures at the time you are assessing the patient's progress. The approach can incorporate such considerations as patients' readiness for change, the environment in which they live, and their social context.

THE IMPORTANCE OF UNDERSTANDING THE PRINCIPLES OF BEHAVIOR CHANGE

It may be a challenge to directly apply research findings while working in community settings, cardiac rehabilitation facilities, school settings, as a personal trainer, or as an exercise physiologist. Therefore, the last part of each subsection provides a clinical application, which essentially transfers the research findings and applies them to real-world examples that a practitioner might encounter in working with patients.

THEORIES OF BEHAVIOR CHANGE

> **1.9.1-HFS: Knowledge of behavioral strategies to enhance exercise and health behavior change (e.g., reinforcement, goal setting, social support).**

> **1.9.1-CES: List and apply behavioral strategies that apply to lifestyle modifications, such as exercise, diet, stress, and medication management.**

THE STAGE OF MOTIVATIONAL READINESS FOR CHANGE MODEL

> **1.9.5-HFS: Knowledge of the states of motivational readiness.**

The stages of motivational readiness for change (SOC) model, or the transtheoretical model (TTM), consists of numerous components, including the stages of change and processes of change. In addition, components of other theories are used in conjunction with the SOC model. These examples include decisional balance from decision-making theory (32) and self-efficacy, which is a key concept of SCT (7), both of which are described in detail in other sections of the chapter.

Stages

The SOC model postulates that individuals move through a series of stages and face common barriers when making behavior changes and that intervention approaches may vary by the patient's identified stage of change (68). Several researchers have applied this model to individuals adopting and maintaining physical activity (21,49). The stages include precontemplation, contemplation, preparation, action, and maintenance The precontemplation stage includes individuals who are

inactive and not thinking about becoming active. Individuals in the contemplation stage are inactive but are thinking about becoming active. The preparation stage includes individuals who are physically active but not at the recommended levels (30 minutes or more of moderate-intensity physical activity on most, preferably all, days of the week [65,83]). The action stage includes individuals who are physically active at the recommended levels but have been active at this level for fewer than 6 months. Individuals in the maintenance stage are physically active at the recommended levels and have been for more than 6 months.

The movement across stages may be conceptualized as cyclic rather than linear, given that it takes many individuals numerous attempts before successfully adopting and maintaining physical activity. A self-report four-item questionnaire is available to identify an individual's stage of change, including such statements as, "I intend to become more physically active in the next 6 months," and "I currently engage in regular physical activity" (51,52) (see Chapter 44 for the recommended questionnaire and scoring information) (85).

Processes of Change

The SOC model also posits that individuals use a variety of processes of change as they progress through the stages. Five behavioral and five cognitive processes have been identified (49). The behavioral processes include rewarding yourself (e.g., doing something nice for yourself when achieving a physical activity goal), substituting alternatives (e.g., participating in physical activity to decrease fatigue and increase energy), committing yourself (e.g., making promises to be physically active), reminding yourself (e.g., posting reminders to be physically active at work), and enlisting social support (e.g., having someone to depend on when having problems sticking with a physical activity program). Cognitive processes include being aware of risks (e.g., thinking that physical inactivity can be harmful), increasing knowledge (e.g., thinking about physical activity information obtained from articles), comprehending benefits (e.g., believing that physical activity would make one healthy), increasing healthy opportunities (e.g., awareness of physical activity programs), and caring about consequences to others (e.g., wondering how inactivity affects family and friends). The use of cognitive processes typically peaks in the preparation stage, and the use of the behavioral processes typically peaks in the action stage. A self-report 40-item measure has been developed to assess the 10 processes of change (see Marcus and Forsyth [51] and Marcus et al. [49]).

Results from a meta-analysis (57) indicated that all 10 processes of change are used across the stages when individuals are actively making behavior changes. The transition from precontemplation to contemplation and from preparation to action was marked by the sharpest increases in the use of behavioral processes.

Integrating the Components of the Stages of Motivational Readiness for Change Model

Although some of the components of the SOC model can be examined separately, research and practice applications are most effective when combining the different components. Therefore, a summary of the research findings that integrate the different aspects of the model and practice applications for integrating the model are presented below.

Research Findings

According to a recent review of 150 studies applying the SOC model to exercise (78), interventions based on the SOC model appear to be effective for exercise promotion. Additionally, authors from this review highlighted that stage-matched interventions led to forward progression on the stages of change, which is important given the large percentage of individuals who are in precontemplation or contemplation for exercise. The authors also concluded that the measures used to assess constructs related to the SOC model, including measures of the processes of change and decisional balance, appear valid and reliable and have been applied to a variety of populations.

An excellent example of research that is guided by the theoretical framework of the SOC is a study by Marcus et al. (47). This study used information that was targeted and information that was tailored to the individual. Targeting refers to defining and intervening with a subgroup of the population based on one common characteristic (e.g., sex) (48). Targeting assumes that individuals have similar enough characteristics to be influenced by the same message (48). Alternatively, tailoring incorporates a higher level of specificity, and interventions that are tailored use information on characteristics unique to an individual person (48,50).

Marcus et al. (47) randomly assigned sedentary individuals (n = 194) to an intervention targeted to stage of change and tailored to other theory-based constructs believed to be important for behavior change or to a standard treatment group not targeted to stage of change. The tailored group reported a significantly greater number of physical activity minutes per week than individuals in the nontailored self-help group at 6 months. This increase in physical activity minutes was also maintained at the 12-month follow-up (15).

A recent study indicates that the Internet is another efficacious channel for delivering tailored physical activity interventions. Specifically, Marcus et al. (46) conducted a randomized controlled trial in which healthy sedentary participants (n = 249) were randomly assigned to one of the following three conditions: (a) individually tailored Internet intervention; (b) individual tailored print intervention; or (c) standard Internet comparison arm. Participants in the tailored Internet intervention completed online questionnaires and received immediate tailored feedback based on responses to the questionnaires. The tailored print arm also completed questionnaires and received tailored feedback; however, the questionnaires and feedback were done through the mail. Results indicated that all three groups increased their physical activity from baseline to 6 and 12 months (46). Another recent study randomly assigned 239 healthy, sedentary adults to (a) telephone-based, individualized feedback; (b) print-based, individualized feedback; or (c) contact control. Both intervention arms were guided by a motivationally tailored, theoretically driven computer expert system based on SCT and TTM constructs (46). At 6 months, both telephone and print arms significantly increased in minutes of moderate-intensity physical activity compared with control, with no differences between the intervention arms. At 12 months, print participants reported a significantly greater number of moderate-intensity minutes than both telephone and control participants. There were no differences between telephone and control participants. Results suggest that both telephone and print enhance the adoption of physical activity among sedentary adults; however, print interventions may be particularly effective in maintaining physical activity in the longer term.

Practice Applications

To follow is a summary of strategies to help individuals increase or maintain physical activity, based on the SOC model. One way to integrate the different components is to provide different types of intervention strategies depending on an individual's stage of change, although there may be some overlap across the stages.

Precontemplation

The precontemplation stage includes individuals who are not active and are not thinking about becoming active. Therefore, the goal for this stage is for the individual to begin thinking about physical activity. The pros and cons of becoming physically active should be discussed with the individual. Specifically, the individual should write down what the benefits of physical activity would be in addition to the disadvantages of physical activity. Specific barriers to physical activity should also be assessed, such as lack of time, lack of energy, environmental constraints (e.g., lack of access to physical activity facilities), and fear of injury.

Another important behavioral strategy for this stage is goal setting. Research indicates that goal setting is important for focusing attention on physical activity behavior change (63). Specifically, a stage-appropriate goal for the precontemplation stage would be to set aside time for reading a pamphlet about physical activity to learn more about the benefits of regular physical activity.

Contemplation

The contemplation stage includes individuals who are not physically active but are thinking about becoming active. The aim for this stage is for the individual to begin taking steps to become physically active and to think about setting goals. Individuals in this stage should also weigh the pros and cons of physical activity as well as read materials describing how to start a physical activity program. The individual can then make specific physical activity goals after he decides on which physical activity he would most prefer. Personal preference for specific activities as well as positive experience with certain activities should be considered when developing a program. The individual should also implement a reinforcement program in which he rewards himself for meeting his specific physical activity goals. Because research indicates that social support is important for becoming physically active (4), individuals might identify one or two people who could be supportive and enlist their support for starting and maintaining a physical activity program.

Preparation

The preparation stage includes individuals who are currently engaging in some physical activity but not at the recommended level (49,51). The goal for this stage is to increase physical activity behavior to the recommended level. Specifically, the goal is to engage in physical activity of at least moderate intensity on most, preferably all, days of the week for 30 minutes or more each day. Several of the strategies used in the previous stages can also be used in this stage, including weighing the pros and cons of physical activity, choosing an appropriate physical activity program, and implementing a reinforcement schedule. Identifying and overcoming the barriers that prevent the individual from increasing their physical activity to the recommended level is the key for this stage. Goal setting can play an instrumental role in gradually increasing physical activity to the intended level.

Action

The action stage includes individuals who are physically active at the recommended level but have been for fewer than 6 months. The goal of this stage is to continue to make physical activity a regular part of the patient's life. Important strategies for this stage include setting up a plan for self-monitoring physical activity and making short-term goals (e.g., "I will walk on Monday, Wednesday, and Friday after work with my coworkers and then walk on Saturday and Sunday with my husband"). In addition, it might be helpful to suggest that your patient try a new activity or find a walking or running race that is going to take place in the future for which your patient can train. Talking with your patient about relapse prevention (discussed later in this chapter) is also very useful at this stage.

Maintenance

The maintenance stage includes individuals who have been physically active at the recommended level and have been for 6 or more months. The goal for this stage is to prepare for future setbacks and to continue to increase enjoyment for physical activity. Therefore, some of the same suggestions that apply to individuals in the action stage will also apply to individuals in the maintenance phase. It is important to continue to help your patients find ways to avoid boredom, either by trying out new activities or by enlisting social support (e.g., walking with a neighbor). Also, it might be helpful to have your patients reflect on the benefits they have already achieved from physical activity because these might be powerful rewards.

DECISION-MAKING THEORY

Decision-making theory postulates that individuals decide whether to engage in a particular behavior based on their comparison of the perceived benefits versus the perceived costs of the behavior (32). Specifically, individuals are more likely to be physically active if they perceive that the benefits (e.g., sleeping better) outweigh the costs (e.g., time lost to other activities [32,76]). Decisional balance is another important component that is used in conjunction with the SOC model (55). Research has shown that in later stages of motivational readiness for behavior change (e.g., action, maintenance), individuals perceive more benefits for being physically active. In contrast, individuals who are in earlier stages (e.g., precontemplation) perceive that there are more disadvantages than advantages (55). An example of an advantage of physical activity is, "I would have more energy for my family and friends if I were regularly physically active," and an example of a disadvantage is, "I think I would be too tired to do my daily work after being physically active." A 16-item self-report measure has been developed to assess decisional balance. Examples of these include: "I would feel more confident if I were regularly physically active" and "Regular physical activity would take up too much of my time" (51,55).

Research Findings

An intervention study of 355 patients participating in a physician-based counseling intervention (intervention n = 181; control n = 184; mean age, 65.6 years) was conducted (28). The intervention was based on the SOC model and incorporated components of SCT and health education theory. After 6 weeks of intervention, the intervention group had significant changes in decisional balance, self-efficacy, and processes of change. Specifically, individuals increased their view of the benefits of physical activity, were more confident about their ability to perform the behavior, and were using more strategies to assist them in their behavior change. Therefore, intervention studies that are grounded in SOC theory show intermediate changes in variables such as decisional balance.

SOCIAL COGNITIVE THEORY

Social cognitive theory has had the most success in its application to changing physical activity behavior (7,9,82). This model states that behavior change is influenced by the interactions between the environment, personal factors, and the behavior itself (7,9). This is called the model of reciprocal determinism (9). Components of this model are shown in Figure 43-1.

Self-Efficacy

An important construct of SCT is self-efficacy. Self-efficacy is one's beliefs about his or her capabilities to exercise control over particular or specified life events (6,7). For example, someone with high self-efficacy for physical activity would endorse having the confidence to continue to exercise despite barriers (e.g., feeling tired). Efficacy beliefs influence health behavior choices in that people tend to pursue tasks that they feel competent to perform and avoid those about which they feel incompetent (9,44). The most commonly measured and cited type of self-efficacy, barriers self-efficacy, is related to the level of effort and persistence expended when faced with adverse situations or barriers to attaining the desired outcome. Self-efficacy to perform the behavior itself (e.g., how confident are you that you can walk 30 minutes five times per week) has also been measured. Research indicates that self-efficacy level predicts participation in physical activity (18,59).

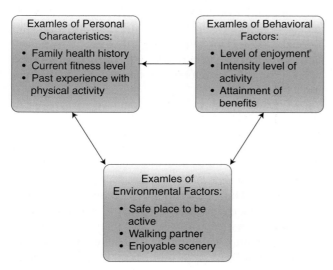

FIGURE 43-1. Components of social cognitive theory. (Adapted with permission from Marcus BH, Forsyth LH. *Motivating People to be Physically Active.* Champaign [IL]: Human Kinetics; 2003.) (51)

Differences in self-efficacy have been found for individuals in different stages of change (53,54). Cross-sectional studies indicate that as the stages of change progress from precontemplation to maintenance, a corresponding increase in self-efficacy for physical activity takes place. A five-item self-report measure has been developed to examine self-efficacy for physical activity in different situations (e.g., feeling fatigued, inclement weather) (51,54).

Bandura (9) has listed the four influences on self-efficacy as performance of mastery experiences, vicarious experiences, verbal persuasion regarding one's capabilities, and inferences from physiologic and affective responses. The two that are discussed in this chapter are performance accomplishments and vicarious experience. The sense of efficacy that arises from performance accomplishments is based on personal mastery experiences—that is, success increases feelings of mastery, which, in turn, promotes the behavior and increases the likelihood of setting new and more challenging goals. Also, setting smaller, accomplishable goals helps a person feel more confident (or self-efficacious) and helps build more challenging goals. Personal experience is the strongest influence on feelings of self-efficacy. For example, if a person is able to be physically active again after an illness, he or she should have a resulting increase in self-efficacy.

The second influence on self-efficacy, vicarious experience or modeling, involves improvements in self-efficacy caused by observing others perform the activity (e.g., watching a demonstration or video). Individuals increase their self-efficacy by observing others succeed at being physically active. This type of efficacy expectation is of particular interest in group sessions: if one participant is doing extraordinarily well, this can improve the self-efficacy of the others and further motivate them. For example, in a cardiac rehabilitation setting, if one patient is doing well with her physical activity program, then this might serve to increase the self-efficacy of others in that setting.

Outcome Expectations

Another important SCT construct is outcome expectations, which refers to the potential results that one anticipates after performing a particular behavior (7). This distinction is exemplified in that an individual can anticipate or understand that exercise will have positive health consequences (e.g., more energy) yet not have the self-efficacy to execute the behavior (e.g., exercise regularly to accrue benefits). As would be expected, the extent to which individuals perceive they will be able to perform a behavior is related to the outcomes they anticipate. Three major forms of outcome expectations have been identified: positive and negative physical effects, positive and negative social effects, and positive and negative self-evaluative reactions to the change in behavior (9). Within each major form, positive expectations function as incentives and the negative expectations function as disincentives toward making behavior change.

Self-Regulatory Strategies

Self-regulation is the ability to mobilize oneself to perform a behavior regularly in the face of a variety of personal, situational, or social barriers. Bandura (7) postulates that the major process of self-regulation includes self-monitoring, proximal goal setting, strategy development, and self-motivating incentives. A person's self-regulatory efficacy is crucial for adherence to a behavior such as exercise in that those with low self-regulatory efficacy tend to drop out of programs more quickly and are less able to exercise at the intensity, duration, and frequency needed to accrue health benefits.

According to Bandura (7), goals do not directly regulate motivation and action. Instead, self-efficacy beliefs influence people's choices of goals and persistence of behavior when they face challenges and obstacles (9). Goals provide direction and reference points against which people can monitor their progress (44). Through self-monitoring, people can develop efficacy beliefs about their current level of competence and expectancies regarding their rate of improvement (43). Bandura (7) states that goal specificity, challenge, and proximity are the most important qualities of goals to enhance motivation and persistence.

Research Findings

Although studies have examined the efficacy of SCT-based interventions (83), most research focuses on the SCT construct of self-efficacy. Therefore, research on self-efficacy is the primary focus of this section.

As already mentioned, SCT incorporates personal influences, cognitions, and environmental factors as variables that influence each other as well as influence behavior (77). Hofstetter et al. (31) investigated correlates of exercise self-efficacy to study the extent to which childhood experience with exercise would affect exercise self-efficacy later in life. They found that environmental variables (e.g., barriers to exercise, the availability of home equipment, facilities), cognitive variables (e.g., benefits and barriers, normative beliefs), and social variables (e.g., social support) all influenced self-efficacy. Therefore, this research supports the notion that self-efficacy is malleable and can be influenced by additional factors, such as the context in which the individual is located.

McAuley et al. (58) conducted a study to examine the effect of walking and stretching on changes in self-efficacy in 184 previously sedentary older adults (mean age, 65.5 years). Results indicated that there was no change in barriers for self-efficacy from baseline to month 2, but it declined at months 4 and 6. For exercise self-efficacy,

there was a reported decline over the four time points (week 2, month 2, month 4, and month 6). It is interesting that efficacy cognitions declined in the context of an exercise intervention rather than increased. These results highlight the temporal relationship of self-efficacy and show that it can vary during the course of an exercise program. The authors conclude that it is important to target different sources of efficacy information (e.g., one's beliefs about exercise, such as "I might become injured if I exercise"; or the barriers related to exercise, such as not having enough time or the weather, which might have implications for the long-term maintenance of physical activity). One area that may be important to target is assessing feelings of confidence and working to build self-efficacy at the end of a program to help individuals maintain their behavior changes. In a recent follow-up study conducted five years following the start of this intervention, McCauley et al. (59) found self-efficacy at 2 years to be an important predictor of physical activity at 5 years. This study indicates that self-efficacy may be particularly important for long-term maintenance of physical activity.

Practice Implications

The research findings cited above underscore the importance of helping patients make intermediate steps toward behavior change. Some of these intermediate steps include increasing self-efficacy, learning how to set goals, planning for physical activity, and having realistic expectations for behavior change.

Self-efficacy is a powerful component of SCT, and it can be influenced in two primary ways: performance accomplishments and vicarious experience or modeling (8). Thus, one way for SCT to be applied to clinical practice is to assist patients in improving their self-efficacy. Someone who has had a cardiac event might learn to make exercise a part of his life by watching others like himself participate in cardiac rehabilitation. Another way to help a person increase her self-efficacy is to set small goals and "try out" activities. Therefore, for someone who does not exercise, the strategy might be to have her begin to walk for 2 minutes at a time. As soon as this patient begins to feel confident with the short duration of a walking bout, her self-efficacy is likely to increase, and then she might have the confidence to walk for an even longer distance.

An outcome expectation is a person's belief that certain behaviors will lead to specific outcomes. Therefore, another way to assist your patients in becoming more physically active is to work on developing realistic expectations of physical activity behavior change. For example, it might be helpful to educate your patient about the short-term benefits of being physically active (e.g., having more energy, sleeping better), as well as some of the long-term benefits (e.g., prevention of cardiovascular disease). In addition, many people have an outcome expectation that significant weight loss will result from being physically active. To establish realistic outcome expectations, it might be important to talk with your patient about the synergy between physical activity and diet, in that dietary changes in conjunction with physical activity are usually necessary for weight changes.

HEALTH BELIEF MODEL

The HBM was designed to explain and predict why people engage in preventive health practices (11,73). Generally, the HBM hypothesizes that the extent to which individuals engage in a health action is determined by their readiness to take action coupled with their belief of the threat of not taking action. There are four main components of the HBM that serve to explain a system of beliefs individuals hold while attempting to avoid disease: (a) the person perceives being susceptible to a particular disease; (b) the consequences of the disease appear serious enough to warrant action; (c) there are benefits to taking action; and (d) there would not be insurmountable barriers, such as cost, inconvenience, pain, or embarrassment, associated with taking action (11,72). In 1984, Janz and Becker (33) modified the HBM to incorporate self-efficacy into the barriers component of the HBM, which some researchers have suggested as a positive move because it places limits on the barriers dimension, which tended to be a "catch-all" category, and it suggests more areas for future research (73).

Research Findings

The HBM has not received as much consistent research support as the SCT and SOC models (76). A recent cross-sectional study examined constructs of SOC and the HBM (35) in 233 African American women. Those who were inactive reported higher perceived barriers but lower perceived self-efficacy and susceptibility to severity of disease. They also had fewer cues to action than those who reported being physically active. Other evidence has been found for the use of the HBM in predicting health actions. For example, the HBM has been used to predict compliance with a cardiac rehabilitation program. Oldridge and Streiner (64) found that after a 6-month exercise rehabilitation program for cardiac patients, the only difference in HBM factors between individuals who complied and those who dropped out (52% dropout rate) was that the compliers had greater scores on perceived severity. Other components of the HBM also have provided predictive usefulness. For example, two studies of postsurgery coronary artery disease patients found that a significant portion of the variance in exercise compliance was accounted for by the concept of perceived barriers (financial costs, side effects) (71,81). Another study investigated which components of the HBM were associated with attendance at a supervised exercise program for the prevention,

detection, and treatment of coronary heart disease. General health motivation and perceived severity of cardiovascular disease were associated with attendance at the program. However, perceived benefits were negatively associated, with higher benefits associated with lower attendance rates (61). Therefore, overall, the HBM has not received consistent support as a useful model for intervention studies of physical activity, although subcomponents of the model have shown potential utility.

Practice Implications

It may be useful for practitioners to assess the components of the HBM in working with their patients (73). One way to do this is to first assess the educational needs of your patients. Is your patient interested in health matters? Does your patient feel susceptible to serious health problems? Does your patient believe threat could be reduced by engaging in preventive health practices? Does your patient believe that there are major barriers to making behavior changes? These needs assessments are important for understanding patients' perceptions of risk and their likelihood of engaging in and maintaining preventive health behaviors. It is important for the practitioner to ask these types of questions to better understand the perceptions and beliefs that are held by their patients. For instance, the practitioner may think that given a patient's family history of cardiovascular disease and the patient's own individual risk factors, the patient is susceptible to developing some form of cardiovascular disease. However, without assessing the patient's own perceptions, the practitioner would not know if the patient held these same beliefs, which might influence the strength and conviction with which a person would opt to make behavior changes. There has been little intervention research on the HBM in healthy populations. It appears that the HBM has most of its utility for understanding the beliefs that patients hold and for helping them set goals based on their health beliefs.

SOCIAL ECOLOGY THEORY

Social ecology theory underscores the importance of the constant interaction between an individual's behavior and his or her environment. It emphasizes multiple influences on behavior, such as sociocultural factors and the qualities of the individual's environment, and suggests that the most successful programs are the ones that combine and target these multiple influences on behavior. Therefore, it is important to develop individual skills for changing behavior as well as having physical environments and policies that are supportive of physical activity. By also changing the environment to make it more "activity friendly," this influences everyone living in that neighborhood and is a more permanent change than an individual physical activity promotion program having limited availability (36).

Research Findings

Intrapersonal Factors

Intrapersonal factors related to physical activity have been researched extensively. Some examples of these factors are demographic factors (e.g., age, sex, race, health status), personal barriers (e.g., motivation level, child care), cognitive perceptions (e.g., perceived lack of time, self-efficacy), and behavioral factors (80).

Population-based, cross-sectional studies have examined correlations among perceived environmental and policy variables and physical activity behavior (19,75). These studies have found that the intrapersonal barriers that were inversely related to physical activity included having too little time, being too tired, lacking energy, lacking motivation, having less education, and not liking physical activity. One interesting study examined the psychological benefit afforded to women when exercising in different environments (67). In the first experiment of this study, 128 female college students were assigned different people with whom to exercise (alone, stranger, close friend). Women were found to be most calm when exercising alone. In the second experiment, women walked either alone or with a friend inside or outside (four conditions). Results were that those who exercise outdoors were more satisfied and enjoyed the exercise more regardless of social contact (67).

Interpersonal Factors

To a lesser degree, interpersonal factors have begun to be researched. Interpersonal factors such as one's living area (where many people exercise), friends who encouraged exercise, and having at least one friend with whom to exercise have been shown to be related to physical activity (19). Similarly, another study (37) found the infrequent observation of others exercising in one's neighborhood was associated with inactivity. Additionally, policy factors were examined in relation to physical activity, and most of the respondents were supportive of policies that supported physical activity promotion (19). For example, 71% of respondents believed the employers should provide time during the workday for employees to exercise, and 95% believed physical education should be required in schools. The policy variables that were positively associated with physical activity believed one's employer should provide time for exercise and supporting the use of local government funds for walking and jogging trials.

Physical Environment

The relationships between environmental settings and support for physical activity are not as well understood as personal, cognitive, social, and physiologic barriers (16). However, several studies show that environmental characteristics have an effect on physical activity behaviors (16,19). The presence of sidewalks, heavy traffic, hills, enjoyable scenery (38), and malls (60) were positively associated with physical activity, whereas crime or fear of crime and the lack of enjoyable scenery and hills (37) have been shown to be negatively related to activity behavior (66).

Practice Implications

Researchers postulate that to maximize the efficacy of interventions, programs need to combine environmental components with individual and community-based physical activity promotion efforts (69,75). Understanding patients' social and physical environments as well as assisting them in understanding these factors can help you to work with them toward maximizing their activity. For instance, many people might not recognize that their social and physical environments can function as a facilitator or a barrier to making behavior changes. Therefore, it may be helpful to point out ways that individuals can work within their social structures, such as finding social support to walk in a neighborhood, or within the parameters of their community.

THE THEORY OF REASONED ACTION

The TRA was developed as a way of understanding and predicting an individual's behavior (22,23). For the purposes of this theory, the behavior must be clearly specified, volitional in nature, and performed in a specific situation. This theory postulates that a person who believes that a given behavior will result in a positive outcome will most likely hold a favorable attitude toward performing that behavior. According to the TRA, intention is the sole and immediate predictor of behavior (22), and intention mediates the effect of attitude toward the behavior and the subjective normative beliefs (NBs) toward the behavior (3,29).

There has been limited support of the TRA when applied to physical activity (26,76,82). To date, it has been found that the basic variables in this model only account for a fraction of the variance in exercise behavior (26). Also, the TRA has been found to be most useful (1,2) when behaviors are completely under volitional control, meaning no practical constraints or barriers to executing the behavior are present. One recent study found a higher degree of predictive utility of the TRA constructs (20). This study, which examined 63 low-income postpartum women, found that attitude and subjective norms accounted for 66% of the variance in intention to exercise, whereas perceived behavioral control was not a significant predictor (20). It has been shown that for exercise, perceived barriers are variables that influence exercise intention and behavior (54,74), which may help to explain the lack of support of the TRA within the physical activity literature.

THE THEORY OF PLANNED BEHAVIOR

The theory of planned behavior (TPB) (42) is an extension of the TRA that includes perceived behavioral control as a third exogenous variable. Perceived behavioral control is similar to the concept of self-efficacy (8,10) because it reflects one's belief as to the likelihood of difficulty to be encountered when adopting a particular behavior and the perceived availability of resources and opportunities that may be beneficial in adopting a particular behavior. It has been stated that the TPB is most useful for describing behaviors that are entirely under volitional control, or ones with no perceived barriers present (1,2). Alternatively, a lack of control exists when adoption of the behavior requires opportunities, resources, or skills that are not readily available to the individual. Intuitively, most behaviors (including exercise) fall somewhere on the continuum between total control to complete lack of control (22,25). Figure 43-2 is a representation of this model.

Thus, perceived behavioral control has a direct and indirect (through behavioral intention) effect on behavior. The theory postulates that perceived behavioral control can affect behavioral intention through motivation. The TPB also proposes that individuals intend to perform a behavior if they evaluate it positively, believe that others think it is important, and perceive the behavior to be under their control (1). Some have suggested that applications of the TPB and the HBM should also include affective (e.g., enjoyment, boredom) components and not solely rely on instrumental components (e.g., negative health consequences of being inactive) (24,40).

Research Findings

Although research has indicated that the inclusion of perceived behavioral control as an exogenous variable enhances the prediction of intentions and target behaviors (42), the research applying the TRA and the TPB to physical activity has been limited. Most of the studies to date have tended to combine or compare the efficacy of the two theories rather than directly test their predictive utility or examine the mediation role of intention and stage of change in predicting activity behavior (41,76,82).

In a literature review of studies on the predictive utility of the TRA and TPB for exercise between the years 1980 and 1995, Blue (14) cited 16 studies that used the TRA and seven studies that used the TRB. Cross-sectional designs were used most frequently, and the majority of studies conducted used young, healthy middle-aged adults. Findings from this review indicate that the TRB was better than the TRA for predicting exercise behavior. According to Blue (14), this was because the TPB has more predictive qualities for exercise intention and the TPB does not assume that the exercise behavior is entirely under the volitional control of the individual. Blue does state, however, that this finding should be interpreted with caution because of the limited number of studies in this area. These findings are consistent with meta-analyses, which have found perceived behavioral control to be associated with exercise behavior (29,30).

Godin et al. (27) conducted two similar studies in different populations to evaluate the utility of the construct of perceived behavioral control for predicting exercising behavior in a group of healthy adults (130 men and 218 women) and in 136 pregnant women. The pertinent TPB variables (i.e., exercise behavior, intention, attitude, subjective social norm, and perceived behavioral control) were measured in both samples. The healthy adults were followed for 6 months after initial assessments, and the pregnant women were followed 8 to 9 months after baseline, at which time they completed behavioral measures to assess how many times within that time frame they had engaged in one or more physical activities for at least 20 minutes per session. Structural equation modeling was used to analyze the data. For the healthy adults, results indicate that intention to exercise directly influenced exercise behavior. Perceived behavioral control influenced exercise behavior only through the effects it had on intention. For the pregnant women, none of the TPB constructs were associated with exercising behavior. These two studies provide mixed support for utility of using the TPB for predicting exercise behavior.

A recent study examined the TPB constructs related to different types of activities (e.g., endurance, strength, and flexibility) in 185 undergraduates and found endurance type activity was influenced by behavioral beliefs, flexibility was influenced by normative and control beliefs, and strength was influenced by behavioral, normative, and control beliefs (70).

Another study (13) examined the utility of the TPB for understanding exercise adherence during phase II cardiac rehabilitation. In this study, 215 patients completed

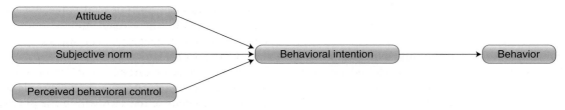

FIGURE 43-2. Representation of the theory of planned behavior.

questionnaires that included TBP constructs before beginning phase II cardiac rehabilitation. The results of this study indicated that the TBP constructs of attitude, subjective norm, and perceived behavioral control accounted for 30% of the variance in exercise intention. Exercise intention accounted for 12% of the variance in explaining exercise adherence (i.e., number of sessions prescribed divided by the number of sessions attended). Although this study provided some support for the predictive utility of the TBP for use in understanding adherence to cardiac rehabilitation, overall, the model only accounted for a small portion (12%) of the variance in explaining exercise behavior. A recent study also examined the TBP to predict health behaviors among 597 patients diagnosed with coronary artery disease (34). Perceived behavioral control predicted exercise, distance walked, and smoking cessation; however, intention itself was not a reliable predictor of health behavior. Despite these results, for physical activity, the total variance in the model explained by perceived behavioral control ranged from 9% to 20%.

Another study examined constructs from TPB in a 12-week longitudinal study of 94 individuals (ages 16–65) enrolling in a fitness facility (5). Both subjective norms and perceived behavioral intentions were significantly predictive of behavioral intention, whereas only perceived behavioral control was significantly associated with physical activity behavior (i.e., attendance).

The results of the present studies have indicated mixed findings with respect to the usefulness of the TRA or TPB in the area of intervening on exercise behaviors; however, more recent studies (5,20) have found greater research applicability of these models. The TRA and TPB have provided some theoretical information for understanding health behaviors, such as exercise, and the postulated relationships between the variables have been supported (29,30). The theories, however, are limited in their applicability to interventions related to changing physical activity behavior. Intentions may be an important prerequisite for exercise adoption, but they are not solely sufficient for predicting regular physical activity. In sum, the TRA and TPB intuitively have some merit but have limitations in their application for the field of exercise adoption and maintenance.

Practice Applications

Although the research findings relating to the TRA and TPB have been mixed, components of these theories may be useful for assisting patients in making changes in their physical activity. For instance, in helping a patient make behavior change, the first step is to typically understand the framework under which the individual is operating. For example, it is helpful to understand patients' attitudes toward physical activity, the value that they and other people in their lives place on physical activity, and their sense or belief that they have control over the behavior. It is possible that a patient may hold certain beliefs toward exercise (e.g., "I have never been athletic, so I can't exercise") or their family members may not understand the importance of being physically active and, therefore, not value it, which may negatively affect your patient. By assessing these factors initially, the practitioner can help anticipate potential barriers and help the patient problem solve to address those barriers.

Additionally, an important component of the TPB is perceived behavioral control, which is similar to the concept of self-efficacy. The methods for helping patients improve their self-efficacy are similar to those that could be used for helping them increase their sense of perceived behavioral control. For instance, patients could be encouraged to think about the realistic barriers they might encounter when making behavior changes and about the resources available to them for helping overcome those barriers. An example is a patient who thinks she does not have a safe place to exercise. The practitioner could help the patient think about other options for overcoming this barrier, including finding a walking "buddy," finding a mall in which to walk indoors, or finding other locations (e.g., a YMCA).

RELAPSE PREVENTION

The relapse prevention (RP) model was developed to help understand relapse behavior in individuals who were seeking to remain abstinent from a negative health behavior (e.g., smoking, drinking). However, the components of the RP model can be applied to other health behaviors, such as at the beginning of a physical activity program. The overall goal of RP is to assist individuals in maintaining long-term behavior change by anticipating potentially high-risk situations and devising strategies to cope with these high-risk situations (55,56). The RP model is a combination of behavioral skills training, cognitive intervention, and lifestyle change. Therefore, it is an important model for use with physical activity behavior maintenance. The RP model makes two very important distinctions in defining the terms *lapse* and *relapse*. Whereas *lapse* is defined as a slight error or slip (e.g., missing one exercise session), *relapse* is a return to former behavior patterns (e.g., not being physically active for an extended period of time).

The RP model cautions against viewing behavior change as either a complete success or a complete failure. This dichotomous approach ignores the potential influence of situational and psychological factors as determinants in relapse and reinforces the idea that someone who experiences a relapse lacks personal control (56). Furthermore, establishing the dichotomy of success (e.g., exercising 5 days per week for 30 minutes each time) or failure (e.g., not exercising at all) can also set up an individual for a "abstinence violation effect," which is one's tendency to give up if even a small slip has occurred. For instance, if someone has missed her exercise sessions for the week because of work demands, she may think, "Why should I bother now? I am already out of my routine." Instead, the RP model encourages people to view a lapse as a "fork in the road" (56) that could either lead back to successful behavior maintenance or a return to earlier behavior patterns. For example, someone would be using RP strategies if he or she thought in advance about a high-risk situation such as a vacation and devised a plan for exercising during the vacation (i.e., locating a walking path near the hotel).

Research Findings

Although many experts cite the importance of RP strategies for helping individuals maintain behavior changes, little research has focused specifically on RP for physical activity. A large body of literature focuses on RP for weight loss (17); however, for physical activity, the focus on RP tends to be incorporated with a variety of other strategies (62,84). One study investigated the use of RP to promote exercise adherence among 120 women who were previously sedentary (45). In this study, subjects were randomly assigned to either a control group or one of two experimental groups (RP or reinforcement/lottery); all groups participated in an 18-week exercise program. The RP group consisted of focusing on potential high-risk situations, developing coping responses, and using a planned relapse. The reinforcement group consisted of rewarding participants for consistent attendance. Results indicated that compared with the control group, the RP group attended significantly more sessions during the first 9 weeks of the program; the reinforcement group was not significantly different from the control group. However, by 18 weeks and at the 2-month posttreatment assessment, there were no differences between the groups. Marcus and Stanton (45) cite some potential considerations when examining the RP approach for physical activity. They state that factors such as the convenience of class schedule, group cohesion, and the strength of the intervention may have been mitigating factors to help explain the lack of longer-term efficacy of the RP approach.

A recent study examined RP strategies among 65 long-term exercisers who identified high-risk situations as bad weather, inconvenient time of day, being alone, negative emotions, and being tired (79). Positive cognitive coping strategies, such as problem solving and positive reappraisal, were employed by 43% of the sample; the positive behavioral coping strategy of having a pre-exercise ritual was used by 22% of the men, but only 3% of the women. These findings have implications for practice and the suggestion of ways of coping with different types of high-risk situations.

Practice Implications

Relapse prevention is an important aspect of any behavior change program. Marlatt and Gordon (56) stress the importance of establishing a collaborative relationship with the patient and focusing on using a few techniques at a time rather than trying to incorporate all techniques at once. The research of Marcus and Stanton (45) provide an excellent framework for practitioners who are working with patients trying to maintain physical activity behavior change. The RP model has a series of strategies that can be used by patients to learn how to anticipate and cope with the possibility of relapse. In the study conducted by Nies et al. (62), women were asked to identify what they could do to prevent a relapse in their walking program and to consider the use of social support, cognitive restructuring, and identifying personal benefits as potential strategies. The first step in RP helps patients reflect on the importance of regular exercise and the importance of being flexible in their thinking regarding the need to miss a session, if necessary. In addition, the next phase is to work with patients to help them identify situations in which they were able to successfully overcome a potential barrier and the challenges faced when they were not successful. Reflecting on a situation in which the patient was successful can help them understand that they have a skill set, or a "tool-box" of skills, that they have successfully engaged in the past.

Next, it is important to teach patients how to identify high-risk situations that may trigger a relapse. It may be helpful in this step to identify some examples of potential relapse situations, which can be combined into two main categories: intrapersonal and interpersonal (75). Examples of intrapersonal determinants include negative emotional states, negative physical states, and positive emotional states. Interpersonal determinants include social pressure and interpersonal conflict. One intrapersonal state that tends to be common is stress. Patients who have difficulty managing stress should be encouraged to take a walk or do some other physical activity. Even if the patient only has 10 minutes between scheduled meetings during a busy day, a brisk walk can help clear the mind, provide some relaxation, and reduce stress. An interpersonal state that patients might identify is having many demands on their time and feeling unable to devote the time to being physically active. One suggestion that might assist patients with these types of high-risk situations is to see if the patient might be able to fit in shorter bouts of activity (e.g., 10 minutes in length three times a day) rather than trying to block out a full 30 minutes each day. By dividing the time into smaller bouts, this can help patients feel like they have more control over ways to "fit in" the activity.

After identifying high-risk situations, the next step is to anticipate those situations, and problem solve around effective coping strategies. Using the example above, you might suggest to a patient who has multiple demands that if she is feeling unsure about how to fit in physical activity that she can try to do 10 minutes first thing in the morning, 10 minutes at lunch, and 10 minutes right after dinner. By dividing a longer bout into smaller pieces, this can be an effective coping strategy to address a potential high-risk situation and avoid a relapse.

SUMMARY

This chapter has provided an overview of the theories of behavior change that have been applied most successfully to physical activity. This information should be useful for helping to understand the factors that influence the complicated process through which individuals decide to begin and maintain a physical activity program. This chapter has provided you with several theoretical frameworks for understanding the strategies and skills associated with adopting a new behavior and with some ways to help your patients prevent relapse. This chapter also has provided you with the research applications of these theories, as well as practical implications for everyday interactions with individuals wanting to become more physically active. The information provided in this chapter should serve as a reference point for helping individuals become and stay physically active to live a healthier lifestyle and prevent disease.

REFERENCES

1. Ajzen I. *Attitudes, Personality and Behavior*. Chicago: Dorsey Press; 1988. p. 32–3, 116–27, 132–43.
2. Ajzen I. From intentions to actions: a theory of planned behavior. In: Kuhl J, Beckman J, editors. *Action-Control: From Cognition to Behavior*. New York: Springer; 1985. p. 11–39.
3. Ajzen I, Fishbein M. *Understanding Attitudes and Predicting Social Behavior*. Englewood Cliffs (NJ): Prentice-Hall; 1980. p. 4–11.
4. Anderson ES, Wojcik JR, Winett RA, Williams DM. Social-cognitive determinants of physical activity: the influence of social support, self-efficacy, outcome expectations, and self-regulation among participants in a church-based health promotion study. *Health Psychol.* 2006;25(4):510–20.
5. Armitage CJ. Can the theory of planned behavior predict the maintenance of physical activity? *Health Psychol.* 2005;24(3):235–45.
6. Bandura A. Exercise of personal agency through the self-efficacy mechanism. In: Schwarzer R, editor. *Self-Efficacy: Thought Control of Action*. Washington (DC): Hemisphere; 1992. p. 3–38.
7. Bandura A. *Self-Efficacy: The Exercise of Control*. New York: W. H. Freeman; 1997. p. 3–36, 128–37.
8. Bandura A. Self-efficacy: toward a unifying theory of behavior change. *Psychol Rev.* 1977;84:192–215.
9. Bandura A. *Social Foundations of Thought and Action: A Social Cognitive Theory*. Englewood Cliffs (NJ): Prentice-Hall; 1986. p. 18–30, 335–50, 390–414, 435–9.
10. Bandura A. *Social Learning Theory*. Englewood Cliffs (NJ): Prentice Hall; 1977. p. 79–85.
11. Becker MH, editor. The health belief model and personal health behavior. *Health Educ Monogr.* 1974;2:324–508.
12. Biddle SJH, Nigg NR. Theories of exercise behavior. *Int J Sport Psychol.* 2000;31(2):290–304.
13. Blanchard CM, Courneya KS, Rodgers WM, et al. Is the theory of planned behavior a useful framework for understanding exercise adherence during phase II cardiac rehabilitation? *J Cardiopulm Rehabil.* 2003;23(1):29–39.
14. Blue CL. The predictive capacity of the theory of reasoned action and the theory of planned behavior in exercise research: an integrated literature review. *Res Nurs Health.* 1995;18(2):105–21.
15. Bock BC, Marcus BH, Pinto B, Forsyth L. Maintenance of physical activity following an individualized motivationally-tailored intervention. *Ann Behav Med.* 2001;23(2):79–87.
16. Booth ML, Owen N, Bauman A, Clavisi O, Leslie E. Social-cognitive and perceived environment influences associated with physical activity in older Australians. *Prev Med.* 2000;31(1):15–22.
17. Bray SR. Self-efficacy for coping with barriers helps students stay physically active during transition to their first year at a university. *Res Q Exerc Sport.* 2007;78(2):61–70.
18. Brownell KD, O'Neil PM. Obesity. In: Barlow D, editor. *Clinical Handbook of Psychological Disorders*. New York: Guilford Press; 1993. p. 318–61.
19. Brownson RC, Baker EA, Houseman RA, Brennan LK, Bacak SJ. Environmental and policy determinants of physical activity in the United States. *Am J Public Health.* 2001;91(12):1995–2003.
20. Downs DS. Understanding exercise intention in an ethnically diverse sample of postpartum women. *J Sport Exerc Psychol.* 2006;28(2):159–80.
21. Dunn AL, Marcus BH, Kampert JB, Garcia ME, Kohl HW, Blair SN. Reduction in cardiovascular disease risk factors: 6-month results from Project ACTIVE. *Prev Med.* 1997;26(6):883–92.
22. Fishbein MA. Theory of reasoned action: some applications and implications. *Nebr Symp Motiv.* 1979;27:65–116.
23. Fishbein M. *Belief, Attitude, Intention, and Behavior*. Boston: Addison-Wesley; 1975.
24. French DP, Sutton S, Hennings SJ, et al. The importance of affective beliefs and attitudes in the theory of planned behavior: predicting intention to increase physical activity. *J Appl Soc Psych.* 2005;35(9): 1824–48.
25. Godin G. Social-cognitive models. In: Dishman RK, editor. *Advances in Exercise Adherence*. Champaign (IL): Human Kinetics; 1994. p. 113–36.
26. Godin G. Theories of reasoned action and planned behavior: usefulness for exercise promotion. *Med Sci Sports Exerc.* 1994;26(11): 1391–4.
27. Godin G, Valois P, Lepage L. The Miriam Hospital pattern of influence of perceived behavioral control upon exercising behavior: an application of Ajzen's theory of planned behavior. *J Behav Med.* 1993;16:81–101.
28. Goldstein MG, Pinto BM, Marcus BH, et al. Physician-based physical activity counseling for middle-aged and older adults: a randomized trial. *Ann Behav Med.* 1999;21(1):40–7.
29. Hagger MS, Chatzisarantis NLD, Biddle SJH. A meta analytic review of the theories of reasoned action and planned behavior in physical activity: predictive validity and the contribution of additional variables. *J Sport Exerc Psychol.* 2002;24(1):3–32.
30. Hausenblas HA, Carron AV, Mack DE. Application of the theories of reasoned action and planned behavior to exercise behavior: a meta-analysis. *J Sport Exerc Psychol.* 1997;19(1):36–51.
31. Hofstetter CR, Hovell MF, Sallis JF. Social learning correlates of exercise self-efficacy: early experiences with physical activity. *Soc Sci Med.* 1990;31(10):1169–86.
32. Janis IL, Mann L. *Decision Making: A Psychological Analysis of Conflict, Choice and Commitment*. New York: Free Press; 1977. p. 10–4, 147–69.
33. Janz NK, Becker MH. The health belief model: a decade later. *Health Education Quarterly.* 1984;11(1):1–47.
34. Johnston DW, Johnston M, Pollard B, Kinmonth A, Mant D. Motivation is not enough: prediction of risk behavior following diagnosis of coronary heart disease from the theory of planned behavior. *Health Psychol.* 2004;23:533–8.
35. Juniper KC, Oman RF, Hamm RM, Kerby DS. The relationships among constructs in the health belief model and the transtheoretical model among African-American college women for physical activity. *Am J Health Promot.* 2004;18:354–7.
36. Kelly CM, Hoehner CM, Baker EA, Ramirez LKB, Brownson RC. Promoting physical activity in communities: approaches for

successful evaluation of programs and policies. *Evaluation and Program Planning*. 2006;29(3):280–92.

37. King AC, Castro C, Wilcox S, Eyler AA, Sallis JF, Brownson RC. Personal and environmental factors associated with physical inactivity among different racial-ethnic groups of U.S. middle-aged and older-aged women. *Health Psychol*. 2000;19(4):354–64.

38. King AC, Toobert D, Ahn D, et al. Perceived environments as physical activity correlates and moderators of intervention in five studies. *Am J Health Promot*. 2006;21(1):24–35.

39. Kinzie MB. Instructional design strategies for health behavior change. *Patient Educ Couns*. 2005;56(1):3–15.

40. Kiviniemi MT, Voss-Humke AM, Seifert AL. How do I feel about the behavior? The interplay of affective associations with behaviors and cognitive beliefs as influences on physical activity behavior. *Health Psychol*. 2007;26(2):152–8.

41. Kosma M, Ellis R, Cardinal BJ, Bauer JJ, McCubbin JA. The mediating role of intention and stages of change in physical activity among adults with physical disabilities: an integrative framework. *J Sport Exerc Psychol*. 2007;29(1):21–38.

42. Madden TJ, Ellen PS, Ajzen I. A comparison of the theory of planned behavior and the theory of reasoned action. *Pers Soc Psychol Bull*. 1992;18(1):3–9.

43. Maddux JE. *Self-Efficacy, Adaptation, and Adjustment: Theory, Research, and Application*. New York: Plenum Press; 1995.

44. Maibach EW, Cotton D. Moving people to behavior change: a staged social cognitive approach to message design. In: Maibach E, Parrot RL, editors. *Designing Health Messages: Approaches from Communication Theory and Public Health Practice*. Thousand Oaks (CA): Sage Publications; 1995.

45. Marcus BH, Stanton AL. Evaluation of relapse prevention and reinforcement interventions to promote exercise adherence in sedentary females. *Res Q Exerc Sport*. 1993;64(4):447–52.

46. Marcus BH, Lewis BA, Williams DM, et al. Step into Motion: A randomized trial examining the relative efficacy of Internet vs. print-based physical activity interventions. *Contemp Clin Trials*. 2007; 28(6):737–47.

47. Marcus BH, Bock BC, Pinto BM, Forsyth LH, Roberts MB. Efficacy of an individualized, motivationally-tailored physical activity intervention. *Ann Behav Med*. 1998;20(3):184–8.

48. Marcus BH, Nigg CR, Riebe D, Forsyth LH. Interactive communication strategies: implications for population-based physical activity promotion. *Am J Prev Med*. 2000;19(2):121–6.

49. Marcus BH, Rossi JS, Selby VC, Niaura RS. The stages and processes of exercise adoption and maintenance in a worksite sample. *Health Psychol*. 1992;11(6):386–95.

50. Marcus BH, Emmons KM, Simkin-Silverman LR, et al. Evaluation of motivationally tailored vs. standard self-help physical activity interventions at the workplace. *Am J Health Promot*. 1998;12(4): 246–53.

51. Marcus BH, Forsyth LH. *Motivating People to be Physically Active*. Champaign (IL): Human Kinetics; 2003. p. 11–40.

52. Marcus BH, Simkin LR. The stages of exercise behavior. *J Sports Med Phys Fitness*. 1993;33(1):83–8.

53. Marcus BH, Owen N. Motivational readiness, self-efficacy, and decision-making for exercise. *J Appl Soc Psychol*. 1992;22(1):3–16.

54. Marcus BH, Selby VC, Niaura RS, Rossi JS. Self-efficacy and the stages of exercise behavior change. *Res Q Exerc Sport*. 1992;63(1): 60–6.

55. Marcus BH, Rakowski W, Rossi RS. Assessing motivational readiness and decision-making for exercise. *Health Psychol*. 1992;11(4): 257–61.

56. Marlatt GA, Gordon JR. *Relapse Prevention: Maintenance Strategies in the Treatment of Addictive Behaviors*. New York: Guilford Press; 1985. p. 3–67.

57. Marshall SJ, Biddle SJH. The transtheoretical model of behavior change: a meta-analysis of applications to physical activity and exercise. *Ann Behav Med*. 2001;23(4):229–46.

58. McAuley E, Jerome JG, Marquez DX, Elavsky S, Blissmer B. Exercise self-efficacy in older adults: social affective and behavioral influences. *Ann Behav Med*. 2003;25(1):1–7.

59. McAuley E, Morris KS, Motl RW, Hu L, Konopack JF, Elavsky S. Long-term follow-up of physical activity behavior in older adults. *Health Psychol*. 2007;26(3):375–80.

60. Michael Y, Beard T, Choi D, Farquhar S, Carlson N. Measuring the influence of built neighborhood environments on walking in older adults. *J Aging Phys Act*. 2006;14(3):302–12.

61. Mirotznik J, Feldman L, Stein R. The health belief model and adherence with a community center-based supervised coronary heart disease exercise program. *J Community Health*. 1995;20(3):233–47.

62. Nies MA, Reisenberg CE, Chruscial HL, Artibee K. Southern women's response to a walking intervention. *Public Health Nurs*. 2003;20:146–52.

63. Nothwehr F, Yang J. Goal setting frequency and the use of behavioral strategies related to diet and physical activity. *Health Educ Res*. 2007;22(4):532–8.

64. Oldridge NB, Streiner DL. The health belief model: predicting compliance and dropout in cardiac rehabilitation. *Med Sci Sports Exerc*. 1990;22(5):678–83.

65. **Pate RR, Pratt M, Blair SN, et al. Physical activity and public health: a recommendation from the Centers for Disease Control and Prevention and the American College of Sports Medicine. *JAMA*. 1995;273(5):402–7.**

66. Piro FN, Noess O, Claussen B. Physical activity among elderly people in a city population: the influence of neighbourhood level violence and self perceived safety. *J Epidemiol Community Health*. 2006;60(7):626–32.

67. Plante TG, Gores C, Brecht C, Carrow J, Imbs A, Willemsen E. Does exercise environment enhance the psychological benefits of exercise for women? *International Journal of Stress Management*. 2007; 14(1):88–9.

68. Prochaska JO, DiClemente CC. Stages and processes of self-change in smoking: towards an integrative model of change. *J Consul Clin Psychol*. 1983;51(3):390–5.

69. Reger-Nash B, Adrian B, Cooper L, Chey T, Simon KJ. Evaluating communitywide walking interventions. *Evaluation and Program Planning*. 2006;29(3):251–9.

70. Rhodes RE, Blanchard CM, Matheson DH. Motivational antecedent beliefs of endurance, strength, and flexibility activities. *Psychology, Health & Medicine*. 2007;12(2):148–62.

71. Roberston D, Keller C. Relationships among health beliefs, self-efficacy and exercise adherence in patients with coronary artery disease. *Heart Lung*. 1992;21(1):56–63.

72. Rosenstock IM. Historical origins of the health belief model. *Health Educ Monogr*. 1974;2:328–35.

73. Rosenstock IM, Strecher VJ, Becker MH. Social learning theory and the health belief model. *Health Educ Q*. 1988;15(2):175–83.

74. Sallis JF, Hovell MF, Hofstetter CR, et al. A multivariate study of determinants of vigorous exercise in a community sample. *Prev Med*. 1989;18(1):20–34.

75. Sallis JF, Owen N. Ecological models of health behavior. In: Glanz K, Rimer BK, Lewis FM, editors. *Health Behavior and Health Education: Theory, Research and Practice*. 3rd ed. San Francisco: Jossey-Bass; 2002. p. 161–5, 185–210, 275–9.

76. Sallis JF, Owen N. *Physical Activity and Behavioral Medicine*. Thousand Oaks (CA): Sage Publications; 1999. p. 108–33.

77. Schwarzer R. Self-efficacy in the adoption and maintenance of health behaviors: theoretical approaches and a new model. In: Schwarzer WR, editor. *Self-Efficacy: Thought Control of Action*. Washington (DC): Hemisphere; 1992. p. 218–42.

78. Spencer L, Adams TB, Malone S, Roy L, Yost E. Applying the transtheoretical model to exercise: a systematic and comprehensive review of the literature. *Health Promot Pract*. 2006;7(4):428–43.

79. Stetson BA, Frommelt SJ, Boutelle KN, Cole JD, Ziegler CH, Looney SW. Exercise slips in high-risk situations and activity patterns in

long-term exercisers: an application of the relapse prevention model. *Ann Behav Med.* 2005;30(1):25–35.

80. Stokols D. Establishing and maintaining healthy environments: toward a social ecology of health promotion. *Am Psychol.* 1992;47(1):6–22.

81. Tirrell BE, Hart LK. The relationship of health beliefs and knowledge to exercise compliance in patients after coronary bypass. *Heart Lung.* 1980;9(3):487–93.

82. Trost SG, Owen N, Bauman AE, Sallis JF, Brown W. Correlates of adults' participation in physical activity: review and update. *Med Sci Sports Exerc.* 2002;34(12):1996–2001.

83. **U.S. Department of Health and Human Services. *Physical Activity and Health: A Report of the Surgeon General.* Atlanta: U.S. Department of Health and Human Services, Centers for Disease Control and Prevention, National Center for Chronic Disease Prevention and Health Promotion; 1996. p. 209–43.**

84. Vickers KS, Nies MA, Patten CA, Dierkhising R, Smith SA. Patients with diabetes and depression may need additional support for exercise. *Am J Health Behav.* 2006;30(4):353–62.

85. Whitely JA, Lewis BA, Napolitano MA, Marcus BH. Health behavior counseling skills. In: Ehrman JK, editor. *Resource Manual for Guidelines for Exercise Testing and Prescription,* 6th ed. Champaign: Human Kinetics; 2009. p. 723–733.

SELECTED REFERENCES FOR FURTHER READING

Anshell MH. *Applied Exercise Psychology: A Practitioner's Guide to Improving Client Health and Fitness.* New York: Springer Publishing; 2005.

Conn VS, Minor MA, Burkes KJ, Rantz MJ, Pomeroy SH. Integrative review of physical activity interventions with aging adults. *J Am Geriatr Soc.* 2003;51(8):1159–68.

Glantz K, Rimer BK, Lewis FM. *Health Behavior and Health Education: Theory, Research, and Practice.* San Francisco: Jossey-Bass; 2002.

Hagger MS, Chatzisarantis NLD, Biddle SJH. Meta-analysis of the theories of reasoned action and planned behavior in physical activity: an examination of predictive validity and the contribution of additional variables. *J Sport Exerc Psychol.* 2002;24:3–32.

Marcus BH, Forsyth LH. *Motivating People to be Physically Active.* Champaign (IL): Human Kinetics; 2003.

Marlatt GA, Donovan DM . *Relapse Prevention, Second Edition: Maintenance Strategies in the Treatment of Addictive Behaviors.* New York: Guilford Press; 2005.

Reger-Nash B, Bauman A, Cooper L, Chey T, Simon KM. Evaluating communitywide walking interventions. *Evaluation and Program Planning.* 2006;29(3):251–9.

Sallis JF, Owen N. Ecological models of health behavior. In: Glanz K, Rimer BK, Lewis FM, editors. *Health Behavior and Health Education: Theory, Research and Practice.* 3rd ed. San Francisco: Jossey-Bass; 2002.

INTERNET RESOURCES

- Centers for Disease Control and Prevention. Understanding and promoting physical activity. In: *Physical Activity and Health*: www.cdc.gov/nccdphp/sgr/chap6.htm.
- Edwards P. Evidence-based strategies for increasing participation in physical activity in community recreation, fitness and sport.: www.lin.ca/resource/html/mm83.htm.
- Grizzell J. Behavior change theories and models.: www.csupomona.edu/~jvgrizzell/best_practices/bctheory.html.
- Marcus BH, Lewis BA. Physical activity and the stages of motivational readiness for change model. *Research Digest*: http://fitness.gov/Reading_Room/Digests/march2003digest.pdf.
- Sallis JF, Kerr J. Physical activity and the built environment. *Research Digest*: http://fitness.gov/digests/December2006Digest.pdf.

This chapter discusses some fundamental counseling skills and steps for applying them with patients. In doing so, the chapter borrows from several of the theoretical principles described in Chapter 43 (23). Practical application strategies are provided in more detail for the transtheoretical model (26), social cognitive theory (2,3), and the relapse prevention model (20). In addition, the chapter introduces some strategies from motivational interviewing, a counseling technique in which motivation for change is elicited and enhanced from the patient, rather than imposed upon externally by the health professional (4,7,12,22,27). The intention is to teach strategies that help practitioners to better understand how to communicate with their patients by applying the theoretical strategies presented in Chapter 43 (23). The communication techniques discussed in this chapter will blend a patient-centered approach (10,12,28,29), in which the counselor listens and follows what the patients say, and a directive approach, in which the counselor leads constructive discussions regarding behavior change (29). The strategies provided here do not include giving advice. Advice giving, although effective in some instances, can be detrimental to behavior change in others (9,29). Some patients may perceive advice giving as condescending or presumptuous, in that the patient might perceive they are being told what to do, thereby undermining their autonomy and possibly generating resistance (29). Instead, this chapter focuses on a patient-centered approach that

> > > KEY TERMS

Active listening: A process whereby a practitioner tries to understand the underlying meaning of what a patient is saying.

Decisional balance: The comparison of the benefits versus the costs of making a behavior change.

Empathy: The understanding that is conveyed by a counselor to a patient.

Open-ended questions: Questions that allow the patient to provide expansive responses beyond a simple yes or no in which they can explore their thoughts and feelings.

Motivational interviewing: A patient-centered counseling method in which the patient's own motivation for change is elicited and enhanced by exploring and resolving ambivalence to change.

Patient-centered approach: A counseling style that takes the patient's perspective into account, features collaboration between the patient and counselor, and includes genuine respect for the patient's opinions.

Processes of change: The strategies that individuals use as they are adopting and maintaining behavior

changes; five behavioral (e.g., obtaining social support) and five cognitive processes (e.g., increasing knowledge) have been identified.

Rapport: The positive relationship counselors establish with their patients.

Reflective statements: Statements that repeat back to the patient what the counselor has heard and understood the patient to say. If done in conjunction with active listening, these statements reflect the underlying meaning and/or feeling of what the patient is saying.

Relapse prevention: The process by which one maintains long-term behavior change by anticipating potentially high-risk situations and devising strategies to cope with these situations.

Self-efficacy: An individual's belief and confidence about his or her ability to make specific behavior changes.

Stages of change: A model that postulates that individuals move through a series of stages and face common barriers when making a behavior change.

incorporates the counseling skills of rapport building, active listening, reflective listening, and empathy, all of which are motivational interviewing skills (22,29). These counseling skills can then be the tools that are used with a directive approach in which discussions regarding self-monitoring, benefits and barriers, confidence, feedback, and relapse prevention can take place.

HEALTH COUNSELING TECHNIQUES

> **1.9.2-HFS: Knowledge of the important elements that should be included in each behavior modification session.**

> **1.9.6-HFS: Knowledge of approaches that may assist less motivated patients to increase their physical activity.**

> **1.9.10-CES: Facilitation of effective and contemporary motivational and behavior modification techniques to promote behavioral change.**

The "**patient-centered approach**" (6,9–12,28,29,33) takes the patient's perspective into account when making decisions about behavior change. Box 44-1 lists what Stewart et al. (33) have described as several of the key elements of the patient-centered approach. This approach, when used by physicians, has been shown to be related to higher patient satisfaction, increased medication compliance, a reduction in patients' concerns, and a reduction in actual symptoms, such as raised blood pressure (33).

Rollnick et al. (29) summarize the goals of the patient-centered approach as encouraging patients to express

BOX 44-1	KEY ELEMENTS OF THE PATIENT-CENTERED APPROACH

- Approach the patient with unconditional positive regard.
- Behavior change is based on a genuine, respectful relationship.
- Assessment of the patient occurs when the practitioner seeks to enter the world of the patient to understand his or her unique perspective.
- The patient and the practitioner work together to define the problem and to establish the goals and the roles of the patient and practitioner.
- Each contact between the practitioner and the patient is an opportunity to build the therapeutic relationship for health promotion.

Adapted from Stewart M, Stewart M, Belle Brown J, et al. *Patient-Centered Medicine: Transforming the Clinical Method.* (33)

concerns, helping them to be more active in the consultation, allowing them to state what information they need, giving them more control of the decision making, and reaching joint decisions. One caveat to this approach is that there is typically a very limited amount of time with a patient (e.g., one 15-minute consultation), which makes the patient-centered approach more difficult. In this case, you may need to be more direct. However, whenever possible, we recommend trying to incorporate the techniques discussed in this chapter.

To achieve these goals, the practitioner needs to adopt a set of counseling skills that are nonjudgmental. Practitioners need to establish rapport, be encouraging, be interested in the patient's perspective, ask open-ended questions, and be good active listeners.

ESTABLISHING RAPPORT

> **1.9.10-CES: Facilitation of effective and contemporary motivational and behavior modification techniques to promote behavioral change.**

The first important aspect in using the patient-centered approach in working with patients is establishing **rapport**. Rapport is the relationship established with a patient. It is built on trust and mutual respect. If a strong therapeutic relationship is established from the beginning, the behavior change process is more likely to succeed. One strategy for establishing rapport is to ask the patient **open-ended questions**. For example, Rollnick et al. (29) suggest asking patients "Can you please describe what a typical day is like for you?" This question is also part of the dialogue presented in Box 44-2.

This is meant to allow patients to tell about activities that occur throughout their day while providing several facts regarding how they spend their time. This may be helpful in identifying opportunities for decreasing sedentary behavior and increasing active behavior.

INTEREST AND EMPATHY

> **1.9.10-CES: Facilitation of effective and contemporary motivational and behavior modification techniques to promote behavioral change.**

Conveying interest and **empathy** also helps to establish rapport (29). The process of listening and conveying understanding, or empathy, is not a passive process. When listening carefully to a patient, one can convey what is heard by either reflecting or repeating the information, summarizing their statements, or asking questions for clarification. Examples of empathy are provided in the dialogue in Box 44-2. Using empathy demonstrates listening and gives a chance to make sure all is understood. This helps to build rapport with a patient.

BOX 44-2   CASE STUDY

Case: A 43-year-old woman has come to your fitness facility looking to get in shape. From her initial paperwork you learn that she was active in sports as a child but has not had the time to fit regular activity into her daily life. She has a part-time job and is the mother of three children.

Dialogue	Health Behavior Counseling Skills
Fitness Professional: Hello, Jane. It's great to meet you. Why don't you tell me a little bit about why you are here today?	Rapport building and an open-ended question
Patient: Well, I need to lose a little weight and I would like to be fit again.	
Fitness Professional: Okay, so, you would like to get in shape and lose weight. Can you tell me more about that? What else is there?	Active listening with a reflective statement, open-ended question
Patient: Sure. I used to be very active in high school. I played sports and loved it. Now I just can't seem to find the time to exercise. Yes, I have three kids and I work part-time. I am always running them to after school activities and feel like a chauffeur more than anything most days. *(Sighs and slumps her shoulders.)* It's been so long since I was active I'm not sure I'll be good at it or enjoy it, I'm also not sure I can find the time to exercise.	
Fitness Professional: It sounds like you are a little apprehensive about exercising right now. This is common when you haven't been active in awhile. Let me just make sure I am following you, Jane. You played sports as a child, but as you have gotten older and have more responsibilities with your job and family, you have had less time to be active. It also sounds like you aren't sure if you will enjoy it anymore. Is that right?	Active listening, reflective statement, empathetic statement, summary statement, verification
Patient: That pretty much sums it up.	
Fitness Professional: Why don't you tell me what a typical day is like for you?	Open-ended question to build rapport and gather information

ACTIVE LISTENING

> **1.9.10-CES: Facilitation of effective and contemporary motivational and behavior modification techniques to promote behavioral change.**

Another patient-centered technique is called **active listening** (9,29). Active listening is a process wherein the practitioner tries to understand the *underlying meaning* of what the patient is saying. The practitioner then makes **reflective statements** to convey that she has heard and understood this underlying meaning. This is a more advanced counseling skill and typically takes some practice to use naturally. Reflecting back the underlying meaning can help to establish rapport and empathy in that it demonstrates understanding of the patient's perspective. Summarizing statements can also be used to summarize content over a longer period of time, and elucidating themes of which the patient might not be aware can also demonstrate an understanding of the patient's perspective

as well as help to keep the session focused (9). **Open-ended questions** permit an expansion of the dialogue by allowing patients to continue the conversation and clarify their thoughts or meaning (9). Attending to the patient's nonverbal communications, such as his or her posture and facial expressions, can also be important to fill in the gaps between what the patient might be saying and what he or she is feeling (9). The dialogue in Box 44-2 illustrates how reflective statements, summarizations, open-ended questions, and attendance to verbal cues allow for an understanding of the patient's motives and barriers to change.

SUMMARY OF HEALTH COUNSELING TECHNIQUES

Through the use of a few patient-centered counseling techniques, one can increase satisfaction and compliance with patients. Rollnick et al. (29) summarize these techniques found in Box 44-3. To learn if these techniques performed properly, a few clues from the patient are summarized in Box 44-4 (29).

BEHAVIOR CHANGE STRATEGIES

 1.9.1-HFS: Knowledge of behavioral strategies to enhance exercise and health behavior change (e.g., reinforcement, goal setting, social support).

 1.9.2-HFS: Knowledge of the important elements that should be included in each behavior modification session.

 1.9.4-HFS: Knowledge of extrinsic and intrinsic reinforcement and give examples of each.

 1.9.9-CES: Implement tools for assessment of behavioral change such as the transtheoretical

model (i.e., readiness for change), quality-of-life questionnaires (e.g., Short Form 8, 12, or 36, Kansas City Cardiomyopathy Questionnaire).

 1.9.10-CES: Facilitation of effective and contemporary motivational and behavior modification techniques to promote behavioral change.

The health counseling skills described previously can be used within the framework of behavior change strategies. These strategies are more direct but can be accomplished through conversations using the patient-centered techniques of summarizing, clarifying, active listening, reflective statements, summarizing statements, and empathy. To maximize patient success, it is important to use techniques and strategies that are effective. Thus, the behavior change strategies presented here offer methods to work with patients to assess readiness for behavior change, determine strategies appropriate for a given stage of change, track progress, and set goals to achieve progress.

STAGES OF CHANGE

 1.9.5-HFS: Knowledge of the stages of motivational readiness.

 1.9.6-HFS: Knowledge of approaches that may assist less motivated patients to increase their physical activity.

 1.9.9-CES: Implement tools for assessment of behavioral change such as the transtheoretical model (i.e., readiness for change), quality-of-life questionnaires (e.g., Short Form 8, 12, or 36, Kansas City Cardiomyopathy Questionnaire).

 1.9.10-CES: Facilitation of effective and contemporary motivational and behavior modification techniques to promote behavioral change.

As is described in Chapter 43 (23), the transtheoretical model offers both a means of assessing readiness to change as well as several cognitive and behavioral processes to promote behavior change with your patients. In brief, the transtheoretical model postulates that individuals move through a series of stages as they become physically active (16,26,30). As participants move through the **stages of change**, they engage in cognitive and behavioral processes.

Although there are a few different versions of how to assess the stages of change, we recommend using the version in Box 44-5 (16). Moderate-intensity physical activity is defined for the individuals. Then patients indicate a "yes" or "no" to four statements about their physical activity behavior and intentions. The algorithm shown in Box 44-5 is used to identify the stage for a specific individual. In working with your patient, you could ask these questions conversationally to assess the patient's motivational readiness, or you might have the patient fill out the questionnaire.

BOX 44-5   ASSESSING PHYSICAL ACTIVITY STAGES OF CHANGE

PHYSICAL ACTIVITY STAGES OF CHANGE

INSTRUCTIONS: For each question below, please fill in the square Yes or No. Please be sure to follow the instructions carefully.

	Yes	No
1. I am currently physically active.	Y	N
2. I intend to become more physically active in the next 6 months.	Y	N

For activity to be regular, it must add up to a total of 30 or more minutes per day and be done at least 5 days per week. For example, you could take one 30-minute walk or three 10-minute walks each day.

	Yes	No
3. I currently engage in regular physical activity.	Y	N
4. I have been regularly physically active for the past 6 months.	Y	N

Stage	ITEM			
	1	2	3	4
Precontemplation	No	No	—	—
Contemplation	No	Yes	—	—
Preparation	Yes	—	No	—
Action	Yes	—	Yes	No
Maintenance	Yes	—	Yes	Yes

Modified with permission from Marcus BH, Forsyth LH. *Motivating People to be Physically Active.* Champaign (IL): Human Kinetics; 2003.

Knowing a person's stage of change suggests different strategies for working with that particular person. It is possible to target an intervention to an individual's stage of change (15,17–19). It has been shown that individuals who are in the earlier stages of change—precontemplation and contemplation—are more likely to use the cognitive processes of change, such as increasing knowledge and comprehending the benefits. As people move into the later stages, they start to use more behavioral processes of change, such as enlisting social support and substituting alternatives. Matching the change processes to the participant's stage is another important component of a patient-centered approach. This conveys that you understand how ready a patient is to change.

TRACKING ACTIVITY

> **1.9.1-HFS: Knowledge of behavioral strategies to enhance exercise and health behavior change (e.g., reinforcement, goal setting, social support).**

> **1.9.2-HFS: Knowledge of the important elements that should be included in each behavior modification session.**

> **1.9.10-CES: Facilitation of effective and contemporary motivational and behavior modification techniques to promote behavioral change.**

> **1.1.1-CES: List and apply behavioral strategies that apply to lifestyle modifications, such as exercise, diet, stress, and medication management.**

Another strategy to assess daily activities is to have your patients track their daily behaviors on self-monitoring forms (8,13,18,19). There are many ways to do this, and you can tailor the tracking form to an individual's needs. For example, if a patient is in contemplation, she may need to track how she spends her time on a daily basis. This means writing down her activities, including sedentary activities (e.g., time spent watching television, driving, sitting while eating, sitting at the computer) and the time spent at each activity. Box 44-6 provides an example of a self-monitoring log.

If the patient keeps track of this for several days over the course of the week, you can review the monitoring form together the following week. This provides a directive framework for your discussion while still using your patient-centered counseling strategies. It is important to

BOX 44-6 TRACKING FORM

EXAMPLE

Date: _____

TIME	ACTIVITY	MINUTES SPENT DOING	NOTES
7:00 a.m.	Got ready for work	60	
8:00 a.m.	Drove to work	45	
8:45 a.m.	Walked in to work	3	Walked slowly
8:50 a.m.	At my desk for computer work	180	Wow!

identify opportunities for decreasing sedentary behavior and increasing physical activity, and what the benefits and barriers might be for both. For instance, if the patient is sitting at a computer for many hours at a time, it may be possible to encourage incorporating short walks to break up this computer time. From a patient-centered perspective, you would initiate a conversation about how computer time exemplifies physical inactivity that may lead the patient to recognize this as an opportunity for change. Finding small instances for the patient to become less sedentary can provide the first building block of activity for an individual who has been inactive.

In contrast, if a person is in the preparation stage, the tracking might be quite different. Individuals in the preparation stage may not need to record their activity throughout the day but may focus instead on their bouts of moderate or vigorous activity and identify opportunities for increasing these behaviors. This self-monitoring form would be used to log the type of activity, days and times performed, perceived intensity, and even their enjoyment level during the physical activity bouts. Again, the self-monitoring form can provide the framework for a discussion regarding physical activity. You can review with your patient any patterns of behavior that may arise and work with him to think of ways to increase his activity level. For instance, in tracking his activity, a patient may have 2 days when he was physically active. In an attempt to clarify and understand this, you may ask, "What is different about the days when you weren't physically active versus the days you were?" The patient may then describe that on the days when he was inactive; he had planned to go to the fitness facility *after work* rather than before work. However, he often found he was too tired and went home instead. Thus, he may recognize that he was more successful going to the fitness center before work. The natural tendency is to advise the patient based on this information. However, using the patient-centered approach, it would be important for the patient to come to his own realizations about changing his behavior. By listening carefully, reflecting, and emphasizing the positive, the patient might make the connections that you hope he will make (i.e., "I should be physically active in the mornings or make a plan to go the gym even if I am tired"). In some cases, the patient may understand what is not working but is unsure of what to do to change the situation. In these situations, the technique of problem solving, as described later, may be used.

DECISIONAL BALANCE

> **1.9.1-HFS: Knowledge of behavioral strategies to enhance exercise and health behavior change (e.g., reinforcement, goal setting, social support).**

> **1.9.2-HFS: Knowledge of the important elements that should be included in each behavior modification session.**

> **1.9.6-HFS: Knowledge of approaches that may assist less motivated patients to increase their physical activity.**

> **1.1.1-CES: List and apply behavioral strategies that apply to lifestyle modifications, such as exercise, diet, stress, and medication management.**

> **1.9.10-CES: Facilitation of effective and contemporary motivational and behavior modification techniques to promote behavioral change.**

Another strategy for motivating behavior change is to have patients identify the benefits and barriers of being physically active that reflect **decisional balance** (18,19). To do this, you might have an open-ended conversation about this, or you can have your patient list their perceived benefits (pros) and perceived barriers (cons) for physical activity. The list must reflect what is important to the patient and not just a list of general benefits of physical activity. For example, a patient may know that one of the benefits of physical activity is decreasing the risk of osteoporosis, but this might not be personally important. However, feeling less fatigued may be a more motivating factor for this particular patient. Information obtained from this list can provide the framework for another conversation about behavior change while continuing to use your counseling techniques. Another resource for a similar measure is the decisional balance questionnaire, which is found in Marcus and Forsyth (16).

Benefits

This list of benefits, or pros, can be important to discuss as a means of affirming the reasons why the patient is interested in behavior change (8,18,19,24). This list can also be important to keep in mind when working with your patient if his motivation or behavior is low in the future. You can ask your patient to recount why he would like to be physically active. For a patient who feels tired after work, remembering that one of the pros he listed was increased energy and that he will feel more energetic after exercising may give him the motivation he needs to make that decision in the moment. In addition, if you are working with a patient over time, you can emphasize progress with positive statements that will help to reinforce or increase the behavior. For example, if you see the patient looking less fatigued, you might comment, "It looks like you have more energy these days." This helps to reaffirm the benefits of his activity that you knew were important to him from his initial list of pros and cons.

Barriers

The list of barriers, or cons, is important to address to determine the obstacles that may stand in the way of your patient's making progress (8,18,19). If your patient is having difficulty identifying her barriers or it seems the list is incomplete, you may find that self-monitoring provides insight into the patient's barriers. For example, if the patient takes a walk only on the days her neighbor is available to walk with her but not on the days when she would need to walk alone, you might have a discussion about this. As mentioned earlier, you should find a way to allow the patient to come to her own conclusion. Examples of what you might say include: "It seems as though you really enjoy walking with your neighbor" or "What do you enjoy about your walks with your neighbor?" In this way, you may be able to gently direct the patient to realize that walking alone is a barrier and having someone to walk with is a facilitator to being active. The goal is to work with your patient to determine her unique barriers to increase physical activity. In doing so, you may need to refer to the self-monitoring form, and you may need to help the patient determine which barriers are more or less difficult to overcome. It is particularly

important to be nonjudgmental in this process so that the patient feels comfortable and confident to problem solve solutions to the barriers.

PROBLEM SOLVING

> **1.9.1-HFS: Knowledge of behavioral strategies to enhance exercise and health behavior change (e.g., reinforcement, goal setting, social support).**

> **1.9.2-HFS: Knowledge of the important elements that should be included in each behavior modification session.**

> **1.9.10-CES: Facilitation of effective and contemporary motivational and behavior modification techniques to promote behavioral change.**

> **1.1.1-CES: List and apply behavioral strategies that apply to lifestyle modifications, such as exercise, diet, stress, and medication management.**

After the barriers have been determined, an important skill to help your patient develop is problem solving. Problem solving can be done to determine solutions for the barriers that your patient has identified (8,14,16). The *process* of problem solving is more important to learn than a set of solutions for any one barrier, so that the patient will know how to tackle barriers in the future. Problem solving, therefore, fosters independent thinking and self-confidence in one's abilities to remain physically active. Problem solving involves several different steps (16). The acronym IDEA has been developed to identify the four steps of *I*dentifying the problem, *D*eveloping a list of solutions, *E*valuating the solutions, and *A*nalyzing how well the plan worked. Box 44-7 provides an example of this problem-solving technique.

The first step involves identifying the problem. From the list of barriers that your patient has been able to identify, have your patient pick one that is most pressing. In identifying the problem, it will be important to think through the problem fully to determine the key element or elements. In our example above of the woman who only walked when her neighbor was available, you should ask her to identify why this occurred. As the patient starts to talk about this, she may realize that she needs social support to be active. There are often many layers to any one problem, and it may be necessary to probe further to determine what about obtaining social support is important. In doing so, you may learn that walking with her neighbor is enjoyable, the time passes quickly, she feels safer, and she feels more motivated because she knows her friend is going to be meeting her.

The second step is to develop a list of solutions. This is a brainstorming session in which the patient thinks of any and all solutions while withholding any evaluation of them until later. This is a time to be creative. You may help your patient with a few if he or she is having trouble

BOX 44-7   **PROBLEM-SOLVING WORKSHEET IDEA**

1. Identify the problem.
2. Develop solutions.
3. Evaluate the solutions.
4. Analyze the plan.

EXAMPLE
1. Identify the problem: Don't want to exercise by myself.
   Details of the problem: Prefer the company, need the accountability, feel safer.
2. Develop solutions.

SOLUTIONS	EVALUATION	SELECT
Walk with my neighbor		
Walk with other friends		
Join an aerobics class		

3. Evaluate the solutions.

SOLUTIONS	EVALUATION	SELECT
Walk with my neighbor	She is too busy	
Walk with other friends	Offers company, safety, accountability	X
Join an aerobics class	Offers company, safety, and accountability but is too expensive	

4. Analyze the solution: Two friends agreed and I went on one walk with one friend and two walks with another friend. Seems to be working._____

YOUR TURN:
1. Identify the problem:_____
   Details of the problem:_____
   _____

2. Develop solutions.
3. Evaluate solutions.

SOLUTIONS	EVALUATION	SELECT

4. Analyze plan:_____

Modified with permission from Marcus BH, Forsyth LH. *Motivating People to be Physically Active*. Champaign (IL): Human Kinetics; 2003.

getting started. It is likely that you will need to remind your patient that you do not evaluate the ideas at this stage. Have the patient write down all of the solutions that are generated. Possible solutions for the female walker include seeing if her neighbor can walk more often, joining a class at a gym, walking with her spouse, starting a walking club, or finding other friends who are available on other days.

The third step is to evaluate the solutions. Some solutions will be more realistic and address more of the details of the problems than others. You can work with your patient to determine which of the solutions seem most appropriate. It may be that starting a walking club is too daunting but asking her neighbor to walk more often seems feasible. Whatever the solutions, work with your patient to set goals and make a concrete plan about how the solution will be implemented.

The final step is to analyze how well the plan worked. If a plan worked well, then praise the patient for a job well done. Many times, however, the plan will not have worked as was intended. It is important to emphasize that problem solving is a process that allows for learning and it is not uncommon to fine-tune the solution. In some cases, attempts to implement a solution elicit new details regarding the problem or new barriers. This information is critical to correctly identifying all of the important aspects of a problem and searching for a solution that addresses these aspects. Patients may be discouraged with their progress. It is important to emphasize the positive of what the patient did accomplish, emphasize the importance of learning from what does not work, and work together to generate new solutions and plans.

GOAL SETTING

> **1.9.1-HFS: Knowledge of behavioral strategies to enhance exercise and health behavior change (e.g., reinforcement, goal setting, social support).**

> **1.9.2-HFS: Knowledge of the important elements that should be included in each behavior-modification session.**

> **1.9.10-CES: Facilitation of effective and contemporary motivational and behavior-modification techniques to promote behavioral change.**

> **1.1.1-CES: List and apply behavioral strategies that apply to lifestyle modifications, such as exercise, diet, stress, and medication management.**

Another important skill for patients to develop is the ability to set goals (1,24,25,30). It is important to identify several characteristics of goal setting, including setting goals that are specific, short term, and challenging yet realistic (3). It also is also important to make goals measurable, develop a way to track goals through self-monitoring, and provide feedback regarding success or failure to achieve

goals. A popular model for framing a patient's goal is provided by the acronym SMART—goals that are Specific, Measurable, Action-oriented, Realistic, and Timely (30). In the context of the stages of change, the goals that are appropriate for patients vary by stage. For example, a person in precontemplation may read about the benefits of physical activity over the coming week, whereas a person in preparation may set a physical activity goal of walking four times per week for 30 minutes each time.

Setting goals that are specific is the first important characteristic of a goal. This might initially require some coaching. Patients may set a goal of "I will try to be more physically active." Although this is a good start and should be reinforced, getting the patient to fill in the details increases the likelihood of success. Therefore, work with your patient to establish specific and realistic goals related to physical activity that includes frequency, intensity, time, and type of activity. Consider individual circumstances and possible physical limitations. Help your patient set a short-term goal that is limited to the following week and realistic to achieve. For example, if a patient knows travel for business is scheduled in the following week, it may not be realistic to set a goal that is more achievable during a routine week at home. Accomplishing goals increases self-confidence and the likelihood that a patient will set more challenging goals in the future. On the other hand, it is also important to make sure that the goal is challenging and not too easy to accomplish because more difficult goals can provide increased motivation.

Writing down the goal and then recording activity is an important way for the patient to see his or her progress and to continue to identify barriers. The monitoring sheets provide feedback to the patient (Box 44-6) and an opportunity to reinforce any positive changes that the patient was able to make, even if all of the established goals were not met. Ideally, patients will learn how to give themselves feedback and feel proud of their accomplishments. In addition, the monitoring forms can provide opportunities for identifying barriers and problem-solving opportunities and serve as cues, or reminders, to be active.

CONFIDENCE

> **1.9.1-HFS: Knowledge of behavioral strategies to enhance exercise and health behavior change (e.g., reinforcement, goal setting, social support).**

> **1.9.2-HFS: Knowledge of the important elements that should be included in each behavior modification session.**

> **1.9.4-HFS: Knowledge of extrinsic and intrinsic reinforcement and give examples of each.**

> **1.9.10-CES: Facilitation of effective and contemporary motivational and behavior modification techniques to promote behavioral change.**

> **1.1.1-CES: List and apply behavioral strategies that apply to lifestyle modifications, such as exercise, diet, stress, and medication management.**

Self-efficacy, or confidence in one's abilities to be physically active, is very important for behavior change (1,3,5,8,14,21,24). Confidence can be increased in several ways: (a) through verbal praise and reinforcement, (b) by watching others be successful at the behavior, (c) by correctly interpreting the body's physiologic reaction to physical activity, and (d) through guided mastery experiences (3). The exercise professional can help patients with all of these components by encouraging their successes and by having them think of others who were successful. Additionally, the exercise professional can encourage patients to think about other areas in their lives in which they are successful and about how information from these experiences can help them with this new behavior change by guiding them to self-monitor, problem solve, set goals, and receive feedback. In this way, patients increase their confidence and become better equipped to problem solve new obstacles. The use of a patient-centered approach and matching the activity to patients' particular stages of change also help in increasing patients' confidence in being physically active. See Marcus and Forsyth (16) for a self-efficacy assessment and Brehm's and Griffin's books listed in the Selected References at the end of this chapter for more information about implementing strategies to improve your patients' self-efficacy.

RELAPSE PREVENTION

> **1.9.10-CES: Facilitation of effective and contemporary motivational and behavior modification techniques to promote behavioral change.**

> **1.1.1-CES: List and apply behavioral strategies that apply to lifestyle modifications, such as exercise, diet, stress, and medication management.**

> **1.9.5-CES: Recognize observable signs and symptoms of anxiety or depressive symptoms and the need for a psychiatric referral.**

Another area that can be helpful in working with your patients is that of **relapse prevention** (8,20,24,32). Preventing relapse (i.e., reverting to inactivity) is a proactive approach to problem solving future obstacles or for managing temporary lapses (i.e., temporary periods of inactivity). If you have a patient who has a life event coming up during which it will be difficult to remain active, you can identify the problem and engage in problem solving just as you would any other barrier. These times are often referred to as *high-risk situations*. Examples include times of bad weather, injury, losing an exercise partner, vacations, visitors, holiday gatherings, or other situations that might make it difficult to engage in physical activity.

There may also be times when you notice that your patient's activity level has dropped. Helping your patient see this as a temporary lapse and not a relapse can be helpful in getting the patient back into a routine of activity. To do this, you can problem solve and set goals but also let the patient know that although it is not unusual to have times of decreased activity, it is important to get back on track as soon as possible.

There may be times, however, when a patient is experiencing difficulties that are making physical activity difficult to accomplish. In some cases, a person may be experiencing depression, anxiety, or other mental health issues. Some of the symptoms of depression and anxiety are lack of energy and difficulty concentrating, both of which make attending to physical activity difficult. In these cases, it may be important to determine if there is a need to refer the person for additional help. For suspected depression, simply ask, "Are you feeling so sad or down that it is making it difficult to perform your daily activities?" For anxiety, the question "Are you feeling so nervous or anxious that it is making it difficult to perform your daily activities?" is appropriate. If the patient answers yes, then it is appropriate to recommend seeking help from a physician or a mental health professional.

SUMMARY

Health counselors have the opportunity to develop rapport and facilitate behavior change with their patients. This chapter discussed the patient-centered approach, which emphasizes techniques such as empathy, listening, active listening, and reflective statements (4,6,7,9–12,27–29,33). These skills can be used by counselors to understand the perspective of their patients. These counseling techniques can also be used when using behavior change techniques, such as tracking progress, solving problems, increasing confidence, setting goals, and providing feedback. Long-term success for patients will be enhanced as they become increasingly self-sufficient with these behavior change strategies. We would also like to encourage the use of print materials, the phone, and the Internet to maintain contact with your patients in addition to in-person sessions (15,16,18,19).

REFERENCES

1. Anderson ES, Wojcik JR, Winett RA, Williams DM. Social-cognitive determinants of physical activity: the influence of social support, self-efficacy, outcome expectations, and self-regulation among participants in a church-based health promotion study. *Health Psychol.* 2006;25(4):510–20.
2. Bandura A. *Social Foundations of Thought and Action: A Social Cognitive Theory.* Englewood Cliffs (NJ): Prentice Hall; 1986.
3. Bandura A. *Self-Efficacy: The Exercise of Control.* New York: W. H. Freeman and Company; 1997.
4. Bennett JA, Lyons KS, Winters-Stone K. Motivational interviewing to increase physical activity in long-term cancer survivors: a randomized controlled trial. *Nurs Res.* 2007;56(1):18–27.

5. Bray SR. Self-efficacy for coping with barriers helps students stay physically active during transition to their first year at a university. *Res Q Exerc Sport*. 2007;78(2):61–70.

6. Brehm BA. *Successful Fitness Motivation Strategies*. Champaign (IL): Human Kinetics; 2004.

7. Carels R, Darby L, Cacciapaglia, HM. Using motivational interviewing as a supplement to obesity treatment: a stepped-care approach. *Health Psychol*. 2007;26(3):369–74.

8. Dunn AL, Marcus BH, Kampert JB, Garcia ME, Kohl HW, Blair SN. Reduction in cardiovascular disease risk factors: 6-month results from Project ACTIVE. *Prev Med*. 1997;26(6):883–92.

9. Gavin J. *Lifestyle Fitness Coaching*. Champaign (IL): Human Kinetics; 2005.

10. Griffin JC. *Client-Centered Exercise Prescription*. 2nd ed. Champaign (IL): Human Kinetics; 2006.

11. Grueninger UL, Duffy FD, Goldstein MG. Patient education in the medical encounter: how to facilitate learning, behavior change, and coping. In: Lipkin M, Putnam S, Lazare A, editors. *The Medical Interview*. New York: Springer-Verlag; 1995.

12. Hardcastle S, Taylor A, Bailey M. A randomized controlled trial on the effectiveness of a primary health care based counseling intervention on physical activity, diet and CHD risk. *Patient Ed Counsel*. 2008;70(1):31–9.

13. Heesch KC, Mâss LC, Dunn AL. Does adherence to a lifestyle physical activity intervention predict changes in physical activity? *J Behav Med*. 2003;26(4):333–48.

14. Hughes SL, Seymour RB, Campbell RT. Long-term impact of Fit and Strong! on older adults with osteoarthritis. *Gerontologist*. 2006; 46(6):801–14.

15. Marcus BH, Emmons KM, Simkin-Silverman LR, et al. Evaluation of motivationally tailored vs. standard self-help physical activity interventions at the workplace. *Am J Health Promot*. 1998;12(4): 246–53.

16. Marcus BH, Forsyth LH. *Motivating People to be Physically Active*. Champaign (IL): Human Kinetics; 2003.

17. Marcus BH, Lewis BA. Stages of motivational readiness to change physical activity behavior. *President's Council on Physical Fitness and Sports Research Digest*. 2003;4:1–8.

18. Marcus BH, Lewis B, Williams DM, et al. Step into Motion: a randomized trial examining the relative efficacy of Internet vs. print-based physical activity interventions. *Contemp Clin Trials*. 2007; 28(6):737–47.

19. Marcus B H, Napolitano MA, King AC, et al. Telephone versus print delivery of an individualized motivationally-tailored physical activity intervention: Project STRIDE. *Health Psych*. 2007;26(4):401–9.

20. Marlatt GA, Gordon JR. *Relapse Prevention: Maintenance Strategies in the Treatment of Addictive Behaviors*. New York: Guilford Press; 1985.

21. McAuley E, Morris KS, Motl RW, Hu L, Konopack JF, Elavsky S. Long-term follow-up of physical activity behavior in older adults. *Health Psychol*. 2007;26(3):375–80.

22. Miller WR, Rollnick S. *Motivational Interviewing: Preparing People to Change Addictive Behavior*. New York: Guilford Press; 1991.

23. Napolitano MA, Lewis BA, Whitely JA, Marcus BH. Principles of health behavior change. In: Ehrman JK, editor. *Resource Manual for Guidelines for Exercise Testing and Prescription*, 6th ed. Champaign: Human Kinetics; 2009, p. 709–722.

24. Nies MA, Reisenberg CE, Chruscial HL, Artibee K. Southern women's response to a walking intervention. *Public Health Nurs*. 2003;20:146–52.

25. Nothwehr F, Yang J. Goal setting frequency and the use of behavioral strategies related to diet and physical activity. *Health Educ Res*. 2007;22(4):532–8.

26. Prochaska JO, DiClemente CC. Stages and processes of self-change of smoking: towards an integrative model of change. *J Consult Clin Psychol*. 1983;51:390–5.

27. Resnicow K, Jackson A, Blissett D. Results of the Healthy Body Healthy Spirit Trial. *Health Psychol*. 2005;24(4):339–48.

28. Rogers CT. A theory of therapy, personality, and interpersonal relationships as developed in the client-centered framework. In: Kock S, editor. *Psychology: The Study of a Science, vol. 3. Formulations of the Person and the Social Context*. New York: McGraw Hill; 1959.

29. Rollnick S, Mason P, Butler C. *Health Behavior Change: A Guide for Practitioners*. New York: Churchill Livingstone; 1999.

30. Shilts MK, Horowitz M, Townsend MS. Goal setting as a strategy for dietary and physical activity behavior change: a review of the literature. *Am J Health Promot*. 2004;19(2):81–93.

31. Smith HW. *The 10 Natural Laws of Successful Time and Life Management: Proven Strategies for Increased Productivity and Inner Peace*. New York: Warner; 1994.

32. Stetson BA, Frommelt SJ, Boutelle KN, Cole JD, Ziegler CH, Looney SW. Exercise slips in high-risk situations and activity patterns in long-term exercisers: an application of the relapse prevention model. *Ann Behav Med*. 2005;30(1):25–35.

33. Stewart M, Stewart M, Belle Brown J, et al. *Patient-Centered Medicine: Transforming the Clinical Method*. Thousand Oaks (CA): Sage Publications; 1995.

SELECTED REFERENCES FOR FURTHER READING

American College of Sports Medicine. *ACSM Fitness Book* 3rd ed. Champaign (IL): Human Kinetics; 2003.

Brehm BA. *Successful Fitness Motivation Strategies*. Champaign (IL): Human Kinetics; 2004.

Gavin J. *Lifestyle Fitness Coaching*. Champaign (IL): Human Kinetics; 2005.

Griffin JC. *Client-Centered Exercise Prescription*. 2nd ed. Champaign (IL): Human Kinetics; 2006.

Marcus BH, Forsyth LH. *Motivating People to be Physically Active*. Champaign (IL): Human Kinetics; 2003.

Marcus BH, Lewis BA. Stages of motivational readiness to change physical activity behavior. *President's Council on Physical Fitness and Sports Research Digest*. 2003;4:1–8.

Rollnick S, Mason P, Butler C. *Health Behavior Change: A Guide for Practitioners*. New York: Churchill Livingstone; 1999.

Stewart M, Stewart M, Belle Brown J, et al. *Patient-Centered Medicine: Transforming the Clinical Method*. Thousand Oaks (CA): Sage Publications; 1995.

INTERNET RESOURCES

- American Heart Association (exercise [physical activity] counseling): www.americanheart.org/presenter.jhtml?identifier=4534
- Cancer Control Planet (Physical Activity: 5 Steps to Effective Cancer Control Planning): http://cancercontrolplanet. cancer.gov/physical_activity.html
- Centers for Disease Control and Prevention, National Center for Chronic Disease Prevention and Health Promotion (Nutrition and Physical Activity): www.cdc.gov/nccdphp/dnpa/physical/index.htm

Channels for Delivering Behavioral Programs

An important consideration when developing a behavioral program for physical activity promotion relates to how it will reach the target population. *Reach* refers to the extent to which the message or program is delivered to the target population. The greater the reach, the greater the potential for affecting health. This chapter focuses on the modes or channels for delivering behavioral programs.

Only very motivated or strongly encouraged individuals seek out information and training from exercise professionals. More commonly, exercise professionals use one or more communication strategies to attract and engage the target population. Program objectives may include increasing the demand for, availability of, and access to physical activity programs as well as enhancing social norms that promote a physically active lifestyle.

With advances in technology and interactive communications, a multitude of channels for delivering health messages (e.g., personal, print, or electronic media) are available (Table 45-1). A communication framework can help select the most effective channel in delivering a message when considering important factors. Factors that influence the choice of channel delivery include the message and program objectives, the source, the target audience, and the context or setting.

The message may focus on health-supporting (e.g., walking, aerobic activity, strength training, stretching) or potentially health-compromising (e.g., excessive sedentary behaviors associated with television watching, video gaming) behavior. The source of the message may be an authoritative voice (e.g., exercise professional, teacher, physician) or organization (e.g., American College of Sports Medicine [ACSM], Centers for Disease Control and Prevention [CDC]), a famous figure (e.g., athlete, actor), or a layperson (e.g., peers). The target audience is the receiver of the message and may be defined by demographic (e.g., age, sex), geographic, social, cultural, or psychological factors. The message or program may occur in a variety of contexts or settings, such as a school, home, or work.

Characteristics of each factor influence the strategies chosen in delivering behavioral programs. Ideally, the selected channel should reflect the target audience's preferred format and context. It should also provide a feasible medium for delivering the message or program. For example, a program to increase vigorous physical activity (message) among adolescents (target audience) at school (context) might be delivered via the Internet, a text message, or an after-school program (channels). But a program developed for disabled older adults (target audience) to promote strength training (message) in assisted living programs (context) may select a very different delivery channel (e.g., individualized personal training, video).

This chapter focuses on channels for delivering behavioral programs and health promotion messaging.

TABLE 45-1. OPTIONS FOR APPLYING A COMMUNICATIONS MODEL

SOURCE	DELIVERY CHANNEL	TARGET AUDIENCE	CONTEXT/SETTING
• Celebrity • Health professional • Peer • Organization	• Personal (individual, group, curricula) • Print (brochures, books, tip sheets) • Electronic (telephone, radio, video, television, computer, cell phone, personal digital assistant)	• Age based • Race or ethnicity based • Geography based (e.g., city, neighborhood) • Culturally based • Psychological profile based (e.g., readiness to change)	• Home • School • Work site • Community organization • Religious institution

Individual delivery channels are presented by modality followed by a discussion of approaches for integrating them across multiple channels. Repeated presentation of information and behavior change strategies is often key to the adoption and maintenance of physical activity, and a multilevel approach is recommended. As much as possible, the strategies presented are evidence-based—that is, they are drawn from the research literature.

CHANNELS FOR HEALTH BEHAVIOR CHANGE

> **1.9.3-HFS: Knowledge of specific techniques to enhance motivation (e.g., posters, recognition, bulletin boards, games, and competitions).**

> **1.9.10-CES: Facilitation of effective and contemporary motivational and behavior modification techniques to promote behavioral change.**

PERSONAL COMMUNICATION

The oldest, most traditional channel is personal communication delivered individually in small groups, to organizations, or to entire communities. Program objectives often include teaching participants specific behavioral skills to incorporate regular physical activity participation into their daily routines. Personal communications may be delivered in a variety of contexts, including an individual's home, school, work site, church, community or commercial agency, primary care setting, or health fair.

In developing the U.S. *Guide to Community Preventive Services,* an extensive review was conducted of physical activity programs organized by channel delivery (8). The document reported strong evidence in support of individually based health behavior change programs, school-based physical education, and social support interventions in community settings. School-based physical education programs have been effective at increasing the amount of class time students spend engaged in physical activity with the benefit of reaching large groups of youths. Programs encouraging a decrease in sedentary activity (e.g., television watching, video games) also show promise. Strong evidence supports the use of inter-

ventions in community settings that focus on building, strengthening, and maintaining social networks for supporting physical activity involvement—examples include setting up "buddy" systems with peers, community walking groups, and social contracts. Insufficient evidence was found for classroom-based health education focused on information provision, college-based health education and physical education, or family-based social support programs.

An example of a physical activity program that centers on personal communication is the Community Healthy Activities Model Program for Seniors (CHAMPS II), an individually tailored, choice-based physical activity program for adults 65 years or older. The program guides participants in creating a physical activity regimen matched to their preferences, health, ability, and resources. The program includes an individual planning meeting, regular telephone contacts, and 10 monthly group workshops over a year's time. From baseline to 1-year follow-up, the program resulted in increased energy expenditure in moderate and overall physical activity as well as reductions in body mass index (23).

Personal communications are often the most effective of delivery channels, but are also time intensive. The result is often limited reach and costly dissemination. To reach a greater number of individuals, print and electronic media can be used alone or as an adjunct to personal communications.

PRINT MEDIA

Print media can take the form of informational pamphlets and brochures, newsletters, articles and newspaper inserts, advertisements, self-help materials and books, exercise diaries, direct mailings, and poster and billboard displays (Fig. 45-1).

Messages can be informative, persuasive, or promote the use of specific behavioral strategies (e.g., self-monitoring, personal fitness contracts). A variety of print materials are available free or at low cost from professional organizations such as the ACSM, the CDC, and other fitness, sport, or physical activity agencies.

A simple form of print media with demonstrated efficacy is the use of point-of-decision prompts that encourage people to use the stairs instead of elevators

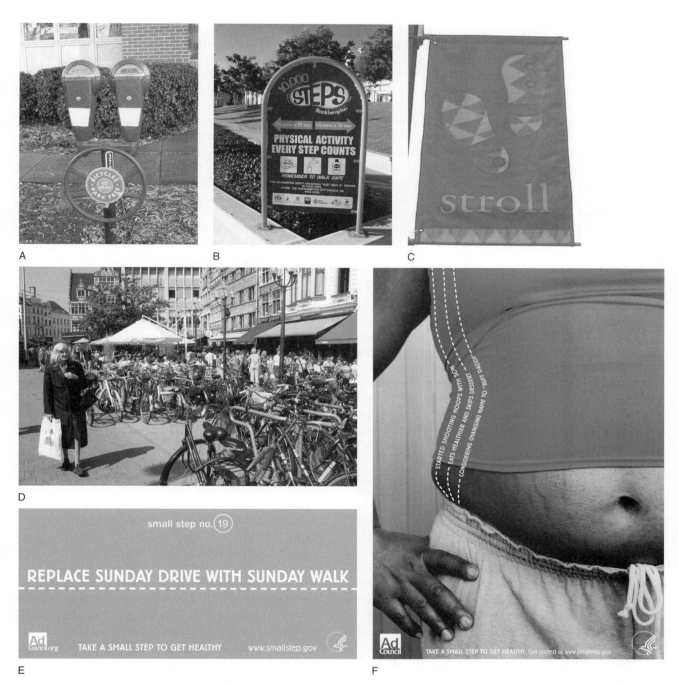

FIGURE 45-1. A: A sign supporting a policy of free parking for bicycles shows one of the multiple roles of communication. **B:** A multifaceted community intervention in Rockhampton, Australia, included this informational sign. **C:** A banner on a light pole in the Dupont Circle section of Washington, D.C. **D:** A communications program may work better in a culture that supports physical activity and in an environment that makes it easy to bike and walk. **E** and **F:** The Small Steps campaign included television and print advertisements. (Photo credit for A–D, James Sallis; image credit for E, F, public campaign of the Ad Council and the U.S. Department of Health and Human Services.)

and escalators. In five studies reviewed, increases in stair climbing exceeded 50% (8). Collaborations with local news agencies and commercial entities are another method of disseminating health messaging and program promotion. An innovative example is the ACSM's partnership with General Mills to promote physical activity messaging on the back of millions of Wheaties cereal

boxes. Importantly, print media can be used as a "pull" strategy, creating interest and consumer demand, in concert with a "push" strategy delivered by exercise professionals or interactive media channels.

Whereas traditional print mass media campaigns once took a one-size-fits-all approach, more recent efforts have focused on the development of targeted or tailored print communications. Targeted messages and materials are directed at a specific segment of the population, usually defined by one or more demographic or other shared characteristics, such as age, sex, race or ethnicity, or disease group. Tailored communications, on the other hand, are designed to reach specific individuals based on an assessment of their unique characteristics. As one moves from print mass media to targeted and tailored print communications, the message salience and relevance increases along with the program complexity and associated costs. Although tailored communications can be delivered as print media—a personalized handwritten prescription is a simple example—the advance of interactive technologies has made tailoring of health messages more feasible and cost effective.

ELECTRONIC MEDIA

Electronic media include radio, video, telephone, and computers. Recent years have seen a dramatic growth in the variety of electronic media channels available, including e-mail, the Internet, chat rooms, instant messaging and text paging, mobile phones, personal digital assistants, Web-enabled television, and other emerging technologies. The immediate advantage of electronic media is the potential for mass distribution to maximize reach. Interactive media also allows for dynamic tailoring of messages based on assessment of the target audience's characteristics and individual needs.

The most ambitious and well-funded physical activity promotion in the United States was VERB (which drew its name from the meaning of the word "verb" as the **grammatical** term for action), a national, multicultural, social marketing campaign targeting 9- to 13-year-old children. This CDC program had a $125 million budget in the first year to buy prime-time advertising. The media campaign was coordinated with local programs and events. In just 1 year, the program achieved a very high (74%) brand awareness, and youth exposed to the program increased their physical activity much more than those not exposed (6).

Twenty clinical trials have been conducted with demonstrated success to evaluate use of telephone-assisted counseling for physical activity promotion, some in conjunction with a dietary intervention (2). Diverse population groups have been studied, including healthy adults, men with uncomplicated postmyocardial infarction, older female caregivers of relatives with dementia, and adults with knee osteoarthritis. Telephone-based programs have the advantage of convenience, time efficiency, ready availability, and reduced burden associated with travel. In actuality, most programs have included telephone counseling as an adjunct or follow-up to an initial face-to-face contact. Whether used alone or in conjunction with other channels, the evidence supports telephone delivery of physical activity programming. The

California Department of Health Services is translating research into public health practice, funding more than 15 communities to develop and deliver local telephone-based physical activity programs throughout the state. The next generation of telephone-mediated physical activity programs is examining the use of automated systems using keypad data entry for assessment of participants' exercise goals and progress over time (2).

An example of interactive computer-mediated technologies is the Patient-Centered Assessment and Counseling for Exercise Plus Nutrition (PACE+) programs developed for adolescents and adults (17). The programs, delivered over the Internet, include a brief assessment of current physical activity involvement, as well as perceived benefits and barriers. Participants are then guided to develop an individually tailored plan for increasing their physical activity participation; relapse prevention plans are created by participants already meeting recommended levels of physical activity. The plan is printed for review with participants' healthcare providers. Follow-up to support identified goals can occur by mail and/or via telephone counseling. Evaluation of this program with 878 adolescent boys and girls indicated significant reductions in sedentary behaviors for boys and girls and significant increase in days of activity for boys (13). Computer-based delivery channels can be a useful mode of efficiently assessing individual needs and providing personally relevant recommendations. With the capacity to add e-mail messaging and hosted chat rooms, delivery channels such as the Internet expand the possibilities for communication between exercise professionals and their patients.

In 2005, 68% of American adults reported using the Internet, up from 63% in 2004 (14). A 2006 survey reported that 80% of American Internet users, or some 113 million adults, have used the Web to get information on at least one of seventeen health topics, with 44% searching for information on exercise or fitness (16). Limited access to new technologies, however, can reduce reach and contribute to health disparities. Commonly referred to as the "digital divide," persons with less education, certain racial and ethnic groups, people with low income, aging populations, and those residing in rural households are less likely to have Internet access. A 2006 survey reported that 56% of Latinos reported use of the Internet compared with 71% of non-Hispanic whites and 60% of non-Hispanic blacks (15). An identified goal for the nation is to increase the proportion of households with Internet access at home from 26% in 1998 to 80% by 2010 (26). Last, the explosion of growth and the popularity of the Internet increase the risk of poor quality health information (1) as well as risks to privacy and confidentiality of personal health information. As with other channels of delivery, use of electronic media requires careful consideration of message development and characteristics of the target population.

INTEGRATING ACROSS MULTIPLE CHANNELS

Because inactive lifestyles are so common, and specific programs reach only a minority of people, it is widely believed that coordinated, long-term community-wide intervention approaches are needed to increase physical activity levels in the population (9). There is no standard approach to community-wide programs, but they provide opportunities for integrating interventions using a variety of communication channels, in several settings, to reach numerous subgroups of people. The most extensive community-wide physical activity interventions were the heart disease prevention programs conducted during the 1980s in the United States (3,11,27). The studies provide examples of ways to integrate physical activity messages across multiple channels.

All the programs used extensive print media that included booklets, books, self-help kits, tip sheets to post on refrigerators, newspaper columns and stories, billboards, and advertising to promote products, programs, and events. Some of the studies used television ads, programs, and news stories extensively. Radio was used to target specific subgroups, such as Spanish speakers, with ads, news stories, and even health-related soap operas. Personal communication was delivered in health counseling sessions, lectures to community groups, at health fairs, and in courses in schools and colleges. The projects engaged media experts to coordinate the development and delivery of messages, and investigators assured the relevance of the materials by pretesting drafts. Other staff worked with representatives of work sites, schools, and community organizations to deliver information and programs in various settings.

The Stanford Five-City Project (FCP) relied heavily on electronic and print mass media, along with face-to-face activities such as classes. Examples of interventions included a self-help "Walking Kit" and physical activity contests between companies. Young et al. reported modest but statistically significant changes in physical activity (27). The Minnesota Heart Health Program (MHHP) concentrated more on promoting physical activity through local health professionals and community organizations. Large proportions of the communities participated in risk factor screenings, followed by feedback, personal counseling, and printed materials. The MHHP found small but significant physical activity intervention effects over the first 3 years of the program (11). The Pawtucket Heart Health Project (PHHP) was built around partnerships with community organizations, churches, schools, and work sites. One example was the ExerCity program, run by the Department of Recreation, which provided training of activity leaders and promoted use of community resources (e.g., trails) for activity. PHHP did not have any significant effects on physical activity in the population (3). The somewhat disappointing results of all three studies may be partly explained by the modest investment in physical activity promotion compared with other goals, resulting in insufficient numbers of people who were exposed to the materials or participated in programs. The complexity of intervening on multiple risk factors in multiple communities was found to present many challenges to the investigators. Thus, subsequent community interventions have had more modest goals and have identified carefully defined target communities.

A project in Wheeling, West Virginia, was built around paid media advertising but used several other media in a coordinated fashion. The target population was older adults in a small town, and the target behavior was walking, making the intervention more focused than the earlier community interventions. Two paid television ads were shown 683 times over an 8-week period, radio ads were broadcast 1,988 times, and newspaper ad space was bought. Weekly press conferences and coverage of campaign-related events created an even greater media presence. Printed information on walking was distributed at work sites, a Web site allowed people to log their walking, prescription pads for walking were distributed to physicians, and lectures were given to community organizations. Because the media market was small, the project was able to buy enough ads so the average household was exposed more than 50 times to the walking message. Among initially sedentary older adults, 32% in the intervention community met physical activity guidelines at the end of the campaign, compared with 18% in a control community (18). This study may have had stronger effects than previous community interventions because of the high intensity of the media campaign and the limited focus of the targeted behavior (walking) and population (older adults).

Agita Mundo (meaning "shake or move the world") is an approach to physical activity promotion that has had global impact in just a few years. The program began as *Agita Sao Paulo* in Brazil, with interventions targeted to three audiences: schoolchildren, workers, and older adults. *Agita* uses extensive partnerships to extend limited resources, and print materials create brand awareness and deliver the 30-minute-per-day message. Massive public events in schools, work sites, and senior centers generate extensive free press coverage, so program reach is very high in a state of 36 million people (12). The approach was quickly adopted throughout Brazil, then by other countries in Latin America. The World Health Organization used *Agita* as the model for annual Move for Health Days.

POLICY AND ENVIRONMENTAL APPROACHES

Ecologic models of health behavior state that because there are multiple levels of influence on behavior, the most effective interventions should change all levels of influences, including psychological, social, policy, and environmental factors (21). Policy and environmental changes are now seen as essential components of physical activity promotion that complement communications approaches. Motivating people to become more active is not likely to be effective if safe, convenient, pleasant, and affordable places for physical activity are lacking. Physical activity must be done in specific places, and the characteristics of those places matter. Places can be seen as modes of communication. As mentioned earlier, signs by stairways increase stair use (8). Adding markings to playgrounds increases children's physical activity at recess by communicating this is a good place to play a game (24). People who have exercise equipment at home or live near parks or health clubs are more likely to be physically active than those lacking such resources (7,20), partially because these environments provide cues to be active.

The design of neighborhoods seems to have communications value. Fear of crime is higher when potential criminals have many places to hide and potential victims cannot be seen by others (10). People are more active in neighborhoods designed for pedestrians, with nearby shops and services built up to the sidewalk, so the views constantly change as people walk. Neighborhoods built to maximize automobile traffic can discourage walking through having no nearby destinations, discomfort from fast traffic, and boredom from passing by large parking lots (4). Expert panels concluded there is substantial evidence that people who live in "walkable" neighborhoods are more physically active than those who live in automobile-oriented suburbs (5,25).

The Active Living by Design program supports 25 communities around the United States to take a comprehensive approach to physical activity promotion that includes projects to improve the physical environment as well as education programs targeting individuals. The partnerships directing each community program often have representatives from the fields of recreation, planning, and transportation who can engage those sectors in physical activity change efforts.

Policies reflect decisions made by governments and private groups that can affect physical activity (22). Policies control incentives for behavior. Incentives for physical activity could be insurance discounts for active individuals or similar reimbursement for workers who drive or ride bikes for company business. Policies also control the physical environment. Relevant policies may include requiring parks and playgrounds in new developments, mandating a percentage of transportation funds be spent on pedestrian and cycling facilities, and requiring schools to be opened for community use in the evenings and on weekends.

Communication approaches can be useful in achieving policy and environmental changes, though the target audiences and messages need to be expanded. The same communication channels of print, electronic media, and personal interaction still apply. Communication to the lay public can provide information on the benefits of changing policies as well as to motivate advocacy of these changes to policy makers. Policy makers in government and industry become critical audiences for communication. Because policies that affect physical activity can be made by those with responsibility for transportation, real estate, public safety, recreation, education, and healthcare (9,19), there are many target audiences of policy makers.

Physical activity professionals are involved in advocating for policy and environmental changes to promote physical activity. ACSM has several policy initiatives and is one of the primary sponsors of the National Coalition for Promoting Physical Activity, whose mission is to advocate for physical activity. Smart Growth America advocates for walkable communities, and the Surface Transportation Policy Project advocates for transport investments to support walking and cycling.

Those designing physical activity interventions are challenged to expand the messages to include motivation and skills instruction for behavior change as well as advocacy for policy and environment change. For substantial population improvements in physical activity, it may be necessary for those designing interventions to communicate not only with target audiences in the general public but also with policy makers in government and the private sector.

SUMMARY

Channels through which physical activity messages and programs are transmitted can take multiple pathways. Formats include print and electronic media and personal communications. Channel selection is guided by consideration of the target audience's preferred format and context, as well as characteristics of the program to be delivered. With the dramatic increases in communication technology, a wide variety of delivery channels is available. To increase physical activity in large populations, it is necessary to use a variety of communication channels to deliver an array of messages to multiple target audiences. Supplementing communications with other intervention strategies and advocating for policy and environmental changes are important adjuncts to consider.

This chapter provided examples of how different communication channels can be integrated in a coordinated approach. Communications can be used for multiple purposes, including motivating and educating individuals, promoting other physical activity interventions, and encouraging individuals to advocate for policy and environmental changes. To maximize the reach of behavioral programs, the use of multiple channels is encouraged. With greater expansion of delivery channels, however, there comes the greater potential for inaccurate or poor-quality messaging. When multiple channels are used, monitoring the consistency, reliability, and credibility of delivered program content is crucial.

REFERENCES

1. Doshi A, Patrick K, Sallis JF, Calfas K. Evaluation of physical activity web sites for use of behavior change theories. *Ann Behav Med.* 2003;25:105–11.
2. Eakin EG, Lawler SP, Vandelanotte C, Owen N. Telephone interventions for physical activity and dietary behavior change. *Am J Prev Med.* 2007;32:419–34.
3. Eaton CB, Lapane KL, Garber CE, Gans KM, Lasater TM, Carleton RA. Effects of a community-based intervention on physical activity: the Pawtucket Heart Health Program. *Am J Public Health.* 1999;89: 1741–4.
4. Frank LD, Engelke PO, Schmid TL. Health and community design: the impact of the built environment on physical activity. Washington (DC): Island Press; 2003. 250 p.
5. Heath GW, Brownson RC, Kruger J, et al. The effectiveness of urban design and land use and transport policies and practices to increase physical activity: a systematic review. *J Phys Activity Health.* 2006;3(Suppl 1):S55–76.
6. Huhman M, Potter LD, Wong FL, Banspach SW, Duke JC, Heitzler CD. Effects of a mass media campaign to increase physical activity among children: year-1 results of the VERB campaign. *Pediatrics.* 2005;116:e277–84.
7. Humpel N, Owen N, Leslie E. Environmental factors associated with adults' participation in physical activity: a review. *Am J Prev Med.* 2002;22:188–99.
8. Kahn EB, Ramsey LT, Brownson RC, et al. The effectiveness of interventions to increase physical activity. *Am J Prev Med.* 2002; 22(Suppl):73–107.
9. King AC, Stokols D, Talen E, Brassington GS, Killingsworth R. Theoretical approaches to the promotion of physical activity: forging a transdisciplinary paradigm. *Am J Prev Med.* 2002;23(Suppl 2): 15–25.
10. Loukaitou-Sideris A, Eck JE. Crime prevention and active living. *Am J Health Promot.* 2007;21(Suppl):380–9.
11. Luepker RV, Murray DM, Jacobs DR, et al. Community education for cardiovascular disease prevention: risk factor changes in the Minnesota Heart Health Program. *Am J Public Health.* 1994;84: 1383–93.
12. Matsudo SM, Matsudo VR, Andrade DR, et al. Physical activity promotion: experiences and evaluation of the Agita Sao Paulo program using the ecological mobile model. *J Phys Activity Health.* 2004;1: 81–97.
13. Patrick K, Calfas KJ, Norman GJ, et al. Randomized controlled trial of a primary care and home-based intervention for physical activity and nutrition behaviors: PACE+ for adolescents. *Arch Pediatr Adolesc Med.* 2006;160:128–36.
14. Pew Internet and American Life Project. Digital divisions. Available from: www.pewinternet.org/pdfs/PIP_Digital_Divisions_Oct_5_2005. pdf. Accessed September 19, 2007.
15. Pew Internet and American Life Project. Digital divisions: Latinos online. Available from: www.pewinternet.org/pdfs/Latinos_Online_March_14_2007.pdf. Accessed September 19, 2007. Accessed September 19, 2007.
16. Pew Internet and American Life Project. Online health search 2006. Available from: www.pewinternet.org/pdfs/PIP_Online_Health_2006.pdf
17. Prochaska JJ, Zabinski MF, Calfas KJ, Sallis JF, Patrick K. PACE+: Interactive communication technology for behavior change in clinical settings. *Am J Prev Med.* 2000;19:127–31.
18. Reger B, Cooper L, Booth-Butterfield S, et al. Wheeling Walks: A community campaign using paid media to encourage walking among sedentary older adults. *Prev Med.* 2002;35:285–92.
19. Sallis JF, Cervero RB, Ascher W, Henderson KA, Kraft MK, Kerr J. An ecological approach to creating active living communities. *Annu Rev. Public Health.* 2006;27:297–322.
20. Sallis JF, Kerr J. Built environment and physical activity. *PCPFS Research Digest.* 2006;7(4):1–8.
21. Sallis JF, Owen N. Ecological models of health behavior. In: Glanz K, Rimer BK, Lewis FM, editors. *Health Behavior and Health Education: Theory, Research, and Practice.* 3rd ed. San Francisco: Jossey-Bass; 2002. p. 462–84.
22. Schmid TL, Pratt M, Witmer L. A framework for physical activity policy research. *J Phys Activity Health.* 2006;3(Suppl 1):S20–9.
23. Stewart AL, Verboncoeur CJ, McLellan BY, et al. Physical activity outcomes of CHAMPS II: a physical activity promotion program for older adults. *J Gerontology.* 2001;56A(8):M465–70.
24. Stratton G, Mulla En. The effect of multicolor playground markings on children's physical activity level during recess. *Prev Med.* 2005; 41:828–33.
25. **Transportation Research Board and Institute of Medicine. *Does the Built Environment Influence Physical Activity? Examining the Evidence.* Washington (DC): National Academies Press; 2005.**
26. U.S. Department of Health and Human Services. *Healthy People 2010: Understanding and Improving Health.* 2nd ed. Washington (DC): U.S. Government Printing Office; 2000.
27. Young DR, Haskell WL, Taylor CB, Fortmann SP. Effect of community health education on physical activity knowledge, attitudes, and behavior: the Stanford five-city project. *Am J Epidemiol.* 1996;144: 264–74.

SELECTED REFERENCES FOR FURTHER READING

Heath GW, Brownson RC, Kruger J, Miles R, Powell KE, Ramsey LT, and the Task Force on Community Preventive Services. The effectiveness of urban design and land use and transport policies and practices to increase physical activity: a systematic review. *J Phys Activity Health.* 2006;3(suppl 1):S55–76.

Heath GW, SL Martin, editors. *Promoting Physical Activity: A Guide to Community Action.* 2nd ed. Champaign (IL): Human Kinetics; 2008.

Hillsdon M, Foster C, Thorogood M. Interventions for promoting physical activity. *Cochrane Database Syst Rev.* 2005;25(1): CD003180.

Kroeze W, Werkman A, Brug J. A systematic review of randomized trials on the effectiveness of computer-tailored education on physical activity and dietary behaviors. *Ann Behav Med.* 2006;31 :205–23.

Marcus BH, Williams DM, Dubbert PM, et al. Physical activity intervention studies: what we know and what we need to know. *Circulation.* 2006;114:2739–52.

Sallis JF, Owen N. Interventions to promote physical activity in communities and populations. In: *Physical Activity & Behavioral Medicine.* Thousand Oaks (CA): Sage Publications; 1999. p. 153–74.

Weinreich NK. *Hands-On Social Marketing: A Step-by-Step Guide.* Thousand Oaks (CA): Sage Publications; 1999. 255 p.

INTERNET RESOURCES

- Active Living by Design: www.activelivingbydesign.org
- Active Living Network: Communications Toolkit: www.activeliving.org/index.php/Communications_Toolkit/80
- *Agita Mundo* (meaning "shake or move the world"): www.agitasp.com.br
- Centers for Disease Control and Prevention Community Guide (Task force recommendations on increasing physical activity with links to sample evidence-based programs focused on informational approaches, behavioral and social approaches, and environmental and policy approaches): www.thecommunityguide.org/pa/default. htm
- National Coalition for Promoting Physical Activity (Resource Guide): www.ncppa.org/resources.asp
- Smart Growth America: www.smartgrowthamerica.org
- Surface Transportation Policy Project: www.stpp.org
- VERB Campaign, Centers for Disease Control and Prevention: www.cdc.gov/youthcampaign

The evolution in medicine has contributed immensely to the early detection and treatment of chronic diseases, especially cardiovascular diseases (CVDs). A substantial decrease in CVD mortality rates are primarily because of the advances in medical technology, pharmacologic therapies, and preventive/rehabilitative strategies (19). Although improved detection and treatment of chronic diseases have resulted in declining mortality rates, this has led to a growing population of individuals requiring additional healthcare resources to effectively manage their chronic disease. Furthermore, the explosive birth rates that occurred following World War II (1946–1960) is leading to a sharp increase in today's aging population; the first wave of baby boomers are now older than 60 years of age. The higher prevalence of chronic diseases and an expanding aging population has major implications for healthcare and associated healthcare costs (24). However, the actual causes of death and disability from chronic diseases remain largely preventable. In 2000, the top leading causes of preventable death in the United States were attributed to tobacco use, poor diet, and physical inactivity (27). Public health and healthcare systems are challenged with a sense of urgency to develop and deliver more effective interventions that will help address the negative health behaviors that contribute to the disease burden on our nation. Physical activity recommendations are based on the increasing scientific evidence that demonstrates the health benefits of physical activity and exercise for improving physical fitness and reducing the risk of chronic diseases and disabilities (22). Because exercise is also effective in the treatment of many chronic diseases, especially CVDs, healthcare providers are expected to include exercise counseling in their treatment plans (35). As such, there is a growing need for well-qualified exercise professionals in preventive and rehabilitative settings.

This chapter defines the roles and scope of practice of the various levels of American College of Sports Medicine (ACSM) certifications available to the exercise professional. Eligibility criteria based on academic background and practical experience is provided for each of the respective credentials.

EXERCISE AS MEDICINE

Healthcare professionals, including physicians, are encouraged to prescribe physical activity for health and disease management (16). Individuals with chronic disease (e.g., cardiovascular, pulmonary, and/or metabolic) are

> > > KEY TERMS

Ability: The translation of knowledge and skills into behaviors and actions that lead to desired outcomes.

Accreditation: Approval of an educational program according to defined standards.

Certification: A process, often voluntary, by which individuals who have demonstrated the level of knowledge and skill required in the profession, occupation, or role are identified to the public and other stakeholders (28).

Competence: Multifaceted and dynamic concept that encompasses knowledge, skills (i.e., technical,

interpersonal, and problem solving), attitudes, and values that are identified as essential in meeting performance expectations (38).

Knowledge: Facts and information acquired by a person through education and/or experience and practical understanding of a subject.

Skill: A technique or strategy that is usually learned and acquired through training to perform a specific action or a defined set of actions (skill set).

commonly challenged by reduced functional capacity. An inactive lifestyle can exacerbate the associated disease-specific sequelae, causing many individuals to experience secondary complications, such as muscle atrophy, fatigue, weakness and frailty, which leads to continued functional decline. Evidence continues to support the role of exercise on improving the health and fitness or improving the recovery of individuals who are coping with chronic diseases (34). "Exercise as medicine" is an emerging theme that healthcare professionals are incorporating into their treatment strategies. Numerous professional organizations have responded to the need for evidence-based exercise recommendations and have published position and scientific statements with examples listed in Box 46-1.

Despite the available preventative and rehabilitative exercise recommendations, physical activity promotion in primary care disciplines remains suboptimal. Furthermore, the majority of traditional healthcare professionals (physicians, nurses, etc.) have limited academic training and experience in exercise training, physical activity counseling, or addressing the complexities involved with facilitating behavior change (14). The opportunity for success in using exercise to positively affect the health of individuals increases as there is improved collaboration among multiple health disciplines, including exercise professionals. Effective exercise programs can be provided in a variety of settings (e.g., home, community, commercial, corporate, and rehabilitative) if individuals with the appropriate exercise knowledge and skill sets are included in the intervention team.

MEETING EDUCATIONAL AND TRAINING NEEDS

The current editions of *ACSM's Resource Manual* and *ACSM's Guidelines for Exercise Testing and Prescription* represent the ongoing evolution of science related to exercise since this text was first published in 1975. Paralleling the release of ACSM's first guidelines was the development of a certification process to validate the knowledge, skills, and abilities of the exercise professional. ACSM workshops and certifications have served as the industry's gold standard and have provided opportunities for exercise practitioners to develop and advance as professionals. The provision of standardized educational materials and rigorous examinations by ACSM helps prepare exercise professionals and other healthcare providers to more effectively counsel their patients regarding exercise and the benefits of a physically active lifestyle. A recent advancement by ACSM in preparing exercise professionals in the clinical setting is the establishment of a registry program that defines requirements and competencies for the practice of clinical exercise physiology. The practice of an ACSM Registered Clinical

Exercise Physiologist® (RCEP) is restricted to patients who are referred by and are under the care of a licensed physician. A complete description about ACSM's certification and registry programs is available in the Appendix, which also includes a complete listing of the knowledge, skills, and abilities (KSAs) for each of the respective credentials. The content matter for the ACSM certification and registry programs is shown in Box 46-2.

KNOWLEDGE, SKILLS, AND ABILITIES

The *ACSM's Resource Manual* is designed to provide background information, comprehensive resources, and the scientific evidence that supports the more succinct information that is found in the companion text, *ACSM's Guidelines for Exercise Testing and Prescription*. Because KSAs compose the foundation of ACSM certification and registry examinations, a brief review of the learning domains as described by Bloom (26) is discussed, as it is relevant to ACSM certifications.

The original work of Benjamin Bloom and his educational psychology colleagues identified three domains (or categories) of educational activities (10). The original taxonomy identified the three learning categories as cognitive (knowledge), psychomotor (skills), and affective (attitude). These learning behaviors serve as the goals of the training/educational process and thus are incorporated into the ACSM educational resources and certification/registry examinations.

The *knowledge* category relates to recalling and comprehending information acquired through a variety of venues, which may include academic preparation and systematic study, educational offerings through professional organizations, and guided and/or self-learning opportunities. *Skills* encompass the ability to demonstrate certain psychomotor or technical competence as well as exhibiting appropriate and effective communication/interaction activities that are deemed relevant for a specific task or job requirement. Skills are learned through guided learning in protocol/procedure-based training in laboratory settings and/or supervised practical experiences. Such experiences are usually acquired through student internships associated with academic programs or in conjunction with work experiences guided by mentoring from an experienced professional. Affective learning was originally described by Bloom as *attitude*, which referred to growth in feelings or emotional areas (26). Attitude refers to how things are internalized, such as feelings, values, enthusiasm, motivation, and appreciation. Although ACSM currently uses the term *abilities,* the concept remains true to the original concept in describing affective learning behavior. The ability to translate knowledge and skills into desired actions and performance capabilities requires behavior that is based on internal values, active learning (internally motivated),

BOX 46-1	SELECTED POSITION STANDS AND SCIENTIFIC STATEMENTS RELATED TO PHYSICAL ACTIVITY, FITNESS AND HEALTH

1992:	AHA Recognizes Physical Inactivity as 5th Major Alterable CVD Risk Factor
1992:	AHA Scientific Statement: Statement on Exercise (17)
1994:	ACSM Position Stand: Exercise for Patients with Coronary Artery Disease (2)
1995:	CDC/ACSM Joint Position Statement: Physical Activity and Public Health (31)
1995:	AHA Scientific Statement: Statement on Exercise Standards (16)
1996:	U.S. Surgeon General's Report on Physical Activity and Public Health (37)
1996:	AHA Scientific Statement: Statement on Exercise (18)
1997:	AHA Scientific Statement: How to Implement Physical Activity in Primary and Secondary Prevention (15)
1998:	ACSM Position Stand: Recommendations for the Quantity and Quality of Exercise for Improving and Maintaining Cardiorespiratory and Musculoskeletal Fitness, and Flexibility in Healthy Adults[a] (4)
1998:	ACSM Position Stand: Exercise for Older Adults (3)
2000:	ACSM Position Stand: Exercise and Type 2 Diabetes (5)
2000	AHA Scientific Statement: Resistance Exercise in Individuals with and without Cardiovascular Disease: Benefits, Rationale, Safety, and Prescription (33)
2001:	ACSM Position Stand: Appropriate Intervention Strategies for Weight Loss and Prevention of Weight Regain for Adults (6)
2002:	IOM/NAS Nutritional and Physical Activity Recommendations for Weight Loss and Weight Maintenance (23)
2002	ACSM Position Stand: Progression Models in Resistance Training for Healthy Adults (7)
2003:	AHA Scientific Statement: Exercise and Heart Failure (32)
2003	AHA Scientific Statement: Exercise and Physical Activity in Prevention and Treatment of Atherosclerotic Heart Disease (35)
2003	WHO Global Strategy on Diet, Physical Activity and Health (www.who.int/dietphysicalactivity/en/)
2004:	ACSM Position Stand: Exercise and Hypertension (8)
2004	ACSM Position Stand: Physical Activity and Bone Health (9)
2004	AHA Scientific Statement: Physical Activity and Exercise Recommendations for Stroke Survivors (21)
2005:	USDA: Dietary Guidelines for Americans (Physical Activity and Weight Management) (www.healthierus.gov/dietaryguidelines)
2006:	AHA Scientific Statement: Physical Activity Intervention Studies: What We Know and What We Need to Know (25)
2007:	AHA Scientific Statement: Exercise and Acute Cardiovascular Events: Placing the Risk in Perspective (36)
2007:	ACSM and AHA: Physical Activity and Public Health Update (22)
2007:	ACSM and AHA: Physical Activity and Public Health in Older Adults Update (29)

ACSM, American College of Sports Medicine; AHA, American Heart Association; CDC, Centers for Disease Control; CVD, cardiovascular disease; IOM/NAS, Institute of Medicine/National Academy of Sciences; USDA, U.S. Department of Agriculture; World Health Organization.

[a]Update from the 1978 and 1990 position stands.

Note: This is not an exhaustive list. There are other guidelines and recommendations for establishing clinical competencies, cardiac rehabilitaion programming, exercise testing and assessing functional capacities. In addition, there are other population-specific scientific statements on physical activity and exercise from organizations including the American Association of Cardiovascular and Pulmonary Rehabilitation, American Geriatric Society, American College of Obstetricians and Gynecologists, American Medical Association, American College of Physicians, and American College of Chest Physicians.

listening, and empathetic compassion. This hierarchy of learning behaviors of knowledge, skills, and abilities are interrelated and overlapping, and it is often difficult to designate specific criteria for each category. The ACSM KSAs as listed represent the interdependence of these learning behaviors when defining the recommended competencies in knowledge, skills, and abilities for each of the credentials.

Competence is a multifaceted and dynamic concept that includes the integration of knowledge, skills, and abilities and describes performance attributes in a particular job function or role (30). Competencies reflect the legal, ethical, regulatory, and political influences on the practice of professionals in healthcare that are defined as essential for a practitioner within a specific health discipline. Establishing core competencies to account for professionalism in today's healthcare industry is becoming increasingly important. In healthcare, core competencies are used to define the discipline with a set of measurable indicators required for minimal expectations for performance. The core competencies provide a framework to align practitioners, students, educators, and consumers with expectations for service delivery in accordance with evidence-based standards and performance measures (38). The certification processes established by ACSM are designed to assess competency of eligible candidates through standardized and objective evaluation with respect to the defined measures of knowledge, skills, and abilities attributed to a specific ACSM credential.

DEVELOPING COMPETENT EXERCISE PROFESSIONALS

One of the most important challenges in establishing a quality exercise-based preventive or rehabilitative program is recruiting competent personnel to provide safe and efficacious interventions. Qualified personnel are necessary at multiple levels to fulfill the essential roles in providing exercise services and physical activity interventions in a variety of settings that serve healthy individuals and/or patients with known disease. Academic

preparation and certification processes validate that minimal competency requirements are met by the professionals who are providing the services. The extent of academic preparation, experience, and credentialing that an exercise professional would need to perform his or her job competently depends largely on local, state, and federal regulations; other regulatory organizations (e.g., Centers for Medicare and Medicaid Services, Joint Commission on Accreditation of Hospitals); institutional or organizational policy; services provided; and population served.

ACADEMIC PREPARATION

Major advances were recently realized in establishing standards and guidelines in the academic preparation of exercise professionals under the auspices of the Commission on Accreditation of Allied Health Programs (CAAHEP) (13). The CAAHEP program accreditation is an effort to assess the quality of academic institutions and programs by measuring them against agreed-upon standards developed by professionals involved in specific disciplines. For exercise disciplines, the Committee on Accreditation for the Exercise Sciences (CoAES) developed these standards and guidelines. CoAES consists of leadership members representing key professional organizations related to exercise and fitness; they are listed in Box 46-3 (11).

The standards and guidelines are intended to reflect what a professional needs to know and be able to do to function successfully within that profession. The standards and guidelines are used for the development, evaluation, and self-analysis of programs that offer academic degrees in exercise-related fields. Accreditation serves an important function for students seeking qualified programs and also serves an important public interest to inform employers and consumers of expectations from qualified exercise professionals. Accreditation of academic programs in preparing the exercise professionals are defined for the disciplines of personal fitness training, exercise science, and exercise physiology, as described in Table 46-1. Additional information on CAAHEP and

BOX 46-3	COMMITTEE ON ACCREDITATION FOR THE EXERCISE SCIENCES (CoAES) PARTICIPATING ORGANIZATIONAL SPONSORS

American Alliance for Health, Physical Education, Recreation, and Dance: www.aahperd.org

American Association of Cardiovascular and Pulmonary Rehabilitation: www.aacvpr.org

American College of Sports Medicine: www.acsm.org

American Council on Exercise: www.acefitness.org

American Kinesiotherapy Association: www.akta.org

Cooper Institute: www.cooperinst.org

Medical Fitness Association: www.medicalfitness.org

National Academy of Sports Medicine: www.nasm.org

National Strength and Conditioning Association: www.nsca.com

CoAES and accreditation processes can be found at their Web sites.

SKILLS AND ABILITIES

Exercise professionals need to combine art and science to successfully guide interventions that will help their patients achieve optimal outcomes. There are specific desired traits and skills that are common among all professionals who are responsible for providing services that are known to influence the health and well-being of individuals and groups (Table 46-2). Working well within a multidisciplinary team and establishing positive relationships between the exercise leader and participant appear to be particularly important (20). Facilitating

desired behavior change is complex, and exercise professionals must gain understanding and proficiency in implementing effective behavioral strategies for lifestyle modification, including exercise.

LEARNING EXPERIENCES IN THE REAL WORLD

Developing competencies for the exercise practitioner requires opportunities to practice necessary skill sets. The value of "real-world" experiences that students gain by participating in internships or by being precepted by experienced exercise professionals during on-the-job training is fundamental in developing competencies. Various skill sets

TABLE 46-1. SUMMARY DESCRIPTIONS OF THE EXERCISE PROFESSIONS

EXERCISE PROFESSION	DESCRIPTION
Personal Fitness Trainer	• Skilled practitioners who work with a wide variety of patient demographics in one-to-one and small group environments • Familiar with multiple forms of exercise used to improve and maintain health-related components of physical fitness and performance • Knowledgeable in basic assessment and development of exercise recommendations • Proficient in leading and demonstrating safe and effective methods of exercise, motivating individuals to begin and continue with healthy behaviors • Consult with and refer to other appropriate allied health professionals when patient conditions exceed the personal trainer's education, training, and experiences
Exercise Science	• Academically prepared with a Bachelor's degree • Trained to assess, design, and implement individual and group exercise and fitness programs for individuals who are apparently healthy and those with controlled disease • Skilled in evaluating health behaviors and risk factors, conducting fitness assessments, writing appropriate exercise prescriptions, and motivating individuals to modify negative health habits and maintain positive lifestyle behaviors for health promotion • Demonstrated competence as a leader of health and fitness programs in the university, corporate, commercial, or community settings in which their patients participate in health promotion and fitness-related activities
Exercise Physiology • Applied Exercise Physiology • Clinical Exercise Physiology	• Academically prepared with a Master's degree • Manage programs to assess, design, and implement individual and group exercise programs for apparently healthy individuals and those with controlled disease • Work under the direction of a physician in the application of physical activity and behavioral interventions in clinical situations in which they have been scientifically proven to provide therapeutic or functional benefit

From the Commission on Accreditation for the Exercise Sciences Web site. Available from: www.CoAES.org. Accessed July 1, 2007.

TABLE 46-2. TRAITS AND SKILLS OF SUCCESSFUL EXERCISE PROFESSIONALS

TRAITS	SKILLS
Models healthy lifestyle	Application of knowledge
Dependable and accountable	Technically competent
Ethical	Empathetic listening
Positive and self-confident	Behavior change counseling
Compassionate and tactful	Articulate in communication (oral, written, and group presentations)
Energetic and enthusiastic	Setting priorities, organized
Creative and innovative	Problem solving
Team player, maintains good rapport with coworkers	Provides leadership
Flexible and adaptable, receptive to constructive suggestions	Motivating
Responds calmly and effectively under pressure	Evaluate and interpret data to guide interventions
Alert to social environment and sensitive to diversity	Critical thinking

and experiential activities are needed for students to attain the technical competencies and critical thinking abilities that are required to effectively implement strategies in risk assessment, interventions, and outcome evaluation.

Some colleges and universities have established curriculum-based outreach programs to combine academic learning, practical experience, and community outreach as part of an overall effort to improve the real-world training for their students. This approach also provides an opportunity to improve the health and fitness of the surrounding community. Students training to become exercise professionals benefit by having an opportunity to practice their knowledge, skills, and abilities while serving as technicians in the health appraisal and/or exercise programming process. In many programs, students are able to work closely with physicians and other healthcare professionals. These university-based programs provide experiences that enable students to gain a tremendous professional advantage as they compete for internships and jobs in hospital-based clinical programs, corporate wellness, and commercial fitness settings.

INTERNSHIPS

Internship programs offered through qualified institutions or healthcare systems are ideal opportunities to create win-win situations for students, academic programs, and participating work sites. Students have opportunities to apply their knowledge and advance their skill sets in a real-world environment under the supervision of experienced professionals. Academic programs have the opportunity to collaborate with practicing exercise professionals to better prepare their students in developing, assessing, and validating proficiencies. Participating workplaces benefit by integrating contemporary knowledge brought by students into their practice. Additionally, students provide an ideal pool of candidates from which organizations can recruit and hire because the students are already knowledgeable about program services, policies and procedures, and have worked with existing staff and patients.

Successful internship experiences require careful planning with clear expectations agreed upon by the faculty advisor, the work-site preceptor or supervisor, and the student. A contract agreement between the academic institution and agency/institution is required that defines expectations related to supervision and monitoring, learning objectives, and evaluation criteria. The KSAs for ACSM certification provide an ideal outline structure to guide experiential learning experiences for skill-based activities during the internship experience. For example, a set of KSAs previously agreed upon by the internship supervisor and the work-site preceptor could comprise a checklist for evaluating interns in each of the categories listed in section C of Figure 46-1. Well-documented learning objectives provide clear direction and targeted goals for the intern while providing objective measurement criteria for the preceptor and advisor. Ideally, the supervising preceptor at the work site is a certified exercise professional familiar with the KSAs and experienced in the required skills sets. The training nature of an internship requires sufficient supervision that includes assignment of special projects that will stimulate professional growth through real-world experiences. Because of the multidisciplinary approach of healthcare services, the preceptor may need to arrange additional learning activities with collaborating professionals who are proficient with desired skill sets that may not be routinely performed in one department. For example, an applied exercise physiology student may intern within a cardiac rehabilitation program, but the clinical exercise testing may be conducted in another department. In this example, the student may be assigned for observational and practice activities under the supervision of a skilled professional in the clinical exercise testing area. Documentation and constructive feedback of specific objectives are very important for achieving effective learning. Preceptors should take time to evaluate both the student's positive accomplishments and provide suggestions for improvement. Figure 46-1 summarizes some evaluation points for preceptors or supervisors to consider when

5 -exceeds expectations; 4-often meets expectations; 3-regularly meets expectations; 2-sometimes doesn't meet expectations; 1-seldom meets expectations; NA=not applicable						
A. Attendance and Punctuality						
1. Arrives to work prepared and on time, with few absences	5	4	3	2	1	NA
2. Proves to be responsible when completing assigned tasks	5	4	3	2	1	NA
B. Professionalism, Judgment, and Attitude						
1. Exhibits self-direction and responsibility for actions	5	4	3	2	1	NA
2. Demonstrates compassion for the client/patient; maintains confidentiality	5	4	3	2	1	NA
3. Exhibits enthusiasm and interest toward work	5	4	3	2	1	NA
4. Establishes and maintains good rapport with coworkers	5	4	3	2	1	NA
5. Recognizes the value of teamwork and functions well as a member of the team	5	4	3	2	1	NA
6. Exhibits a strong sense of ethical behavior	5	4	3	2	1	NA
7. Is receptive to constructive suggestions or corrections	5	4	3	2	1	NA
8. Responds calmly and effectively under pressure	5	4	3	2	1	NA
9. Observes rules of safety	5	4	3	2	1	NA
10. Adjusts well to new tasks and situations	5	4	3	2	1	NA
11. Participates in continuing education and professional development	5	4	3	2	1	NA
C. Knowledge, Skills and Abilities: Demonstrates a working knowledge of the following principles						
1. Exercise Physiology and Related Exercise Science	5	4	3	2	1	NA
2. Pathophysiology and Risk Factors	5	4	3	2	1	NA
3. Health Appraisal, Fitness, and Clinical Exercise Testing	5	4	3	2	1	NA
4. Electrocardiography and Diagnostic Techniques	5	4	3	2	1	NA
5. Patient Management and Medications	5	4	3	2	1	NA
6. Exercise Prescription and Programming	5	4	3	2	1	NA
7. Nutrition and Weight Management	5	4	3	2	1	NA
8. Human Behavior and Counseling	5	4	3	2	1	NA
9. Safety, Injury Prevention, and Emergency Procedures	5	4	3	2	1	NA
10. Program Administration, Quality Assurance, and Outcome Assessment	5	4	3	2	1	NA

FIGURE 46-1. Example of an employer evaluation survey of an exercise professional.

assessing student or employee progress in achieving the learning objectives (12).

CERTIFICATION OF EXERCISE PROFESSIONALS

The primary purpose for certifying practitioners is to protect the public. This is accomplished by establishing standards related to a profession and insuring that practitioners demonstrate minimal competencies within the specific discipline or scope of practice. The National Commission for Certifying Agencies (NCCA), which serves under the auspices of the National Organization for Competency Assurance (NOCA), is and example of an accreditation organization that "credentials the credentials" (28). Although there are numerous organizations that provide certification opportunities for exercise professionals, it is important for practitioners to choose a credentialing process that is most appropriate for their work setting.

The resource information provided in this manual is directed toward preparing eligible exercise professionals for certification as ACSM Health/Fitness Specialist (HFS)® and ACSM Clinical Exercise Specialist (CES)®. Additional resources are available on the ACSM Web site to help prepare professionals interested in ACSM certification for Personal Trainer® and the Registered Clinical Exercise Physiologist®.

Certified HFSs and CESs have demonstrated competencies to function independently and within teams that include services related to physical activity promotion, exercise testing, prescription, training, and other lifestyle behavior changes. Table 46-3 provides a summary of ACSM's criteria for minimal recommendations for certification as HFS or CES plus some potential roles and career opportunities within each level of certification.

HEALTH FITNESS SPECIALIST

A Health Fitness Specialist® (HFS) is a healthcare professional with the background and training necessary to conduct and manage individual and group exercise and fitness programs for apparently healthy individuals and those with controlled disease. The HFS® is capable of evaluating health behaviors and risk factors, conducting pre-exercise evaluations, making fitness assessments, developing exercise prescriptions, and monitoring exercise sessions. In addition, the HFS® is qualified to provide health promotion educational programming and motivate individuals to adopt, practice, and maintain positive lifestyle behaviors. HFS-certified individuals employed as work-site wellness

TABLE 46-3. CRITERIA AND POTENTIAL ROLES OF PROFESSIONALS SEEKING ACSM CERTIFICATION IN HEALTH FITNESS SPECIALIST® AND CLINICAL EXERCISE SPECIALIST®

	HEALTH/FITNESS SPECIALIST® (HFS)	CLINICAL EXERCISE SPECIALIST® (CES)
Academic preparation	Associate's degree or a Bachelor's degree in a health-related field from a regionally accredited college or university	A Bachelor's degree in a health-related field from a regionally accredited college or university
Knowledge	Demonstrate knowledge of exercise science, kinesiology, functional anatomy, exercise physiology, nutrition, program administration, injury prevention, risk-factor and health-status identification, exercise prescription, and psychology	In addition to demonstrating attainment of knowledge as described for HFS®, the CES will demonstrate more extensive knowledge of functional anatomy, exercise physiology, pathophysiology, electrocardiography, human behavior/psychology, gerontology, graded exercise testing for apparently healthy and diseased populations, exercise supervision/leadership, counseling, and emergency procedures related to exercise testing and training
Skills	Demonstrate competence in defined skill sets required within the health and fitness field	Demonstrate competence in defined skill sets required within community and/or healthcare settings that serve a broader population with established disease or at high risk for developing chronic disease
Abilities	Demonstrate ability to synthesize knowledge and skills through delivery of suitable services designed to achieve desired outcomes for improved function and lifestyle behaviors among groups and/or individuals	Demonstrate ability to synthesize knowledge and skills through delivery of suitable services designed to achieve desired outcomes for improved function and lifestyle behaviors among apparently healthy individuals with multiple risk factors and those with established disease
Clinical hour requirement	No minimal hours required	Minimum 600 hours of practical experience in a clinical exercise program
Other certification requirements	Current adult cardiopulmonary resuscitation (CPR) that has a practical examination component (available through the AHA or the ARC)	Current certification as a basic life support (BLS) provider for the professional rescuer (available through the AHA or the ARC)
Certified	A professional who meets the requirements and demonstrates minimal competencies in the KSAs for HFS® certification as defined by ACSM	A healthcare professional who meets the requirements and has demonstrated minimal competencies in the KSAs for CES® certification as defined by ACSM
Role	HFS® is qualified to assess, design, and implement individual and group exercise and fitness programs for low-risk individuals and individuals with controlled disease.	CES® is qualified to deliver a variety of exercise assessment, training, rehabilitation, risk-factor identification and lifestyle-management services to individuals with or at risk for cardiovascular, pulmonary, and metabolic disease(s).
Potential career opportunities	Health and fitness facilities Work-site wellness programs Community health promotion agencies or organizations Research program related to exercise promotion in apparently healthy populations	Cardiac and pulmonary rehabilitation Multidisciplinary teams providing lifestyle and risk-reduction services: preventive cardiology, chronic disease management (e.g., heart failure, diabetes, obesity, metabolic syndrome, peripheral artery disease) Research program related to exercise in special populations

ACSM, American College of Sports Medicine; AHA, American Heart Association; ARC, American Red Cross; KSAs, knowledge, skills, and abilities.

coordinators, fitness directors, and program managers should also have some training and experience in management, marketing, accounting, and finance.

CLINICAL EXERCISE SPECIALIST®

A Clinical Exercise Specialist® is qualified to deliver a variety of exercise assessment, training, rehabilitation, risk-factor identification, and lifestyle-management services to individuals with or at risk for cardiovascular, pulmonary, and metabolic disease(s). The most common professional role for the CES® is working within a multidisciplinary healthcare team in a cardiac and/or pulmonary rehabilitation program. The healthcare team is generally the first interface with patients, family, and physicians in the application of these exercise and risk-reduction services. Clinical Exercise Specialists® often work within a multidisciplinary health team. The number, disciplinary background, and professional specialization of the team may include licensed and unlicensed healthcare professionals, depending on the nature and size of the program. Nevertheless, the collective knowledge base of those assigned to provide diagnostic testing or exercise treatment services must include a comprehensive and up-to-date understanding of varied topic areas described previously within the KSAs (see Box 43.2). The professions most frequently represented in preventive and rehabilitative exercise programs include physicians (e.g., cardiologists, pulmonologists, internists, family practitioners, physiatrists), specially trained nurses, exercise specialists, clinical exercise physiologists, nutritionists, health educators, health psychologists, social workers, vocational rehabilitation counselors, physical or occupational therapists, and pharmacists. The minimum and preferred experience and educational qualifications for these disciplines are available in previously published sources (1) and in the clinical exercise program chapter of this manual (Chapter 49) (39). In smaller programs with only a few individuals assigned to services on a full- or part-time basis, it is important for team members to cross-train and assume multiple roles (within their scope of practice) to effectively deliver exercise-related services according to evidence-based guidelines. Common responsibilities assumed by a Clinical Exercise Specialist® in a healthcare setting include clinical exercise testing, exercise prescriptions for high-risk populations, patient education and risk-factor counseling, and assumption of the role of a cardiopulmonary rehabilitation specialist.

CONTINUED EDUCATION RESOURCES AND OPPORTUNITIES

It is important for healthcare professionals to participate in continuing education activities related to all facets of their scope of work (e.g., exercise, nutrition) to keep current with the latest scientific evidence and care practices.

Continuing education may also be required for ongoing certification and/or licensure. Examples of professional organizations that provide continuing education and resources that may be relevant to health professionals providing exercise services in healthcare settings are listed in the Internet Resource list at the end of this chapter.

SUMMARY

Exercise professionals have the responsibility to provide safe, effective, and enjoyable forms of physical activity to the patients they serve. To this end, exercise professionals must possess a thorough knowledge of exercise and accompanying physiologic responses, recognize individual differences and adapt exercise interventions as needed, and motivate participants to engage in healthy behaviors. Exercise professionals play a critical role in favorably affecting physical activity and health outcomes among the persons they serve.

REFERENCES

1. American Association of Cardiovascular and Pulmonary Rehabilitation. *Guidelines for Cardiac Rehabilitation and Secondary Prevention Programs*. 4th ed. Champaign (IL): Human Kinetics; 2004. p. 193–6.
2. American College of Sports Medicine. Exercise for patients with coronary artery disease. *Med Sci Sports Exerc.* 1994;26(3):i–v.
3. American College of Sports Medicine. Position Stand: Exercise for older adults. *Med Sci Sports Exerc.* 1998;30(6):992–1008.
4. American College of Sports Medicine. Position Stand: Recommendations for the quantity and quality of exercise for improving and maintaining cardiorespiratory and musculoskeletal fitness in health adults. *Med Sci Sports Exerc.* 1998;30:975–91.
5. American College of Sports Medicine. Position Stand: Exercise and type 2 diabetes. *Med Sci Sports Exerc.* 2000;32(7):1345–60.
6. American College of Sports Medicine. Position Stand: Appropriate intervention strategies for weight loss and prevention of weight regain for adults. *Med Sci Sports Exerc.* 2001;33(12):2145–56.
7. American College of Sports Medicine. Position Stand: Progression models in resistance training for healthy adults. *Med Sci Sports Exerc.* 2002;34(2):364–80.
8. American College of Sports Medicine. Position Stand: Exercise and hypertension. *Med Sci Sports Exerc.* 2004;36(3):533–53.
9. American College of Sports Medicine. Position Stand: Physical activity and bone health. *Med Sci Sports Exerc.* 2004;36(11):1985–96.
10. Bloom BS. *Taxonomy of Educational Objectives, Handbook 1: Cognitive Domain.* Boston: Addison Wesley Publishing Co.; 1956; p. 25–39.
11. Commission on Accreditation for the Exercise Sciences Web site. Available from: www.CoAES.org. Accessed July 1, 2007.
12. Commission on Accreditation for the Exercise Sciences Web site. Self-Study Application Forms and Instructions. Part B., 14. Available from: www.CoAES.org. Accessed July 1, 2007.
13. Commission on Accreditation of Allied Health Programs Web site. Available from: www.caahep.org. Accessed July 1, 2007.
14. Estabrooks PA, Glasgow RE, Dzewaltowski DA. Physical activity promotion through primary care. *JAMA.* 2003;289(22):2913–16.
15. Fletcher GF. How to implement physical activity in primary and secondary prevention: a statement for healthcare professionals from the Task Force on Risk Reduction, American Heart Association. *Circulation.* 1997;96:355–7.
16. Fletcher GF, Balady G, Froelicher VF, Hartley LH, Haskell WL, Pollock ML. Exercise standards: a statement for health care

professionals from the American Heart Association Writing Group. Circulation. 1995;91:580–615.

17. Fletcher G, Blair S, Blumenthal C, et al. Statement on exercise: benefits and recommendations for physical activity programs for all Americans. A statement for health professionals by the Committee on Exercise and Cardiac Rehabilitation of the Council on Clinical Cardiology, American Heart Association. *Circulation.* 1992;86:340–4.

18. Fletcher GF, Blair S, Blumenthal C, et al. Statement on exercise: benefits and recommendations for physical activity programs for all Americans. A statement for health professionals by the Committee on Exercise and Cardiac Rehabilitation of the Council on Clinical Cardiology, American Heart Association. *Circulation.* 1996;94: 857–62.

19. Ford ES, Ajani U, Croft JB, et al. Explaining the decrease in U.S. deaths from coronary disease, 1980–2000. *N Engl J Med.* 2007; 356(23):2388–98.

20. Franklin B. Program factors that influence exercise adherence: practical adherence skills for the clinical staff. In: Dishman R, editor. *Exercise Adherence: Its Impact on Public Health.* Champaign (IL): Human Kinetics; 1988. p. 237–58.

21. Gordon N, Gulanik M, Costa F, et al. AHA Scientific Statement: Physical activity and exercise recommendations for stroke survivors: an American Heart Association Scientific Statement from the Council on Clinical Cardiology, Subcommittee on Exercise, Cardiac Rehabilitation, and Prevention; the Council on Cardiovascular Nursing; the Council on Nutrition, Physical Activity, and Metabolism; and the Stroke Council. *Circulation.* 2004;109:2031–41.

22. Haskell W, Lee I, Pate R, et al. Physical activity and public health: updated recommendation for adults from the American College of Sports Medicine and the American Heart Association. *Med Sci Sports Exerc.* 2007;39(8):1423–34.

23. Institute of Medicine. Physical activity. In: Institute of Medicine, editor. *Dietary Reference Intakes for Energy, Carbohydrate, Fiber, Fatty Acids, Cholesterol, Protein and Amino Acids.* Washington (DC): National Academies Press; 2005. p. 880–935.

24. Jemal A, Ward E, Hao Y, Thun M. Trends in the leading causes of death in the United States, 1970–2002. *JAMA.* 2005;294(10):1255–9.

25. Marcus B, Williams D, Dubbert P, et al. AHA Scientific Statement: Physical activity intervention studies: what we know and what we need to know. A Scientific Statement from the American Heart Association Council on Nutrition, Physical Activity, and Metabolism (Subcommittee on Physical Activity); Council on Cardiovascular Disease in the Young; and the Interdisciplinary Working Group on Quality of Care and Outcomes Research. *Circulation.* 2006;114: 2739–52.

26. Martin J. Encyclopedia of Educational Technology Web site. Available from: http://coe.sdsu.edu/eet/articles/BloomsLD/. Accessed July 1, 2007.

27. Mokdad AH, Marks JS, Strou DF, Gerberding JL. Actual causes of death in the United States, 2000. *JAMA.* 2004;291(10):1238–45.

28. National Organization for Competency Assurance Web site. Available from: www.info@noca.org. Accessed July 1, 2007.

29. Nelson M, Rejeski J, Blair S, et al. Physical activity and public health in older adults: recommendations from the American College of Sports Medicine and the American Heart Association. *Med Sci Sports Exerc.* 2007;39(8):1435–45.

30. Neufeld VR. *Assessing Clinical Competence.* New York: Springer; 1985. p. 330–41.

31. Pate R, Pratt M, Blair S. Physical activity and public health. *JAMA.* 1995;273:402–7.

32. Pina I, Apstein C, Balady G, et al. AHA Scientific Statement: Exercise and heart failure. Circulation. 2003;107:1210–25.

33. Pollock M, Franklin B, Balady G, et al. AHA Scientific Statement: Resistance exercise in individuals with and without cardiovascular disease: benefits, rationale, safety, and prescription. *Circulation.* 2000;101:828–33.

34. Taylor RS, Brown A, Ebrahim S, et al. Exercise-based rehabilitation for patients with coronary heart disease: systematic review and meta-analysis of randomized controlled trials. *Am J Med.* 2004;116(10):682–92.

35. Thompson P, Buchner D, Pina I, et al. AHA Scientific Statement: Exercise and physical activity in prevention and treatment of atherosclerotic heart disease. A Statement from the Council on Clinical Cardiology (Subcommittee on Exercise, Rehabilitation, and Prevention) and the Council on Nutrition, Physical Activity, and Metabolism (Subcommittee on Physical Activity). *Circulation.* 2003;107:3109–16.

36. Thompson P, Franklin B, Balady G, et al. AHA Scientific Statement: Exercise and acute cardiovascular events placing the risks into perspective: a scientific statement from the American Heart Association Council on Nutrition, Physical Activity, and Metabolism and the Council on Clinical Cardiology; American College of Sports Medicine. *Circulation.* 2007;115:2358–68.

37. U.S. Department of Health and Human Services. *Physical Activity and Health: A Report of the Surgeon General.* Atlanta, GA. U.S Department of Health and Human Services, Centers for Disease Control & Prevention, and National Center for Chronic Disease Prevention & Health Promotion; Washington DC; 1996.

38. Verma S, Paterson M, Medves J. Core competencies for health professionals: what medicine, nursing, occupational therapy and physiotherapy share. *J Allied Health.* 2006;35:109–15.

39. Verrill DE, Savage P, Sanderson B. Clinical exercise program development and operation. In Ehrman JK, editor. *Resource Manual for Guidelines for Exercise Testing and Prescription,* 6th ed. Champaign: Human Kinetics; 2009 p. 777–788.

INTERNET RESOURCES

- American Association of Cardiovascular and Pulmonary Rehabilitation (AACVPR): www.aacvpr.org
- American College of Cardiology (ACC): www.acc.org
- American College of Sports Medicine (ACSM): www.acsm.org
- American Council on Exercise (ACE): www.acefitness.org
- American Diabetic Association (ADA): www.diabetes.org/home.jsp
- American Heart Association (AHA): www.americanheart.org
- Commission on Accreditation of Allied Health Programs (CAAHEP): www.caahep.org
- Commission on Accreditation for the Exercise Sciences (CoAES): www.coaes.org
- National Academy of Sports Medicine (NASM): www.nasm.org
- Preventive Cardiology Nurses Association (PCNA): www.pcna.net
- Society of Behavioral Medicine (SBM): www.sbm.org

CHAPTER 47

Community Physical Activity Interventions

COMMUNITY PHYSICAL ACTIVITY INTERVENTIONS: PLANNING AND EVALUATION

In this chapter, research that underlies community programs for the promotion of physical activity (PA) was examined with a particular focus on those that used ecological approaches (i.e., addressed both environmental and individual level strategies). The purpose was to address issues of planning and evaluation to ensure that a community intervention achieves the best possible public health impact. The content of the chapter includes four primary sections: (a) community intervention terminology, (b) types of community interventions (i.e., site-based interventions; community-wide), (c) principles for planning and evaluation of community PA interventions, and (d) recommendations for planning and evaluation to heighten the public health impact of community PA programs.

COMMUNITY INTERVENTION TERMINOLOGY

What is a community PA intervention? A logical starting point might be to check with the *Guide to Community Preventives Services* ("the Guide"), written by a body that completes systematic reviews of the literature and pro-vides recommendations for community intervention across a variety of behaviors (35). In 2002, the Guide provided several conclusions and recommendations related to effective PA interventions that ranged from placing signs that promote stair use to providing individually tailored interventions (Box 47-1) (35). Yet the content and reports from the Guide suggest a range of strategies that can be used, but does not clarify the question of the boundaries of what should be considered as a "community" intervention. That is, the recommendations, while valuable, do not provide an explanation of or definition for community or community intervention.

One issue is that there are several definitions of community (74). For example, a community can be defined as an aggregate of people who share a common identity, set of values, or institution (3). This could include, among others, communities based on racial background (e.g., the Latino community), sexual preference (e.g., the gay community), or educational status (e.g., the academic community). Communities may also be defined to include a spatial component that refers to the location of groups of people or institutions, such as work sites or faith-based organizations. Finally, communities may be linked based on social norms, belief structures, and personal attachments (56).

A second issue is that community PA interventions can be operationalized in several different ways. For

> > > KEY TERMS

Adoption: The participation rate of organizations that will ultimately implement the intervention, policy, or environmental change and the representativeness of those organizations to the population that could implement the intervention.

Community intervention: A place-based focus that is defined by a geographic boundary that can be narrowed (e.g., local community health center) or expanded (e.g., one state within a country) based on the planned intervention strategy.

Implementation: The degree to which an intervention is implemented as intended. Finally, maintenance is defined at both the individual and organizational level.

Reach: The participation rate and representativeness of participants who engage in an intervention or are exposed to a policy or environmental change.

Sustainability: The continued delivery of a given intervention or the institutionalization of an intervention within typical community settings.

BOX 47-1	THE GUIDE TO COMMUNITY PREVENTIVE SERVICES RECOMMENDED APPROACHES TO INCREASE PHYSICAL ACTIVITY

- Point-of-decision prompts
- Community-wide campaigns
- School-based physical education
- Social support interventions in community settings

- Individually adapted health behavior change programs
- Creation of or enhanced access to places for physical activity combined with informational outreach activities

example, the Stanford Five-City Project, which included policy, program, and environmental changes across several boroughs, is considered a community intervention (23). In contrast, the Rockford CHIP program—which provided an intensive educational curriculum to employees and community residents that included 2-hour sessions 5 days a week for a month through the Center for Complementary Medicine—is also described as a community intervention (16).

Clearly, the Stanford Five-City Project and Rockford CHIP are very different interventions, but both are legitimate community interventions. To reconcile these disparate interventions into a consistent genre of health promotion, a useful definition of community for the purposes of intervention implementation and evaluation is a place-based focus that is defined by a geographic boundary that can be narrowed (e.g., local community health center) (5) or expanded (e.g., one state within a country) (46) based on the planned intervention strategy. This definition allows for the inclusion of the Stanford and Rockford interventions and the preventive strategies suggested by the Guide. Point-of-decision prompts, community-wide campaigns, school-based interventions, increased access to PA resources, and even individually adapted behavior change programs can fit within the definition of community through reference to a specified geographic area of intervention. The following discussion of community PA interventions uses a place-based focus to categorize previous research and demonstration projects as site-based or community-wide interventions—all with the consistent characteristic of targeting a specified geographic locale.

TYPES OF COMMUNITY PHYSICAL ACTIVITY INTERVENTIONS

> **1.9.1-HFS: Knowledge of behavioral strategies to enhance exercise and health behavior change (e.g., reinforcement, goal setting, social support).**

> **1.11.4-HFS: Knowledge of the importance of tracking and evaluating member retention.**

> **1.11.7-HFS: Ability to develop marketing materials for the purpose of promoting fitness-related programs.**

> **1.11.9-HFS: Ability to develop and administer educational programs (e.g., lectures, workshops) and educational materials.**

> **1.11.11-HFS: Knowledge of networking techniques with other healthcare professionals for referral purposes.**

> **1.9.10-CES: Facilitation of effective and contemporary motivational and behavior modification techniques to promote behavioral change.**

A recent trend in the literature (over the past 10 years) has been to use ecological models that, like the geographic definition of community, can be narrowed to guide intervention strategies in specific settings such as schools, clinics, work sites, or churches and expanded to identify strategies across numerous settings within a larger community-wide initiative (12,13,18,23,46,57, 60,65,71,73,77,80). A basic ecological theory proposition is that the characteristics and attributes of an individual interact with the characteristics and attributes of the surrounding social and physical environment (80). Ecological models can include variables that range from biological and genetic factors that influence behavior to municipal policies to the built form of the environment (73). Because of the comprehensive nature of these models, interventions that are based in ecological theory often limit the range of strategies to some combination of individual and environmental strategies.

SITE-BASED INTERVENTIONS

School Physical Activity Interventions

The tradition of providing American children with opportunities for PA and physical education at school can be dated to the late 1800s (55). Daily PA was readily accumulated through recess time, physical education classes, intra- and extramural sports, and active transportation to and from school (84). Unfortunately, the current opportunities for PA in schools are not as widespread. Despite a wide range of bodies providing recommendations for increased PA promotion in schools (8,10,55), federal policies such as No Child Left Behind increase the focus on instructional time, thereby creating an unintended consequence of reduced physical education and recess time as well as extending instructional time into the after-school hours—a prime time for children and youth to be physically active.

Recently, the National Association for Sport and Physical Education's Shape of the Nation report documented the reduction in the percentage of students attending physical education classes on a daily basis between 1991 and 2003—from 42% to 28% (52). The report also highlights that approximately 30% of states do not mandate physical education for elementary and middle school students, and almost a quarter of states allow physical education to be completed using online course work (52). In addition, the proportion of schools that provide daily physical education or the recommended amount of time per week of physical education is only approximately 8% for elementary and 6% for middle and high schools (5). Even when physical education is offered, it is typical that less than 40% of the class time is used for moderate to vigorous PA (47,75).

Fortunately, there is some evidence to support the promise for school-based interventions to successfully increase student participation in PA (43,48,49,51,60, 72,82). An early and seminal example is SPARK (Sports, Play, and Active Recreation for Kids). SPARK included two general intervention components: changes to the physical education environment and student self-management. These components reflected an ecological interplay between enhancing student perceptions and confidence for PA while modifying the physical education class environment to include a greater opportunity for regular PA. The physical education component was designed to foster high levels of PA, teach movement skills, and be fun for the students. The self-management component taught children general behavior change skills (e.g., self-monitoring, goal setting, and problem solving) to increase PA outside of school time (72).

The initial randomized controlled trial of SPARK demonstrated that the program successfully increased PA during physical education classes and improved some fitness indices (49,72). Follow-up to this trial provided evidence that teachers who were trained in the SPARK curriculum were able to sustain the delivery 18 months after the training occurred (49). Increased student PA during classes was also sustained (49). Although SPARK did not significantly increase PA outside of school time, another trial, CATCH (Child and Adolescent Trial for Cardiovascular Health), which used a more comprehensive approach (60) but had similar curricular principles, was able to influence both in class and outside of school PA (77). These effects were sustained at 2-year follow-up (51).

The Middle School Physical Activity and Nutrition (M-SPAN) (71), the Healthy Youth Places Project (13), and the Lifestyle Education for Activity Program (LEAP) (57) all used comprehensive multicomponent strategies based on ecological theory and were successful in increasing PA. In M-SPAN and Healthy Youth Places, the students were the primary drivers of activities and were provided with ideas for policy and environmental changes that could facilitate increased PA. Another innovation used consistently across these interventions was social marketing and communications strategies. In the Healthy Youth Places project, students were provided with computers, software, and cameras, which they used to develop public service videos played over the school announcement and multimedia systems.

Pate et al. summarized the current body of literature and provided nine recommendations for PA policy and practice in school settings (Box 47-2) (55). First, schools are recommended to ensure that all students participate daily in at least 30 minutes of moderate to vigorous PA. Second, evidence-based health-related physical

---

BOX 47-2   SCHOOL-BASED POLICY AND PRACTICE RECOMMENDATIONS TO INCREASE PHYSICAL ACTIVITY

- All children participate in a minimum of 30 minutes of moderate to vigorous physical activity during each school day.
- Evidence-based physical education programs should be used.
- Physical education should be taught by certified physical education teachers.
- State policy should hold schools accountable for meeting national physical education standards.
- Schools should expand physical activity opportunities beyond physical education.

- Schools should promote active transportation to and from school.
- Child development and elementary schools should provide 30 minutes of recess every day.
- Schools should provide evidence-based health education that emphasizes behavioral skills to increase physical activity and decrease sedentary behavior.
- University training programs should provide professional preparation so that qualified teachers are available to deliver evidence-based physical and health education.

Adapted from Estabrooks PA, Bradshaw MH, Dzewaltowski DA, Smith-Ray RL. Determining the impact of Walk Kansas: applying a team-building approach to community physical activity promotion. *Ann Behav Med*. 2008;36:1–12.

education should be delivered that meets national standards for students across all school levels. These classes should provide at least 50% of the time to moderate-to-vigorous PA and train students in the skills needed to engage in lifelong PA. Third, schools should increase opportunities for active living by arranging clubs and intramural and extramural sports so that there are options available that match the needs and interests of all students—and not just those who are typically drawn to sporting activities. Fourth, schools should systematically address issues that will improve the likelihood that children will walk or bike to school. Fifth, preschools and elementary schools should implement at least 30 minutes of daily recess. Sixth, evidence-based health education programs that emphasize behavioral training to increase PA and decrease sedentary behaviors should be delivered.

Recommendations for school districts and states include the following: (a) states and school districts should implement and enforce policy that requires certified and highly qualified professionals to lead physical education classes; (b) states should include physical education in their core educational accountability system and direct schools to deliver 150 minutes of physical education per week for children in kindergarten through eighth grade or for 225 minutes per week for grades 9 through 12; and (c) training institutions (i.e., colleges and universities) should provide appropriate preparation so that teachers are highly qualified and prepared to deliver evidence-based health and physical education curriculum.

Work-Site Physical Activity Interventions

There are several practical reasons for delivering PA prevention programs in work sites (19). First, most American adults spend a large proportion of their waking hours at work. Second, policy, organizational, and individual behavior change strategies can be combined into an ecologically informed intervention that is more powerful than any one type of strategy in isolation (26,78). Third, the opportunities for cooperation, communication, and friendly competition among employees provide a strong foundation for various forms of social support strategies such as group rewards, participatory employee wellness teams, and incentive programs. Fourth, work-site programs can reach a broader population and encourage many persons to take advantage of PA programs who may not otherwise participate (27). Finally, comprehensive worksite wellness programs can increase employee recruitment and retention, reduce healthcare costs and absenteeism, and enhance employee morale and productivity (59,69).

Physical activity professionals should also be aware of complexities of work-site PA interventions. Even if support from top management at a work site (79) is obtained, midlevel supervisors may not be supportive or provide workers with the time necessary to participate. Somewhat related to this is the desire for work sites to de-velop comprehensive wellness policies and programs—and to receive all components from a given program or vendor. Therefore, packaging PA promotion within a broader milieu of lifestyle behavior self-management will be more likely to achieve buy-in from work sites when compared with, for example, a simple 12-week pedometer program (79). Finally, competing demands, availability of appropriate space for intervention components, and the logistics of including part-time and night-shift employees highlight reasons why interventions that focus on class-based corporate fitness or health education programs do not effectively reach a large proportion of employees or result in sustained behavior change (45).

In 1998, Dishman et al. completed a systematic review of the literature examining work-site PA promotion (11). The review documented that the mean effect size across the 26 studies included in the analysis was small (i.e., average r = 0.11). It is of note that three of the studies included a more ecological approach to PA promotion by making work-site environmental changes (e.g., public signage documenting participant success, employee contests, and awards or providing on-site exercise facilities) *in addition* to providing behavioral skills training (36,40,54). In comparison to the small overall effect reported in the review, these studies demonstrated a medium-sized effect (i.e., average r = 0.41), suggesting the importance of addressing both individual and environmental strategies. Similarly, a recent American Heart Association Scientific Statement provided an updated summary of the current state of work-site PA intervention research that suggests that work-site PA promotion should be based on a comprehensive approach that includes both individually and environmentally tailored strategies (44).

Research on the effectiveness of comprehensive work-site health promotion (i.e., target multiple behavior change) programs that include PA provide additional findings that are important for a PA professional attempting to intervene at the work site. This literature demonstrated that behavior modification and incentives were used regularly, whereas competitions and capitalizing on the work-site organizational characteristics were used less frequently (32,50). Yet, strategies such as promoting friendly competition increased healthy eating, PA, and work-site smoking cessation rates *without* the unintended consequence of increasing PA at an unsafe rate (39,58). Interactive computer technologies, such as automated telephone support, Internet and e-mail support, and tailored print strategies to develop lifestyle behavior skills, may be as effective as time-intensive and costly individual face-to-face sessions (31). Studies that used employee wellness teams demonstrated improved delivery of health programs on site, and an increased number of employees found the programs appealing (33).

Using the body of research on work-site health promotion and the tacit knowledge of work-site health

---

BOX 47-3	THE WELLNESS COUNCILS OF AMERICA BENCHMARKS TO WORK-SITE INTERVENTION SUCCESS

- Obtain senior level support.
- Create cohesive wellness teams.
- Collect data to drive health efforts.
- Craft an operating plan.
- Choose appropriate interventions.
- Create a supportive environment.
- Consistently evaluate outcomes.

---

professionals, the Wellness Councils of America (WEL-COA) developed a set of seven benchmarks necessary for the successful implementation, effectiveness, and sustainability of work-site wellness initiatives (Box 47-3) (86). The first benchmark is to obtain senior level support by matching the wellness policy to (a) the organizations' short- and long-term priorities, (b) expectations from a wellness initiative (and level of value placed on health promotion), and (c) pressures and demands on leadership that could influence support. Once senior level support is achieved, a cohesive wellness team should be developed to include employees from all sectors of the organization (about 8 to 15 members in total). Volunteer members are likely to be more energetic about the initiative, but it is necessary to work the wellness team responsibilities into the performance goals of the employees involved to reduce the likelihood of burnout.

The wellness team becomes integral in carrying out the remaining benchmarks for success. First, a brief needs assessment is conducted, which includes determining what the business needs to get out of the wellness efforts and, equally as important, what the employees want. Second, the team should develop a work-site wellness operating plan that includes a vision for the health of employees, goals and objectives, specific timelines, marketing strategies, budget needs, and methods to evaluate whether the goals and objectives are being achieved. Third, concurrently with the development of the operating plan, the wellness team should identify and select appropriate intervention components. The selection should be informed by the needs assessment and vision of the organization for its wellness initiative. The wellness team is directed to use evidence-based interventions when available or to base the strategies on the best evidence that is available. Fourth, the team should implement strategies to develop an environment that supports healthy lifestyle behaviors. Recommended strategies to develop a supportive environment includ creating proactive policies that make the healthy decision the easy decision (e.g., implement "walk-and-talk" meetings), creating incentive programs, increasing manager role

modeling of healthy behaviors, and integrating healthy messages into company communications. Fifth, the team should evaluate outcomes that are important to the organization and employees—and that can demonstrate success or the need to modify the wellness plan.

Clinical Interventions

There is a strong rationale for promoting PA during medical visits. First, community health clinics and family medicine clinics are geographically distributed across the United States and have contact with a large proportion of the population (9,30,88). Second, physicians are considered by patients to be experts in health-related information (30). The credibility that physicians bring to a patient visit is highlighted by a recent finding that indicated as many as 90% of patients would consider registering for a PA intervention through a medical office (34). Based on this rationale, several physician-delivered PA counseling interventions have been developed (2,15,62,64,83,85). However, a review of that literature by the United States Preventive Services Task Force (USPSTF) documented that the findings of efficacy were inconsistent (15).

What is clear from the USPSTF findings is that it is difficult to document consistent effects of clinical PA interventions when they rely primarily on interactions between the physician and the patient. That is, simply asking about patients' PA and advising them to do more will not lead to sustained behavior change (25,61,63). Similar to other site-specific community interventions, the use of an ecological approach that uses the entire social and physical environment of a clinic (and, optimally, the surrounding community) and a more comprehensive model for PA promotion that moves beyond the exclusive domain of physician-patient interactions is necessary (18).

The literature supports that when the role of the physician is reduced to a short period of time to provide brief advice (e.g., >3 minutes) and coupled with intervention strategies delivered by other clinical staff (particularly an exercise professional) or community organizations, significant increases in patients' PA can be achieved (1,63). Personnel that can be used to deliver other intervention components include health educators, exercise professionals, community personnel (e.g., YMCA staff), or other clinical staff (e.g., nurses, front desk staff) (1,14,42,63). Finally, a promising path to improve the maintenance of clinical PA intervention effects to is to integrate counseling with the identification of community opportunities for PA support (1,4,35,63,73).

Based on recent PA studies and clinical smoking cessation intervention literature, effective clinical PA interventions can likely be operationalized using the 5 A's of behavior change (20,29,63,64): (a) *Assessing* patient PA level, ability, and readiness to change; (b) providing PA *Advice* relative to personalized benefits and recommended guidelines; (c) *Agreeing* with a patient on a

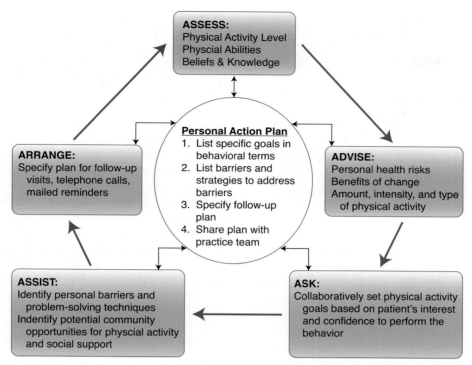

FIGURE 47-1. The 5 A's model applied to physical activity promotion in clinical settings.

collaboratively developed plan of action; (d) *Assisting* patients with barrier resolution and problem solving to aid in the successful completion of the action plan; and (e) *Arranging* for a positive feedback loop through designated follow-up periods and links to environmental resources for active living (20,81,87). Figure 47-1 provides a pictorial representation of the 5 A's process as it may be delivered in a primary-care setting.

Church-Based Interventions

Reported ethnic disparities in cancer-related morbidity and mortality and the associated risk factors (e.g., poor diet quality and low activity levels) underlie a recent scientific movement to target culturally tailored interventions for African Americans within faith organizations (3). Churches serve several social, organizational, and religious functions and offer unique opportunities for promoting healthy behaviors among African Americans (67). Of particular interest for PA professionals wishing to engage churches as a local for health promotion is the National Cancer Institute and American Cancer Society program Body & Soul, which includes several free resources and practical instructions for implementing church-based healthy eating and, more recently, PA promotion (53).

The genesis of Body & Soul began with two efficacy trials: Black Churches United for Better Health (6) and Eat for Life (68). Taking the information and content

from the interventions tested in these trials, representatives from the National Cancer Institute, the American Cancer Society, and the respective intervention development groups identified the core behavioral principals that lead to efficacy and adapted them to a program that could be widely disseminated. Both the Black Churches United for Better Health and Eat for Life targeted nutrition rather than PA behaviors. However, in 2004, the Healthy Body/Healthy Spirit trial (66,67) was completed based on the same underlying principles, and it targeted both nutrition and PA behavior. Healthy Body/Healthy Spirit demonstrated that churches could focus on both behaviors simultaneously and achieve significant dietary and PA changes (66).

The principles and content of these church-based interventions were adapted for dissemination by operationalizing the four pillars of church-based lifestyle behavior change programs (Box 47-4) (53). As with the other site-specific interventions reviewed, Body & Soul includes components that address the church ecology to ensure that strategies were comprehensive and appropriate for a given locale. The first pillar indicates that it is necessary to have a pastor or church leader who is committed and engaged with the program. Pastors are encouraged to begin the program with a kickoff event, be a role model, and integrate health behavior messages in sermons, church bulletins, and newsletters (53).

Church activities that promote healthy eating and active living reflect the second pillar of Body & Soul (53).

BOX 47-4	THE FOUR PILLARS OF CHURCH-BASED LIFESTYLE BEHAVIOR CHANGE PROGRAMS

- A pastor who is committed to, and involved with, physical activity and healthy eating
- Church activities that promote healthy eating and active living
- A church environment that promotes healthy eating and active living
- Peer counseling to motivate healthy lifestyle behavior change

Three general activity categories are proposed. First, the Body & Soul kickoff event introduces the program to the congregation, inspires member engagement, and creates a sense of excitement for upcoming program components. Second, ongoing church activities should include workshops and skill-building strategies on healthy dietary and PA behaviors. Tours of a local grocery store, cooking demonstrations, and taste testing are promoted and communicated through church newsletters and bulletins. Third, activities that celebrate success are suggested to recognize the planning team and program participants (53).

The third pillar has some overlap with the first two pillars in that all activities completed by the pastor or during ongoing activities reflect changes to the church's social and physical environment (53). Changing the environment to support healthy eating and PA can also include components that guide members to bring healthier food to church functions or to make the church space available for PA in areas where weather or safety limit opportunities for outdoor activities (53).

A fourth pillar is peer counseling to motivate church members (53). To achieve this pillar, a group of church members volunteer and are trained in motivational interview skills. The focus is on helping less physically activity members to self-identify problem-solving strategies to aid in achieving PA goals. The use of lay leaders for peer counseling appears to be almost as effective as when delivered by trained research staff (68).

COMMUNITY-WIDE INTERVENTIONS

In contrast to site-specific interventions, community-wide interventions typically include a multilevel and multisector approach. Community-wide interventions can include several site-specific interventions that may or may not be interwoven into a broad community action plan that attempts to increase the PA (or other health behaviors) across the entire population rather than singularly focusing on students, employees, patients, or congregation members. Community-wide interventions

are also often inherently based on ecological models and include a range of policy, environmental, and program components (23,41,46).

The Stanford Five-City Project is a well-known example of a successful community-wide intervention (23). Briefly, the project used mass media, which included television public service announcements, news stories, and newspaper articles—in Spanish and English—to promote cardiovascular risk reduction via lifestyle behavior changes. Community and scientific representation was used to determine the range of interpersonal contacts, classes, seminars, and other group interventions that would be implemented. Ultimately, each of the community programs were offered in several settings and delivered through a variety of community agencies (e.g., the health department, colleges, hospitals, nonprofit organizations). Assessments of PA indicated that there was a positive treatment effect for men in estimated daily energy expenditure and percent participation in vigorous activities. Similarly, women in the intervention communities engaged in significantly more moderate physical activities than those in the control community.

The Naval Community Project in California (41) is worthy of note to provide some practical examples of community changes that can be made within a controlled community, such as a naval base. This project used an array of environmental and policy strategies to improve PA and healthy eating on a military base. During the project, the intervention community constructed bicycle paths along pre-existing roads, purchased new equipment for the gymnasium, opened a women-only fitness center, and marked out multiple 1.5-mile running routes around the base. In addition, social environmental changes were implemented, including the development of jogging clubs and other athletic events. Policy approaches included extending the hours the base recreation center was open and integrating—into structured communications between superiors and subordinates—the expectation that all personnel on the base should participate in regular exercise (41).

The Naval Community Project resulted in significant improvements in fitness and body composition for personnel on the intervention base when compared with a control base and the population of navy personnel (41). The benefits of the intervention demonstrated the value of comprehensive community-wide strategies in that the improvements in fitness occurred in both men and women, officers and enlisted personnel, and within each age category. That is, all segments of the population on the base benefited from the project, highlighting the value of integrating physical and social environmental changes with policy approaches to increasing PA (37).

Building on these and other community-health promotion studies, Agita Sao Paulo developed an elegant yet comprehensive strategy for community-wide PA promotion for a Brazilian state of 645 municipalities with 40 million residents (46). Agita is arguably the first community-wide intervention to be developed on a specified ecological model with linked strategies across intrapersonal, social environment, and physical environment categories while being implemented with the active participation and sponsorship of the region's highest government health authority (the state health secretariat). The program has a simply stated goal: to change the PA of the population (46).

The driving strategic principle of Agita Sao Paulo is a "mobile management" approach to strategies that fall under the umbrella of intrapersonal, social environment, and physical environment (Table 47-1). Specifically, "the multi-level components of the ecological model are distributed three-dimensionally in a dynamic balance as in a mobile" (46). The mobile management approach recom-

mends that strategies across the ecological model be addressed concurrently to facilitate a balanced approach; thus, Agita Sao Paulo engaged with several partnership institutions and a coalition of more than 300 members. To ensure a sharing of the workload as strategies were identified, the central organizing committee also identified the appropriate partner institution to lead the planning and implementation. Although Agita Sao Paulo is clearly a Herculean effort and may seem overwhelming to a community PA professional, the principle of development and delivery can be generalized to small or large community-wide initiatives. That principle is that strategies should be balanced across the ecological framework and matched to the appropriate partner for implementation. Also, it is clearly seen from the model that no one person or organization can plan, implement, and sustain a community-wide initiative.

TABLE 47-1. THE ECOLOGICAL CATEGORIES AND EXAMPLE COMMUNITY-WIDE INTERVENTION STRATEGIES USED IN AGITA SAO PAULO

PRIMARY ECOLOGICAL CATEGORY	ECOLOGICAL SUBCATEGORY	INTERVENTION STRATEGY
Intrapersonal	Demographic	Physical activity promotion materials tailored for specific age and socioeconomic groups
	Cognitive/affective	Behavioral skills–based activities that will lead to the initiation of an active lifestyle: courses, print materials, talks
	Biological	Adapt physical activity materials to address men and women and other special groups (handicapped, chronic disease)
	Behavioral	Stage-based messages to encourage sedentary people to become a little more active, insufficiently active people to become regularly active, and regularly active people to maintain their behavior
Social Environment	Culture	Incentives for local executive committees to form within each municipality; allow local adaptation of logo, mascot, and icons to be culturally relevant
	Social climate	Developed executive committee that unites the representatives of government, private, and social spheres to discuss permanent intervention actions
	Supportive behaviors	Engage employers, government entities, school leaders, and healthcare providers to implement incentives for physical activity
	Policies governing resources	Define human, material, structural, logistic, and financial resources necessary to execute physical activity promotion; use unpaid media to promote action and results of the program
	Policies governing incentives	The establishment of policies, statutes, and laws to provide incentives and practice of physical activity promotion; healthcare discounts for the regularly active
Physical Environment	Natural environment: geography	Establish practices that use the naturally occurring environment as much as possible
	Natural environment: weather	Adapt intervention strategies specific to the seasons
	Constructed environment: architectural	Construct new sidewalks, tracks, trails where necessary; use school grounds and resources for weekend activities and increase maintenance efforts for existing parks
	Constructed environment: entertainment	Create specific physical activity groups for diverse social groups, including children, adolescents, and the elderly
	Constructed environment: transport	Improve storage and parking of bikes; develop or improve private and public policies to support active transportation to work or school

PRINCIPLES FOR PLANNING AND EVALUATING COMMUNITY PHYSICAL ACTIVITY INTERVENTIONS

> **1.11.13-HFS. Knowledge of the importance of tracking and evaluating health promotion program results.**

THE RE-AIM FRAMEWORK

Consider this scenario: A local PA professional is interested in helping every child in her state to become active at the recommended levels. She picks up the current issue of *Medicine and Science in Sports and Exercise* and reads about a fantastic new intervention that takes only 15 minutes a day, is offered during an after-school program, and helped half of the sedentary and insufficiently active children who received it to meet the recommended

guidelines within a month. Further, when the researchers went back and checked on the children 6 months later, half of those who saw the original benefit were still meeting recommended guidelines. When she reads further, she finds that the intervention needs to be delivered by a trained and certified physical education teacher. The PA professional takes the information with her and successfully lobbies her state's governor to strongly recommend that all schools implement the new intervention.

The above scenario would be exciting for all involved. The researchers would be excited about the large effect size. The PA professional would be excited because the intervention will be implemented. The governor would be excited because of all of the good press. But let's take the scenario a little further. Follow along with Figure 47-2. You will note at the top of the figure a group of clip-art people that represent the total population of students within the school system of the state in question. Following the

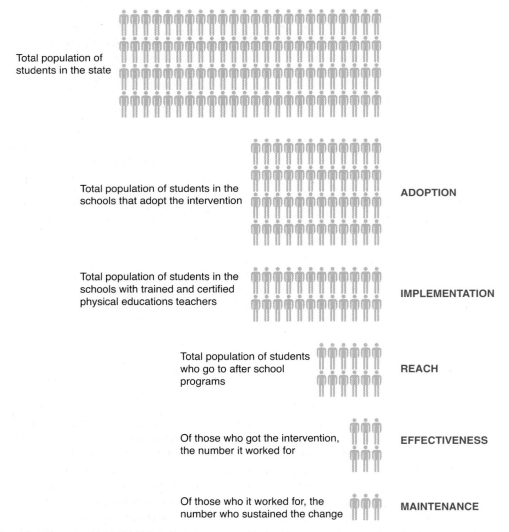

FIGURE 47-2. Applying RE-AIM to the potential public health impact of a new after-school program physical activity intervention.

governor's strong recommendation, a resounding 50% of the schools adopt the program; these schools reflect 50% of the student population (Fig. 47-2: Adoption). However, only half of the schools have a certified teacher who can lead the program, so they use volunteers. Unfortunately, the volunteers can't implement the program with the same fidelity as certified teachers, and the intervention doesn't work in those sites—now 25% of the student population receives the intervention (Fig. 47-2: Implementation). In the schools that are offering the program, only half of the students in their school attend the after-school program—down to 12.5% of the student population receiving the intervention (Fig. 47-2: Reach). Based on the efficacy data, half of the children increased activity to recommended guidelines, or 6.25% of the state population of students (Fig. 47-2: Effectiveness), and half of those (about 3% of the total population) sustain that level of activity (Fig. 47-2: Maintenance).

This scenario highlights the need for evaluation and planning efforts that address several different issues, beyond simply determining if an intervention "works." Each step of the described scenario relates to a dimension of the RE-AIM planning and evaluation framework (www.re-aim.org) (21,28). One purpose of the RE-AIM framework is to increase attention to both individual and organizational level indicators with an effort to either predict or document the public health impact of a given intervention.

RE-AIM is an acronym that stands for *Reach, Effectiveness, Adoption, Implementation,* and *Maintenance. Reach* is defined as the participation rate and representativeness of participants who engage in an intervention. *Effectiveness* is defined as the extent to which the intervention achieves targeted outcomes in real-world contexts and also includes assessing for potential negative consequences. *Adoption* can be defined as the participation rate of organizations that will ultimately implement the intervention and the representativeness of those organizations to the population that could implement the intervention. *Implementation* is defined as the degree to which an intervention is implemented as intended. Finally, *maintenance* is defined at both the individual and organizational level. For individuals, *maintenance* is defined as sustained behavior change for more than 6 months; at the organizational level, *maintenance* is defined as the sustained delivery of a given intervention or the institutionalization of an intervention within typical community settings.

An example of a community PA intervention that used the RE-AIM framework for evaluation is Walk Kansas (17,22). Walk Kansas was developed by a team that was organized to respond to the need to increase the rates of PA in rural Kansas. The conceptual model, developed by Carron and Spink (7), uses group dynamic principles and was applied within the PA promotion program. Walk Kansas aimed to develop a sense of group distinctiveness,

target norms through group goal setting, form groups of individuals within geographic proximity, and foster ongoing group interactions and communication to provide feedback, information sharing, and collective problem solving. In addition, the program was developed to be delivered through the cooperative extension system, which included representatives in each of the 105 counties in Kansas (17). Table 47-2 describes the metrics used to assess each dimension of the RE-AIM framework.

RE-AIM IMPLICATIONS FOR PLANNING

One of the broad appeals of community interventions is the potential to improve the PA of a large proportion of the population. Schools, work sites, clinics, churches, and community-wide interventions share the commonality that by intervening through them, a large proportion of the population can be influenced. Using RE-AIM in the planning process for community PA programs begins with a series of questions related to each dimension that will help PA professionals realize the positive potential for community change (38). By addressing the questions, PA professionals can prepare an initiative to reach a broad cross-section of the target population, increase and sustain PA for those reached, and successfully adapt PA interventions to different settings. Four primary questions are helpful when beginning to plan a community PA intervention.

1. For which individuals or groups do you intend to increase PA as a result of the intervention?
2. Who or what organization will need to be involved in decision making and planning?
3. Who will be responsible for delivering or implementing the strategies?
4. What organization or institution will be needed to ensure sustainability?

By answering these questions, a PA professional can determine who else needs to be involved before comprehensive planning begins (24). Answering these questions and getting the appropriate partners at the table is the first step in the planning process. Once a partnership is formed, careful planning around each RE-AIM dimension will enhance the impact of the community initiative.

When planning to improve the reach of a community, PA intervention it is important to define a target population and have a clear understanding of its denominator. For example, if a community program attracted 500 participants, one might consider this a success. However, if the denominator of the target population was a community of 50,000, then 500 participants is not a success. Conversely, if the program targeted a small rural community of 1,000 people, then 500 participants would be exceptional. Once the denominator is clarified, building relationships with members of the target population and those who provide services to them can help to determine

TABLE 47-2. OPERATIONALIZING THE RE-AIM FRAMEWORK: WALK KANSAS

RE-AIM DIMENSION	INDICATOR	OUTCOME
Reach	Number of participants	Ranged from approximately 6,000 participants in 2002 to 20,000 in 2006
	Percent of county population that participated	Ranged from approximately 3% in 2002 to 5% in 2006
	Representativeness of participants to county populations based on sex, ethnicity, age	Walk Kansas participants were more likely to be female and older than the general population, but representative on ethnicity
Effectiveness	Pre-/postevaluation on subsample of 1,400 program participants divided by baseline activity level (active, inactive, insufficiently active)	Active participants maintained activity levels over the course of the program; inactive and insufficiently active increased moderate-intensity physical activity by approximately 150 minutes per week
Adoption	Number of counties that participated out of 105 eligible	Ranged from 48 in 2002 to 97 in 2006
	Percent of counties that participated	Ranged from 46% in 2002 to 92% in 2006
	Representativeness of counties within the state based on population, proportion female, proportion minority	Counties were representative of the state across variables until 2006, when counties with small populations were less likely to participate (i.e., 8% of the counties)
Implementation	Proportion that delivered core components (i.e., used teams, goal setting, and feedback)	100% of the counties reported delivering the core components
	Proportion that used task force	Approximately 50% used a task force to market and implement the program; the remaining used their own office staff
Maintenance: individual	Random selection of 225 participants surveyed on physical activity 6 months postintervention completion	On average, participants sustained 150 minutes of moderate physical activity each week
Maintenance: organizational	Percent of counties that sustained delivery for 2, 3, 4, or 5 years	Approximately 42% of counties delivered the program for all 5 years, 35% for 4 years, 10% for 3 years, and 5% each delivered the program for 2, 1, or zero years

strategies that will be the most salient in that community. The partnership with community members can also aid in the development of population-specific recruitment materials and strategies. Finally, to ensure a broad reach into the population, go to where the target population is to deliver the intervention and distribute recruitment materials.

As suggested by WELCOA, planning for effectiveness and individual maintenance of behavior begins by understanding the evidence base (86). However, for many community contexts, there are few evidence-based interventions or specific recommendations. In these cases, development of community PA programs should be based on the best available evidence or developed to match the underlying principles of an efficacious intervention (70).

Planning to enhance the adoption of a community intervention begins with the same process that is used when planning for reach—by determining the denominator and characteristics of the settings that will ultimately deliver the intervention (38). As highlighted in the recommendations and processes reviewed for school, work site, clinic, church, and community-wide strategies, using a participatory model of development can enhance the perceived community ownership of a program and help ensure that the end product is consistent with the needs of the potential participants and delivery sites. It is

critical to understand the system that you anticipate will use the program or implement a policy. The organizational mission, flow of day-to-day operations, and available resources are all factors that can either facilitate or impede adoption. Finally, when meeting with a new organization, have data that demonstrate the program's reach, effectiveness, ease of implementation (including cost), and relative advantage (70).

Inevitably, community PA interventions will be adapted over time by those who deliver them (70). This can either be a positive or negative outcome. A positive adaptation would be to make the program easier to deliver while adhering to the principles that made it effective (76). A negative adaptation would be to drop the intervention components that are most difficult but integral to intervention success and deliver only those that are easy to implement. To avoid negative adaptation, program developers should identify and market the functioning principles of the intervention or core components of policy and allow for local adaptation. Manualized programs are also more likely to facilitate fidelity to the intervention program, as are training and technical support during early stages of implementation (38).

Organizational sustainability of community PA programs can be challenging. Issues of program cost and organizational climate can result in the abandonment of new and effective programs. To optimize the chances for a sustained program, collect information on the effectiveness of the program, including reach, implementation, and impacts on both PA behavior and other things, such as participant satisfaction and program costs. Foster program champions at multiple levels who can advocate for the program and provide resources. Program champions are people who really believe in the program and its positive outcomes. Previous participants can be excellent advocates for both the future reach of the program and for sustained funding. It is also important to identify a program sponsor within the organization that is delivering the program. An organizational level program sponsor will be most effective if the organization holds some decision-making authority. Also, programs that have the perception of broad-based local ownership are much more likely to be sustained than those that are considered to be from a research shop that has little understanding of local needs and barriers. Finally, integrate the program into the regular service of the organization that is delivering the program.

RECOMMENDATIONS FOR PLANNING AND EVALUATING COMMUNITY PHYSICAL ACTIVITY INTERVENTIONS

This chapter has reviewed a variety of community PA interventions and provided suggestions on how to assess the potential or actual impact of those interventions. Through this review, several commonalities arose that can be used to provide some recommendations for PA professionals who are interested in developing and delivering community interventions.

First, interventionists should use a broad ecological model as the basis of strategy development. This includes understanding the characteristics of potential participants and the social and physical environmental contexts of the places they reside, work, and spend leisure time. Defining the target population and completing assessments of the target population's perception of need for a PA program and preferences for format and content should improve the chances that the program will reach a broad audience and have intended positive effects. Addressing the social environment in terms of policy, group activities, and social marketing can provide a foundation for successful programming. Finally, ensuring that the physical environment is supportive of regular PA or highlighting existing community resources are promising directions for strategy development.

Second, and related to the first point, use a balanced approach to ensure that all domains in an ecological approach are addressed. The Agita Sao Paulo's mobile management system is an excellent method to ensure that there is a balanced approach to individual, social, and physical environment components. Also implicitly balanced in the Agita approach were the components of the intervention that were based on programs and policies.

This balance has applicability regardless of the type of community intervention being completed. That is, even for an intervention that targets a single school, workplace, church, or clinic, the intervention should include strategies that affect individual, social, and environmental factors to optimize the likelihood of success.

Third, to be successful, community PA interventions should be conceptualized, developed, delivered, and monitored by a partnership that includes representatives of those intended to benefit from the intervention, those intended to deliver it, and those intended to provide support for it. This crosscutting of issues is critical to improve the reach, implementation, and sustainability of community PA interventions. Working with a group that includes all the key stakeholders within a community setting will facilitate the identification of individual, organizational, and contextual barriers that could arise over the course of the program. More importantly, such a group can aid in resolving barriers before they arise.

Fourth, evaluation of community PA interventions should include a variety of outcomes in addition to assessing the potential effectiveness of the program. As demonstrated in Figure 47-2, there are several points in the life course of a behavioral intervention when, without careful planning, large proportions of the target population can be lost. By assessing the outcomes across the RE-AIM framework, one can identify and market individual and organizational success.

REFERENCES

1. Ackermann RT, Deyo RA, LoGerfo JP. Prompting primary providers to increase community exercise referrals for older adults: a randomized trial. *J Am Geriatr Soc.* 2005;53:283–9.
2. Activity Counseling Trial Writing Group. Effects of physical activity counseling in primary care: the Activity Counseling Trial: a randomized controlled trial. *JAMA.* 2001;286(6):677–87.
3. Baskin M, Resnicow K, Campbell M. Conducting health interventions in black churches: a model for building effective partnerships. *Ethn Dis.* 2001;11:823–33.
4. Brownson RC, Housemann RA, Brown DR, et al. Promoting physical activity in rural communities: walking trail access, use, and effects. *Am J Prev Med.* 2000;18(3):235–41.
5. Burgeson CR, Wechsler H, Brener ND, Young JC, Spain CG. Physical education and activity: results from the School Health Policies and Programs Study 2000. *J Sch Health.* 2001;71(7):279–93.
6. Campbell MK, Motsinger BM, Ingram A, et al. The North Carolina Black Churches United for Better Health Project: intervention and process evaluation. *Health Educ Behav.* 2000;27:241–53.
7. Carron AV, Spink KS. Team building in an exercise setting. *The Sport Psychologist.* 1993;7:8–18.
8. **Centers for Disease Control and Prevention. Guidelines for School Health Promotion Programs to Promote Lifelong Healthy Eating. *MMWR Morb Mortal Wkly Rep.* 1996;45(RR-9):1–33.**
9. Chin MH, Cook S, Jin L, et al. Barriers to providing diabetes care in community health centers. *Diabetes Care.* 2001;24:268–74.
10. Council of Sports Medicine and Fitness and Council on School Health. Active healthy living: prevention of childhood obesity through increased physical activity. *Pediatrics.* 2006;117:1834–42.
11. Dishman RK, Oldenburg B, O'Neal H, Shephard RJ. Worksite physical activity interventions. *Am J Prev Med.* 1998;15(4):344–61.

12. Dzewaltowski DA. The ecology of physical activity and sport: merging science and practice. *J Appl Sport Psych.* 1997;9:254–76.

13. Dzewaltowski DA, Estabrooks PA, Johnston JA. Overview of the Healthy Youth Places Project: a child and adolescent fruit and vegetable consumption and physical activity intervention. *Health Ed Res.* 2002;17:541–51.

14. Eakin EG, Glasgow RE, Riley KM. Review of primary care-based physical activity intervention studies: effectiveness and implications for practice and future research. *J Fam Pract.* 2000;49:158–68.

15. Eden KB, Orleans T, Mulrow CD, Pender NJ, Teutsch SM. Does counseling by clinicians improve physical activity? A summary of the evidence for the U.S. Preventive Services Task Force. *Ann Intern Med.* 2002;137(3):208–15.

16. Englert HS, Diehl HA, Greenlaw RL, Willich SN, Aldana SG. The effect of a community-based coronary risk reduction: the Rockford CHIP. *Prev Med.* 2007;44:513–9.

17. Estabrooks PA, Bradshaw MH, Dzewaltowski DA, Smith-Ray RL. Determining the impact of Walk Kansas: applying a team-building approach to community physical activity promotion. *Ann Behav Med.* 2008;36:1–12.

18. Estabrooks PA, Glasgow RE. Translating effective clinic-based physical activity interventions into practice. *Am J Prev Med.* 2006; 31:45–56.

19. Estabrooks PA, Glasgow RE. Worksite interventions. In: Baum A, Newman S, Weinman J, West R, McManus C, editors. *Cambridge Handbook of Psychology, Health and Medicine.* 2nd ed. Cambridge, UK: Cambridge University Press; 2007. p. 264–8.

20. Estabrooks PA, Glasgow RE, Dzewaltowski DA. Physical activity promotion through primary care. *JAMA.* 2003;289:2913–6.

21. Estabrooks PA, Gyurcsik NC. Evaluating the public health impact of physical activity interventions. *Psych Sport Exerc.* 2003;4: 41–55.

22. Estabrooks PA, Bradshaw M, Fox EH, Berg J, Dzewaltowski DA. The relationship between delivery agents' physical activity level and the likelihood of implementing a physical activity program. *Am J Health Promot.* 2004;18:350–3.

23. Farquhar JW, Fortmann P, Maccoby N, et al. The Stanford Five-City Project: design and methods. *Am J Epidemiol.* 2000;122(2): 323–34.

24. Glasgow RE, Bayliss EA, Estabrooks PA. Translation research in diabetes: asking broader questions. In: Montori VM, editor. *Evidence-based Endocrinology.* New York: Humana Press: 2006 p. 241–56.

25. Glasgow RE, Eakin EG. Medical office-based interventions. In: Snoek FJ, Skinner CS, editors. *Psychology in Diabetes Care.* London: John Wiley and Sons, Ltd.; 2002. p. 141–168.

26. Glasgow RE, Hollis JF, Ary DV, Lando HA. Employee and organizational factors associated with participation in an incentive-based worksite smoking cessation program. *J Behav Med.* 1990;13(4): 403–18.

27. Glasgow RE, McCaul KD, Fisher KJ. Participation in worksite health promotion: a critique of the literature and recommendations for future practice. *Health Educ Q.* 1993;20(3):291–408.

28. Glasgow RE, Vogt TM, Boles SM. Evaluating the public health impact of health promotion interventions: the RE-AIM framework. *Am J Public Health.* 1999;89:1322–37.

29. Goldstein MG, Whitlock EP, DePue J. Multiple health risk behavior interventions in primary care: summary of research evidence. *Am J Prev Med.* 2004;27:61–79.

30. Green LA, Dodoo MS, Ruddy G, et al. *Physician Workforce of the United States: A Family Medicine Perspective.* Washington (DC): Robert Graham Center; 2004.

31. Harvey-Berino J, Pintauro S, Buzzell P, Gold EC. Effect of Internet support on the long-term maintenance of weight loss. *Obes Res.* 2004;12(2):320–9.

32. Hennrikus D, Jeffery RW. Worksite intervention for weight control: a review of the literature. *Am J Health Promot.* 1996;10(6): 471–98.

33. Hunt MK, Lederman R, Potter S, Stoddard A, Sorensen G. Results of employee involvement in planning and implementing the Treatwell 5-a-Day Work-Site Study. *Health Educ Behav.* 2000;27(2):223–31.

34. Jimmy G, Martin BW. Implementation and effectiveness of a primary care based physical activity counseling scheme. *Patient Educ Counsel.* 2005;56(3):323–1.

35. Kahn EB, Ramsey LT, Brownson RC, et al. The effectiveness of interventions to increase physical activity: a systematic review. *Am J Prev Med.* 2002;22(4s):73–107.

36. King AC, Carl F, Birkel L, Haskell WL. Increasing exercise among blue-collar employees: the tailoring of worksite programs to meet specific needs. *Prev Med.* 1988;17:357–65.

37. King AC, Jeffery RW, Fridinger F, et al. Environmental and policy approaches to cardiovascular disease prevention through physical activity: issues and opportunities. *Health Educ Q.* 1995;22(4):499–511.

38. Klesges LM, Estabrooks PA, Dzewaltowski DA, Bull SS, Glasgow RE. Beginning with the application in mind: designing and planning health behavior change interventions to enhance dissemination. *Ann Behav Med.* 2005;29(2Suppl):66–75.

39. Klesges RC, Vasey MM, Glasgow RE. A worksite smoking modification competition: potential for public health impact. *Am J Public Health.* 1986;76:198–200.

40. Larsen P, Simmons N. Evaluating a federal health and fitness program: indicators of improving health. *AAOHN J.* 1993;41(3):143–8.

41. Linenger JM, Chesson CV, Nice DS. Physical fitness gains following simple environmental change. *Am J Prev Med.* 1991;7(5):298–310.

42. Lobo CM, Frijling Bd, Hulscher ME, et al. Improving quality of organizing cardiovascular preventive care in general practice by outreach visitors: a randomized controlled trial. *Prev Med.* 2002;35: 422–9.

43. Luepker RV, Perry CL, McKinlay SM, et al. Outcomes of a field trial to improve children's dietary patterns and physical activity: the child and adolescent trial for cardiovascular health (CATCH). *JAMA.* 1996;275(10):768–76.

44. **Marcus BH, Williams DM, Dubbert PM, et al. Physical activity intervention studies: what we know and what we need to know. A scientific statement from the American Heart Association Council on Nutrition, Physical Activity, and Metabolism; Council on Cardiovascular Disease in the Young; and the Interdisciplinary Working Group on Quality of Care and Outcomes Research.** *Circulation.* 2006;114:2739–52.

45. Marshall AL. Challenges and opportunities for promoting physical activity in the workplace. *J Sci Med Sport.* 2004;7:60–6.

46. Matsudo SM, Matsudo VKR, Andrade DR, Araujo TL, Pratt M. Evaluation of a physical activity promotion program: the example of Agita Sao Paulo. *Evalprogplan.* 2006;29:301–11.

47. McKenzie TL, Feldman H, Woods SE, et al. Children's activity levels and lesson context during third-grade physical education. *Res Q Exerc Sport.* 1995;66:184–93.

48. McKenzie TL, Nader PR, Strikmiller PK, et al. School physical education: effect of the Child and Adolescent Trial for Cardiovascular Health. *Prev Med.* 1996;25:423–31.

49. McKenzie TL, Sallis JF, Kolody B, Faucette FN. Long-term effects of a physical education curriculum and staff development program: SPARK. *Res Q Exerc Sport.* 1997;68:280–91.

50. McTigue KM, Harris R, Hemphill B, Lux L, Sutton S. Screening and interventions for obesity in adults: summary of the evidence for the U.S. Preventive Services Task Force. *Ann Intern Med.* 2003;139: 933–49.

51. Nader PR, Stone EJ, Lytle LA, et al. Three-year maintenance of improved diet and physical activity: the CATCH cohort. *Arch Pediatr Adolesc Med.* 1999;153(7):695–704.

52. National Association for Sport and Physical Education and American Heart Association. *Shape of the Nation Report: Status of Physical Education in the USA.* Reston (VA): National Association for Sport and Physical Education and American Heart Association; 2006.

53. National Cancer Institute. Body & Soul: a celebration of healthy eating & living. *National Cancer Institute* 2009; Available at: URL: www.bodyandsoul.nih.gov. Accessed November 25, 2008.

54. Oden G, Crouse SF, Reynolds C. Worker productivity, job satisfaction, and work-related stress: the influence of an employee fitness program. *Fitness Business.* 1989;4:198–204.

55. Pate RR, Davis MG, Robinson TN, Stone EJ, McKenzie TL, Young JC. Promoting physical activity in children and youth: a leadership role for schools. *Circulation.* 2006;114:1214–24.

56. Pate RR, Trost SG, Mullis R, Sallis JF, Wechsler H, Brown DR. Community interventions to promote proper nutrition and physical activity among youth. *Prev Med.* 2000;31:S138–S149.

57. Pate RR, Ward DS, Saunders RP, Felton G, Dishman RK, Dowda M. Promotion of physical activity in high school girls: a randomized controlled trial. *Am J Public Health.* 2005;95:1582–7.

58. Patterson RE, Kristal AR, Glanz K, et al. Components of the Working Well Trial Intervention associated with adoption of healthful diets. *Am J Prev Med.* 1997;13:271–6.

59. Pelletier KR. A review and analysis of the clinical- and cost-effectiveness studies of comprehensive health promotion and disease management programs at the worksite: 1998-2000 update. *Am J Health Promot.* 2001;16(2):107–16.

60. Perry CL, Stone EJ, Parcel GS, et al. School-based cardiovascular health promotion: the Child and Adolescent Trial for Cardiovascular Health (CATCH). *J Sch Health.* 1990;60:406–13.

61. Petrella R, Koval J, Cunningham D, Paterson D. Can primary care doctors prescribe exercise to improve fitness? *Am J Prev Med.* 2003; 24(4):316–22.

62. Pfeiffer BA, Clay SW, Conatser RR. A green prescription study: does written exercise prescribed by a physician result in increased physical activity among older adults? *J Aging Health.* 2001;13(4): 527–38.

63. Pinto BM, Goldstein MG, Ashba J, Sciamanna C, Jette A. Randomized controlled trial of physical activity counseling for older primary care patients. *Am J Prev Med.* 2005;29(4):247–55.

64. Pinto BM, Lynn H, Marcus BH, DePue J, Goldstein MG. Physician-based activity counseling: intervention effects on mediators of motivational readiness for physical activity. *Ann Behav Med.* 2001; 23(1):2–10.

65. Resincow K, Campbell MK, Carr C, et al. Body and soul: a dietary intervention conducted through African-American churches. *Am J Prev Med.* 2004;27:97–105.

66. Resnicow K, Jackson A, Blissett D, et al. Results of the Healthy Body Healthy Spirit Trial. *Health Psych.* 2005;24:339–48.

67. Resnicow K, Jackson A, Braithwaite RL, et al. Healthy Body/Healthy Spirit: a church-based nutrition and physical activity intervention. *Health Educ Res.* 2002;17:562–73.

68. Resnicow K, Jackson A, Wang T, et al. A motivational interviewing intervention to increase fruit and vegetable intake through black churches: results of the Eat for Life trial. *Am J Public Health.* 2001; 91:1686–93.

69. Riedel JE, Lynch W, Baase C, Hymel P, Peterson KW. The effect of disease prevention and health promotion on workplace productivity: a literature review. *Am J Health Behav.* 2001;15(3): 167–91.

70. Rogers EM. *Diffusion of Innovations.* 5th ed. New York: Free Press; 2003.

71. Sallis JF, McKenzie TL, Conway TL, et al. Environmental interventions for eating and physical activity: a randomized controlled trial in middle schools. *Am J Prev Med.* 2003;24(3):209–17.

72. Sallis JF, McKenzie TL, Alcarez JE, et al. The effects of a 2-year physical education program (SPARK) on physical activity and fitness in elementary school students. *Am J Public Health.* 1997;87(8): 1328–34.

73. Sallis JF, Owen N. *Physical Activity and Behavioral Medicine.* Thousand Oaks (CA): Sage Publications; 1998.

74. Sharpe PA. Community-based physical activity intervention. *Arthritis Rheum.* 2003;49:455–62.

75. Simons-Morton BG, Taylor WC, Snider SA, Huang IW, Fulton JE. Observed levels of elementary and middle school children's activity during physical education classes. *Prev Med.* 1994;23: 437–41.

76. Smith-Ray RL, Almeida FA, Bajaj J, et al. Translating efficacious behavioral principles for diabetes prevention into practice. *Health Promotion Pract.* 2007-hpp.sagepub.com.

77. Sorensen G, Barbeau E, Hunt MK, Emmons K. Reducing social disparities in tobacco use: a social-contextual model for reducing tobacco use among blue-collar workers. *Am J Public Health.* 2004;94: 230–9.

78. Sorensen G, Stoddard A, LaMontagne AD, et al. A comprehensive worksite cancer prevention intervention: behavior change results from a randomized controlled trial (United States). *J Public Health Policy.* 2000;24(1):5–25.

79. Sorensen G, Thompson B, Glanz K, et al. Work site-based cancer prevention: primary results from the Working Well Trial. *Am J Public Health.* 1996;86:939–47.

80. Spence JC, Lee RE. Toward a comprehensive model of physical activity. *Psych Sport Exerc.* 2003;4:7–24.

81. Stange KC, Woolf SH, Gjeltema K. One minute for prevention: the power of leveraging to fulfill the promise of health behavior counseling. *Am J Prev Med.* 2002;22(4):320–3.

82. Stone EJ, McKenzie TL, Welk GJ, Booth ML. Effects of physical activity interventions in youth: review and synthesis. *Am J Prev Med.* 1998;15(4):298–315.

83. Swinburn BA, Walter LG, Arroll B, Tilyard MW, Russell DG. The green prescription study: a randomized controlled trial of written exercise advice provided by general practitioners. *Am J Public Health.* 1998;88(2):288–91.

84. Wuest DA, Bucher CA. Historical foundations of physical education and sport. In: Wuest DA, Bucher CA, editors. *Foundations of Physical Education Sport.* 13th ed. Boston: WCB/McGraw Hill; 1999. p. 146–93.

85. Whitlock EP, Orleans CT, Pender N, Allan J. Evaluating primary care behavioral counseling interventions: an evidence-based approach. *Am J Prev Med.* 2002;22(4):267–84.

86. Wellness Councils of America. Seven benchmarks for success: worksite wellness. *The Worksite Wellness Councils of America* 2007. Available at: http://www.welcoa.org/wellworkplace/index.php?category=2. Accessed May 15, 2007.

87. Yarnell KSH, Pollak KI, Ostbye T, Krause KM, Michener JL. Primary care: Is there enough time for prevention? *Am J Public Health.* 2003;93(4):635–41.

88. Zuvekas A. Health centers and the healthcare system. *J Ambul Care Manage.* 2005;28:331–9.

Health and Fitness Program Development and Operation

The numerous benefits of a physically active lifestyle are well documented in the literature and often referred to in both the broadcast and print media. As a consequence, most individuals are aware that fitness is important and that engaging in an exercise program on a regular basis can have multiple positive effects in their lives. Although recent evidence (3) indicates a slight increase in self-reported regular physical activity, fewer than half the adult United States population engaged in recommended levels of physical activity. Obviously, it is not sufficient to merely be aware of the importance of a physically active lifestyle; benefits can only be realized when individuals incorporate healthy lifestyle behaviors into their daily routine. Having access to a well-designed, safe, and operationally efficient health and fitness program may increase the likelihood that more adults would engage in regular physical activity. This chapter presents an overview of the critical factors that health and fitness professionals should consider when developing and operating health and fitness programs. The chapter also reviews individual attitudes and behaviors toward health and fitness as they relate to health and fitness programming.

HEALTH/FITNESS FACILITY SETTINGS

The health and fitness marketplace is composed of a diverse array of facility settings. Each setting tends to be differentiated by a relatively unique combination of key factors, including business model, location, staffing, facilities, and equipment. In each instance, these factors affect the menu of programs and services offered within that particular facility setting.

Cumulatively, the number of individuals who engage in organized health and fitness programs tends to vary from country to country. In the United States, approximately 16% of the population are members of a health and fitness facility, compared with nations such as the Netherlands with 15%, United Kingdom with 13%, Australia 9%, Germany 8.5%, and Japan 2.7%. In this

---

> > > **KEY TERMS**

Financial plan: A written statement that addresses the financial issues for a particular organization or program, including financial objectives and priorities (both short and long term), budget benchmarks, and the identification of actual and projected sources of revenue. A financial plan is often referred to as a budget or pro forma.

Retention strategy: A systematic plan that involves actions and steps that should be undertaken to enhance the likelihood that individuals who currently belong to a facility will retain their membership.

Risk management: A concerted effort to undertake specific steps to minimize risk of injury to a facility's participants and employees, identify and address any potentially unsafe conditions, and maximize the ability of facility personnel to respond appropriately to emergency situations.

Strategic plan: A planning tool that is designed to address strategic decisions concerning key issues, such as (a) short- and long-term goals for the organization, (b) steps needed to be undertaken to achieve each particular goal, (c) a timeline for reaching each goal, and (d) an allocation and prioritization of time, energy, and resources to each goal. Typically, a strategic plan includes a 5-year timeline.

Target audience: A well-defined, specific segment of the population to whom an organization attempts to market and promote a particular service, product, or program offering.

regard, more than 41 million individuals are members of health and fitness facilities in the United States and more than 103 million are members of health and fitness facilities worldwide (7).

By far the largest segment of health and fitness facilities in the United States are commercial clubs (an estimated 50% of all facilities) (7). In the past two decades, the number of commercial health and fitness clubs in the United States has grown threefold, from just more than 9,000 to slightly more than 29,000. Following commercial health and fitness clubs, the next 10 largest U.S. fitness settings are community centers such as Young Men's Christian Associations (YMCAs) and Jewish Community Centers (JCCs) (17%), university-based centers (6%), hospital-based centers (5%), residential centers (5%), corporate-based facilities (4%), municipal centers (4%), military facilities (2%), country clubs (2%), hotels and resorts (1%), and private studios (1%). Despite their comparatively low numbers, membership in residential, municipal, university-based, and hotel and resort fitness facilities has increased substantially in the past few years (10).

UNDERSTANDING HEALTH AND FITNESS CONSUMERS

Health and fitness programming exists in a variety of facility settings. The reasons people choose to exercise in a specific setting are affected by several factors, including cost, convenience, value, interest, and need. Likewise, individuals may stop exercising for any number of reasons that include both personal and facility factors. A key point is that health and fitness professionals must learn to understand consumer behavior. By recognizing the importance of consumer-driven decisions, exercise professionals will be more prepared to develop and operate well-conceived health and fitness facilities and programs. Furthermore, understanding the needs and interests of the target market will provide further advantages when developing strategies to enhance membership retention.

Demographically, the composition of individuals who join health and fitness facilities has changed considerably in recent years. Being aware of and reacting to these changes can aid health and fitness professionals in their efforts to develop and operate successful health and fitness facilities and programs. The following summarizes some pertinent demographic trends in fitness membership (9):

- Women compose 57% of health and fitness membership. In just the past 10 years, the number of women who have joined health/fitness facilities has increased by 130%, whereas the number of men who use health/fitness facilities has increased by 92%.
- Membership among individuals who are 55 years or older has increased from 9% in the late 1980s to slightly more than 19% in 2006. This trend is likely to increase as the baby boomer population ages.

Furthermore, the population aged 55 years and older is the most active user group of health and fitness facilities, with an average of 97 visits per person per year.

- Individuals who are 35 to 54 years old compose the largest membership segment (37%), which represents a 143% increase since 1987.
- Individuals aged 18 to 34 years have shown the least growth in membership over the past 25 years but still represent 36% of the total industry membership. However, individuals younger than age 18 years have increased by more than 58% in the past 5 years.
- For men, the highest membership rates are for those 25 to 34 years old; for women, it is 35 to 44 years old.
- The average household income for those with a fitness membership is $82,900 and 50% of all facility members earn more than $75,000. This compares with an average U.S. household annual income of $42,000.
- For education level, 55% of facility members have at least a 4-year degree (compared with 20% of the U.S. population).
- Geographically, the west north-central and mountain regions have experienced the fastest growth rates in membership (189% and 156%, respectively), and the state with the highest concentration of club members is Colorado.

LEARNING WHAT INDIVIDUALS WANT

At least four primary tools exist for health and fitness professionals to develop meaningful insight into what their patients (actual and prospective) want from their involvement in a health and fitness facility. These tools are focus groups, surveys, in-depth interviews, and feedback systems. The ways health and fitness professionals use the information gained from these tools can affect their ability to attract, serve, and retain members.

Focus Groups

Focus groups provide a qualitative approach to learning about the attitudes, behaviors, and needs of a particular market. As a rule, focus groups serve to: gain an understanding of individual attitudes and where they originate, generate ideas, test ideas, uncover problems, and help design and develop pertinent questions for a survey tool. To maximize the effectiveness of conducting focus groups, the following steps are important:

- Assign a moderator who is impartial and able to manage group process (i.e., someone who has experience facilitating groups and who has no vested interest in the outcomes).
- Invite 10 to 15 individuals to the focus group with the goal of having at least eight to 10 agree to participate.
- To obtain a variety of ideas and input, ensure that the individuals invited to participate in the focus group appropriately reflect diversity.

- Conduct a minimum of three sessions on any one particular topic.
- Conduct the sessions at times that is convenient for the participants.
- Keep each focus group sessions to 90 minutes or less.
- Hold the sessions in a private area. However, some focus groups allow selected individuals to observe the sessions from a distance, as long as they do not get involved.
- Focus on open-ended questions that cannot be answered with a "yes" or "no."
- Document clearly what is communicated (noting specific language as well as take-away message), and note patterns of responses.
- Identify the most common themes and consider opportunities for generating additional inquiries/surveys. Realize that the comments made by the focus group participants do not necessarily represent universal opinion, but do provide a foundation for greater understanding of perceptions about the topic.
- Send thank-you notes to each participant.

Surveys

Surveys provide a quantitative approach that can collect information about specific markets, which can be valuable when developing a business plan. In this regard, surveys can serve several purposes: assessing participant interest; gaining perspective on programmatic issues, such as pricing, hours of operation, and program choices; and gaining insight on information that will be vital when developing the business plan.

The following factors should be considered when conducting surveys:

- Include an adequate sample size of the target audience. If the number of individuals to be surveyed is beyond the scope of available resources, consider surveying a random sample of the target population.
- If a written survey or an e-mail survey is used, provide an introductory statement.
- If the process involves a written survey, provide a convenient, easy way for participants to return the completed survey at no cost.
- Web-based surveys have become more common because of being user friendly, able to reach large audiences, and easy to analyze/interpret responses.
- Use incentives to help gain greater rates of return.
- Focus on closed-end questions, such as multiple choice and true-or-false questions. Always leave at least one part of the survey available for users to write in comments.
- Keep questions to those areas that are of greatest importance and interest.

To help evaluate the survey results, consider the following:

- Tabulate the results in easily understandable constructs, such as averages, percentages, and frequencies. Consult a statistician if you are not familiar with statistical methods or statistical software programs.
- Review the survey results with others who are knowledgeable in the field and, if available, compare the results with similar surveys. This will help guide decisions in developing a business model that includes the target audience's needs and interests.

In-Depth Interviews

In-depth interviews offer a comprehensive and highly personal approach to learning specific attitudes, behaviors, and needs of patients (actual and prospective). Typically, interviews are conducted by professionals who are trained in the process of obtaining group-oriented information through personal interviewing.

Among the factors that health and fitness professionals should consider when conducting in-depth interviews are the following:

- Have a predetermined strategic plan on how the information obtained from the interviews is to be analyzed and used.
- Plan relevant, pertinent questions that will collectively elicit the desired information.
- Conduct the interviews at an appropriate time that is convenient for those being interviewed and within a reasonable time frame.
- Be clear, direct, and articulate when conducting interviews.
- Take accurate notes, and be careful not to make misinterpretations. If permission is granted, tape the sessions.
- Follow up with a thank-you note to the individuals who participated in the interview process.

Feedback Systems

Feedback systems can be implemented through a variety of approaches to gain input from consumers in a nonintimidating, personal manner. One approach is to establish a Web-based comment blog, to which individuals are invited to provide feedback in an anonymous manner. Those responsible for administering this system could post the feedback to the questions and suggestions. Another approach is using a standardized comment card, in which consumers fill out a form and leave it in a conveniently located receptacle. Management should review the suggestions and feedback from customers and develop a means to provide timely responses as needed.

WHY CONSUMERS JOIN HEALTH AND FITNESS FACILITIES

Understanding why individuals join health and fitness facilities will greatly affect business decisions from the inclusion of activities to the implementation of operational guidelines.

TOP REASONS CONSUMERS JOIN HEALTH AND FITNESS FACILITIES

TOP OVERALL REASONS	TOP SPECIFIC REASONS
To get in shape (84%)	To get in shape (64%)
To stay in shape (79%)	Need a place to exercise (54%)
Need a place to exercise (73%)	To stay in shape (49%)
Equipment availability (72%)	Equipment availability (40%)
Liked facility (71%)	Need motivation (33%)
Friendly staff (63%)	Liked facility (30%)
Good price (61%)	Good price (29%)
Need motivation (60%)	Friendly staff (22%)

TABLE 48-1. THE TOP REASONS FOR JOINING HEALTH AND FITNESS FACILITIES

REASONS	MEN (%)	WOMEN (%)
Place to exercise	60	50
Need motivation	28	38
Friendly staff	17	26
Friends joined	17	25
Participate in classes	4	20

From the Fitness Industry Association. *Winning the Retention Battle* (Parts 1–3). Boston: Fitness Industry Association; 2001.

Box 48-1 presents an overview of some important reasons that individuals join health and fitness facilities. It is common for consumers to identify several reasons for joining a particular facility. The level of importance placed on a particular reason will vary from person to person and circumstance to circumstance (5).

Gender may influence decision-making relative to joining health and fitness facilities, as illustrated in both Box 48-2 and Table 48-1. Differences between men and women do exist in reasons for joining health and fitness facilities in general and, more specifically, affect the decisions made in joining a particular facility.

WHY AN INDIVIDUAL QUITS A HEALTH AND FITNESS FACILITY

 1.11.4-HFS: Knowledge of the importance of tracking and evaluating member retention.

For a variety of reasons, more than 31% of the individuals who belong to a health and fitness facility discontinue their membership each year (4,8). The most frequently reported reasons for terminating memberships are affordability (30%), overcrowded facility (27%), lack of time (26%), inconvenient location (18%), lost interest (17%), change in residence (16%), and changing to alternative exercise setting, such as exercising outdoors (15%). As Box 48-3 illustrates, the reasons for discontinuing a health and fitness program membership vary and can be because of personal or facility factors.

WHY MEMBERS STAY

1.11.8-HFS: Ability to create and maintain records pertaining to participant exercise adherence, retention, and goal setting.

There are factors that can have a meaningful effect on the decision-making processes for membership retention (2,6,9):

- Positive first impressions with the facility and the staff
- Social connection with other members that results in early connection and integration within the facility over the first 90 days
- Lower staff-to-member ratio

DIFFERENCES BETWEEN MEN AND WOMEN IN MAKING DECISIONS FOR JOINING HEALTH AND FITNESS FACILITIES

MEN	WOMEN
Location, location, location (fitness facility needs to be within 12–15 minutes of home or work)	Location, location, location (within 2–15 minutes of home or work)
Convenience	Convenience
Quality and quantity of facilities and equipment	Cleanliness of the facility
Price–value equations	Group exercise programs
Availability of equipment	Friends are members
Staff quality and service delivery	Nonintimidating environment
Competitive environment	Staff quality and service delivery
	Program for kids
	Price–value equation

Information from American Sports Data. *Sports Participation Report.* Boston: American Sports Data; 2003. Centers for Disease Control and Prevention. Prevalence of regular physical activity among adults: United States, 2001 and 2005. *MMWR Morb Mortal Wkly Rep.* 2007;56(46);1209–12.

BOX 48-3	FACILITY-DRIVEN AND PERSONAL REASONS FOR QUITTING HEALTH AND FITNESS FACILITIES

FACILITY-DRIVEN REASONS	PERSONAL REASONS
Overcrowding	Did not make enough use of the facility
Dissatisfied with staff	Lost interest or motivation
Lack of attention by staff	Did not have a partner
Unresponsive management	Switched to home exercise
Favorite staff member left	Switched to exercising outdoors
Facility was not clean	Did not achieve desired results
Culture of the facility	
Equipment was not well kept	
Dishonest business practices	

- Regular and frequent attendance during the first 90 days
- Age and education: older and more educated members more likely to remain
- Financial: a higher enrollment fee associated with higher retention
- Contract term: annual membership versus a month-to-month membership associated with higher retention
- Members achieving their expressed fitness and health goals leads to better retention

There may be a disconnect between what patients believe are their reasons for joining a fitness facility versus their actual reasons. Box 48-4 illustrates how this disconnect can have important decision-making implications for individuals who manage health and fitness facilities.

The following strategies are suggestions that may help improve member retention:

- Provide each member with an immediate connection and orientation to the facility's programs, services, staff, and other members.
- Personalize the orientation around the member's needs and interests with special attention to sex, age, and culture.

- Help establish realistic goals for members, and then provide a program that optimizes the potential for success.
- Provide extra staff interaction and follow-up, especially during the initial 90 days of membership.
- Track member's use of the facility. Contact nonusers and low users with special attention during the first 90 days of membership.
- Survey members regularly to ensure that the facility is offering appropriate services and programs.
- Create member-driven activities so social connections with other members are enhanced.
- Recognize the success and accomplishments of the members through newsletters, bulletin board postings, member blogs, and awards.
- Provide a clean and neat facility, and ensure adequate and proper functioning equipment.
- Keep membership recruitment and enrollment goals compatible with available resources.
- Price membership fees at market value commensurate with consumers' perceived value.
- Designate a portion of the facility that may portray a less intimidating environment for less-fit or other participants with special needs.

BOX 48-4	THE DISCONNECT BETWEEN PERCEPTION AND REALITY CONCERNING WHY INDIVIDUALS JOIN AND QUIT HEALTH AND FITNESS FACILITIES

PERCEPTION OF FACILITY	JOIN FOR	LEAVE FOR
Worth the money	Good price	Overcrowded
Fun	Available equipment	Lost interest
Knowledgeable staff	Get in shape or stay in shape	Could not afford
For fit people	Staff quality or service	No partner
For young people	Cleanliness (women)	Results not achieved
Overcrowded	Friends are members (women)	Lack of attention by staff
	Nonintimidating environment	Culture of club
	Group exercise program (women)	Poor programs
		Dissatisfied with staff; No connection

- Make sure that everything in the facility is convenient, and take steps to implement areas that need improving.
- Encourage member feedback and respond appropriately and quickly to special requests or issues.
- Provide an environment that is welcoming and personal. Greet members by name, and let them know you care.

DEVELOPING A HEALTH AND FITNESS PROGRAM

> **1.11.1-HFS: Knowledge of the health/fitness instructor's role in administration and program management within a health/fitness facility.**

> **1.11.3-HFS: Knowledge of how to manage a fitness department (e.g., working within a budget, interviewing and training staff, scheduling, running staff meetings, staff development).**

Several factors should be taken into consideration when developing a health and fitness program. None is more important than designing a program that is consistent with the strategic plan of the facility or organization. Providing people with the opportunity to achieve the innumerable benefits of exercise is undeniably a worthy undertaking. Detailed planning is required to make sure appropriate attention to the facility's health and fitness program is provided.

ENHANCING THE FACILITY'S OPPORTUNITY FOR SUCCESS

A sound plan for developing a health and wellness program should address several factors, including finances, staffing, necessary facilities, equipment, risk management, and target markets. After the plan is developed, the decisions relating to the health and wellness program become an integral part of the health and fitness facility's business plan.

A business plan for a health and fitness facility should have a vision of the future for that facility and a plan for how that vision will be achieved. To be viable, the vision must meet several criteria. First and foremost, it must be compelling to those charged with executing the vision. It must also be tangible and realistic. Finally, it must meet the expectations of those responsible for the future of the facility. The business plan should also have a mission or clearly stated purpose. The mission succinctly articulates for every employee what business they are in and the purpose behind the experiences they are delivering. Next, the business plan should detail the parameters of the path that the facility will take in achieving its articulated vision and fulfilling its mission. In this regard, the two most commonly used guideposts are goals and objectives. As a rule, goals are positive statements that delineate what needs to be ac-

complished over the long run to achieve the vision of the facility, and objectives are clear, relatively specific statements or targets, the completion of which will lead to the achievement of the facility's goals. Unlike objectives, goals are purposely stated in generalities (e.g., to be the largest health and fitness facility in town within 5 years). Objectives, on the other hand, are generally short-range, challenging (but realistic) statements of a facility's intentions that focus on immediate accomplishments that are consistent with an organization's long-range goals (e.g., achieve a 4% net growth in the facility's membership in the current fiscal year).

A responsible business plan specifies a financial plan or budget that specifies the resources needed to keep the facility viable in reaching the goals. This budget projection includes detailing the specific resources needed (currently and in the future) and where those resources will be allocated. An appropriate business plan also outlines the strategic steps for implementing the plan, including cataloging what the facility will do if things do not go as planned (a process typically referred to as *contingency planning*).

IDENTIFYING TARGET AUDIENCES

The health and fitness program offering in some organizational settings (e.g., YMCAs, JCCs, hospital-based groups) is influenced by the expressed mission of the organization involved. For those organizations, the mission essentially defines the facility's menu of services and activities. The family orientation of YMCAs, for example, mandates that YMCAs offer a significant number of activities that are geared toward families, particularly children. In the same regard, hospital-based programs tend to focus primarily on secondary prevention and rehabilitation-directed services.

Although all health and fitness facilities have a degree of freedom in deciding what services and activities to include in their program offerings, none has more latitude than commercial health and fitness clubs. Strategically, the key issue for health and fitness clubs is to identify target audiences who will be interested in using and paying for the services and activities that are offered. How well clubs executive the strategic plan has a major impact on their ability to succeed.

Health and fitness clubs vary in the way that they evaluate market relevance and appropriateness. A typical approach is to analyze the market by specific demographic and psychographic variables. This analysis allows the clubs to segment the market according to a variable-driven structure. As a rule, three major ways exist to segment a market: geographic (location, density, urban vs. rural), demographic (age, sex, family size, family cycle, household income, occupation, education, religion, race, nationality, social class), and psychographic (lifestyle, personality, benefits sought, user status, user rate, loyalty status, readiness stage).

The majority of commercial health and fitness facilities utilize demographic segmentation to determine their targeted audience (e.g., population density, age mix, average household income). Because psychographic segmentation focuses more on individuals and their attitudes and behaviors, health and fitness clubs should incorporate psychographic metrics into their overall evaluation of their target audience. Recognizing the importance of psychographic factors is effective to help recognize market opportunity and address individual needs. Psychographic portraits of potential patients have potential implications for health and fitness professionals who are responsible for attracting and retaining members. Reports indicate that individuals fall into one of six general categories with some general characteristics (5):

1. Balanced holistics (13%)
   - Take a balanced approach to exercise; exercise regularly; and exercise for both emotional and physical reasons, including "to get centered."
   - Usually feel badly if they do not exercise.
   - Are twice as likely to be health club members than the general population (26% vs. 13%).
   - Describe themselves as socially confidant, goal oriented, intelligent, energetic, and health conscious.
   - Are considered "hard-core" exercisers.
2. Conscientious preventers (8%)
   - Take a balanced approach to exercise and are more focused on exercise as a way to prevent health problems and treat existing medical conditions.
   - Place a high level of importance on fitness.
   - Are twice as likely to be health-club members than the general population (26% vs. 13%).
   - Describe themselves as health conscious, family-oriented, energetic, religious, and perfectionistic.
   - Are also considered "hard-core" exercisers.
3. Social competitors (20%)
   - Prefer social, competitive, and relationship-engaging activities.
   - Equally likely to be a health club member as the general public (13%).
   - Describe themselves as professionally ambitious, competitive, outgoing, risk taking, and a sports fan.
4. "Abracadabras" (14%)
   - Have low fitness levels; do not exercise and have no desire to do so.
   - Dislike exercise; if they do exercise, the reason cited is often to lose weight.
   - Are half as likely to be health club members (6.5%).
   - Describe themselves as energetic, socially skillful, health conscious, and less outgoing.
   - Considered to be an "indifferent" group.
5. "Woulda–shouldas" (12%)
   - Do exercise, but less than general public.
   - Are self-conscious; tend to have low fitness levels.
   - Do not hate exercise; rather, lack self-discipline.

- As likely as the general public to be health club members.
- Describe themselves as emotional, bookish, shy, and professionally ambitious.
- Considered to be part of the "uninitiated believers" group.
6. Sitcom skeptics (12%)
   - Believe that individuals who exercise are self-absorbed.
   - Believe that a good diet and clean living negate the need to exercise.
   - Some do exercise occasionally and are equally likely to be health club members as the general public.
   - Describe themselves as not falling for the fitness craze.
   - Considered to be part of the "indifferent" group.

DETERMINING THE PROGRAM OFFERING

Perhaps no decision has more important ramifications for the ability of a health and fitness facility to fulfill its mission and achieve its vision than to determine appropriate services and activities. Such a decision can affect not only the facility's short-term financial health but also its ability to survive in the long term.

The business plan is the basic foundation underlying the decisions of what to include in the program offerings. Collectively, the offerings must be appropriate for the short- and long-term goals and objectives of the organization. How the offerings address this lofty aspiration may require a strategic balancing act because one decision may be more appropriate than another for the organization in the short term or in a particular set of ever-changing circumstances.

Within the context of adhering to the business plan, the next factor that must be considered when developing a health and fitness program is meeting the needs and interests of the consumers (actual and potential) that the facility is intended to serve. As previously discussed, several tools for helping to determine those needs and interests exist, including surveys, focus groups, and in-depth interviews.

Additional tools that are used to help identify the services and activities offered in a facility's health and wellness program are fitness assessments and preactivity health screening instruments. Properly used, both approaches provide information that can help "personalize" the program offering specifically to an individual's needs. The information gained from the assessments provides insight concerning activity choice and helps health and fitness professionals prioritize specific activities that are most appropriate for that person. The primary aim is to ensure that the programming considers the unique characteristics of participants.

Another factor to consider when determining the offering of services and activities is the dynamic nature of individuals' attitudes over time that may affect their choices for fitness programming. For example, the following macrotrends in fitness activities have occurred in the past decade (8,9):

- Traditional aerobic dancing participation has declined, and group fitness programming has increased.
- High-impact aerobic activity participation has declined, and group fitness classes geared toward functional fitness has increased.
- Mind-body classes such as yoga and Pilates have grown significantly as a reflection of consumers' desire for exercise that is softer and more balanced.
- Treadmill participation has become the most popular form of cardiovascular activity in health/fitness facilities, a growth that corresponds with the aging of the population.
- Stair-climbing participation has declined significantly, and elliptical training has increased.
- Personal training, both individual and group formats, has grown significantly and represents the largest program element in most commercial health and fitness facilities.
- Functional fitness that emphasizes movements to strengthen the "core" and enable more effective performance of everyday activities has become one of the top five trends.
- Fusion fitness is evolving as an important trend, which is the integration of different exercise activities into one exercise program format (e.g., yoga and group cycling, stretching and strengthening, Pilates with yoga).
- Exer-gaming (e.g., fitness movements performed in a reality- or virtual-based game environment) and entertainment options (e.g., equipment with MP3 player integration, equipment with built-in Internet connectivity) are also important elements in current fitness programming.

EVALUATING THE PROGRAM OFFERINGS

> **1.11.13-HFS: Knowledge of the importance of tracking and evaluating health promotion program results.**

A process should be established to evaluate whether the various parts of the health and wellness program (i.e., services and activities) are meeting expectations of the business plan. The following factors are important to consider when evaluating health and wellness programs:

- Identify specific criteria (e.g., performance metrics) that are consistent with the parameters detailed in the business plan (e.g., financial, growth, total participation, community service, retention percentage).
- Define short- and a long-term goals and measurable objectives.
- Consider industry participation trends when evaluating the results.
- Conduct ongoing process evaluation.

OPERATING A HEALTH AND FITNESS BUSINESS

Operating a health and wellness program requires strategic planning, the ability to adapt to circumstances, and having competent management that is accountable and pays keen attention to detail. Administrative matters that health and fitness administrators must be concerned with include staffing, facilities and equipment, finances, marketing and sales, customer service, and risk management.

STAFFING

> **1.11.2-HFS: Knowledge of and the ability to use the documentation required when a patient shows signs or symptoms during an exercise session and should be referred to a physician.**

> **1.11.9-HFS: Ability to develop and administer educational programs (e.g., lectures, workshops) and educational materials.**

Competent staff must be hired to supervise all of the various elements of the health and wellness program. Ideally, overall responsibility for the fitness program is assigned to an individual with a college degree in health and fitness or a related exercise science degree. Preferably, that person will also hold a current certification from a nationally recognized third-party accredited professional organization, such as American College of Sports Medicine (ACSM) certification. All applicable local, state, and federal regulations and laws concerning staffing should be strictly followed, especially those laws that apply to licensing and registration of health and fitness professionals. In addition, professionally trained and certified instructors who have demonstrable expertise in the activity being taught should lead all group exercise classes and periodically monitor all activity areas on a regular basis. Competent personnel who are fully qualified to conduct screening assessments and exercise training are required when working in a health and fitness program.

FACILITIES AND EQUIPMENT

> **1.10.13-HFS: Knowledge of the components of an equipment maintenance/repair program and how it may be used to evaluate the condition of exercise equipment to reduce the potential risk of injury.**

> **1.10.17-HFS: Ability to identify the components that contribute to the maintenance of a safe environment, including equipment operation and maintenance, proper sanitation, safety and maintenance of exercise areas, and overall facility maintenance.**

All activities conducted in facilities should be appropriate for the activity being offered and that meet all local, state, and federal codes, regulations, and laws. All facilities should be well lighted, with an appropriate level of temperature, humidity, and ventilation. Every activity area should be clean, well kept, and regularly inspected to ensure that no condition involving an undue risk of injury to participants exists.

Similar to the facility areas, all equipment used in a particular activity should be appropriate for that activity. To the extent that is feasible and appropriate to the business plan, a variety of equipment should be provided that addresses each of the major components of fitness. Among the criteria that should be considered when purchasing equipment is durability, serviceability, value, appropriate for the intended users, and safety. Equipment should be purchased from reputable companies with demonstrable records of responsible and ethical behavior with regards to making user-friendly equipment and honoring their service commitments.

All equipment should be well maintained (i.e., at a minimum, strictly adhere to the maintenance guidelines prescribed in the owner's manual provided by the equipment's manufacturer) and regularly inspected to ensure that the equipment does not present a potential risk to participants. When necessary, all equipment should have instructional signage posted in an appropriate place (e.g., attached to or adjacent to the particular piece of equipment) that details how to safely use each piece of equipment.

FINANCES

 1.11.6-HFS: Ability to administer fitness-related programs within established budgetary guidelines.

A detailed plan is needed for addressing all of the financial issues involving the health and wellness program (both required operating and capital expenditures and anticipated revenues generated by the program). This step involves formulating a financial plan (e.g., budget) for the facility, evaluating the various elements of the plan that were implemented, and making changes when appropriate. The financial planning process includes establishing financial objectives and priorities (both short and long term), budgeting, and identifying actual and projected sources of funds.

Individuals responsible for the financial health of the organization must be knowledgeable about key financial issues. The information that they have concerning the finances of the organization must be accurate and up to date. They should also be aware of industry benchmarks for revenues and expenses because such information will help them validate their budget assumptions.

MARKETING AND SALES

 1.11.7-HFS: Ability to develop marketing materials for the purpose of promoting fitness-related programs.

 1.11.10-HFS: Knowledge of basic sales techniques to promote health, fitness, and wellness services.

 1.11.11-HFS: Knowledge of networking techniques with other healthcare professionals for referral purposes.

In today's market, establishing a brand strategy and then building a marketing plan to communicate that brand message is important. Promoting a health and wellness facility/program "brand" requires systematic planning. It involves an understanding of the potential markets for the menu of services and programs offered by the program and a concerted, well-conceived effort to reach the targeted markets. Responsibility for each step in the particular effort to promote the program should be specifically defined, including overall accountability for each executed marketing effort.

Depending on the circumstances, a variety of tools can be used to promote a health and wellness program, either as a whole or in part, including direct mail, exterior/interior signage, Web sites, Internet blogs, member incentives, telephone calls, e-mails, radio, television, word of mouth, sponsorships, and endorsements. The choice of tools depends on such factors as the organization's strategic plan, resource availability, accessibility and sophistication of the targeted audiences, and the competition for the attention and resources of the targeted audiences. A key point to remember is that marketing and promotion of a health and wellness program is an ongoing process that directly or indirectly involves everyone in the organization.

Within some health and fitness organizational settings, particularly health clubs, a key focal point of the marketing process is the sale of memberships. As a rule, membership sales tend to follow a three-step pathway. The first stage involves identifying individuals who are referred to as *leads*. Leads are individuals who have demographics or characteristics that match the targeted audience of the health club. Leads have not expressed any interest or been shown to have an interest in becoming a club member.

The second level of the membership pathway involves individuals who are typically known as prospects. Prospects either have shown an interest in the club or have been identified as being more suitable candidates for membership.

The third pathway to membership involves individuals who have decided to actually become members of the club. The obvious goal of the process is to capture leads, turn them into prospects, and ultimately convince them to become members of the club.

Health and fitness clubs use a variety of strategies to build their memberships. Among the more popular steps that are used in this regard are the following:

1. Membership referral
   - This approach is the most focused strategy for generating prospective members.
   - The process involves existing members providing the names of potential new members. This is usually conducted once a year.

- Members are provided with referral cards to hand in the names of prospects. Incentives are typically given to members for providing referrals.
- High-end clubs often make this strategy one of their major sales focuses by using committees and getting referrals from all new members.

2. Lead boxes
   - Lead boxes are placed in business locations that tend to serve customer bases that are demographically similar to the targeted audiences (e.g., sporting good stores, restaurants).
   - Businesses are given awards for allowing the lead boxes to be placed in their locales.
   - Primarily used in low-price and high-volume fitness clubs.
   - This strategy usually does not generate quality leads and produces a low rate of return.

3. Advertising
   - In general, this strategy is a scatter-gun approach to reaching a facility's market (versus a sharp-shooter method) and is designed to enhance the image of the organization, create leads, or occasionally generate prospects.
   - Examples include promotional messages on cable television, Internet advertisements, social Web site videos, radio, newspapers, billboards, and external or internal signage.
   - The most effective type of advertising for generating leads or prospects focuses on engaging the audience to act via such devices as coupons, raffles, and so on.
   - It is important to know the audience before the advertising medium is selected. For example, young adults are more likely to learn of the club through "buzz" marketing, blogs, or chat rooms and other social networking sites on the Internet, whereas older adults are more likely to respond to targeted direct mail pieces and member referral programs.

4. Alliances with Homeowner Associations and Realtors
   - Involves an approach in which homeowner associations (HOAs) and realtors provide the names of new residents to fitness facilities.
   - This strategy is a good source for qualified leads (and even prospects) when the HOAs' and realtors' customers match the organization's target market.
   - This strategy usually involves providing some complementary club memberships or guest passes for the HOAs or realtors to use.
   - Another option is to presell club memberships to the HOA or builder so that when a home is purchased, the new owner is already a member of the club.

5. Direct mail
   - This strategy is primarily a technique for creating leads or turning leads into prospects. It is a more focused technique than advertising.
   - Mailing lists from agencies provide targeted lists to best match the desired market area and demographics of the targeted audience.
   - The message is usually simple, with an attention-grabbing call for action that normally incorporates some incentive into the mailed piece to generate an action response.
   - The return rate for this technique is usually 1% to 2% for mailed pieces and 2% to 5% for e-mails.

6. Community involvement
   - This strategy focuses on creating relationships to find prospects. It involves creating a specific image in the community and becoming recognized as an integral part of the community.
   - An example of this approach is to become active in community organizations, such as the local chambers of commerce, the Rotary, or church groups, or to host community events in the club or sponsor community events at other locations.
   - Service and relationship-driven clubs use this strategy most often.

7. Cold calling
   - This strategy is used to turn leads into prospects and can use general or targeted lists of names.
   - Examples include telemarketing, phone call solicitation, and cold calling on homes. Be aware of the no-call lists that are in effect in most states and the penalties that are associated with cold calling someone whose name appears on a no-call list.
   - This strategy normally includes some incentives to get action-oriented responses.
   - Individuals who are contacted often consider this technique intrusive, and this approach typically gets a low rate of return.

8. Reputation management
   - This strategy is used to enhance the public image of the organization and, over time, can be a great source for prospects.
   - It involves the development of a press kit on the club (e.g., a background, fact sheet) and requires establishing positive relationships with the local media.
   - The approach requires regular issuing of human interest press releases involving the club and following up with the media.

9. Promotional materials
   - This strategy is normally used to assist converting leads to prospects or prospects to members.
   - It involves developing materials that are designed to create a positive image of the club and to help educate consumers on the club.
   - Examples include promotional Web sites, print brochures, and video brochures and materials that are given to leads and more often to prospects.

10. Strategic alliances
    - This strategy is designed to create partnerships between businesses and organizations with similar

target audiences and is useful for bringing in leads and prospects.

- The approach involves cross-marketing between the businesses and focuses on enticing customers of each business to become potential customers for the other partner (alliance group).
- This method is frequently used in an effective, strategic manner by relatively large, multiple-club organizations.

CUSTOMER SERVICE

 1.11.12-HFS: Ability to provide and administer appropriate customer service.

An important factor of health and fitness clubs is to retain customers. Accordingly, every club should make an absolute commitment to customer service. Integral to this commitment is a clean, well-run facility that is responsive to the needs and interests of the members. Furthermore, all staff members should be pleasant, well groomed, appropriately attired, and exhibit an attitude that displays caring attitudes. Communicating with members on a personal level and understanding their interests and needs are hallmarks of an outstanding customer service culture. In addition, every health and fitness facility should implement a specific system for soliciting and responding to feedback provided by the members. A common complaint from members is the inability of management to respond to issues or concerns in a timely manner. If feedback is solicited from membership, one must be prepared to respond promptly and respectfully.

RISK MANAGEMENT

Every health and fitness facility should take specific steps to minimize the risk of unsafe conditions and to maximize the ability of facility personnel to respond to emergency events. Among the actions that can enhance the safety level of the health and fitness program participants are qualified staff, preactivity screening, adequate levels of activity supervision, regular maintenance of all equipment and facilities, attention accorded to physical plant safety issues, appropriate signage, and requiring all activities to be conducted in an appropriate, safety-conscious manner.

Health and fitness facilities must also have emergency plans that ensure that events involving the health or safety of participants are handled in an appropriate manner (1). An emergency plan should be developed and implemented to provide specific guidelines concerning how the staff members should react when emergency incidents occur. Just as importantly, an emergency plan should be rehearsed regularly to ensure that the staff is fully prepared to respond to an untoward or unexpected event. Staff members should conduct

themselves in a manner that minimizes the consequences of the incidents. In practical terms, emergency plans help to ensure that minor incidents do not become major incidents and that major incidents do not lead to fatalities (1,11). Health and fitness facilities should put their emergency plans in writing and ensure that all staff members are fully aware of the emergency procedures.

SUMMARY

Over the years, the health/fitness club industry has matured and expanded. In the process, many of the dynamics of the club business have changed. Three decades ago, the industry was in its infancy—developed, operated, and pushed forward by entrepreneurs who had a passion for fitness and what they were doing. Over time, profitability and financial issues have become a primary focal concern of the industry. This information has had a profound impact on the industry.

Developing and operating a health/fitness facility is a multifaceted process that involves giving due consideration to several factors, particularly the business plan of the health/fitness facility and the needs and interests of the targeted participants. Regardless of the specific circumstances involved in a particular facility, it is essential that the process is undertaken in a systematic, thoughtful manner to ensure that the effort is both appropriate and effective.

REFERENCES

1. **American College of Sports Medicine. Recommendations for cardiovascular screening, staffing, and emergency policies at health/fitness facilities: a joint position statement with the American Heart Association.** *Med Sci Sports Exerc.* 1998;30:1009–18.
2. American Sports Data. *Sports Participation Report.* Boston: American Sports Data; 2003.
3. Centers for Disease Control and Prevention. Prevalence of regular physical activity among adults: United States, 2001 and 2005. *MMWR Morb Mortal Wkly Rep.* 2007;56(46);1209–12.
4. Fitness Industry Association. *Winning the Retention Battle* (Parts 1–3). Boston: Fitness Industry Association; 2001.
5. International Health, Racquet & Sportsclub Association. *2006 Profiles of Success.* Boston: IHRSA; 2006.
6. International Health, Racquet & Sportsclub Association (prepared by Roper Starch). *Fitness American-Style: A Look at How and Why Americans Exercise.* Boston: IHRSA; 2001.
7. International Health, Racquet & Sportsclub Association. *IHRSA Global Report: State of the Health Club Industry 2006.* Supplement to *Club Business International.* Boston: IHRSA; 2006.
8. International Health, Racquet & Sportsclub Association. *Why People Quit.* Boston: IHRSA; 1998.
9. International Health, Racquet & Sportsclub Association. *Why People Stay.* Boston: IHRSA; 2000.
10. International Health, Racquet & Sportsclub Association/ASD. *Health Club Trend Report: 1987–2002.* Boston: IHRSA; 2002.
11. Peterson J, Tharrett S, McInnis K, editors. *ACSM's Health/Fitness Facility Standards and Guidelines.* 3rd ed. Champaign (IL): Human Kinetics; 2006.

SELECTED REFERENCES FOR FURTHER READING

Grantham B, Patton R, York T, Winick M. *Health Fitness Management.* Champaign (IL): Human Kinetics; 1998.

McCarthy J, ed. *IHRSA's Guide to Lenders and Investors.* 2nd ed. Boston: IHRSA; 2003.

Plummer T. *The Business of Fitness: Understanding the Financial Side of Owning a Fitness Business.* Monterey (CA): Healthy Learning; 2003.

Plummer T. *Making Money in the Fitness Business.* Monterey (CA): Healthy Learning; 1999.

Plummer T. *Open a Fitness Business and Make Money Doing It.* Monterey (CA): Healthy Learning; 2007.

Tharrett S. *The Health/Fitness Operators Guide to Recruiting and Retaining Great Employees.* Monterey (CA): Healthy Learning; 2007.

Tharrett S, Peterson J. *Fitness Management.* Monterey (CA): Healthy Learning; 2006.

INTERNET RESOURCES

- American College of Sports Medicine: www.acsm.org
- American Council on Exercise: www.acefitness.org
- Fitness Management: www.fitnessmanagement.com
- IDEA Health & Fitness Association: www.ideafit.com
- International Health, Racquet & Sportsclub Association: www.ihrsa.org

Clinical Exercise Program Development and Operation

Exercise professionals who work in the clinical setting are responsible for a broad range of knowledge, skills, and abilities (KSAs) that address the needs of patients with chronic disease and complex comorbidities. The challenge of clinical program management is to deliver quality care that goes beyond the provision of appropriate exercise assessment and training principles to address other educational, safety, and risk-reduction needs of patients. Furthermore, clinical programs must assure safe and effective treatment strategies that are provided by an appropriately credentialed multidisciplinary team and remain within the parameters (e.g., eligible diagnosis, number of sessions, length of program, allotted reimbursement) defined by third-party payers. Cardiac rehabilitation (CR) and pulmonary rehabilitation (PR) programs are well-established and proven effective clinical models for the treatment of cardiopulmonary disease.

The purpose of this chapter is to provide an overview of cardiopulmonary rehabilitation programs and discuss operational strategies for program administration related to interdisciplinary team roles and responsibilities, intervention components, policies and procedures, program certification, reimbursement issues, and outcome evaluation. Healthcare professionals pursuing a career in cardiopulmonary rehabilitation programs are recommended to acquire the KSAs as defined at the American College of Sports Medicine (ACSM) Clinical Exercise Specialist (CES)® level. The ACSM Registered Clinical Exercise Physiologist (RCEP)® is an ideal candidate to work in CR and PR programs, but advanced academic training and experience is needed to fulfill the requirements of the RCEP® as described in the ACSM RCEP® Certification Resource Manual (8).

CARDIAC REHABILITATION AND SECONDARY PREVENTION PROGRAMS

Coronary artery disease (CAD) is the leading cause of death and disability in the United States. Individuals with established CAD are at high risk for recurrent events. Cardiac rehabilitation programs are secondary prevention services that help to slow, stabilize, or reverse the atherosclerosis process, resulting in a reduction in the risk of future cardiovascular events (1,10,44). Cardiac rehabilitation/secondary prevention (CR/SP) programs provide important resources to optimize physical, vocational, psychological, and social functioning among patients with cardiac disease (3).

Contemporary CR began in the early 1970s when exercise programs were extended beyond hospital discharge

> > > KEY TERMS

Benchmark: A standard or norm for evaluating quality and performance.

Comorbidities: Adverse health-related conditions (in addition to pulmonary disease or coronary heart disease) that have a negative impact on morbidity and mortality and have the potential to alter exercise performance.

Core competencies: The clinical skills, educational training, and knowledge base that ensure quality staffing for the delivery of safe and effective cardiac and pulmonary rehabilitation program services.

Outcome measures: Assessment of the effects or results of treatments and/or services for a particular disease or condition using quantitative methods.

Outcomes matrix: A foundation to guide outcome assessment in cardiac and pulmonary rehabilitation programs that includes measures of health, behavioral, clinical, and service outcomes.

Performance measures: Assessment of the implementation of actions and/or processes that are known to produce a desirable outcome using quantitative methods.

to highly structured, physician-supervised, electrocardiographic (ECG)-monitored exercise programs (44). Originally, CR programs focused almost entirely on exercise training to reverse the physical decline that resulted from prolonged bed rest. During the 1980s, CR evolved to a more comprehensive lifestyle modification model, specifically aimed at secondary prevention (19). In addition to exercise training, risk-factor management was employed in an attempt to help patients slow or slightly reverse the progression of CAD and reducing cardiac events.

Present-day CR programs have evolved from a primarily singular intervention-exercise training to a multifaceted medical and lifestyle treatment for CAD (24,27). The evolution of CR has occurred as our understanding of the atherosclerotic process and the role of risk factors has matured. Cardiac rehabilitation programs play a critical role in acute and chronic care of the patients with CAD and have demonstrated powerful morbidity and mortality benefits. There is a growing body of evidence confirming that aggressive and comprehensive secondary prevention increases survival, reduces recurrent events and the need for interventional procedures, and improves quality of life (40). The mortality reduction with exercise-based rehabilitation is 27% (22), which is comparable to the effects of our most potent pharmacologic agents. Furthermore, it has been demonstrated that CR and medical treatments of cardiovascular risk factors may be superior to percutaneous coronary intervention among some patients regarding the prevention of subsequent cardiovascular events and improvement in exercise tolerance (18).

PROGRAM DESCRIPTION

The aims of CR programs are to optimize cardiovascular risk reduction, promote adoption and adherence to healthy lifestyle behaviors, reduce disability, and promote an active lifestyle for patients with cardiovascular disease (10). Eligible participants for CR programs typically include those with heart-related medical conditions including myocardial infarction, coronary artery bypass grafting, chronic stable angina pectoris, percutaneous coronary intervention, congestive heart disease, heart transplant, valvular surgery, and arrhythmias (41,44,45). Ideally, the care-continuum approach to comprehensive risk reduction through CR services should begin during hospitalization (phase I) and transition to the outpatient setting (phase II).

As structured in-hospital (phase I) CR programs diminish because of shorter hospital stays for patients with acute cardiac events and/or procedures, outpatient CR programs continue to evolve and expand. Many myocardial infarction patients, for example, are now hospitalized for only 3 to 4 days (27), minimizing the negative consequences of prolonged bed rest that occurred in the past. An unfortunate consequence of shorter hospitalizations is that there is minimal opportunity to address comprehensive risk-factor modification during hospitalization. Several important interventions, however, are still needed during the brief hospitalization. First, and most importantly, patients need to be directed to an outpatient (phase II) program. Second, continued smoking cessation and relapse prevention needs to be addressed for individuals who were smoking before their hospitalization. Third, cardiovascular risk factors should be defined and reviewed and follow-up appointments should be scheduled. Because a physician's recommendation is the most important predictor of CR participation, it is important that all physicians (e.g., specialists and primary care) emphasize the importance of secondary prevention that includes optimal medical management and comprehensive lifestyle interventions that will help patients achieve their treatment goals (2). For programs that are affiliated with a hospital, it is beneficial to have a CR team member designated as a liaison between the inpatient and outpatient settings of CR services. Identifying and contacting patients in hospital and developing a computerized referral process to outpatient CR will enhance the likelihood that the individual will participate in CR (17).

CORE COMPONENTS OF CARE

Cardiac rehabilitation services offer a multifaceted and multidisciplinary approach to overall cardiovascular risk reduction that goes beyond exercise training alone. In alignment with the American Heart Association (AHA)/American College of Cardiology (ACC) secondary prevention guidelines (40), the AHA and American Association of Cardiovascular and Pulmonary Rehabilitation (AACVPR) published a scientific statement that detailed the core components of care for programs offering CR services (9). The statement provides detailed recommendations for patient evaluation, interventions, and expected outcomes for services related to patient assessment, risk-factor management, prescribed exercise, and lifestyle counseling (9). The core components of a CR/SP program make up the foundation of a successful program and are summarized in Table 49-1.

The scientific evidence supporting CR/SP services is so strong that performance measures were collaboratively published by AACVPR, ACC, and AHA (42). The purpose of these performance measures is to help improve the delivery of services and provide a focus on care processes known to improve patient outcomes.

CHALLENGES AND FUTURE DIRECTIONS

Despite all the documented benefits, only about 15% of eligible patients in the United States receive CR services (44). Women significantly underutilize CR services despite presenting with a more prominent risk-factor profile and a lower functional capacity than men (2,34,37).

TABLE 49-1. SUMMARY OF PATIENT ASSESSMENT AND OUTCOME EVALUATION IN CARDIAC REHABILITATION AND SECONDARY PREVENTION PROGRAMS[a]

CORE COMPONENT	ASSESSMENT AND OUTCOME EVALUATION
Patient assessment	Review medical history: Diagnoses, interventional procedures, comorbidities, test results, symptoms, risk factors, recent influenza vaccination, and medications. Assess: Vital signs, current clinical status, administer standardized measurement tools to assess status in each component of care. Goal: Develop an individualized, goal-directed treatment plan with achievable short- and long-term goals for cardiovascular risk reduction and improvement in quality of life.
Nutritional counseling	Assess: Current dietary behavior: dietary content of fat, cholesterol, sodium, caloric intake; eating and drinking habits. Goal: Individualized prescribed diet based on needs assessed. Promote adherence.
Weight management	Assess: Weight, height, body mass index, waist circumference. Determine risk (obese >30 kg/m^2, overweight 25–29.9 kg/m^2, waist >40 inches men, >35 inches women) Goal: Weight risk identified: energy deficit of 500–1,000 kcal/day with diet and exercise to reduce weight by at least 10% (1–2 lb/wk). Establish realistic short- and long-term weight loss goals. Promote adherence and weight-loss maintenance.
Hypertension management	Assess: Resting blood pressure, current treatment, and compliance. Goal: <130 mm Hg systolic and <80 mm Hg diastolic blood pressure.
Lipid management	Assess: Lipid profile, current treatment, and compliance. Goal: LDL <100 mg/dL (<70 mg/dL is considered optimal); secondary goals: HDL >35 mg/dL, triglycerides <200 mg/dL.
Diabetes management	Assess: Diabetes present: HbA$_1$C and fasting blood glucose (FBG); current treatment and compliance. Goal: HbA$_1$C <7.0, FBG 80–110 mg/dL.
Smoking cessation	Assess: Smoking status: current, recent (quit <6 months), former, never. If current or recent, assess amount of tobacco/day (or other nicotine) and readiness to quit. Goal: Abstinence from smoking and use of all tobacco products.
Psychosocial management	Assess: Psychological distress (e.g., depression, anxiety, hostility); refer patients with clinically significant distress to appropriate mental health specialists for further evaluation and treatment. Goal: Reduction of psychological distress (if present); coping and stress management skills enhanced.
Exercise training	Assess: Functional capacity (maximal or submaximal), physiologic responses to exercise. Goal: Individualized exercise prescription defining frequency (times/week), intensity (metabolic equivalent [MET] level), duration (minutes), and modality to achieve aerobic, muscular, and flexibility goals. Provide progressive updates. Promote adherence.
Physical activity counseling	Assess: Current (past 7 days) physical activity behavior, include leisure and usual activities (e.g., occupational, domestic). Specify: time (minutes/day), frequency (days/week), and intensity (light, moderate, vigorous). Goal: Accumulate 30–60 minutes/day of moderate-intensity physical activity on ≥5 days/wk; caution patients to avoid unaccustomed vigorous activity. Promote adherence.

[a]Adapted from Balady GJ, Williams MA, Ades PA, et al. Core components of cardiac rehabilitation/secondary prevention programs: 2007 update: a scientific statement from the American Heart Association Exercise, Cardiac Rehabilitation, and Prevention Committee, the Council on Clinical Cardiology; the Councils on Cardiovascular Nursing, Epidemiology and Prevention, and Nutrition, Physical Activity, and Metabolism; and the American Association of Cardiovascular and Pulmonary Rehabilitation. *Circulation.* 2007;115(20):2675–782.

Furthermore, CR benefits are underused among indigent and minority populations (21,26), as well as in populations of developing countries where rates of CAD are increasing (33). There is a multitude of reasons for this remarkably low utilization rate, including geographic inability to access a program (15), inadequate insurance coverage, cost, and work and family conflicts (20). Clearly, a critical examination of how we presently deliver CR services is indicated, and we need to work to expand program utilization.

Equally problematic, for individuals who do participate in CR, only about 50% who complete CR are adhering to an exercise regimen at 1 year (30,34). This lack of adherence to an exercise routine is exacerbated by less-than-ideal compliance with pharmacotherapy (11,46). Provisions for the long-term continuation of risk-factor modification need to be improved.

PULMONARY REHABILITATION

In the United States, chronic obstructive pulmonary disease (COPD) accounted for approximately 120,000 deaths in 2000, ranking as the fourth leading cause of death. It is the only major disease among the top ten in which mortality and morbidity continue to increase. Moreover, death rates from COPD increased 282% for women compared with only 13% for men, making this one of the fastest growing diseases in women (35).

Pulmonary rehabilitation is defined as an evidenced-based, multidisciplinary, and comprehensive intervention for patients with chronic respiratory diseases who are symptomatic and often have decreased daily life activities (28). Integrated into the individualized treatment of the patient, PR is designed to reduce symptoms, optimize functional status, increase participation, and reduce healthcare costs through stabilizing or reversing systemic manifestations of the disease (35).

PROGRAM DESCRIPTION

Participants of PR programs may include those with (a) obstructive lung diseases, including COPD, asthma, cystic fibrosis, bronchiectasis, and emphysema (including alpha-1 antitrypsin deficiency); (b) restrictive lung diseases, including pulmonary fibrosis, interstitial lung disease, sarcoidosis, and occupational or environmental lung disease; (c) chest wall diseases, including kyphoscoliosis and ankylosing spondylitis; and (d) neuromuscular diseases, including Parkinson disease, multiple sclerosis, amyotrophic lateral sclerosis, postpolio syndrome, and posttuberculosis syndrome (4). Patients with other lung conditions—such as pre- or post-lung transplant, lung volume reduction surgery, or thoracic and abdominal surgery (36) and those with obesity-related respiratory diseases (25)—have also been shown to benefit from PR.

In 2007, AACVPR and the American College of Chest Physicians (ACCP) published evidenced-based clinical practice guidelines for PR (35). Although there is insufficient evidence to determine if PR improves survival in COPD patients, important benefits are achieved in this patient population. Pulmonary rehabilitation (a) improves the symptoms of dyspnea, (b) improves health-related quality of life, (c) reduces hospital days and other healthcare utilization measures, and (d) provides psychosocial benefits. Pulmonary rehabilitation was also found to be cost-effective among COPD patients. Based on these findings, PR programs are recommended with a program of exercise training that includes both low- and high-intensity endurance training as appropriate to achieve the desired physiological benefits, resistance training to increase muscle strength and mass, and the use of supplemental oxygen during exercise for patients with exercise-induced hypoxemia. Education should be an integral component of PR, including information on self-management and prevention and treatment of exacerbations. Please refer to the AACVPR/ACCP PR Clinical Practice Guidelines for more specific recommendations and detailed discussion (35).

CORE COMPONENTS OF CARE

Pulmonary rehabilitation services offer a multifaceted and multidisciplinary approach to care. The core components of a successful PR program as defined by AACVPR (4) are outlined in Box 49-1.

ADMINISTRATIVE CONSIDERATIONS: CARDIAC AND PULMONARY REHABILITATION PROGRAMS

The patient population, educational focus, and the format of service delivery may differ between cardiac and pulmonary rehabilitation (CP-R) programs, but the administrative structure and program processes are similar in clinical settings. The following summarizes operational functions that are common in CP-R programs. For more detailed descriptions of operational functions within each program type, please refer to the AACVPR *Guidelines for Cardiac Rehabilitation and Secondary Prevention* (3) and AACVPR *Guidelines for Pulmonary Rehabilitation Programs* (4).

BOX 49-1   CORE COMPONENTS OF PULMONARY REHABILITATION PROGRAMS

- Baseline patient assessment (e.g., assessing the patient's medical history, prescribed medications, physical activity habits, smoking history, oxygen usage, nutritional habits)
- Physical function assessment (e.g., 6-minute walk testing, graded exercise metabolic testing, upper- and lower-body strength testing, flexibility assessment)
- Body composition assessment (e.g., height, weight, body mass index [BMI], abdominal circumference, skinfold analysis)
- Instruction in proper breathing techniques (e.g., pursed-lip and diaphragmatic breathing)
- Instruction in pulmonary hygiene techniques (e.g., postural drainage, Flutter™ or Acapela™ valve, controlled coughing)

- Instruction in respiratory apparatus and modalities (e.g., liquid or compressed oxygen, metered dose inhaler [MDI], peak flow meter, nasal cannula and tubing, nebulizer)
- Psychosocial assessment (e.g., health-related quality of life, depression, anxiety, hostility, panic control)
- Counseling on activities of daily living, home exercise, and methods to improve muscular strength and function, particularly of the respiratory muscles
- Exercise training on a variety of upper- and lower-body aerobic and resistive modalities
- Follow-up assessment (e.g., periodic 6-minute walk testing, increased or decreased oxygen supplementation, quality-of-life [QOL] assessment, changes in body weight/body fat)

FACILITIES AND EQUIPMENT

A CP-R program can be conducted in an inpatient, outpatient, home-based, or community-based setting. The locations of a CP-R program must meet state, federal, and the Joint Commission's safety standards or other regulatory agencies as appropriate. Adequate space should be provided for exercise testing and training, patient consultations, psychosocial evaluations, confidential storage of patient medical records, administrative office assistance, and office space for staff members. The environment should also allow for safe and easy patient movement and flow (e.g., exercise machines spaced far enough apart to discourage patient falls and injuries). More detailed information regarding exercise facility environmental recommendations are published elsewhere (7).

The exercise equipment selection in CP-R programs is individualized to each program and based primarily on the available space, budget guidelines, and the patient's needs and preferences. General exercise equipment typically includes weight-bearing modalities (e.g., treadmills, stairs, stair-steppers, elliptical trainers) and non–weight-bearing modalities (e.g., recumbent cycles, arm ergometers, stationary and wind-resistance cycles, and rowing machines). Other exercise equipment may include resistance-training modalities, such as machine weights, free weights, dumbbells, cuff weights, and wall pulleys.

The provision of a safe exercise environment and trained personnel in emergency procedures is critical when serving patient populations with chronic diseases.

POLICIES, PROCEDURES, AND DOCUMENTATION

The essential requirements for CP-R program documentation should reflect the program structure and detailed description of program operations and care delivery. The AACVPR has a program certification process for both CR and PR. The certification process was established to develop a standard of minimal requirements for program operation to achieve the desired outcomes in a safe environment. A template for the appropriate items to include in CP-R documentation is outlined in Box 49-2. A complete description of the AACVPR certification application requirements is available at www.aacvpr.org.

Since 1998, more than 1,500 programs across the United States have been awarded AACVPR certification. The program certification process is an excellent guide for developing new programs and serves as a periodic program review to update existing programs to current professional standards. Program certification is granted for 3 years, after which time a recertification application process and review must be completed.

HEALTHCARE TEAM

The key to a successful CP-R program is having competent and motivated team members. The collective knowledge, skills, and clinical experience of the staff are essential to building a comprehensive multidisciplinary team. Healthcare professionals typically represented in the CP-R team include clinical exercise physiologists, specially trained nurses, respiratory therapists, dietitians, physical therapists, psychologists, occupational therapists, clinical social workers, and physicians. Other health professionals utilized by some CP-R programs include vocational rehabilitation counselors, physician extenders (e.g., nurse practitioners, physician assistants), home healthcare personnel, psychiatrists, speech and recreational therapists, and chaplain or pastoral care associates. There is a complimentary overlap of skill sets among CP-R professionals, and cross-training of competencies is strongly encouraged. Program efficiency is enhanced by having a multidisciplinary team that is able to provide care within their scope of practice while exhibiting multiple competencies across disciplines related to health education and individual counseling.

BOX 49-2	**AMERICAN ASSOCIATION OF CARDIOVASCULAR AND PULMONARY REHABILITATION PROGRAM CERTIFICATION CATEGORIES**

Program Management

- Personnel: Staff credentials and competencies
- Emergency equipment and supplies
- Documentation of current processes:
  - Policies/procedures
  - Patient medical records
  - Medical emergency plan
  - Program evaluation

Patient Care

- Assessment measures
- Therapeutic/treatment plan
- Intervention/treatment components
- Outcome assessment

Discharge plan

Medical Director

The CP-R medical director is ultimately responsible for the supervision and operation of the program and should be involved in the formation of policies and procedures for the program (23). The primary role of the medical director, as leader of the multidisciplinary team, is to assure that the CP-R program is safe, comprehensive, cost-effective, and medically appropriate for the services provided. Expertise in disease management and experience in exercise testing and training in those with chronic disease are requisites for the CP-R medical director. Also, positive interpersonal skills and an ability to work within the multidisciplinary CP-R team approach are certainly desirable attributes. The CP-R medical director is typically a cardiologist or pulmonologist, although other physicians may serve in this role. Other roles of the CP-R medical director include:

- Responsibility for assuring that policies and procedures are consistent with evidenced-based guidelines and that they comply with certification and regulatory standards
- Responsibility for policies related to patient referral, including inclusion and exclusion criteria
- Recognition of local, regional, and national regulations pertaining to PR/CR reimbursement
- Exercise supervision and program monitoring, including definition and standardization of physician proximity to the exercise area per hospital or clinic guidelines

Program Director/Coordinator

The program director/coordinator has administrative, clinical, and educational duties and works in collaboration with the medical director in all aspects of CP-R management and program operation. The CP-R program director/coordinator's duties include program leadership and administrative responsibilities. Such responsibilities include developing and evaluating programs, developing and monitoring budget, analyzing reimbursement concerns, overseeing personnel (hiring, training, scheduling, and evaluating performance), and participating in program marketing plans. The program director/coordinator also serves as the liaison among the patients, medical director, referring healthcare providers, administration, and the CP-R multidisciplinary team.

Multidisciplinary Health Professionals

Cardiopulmonary rehabilitation team members must possess the knowledge and skills to assess, evaluate, and implement treatment plans for patients with cardiovascular and/or lung disease and any associated comorbidities. Staff members involved in direct patient-care activities and exercise supervision should be proficient

in medical emergency management, be certified in Basic Cardiac Life Support (BLS), and, preferably with select staff members, trained in Advanced Cardiac Life Support (ACLS). All team members are required to participate in periodic employee educational opportunities and staff competency reviews. Staff competencies consist of the ability to provide the core components of care (4,9) and provide emergency response capabilities. Staff competency assessments, training, and education are initiated at orientation and are ongoing; they require annual validation that is documented in the personnel files. A detailed description of competency assessments for CP-R program professionals have been published by AACVPR (29,41). The ACSM CES KSAs also provide an excellent guide to assess staff competencies in CP-R programs.

PROCESS OF CARE

> **1.5.5-CES: Practice disease/case management responsibilities, including daily follow-up concerning patient needs, signs and symptoms, physician appointments, and medication changes for patients with chronic diseases.**

> **1.5.8-CES: Recognize patient clinical need for referral to other (non-ES) allied health professionals (e.g., behavioralist, physical therapist, diabetes educator, nurse).**

> **1.7.4-CES: Design, implement, and supervise individualized exercise prescriptions for people with chronic disease and disabling conditions.**

> **1.7.5-CES: Design a supervised exercise program beginning at hospital discharge and continuing for up to 6 months for the following conditions: myocardial infarction; angina; left ventricular assist device; congestive heart failure; percutaneous coronary intervention; coronary artery bypass surgery; medical management of coronary artery disease; chronic pulmonary disease; weight management; diabetes; metabolic syndrome; and cardiac transplants.**

> **1.9.11-CES: Ability to conduct effective and informative group and individual education sessions directed at primary or secondary prevention of chronic disease.**

Case-management is an integrated approach to provide individualized care for patients with chronic disease, including cardiac (19), pulmonary (12), and other chronic diseases (16). A more detailed description of case management within CP-R programs is described in the AACVPR guidelines (3,4). The patient typically undergoes a comprehensive baseline assessment by a case manager on the rehabilitation team (e.g., nurse, exercise physiologist, respiratory therapist) under the direction of the medical director. Based on the patient assessment, risk stratification, risk-factor profile, and learning needs, a care or treatment plan is developed that outlines realistic short- and long-term goals. It is imperative that the patient is an active participant in this process. The case-management system of patient care allows the staff to develop a rapport with the patient, to monitor and evaluate patient progress, and to facilitate communication among other healthcare providers.

Intake Evaluation

A systematic intake evaluation is necessary to assess a patient's individual risk factors and learning needs. The initial assessment includes, but is not limited to, patient demographics, insurance information, physician referral, informed consent, record of advanced directives, past medical history, symptoms, present health status, comorbidities, medications, employment status, and psychosocial history (Box 49–1). A physical examination and exercise tolerance test should be performed to assess the clinical risk associated with exercise and to develop an individualized exercise prescription. Results should be shared with the patient and other healthcare professionals involved in the individual's care.

Risk Stratification

Guidelines for risk stratification for cardiac patients are available through the AAVCPR (3) and ACSM's GETP8 (6). Cardiac patients in whom high-risk characteristics are identified should participate in a supervised program in which ECG monitoring is available. Individuals at lower to intermediate risk can be considered for less supervised non-ECG monitoring or even a home-based program. For patients with pulmonary disease, oxygen saturation during exercise is assessed to detect exercise-induced hypoxemia and to determine the need for supplemental oxygen therapy (4). Because many pulmonary patients have multiple comorbidities, risk assessment is used to help meet the needs of the patients with other complex medical needs.

Care or Treatment Plan

The intake evaluation allows the clinician and patient to collaboratively identify desired outcomes, develop a plan and timeline to achieve the planned objectives, and to define the outcome measures. The individual care plan should identify the desired outcomes, a plan to achieve the outcomes, and the methods for measuring the outcomes. A care plan describes the individualized exercise prescription, action plans for specific risk-factor intervention, and the timeline for goal achievement (e.g., 3, 6, 12, 18, or 24 months). The care plan includes objectives from the health, clinical, behavioral, and service domains (32,38). The care plan should also be customized for each patient, describing the evaluation, intervention, and follow-up components for each program discipline involved in the care of the patient (e.g., nutrition, psychology, physical function).

Exercise Prescription and Training

Based on the risk assessment and intake evaluation, an exercise prescription is developed that specifies the frequency, intensity, duration, mode, and rate of progression that is most appropriate for the individual patient. A thorough discussion on developing exercise prescriptions is provided for patients with cardiovascular (Chapter 35) (39) and pulmonary (Chapter 36) (14) disease, which supports the specific exercise prescription guidelines detailed in the ACSM GETP8 (6). Beyond a specific exercise prescription, counseling regarding general physical activity and return to work is necessary. The objective is to assist patients to safely progress to the level of physical activity that is associated with health benefits and establish a long-term goal of regular, physical activity on most days of the week.

Education and Counseling

Comprehensive CP-R programs include behavior change strategies that incorporate effective education and counseling interventions to meet the individual's needs. Behavior change is complex, and the needs of the patient vary based on risk factors, personal priorities, psychosocial status, and current health status. Furthermore, the importance of long-term adherence to positive lifestyle habits and pharmacotherapy is critical in achieving expected outcomes. The CP-R team members need to develop competencies in health counseling techniques and employ a variety of patient-centered approaches to enhance the effectiveness of educational strategies.

Patient education may be provided in many forms, including one-to-one counseling, group sessions, written materials, and use of computers and the Internet. A more comprehensive look at education and counseling is provided in the AACVPR guidelines (3,4).

Discharge Plan

The goal of discharge planning is to review the outcomes achieved and develop a specific plan to facilitate patients as they transition from a more intensively monitored situation to a self-management phase. Discharge planning should begin weeks before the actual discharge date so the CP-R team can help patients develop and implement important self-management plans. Many CP-R programs offer a less structured, yet supervised exercise program (phase III) that provides the patient with a convenient opportunity to transition into a long-term maintenance program within familiar surroundings and associated

TABLE 49-2. SAMPLE BUDGET OUTLINE FOR A CARDIOPULMONARY REHABILITATION PROGRAM

VOLUME	YEAR 1	YEAR 2	YEAR 3	YEAR 4	ASSUMPTION
Number of patients (patient units)					
Initial evaluations					
Exercise visits					
PRODUCTIVITY					
Initial evaluations/day					
Exercise visits/month (insurance patients)					
Exercise visits/month (self-pay patients)					
REVENUE					
Program/education fee (self-pay)					
Maintenance exercise fee (self-pay)					
Smoking cessation program (self-pay)					
Psychological evaluations					
6-minute walk tests					
Initial evaluations					
Group exercise classes					
Individualized instruction/1:1 therapy					
Healthy living cookbooks					
Weight loss program					
Sale of elastic bands, pedometers					
EXPENSES					
Salaries					
Benefits					
Equipment purchase and maintenance					
Utilities (gas, electric, water)					
Cleaning service					
Medical supplies					
Travel and education					
Marketing					
Printing, postage, office supplies					
Telephone/Internet					
Special programs (e.g., patient awards)					
Miscellaneous					
CORPORATE					
Amortization/depreciation					
Rent (cost per square foot of used space)					
Debt					
Insurance					
Property taxes					
TOTAL EXPENSES					
NET INCOME					
PROFIT MARGIN					

with CP-R team members. Other possibilities for maintenance exercise programs include local health club facilities or home-based exercise. Regardless of how the patient chooses to do the long-term maintenance program, it is important that the CP-R team works collaboratively with the patient during the discharge planning process. The complete discharge summary documents interventions, patient progress, outcome/goal achievements, satisfaction with the program, discharge exercise prescription, and a plan for maintaining or improving on the goals achieved in the C-PR program. A copy of the discharge summary should be sent to the patient's referring physician, and periodic telephone calls are recommended to promote adherence to positive lifestyle behaviors and monitor progress toward goals.

OUTCOME ASSESSMENT AND QUALITY IMPROVEMENT

> **1.11.1-CES: Discuss the role of outcome measures in chronic disease management programs, such as cardiovascular and pulmonary rehabilitation programs.**

> **1.11.2-CES: Identify and discuss various outcome measurements used in a cardiac or pulmonary rehabilitation program.**

> **1.11.3-CES: Utilize specific outcome collection instruments to collect outcome data in a cardiac or pulmonary rehabilitation program.**

Evaluating patient outcomes and program effectiveness are best achieved through an integrated and systemic assessment of patient and program outcomes. Reviewing outcomes for a particular patient and the program in general allows for a critical assessment of the program's effectiveness in providing patient care and contributes to improving quality of care.

The AACVPR has published recommendations that emphasize a comprehensive approach to outcome measurements (31) with recent recommendations for integrating within routine clinical practice for both CR (38,43) and PR programs (32,43). The specific recommendations include the importance of identifying outcome measures that reflects the care in the following domains: (a) clinical, (b) behavioral, (c) health, and (d) service. Having clear definitions of outcome and performance measures (6) is essential for optimal short- and long-term monitoring of patient progress, quality assurance, and overall CP-R program effectiveness. This information will assist the CP-R team when they present their patient outcomes to physicians, healthcare administrators, JCAHO, insurance providers, and third-party payers in the quest to assure the highest quality of patient care. Measurements for outcome evaluation are typically assessed at the start of the program and repeated at the end of the initial exercise and education phase (e.g., 8–12 weeks). Follow-up as-

sessments are also recommended at 6- or 12-month intervals thereafter. These findings provide valuable information for quality improvement, accreditation, and program reimbursement, and are critical for providing feedback to CP-R participants and their physicians regarding individual progress.

In addition to the position statements on outcome evaluation within CP-R programs (3,4), the AACVPR also provides resources such as the *Outcomes Tools Resource Guide* through their members' Web site (www.aacvpr.org) (5).

REIMBURSEMENT AND FINANCIAL CONSIDERATIONS

Financial considerations are essential with pressure from declining and variable reimbursement rates, increasing costs, and the demand for high-quality services. Justification for dollars spent and goals to enhance financial performance are crucial to support decisions that lead to program success and sustainability. Although exercise and health professionals are primarily concerned with care provided to promote the health and well-being of their patients, this would not be possible over the long term without maintaining a positive bottom line. An outline of budgetary considerations for a CP-R program is provided in Table 49-2.

Typically, clinical CP-R programs are provided through health systems, and patient enrollment requires a physician referral. Payments for CP-R services are usually generated through third-party reimbursement. Continuous changes in healthcare management and reimbursement patterns require constant monitoring because rules and regulations change over time. Before program participation, programs should verify the patient's medical insurance policy to determine whether precertification is required, the level of reimbursement, and the number of available sessions. This information should be communicated to the patient.

Centers for Medicare and Medicaid Services

> **11.4-CES: Understand the most recent cardiac and pulmonary rehabilitation Centers for Medicare Services (CMS) rules for patient enrollment and reimbursement (e.g., diagnostic current procedure terminology [CPT] codes, diagnostic related groups [DRG]).**

The largest payer for CP-R services is the Centers for Medicare and Medicaid Services (CMS). Information regarding CMS coverage for rehabilitation services can be found at www.cms.hhs.gov/center/coverage.asp (13). In July of 2008, the Pulmonary and Cardiac Rehabilitation Act was voted into law, establishing both CR and PR as specific Medicare benefit categories that mandate coverage and payment of services. At this time, discussions are taking place which are exploring the options for a proposal of CPT codes for CP-R services and the reimbursement tied with these codes. The policy goes into effect on January 1, 2010. The current procedural terminology (CPT) codes that are appropriate to CR include:

93793: Physician services for outpatient program without continuous ECG monitoring (note that the use of this code is subject to regional interpretation and not accepted by all intermediaries)
93798: Physician services for outpatient program with continuous ECG monitoring

Pulmonary rehabilitation services are provided under different CMS reimbursement mechanisms. At this time, there are CPT and G-codes (e.g., GO237, GO238, and GO239) that are used for many inpatient or outpatient PR services.

Although CMS is the governing body for establishing payment guidelines for Medicare, these guidelines are distributed to regional offices throughout the United States. Each region is overseen by a fiscal intermediary (FI) that administers the CMS guidelines. Each FI interprets the guidelines and, as a result, coverage is not uniform from region to region. Currently, CMS is converting the FI administration payment plan to Medicare Administrative Contractors (MACs). MACs are divided into territorial jurisdictions across the United States. Each MAC has the authority to impose individual rules and regulations with regard to Medicare reimbursement for services in their particular territory called Local Coverage Determinations (LCD). Thus, a wide variability in decisions regarding payment for rehabilitation remains an issue until the Pulmonary and Cardiac Rehabilitation Act goes into effect in 2010. Because reimbursement regulations are dynamic, the AACVPR Web site (www.aacvpr.org) provides the most up-to-date information on the various national and regional reimbursement guidelines. Other insurance carriers tend to follow the lead of CMS. Therefore, a clinical program based on the published CMS rules will tend to be compliant with other third-party requirements.

Other Insurance Providers

Health insurance coverage provided by private insurance companies is highly variable for both CR and PR services. Plans may provide no coverage, a minimal number of sessions or all that are deemed medically necessary. Additionally, co-payments may or may not apply. Consequently, it is important that the patient and the billing department personnel obtain pre-certification and a determination to the extent of coverage prior to a patient enrolling in a CP-R program.

Expanding Populations and Self-Pay Services

Clinical research supports exercise therapy and aggressive risk-factor management in patients with CAD, other forms of atherosclerotic disease (40), and many chronic diseases and disabilities (1). The incidences of overweight and obesity have increased dramatically over the last few decades, and our population is aging. Rehabilitation professionals are experts in dealing with older patients with comorbid conditions in the course of managing patients with either cardiac or pulmonary disease. Therefore, CP-R programs are ideally suited to take on the challenges posed by other high-risk populations that may benefit from medically supervised exercise programs. Unfortunately, most insurance companies do not reimburse payment for other clinical conditions beyond the traditional cardiac or pulmonary rehabilitation program. A fee-for-service or self-pay model, however, may be designed to meet the needs of other high-risk patient populations while providing an alternative revenue source for a CP-R program. Medically based fitness and wellness centers can provide primary and secondary prevention programs for a diverse patient population while providing health systems an opportunity to promote health within the community.

CP-R programs have evolved dramatically from the historically exercise-based programs to the present-day comprehensive services. Without question, CP-R programs will continue to evolve in the future to best achieve optimal clinical outcomes for program participants. Furthermore, multiple financial challenges exist with increasing patient copayments and decreasing reimbursement options for services rendered. Programs will need to explore cost-effective options that go beyond the traditional CP-R models to better reflect the specific needs of the program participants while maintaining financial viability.

SUMMARY

Cardiopulmonary rehabilitation programs are proven effective strategies to help manage patients with cardiac and pulmonary disease. All patients with a diagnosis of coronary or pulmonary disease should be systematically evaluated and considered for treatment within a CP-R program. Additionally, at a time when chronic disease is at epidemic levels, opportunities abound for the specialized services provided by CP-R professionals. An individualized program, developed in close collaboration between the patient and healthcare providers, is the most effective means by which to deliver optimal care.

The management of clinical CP-R programs requires a multidisciplinary team that understands the clinical parameters for special populations; knows how to develop, implement, and evaluate care plans; understands management principles; maintains financial viability; and adapts to the challenges in today's healthcare environment. Quality care is imperative to CP-R program success, and the pinnacle for quality care is having competent team members to deliver program services. Quality rehabilitation programs have a proven ability to provide services that reduce the risk of future events and assists in returning patients to optimal physical, psychological, and social well-being.

REFERENCES

1. Ades PA. Cardiac rehabilitation and secondary prevention of coronary heart disease. *N Engl J Med*. 2001;345(12):892–902.

2. Ades PA, Waldmann ML, Polk DM, Coflesky JT. Referral patterns and exercise response in the rehabilitation of female coronary patients aged greater than or equal to 62 years. *Am J Cardiol*. 1992;69(17):1422–5.

3. American Association of Cardiovascular and Pulmonary Rehabilitation. *Guidelines for Cardiac Rehabilitation and Secondary Prevention Programs*. 4th ed. Champaign (IL): Human Kinetics; 2004.

4. American Association of Cardiovascular and Pulmonary Rehabilitation. *Guidelines for Pulmonary Rehabilitation Programs*. 3rd ed. Champaign (IL): Human Kinetics; 2004.

5. American Association of Cardiovascular and Pulmonary Rehabilitation (AACVPR) Web site. Outcome Tools Resource Guide, 2002. Available to AACVPR members at: http://www.aacvpr.org. Accessed December 22, 2008.

6. American College of Sports Medicine. *ACSM's Guidelines for Exercise Testing and Prescription*. 8th ed. Philadelphia: Lippincott Williams & Wilkins; 2009.

7. American College of Sports Medicine. *ACSM's Health Fitness Facility Standards and Guidelines*. Champaign (IL): Human Kinetics; 2006. p.1–20.

8. American College of Sports Medicine. *ACSM's Resources for Clinical Exercise Physiology*. 2nd ed. Philadelphia: Lippincott Williams & Wilkins; 2009.

9. Balady GJ, Williams MA, Ades PA, et al. Core components of cardiac rehabilitation/secondary prevention programs: 2007 update: a scientific statement from the American Heart Association Exercise, Cardiac Rehabilitation, and Prevention Committee, the Council on Clinical Cardiology; the Councils on Cardiovascular Nursing, Epidemiology and Prevention, and Nutrition, Physical Activity, and Metabolism; and the American Association of Cardiovascular and Pulmonary Rehabilitation. *Circulation*. 2007;115(20):2675–82.

10. Bittner V, Sanderson B. Cardiac rehabilitation as secondary prevention center. *Coron Artery Dis*. 2006;17(3):211–8.

11. Burke LE, Dunbar-Jacob JM, Hill MN. Compliance with cardiovascular disease prevention strategies: a review of the research. *Ann Behav Med*. 1997;19(3):239–63.

12. Burton GG, Hodgkin JE, Ward JJ. *Respiratory Care—A Guide to Clinical Practice*. 4th ed. Philadelphia: Lippincott; 1997. p. 877–88.

13. Centers for Medicare and Medicaid Services Web site: Medicare Preventive Services. Available from: www.cms.hhs.gov/center/coverage.asp. Accessed January 10, 2008.

14. Cooper CB, Storer TW, Exercise prescription in patients with pulmonary disease. In: Ehrman JK, editor. *Resource Manual for Guidelines for Exercise Testing and Prescription*: 6th ed. Champaign: Human Kinetics;2009. p. 575–599.

15. Currnier DY, Savage PD, Ades PA. Geographic distribution of cardiac rehabilitation programs in the United States. *J Cardiopulm Rehabil*. 2005;25(2):80–4.

16. Durstine JL, Moore GE. *ACSM's Exercise Management for Persons with Chronic Diseases and Disabilities*. Champaign (IL): Human Kinetics; 2003.

17. Grace SL, Scholey P, Suskin N, et al. A prospective comparison of cardiac rehabilitation enrollment following automatic vs usual referral. *J Rehabil Med*. 2007;39(3):239–45.

18. Hambrecht R, Walther C, Mobius-Winkler S, et al. Percutaneous coronary angioplasty compared with exercise training in patients with stable coronary artery disease: a randomized trial. *Circulation*. 2004;109(11):1371–8.

19. Haskell WL, Alderman EL, Fair JM, et al. Effects of intensive multiple risk factor reduction on coronary atherosclerosis and clinical cardiac events in men and women with coronary artery disease. The Stanford Coronary Risk Intervention Project (SCRIP). *Circulation*. 1994;89(3):975–990.

20. Jackson L, Leclerc J, Erskine Y, Linden W. Getting the most out of cardiac rehabilitation: a review of referral and adherence predictors. *Heart*. 2005;91(1):10–4.

21. Jeger RV, Jorg L, Rickenbacher P, Pfisterer ME, Hoffmann A. Benefit of outpatient cardiac rehabilitation in under-represented patient subgroups. *J Rehabil Med*. 2007;39(3):246–51.

22. Jolliffe JA, Rees K, Taylor RS, Thompson D, Oldridge N, Ebrahim S. Exercise-based rehabilitation for coronary heart disease. *Cochrane Database Syst Rev*. 2001;(1):CD001800.

23. King ML, Williams MA, Fletcher GF, et al. Medical director responsibilities for outpatient cardiac rehabilitation/secondary prevention programs. *J. Cardiopulm Rehabil*. 2005;25:315–20.

24. **Leon AS, Franklin BA, Costa F, et al. American Heart Association; Council on Clinical Cardiology (Subcommittee on Exercise, Cardiac Rehabilitation, and Prevention); Council on Nutrition, Physical Activity, and Metabolism (Subcommittee on Physical Activity); American Association of Cardiovascular and Pulmonary Rehabilitation. Cardiac rehabilitation and secondary prevention of coronary heart disease: an American Heart Association scientific statement from the Council on Clinical Cardiology (Subcommittee on Exercise, Cardiac Rehabilitation, and Prevention) and the Council on Nutrition, Physical Activity, and Metabolism (Subcommittee on Physical Activity), in collaboration with the American Association of Cardiovascular and Pulmonary Rehabilitation. *Circulation*. 2005;111(3):369–76.**

25. Marquis K, Maltais F, Duguay V, et al. The metabolic syndrome in patients with chronic obstructive pulmonary disease. *J Cardiopulm Rehabil*. 2005;25:226–32.

26. Mochari H, Lee JR, Kligfield P, Mosca L. Ethnic differences in barriers and referral to cardiac rehabilitation among women hospitalized with coronary heart disease. *Prev Cardiol*. 2006;9(1):8–13.

27. Newby LK, Eisenstein EL, Califf RM, et al. Cost effectiveness of early discharge after uncomplicated acute myocardial infarction. *N Engl J Med*. 2000;342(11):749–55.

28. **Nici L, Donner C, Wouters E, et al. American Thoracic Society/European Respiratory Society Statement on Pulmonary Rehabilitation. *Am J Respir Crit Care Med*. 2006;173:1390–413.**

29. **Nici L, Limberg T, Hilling L, et al. American Association of Cardiovascular and Pulmonary Rehabilitation Position Statement: Clinical competency guidelines for pulmonary rehabilitation professionals. *J Cardiopulm Rehabil Prev*. 2007;27:355–8.**

30. Oldridge NB. Compliance and dropout in cardiac rehabilitation. *J Cardiopulm Rehabil*. 1984;4:166–77.

31. **Pashkow P, Ades P, Emery CF, et al. Outcome measurement in cardiac and pulmonary rehabilitation by the AACVPR Outcomes Committee. *J Cardiopulm Rehabil*. 1995;15:394–405.**

32. **Peno-Green L, Verrill D, McIntyre N, Vitcenda M. AACVPR Outcome Committee Position Statement: Patient-centered outcomes enhance the evaluation of patient performance and program effectiveness in pulmonary rehabilitation. *J Cardiopulm Rehabil*. In press.**

33. Reddy KS. Cardiovascular disease in non-western countries. *N Engl J Med*. 2004;350(24):2438–40.

34. Reid RD, Morrin LI, Pipe AL, et al. Determinants of physical activity after hospitalization for coronary artery disease: the Tracking Exercise After Cardiac Hospitalization (TEACH) Study. *Eur J Cardiovasc Prev Rehabil*. 2006;13(4):529–37.

35. **Ries AL, Bauldoff GS, Carlin BW, et al. Pulmonary rehabilitation: Joint ACCP/AACVPR evidenced-based clinical practice guidelines. *Chest*. 2007;131:4S–42S.**

36. Ries AL, Make BJ, Lee SM, et al. The effects of pulmonary rehabilitation in the National Emphysema Treatment Trial. *Chest*. 2005; 128:3799–809.

37. Sanderson BK, Bittner V. Women in cardiac rehabilitation: outcomes and identifying risk for dropout. *Am Heart J.* 2005;150(5): 1052–8.

38. **Sanderson BK, Southard D, Oldridge N. Writing Group. AACVPR consensus statement. Outcomes evaluation in cardiac rehabilitation/secondary prevention programs: improving patient care and program effectiveness.** *J Cardiopulm Rehabil.* **2004;24(2):68–79.**

39. Schairer JR, Jarvis RA, Keteyian SJ. Exercise prescription in patients with cardiovascular disease. In: Ehrman JK, editor. *Resource Manual for Guidelines for Exercise Testing and Prescription,* 6th ed. Champaign: Human Kinetics; 2009. p.559–574.

40. Smith SC Jr, Allen J, Blair SN, et al. AHA/ACC; National Heart, Lung, and Blood Institute. AHA/ACC guidelines for secondary prevention for patients with coronary and other atherosclerotic vascular disease: 2006 update: endorsed by the National Heart, Lung, and Blood Institute. *Circulation.* 2006;113(19):2363–72.

41. **Southard DR, Cert C, Comoss P, et al. Core competencies for cardiac rehabilitation professionals. Position Statement of the Cardiovascular and Pulmonary Rehabilitation.** *J Cardiopulm Rehabil.* **1994;14:87–92.**

42. **Thomas RJ, King M, Lui K, et al. and the ACC/AHA Task Force Members. AACVPR/ACC/AHA 2007 performance measures on cardiac rehabilitation/secondary prevention services.** *J Cardiopulm Rehabil Prev.* **2007;27:260–290.**

43. **Verrill D, Graham H, Vitcenda M, et al. Measuring behavioral outcomes in cardiopulmonary rehabilitation—An AACVPR Statement.** *J Cardiopulm Rehabil.* **2009;29 (In press).**

44. **Wenger NK, Froelicher ES, Smith LK, et al.** *Cardiac Rehabilitation as Secondary Prevention.* **Agency for Health Care Policy and Research and National Heart, Lung, and Blood Institute.** *Clin Pract Guidel Quick Ref Guide Clin.* **1995;(17):1–23.**

45. Williams MA, Ades PA, Hamm LF, et al. Clinical evidence for a health benefit from cardiac rehabilitation: an update. *Am Heart J.* 2006;152(5):835–41.

46. Willich SN, Muller-Nordhorn J, Kulig M, et al. PIN Study Group. Cardiac risk factors, medication, and recurrent clinical events after acute coronary disease: a prospective cohort study. *Eur Heart J.* 2001;22(4):307–13.

SELECTED REFERENCES FOR FURTHER READING

American Thoracic Society. ATS Statement: Guidelines for the six-minute walk test. *Am J Respir Crit Care Med.* 2002;166:111–7.

Expert Panel on the Identification, Evaluation, and Treatment of Overweight and Obesity in Adults: Executive summary of the Clinical Guidelines on the Identification, Evaluation, and Treatment of Overweight and Obesity in Adults. *Arch Intern Med.* 1998;158: 1855–67.

Global Strategy for the Diagnosis, *Management, and Prevention of COPD.* Global Initiative for Chronic Obstructive Lung Disease (Gold) 2008. Available from: http://www.goldcopd.org. Accessed November 25, 2008.

Joint National Committee on Prevention, Detection, Evaluation, and Treatment of High Blood Pressure. Seventh report of Joint National Committee on Prevention, Detection, Evaluation, and Treatment of High Blood Pressure. *JAMA.* 2003;289:2560–72.

National Cholesterol Education Program (NCEP). Executive summary of the third report of the Expert Panel on Detection, Evaluation and Treatment of High Blood Cholesterol in Adults (Adult Treatment Panel III). *JAMA.* 2001;285:2486–97.

Ries AL. Position paper of the AACVPR: Scientific evidence of pulmonary rehabilitation. *J Cardiopulm Rehabil.* 1990;10:418–41.

Troosters TR, Casaburi R, Gosselink, Decramer R. Pulmonary rehabilitation in chronic obstructive pulmonary disease. *Am J Respir Crit Care Med.* 2005:172:19–38.

United States Department of Health and Human Services, Centers for Disease Control and Prevention. Physical Activity and Health: A Report of the Surgeon General. Washington (DC): National Center for Chronic Disease Prevention and Health Promotion; 1996.

United States Department of Health and Human Services, Public Health Services, Agency for Health Care Policy and Research, and the National Heart, Lung and Blood Institute. Guide for smoking cessation specialists. AHCPR Publication No. 96-0693. Rockville (MD): AHCPR; April 1996.

INTERNET RESOURCES

- American Association of Cardiovascular and Pulmonary Rehabilitation: www.aacvpr.org
- American Lung Association: www.lungusa.org
- The Joint Commission: www.jointcommission.org
- Medicare (CMS): www.medicare.gov
- National Institutes of Health: www.nih.gov
- Preventive Cardiovascular Nurses Association: www.pcna.net

CHAPTER 50

Exercise Program Safety and Emergency Procedures

The risk of sudden cardiac death or other injury during activity is always a concern in both the clinical and health/fitness settings. Although injuries are far more prevalent during exercise, exercise-related deaths can occur. Exercise-related deaths in young persons younger than 30 to 40 years are most often related to hereditary or congenital abnormalities (12). In contrast, coronary artery disease (CAD) is the most common exertion-related cardiovascular event in older individuals. Although studies have demonstrated that the risk of sudden cardiac death is transiently elevated during moderate to vigorous exercise compared with low-intensity activity or no exertion, habitual activity has been shown to modify this transient risk (1,29). In addition, studies of both men and women have shown that regardless of cardiovascular risk factors or the presence of cardiovascular disease that functional capacity is inversely related to both CAD and all-cause mortality rates (19,20). Studies investigating the incidence of exercise-related deaths suggest that with the exception of individuals with heart disease, diagnosed or occult, the benefits of vigorous exercise outweigh the risks (12). Moderate exercise, however, may be appropriate for individuals with heart disease if it does not significantly elevate cardiovascular risk.

Although the benefits of habitual exercise have been shown to outweigh the risks, clinical and fitness facilities, as well as exercise professionals, have an obligation to their patients to provide the safest possible training and testing environments while minimizing the legal and personal liability associated with adverse outcomes. The best approach to management of emergencies is prevention through (a) screening for cardiovascular risk factors, signs, and symptoms, and fall risk before exercise and exercise testing; (b) selection of appropriate exercise testing protocols; (c) participant education to minimize the risk of sudden cardiac death and injury; (d) appropriate participant supervision and monitoring; (e) exercise equipment that is safely designed and positioned in the exercise area; and (f) the development of a data-based exercise prescription for patients. However, given that exercise-related emergencies and injuries are not always preventable, all facilities should have policies and procedures to manage medical emergencies. The purpose of this chapter is to provide recommendations and resources that address the management of both life-threatening (major) and non–life-threatening (minor) medical emergencies.

EMERGENCY PREPAREDNESS

> **1.10.1-HFS: Knowledge of and skill in obtaining basic life support, first aid, cardiopulmonary resuscitation (CPR), and automated external defibrillator (AED) certifications.**

> > > KEY TERMS

Automated external defibrillator (AED): A portable device that identifies heart rhythms amenable to shock, directs the response, and delivers the appropriate shock.

Biphasic defibrillators: These use a biphasic waveform in which current flows in two directions rather than one (as in a conventional monophasic defibrillator).

Implantable cardioverter defibrillator (ICD): A small cardiac defibrillator implanted beneath the skin capable of delivering a shock to the heart if a malignant arrhythmia develops. Most can also provide backup pacing (pacemaker) if the heart rate becomes too slow.

Occult: A medical condition that is hidden or difficult to detect.

Sudden cardiac arrest: A cardiac emergency in which an individual develops an abnormal heart rhythm, preventing the effective pumping of blood.

> **1.10.2-HFS: Knowledge of appropriate emergency procedures (i.e., telephone procedures, written emergency procedures, personnel responsibilities) in a health and fitness setting.**

> **1.10.9-HFS: Knowledge of safety plans, emergency procedures, and first-aid techniques needed during fitness evaluations, exercise testing, and exercise training.**

> **1.10.16-HFS: Skill in demonstrating appropriate emergency procedures during exercise testing and/or training.**

> **1.10.3-CES: Describe the emergency equipment and personnel that should be present in an exercise testing laboratory and rehabilitative exercise training setting.**

> **1.10.4-CES: Describe the appropriate procedures for maintaining emergency equipment and supplies.**

> **1.10.7-CES: Describe the process for developing and updating emergency policies and procedures (e.g., call 911, call code team, call medical director, transport and use defibrillator).**

> **1.10.8-CES: Be aware of the current CPR, AED, and advanced cardiac life support (ACLS) standards to be able to assist with emergency situations.**

EXERCISE FACILITIES

All facilities should have written emergency plans for medical complications. Box 50-1 contains a list of questions to facilitate the preparation of an emergency plan. The plan should list specific responsibilities of each staff member, emergency equipment, and a predetermined contact for emergency response. Emergency plans— including numbers for emergency medical services, police, building security, and the fire department—should be posted next to all telephones. If paramedics or code teams are used for emergency response, it is imperative that they know the location and hours of the facility. First-aid kits, first-responder bloodborne pathogen kits, latex gloves, a blood pressure kit with stethoscope, an automated external defibrillator (AED) or manual defibrillator, oxygen, crash cart with medications and supplies, cardiopulmonary resuscitation (CPR) masks, and resuscitation bags as recommended based on the level of the facility as outlined in the American College of Sports Medicine (ACSM)/American Heart Association (AHA) Joint Position Statement (Table 50-1) must be readily available and transportable (6).

Facilities that perform maximal exercise tests or offer medically supervised cardiac rehabilitation programs should have all emergency equipment and drugs outlined for Level 5 facilities. Defibrillators, AEDs, crash carts (supplies and medication), oxygen tanks, and first-aid kits should be checked daily. Their storage areas must be clearly labeled with appropriate signage. A specific person should be assigned the task of daily equipment maintenance and documentation of all equipment checks.

In most facilities, the medical director or a risk management or safety committee is formed to oversee the development and revision of policies and procedures for medical emergencies. Regular periodic review of the emergency plan is recommended to ensure that all appropriate steps are outlined. The plan should be practiced with both announced and unannounced drills on a quarterly basis or more often, depending on staff turnover. All new employees should receive specific training regarding emergency procedures with documentation of training. Strategies for coping with potential and common injuries in the exercise, rehabilitation, and exercise testing settings should also be rehearsed. During the rehearsal or practice sessions, the supervisor presents a mock emergency, giving the staff information about the victim as the emergency unfolds; drills are practiced until the staff can effectively manage the emergency in a timely manner. All mock codes and other emergencies should be documented on a written report that includes a brief description of the drill, list of staff participating in the drill, documentation of each employee's competence, and any further training required. Each drill should be evaluated and recommendations for change documented and implemented.

Emergency plans should delineate procedures for both minor and major medical incidents. Minor medical events are not life or limb threatening and can be initially managed within the facility but they may be referred to a medical resource. Major medical emergencies that occur in the nonmedical setting require an initial response by the staff followed by immediate transport to a medical facility. In the clinical setting outside the hospital, the physician or other medical staff should determine whether to transport the patient to a hospital. In the health/fitness setting without a physician, if there is any doubt as to the status of the individual, he or she should be transported to a hospital. Emergency plans vary according to the type and size of facility, staff, location (hospital, physician's office, or fitness center), and local emergency response system. At least one staff member trained in the emergency plan and certified in CPR/AED and first aid should be on duty at all times in the health/fitness facility. Both the AHA and American Red Cross (ARC) offer CPR for the layman and healthcare provider. In the clinical setting, at least one staff member should also be certified in advanced cardiac life support (ACLS) and licensed to administer medications (18). ACLS training is available through the AHA. Because a medical emergency may arise at any time and any location, all employees, including secretarial, janitorial, and

BOX 50-1   STRATEGIES FOR DEVELOPING AN EMERGENCY CARE PLAN

- Is an outline of the entire emergency care plan displayed and accessible at a central staff location?
- Are different emergency procedures developed and posted for various areas within the facility (testing areas, pool, weight room, and gymnasium)?
- What care will be provided?
- Who will render care?
- Are all staff and supervisors certified in first aid, CPR, AED, and/or ACLS as appropriate?
- Is staff training documented in personnel files or emergency procedure plan?
- Is all staff familiar with OSHA's bloodborne pathogen guidelines and procedures?
- Are the responsibilities of individual staff members identified (e.g., team leader, captain, and medical liaison)?
- Who will activate EMS? Are telephone numbers for emergency procedures clearly posted?
- Are all staff members familiar with the information to be provided to EMS over the telephone, and is this information posted next to the phone?
  - Type of emergency (injury, illness)
  - Current status of involved or injured individuals
  - Type of assistance being given
  - Exact location of the facility and the afflicted individual within the facility
  - Specific point of entry into the facility
  - Telephone number being used
- Who will supervise the other activity areas if supervisors must leave to assist at an accident scene?
- Who will help with crowd control?
- Who has access to keys for locked areas or doors?
- Who will direct ambulance, EMS, or the code team to the emergency scene?
- Have the facility administrators invited representatives from EMS to become familiar with the floor plan and activities of the facility?
- Are emergency response training sessions conducted regularly (at least once every 3 months) and documented?

- Does emergency training consist of both announced and unannounced mock drills?
- Are emergency drills and training documented and evaluated with recommendations for necessary changes?
- Is EMS involved in the training and conduction of drills?
- Do all staff members know the location and have easy access to first-aid kits, AED, splints, stretchers, fire extinguishers, and other emergency equipment?
- Are emergency equipment and supplies clearly labeled and routinely checked, and do they receive routine maintenance?
- Is the facility conducting and documenting cardiovascular risk screening of all new members, guests, and patients?
- Are persons at high risk directed to seek facilities providing appropriate levels of care and staff supervision?
- Are appropriate documents (health appraisal, physician permission to participate, assumption of risk or waiver, informed consent, emergency information, and advanced directives) completed and accessible to staff in the event of an emergency?
- Have staff members been appropriately informed of orthopedic or other health problems, including cognitive problems such as dementia or Alzheimer disease, that might affect participation?
- Are emergency notification cards on file for each participant that include telephone numbers of family members, physician names, telephone numbers with special instructions, and alternative telephone numbers if primary contacts are unavailable? Patients should be encouraged to update this information on a regular basis.
- Are properly documented injury and accident reports completed and stored in an appropriate secure location for review and follow-up by administration?

ACLS, advanced cardiac life support; AED, automated external defibrillator; CPR, cardiopulmonary resuscitation; EMS, emergency medical system; OSHA, Occupational Safety and Health Administration.

From American College of Sports Medicine. *ACSM's Health/Fitness Facility Standards and Guidelines.* 2nd ed. Champaign (IL): Human Kinetics; 1997.

child-care staff, should be certified in CPR/AED operation through an accredited training organization. Facilities with aquatic areas should require water safety or life guard certification for all exercise instructors and staff working in the area so that someone who is trained to perform a water rescue and is CPR/AED certified is available at all times that the pool is open. Records of current certification and credentials for employees and consultants or contract staff should be kept with the emergency plan and/or personnel files.

TABLE 50-1. EMERGENCY PLANS AND EQUIPMENT FOR HEALTH FITNESS FACILITIES

	LEVEL 1	LEVEL 2	LEVEL 3	LEVEL 4	LEVEL 5
Type of facility	Unsupervised exercise room (e.g., hotel, commercial building)	Single exercise leader	Fitness center for general membership	Fitness center offering special programs for clinical populations	Medically supervised clinical exercise program (e.g., cardiac rehabilitation)
Personnel	None	Exercise leader; recommended: medical liaison	General manager; H/F instructor; exercise leader; recommended: medical liaison	General manager; exercise specialist; H/F instructor; medical liaison	General manager; exercise specialist; H/F instructor; exercise leader; medical liaison
Emergency plan	Present	Present	Present	Present	Present
Emergency equipment	Telephone in room Signs; encouraged: PAD plan with AED as part of the composite PAD plan in the host facility (hotel, commercial building)	Telephone; signs Encouraged: BP kit, stethoscope, PAD plan with AED	Telephone; signs Encouraged: BP kit, stethoscope, PAD plan with AED (the latter is strongly encouraged in facilities with membership >2,500 and those in which EMS response time is expected to be <5 min from recognition of arrest)	Telephone; signs BP kit stethoscope; strongly encouraged: PAD plan with AED	Telephone; signs BP kit, stethoscope, oxygen, crash cart defibrillator

AED, automated external defibrillator; BP, blood pressure; EMS, emergency medical services; H/F, health and fitness; PAD, public access to defibrillation.

Reprinted with permission from American College of Sports Medicine and American Heart Association. Recommendations for cardiovascular screening, staffing, and emergency policies at health/fitness facilities. *Med Sci Sports Exerc.* 1998;30(6):1009–18.

CLINICAL EXERCISE TESTING LABORATORIES

The guidelines for emergency planning outlined above are also applicable to the clinical exercise testing laboratory. However, in addition to standard 12-lead monitoring with or without gas exchange measurements, laboratories that use other cardiac imaging modalities—such as echocardiography and nuclear and pharmacologic studies—should have additional policies and procedures to manage emergencies unique to these modalities. In addition to policies and procedures specific to indications/contraindications for exercise testing, exercise protocol selection, and test termination, protocols for the administration of contrast agents and medications such as dobutamine, atropine, dipyridamole, and adenosine should be outlined with procedures for managing adverse reactions to any of these agents. Exercise testing should be supervised by an appropriately trained physician with ACLS certification. The AHA has established minimal competencies for physicians who supervise and interpret exercise tests (23). Some laboratories require the physician to be present during testing; however, exercise testing may be safely performed by properly trained nurses, exercise physiologists, physician assistants, and nurse practitioners with sufficient knowledge of exercise physiology (16) under the supervision of a physician who is in the immediate vicinity to respond to emergencies.

LIFE-THREATENING EMERGENCIES

> **1.10.11-HFS: Knowledge of potential musculoskeletal injuries (e.g., contusions, sprains, strains, fractures), cardiovascular/pulmonary complications (e.g., tachycardia, bradycardia, hypotension/hypertension, tachypnea), and metabolic abnormalities (e.g., fainting/syncope, hypoglycemia/hyperglycemia, hypothermia/hyperthermia).**

> **1.10.1-CES: Respond appropriately to emergency situations (e.g., cardiac arrest; hypoglycemia and hyperglycemia; bronchospasm; sudden onset hypotension; severe hypertensive response; angina; serious cardiac arrhythmias; implantable cardiac defibrillator [ICD] discharge; transient ischemic attack [TIA] or stroke; myocardial infarction [MI] that might arise before, during, and after administration of an exercise test and/or exercise session).**

> **1.10.2-CES: List medications that should be available for emergency situations in exercise testing and training sessions.**

> **1.10.3-CES: Describe the emergency equipment and personnel that should be present in an exercise testing laboratory and rehabilitative exercise training setting.**

Ventricular Ectopy

Symptomatic?

Yes	No
1. Stop activity.	1. Stop exercise if new ventricular ectopy.
2. Sit patient down.	2. Notify physician if new ventricular ectopy.
3. Check vitals (heart rate, blood pressure, oximetry) and responsiveness and document.	3. Check vitals and document.
	4. Document rhythm.
4. Document rhythm.	5. Observe.
5. Notify physician.	
6. Transfer to Emergency Room if unresolved.	
7. Initiate ACLS tachycardia or pulseless arrest protocol if patient is symptomatic or becomes unconscious.	

ACLS, advanced cardiac life support

FIGURE 50-1. Standing orders for the management of ventricular ectopy.

CLINICAL SETTINGS

In the clinical setting, such as exercise testing laboratories and cardiac rehabilitation programs, standing orders to manage a variety of potentially life-threatening emergencies such as hypotension, hypoglycemia, bronchospasm, arrhythmia, angina, transient ischemic attack, and cardiac arrest should be included in the policies and procedures manual. An example of an emergency standing order is shown in Figure 50-1. Box 50-2 lists equipment required to respond to a variety of life-threatening emergencies; equipment such as defibrillators, oxygen tanks, suction, and glucometers should be checked and documented daily.

Appendix B of ACSM's GETP8 (4) lists ACLS drugs that should be available in the crash cart (8). Expiration dates on ACLS drugs and non-ACLS medications used during stress testing should be checked regularly by staff or pharmacy and discarded and replaced when expired. Table 50-2 outlines common life-threatening emergencies, associated signs and symptoms, and the appropriate acute response.

Appendix B of the ACSM's GETP8 outlines sample emergency protocols for life-threatening situations that can be used as a template for development of protocols specific to the clinical and fitness setting as well as settings without emergency equipment (4). In clinical settings lo-

cated outside of the hospital, the emergency medical system (EMS) may be summoned rather than the code team. Emergency procedure plans will differ between programs depending on staffing, physician availability, hours of operation, access to emergency equipment, and location. For this reason, each area/program within the same facility should have its own emergency plan, i.e., hospital-based cardiac rehabilitation program versus exercise testing laboratory. Many disciplines are involved in the execution of an emergency plan in the clinical setting; each staff member has a specific role to perform. In cardiac rehabilitation programs, a physician should be available for medical consultation or to respond to emergencies within 3 minutes (2). All nursing staff and licensed physical therapists trained in ACLS may perform defibrillation/cardioversion per ACLS protocol and licensing practice acts. The clinical staff, including physicians, nurses, exercise physiologists, and physical therapists, should be trained in ACLS. There should be at least one (preferably two) licensed and trained ACLS personnel and a physician immediately available when high-risk patients are exercising or participating in graded exercise tests. Patient information, including advanced directives, should be readily accessible during an emergency. After an emergency (major or mi-

BOX 50-2   EMERGENCY EQUIPMENT REQUIRED FOR CLINICAL SETTINGS

- Portable, battery-operated defibrillator with monitor (An automated external defibrillator [AED] is an acceptable alternative to a manual defibrillator in most settings. Defibrillator may also be used for transcutaneous pacing.)
- Sphygmomanometer, including aneroid cuff and stethoscope
- Airway supplies, including oral, nasopharyngeal, and/or intubation equipment (only in situations in which licensed and trained personnel are available for use)
- Oxygen, available by nasal cannula and mask
- AMBU bag with pressure release valve
- Suction equipment

- Intravenous fluids and stand
- Intravenous access equipment in varying sizes, including butterfly intravenous supplies
- Syringes and needles in multiple sizes
- Tourniquets
- Adhesive tape, alcohol wipes, gauze pads
- Sharp's container
- Biohazard bags
- 10% bleach—ten parts water to one part bleach to clean up blood or body fluids
- Flashlight with extra batteries
- Emergency documentation forms (code charting form and incident forms)

nor), an accident/incident report should be completed and filed with the appropriate department for review and evaluation. Box 50-3 details items that should be addressed in this report in both clinical and nonclinical settings.

The Association for Cardiovascular and Pulmonary Rehabilitation has published guidelines for cardiac (2) and pulmonary (3) rehabilitation programs that provide sample emergency reports for documentation of mock codes, equipment checks, emergencies, and in-service training.

COMMUNITY SETTINGS

> **1.10.9-HFS: Knowledge of safety plans, emergency procedures, and first-aid techniques needed during fitness.**

Nonclinical settings, such as recreational and fitness facilities without access to a CPR code team or physician, also need a set of emergency procedures to manage life-threatening and non–life-threatening events until an emergency team arrives. Emergency numbers should be posted in areas designated for fitness evaluations as well as exercise training. It is important to provide the 911 operator with a brief description of the problem as an advanced life support unit is dispatched in the event of a cardiac event or respiratory arrest. In non–life-threatening situations, such as seizures or bodily injury, a basic life support unit is often dispatched. The life-threatening emergencies, associated signs and symptoms, and the appropriate acute response in Table 50-2 also apply to the health/fitness setting; however, depending on the availability of emergency equipment, staff training, and licensure, all of the responses to a specific emergency may not be possible or legally appropriate. Box 50-4 lists emergency equipment that should be available in the health/fitness setting.

In addition, the facility should have a signed medical release that provides authorization to release the victim's

medical history and emergency contacts in the event that the emergency renders the victim unresponsive. Medical histories and other healthcare information should be kept in a locked file that is accessible to appropriate staff in the event of an emergency. When possible, a senior staff member should assume control of the emergency response, complete an accident/incident report after the emergency, and file the report with the facility's director. Depending on the type of incident, the facility's insurance carrier may also need to be alerted. The director or senior staff member should follow up with the victim or family regarding the victim's medical status as permitted by law and as the victim and family are willing to disclose information. Any information provided should be documented in the victim's personal file. The Health Insurance Portability and Accountability Act (HIPAA) does not allow private health information to be released to anyone except the medical director unless the victim has signed the appropriate authorization allowing a medical director designate to release the information. As in the clinical setting, an accident/incident report (Box 50-3) should be completed by a senior staff member. ACSM's *Health/Fitness Facility Standards and Guidelines* (5) contains examples of emergency procedures and incident reports specific to the fitness setting that can be used as a template. Daily equipment checks of AEDs and first-aid kits should also be documented.

SUDDEN CARDIAC ARREST

> **1.10.1-CES: Respond appropriately to emergency situations (e.g. cardiac arrest; hypoglycemia and hyperglycemia; bronchospasm; sudden onset hypotension; severe hypertensive response; angina; serious cardiac arrhythmias; ICD discharge; TIA or stroke; MI that might arise before, during, and after administration of an exercise test and/or exercise session).**

TABLE 50-2. ACUTE RESPONSES FOR CARDIOPULMONARY AND METABOLIC CONDITIONS/EMERGENCIES

CONDITION	DEFINITION/SIGNS AND SYMPTOMS	ACUTE CARE
Dizziness/fainting	Disoriented; confused; skin color—pale; rapid, irregular pulse; weak	Determine responsiveness, place supine with legs elevated, administer fluids if conscious, begin emergency breathing or compressions as needed, check blood sugar if patient does not respond immediately. Activate EMS.
Syncope	Temporary loss of consciousness	
Hypoglycemia	Low blood sugar. Profuse sweating, tachycardia, hunger, blurred or double vision, tremors, headache, confusion, seizure, unconsciousness	Check blood sugar, administer 10–30 g of CHO (regular soda, orange juice or 3 glucose tablets) if conscious. If unconscious, place sugar granules under tongue or give glucose gel. When recovery requires more than 1–2 minutes, activate EMS.
Hyperglycemia	Abnormally high blood sugar. Nausea, dizziness, polyuria, blurred vision, lethargy, sweet fruity breath, vomiting, hyperventilation	Stop activity, turn head to side if vomiting, check blood sugar, administer fluids orally if conscious, give insulin to lower blood sugar, activate EMS.
Angina	Pain/pressure in the chest, neck, jaw, arm and/or back, sweating, denial of medical problem, nausea, shortness of breath.	Stop activity, place in seated or supine position (whichever is most comfortable), give nitroglycerin and oxygen per ACLS protocol, activate EMS or physician evaluation (unless patient is diagnosed with chronic stable angina, which is relieved with rest and/or medication).
Sudden cardiac arrest	An abnormal heart rhythm usually caused by lack of oxygen to the heart; victim may be unresponsive without breathing or pulse	Check ABCs; activate EMS; start CPR; when AED/ manual defibrillator is available, defibrillate shockable rhythms; continue CPR as indicated.
Dyspnea	Labored breathing. Hyperventilation, dizziness, wheezing, coughing, loss of coordination	Stop activity. Maintain open airway, administer bronchodilator if prescribed. Try pursed-lip breathing; if no relief, activate EMS and transport.
Tachypnea	Abnormally rapid respiration rate. Hyperventilation	Stop activity. Maintain open airway, treat cause if known, if signs/symptoms persist, activate EMS.
Stroke or TIA	Lack of oxygen to the brain. May cause symptoms such as drowsiness, confusion, severe headache, nausea, or loss of vision and voluntary movement, muscle weakness, slurred speech, loss of coordination, or facial droop	Check ABCs, activate EMS, start CPR if needed and continue. Monitor vitals and signs/symptoms, give oxygen if hypoxic, establish time of onset of symptoms if possible.
Hypertension	High blood pressure—resting SBP >185 or DBP >105. Exercise SBP >250 or DBP >115 without symptoms of stroke or TIA	Stop activity, monitor vitals and signs/symptoms. If BP does not drop quickly, alert physician or take to ER.
Hypotension	Low blood pressure that causes symptoms such as syncope, dizziness, and fatigue	Stop activity. Place in a supine position, elevate legs, assess vital signs, and give oral fluids if conscious. Activate EMS if symptoms do not resolve and BP does not improve. Treat the cause.
Tachycardia	Resting HR ≥100 bpm. Other signs and symptoms, such as dyspnea or angina, may be present	Stop activity. Assess vital signs, secure airway, give oxygen, and identify the rhythm. Activate EMS or obtain physician evaluation, follow ACLS guidelines for tachycardia and treat contributing factors.
Bradycardia	Resting HR <60 bpm with symptoms; it is not unusual for patients on β-blockers or athletic individuals to have slow resting heart rates without symptoms	Stop activity. Maintain airway, check vital signs, give oxygen, and identify rhythm. Check for signs of poor perfusion, activate EMS.
Exertional rhabdomyolysis	Muscle pain, swelling and weakness, dark urine	Activate EMS and transport to hospital immediately, cool, and administer fluids if conscious.
Hyperthermia	Heat injury	
Heat cramps	Involuntary, isolated muscle spasms	Stop activity. Administer chilled oral fluids with electrolytes, and apply direct pressure to spasm and release. Massage cramping area with ice, monitor vitals and hydration status.
Heat exhaustion	Profuse sweating, pale, clammy skin, multiple muscle spasms, headache, nausea, loss of consciousness, dizziness, tachycardia, hypotension	Stop activity and move to cool area; place supine with feet elevated; remove clothes; cool with fans, cold water, or ice but avoid chilling the victim. Administer fluids, monitor core temperature, refer for physician evaluation, or activate EMS if no rapid improvement.
Heat stroke	Hot, dry skin, but can be sweating, dyspnea, confusion; often unconscious	Activate EMS and transport to hospital immediately, move to cool area and remove clothing, dowse with cool water (ice water baths preferred), or wrap in cool wet sheets. Administer fluids if conscious, monitor core temperature and vitals.
Hypothermia	Body temperature falls below 36°C or 97°F; shivering, loss of coordination, muscle stiffness, and lethargy	Activate EMS and move to a warm place. Remove any wet clothing and replace with dry, warm clothing and cover with blankets. Monitor vital signs, give hot liquids.

ABCs, airway, breathing, circulation; ACLS, advanced cardiac life support; AED, automated external defibrillator; BP, blood pressure; CHD, carbohydrate; CPR, cardiopulmonary resuscitation; DBP, diastolic blood pressure; EMS, emergency medical services; ER, emergency room; HR, heart rate; SBP, systolic blood pressure; TIA, transient ischemic attack.

| BOX 50-3 | INFORMATION PERTINENT TO AN INCIDENT REPORT |

- Date, time of the incident
- Location of incident
- Person(s) involved in the incident and contact information
- Witnesses to the incident and contact information
- Details of the incident
- Staff and their actions taken in response to the incident
- Signature of staff person completing the report
- Follow-up communication with the victim or victim's family

Sudden cardiac arrest, which is caused by factors such as heart disease, rhythm disturbances, and congenital abnormalities, results in 330,000 deaths annually (10). It is usually caused by an abnormal heart rhythm called *ventricular fibrillation,* which causes the heart to beat in an uncoordinated fashion. Because blood is not effectively being pumped, the pulse and subsequently the breathing stop. Death can occur within minutes after the first symptoms appear, especially if intervention does not occur. About half of all cardiac-related deaths occur before the victim reaches the hospital (10). If the heart is electrically shocked soon thereafter, normal rhythm may be restored. Cardiopulmonary resuscitation alone can add only a few minutes to the time available for defibrillation. Hence, early defibrillation is the single most important intervention for improving survival in out of

| BOX 50-4 | EMERGENCY EQUIPMENT AND SUPPLIES FOR A HEALTH/FITNESS FACILITY |

- Automated external defibrillator (AED)
- Cardiopulmonary resuscitation (CPR) barrier masks
- Blood pressure kit with aneroid sphygmomanometer and stethoscope
- First-aid kit
- First-responder bloodborne pathogen kits (often part of first-aid kit)
- 10% bleach—ten parts water to one part bleach to clean up blood or body fluids (may be part of bloodborne pathogen kit)
- Flashlight with extra batteries
- Accident report form

hospital cardiac arrests (11). Automated external defibrillators used by trained lay responders provide the best chance of early defibrillation, as it is often difficult for EMS personnel to reach the victim within this time frame, especially in rural areas. For witnessed ventricular fibrillation, survival rates as high as 90% have been reported when defibrillation was administered within the first minute of collapse (11). For every minute that defibrillation is delayed, there is a 7% to 10% reduction in the chance of survival.

Automated External Defibrillators

An AED is a portable device that identifies heart rhythms amenable to defibrillation, uses audiovisual prompts to direct the correct response, and delivers the appropriate shock. Even children can be trained to operate AEDs safely and effectively (17). Courses that incorporate AED training into traditional CPR training are available to the public through the ARC and AHA. The Cardiac Arrest Survival Act extends Good Samaritan protection to AED users. The limited number of trial court verdicts on AEDs suggest that organizations adopting AED programs have a lower risk of liability than those who do not. The ACSM and AHA's joint position statement on automated external defibrillators in health/fitness facilities makes recommendations for the use and purchase of AEDs in both the clinical and fitness settings (11). The position statement recommends that AEDs be placed in health and fitness facilities with more than 2,500 members, facilities that offer programs for clinical or elderly populations, and those with an anticipated response time (from cardiac arrest to delivery of the first shock) greater than 5 minutes. In addition, unsupervised facilities are encouraged to purchase AEDs as part of their emergency plans. AEDs should be placed in well-marked, easily accessible locations near telephones. It should take no more than 3 minutes for a responder to retrieve the AED and reach the victim (25). Optimal response time should determine the number of AEDs placed in a facility. AEDs are not recommended for use in children younger than 8 years (13). As more data become available, recommendations for the use of AEDs will be updated, necessitating periodic revision of policies and procedures for emergencies. Appendix B of the ACSM's GETP8 (4) outlines general guidelines and special considerations regarding AEDs and CPR.

In addition to the use of AEDs in the lay community and outpatient and chronic care units, many medical facilities have replaced conventional manual monophasic defibrillators with combination biphasic waveform defibrillators, which can be used in manual or AED mode. Biphasic defibrillators, as the name implies, use two phases of reversed current flow that adjust for impedance (body's resistance to flow). This allows the use of lower energy levels compared with conventional monophasic waveform shocks. Observational studies suggest that the lower energy shocks of biphasic defibrillators are at least if not more effective than higher-energy monophasic waveform shocks in terminating ventricular fibrillation (9). Given that adverse effects such as myocardial dysfunction and skin burns are related to the use of higher energy levels (30), the lower energy levels used for biphasic defibrillators may offer additional advantages compared with monophasic waveforms. An observational study comparing the use of manual monophasic defibrillators with biphasic defibrillators used in AED mode in the hospital setting and AED placement in all outpatient clinics and chronic care units reported improved survival to discharge in hospitalized patients with cardiopulmonary arrest (31). Some of the currently available AED-only devices are also able to deliver biphasic shock. More research is needed to determine the benefits of biphasic versus monophasic waveforms and if the use of AEDs in clinical/hospital settings will improve survival and outcomes.

All medical devices, including AEDs and manual defibrillators, are subject to malfunction. Data suggest that although the number of AED advisories and AEDs affected by advisories has increased, the total number of device malfunctions is small compared with the number of lives saved (24). However, although medical devices are registered with the manufacturer when implanted in patients, no process exists for AEDs, making it difficult to track devices and end users. Because of the rapid growth in AED use, this presents a challenge for both the Food and Drug Administration (FDA) and manufacturers to develop a reliable reporting system to insure timely and accurate communication to potential users regarding advisory defects. For this reason, it is important for facilities to be vigilant about responding to advisory alerts and performing daily equipment checks.

Implantable Cardioverter Defibrillators and Sudden Cardiac Arrest

Just as an AED recognizes shockable rhythms and delivers a life-saving shock, implantable cardioverter defibrillators (ICDs) can do the same when surgically implanted. The ICD is placed underneath the patient's skin, and lead wires from the device are attached directly to the heart, usually though the subclavian vein. ICDs are used to treat life-threatening arrhythmias in patients with heart failure and other cardiac disease. In addition to the delivery of cardioversion/defibrillation shocks, the ICD can be programmed to provide overdrive pacing to convert sustained ventricular tachycardia or provide backup pacing for bradycardia. According to the American Heart Association, nearly 5 million Americans are living with heart failure, and an additional 550,000 new cases are diagnosed each year (7). To reduce the risk of sudden cardiac death, many patients with heart failure are implanted with ICDs. Given that Medicare and insurance companies reimburse for limited (≤12 weeks) supervised training in a cardiac rehabilitation program, even the health/fitness professional may train patients with ICDs or supervise workout areas where members with ICDs are exercising. For this reason, it is not only important for exercise professionals working in the clinical setting, but also for those working with special populations in the nonclinical setting, to have a basic understanding of ICDs when conducting risk-factor screening, corresponding with clinical healthcare professionals regarding exercise prescriptions, and responding to emergencies.

Although ICDs save lives, they have been reported to fail to deliver appropriate shocks. If an ICD fails, an AED or manual defibrillator should be used to convert pulseless ventricular tachycardia/ventricular fibrillation. Care should be taken to avoid placement of paddles over the ICD. Another concern with ICD malfunction is the delivery of inappropriate shocks when the ICD misinterprets the rhythm. Inappropriate shocks in patients with sinus tachycardia and supraventricular dysrhythmias (28) can induce life-threatening dysrhythmias. Thus, the exercise specialist should have knowledge of each patient's ICD program setting. For pacemakers, the upper rate limit for patients with complete heart block and the type of programmability or rate-responsive pacing should be utilized when developing the exercise prescription. Maximal exercise heart rate should be set at least 10 to 15 beats/minute below the ICD discharge heart rate (2) to reduce the risk of inappropriate shocks. A magnet can be used to terminate inappropriate shocks; however, only a physician/provider with electrophysiology training should decide if the use of a magnet is appropriate. Any ICD malfunction should be immediately reported to the patient's electrophysiologist so it can be interrogated to determine if the settings need to be adjusted or if there are problems with lead displacement (any position change in the pacemaker or leads).

OTHER MEDICAL CONCERNS

FIRST AID

> **1.10.9-HFS: Knowledge of safety plans, emergency procedures, and first-aid techniques needed during fitness evaluations, exercise testing, and exercise training.**

First-aid kits are vital to an appropriate emergency response. The Occupational Safety and Health Administration (OSHA) provides general standards for work-site first-aid kits based on the degree of hazard, location, size, amount of staff training, and availability of professional medical service (26), but does recommend the minimum requirements set forth by the American National Stan-

---

BOX 50-5   SAMPLE CONTENTS OF A FIRST-AID KIT FOR A FITNESS FACILITY

- Sterile first-aid dressings in sealed envelope (2″ × 2″ for small wounds, 4″ × 4″ for larger wounds and for compress to stop bleeding)
- Tongue blades
- Bandage scissors
- Tweezers
- Eyewash solution
- Safety pins
- Ace bandage
- Band-Aids
- Roller bandage 1″ × 5 yards (for finger)
- Roller bandage 2″ × 5 yards to hold dressings in place
- Adhesive tape

- Triangular bandages for a sling or as a covering over a larger dressing
- Cotton balls for cleaning wounds or applying medication
- Splints 1/4″ thick, 1/2″ wide, 12″ to 15″ long for splinting broken arms and legs
- 70% isopropyl alcohol and tincture green soap in a covered container for cleaning
- Ice packs (chemical ice bags) to use to reduce swelling
- Insect bite kit (facilities with outdoor activities)
- Several pairs of disposable gloves
- Waterless hand wash
- First-aid instruction booklet
- Space blanket (facilities with outdoor activities)

---

dards Institute (ANSI) (14). These supplies are required items to treat major wounds, cuts and abrasions, minor burns, and eye injuries. There are three ANSI classifications for first-aid kits, depending on whether the kit is used indoors or outdoors and if it needs to be portable. The contents of first-aid kits in healthcare versus fitness facilities may be quite different, as many of the items in a standard first-aid kit may already be readily available in the medical setting. In the health/fitness setting, first-aid kits are a necessity. The number of kits and amount of supplies should depend on the number of members, types of activities performed that determine types of potential injuries, the layout of the facility, response time, level of staff training, and whether activities are indoors and/or outdoors (26). Box 50-5 lists a sample of kit contents adequate to respond to a variety of injuries and emergencies.

All first-aid kits should also be stocked with CPR barrier masks. The ARC Web site is a good resource for additional recommendations and for first-aid kits tailored for different settings (home vs. work site). The ARC offers various levels of training for first aid, CPR, and bloodborne pathogens. Although it is not necessary to keep an aneroid sphygmomanometer and blood pressure cuff in the first-aid kit, it should be readily accessible to monitor vitals.

BLOODBORNE PATHOGENS

Universal bloodborne pathogen precautions were developed by the Centers for Disease Control and Prevention (CDC) as an aggressive set of guidelines to protect employees from bloodborne pathogens, such as human immunodeficiency virus (HIV) and hepatitis B virus. Recommendations include the use of gloves, masks,

gowns, and other barriers whenever it is possible for an individual to come in contact with blood and other body fluids. OSHA issued a regulation in 1991 requiring the adoption of universal precautions for occupational exposure to bloodborne pathogens (27). The standard also mandates annual training and documentation of training for all employees who potentially could be exposed to bloodborne pathogens.

Staff members should always use latex gloves and appropriate barriers when treating skin wounds and handling items such as mouthpieces, resuscitation bags, and equipment that may have been exposed to bloodborne pathogens or other body fluids. Biohazard kits should be available to all employees who may be exposed to blood, cerebrospinal fluid, pleural fluid, saliva, or any body fluid with visible blood. These kits should contain disposable paper towels, a spray bottle with 10% bleach solution, hydrogen peroxide, assorted sizes of gloves, disposable gauze and towels, red biohazard bags, gowns, masks, and face shields (21). Hands should always be washed according to guidelines established by the CDC's Healthcare Infection Control Practices Advisory Committee (15) immediately after providing any type of care.

MUSCULOSKELETAL INJURIES

> **1.10.3-HFS: Knowledge of and skill in performing basic first-aid procedures for exercise-related injuries, such as bleeding, strains/sprains, fractures, and exercise intolerance (dizziness, syncope, heat and cold injuries).**

> **1.10.12-HFS: Knowledge of the initial management and first-aid techniques associated with open wounds, musculoskeletal injuries, cardiovascular/pulmonary complications, and metabolic disorders.**

TABLE 50-3. ACUTE RESPONSES FOR COMMON MUSCULOSKELETAL INJURIES/EMERGENCIES

INJURY	DESCRIPTION	SIGNS/SYMPTOMS	ACUTE CARE
Blisters/corns	Closed skin wounds	Pain, swelling, infection	Clean with antiseptic soap. Apply sterile dressing, antibiotic ointment.
Lacerations/abrasions	Open skin wounds	Pain, redness, bleeding, swelling, mild fever	Follow universal precautions to prevent the transfer of bloodborne pathogens. Apply pressure and elevate to stop bleeding. Clean with soap or sterile saline, apply sterile dressing, and refer to physician for stitches/tetanus. Wash your hands immediately after providing care.
Strain[a]			
Grade I	A stretch or tear in a muscle, tendon, and/or fascia	Pain, localized tenderness, tightness	RICES (see Table 50-4 for definitions and protocol)
Grade II		Loss of function, hemorrhage	RICES, refer for physician evaluation if impaired function
Grade III		Palpable defect	Immobilization, RICES, prompt physician evaluation
Sprain[a]			
Grade I	A stretch or tear to the ligaments and stabilizing connective tissues of a joint	Pain, point tenderness, strength loss, edema	RICES
Grade II		Hemorrhage, measurable laxity	RICES, physician evaluation.
Grade III		Palpable or observable defect	Immobilization, RICES, prompt physician evaluation.
Stress fracture	Microscopic damage to the bone because of repetitive stress	Insidious onset of pain that persists when attempting activity, tenderness	Physician evaluation, rest, non–weight-bearing activities.
Simple acute fracture	Sudden break of a bone	Swelling, point tenderness, disability, pain, swelling, ecchymosis	Immobilize joint with splint if warranted, physician evaluation, x-rays.

RICES, rest, ice, compression, elevation, stabilization.

[a]Signs and symptoms for each grade include those for the grade below the one listed (i.e., grade II includes those of grades I and II; grade III includes signs and symptoms listed under grades I, II, and III).

Most musculoskeletal injuries seen in the exercise setting are non–life-threatening, although they require a prompt emergency response to optimize outcomes and minimize liability. Injuries may be the result of a single traumatic event or chronic, repetitive, submaximal forces that lead to inflammation and pain. Strains, sprains, and fractures are often caused by an acute event, whereas injuries such as tendonitis, shin splints, plantar fasciitis, and stress fractures are examples of chronic "overuse" injuries. A description of the characteristics and appropriate first-aid procedures for common exercise-related musculoskeletal injuries are outlined in Table 50-3. The RICES protocol outlined in Table 50-4 involves the utilization of rest, ice, compression, elevation, and stabilization and is the appropriate treatment for most acute musculoskeletal injuries (22).

When used properly, the RICES treatment regimen reduces the total amount of tissue damage, decreases swelling and pain, and aids in controlling the inflammatory response, which results in quicker rehabilitation and recovery. Improper care or delay in treatment may cause additional pain, swelling, and damage of healthy tissues, resulting in secondary hypoxic injury (cell death because of lack of oxygen) even after bleeding is controlled. The initial RICES treatment protocol should be continued for 24 to 72 hours after injury.

TABLE 50-4. RICES PROTOCOL FOR ACUTE INJURIES

TREATMENT	PURPOSE	APPLICATION
Rest	Pain control, prevention of reinjury	Complete rest, immobilization, or reduction in training intensity, duration, frequency or non–weight-bearing activities, depending on severity of injury
Ice	Reduction of pain, swelling, inflammation, spasms, and bleeding	Immediately postinjury, every 2 hours: 20–30 minutes plastic bag filled with crushed ice and secured with an elastic bandage; or ice massage for small areas, such as tendons and strains, for 10–20 minutes
Compression	Reduction of swelling	Elastic wrap/compression sleeve
Elevation	Reduction of swelling	Elevate extremity above heart level
Stabilization	Reduce muscle spasm	Use of braces, splints, wraps to stabilize area around joint injury

PREVENTING EXERCISE-RELATED EMERGENCIES

 1.10.4-HFS: Knowledge of basic precautions taken in an exercise setting to ensure participant safety.

One of the major priorities in both the clinical and non-clinical settings is the prevention of emergencies and injuries through the development of policies and procedures that address risk-factor screening, data-based exercise prescription, patient orientation and education, and training and competencies for both staff and consultants relative to patient risk status. The program director and/or office of human resources should verify that staff credentials include certifications and licensure appropriate for the patient/patient population at that facility. Appropriate levels of supervision and staffing relative to the number of members/patients and facility layout and size, as well as equipment maintenance and selection, should also be addressed. The facility floor plan should provide for adequate space and appropriate traffic flow to prevent exercise-related injuries and facilitate a prompt emergency response. For a detailed discussion of these topics, the reader is referred to ACSM's *Health/Fitness Facility Standards and Guidelines* (5). Finally, documentation and referral to an appropriate medical professional is crucial when the exercise professional recognizes early signs and symptoms of potential medical problems or the patient reports them. Because it is impossible to prevent all exercise-related emergencies and injuries, the policies and procedures addressed in this chapter should be utilized as a template for the development of an emergency plan specific to each facility and area within the facility to effectively manage a variety of medical emergencies.

SUMMARY

First and foremost, every clinical, fitness, and recreational facility should have a thorough set of policies and procedures in place and readily accessible to staff in an emergency. They should follow national standards and guidelines, satisfy accrediting organizations, and provide a safe and effective exercise environment for all participants. Policies and procedures should be reviewed and revised on a regular basis. Employee training and rehearsal of procedures for managing both major and minor medical events should be conducted at orientation and on a regular schedule thereafter to maintain optimal skill levels. In addition, all aspects of the emergency plan should be followed and documented to ensure participant safety, meet best practice guidelines, and to limit both professional and personal liability.

REFERENCES

1. Albert CM, Mittleman, MA, Chae CU, et al. Triggering of sudden death from cardiac causes by vigorous exertion. *N Engl J Med.* 2000;343:1355–61.

2. American Association of Cardiovascular and Pulmonary Rehabilitation. *Guidelines for Cardiac Rehabilitation and Secondary Prevention Programs.* 4th ed. Champaign (IL): Human Kinetics; 2004.

3. American Association of Cardiovascular and Pulmonary Rehabilitation. *Guidelines for Pulmonary Rehabilitation Programs.* 3rd ed. Champaign (IL): Human Kinetics; 2004.

4. **American College of Sports Medicine. *ACSM's Guidelines for Exercise Testing and Prescription.* 8th ed. Philadelphia: Lippincott Williams and Wilkins; 2009.**

5. American College of Sports Medicine. *ACSM's Health/Fitness Facility Standards and Guidelines.* 3rd ed. Champaign (IL): Human Kinetics; 2007.

6. **American College of Sports Medicine and American Heart Association. Recommendations for cardiovascular screening, staffing, and emergency policies at health/fitness facilities. *Med Sci Sports Exerc.* 1998;30(6):1009–18.**

7. **American Heart Association. Heart Disease and Stroke Statisics—2007 Update: A Report from the American Heart Association Statistics Committee and Stoke Statistics Committee. *Circulation.* 2007;115:e69–171.**

8. **American Heart Association. Guidelines for cardiopulmonary resuscitation (CPR) and emergency cardiovascular care. *Circulation.* 2005;112(24):1–211.**

9. **American Heart Association. Part 5: Electrical therapies: automated external defibrillators, defibrillation, cardioversion, and pacing. *Circulation.* 2005;112:IV1–35, IV46.**

10. **American Heart Association Web site. Dallas (TX): Scientific position statement: Sudden cardiac death. Available from: www.americanheart.org/presenter.jhtml?identifier54741. Accessed May 28, 2007.**

11. **American Heart Association and American College of Sports Medicine. Automated external defibrillators in health/fitness facilities. *Circulation.* 2002:105:1147–50.**

12. **American Heart Association and American College of Sports Medicine. Exercise and acute cardiovascular events: placing the risks into perspective. A scientific statement from the American Heart Association Council on Nutrition, Physical Activity, and Metabolism and the Council on Clinical Cardiology. *Circulation.* 2007;115: 2358–68.**

13. **American Heart Association and International Liaison Committee on Resuscitation. Guidelines 2000 for cardiopulmonary resuscitation and emergency cardiovascular care. *Circulation.* 2000;102 (Suppl 1):160–76.**

14. **American National Standards Institute. *ANSI Z308.1—2003 Minimum Requirements for Workplace First Aid Kits.* Arlington (VA): International Safety Equipment Association; 2003.**

15. **Centers for Disease Control and Prevention. *Guidelines for Hand-Hygiene in Healthcare Settings. MMWR Morb Mortal Wkly Rep.* 2002;51:RR-16.**

16. **Fletcher GF, Balady GJ, Amsterdam EA, et al. Exercise standards for testing and training: a statement for healthcare professionals from the American Heart Association. *Circulation.* 2001;104(14): 1694–740.**

17. Gundry JW, Comess KA, DeRook FA, Jorgenson D, Bardy GH. Comparison of naïve sixth-grade children with trained professionals in the use of an automated external defibrillator. *Circulation.* 1999;100:1703–7.

18. Kern KB, Halperin HR, Field J. New guidelines for cardiopulmonary resuscitation and emergency cardiac care: changes in the management of cardiac arrest. *JAMA.* 2001;285(10):1267–9.

19. Mora S, Redberg RF, Yadong C, et al. Ability of exercise testing to predict cardiovascular and all-cause death in asymptomatic women. *JAMA.* 2003;290:1600–7.

20. Myers J, Prakash M, Froelicher V, Do D, Partington S, Atwood JE. Exercise capacity and mortality among men referred for exercise testing. *N Engl J Med.* 2002;346:793–801.

21. National Safety Council. *Bloodborne Pathogens*. Boston: Jones & Bartlett; 1993.

22. Prentice WE. *Arnheim's Principles of Athletic Training*. 11th ed. Boston: McGraw Hill; 2003.

23. **Rodgers GP, Ayanian JZ, Balady G, et al. American College of Cardiology/American Heart Association clinical competence statement on stress testing. A report of the American College of Cardiology/American Heart Association/American College of Physicians–American Society of Internal Medicine task force on clinical competence. *Circulation*. 2000;102(14):1726–38.**

24. Shah JS, Maisel WH. Recalls and safety alerts affecting automated external defibrillators. *JAMA*. 2006;296(6):655–60.

25. U.S. Department of Health and Human Services, Federal Occupational Health Web site. Washington (DC): Federal Register: May 23, 2001 (Volume 66, Number 100). Available from: www.foh. dhhs.gov/Public/WhatWeDo/AED/HHSAED.ASP. Accessed on May 28, 2007.

26. U.S. Department of Labor. *Best Practices Guide: Fundamentals of a Workplace First-Aid Program*. Washington (Dc): U.S. Department of Labor, Occupational Safety and Health Administration; 2006. 3317-05n.

27. U.S. Department Of Labor. *The OSHA Bloodborne Pathogens Standard*. Washington (Dc): U.S. Department of Labor, Occupational Safety and Health Administration; 2006. 71 Federal Register 16672 and 16673.

28. Vanhees L, Kornaat M, Defoor J, et al. Effect of exercise training in patients with an implantable cardioverter defibrillator. *Eur Heart J*. 2004;25:1120–6.

29. Whang W, Manson JE, Hu FB, et al. Physical exertion, exercise, and sudden cardiac death in women. *JAMA*. 2006;295:1399–1403.

30. Xie J, Weil MH, Sun S. High-energy defibrillation increases the severity of postresuscitation myocardial dysfunction *Circulation*. 1997;96:683–8.

31. Zafari AM, Zarter SK, Heggen V, et al. A program encouraging early defibrillation results in improved in-hospital resuscitation efficacy. *J Am Coll Cardiol*. 2004;44:846–52.

SELECTED REFERENCES FOR FURTHER READING

American Heart Association Web site. Dallas (TX): American College of Cardiology and American Heart Association Guideline Update for Exercise Testing. Task Force on Practice Guidelines (Committee on Exercise Testing), 2002. Available from www.americanheart.org/downloadable/heart/1032279013658exercise.pdf. Accessed September 24, 2007.

INTERNET RESOURCES

- American Association of Cardiovascular and Pulmonary Rehabilitation: www.aacvpr.org
- American Heart Association: www.americanheart.org
- American Red Cross: www.redcross.org/services/hss/courses/workplace.html
- Occupational Safety and Health Administration: www.osha.gov/

Legal Considerations for Exercise Programming

51

Legal considerations constitute an important matter for those administering fitness evaluations and exercise tests, engaging in physical activity counseling, providing exercise recommendations, and directing fitness programs for apparently healthy adults or individuals with stable chronic diseases. One area of critical concern to personal trainers, health/fitness instructors, and rehabilitation specialists is the professional–patient relationship and the activities performed within the confines of that relationship. Other considerations with special significance when evaluated from a legal perspective include the physical setting, areas in which program activities are conducted, the specific purpose for which exercise services are performed, the equipment used, the techniques applied with patients, and the instruction and supervision provided to those patients.

The law influences exercise professionals in each of these domains, as well as in others. Furthermore, expectations are substantially affected by the exercise environment—recreational, commercial, or clinical by the type of patient being served and by the nature of the services being provided. Regardless of the situation, sensitivity to legal issues, adherence to current professional guidelines, and the rigorous application of risk-management principles may enhance not only the quality of provided service but patient satisfaction as well. Moreover, the use of risk-management techniques may reduce service-related injuries, the likelihood of personal injury litigation, and the extent of damage to the provider in the event of claim and lawsuit.

Laws that affect these matters vary considerably from state to state. Nonetheless, certain legal principles have broad application to pre-exercise screening, exercise testing, exercise program planning, activity supervision, and emergency response considerations. All exercise program personnel should know these principles and endeavor to develop practices aimed at reducing the risks of claims and lawsuits.

In carefully screened and supervised adult populations, the risks of serious cardiovascular accidents in exercise programs are very low. Even for those with some signs of disease who undergo clinical tests, the cardiovascular complication rate appears to be no greater than seven in 10,000 participants, and for aerobic exercise performed by cardiac patients, these rates are less than one in 20,000 (14,33). Recent survey findings indicate that facility readiness, staff training, and practice for serious adverse events in the health and fitness industry are abysmal despite the fact that more and more such facilities accept older patients and those with controlled chronic diseases (8,16,29,30). More than 75% of these facilities reported that they had summoned emergency medical services at

> > > KEY TERMS

Assumption of risk (waiver): An agreement by a patient, provided before beginning participation, to give up, relinquish, or waive the participant's rights to legal remedy (damages) in the event of injury, even when such injury arises as a result of provider negligence.

Informed consent: A process that entails conveying information to a patient to achieve an understanding about the options to choose to participate in a procedure, test, service, or program.

Negligence: A failure to conform one's conduct to a generally accepted standard or duty.

Risk management: An initial and ongoing process to identify relevant risks associated with the delivery of a service and then, through the application of various techniques, to eliminate, reduce, or transfer those risks through the implementation of operational strategies to the program activities designed to benefit the patients and program.

least once in 5 years. This suggests a high potential for personal injury lawsuits (8,16,29,30). Until the 1990s, only a small fraction of all personal injury cases resulted in claims against exercise professionals. In recent years, however, there has been a definite increase in exercise-related claims processed through the legal system, especially claims against health and fitness facilities (27,28). Those dealing with emergency response deficiencies in the industry also appear to be on the increase (21). Although tort reform proposals may help stem this trend, the future portends an ever-increasing risk of claims and lawsuits for healthcare professionals generally; exercise professionals are not likely to escape the same problem.

TERMINOLOGY AND CONCEPTS

Generally, legal claims against exercise professionals center on alleged violations of either contract or tort law. These two broad concepts, along with written and statutory laws, define and govern most legal relationships between individuals, including the interrelationship of exercise professionals with patients.

CONTRACT LAW

The law of contracts defines and governs the undertakings that may be specified among individuals. A contract is simply a promise or performance bargained for and given in exchange for another promise or performance, all of which is supported by adequate consideration (i.e., something of value).

In examining exercise testing procedures and recommendations for structured physical activity provided to patients, it is important for professionals to understand how the law of contracts affects their relationships with patients. Examples are numerous and include patients receiving physical fitness information; recommendations given on intensity, duration, and modalities for exercise training; or even instructions on techniques for exercise participation. Likewise, the professional may perform exercise testing in exchange for payment or some other consideration of value. This contract relationship also encompasses any related activities that occur before and after exercise testing, such as health screening before testing, as well as first aid and emergency care that may arise out of the provision of provider services. If patient expectations during this relationship are not fulfilled, a lawsuit for breach of contract may be instituted. Such potential suits allege nonfulfillment of certain promises or a breach of alleged warranties that the law sometimes imposes on many contractual relationships. Apart from professional–patient relationships, contract law also has implications for interprofessional relations, such as those dealing with equipment companies, independent service contractors, and employees.

INFORMED CONSENT

Aside from breach of contract claims arising from a lack of promise fulfillment, claims against exercise professionals can be based on a type of breach of contract for failure to obtain adequate informed consent from exercise participants. Although claims based on lack of informed consent, founded upon contract principles, are somewhat archaic today, suits based on such failures are still put forth in some jurisdictions. More frequently today, however, such claims are brought forth in connection with negligence actions rather than breach-of-contract suits. Before an exercise professional administers a specific exercise procedure with a patient, the individual must give informed consent to participate in the procedure. Informed consent is intended to ensure that the patient entered into the procedure with adequate knowledge of the relevant material risks, any alternative procedures that might satisfy certain of the objectives, and the benefits associated with that activity. This consent can be express (written) or implied by law simply as a function of how the two parties to the procedure conducted themselves. To give valid consent to a procedure, the person must be of legal age, not be mentally incapacitated, know and fully understand the importance and relevance of the material risks and benefits, and give consent voluntarily and not under any mistake of fact or duress (22). Written consent is certainly preferable to any oral or implied form of consent; and of great importance, it expressly demonstrates the process if questions arise later as to whether that was the case.

In many states, adequate information must be provided to ensure that the participant knows and understands the risks and circumstances associated with a procedure before informed consent can be given. In such states, a so-called subjective test is used to determine whether that person understood and comprehended the risks and procedures associated with the matter at hand. Other states have adopted a less rigid rule and provide an objective test to determine consent to a procedure or treatment. Under this test, the determination centers on whether the participant, as a reasonable and ordinary person, understood the facts and circumstances associated with the procedure so as to give voluntary consent. Although some states do not require the use of informed consent for nonsurgical procedures or when a test is performed for non–healthcare-related purposes, adherence to the process is a desired approach and an apparent part or expectation associated with the applicable standard of case for the profession. Examples of informed consent documents for exercise testing and training programs are available elsewhere (2–4,22).

In lawsuits arising out of the informed consent process, an injured party commonly claims that a professional was negligent in the explanation of the procedure, including the risks, and that the participant would not, if not for the negligence of the professional, have undergone the procedure. These cases are often decided upon the testimony of expert witnesses who express opinions on the issue of whether the professional engaged in substandard conduct in securing the informed consent. These cases can involve claims related to contract law, warranties, negligence, and malpractice. Lawsuits arising from alleged deficiencies in the informed consent process related to testing, exercise prescription, or physical activity supervision have become more commonplace. The law is moving toward a broadening requirement for disclosure of risk to participants. Some courts have even gone so far as to require the disclosure of all possible risks, as opposed to those that are simply material (15). Such a requirement imposes unusual burdens on programs and raises substantial medicolegal concerns (17). These concerns require individual analysis and response by legal counsel.

One element of the informed consent process relates to confidentiality and disclosure of personal and sensitive information that may be gathered from the patient in the course of evaluating his or her health status or delivering services. Provision should be made in the informed consent or other documentation to secure the written authorization from patients to disclose specific test results, exercise progress reports, and so on, to healthcare professionals who have a need to know, such as a primary care physician. Written authorization may also be secured from patients if there is intent to use data in reporting group statistics for program evaluation or research purposes, even when such information is only to be presented in ways not identifiable with the patient. Many states and the federal government have promulgated privacy statutes that may affect the release of personally identifiable material regarding a program participant that requires the creation and adoption of privacy policies as well as consents or authorizations for the disclosure of information.

A relatively new federal privacy law, the Health Information Portability and Accountability Act (HIPAA), became effective in early 2003 (32). The HIPAA law was enacted for several purposes, including the promotion of access for consumers to health insurance, protecting the privacy of healthcare data, and to standardize and promote efficiency of billing and insurance claims processing in the healthcare industry. Its provisions for protecting the rights of individual consumers define what providers and others must do to safeguard patients' personal medical and health information. The rule assures patient's access to their own health information and, at the same time, eliminates inappropriate uses. It applies to healthcare providers, medical claims clearinghouses, and health insurance carriers. Health and fitness and rehabilitative exercise professionals who interact with physicians, nurses, medical technicians, and billing clerks and who access a patient's medical records in conjunction

with delivery of their services are affected by the HIPAA requirements. Just a few of the several important provisions include (a) individual patients must be provided with copies of the HIPAA privacy rule, (b) patients' prior written authorization must be obtained before information disclosure or use by any third party, and (c) the purposes for which the information is to be used and the time limits of the authorization must be provided to the patient.

Most states have enacted laws to clarify and complement the HIPAA provisions, and these vary among jurisdictions. There are many examples of information routinely collected and maintained by health and fitness and exercise rehabilitation professionals, the uses and disclosure of which are affected by HIPAA. These include not only data collected in the exercise service setting, such as clinical exercise test results, blood pressure, and electrocardiographic records, but also untoward outcome events. With equal certainty, the rule affects the release of information to an exercise professional by healthcare professionals when the former seeks data needed for safeguarding patients in the process of delivering exercise services (e.g., medical history and laboratory data for pre-exercise screening or results of clinical exercise tests). The extent to which the HIPAA provisions apply to exercise professionals should be determined through consultation with risk managers and local legal counsel. Nonetheless, all should review and understand the rule, the content of which may be accessed on the Internet at the Health Resources and Services Administration's (USDHHS) Web site. The HIPAA provisions may be subject to revision or updating, as may the target Web site reference for related U.S. government information. At the time of this writing, the Web site containing this information may be found at www.hhs.gov/ocr/hipaa/. The application of these laws to a program and rights to release information depends on a variety of factors that only individual counsel can properly address.

TORT LAW

A tort is simply a civil wrong. Most tort claims affecting exercise professionals are based on allegations of negligence or malpractice causing personal injury or death.

NEGLIGENCE

Although negligence has no precise definition in law, it is regarded as failure to conform one's conduct to a generally accepted standard or duty. A legal cause of action based on claims of negligence may be established given proof of certain facts, specifically, that one person failed to provide due care to protect another to whom the former owed some duty or responsibility and that such failure proximately caused some injury to the latter person

(22). Thus, the validity of negligence claims is typically established through a specific process that examines certain facts and establishes whether:

- A defendant owed a particular duty or had specific responsibilities to some person who has asserted a claim of negligence
- One or more failures (breaches) occurred in the performance of that duty compared with a particular set of behaviors that were expected (due care, standard of care)
- The injury or damage in question was attributable to an established act or a failure to perform (i.e., a negligent act or omission was the proximate cause of the injury or damage)

When negligence claims are asserted, the critical question centers on whether an exercise professional provided service in accordance with the so-called standard of care. After a duty is established, the nature and scope of expected performance are usually determined by one or more expert witnesses' references to published standards and guidelines from peer professional associations. Although standards of care are discussed in a different section of this chapter, ultimately, the most effective shield against claims of negligence may be the daily pattern of delivering services to patients and documenting fulfillment so as to show compliance with the most rigorous published guidelines that are relevant to the established activity.

MALPRACTICE

Malpractice is a specific type of negligence action involving claims against defined professionals. Malpractice actions generally involve claims against professionals who have been provided with public authority to practice (arising from specific state statutes) for alleged breaches of professional duties and responsibilities toward patients or other persons to whom they owed a particular standard of care or duty (22). Historically, malpractice claims have been confined to actions against physicians and lawyers. By statute or case law, however, some states have expanded this group to include nurses, physical therapists, dentists, psychologists, and other health professionals. In 1995, Louisiana became the first state to pass legislation to license and regulate exercise practitioners who work under the authority of physicians with patients in cardiopulmonary rehabilitation treatment programs (23,26). The Louisiana State Board of Medical Examiners now provides regulatory management for this practitioner group. Other states in recent years, such as Maryland, Massachusetts, and California, have also examined legislative proposals with various provisions to publicly regulate health and fitness and clinical exercise professionals, but no statutes have yet been enacted in jurisdictions beyond Louisiana. To date, no published reports have addressed the effect of this relatively new public regulation on cardiac rehabilitation professionals in Louisiana. The more obvious possibilities of the effect include the level of autonomy in practice, changes in provisions of liability insurance, costs of such insurance, and exposure to claims of malpractice. The advantages and disadvantages of licensure for exercise practitioners have been debated for many years. The issues are complex and involve divergent perspectives from different stakeholders (e.g., those who have the goal of improving quality of service and safety for patients). Imposing added regulatory costs in an era of scarce public resources, intensifying competition with established licensed professions, raising the costs of credentialing and liability insurance for practitioners, and increasing negligence-type claims and suits are by-products of licensure and are not in the best interests of the profession. It remains to be seen whether the advent of licensure for exercise physiologists in Louisiana has generally succeeded in areas originally of greatest concern to the advocates.

DEFENSES TO NEGLIGENCE OR MALPRACTICE ACTIONS

The proper conduct of the informed consent process can sometimes be used as defense against legal claims based on either tort or contract principles. In such cases, defense counsel may seek to characterize consent as an assumption of risk by the plaintiff. Assumption of risk to a procedure, however, is often difficult to establish without an explicit written statement or clear conduct that demonstrates such an assumption. In addition, an assumption of risk never relieves the exercise professional of the duty to perform in a competent and professional manner. Even when a valid informed consent with assumption of risk is obtained from a patient, a spouse, children, or heirs can sometimes independently file suits against the exercise professional for loss of consortium-type claims, even when the participant could not have asserted these claims because of his or her own assumption of risk (11). In some jurisdictions, it may be advisable or even necessary to obtain consent from a participant, a spouse, and, perhaps, in a limited number of states, to make it binding on any children or the executor, administrators, and heirs to an estate. Certainly, such consents should be binding on estates if certain of these negligence and malpractice claims from some such parties are to be successfully avoided (24,25). Thus, exercise professionals need to secure individual advice from legal counsel and, if applicable, their institutional risk managers to determine the legally sufficient elements of informed consent that must be presented to patients in their settings and the extent to which "loss of consortium" issues should be addressed.

Informed consent often is confused with so-called releases. Releases are statements sometimes written into consent-type documents that contain exculpatory language—that is, wording that relieves the provider of legal responsibility in the event of an injury or death caused by any error, omission, or even negligence. Release documents, sometimes called prospective waivers of liability or responsibility, are disfavored in some states. Moreover, in a medical setting, the use of such releases, with certain limited exceptions, has been declared invalid and against public policy. In nonmedical settings, however, particularly with certain ultrahazardous activities, such as auto racing, skydiving, and even exercise-related activities, the use of such releases may be valid in some jurisdictions, under certain circumstances, if they are properly drafted and used. In fact, when they are well defined and properly written, such documents may have substantial benefit to programs. In recent years, there has been a definite trend toward the increased use of waivers and judicial "approval" of such documents in health and fitness and recreational exercise settings to reduce providers' exposure to damage and loss arising from negligence actions. Improperly developed waivers can fail to protect providers. Consequently, a qualified attorney with a license in the jurisdiction should be consulted to determine their applicability and to prepare these documents. Materials are available to assist in the drafting and application of waivers (12).

Several other defenses to claims of negligence or malpractice are also available. In some states, for example, proof of negligence committed by the participant, referred to in law as *contributory negligence,* can preclude any recovery of damages from a defendant. In many states, however, this rule has been modified by adoption of a so-called system of comparative negligence. Under this rule, negligence of the injured party is compared with negligence of all defendants in the case. Then, if the negligence of the injured party is found to be less than that of all defendants in the case (or in some states, of any defendant in the case), the plaintiff is allowed to recover, albeit in an amount reduced by the contribution of negligence by the injured party (22).

Liability insurance is an effective mechanism to protect against financial loss in the event of claims and lawsuits. Such insurance policies pay for defense of any covered claims and lawsuits and provide indemnification from any judgment or settlement that is not excluded from the terms of coverage, up to the limits of coverage defined by the provisions of the policy. Proper professional liability insurance, which covers the activities and personnel in question, is readily available through individual purchase or many professional associations as a fee-based option for qualified members (13). In some cases, these liability policies may include special categories, provisions, and pricing for members who hold special credentials (e.g., certification). The extent of liability policy coverage considered sufficient for a given exercise professional depends on individual judgment, exposure incurred in the delivery of service, and the advice of insurance professionals. The decision on the purchase of insurance also should be affected by whether the professional is self-employed, employed by an organization that extends coverage to the professionals who engage only in services on behalf of the organization, or function in both contexts at the same time.

STANDARDS OF PRACTICE

Standards of practice (or care) express how contemporary services should be delivered to give reasonable assurance that desired outcomes will be achieved in a safe manner. In most professions, such standards are developed and periodically revised by consensus among professionals or national associations of providers. Standards documents address what are considered to be benchmark methods, procedures, processes, and protocols that are applied in almost all settings regardless of location, resources, or training of the provider.

In reality, the prevailing or applicable national standard of practice is influenced by a variety of sources, including published statements from professional associations, research findings, government policies, state and national government regulations, litigation, prevailing professional practices in the field, and other factors. In recent years, the promulgation of standards for fitness and healthcare has increased dramatically. These circumstances mandate that professionals stay abreast of new pronouncements and regulations. Without knowledge of the most relevant and current standards and incorporation of these tenets into the operating protocols and records of service fulfillment, individual practitioners become vulnerable to damage and loss in the event of legal challenges arising from personal injury or wrongful death lawsuits.

In negligence actions, courts rely heavily on interpretations of standards from expert witnesses to determine what should or what should not have been done in particular cases. The use of these standards in certain cases dealing with exercise testing and exercise leadership has already occurred (28).

In recent years, there has been a tendency for certain healthcare and fitness-related professionals to favor couching their pronouncements on how care should be delivered in the framework of "guidelines," as opposed to "standards" documents. The latter term implies an immutable requirement for practice and implies no flexibility or exceptions in individual applications. A "guideline" should be interpreted to mean a highly recommended method, procedure, or way of providing service that is advocated by leaders of the field or their consensus. The motivation for the "guidelines" approach is that although it may have clarity and specificity, it is also written to express the importance of individual practitioners' being able to apply sound judgment in how they implement practice parameters for a particular situation or patient without incurring increased risk of claim and lawsuit in the event of an untoward outcome. Although a profession-wide shift toward practice parameters that are defined as guidelines or recommendations rather than standards may have a solid rationale from a professional perspective, the extent to which this may add a margin of provider protection in the event of negligence-type lawsuits is difficult to predict. In the past, the absence of definitive standards of practice may have led to an increased legal vulnerability for defendants. This has been because in the absence of clear and uniform standards from the profession, the opinions of individual expert witnesses brought by the plaintiff can have increased sway in the legal determination of what care was expected for a particular patient who suffered a personal injury in a given situation.

Many organizations have published documents that influence the legal standard of care in the health, fitness, exercise, and rehabilitation fields. Some of the most important are those of the American College of Sports Medicine (ACSM) (4,9), American Heart Association (AHA) (5–9), American Association of Cardiovascular and Pulmonary Rehabilitation (AACVPR) (1–3), Agency for Health Care Policy and Research, American College of Cardiology, American Medical Association, International Health Racquet and Sportsclub Association, Aerobics and Fitness Association of America, and National Strength and Conditioning Association (31) (also see "Internet Resources"). Documents from these organizations vary in their scope and applicability. Professionals should carefully examine the services, uses of technologies and procedures, and types of patients before deciding which standards and guidelines are most applicable to their own programs or situations.

Published guidelines may be incomplete or not entirely uniform. In the event of injury or death of a participant, such deficits may create confusion rather than define the professional behavior expected in a specific setting. In the area of exercise testing, standards of the ACSM, AACVPR, and AHA are inconsistent with regard to the need for significant involvement of a physician during graded exercise testing (2–7).

On the matter of exercise prescription, one AHA publication (6) explicitly identifies a nurse as an individual who may "assess physical activity habits, prescribe exercise, and monitor responses in healthy persons and cardiac patients." Another contemporary AHA source (5) acknowledges that exercise by cardiac patients may be appropriately supervised by physicians, nurses, or exercise physiologists, as long as supervisors are trained and their duties are consistent with state statutes governing the practice of medicine and certain other allied healthcare professions. If deficiencies or disparities in the published guidelines have implications for safety and legal

exposure in a particular situation, the development of low-risk protocols and procedures may be a matter of critical importance that requires the advice of local counsel.

Healthcare professions are in the midst of a movement that may eventually see written standards and guidelines covering nearly every major dimension of care. Fitness and rehabilitation professionals are in similar circumstances and must keep up to date with consensus publications that affect services. To reduce medicolegal risks, it is prudent to adopt the most stringent standards possible. Fulfillment is equally important: Practitioners should not only update program operating manuals to verify adoption of current standards but also document day-to-day patient records of service delivery to show what was done and how it was done.

In fact, documentation is vital to many aspects of risk management, not just verification of adherence to standards. Documentation should include contemporaneous recording of critical response levels that arise in exercise testing or training (e.g., important symptoms, estimations of effort, and activity demand, along with signs suggesting myocardial ischemia or poor ventricular response) and annotations about how these occurrences are referred to appropriate healthcare providers in a timely way. It also encompasses notations on program incidents, especially care delivered in emergencies (perhaps the most important setting in which to demonstrate, after the fact, what and when the essential steps were performed). Follow-up should always be performed and program records maintained to verify the outcome of the situation whenever emergency and nonemergency incidents occur.

> **1.10.10-HFS: Knowledge of the health/fitness instructor's responsibilities and limitations, and the legal implications of carrying out emergency procedures.**

> **1.10.14-HFS: Knowledge of the legal implications of documented safety procedures, the use of incident documents, and ongoing safety training documentation for the purposes of safety and risk management.**

In 1998, the AHA and ACSM released a joint position statement recommending certain basic policies and procedures for pre-exercise screening and emergency readiness in all health and fitness facilities, even in hotels offering only unsupervised access (9). These recommendations of AHA/ACSM were expanded and updated in 2002 to delineate emergency response capabilities that include automated external defibrillation (AED) (10). Every health club and recreational fitness center should evaluate the key features of their organizations and patients, finding how best to structure written policies, procedures, and fulfillment relative to these important safety functions so as to adhere to this new recommendation (9). From a risk management point of view, the adequacy of any policy or procedure is a function of its being committed to written form, kept up to date relative to changing professional guidelines, and linked to ongoing evidence of fulfillment (20). With regard to emergency readiness, fulfillment may be partially shown by keeping dated records of regular emergency drills. Another dimension of documenting fulfillment may be achieved by maintaining records that show the names of staff members who practiced in emergency drills and notations on staff performance and any improvements made in the emergency drills. These formal drills prepare staff members for rapid and effective response when a genuine emergency arises. If a legal challenge should ever occur, this record of fulfillment may be quite helpful in establishing that a particular standard of care was adopted and routinely followed (19).

Forms may also be developed for staff members to use routinely in ensuring standardization in operational areas in which injury or legal risks are considered significant. Examples of these situations include forms for pre-exercise screening and consultation, instruction of new patients in exercise routines, specific cautions for avoidance of injury to patients, and staff inspection of equipment and facilities. Effective forms demonstrate how a facility has linked an important standard to a critical area of service. Use of such forms, along with routine annotation of patient records, shows consistency of fulfillment.

UNAUTHORIZED PRACTICE OF MEDICINE AND ALLIED HEALTH PROFESSIONAL STATUTES

In recent years, the growing prominence of exercise testing and other health and fitness services increasingly places exercise professionals in collaborative roles with licensed healthcare providers. This evolution has stimulated a variety of initiatives to clarify roles and responsibilities, promote professionalism, and increase professional opportunities. Competency credentials of the ACSM (e.g., ACSM Clinical Exercise Specialist®, ACSM Health/Fitness Specialist®, and ACSM Registered Clinical Exercise Physiologist®), the AACVPR's core competency position statement for cardiac rehabilitation specialists, and efforts to establish licensure are illustrations of initiatives that affect the positioning of specialists and greater role delineation (1,23).

Providing exercise services with some degree of independence in collaboration with licensed providers can create legally precarious circumstances for exercise professionals. A prime example of confusion in this area is reflected in questions that often arise about the competency and legal authority needed to provide emergency cardiac care in community- or clinic-based settings in exercise settings where the purpose of the exercise services may be defined as treatment for diagnosed or suspected cardiovascular or other major chronic diseases.

The standard for emergency response in this situation is clear and universal. It calls for a defibrillator; a crash cart with artificial airways, suction pump, and emergency drugs; and the competency of an on-site provider who can administer the AHA's advanced cardiac life support (ACLS) skills when needed (2,3,7). This provider, however, must understand that he or she cannot assume such duties unless the physician in charge has given written standing orders to that effect or the individual also has legal authorization under state statutes to accept such standing orders or to otherwise carry out the activity. This is almost never the case for unlicensed exercise professionals who provide exercise services within the healthcare setting, such as a hospital-based exercise testing or cardiac rehabilitation program, with or without current ACLS training. Thus, there is no legal authority for an exercise professional to evaluate the need for or perform defibrillation on a patient in these circumstances, *unless* he or she has independently completed training and licensure requirements to perform these procedures in the jurisdiction.

Recent advances in technology and new state and federal statutes are changing public expectations regarding use of AEDs. This evolution may soon alter the standard of care for emergency service in the health and fitness setting (20). It is expected, because of the ongoing development of published statements from professional organizations (4,34) and continuing litigation as to AED issues (18), that the use of AEDs is fast reaching the point that it has become the standard of care owed by health and fitness facilities toward their patrons. This time may have already come (4).

The continuing evolution of healthcare reform further confuses the roles of healthcare providers. This may often be problematic for exercise professionals working in diagnostic exercise laboratories or rehabilitation centers. A significant part of this evolution has been aimed at reducing costs by using paraprofessionals in increasingly important clinical roles. In fact, various states have undertaken efforts to expand nursing practice and other provider practice laws beyond mere observation, reporting, and recording of a patient's signs and symptoms. Various physician assistant and similar paraprofessional practice laws provide expanded treatment authority to nonphysicians.

Until healthcare reform is complete, however, some nonphysicians will continue to be engaged in certain practices that might be characterized as the practice of medicine or some other statutorily defined and controlled allied health profession. In such situations, the unlicensed provider runs the risk of engaging in unauthorized practices that could lead to both criminal and civil sanctions. Many states have defined the practice of medicine broadly so that persons engaged in exercise testing and prescription activities could, under some circumstances, fall within the range of such statutes.

BOX 51-1 TIPS FOR EXERCISE PROFESSIONALS

Some tips for exercise professionals regarding legal matters include:

1. Know and apply in practice the most rigorous and current peer-developed guidelines applicable to your services, patients, and organization or environment.
2. Maintain credentials relevant to your service (e.g., personal certification or public licensure) and professional liability insurance coverage.
3. Use appropriate informed consent for all services in which such consent is relevant (consult with qualified attorney and risk manager).
4. Instruct patients in techniques of participation and limitations relevant to their health and physical capabilities, observe their related participation, correct problems, and follow up to verify that they

manage their own participation safely and effectively.

5. Document fulfillment of your service in a manner consistent with standard of care and your written program policies and procedures.
6. Communicate critical information in a timely way to authorized parties.
7. Develop emergency response plans, rehearse for emergencies, document and upgrade procedures based on rehearsal experiences, and institute automated external defibrillation programs as applicable.
8. Report incidents and follow up to continuously improve emergency readiness and performance.
9. Maintain equipment and inspect facilities on a frequent and regular basis.

As previously indicated in this chapter, published standards are not always definitive in expressing the roles and responsibilities for exercise professionals, particularly with regard to the delivery of services for patients with documented diseases or even those with no outward signs of disease (e.g., silent myocardial ischemia). Thus, without the presence or assistance of a licensed physician or other allied health professional for certain aspects of the provision of exercise services, claims as to the unauthorized practice of medicine or some other provider practice could be put forth. Under some of these state statutes, such practices are often classified as crimes, usually misdemeanors, punishable by imprisonment for less than 1 year, a fine, or both. In some jurisdictions, felony classification for such offenses has been established with greater potential punishment.

In addition, a person found to have engaged in the unauthorized practice of medicine or some other allied health profession faces (after the fact) the legal expectation that he or she should have provided an elevated standard of care in the event of injury to or death of a participant. Under this rule, the actions of an exercise professional would be compared with the presumed standard of care of a physician or other allied health professional acting under the same or similar circumstances. In the event that the actions do not meet this standard (which the nonphysician or allied health professional cannot meet because of inadequacies of knowledge, skill, authorization, and experience), liability may result (Box 51-1).

SUMMARY

More and more individuals are becoming exposed to organized exercise programs. Exercise professionals and fitness facility operators should note that middle-aged and

older adults represent one of the fastest growing segments of their membership. These individuals tend to have more chronic disease risk factors, medical considerations affecting exercise participation, and likely a higher occurrence of undiagnosed diseases than any other group that might enter their programs. Therefore, the actual number of untoward events in exercise programs, avoidable or otherwise, will inevitably increase. Increased numbers of these occurrences will result in negligence claims that will ultimately find resolution in court. The probabilities of such traumatic actions are low, particularly for individuals and organizations that operate programs in a manner commensurate with accepted professional standards. Awareness of the areas of special legal vulnerability and adoption of legally sensitive practices, however, will keep the risks of litigation low and lead to safer and more efficacious programs. Professionals are advised to keep current concerning developments in this ever-changing medicolegal field (22).

REFERENCES

1. American Association for Cardiovascular and Pulmonary Rehabilitation. Core competencies for cardiac rehabilitation specialists. *J Cardiopulm Rehabil.* 1994;14:87.
2. American Association for Cardiovascular and Pulmonary Rehabilitation. *Guidelines for Cardiac Rehabilitation and Secondary Prevention Programs.* 4th ed. Champaign (IL): Human Kinetics; 2004.
3. American Association for Cardiovascular and Pulmonary Rehabilitation. *Guidelines for Pulmonary Rehabilitation Programs.* 3rd ed. Champaign (IL): Human Kinetics; 2004.
4. American College of Sports Medicine. *ACSM's Health/Fitness Facility Standards & Guidelines.* 3rd ed. Champaign (IL): Human Kinetics; 2006.
5. American Heart Association. Scientific Statement from the Council on Clinical Cardiology (Subcommittee on Exercise, Cardiac Rehabilitation, and Prevention) and the Council on Nutrition, Physical

Activity, and Metabolism (Subcommittee on Physical Activity), in collaboration with the American Association of Cardiovascular and Pulmonary Rehabilitation. Cardiac rehabilitation and secondary prevention of coronary heart disease. *Circulation*. 2005;111(3): 369–76.

6. American Heart Association. Scientific statement in collaboration with the American College of Sports Medicine. Exercise and acute cardiovascular events: placing the risks into perspective. *Circulation*. 2007;115:2358–68.

7. American Heart Association. Guidelines for cardiopulmonary resuscitation (CPR) and emergency cardiovascular care. *Circulation*. 2005;112(24):1–211.

8. American Heart Association. Health clubs not fit for cardiac emergencies [news release]. November 13, 2000.

9. Balady GJ, Chaitman B, Driscoll D, et al. American College of Sports Medicine and American Heart Association joint position statement: Recommendations for cardiovascular screening, staffing, and emergency policies at health/fitness facilities. *Circulation*. 1998;97:2283.

10. Balady GJ, Chaitman B, Foster C, et al. Automated external defibrillators in health/fitness facilities: supplement to the AHA/ACSM recommendations for cardiovascular screening, staffing, and emergency policies at health/fitness facilities. *Circulation*. 2002;105: 1147.

11. Child sues for "loss of consortium." *Lawyers Alert*. 1984;3:249.

12. Cotten D, Cotten MB. *Legal Aspects of Waivers in Sport, Recreation, and Fitness Activities*. Canton (OH): PRC Publishing; 1997.

13. Eickhoff-Shemek J. Distinguishing "general" and "professional" liability insurance. *ACSM's Health & Fitness Journal*. 2003;7:28.

14. Foster C, Porcari JP. The risks of exercise training. *J Cardiopulm Rehabil*. 2001;21:347–52.

15. Hedgecorth v. United States. 618 F. Supp.627 (E.D. Mo, 1985).

16. Herbert DL. Health clubs may not be meeting standards of care. *Exercise Standards and Malpractice Reporter*. 2002;15:12.

17. Herbert DL. Informed consent documents for stress testing to comport with Hedgecorth v. United States. *Exercise Standards and Malpractice Reporter*. 1987;1:81.

18. Herbert DL. Lives, liabilities and lawsuits on the line: defibrillators are becoming part of the "standard of care" for recreation facilities. *Recreation Management*. 2003;10. Available at: www. remanagement.com/200301gc01.php. Accessed November 24, 2008.

19. Herbert DL. Plan to save lives: create and rehearse an emergency response plan. *ACSM's Health & Fitness Journal*. 1997;1:34.

20. Herbert DL. Standards of care for health and fitness facilities are ever evolving. *ACSM's Health & Fitness Journal*. 2000;4:18.

21. Herbert DL. Working out the risks: inadequate response to emergencies by fitness center employees has led to lawsuits. Widespread use of defibrillators could avert tragedies and reduce claims. *Best's Review*. 2000;99.

22. Herbert DL, Herbert WG. *Legal Aspects of Preventive, Rehabilitative and Recreational Exercise Programs*. 4th ed. Canton (OH): PRC Publishing; 2002.

23. Herbert WG. Licensure of clinical exercise physiologists: impressions concerning the new law in Louisiana. *Exercise Standards and Malpractice Reporter*. 1995;9:65.

24. Herbert WG, Herbert DL. Exercise testing in adults: legal and procedural considerations for the physical educator and exercise professionals. *Journal of Health, Physical Education and Recreation*. 1975;46:17.

25. Koeberle BE. Legal aspects of personal fitness training. *Professional Reports*. 1990;35–8.

26. Louisiana licenses clinical exercise physiologists [editorial]. *Exercice Standards and Malpractice Report*. 1995;9:56.

27. Mandel v. Canyon Ranch, Inc., et al: Superior Court of the State of Arizona, Puma County, Case No.3122777; 1998.

28. Mathis v. New York Health Club, Inc. 690 N.Y.S.2d 433; 1999.

29. McInnis KJ, Hayakawa S, Balady GJ. Cardiovascular screening and emergency procedures at health clubs and fitness centers. *Am J Cardiol*. 1997;80:380.

30. McInnis KJ, Herbert W, Herbert D, et al. Fitness clubs fail to adhere to AHA emergency standards. *Circulation*. 2000;102(suppl II):394.

31. National Strength and Conditioning Association. Strength and Conditioning Professional Standards and Guidelines; May 2001. Available at: www.nsca-lift.org/Publications/Standards.shtml. Accessed November 25,2008.

32. Public Law 104-191, August 21, 1996.

33. Rochmis P, Blackburn H. Exercise tests: a survey of procedures, safety and litigation experience in approximately 170,000 tests. *JAMA*. 1971;217:1061.

SELECTED REFERENCES FOR FURTHER READING

Herbert DL, Herbert WG. *Legal Aspects of Preventative, Rehabilitative, and Recreational Exercise Programs*. 4th ed. Canton (OH): PRC Publishing; 2002.

Koeberle BE. *Legal Aspects of Personal Fitness Training*. 2nd ed. Canton (OH): Professional Reports; 1998.

INTERNET RESOURCES

- Aerobics and Fitness Association: www.afaa.com
- Agency for Healthcare Research and Quality: www.ahrq.gov
- American Association of Cardiovascular and Pulmonary Rehabilitation: www.aacvpr.org
- American College of Cardiology: www.acc.org
- American Heart Association: www.americanheart.org
- American Medical Association: www.ama-assn.org
- International Health, Racquet and Sportsclub Association: www.ihrsa.org
- National Strength and Conditioning Association: www.nsca-lift.org

This appendix details information about American College of Sports Medicine (ACSM) Certification and Registry Programs and gives a complete listing of the current knowledge, skills, and abilities (KSAs) that compose the foundations of these certification and registry examinations. The mission of the ACSM Committee on Certification and Registry Boards is to develop and provide high-quality, accessible, and affordable credentials and continuing education programs for health and exercise professionals who are responsible for preventive and rehabilitative programs that influence the health and well-being of all individuals.

ACSM CERTIFICATIONS AND THE PUBLIC

The first of the ACSM clinical certifications was initiated more than 30 years ago in conjunction with publication of the first edition of *Guidelines for Exercise Testing and Prescription*. That era was marked by rapid development of exercise programs for patients with stable coronary artery disease (CAD). ACSM sought a means to disseminate accurate information on this healthcare initiative through expression of consensus from its members in basic science, clinical practice, and education. Thus, these early clinical certifications were viewed as an aid to the establishment of safe and scientifically based exercise services within the framework of cardiac rehabilitation.

Over the past 30 years, exercise has gained widespread favor as an important component in programs of rehabilitative care or health maintenance for an expanding list of chronic diseases and disabling conditions. The growth of public interest in the role of exercise in health promotion has been equally impressive. In addition, federal government policy makers have revisited questions of medical efficacy and financing for exercise services in rehabilitative care of selected patients. Over the past several years, recommendations from the U.S. Public Health Service and the U.S. Surgeon General have acknowledged the central role for regular physical activity in the prevention of disease and promotion of health.

The development of the health/fitness certifications in the 1980s reflected ACSM's intent to increase the availability of qualified professionals to provide scientif-ically sound advice and supervision regarding appropriate physical activities for health maintenance in the apparently healthy adult population. Since 1975, more than 35,000 certificates have been awarded. With this consistent growth, ACSM has taken steps to ensure that its competency-based certifications will continue to be regarded as the premier program in the exercise field.

The ACSM Committee on Certification and Registry Boards (CCRB) Publications Sub-Committee publishes *ACSM's Certified News*, a periodical addressing professional practice issues; its target audience is those who are certified. The CCRB Continuing Professional Education Sub-Committee has oversight of the continuing education requirements for maintenance of certification and auditing renewal candidates. Continuing education credits can be accrued through ACSM-sponsored educational programs, such as ACSM workshops (ACSM Certified Personal Trainer[SM], ACSM Certified Health Fitness Specialist, ACSM Certified Clinical Exercise Specialist, ACSM Registered Clinical Exercise Physiologist[®]), regional chapter and annual meetings, and other educational programs approved by the ACSM Professional Education Committee. These enhancements are intended to support the continued professional growth of those who have made a commitment to service in this rapidly growing health and fitness field.

In 2004, ACSM was a founding member of the multiorganizational Committee on Accreditation for the Exercise Sciences (CoAES) and assisted with the development of standards and guidelines for educational programs seeking accreditation under the auspices of the Commission on Accreditation of Allied Health Education Programs (CAAHEP). Additional information on outcomes-based, programmatic accreditation can be obtained by visiting www.caahep.org, and specific information regarding the standards and guidelines can be obtained by visiting www.coaes.org. Because the standards and guidelines refer to the KSAs that follow, reference to specific KSAs as they relate to given sets of standards and guidelines will be noted when appropriate.

ACSM also acknowledges the expectation from successful candidates that the public will be informed of the high standards, values, and professionalism implicit in meeting these certification requirements. The college has formally organized its volunteer committee structure and national office staff to give added emphasis to informing the public, professionals, and government agencies about issues of critical importance to ACSM. Informing these constituencies about the meaning and value of ACSM certification is one important priority that will be given attention in this initiative.

ACSM CERTIFICATION PROGRAMS

The ACSM Certified Personal Trainer^{SM} is a fitness professional involved in developing and implementing an individualized approach to exercise leadership in healthy populations and/or those individuals with medical clearance to exercise. Using a variety of teaching techniques, the CPT is proficient in leading and demonstrating safe and effective methods of exercise by applying the fundamental principles of exercise science. The CPT is familiar with forms of exercise used to improve, maintain, and/or optimize health-related components of physical fitness and performance. The CPT is proficient in writing appropriate exercise recommendations, leading and demonstrating safe and effective methods of exercise, and motivating individuals to begin and to continue with their healthy behaviors.

The ACSM Certified Health Fitness Specialist (HFS) is a degreed health and fitness professional qualified for career pursuits in the university, corporate, commercial, hospital, and community settings. The HFS has knowledge and skills in management, administration, training, and in supervising entry-level personnel. The HFS is skilled in conducting risk stratification, conducting physical fitness assessments and interpreting results, constructing appropriate exercise prescriptions, and motivating apparently healthy individuals and individuals with medically controlled diseases to adopt and maintain healthy lifestyle behaviors.

The ACSM Certified Clinical Exercise Specialist (CES) is a healthcare professional certified by ACSM to deliver a variety of exercise assessment, training, rehabilitation, risk-factor identification, and lifestyle management services to individuals with or at risk for cardiovascular, pulmonary, and metabolic disease(s). These services are typically delivered in cardiovascular/pulmonary rehabilitation programs, physicians' offices, or medical fitness centers. The ACSM Certified Clinical Exercise Specialist is also competent to provide exercise-related consulting for research, public health, and other clinical and nonclinical services and programs.

The ACSM Registered Clinical Exercise Physiologist$^{®}$ (RCEP) is an allied health professional who works in the application of physical activity and behavioral interventions for those clinical conditions for which they have been shown to provide therapeutic and/or functional benefit. Persons for whom RCEP services are appropriate may include, but are not limited to, those individuals with cardiovascular, pulmonary, metabolic, orthopedic, musculoskeletal, neuromuscular, neoplastic, immunologic, or hematologic disease. The RCEP provides primary and secondary prevention strategies designed to improve fitness and health in populations ranging from children to older adults. The RCEP performs exercise screening, exercise and fitness testing, exercise prescription, exercise and physical activity counseling, exercise supervision, exercise and health education/promotion, and measurement and evaluation of exercise and physical activity related outcome measures. The RCEP works individually or as part of an interdisciplinary team in a clinical, community, or public health setting. The practice and supervision of the RCEP is guided by published professional guidelines, standards, and applicable state and federal regulations.

Certification at a given level requires the candidate to have a knowledge and skills base commensurate with that specific level of certification. In addition, the HFS level of certification incorporates the KSAs associated with the ACSM Certified Personal Trainer^{SM} certification, the CES level of certification incorporates the KSAs associated with the CPT and HFS certification, and the RCEP level of certification incorporates the KSAs associated with the CPT, HFS, and CES levels of certification, as illustrated in Figure 1. In addition, each level of certification has minimum requirements for experience, level of education, or other certifications.

ACSM also develops specialty certifications to enhance the breadth of knowledge for individuals working in a health, fitness, or clinical setting. For information on KSAs, eligibility, and scope of practice for ACSM specialty certifications, visit www.acsm.org/certification or call 1-800-486-5643.

HOW TO OBTAIN INFORMATION AND APPLICATION MATERIALS

The certification programs of ACSM are subject to continuous review and revision. Content development is entrusted to a diverse committee of professional volunteers with expertise in exercise science, medicine, and program management. Expertise in design and procedures for competency assessment is also represented on this committee. The administration of certification exams is conducted through Pearson VUE authorized testing centers. Inquiries regarding exam registration can be made to Pearson VUE at 1-888-883-2276 or online at www.pearsonvue.com/acsm.

For general certification questions, contact the ACSM Certification Resource Center:

1-800-486-5643
Web site: www.acsm.org/certification
E-mail: certification@acsm.org

FIGURE 1

LEVEL	REQUIREMENTS	RECOMMENDED COMPETENCIES
ACSM Certified Personal Trainer[SM]	• 18 years of age or older • High school diploma or equivalent (GED) • Possess current adult CPR certification that has a practical skills examination component (such as the American Heart Association or the American Red Cross)	• Demonstrate competence in the KSAs required of the ACSM Certified Personal Trainer™ as listed in the current edition of the *ACSM's Guidelines for Exercise Testing and Prescription* • Adequate knowledge of and skill in risk-factor and health-status identification, fitness appraisal, and exercise prescription • Demonstrate ability to incorporate suitable and innovative activities that will improve an individual's functional capacity Demonstrate the ability to effectively educate and/or communicate with individuals regarding lifestyle modification
ACSM Certified Health Fitness Specialist	• Associate's degree or a bachelor's degree in a health-related field from a regionally accredited college or university (one is eligible to sit for the exam if the candidate is in the last term of their degree program); AND • Possess current adult CPR certification that has a practical skills examination component (such as the American Heart Association or the American Red Cross)	• Demonstrate competence in the KSAs required of the ACSM Certified Health Fitness Specialist In as listed in the current edition of the *ACSM's Guidelines for Exercise Testing and Prescription* • Work-related experience within the health and fitness field • Adequate knowledge of, and skill in, risk-factor and health-status identification, fitness appraisal, and exercise prescription • Demonstrate ability to incorporate suitable and innovative activities that will improve an individual's functional capacity • Demonstrate the ability to effectively educate and/or counsel individuals regarding lifestyle modification • Knowledge of exercise science including kinesiology, functional anatomy, exercise physiology, nutrition, program administration, psychology, and injury prevention
ACSM Certified Clinical Exercise Specialist	• Bachelor's degree in an allied health field from a regionally accredited college of university (one is eligible to sit for the exam if the candidate is in the last term of their degree program); AND • Minimum of 600 hours of observational and active patient/client care in a clinical exercise program (e.g., cardiac/pulmonary rehabilitation programs; exercise testing; exercise prescription; electrocardiography; patient education and counseling; disease management of cardiac, pulmonary, and metabolic diseases; and emergency management); AND • Current certification as a basic life support provider or CPR for the professional rescuer (available through the American Heart Association or the American Red Cross)	• Demonstrate competence in the KSAs required of the ACSM Certified Clinical Exercise Specialist and Certified Health Fitness Specialist, as listed in the current edition of *ACSM's Guidelines for Exercise Testing and Prescription* • Ability to demonstrate extensive knowledge of functional anatomy, exercise physiology, pathophysiology, electrocardiography, human behavior/psychology, gerontology, graded exercise testing for healthy and diseased populations, exercise supervision/leadership, patient counseling, and emergency procedures related to exercise testing and training situations
ACSM Registered Clinical Exercise Physiologist®	• Master's degree in exercise science, exercise physiology, or kinesiology from a regionally accredited college or university • Current certification as a basic life support provider or CPR for the professional rescuer (available through the American Heart Association or the American Red Cross) • Minimum of 600 clinical hours or alternatives as described in the current issue of ACSM's *Certification Resource Guide* (hours may be completed as part of a formal degree program) • Recommendation of hours in clinical practice areas: cardiovascular—200; pulmonary—100 ; metabolic—120; orthopedic/ musculoskeletal—100; neuromuscular—40; immunologic/hematologic—40	• Demonstrate competence in the KSAs required of the ACSM Registered Clinical Exercise Physiologist®, ACSM Certified Clinical Excercise Specialist, ACSM Certified Health Fitness Specialist, and ACSM Certified Personal Trainer[SM] as listed in the current edition of *ACSM's Guidelines for Exercise Testing and Prescription*

KNOWLEDGE, SKILLS, AND ABILITIES (KSAs) UNDERLINING ACSM CERTIFICATIONS

Minimal competencies for each certification level are outlined below. Certification examinations are constructed based on these KSAs. For the ACSM Certified Health Fitness Specialist and the ACSM Certified Clinical Exercise Specialist credentials, two companion ACSM publications, *ACSM's Resource Manual for Guidelines for Exercise Testing and Prescription,* sixth edition, and *ACSM's Certification Review Book,* third edition, may also be used to gain further insight pertaining to the topics identified here. For the ACSM Certified Personal Trainer^{SM}, candidates should refer to *ACSM's Resources for the Personal Trainer,* current edition, and *ACSM's Certification Review Book,* third edition. For the ACSM Registered Clinical Exercise Physiologist®, candidates should refer to ACSM's *Resources for Clinical Exercise Physiology,* current edition, and *ACSM's Resource Manual for Guidelines for Exercise Testing and Prescription,* sixth edition. However, neither the *ACSM's Guidelines for Exercise Testing and Prescription* nor any of the above-mentioned resource manuals provides all of the information upon which the ACSM Certification examinations are based. Each may prove to be beneficial as a review of specific topics and as a general outline of many of the integral concepts to be mastered by those seeking certification.

CLASSIFICATION/NUMBERING SYSTEM FOR KNOWLEDGE, SKILLS, AND ABILITIES (KSAs)

All the KSAs for a given certification/credential are listed in their entirety across a given practice area and/or content matter area for each level of certification. Within each certification's/credential's KSA set, the numbering of individual KSAs uses a three-part number as follows:

- First number: denotes practice area (1.x.x)
- Second number: denotes content area (x.1.x)
- Third number: denotes the sequential number of each KSA (x.x.1) within each content area. If there is a break in numeric sequence, it indicates that a KSA was deleted in response to the recent job-task analysis from the prior version of the KSAs. From this edition forward, new KSAs will acquire a new KSA number.

The practice areas (the first number) are numbered as follows:

1.x.x General population/core
2.x.x Cardiovascular
3.x.x Pulmonary
4.x.x Metabolic
5.x.x Orthopedic/musculoskeletal
6.x.x Neuromuscular
7.x.x Neoplastic, immunologic, and hematologic

The content matter areas (the second number) are numbered as follows:

x.1.x Exercise physiology and related exercise science
x.2.x Pathophysiology and risk factors
x.3.x Health appraisal, fitness, and clinical exercise testing
x.4.x Electrocardiography and diagnostic techniques
x.5.x Patient management and medications
x.6.x Medical and surgical management
x.7.x Exercise prescription and programming
x.8.x Nutrition and weight management
x.9.x Human behavior and counseling
x.10.x Safety, injury prevention, and emergency procedures
x.11.x Program administration, quality assurance, and outcome assessment
x.12.x Clinical and medical considerations (ACSM Certified Personal Trainer^{SM} only)

EXAMPLES BY LEVEL OF CERTIFICATION/CREDENTIAL

ACSM CERTIFIED PERSONAL TRAINER^{SM} KSAs

1.1.10 Knowledge to describe the normal acute responses to cardiovascular exercise.

In this example, the practice area is *general population/core*; the content matter area is *exercise physiology and related exercise science*; and this KSA is the tenth KSA within this content matter area.

ACSM CERTIFIED HEALTH FITNESS SPECIALIST KSAs

1.3.8 Skill in accurately measuring heart rate, blood pressure, and obtaining rating of perceived exertion (RPE) at rest and during exercise according to established guidelines.

In this example, the practice area is *general population/core*; the content matter area is *health appraisal, fitness, and clinical exercise testing*; and this KSA is the eighth KSA within this content matter area.

ACSM CERTIFIED CLINICAL EXERCISE SPECIALIST KSAs^a

1.7.17 **Design strength and flexibility programs for individuals with cardiovascular, pulmonary, and/or metabolic diseases; the elderly; and children.**

In this example, the practice area is *general population/core*; the content matter area is *exercise prescription and programming*; and this KSA is the seventeenth KSA within this content matter area. Furthermore, because this specific KSA appears in bold, it covers multiple practice areas and content areas.

ACSM REGISTERED CLINICAL EXERCISE PHYSIOLOGIST® KSAs

7.6.1   List the drug classifications commonly used in the treatment of patients with a neoplastic, immunologic, and hematologic (NIH) disease, name common generic and brand-name drugs within each class, and explain the purposes, indications, major side effects, and the effects, if any, on the exercising individual.

In this example, the practice area is *neoplastic, immunologic, and hematologic*; the content matter area is *medical and surgical management*; and this KSA is the first KSA within this content matter area.

ACSM CERTIFIED PERSONAL TRAINER^SM KNOWLEDGE, SKILLS, AND ABILITIES (KSAs)

GENERAL POPULATION/CORE: EXERCISE PHYSIOLOGY AND RELATED EXERCISE SCIENCE

1.1.1   Knowledge of the basic structures of bone, skeletal muscle, and connective tissue.

1.1.2   Knowledge of the basic anatomy of the cardiovascular system and respiratory system.

1.1.3   Knowledge of the definition of the following terms: inferior, superior, medial, lateral, supination, pronation, flexion, extension, adduction, abduction, hyperextension, rotation, circumduction, agonist, antagonist, and stabilizer.

1.1.4   Knowledge of the plane in which each muscle action occurs.

1.1.5   Knowledge of the interrelationships among center of gravity, base of support, balance, stability, and proper spinal alignment.

1.1.6   Knowledge of the following curvatures of the spine: lordosis, scoliosis, and kyphosis.

1.1.8   Knowledge of the biomechanical principles for the performance of common physical activities (e.g., walking, running, swimming, cycling, resistance training, yoga, Pilates, functional training).

1.1.9   Ability to distinguish between aerobic and anaerobic metabolism.

1.1.10   Knowledge to describe the normal acute responses to cardiovascular exercise.

1.1.11   Knowledge to describe the normal acute responses to resistance training.

1.1.12   Knowledge of the normal chronic physiologic adaptations associated with cardiovascular exercise.

1.1.13   Knowledge of the normal chronic physiologic adaptations associated with resistance training.

1.1.14   Knowledge of the physiologic principles related to warm-up and cool-down.

1.1.15   Knowledge of the common theories of muscle fatigue and delayed onset muscle soreness (DOMS).

1.1.16   Knowledge of the physiologic adaptations that occur at rest and during submaximal and maximal exercise following chronic aerobic and anaerobic exercise training.

1.1.17   Knowledge of the physiologic principles involved in promoting gains in muscular strength and endurance.

1.1.18   Knowledge of blood pressure responses associated with acute exercise, including changes in body position.

1.1.19   Knowledge of how the principle of specificity relates to the components of fitness.

1.1.20   Knowledge of the concept of detraining or reversibility of conditioning and its implications in fitness programs.

1.1.21   Knowledge of the physical and psychological signs of overtraining and to provide recommendations for these problems.

1.1.22   Knowledge of muscle actions, such as isotonic, isometric (static), isokinetic, concentric, eccentric.

1.1.23   Ability to identify the major muscles. Major muscles include, but are not limited to, the following: trapezius, pectoralis major, latissimus dorsi, biceps, triceps, rectus abdominis, internal and external obliques, erector spinae,

---

^a*A special note about ACSM Certified Clinical Exercise Specialist KSAs*

Like the other certifications presented thus far, the ACSM Certified Clinical Exercise Specialist KSAs are categorized by content area. However, some CES KSAs cover multiple practices areas within each area of content. For example, several of them describe a specific topic with respect to both exercise testing and training, which are two distinct content areas. Rather than write out each separately (which would have greatly expanded the KSA list length), they have been listed under a single content area. When reviewing these KSAs, please note that KSAs in bold text cover multiple content areas. Each CES KSA begins with a l as the practice area. However, where appropriate, some KSAs mention specific patient populations (i.e., practice area). If a specific practice area is not mentioned within a given KSA, then it applies equally to each of the general population, cardiovascular, pulmonary, and metabolic practice areas. Note that "metabolic patients" are defined as those with at least one of the following: overweight or obese, diabetes (type I or II), or metabolic syndrome. Each KSA describes either a single or multiple knowledge (K), skill (S), or ability (A)—or a combination of K, S, or A—that an individual should have mastery of to be considered a competent ACSM Certified Clinical Exercise Specialist.

gluteus maximus, quadriceps, hamstrings, adductors, abductors, and gastrocnemius.

1.1.24 Ability to identify the major bones. Major bones include, but are not limited to, the clavicle, scapula, sternum, humerus, carpals, ulna, radius, femur, fibula, tibia, and tarsals.

1.1.25 Ability to identify the various types of joints of the body (e.g., hinge, ball, and socket).

1.1.26 Knowledge of the primary action and joint range of motion for each major muscle group.

1.1.27 Ability to locate the anatomic landmarks for palpation of peripheral pulses.

1.1.28 Knowledge of the unique physiologic considerations of children, older adults, persons with diabetes (type 2), pregnant women, and persons who are overweight and/or obese.

1.1.29 Knowledge of the following related terms: hypertrophy, atrophy, and hyperplasia.

GENERAL POPULATION/CORE: HEALTH APPRAISAL, FITNESS, AND CLINICAL EXERCISE TESTING

1.3.1 Knowledge of and ability to discuss the physiologic basis of the major components of physical fitness: flexibility, cardiovascular fitness, muscular strength, muscular endurance, and body composition.

1.3.2 Knowledge of the components of a health/medical history.

1.3.3 Knowledge of the value of a medical clearance before exercise participation.

1.3.4 Knowledge of the categories of participants who should receive medical clearance before administration of an exercise test or participation in an exercise program.

1.3.5 Knowledge of relative and absolute contraindications to exercise testing or participation.

1.3.6 Knowledge of the limitations of informed consent and medical clearance.

1.3.7 Knowledge of the advantages/disadvantages and limitations of the various body composition techniques including, but not limited to, skinfolds, plethysmography (BOD POD®), bioelectrical impedance, infrared, dual-energy x-ray absorptiometry (DEXA), and circumference measurements.

1.3.8 Skill in accurately measuring heart rate and obtaining rating of perceived exertion (RPE) at rest and during exercise according to established guidelines.

1.3.9 Ability to locate body sites for circumference (girth) measurements.

1.3.10 Ability to obtain a basic health history and risk appraisal and to stratify risk in accordance with ACSM Guidelines.

1.3.11 Ability to explain and obtain informed consent.

1.3.13 Knowledge of preactivity fitness testing, including assessments of cardiovascular fitness, muscular strength, muscular endurance, flexibility, and body composition.

1.3.14 Knowledge of criteria for terminating a fitness evaluation and proper procedures to be followed after discontinuing such a test.

1.3.15 Knowledge of and ability to prepare for the initial client consultation.

1.3.16 Ability to recognize postural abnormalities that may affect exercise performance.

1.3.17 Skill in assessing body alignment.

GENERAL POPULATION/CORE: EXERCISE PRESCRIPTION AND PROGRAMMING

1.7.1 Knowledge of the benefits and risks associated with exercise training and recommendations for exercise programming in children and adolescents.

1.7.2 Knowledge of the benefits and precautions associated with resistance and endurance training in older adults and recommendations for exercise programming.

1.7.3 Knowledge of specific leadership techniques appropriate for working with participants of all ages.

1.7.4 Knowledge of how to modify cardiovascular and resistance exercises based on age and physical condition.

1.7.5 Knowledge of and ability to describe the unique adaptations to exercise training with regard to strength, functional capacity, and motor skills.

1.7.6 Knowledge of common orthopedic and cardiovascular considerations for older participants and the ability to describe modifications in exercise prescription that are indicated.

1.7.7 Knowledge of selecting appropriate training modalities according to the age and functional capacity of the individual.

1.7.8 Knowledge of the recommended intensity, duration, frequency, and type of physical activity necessary for development of cardiorespiratory fitness in an apparently healthy population.

1.7.9 Knowledge to describe and the ability to safely demonstrate exercises designed to enhance muscular strength and/or endurance.

1.7.10 Knowledge of the principles of overload, specificity, and progression and how they relate to exercise programming.

1.7.11   Knowledge of how to conduct and the ability to teach/demonstrate exercises during a comprehensive session that would include pre-exercise evaluation, warm-up, aerobic exercise, cool-down, muscular fitness training, and flexibility exercise.

1.7.12   Knowledge of special precautions and modifications of exercise programming for participation at altitude, different ambient temperatures, humidity, and environmental pollution.

1.7.13   Knowledge of the importance and ability to record exercise sessions and performing periodic evaluations to assess changes in fitness status.

1.7.14   Knowledge of the advantages and disadvantages of implementation of interval, continuous, and circuit training programs.

1.7.15   Knowledge of the concept of activities of daily living (ADLs) and its importance in the overall health of the individual.

1.7.16   Knowledge of progressive adaptation in resistance training and its implications on program design and periodization.

1.7.17   Knowledge of interpersonal limitations when working with clients one on one.

1.7.19   Skill to teach and demonstrate appropriate modifications in specific exercises and make recommendations for exercise programming for the following groups: children, older adults, persons with diabetes (type 2), pregnant women, persons with arthritis, persons who are overweight and/or obese, and persons with chronic back pain.

1.7.20   Skill to teach and demonstrate appropriate exercises for improving range of motion of all major joints.

1.7.21   Skill in the use of various methods for establishing and monitoring levels of exercise intensity, including heart rate, RPE, and metabolic equivalents (METs).

1.7.22   Knowledge of and ability to apply methods used to monitor exercise intensity, including heart rate and rating of perceived exertion.

1.7.24   Ability to differentiate between the amount of physical activity required for health benefits and the amount of exercise required for fitness development.

1.7.25   Ability to determine training heart rates using two methods: percent of age-predicted maximum heart rate and heart rate reserve (Karvonen).

1.7.26   Ability to identify proper and improper technique in the use of resistive equipment, such as stability balls, weights, bands, resistance bars, and water exercise equipment.

1.7.27   Ability to identify proper and improper technique in the use of cardiovascular conditioning equipment (e.g., stair-climbers, stationary cycles, treadmills, and elliptical trainers).

1.7.28   Ability to teach a progression of exercises for all major muscle groups to improve muscular fitness.

1.7.29   Ability to modify exercises based on age and physical condition.

1.7.30   Ability to explain and implement exercise prescription guidelines for apparently healthy clients or those who have medical clearance to exercise.

1.7.31   Ability to adapt frequency, intensity, duration, mode, progression, level of supervision, and monitoring techniques in exercise programs for apparently healthy clients or those who have medical clearance to exercise.

1.7.34   Ability to evaluate, prescribe, and demonstrate appropriate flexibility exercises for all major muscle groups.

1.7.35   Ability to design training programs using interval, continuous, and circuit training programs.

1.7.36   Ability to describe the advantages and disadvantages of various types of commercial exercise equipment in developing cardiorespiratory and muscular fitness.

1.7.37   Ability to safely demonstrate a wide variety of conditioning exercises involving equipment, such as stability balls, BOSU® balls, elastic bands, medicine balls, and foam rollers.

1.7.38   Ability to safely demonstrate a wide range of resistance-training modalities, including variable resistance devices, dynamic constant external resistance devices, static resistance devices, and other resistance devices.

1.7.39   Ability to safely demonstrate a wide variety of conditioning exercises that promote improvements in agility, balance, coordination, reaction time, speed, and power.

1.7.40   Knowledge of training principles, such as progressive overload, variation, and specificity.

1.7.41   Knowledge of the Valsalva maneuver and the associated risks.

1.7.42   Knowledge of the appropriate repetitions, sets, volume, repetition maximum, and rest periods necessary for desired outcome goals.

1.7.43   Ability to safely demonstrate a wide variety of plyometric exercises and be able to determine when such exercises would be inappropriate to perform.

1.7.44 Ability to apply training principles so as to distinguish goals between an athlete and an individual exercising for general health.

1.7.45 Knowledge of periodization in exercise in aerobic and resistance-training program design.

GENERAL POPULATION/CORE: NUTRITION AND WEIGHT MANAGEMENT

1.8.1 Knowledge of the role of carbohydrates, fats, and proteins as fuels.

1.8.2 Knowledge to define the following terms: obesity, overweight, percent fat, body mass index (BMI), lean body mass, anorexia nervosa, bulimia nervosa, and body fat distribution.

1.8.3 Knowledge of the relationship between body composition and health.

1.8.4 Knowledge of the effects of diet plus exercise, diet alone, and exercise alone as methods for modifying body composition.

1.8.5 Knowledge of the importance of an adequate daily energy intake for healthy weight management.

1.8.6 Knowledge of the importance of maintaining normal hydration before, during, and after exercise.

1.8.7 Knowledge and understanding of the current Dietary Guidelines for Americans, including the USDA Food Pyramid.

1.8.8 Knowledge of the female athlete triad.

1.8.9 Knowledge of the myths and consequences associated with inappropriate weight loss methods (e.g., saunas, vibrating belts, body wraps, electric simulators, sweat suits, fad diets).

1.8.10 Knowledge of the number of kilocalories in one gram of carbohydrate, fat, protein, and alcohol.

1.8.11 Knowledge of the number of kilocalories equivalent to losing one pound of body fat.

1.8.12 Knowledge of the guidelines for caloric intake for an individual desiring to lose or gain weight.

1.8.13 Knowledge of common ergogenic aids, the purported mechanism of action, and potential risks and/or benefits (e.g., anabolic steroids, caffeine, amino acids, vitamins, minerals, creatine monohydrate, adrostenedione, DHEA).

1.8.14 Ability to describe the health implications of variation in body-fat distribution patterns and the significance of the waist-to-hip ratio.

1.8.15 Ability to describe the health implications of commonly used herbs (e.g., echinacea, St. John's wort, ginseng).

GENERAL POPULATION/CORE: HUMAN BEHAVIOR AND COUNSELING

1.9.1 Knowledge of behavioral strategies to enhance exercise and health behavior change (e.g., reinforcement, goal setting, social support).

1.9.2 Knowledge of the stages of motivational readiness and effective strategies that support and facilitate behavioral change.

1.9.3 Knowledge of the three stages of learning: cognitive, associative, autonomous.

1.9.4 Knowledge of specific techniques to enhance motivation (e.g., posters, recognition, bulletin boards, games, competitions). Define extrinsic and intrinsic reinforcement and give examples of each.

1.9.5 Knowledge of the different types of learners (auditory, visual, kinesthetic) and how to apply teaching and training techniques to optimize a client's training session.

1.9.6 Knowledge of the types of feedback and ability to use communication skills to optimize a client's training session.

1.9.7 Knowledge of common obstacles that interfere with adherence to an exercise program and strategies to overcome these obstacles.

1.9.8 Ability to identify, clarify, and set behavioral and realistic goals with the client (i.e., SMART goals).

1.9.9 Knowledge of basic communication and coaching techniques that foster and facilitate behavioral changes.

1.9.10 Knowledge of various learning theories (e.g., motivation theory, attribution theory, transfer theory, retention theory, and goal theory).

1.9.11 Knowledge of attributes or characteristics necessary for effective teaching.

GENERAL POPULATION/CORE: SAFETY, INJURY PREVENTION, AND EMERGENCY PROCEDURES

1.10.1 Knowledge of and skill in obtaining basic life support, automated external defibrillators (AEDs), and cardiopulmonary resuscitation certification.

1.10.2 Knowledge of appropriate emergency procedures (i.e., telephone procedures, written emergency procedures, personnel responsibilities) in a health and fitness setting.

1.10.3 Knowledge of basic first-aid procedures for exercise-related injuries, such as bleeding, strains/sprains, fractures, and exercise intolerance (dizziness, syncope, heat injury).

1.10.4   Knowledge of basic precautions taken in an exercise setting to ensure participant safety.

1.10.5   Knowledge of the physical and physiologic signs and symptoms of overtraining.

1.10.6   Knowledge of the effects of temperature, humidity, altitude, and pollution on the physiologic response to exercise.

1.10.7   Knowledge of the following terms: shin splints, sprain, strain, tennis elbow, bursitis, stress fracture, tendonitis, patello-femoral pain syndrome, low back pain, plantar fasciitis, and rotator cuff tendonitis.

1.10.8   Knowledge of hypothetical concerns and potential risks that may be associated with the use of exercises such as straight-leg sit-ups, double leg raises, full squats, hurdler's stretch, yoga plow, forceful back hyperexten-sion, and standing bent-over toe touch.

1.10.10   Knowledge of the Certified Personal Trainer's^{SM} responsibilities, limitations, and the legal implications of carrying out emergency procedures.

1.10.11   Knowledge of potential musculoskeletal injuries (e.g., contusions, sprains, strains, fractures), cardiovascular/pulmonary complications (e.g., tachycardia, bradycardia, hypotension/hypertension, tachypnea), and metabolic abnormalities (e.g., fainting/syncope, hypoglycemia/hyperglycemia, hypothermia/hyperthermia).

1.10.12   Knowledge of the initial management and first-aid techniques associated with open wounds, musculoskeletal injuries, cardiovascular/pulmonary complications, and metabolic disorders.

1.10.13   Knowledge of the components of an equipment service plan/agreement and how it may be used to evaluate the condition of exercise equipment to reduce the potential risk of injury.

1.10.14   Knowledge of the legal implications of documented safety procedures, the use of incident documents, and ongoing safety training.

1.10.15   Skill in demonstrating appropriate emergency procedures during exercise testing and/or training.

1.10.16   Ability to identify the components that contribute to the maintenance of a safe exercise environment.

1.10.17   Ability to assist or spot a client in a safe and effective manner during resistance exercise.

GENERAL POPULATION/CORE: PROGRAM ADMINISTRATION, QUALITY ASSURANCE, AND OUTCOME ASSESSMENT

1.11.1   Knowledge of the Certified Personal Trainer's^{SM} scope of practice and role in the administration/program management within a health/fitness facility.

1.11.2   Knowledge of and the ability to use the documentation required when a client shows abnormal signs or symptoms during an exercise session and should be referred to a physician.

1.11.3   Knowledge of professional liability and most common types of negligence seen in training environments.

1.11.4   Understanding of the practical and legal ramifications of the employee versus independent contractor classifications as they relate to the Certified Personal Trainer^{SM}.

1.11.5   Knowledge of appropriate professional responsibilities, practice standards, and ethics in relationships dealing with clients, employers, and other allied health/medical/fitness professionals.

1.11.6   Knowledge of the types of exercise programs available in the community and how these programs are appropriate for various populations.

1.11.7   Knowledge of and ability to implement effective, professional business practices and ethical promotion of personal training services.

1.11.8   Ability to develop a basic business plan, which includes establishing a budget, developing management policies, marketing, sales, and pricing.

GENERAL POPULATION/CORE: CLINICAL AND MEDICAL CONSIDERATIONS

1.12.1   Knowledge of cardiovascular, respiratory, metabolic, and musculoskeletal risk factors that may require further evaluation by medical or allied health professionals before participation in physical activity.

1.12.2   Knowledge of risk factors that may be favorably modified by physical activity habits.

1.12.3   Knowledge of the risk-factor concept of coronary artery disease (CAD) and the influence of heredity and lifestyle on the development of CAD.

1.12.4   Knowledge of how lifestyle factors—including nutrition, physical activity, and heredity—influence blood lipid and lipoprotein (i.e., cholesterol: high-density lipoprotein and low-density lipoprotein) profiles.

1.12.5   Knowledge of cardiovascular risk factors or conditions that may require consultation with medical personnel before testing or training, including inappropriate changes of resting or exercise heart rate and blood pressure; new onset discomfort in chest, neck, shoulder, or arm; changes in the pattern of discomfort during rest or exercise; fainting or dizzy spells; and claudication.

1.12.6   Knowledge of respiratory risk factors or conditions that may require consultation with medical personnel before testing or training, including asthma, exercise-induced bronchospasm, extreme breathlessness at rest or during exercise, bronchitis, and emphysema.

1.12.7   Knowledge of metabolic risk factors or conditions that may require consultation with medical personnel before testing or training, including body weight more than 20% above optimal, BMI >30, thyroid disease, diabetes or glucose intolerance, and hypoglycemia.

1.12.8   Knowledge of musculoskeletal risk factors or conditions that may require consultation with medical personnel before testing or training, including acute or chronic back pain, arthritis, osteoporosis, and joint inflammation.

1.12.10   Knowledge of common drugs from each of the following classes of medications and ability to describe their effects on exercise: antianginals, anticoagulants, antihypertensives, antiarrhythmics, bronchodilators, hypoglycemics, psychotropics, vasodilators, and over-the-counter medications such as pseudoephedrine.

1.12.11   Knowledge of the effects of the following substances on exercise: antihistamines, tranquilizers, alcohol, diet pills, cold tablets, caffeine, and nicotine.

ACSM CERTIFIED HEALTH FITNESS SPECIALIST KNOWLEDGE, SKILLS, AND ABILITIES (KSAs)

The ACSM Certified Health Fitness Specialist is responsible for the mastery of the ACSM Certified Personal Trainer^{SM} KSAs and the following ACSM Certified Health Fitness Specialist KSAs.

NOTE: The KSAs listed here for the ACSM Certified Health Fitness Specialist are the same KSAs for educational programs in Exercise Science seeking undergraduate (Bachelor's) academic accreditation through the CoAES. For more information, please visit www.coaes.org.

GENERAL POPULATION/CORE: EXERCISE PHYSIOLOGY AND RELATED EXERCISE SCIENCE

1.1.1   Knowledge of the structures of bone, skeletal muscle, and connective tissues.

1.1.2   Knowledge of the anatomy and physiology of the cardiovascular system and pulmonary system.

1.1.3   Knowledge of the following muscle action terms: inferior, superior, medial, lateral, supination, pronation, flexion, extension, adduction, abduction, hyperextension, rotation, circumduction, agonist, antagonist, and stabilizer.

1.1.4   Knowledge of the plane in which each movement action occurs and the responsible muscles.

1.1.5   Knowledge of the interrelationships among center of gravity, base of support, balance, stability, posture, and proper spinal alignment.

1.1.6   Knowledge of the curvatures of the spine including lordosis, scoliosis, and kyphosis.

1.1.7   Knowledge of the stretch reflex and how it relates to flexibility.

1.1.8   Knowledge of biomechanical principles that underlie performance of the following activities: walking, jogging, running, swimming, cycling, weight lifting, and carrying or moving objects.

1.1.9   Ability to describe the systems for the production of energy.

1.1.10   Knowledge of the role of aerobic and anaerobic energy systems in the performance of various physical activities.

1.1.11   Knowledge of the following cardiorespiratory terms: ischemia, angina pectoris, tachycardia, bradycardia, arrhythmia, myocardial infarction, claudication, dyspnea, and hyperventilation.

1.1.12   Ability to describe normal cardiorespiratory responses to static and dynamic exercise in terms of heart rate, stroke volume, cardiac output, blood pressure, and oxygen consumption.

1.1.13   Knowledge of the heart rate, stroke volume, cardiac output, blood pressure, and oxygen consumption responses to exercise.

1.1.14   Knowledge of the anatomic and physiologic adaptations associated with strength training.

1.1.15   Knowledge of the physiologic principles related to warm-up and cool-down.

1.1.16   Knowledge of the common theories of muscle fatigue and delayed onset muscle soreness (DOMS).

1.1.17   Knowledge of the physiologic adaptations that occur at rest and during submaximal and maximal exercise following chronic aerobic and anaerobic exercise training.

1.1.18   Knowledge of the differences in cardiorespiratory response to acute graded exercise between conditioned and unconditioned individuals.

1.1.19   Knowledge of the structure and function of the skeletal muscle fiber.

1.1.20   Knowledge of the characteristics of fast- and slow-twitch muscle fibers.

1.1.21   Knowledge of the sliding filament theory of muscle contraction.

1.1.22   Knowledge of twitch, summation, and tetanus with respect to muscle contraction.

1.1.23   Knowledge of the principles involved in promoting gains in muscular strength and endurance.

1.1.24   Knowledge of muscle fatigue as it relates to mode, intensity, duration, and the accumulative effects of exercise.

1.1.26   Knowledge of the response of the following variables to acute static and dynamic exercise: heart rate, stroke volume, cardiac output, pulmonary ventilation, tidal volume, respiratory rate, and arteriovenous oxygen difference.

1.1.27   Knowledge of blood pressure responses associated with acute exercise, including changes in body position.

1.1.28   Knowledge of and ability to describe the implications of ventilatory threshold (anaerobic threshold) as it relates to exercise training and cardiorespiratory assessment.

1.1.29   Knowledge of and ability to describe the physiologic adaptations of the pulmonary system that occur at rest and during submaximal and maximal exercise following chronic aerobic and anaerobic training.

1.1.30   Knowledge of how each of the following differs from the normal condition: dyspnea, hypoxia, and hyperventilation.

1.1.31   Knowledge of how the principles of specificity and progressive overload relate to the components of exercise programming.

1.1.32   Knowledge of the concept of detraining or reversibility of conditioning and its implications in exercise programs.

1.1.33   Knowledge of the physical and psychological signs of overreaching/overtraining and to provide recommendations for these problems.

1.1.34   Knowledge of and ability to describe the changes that occur in maturation from childhood to adulthood for the following:

skeletal muscle, bone, reaction time, coordination, posture, heat and cold tolerance, maximal oxygen consumption, strength, flexibility, body composition, resting and maximal heart rate, and resting and maximal blood pressure.

1.1.35   Knowledge of the effect of the aging process on the musculoskeletal and cardiovascular structure and function at rest, during exercise, and during recovery.

1.1.36   Knowledge of the following terms: progressive resistance, isotonic/isometric, concentric, eccentric, atrophy, hyperplasia, hypertrophy, sets, repetitions, plyometrics, Valsalva maneuver.

1.1.37   Knowledge of and skill to demonstrate exercises designed to enhance muscular strength and/or endurance of specific major muscle groups.

1.1.38   Knowledge of and skill to demonstrate exercises for enhancing musculoskeletal flexibility.

1.1.39   Ability to identify the major muscles. Major muscles include, but are not limited to, the following: trapezius, pectoralis major, latissimus dorsi, biceps, triceps, rectus abdominis, internal and external obliques, erector spinae, gluteus maximus, quadriceps, hamstrings, adductors, abductors, and gastrocnemius.

1.1.40   Ability to identify the major bones. Major bones include, but are not limited to, the clavicle, scapula, sternum, humerus, carpals, ulna, radius, femur, fibia, tibia, and tarsals.

1.1.41   Ability to identify the joints of the body.

1.1.42   Knowledge of the primary action and joint range of motion for each major muscle group.

1.1.43   Ability to locate the anatomic landmarks for palpation of peripheral pulses and blood pressure.

GENERAL POPULATION/CORE: PATHOPHYSIOLOGY AND RISK FACTORS

1.2.1   Knowledge of the physiologic and metabolic responses to exercise associated with chronic disease (heart disease, hypertension, diabetes mellitus, and pulmonary disease).

1.2.2   Knowledge of cardiovascular, pulmonary, metabolic, and musculoskeletal risk factors that may require further evaluation by medical or allied health professionals before participation in physical activity.

1.2.3   Knowledge of risk factors that may be favorably modified by physical activity habits.

1.2.4   Knowledge to define the following terms: total cholesterol (TC), high-density lipoprotein cholesterol (HDL-C), TC/HDL-C ratio, low-density lipoprotein cholesterol (LDL-C), triglycerides, hypertension, and atherosclerosis.

1.2.5   Knowledge of plasma cholesterol levels for adults as recommended by the National Cholesterol Education Program.

1.2.6   Knowledge of the risk-factor thresholds for ACSM risk stratification, which includes genetic and lifestyle factors related to the development of CAD.

1.2.7   Knowledge of the atherosclerotic process, the factors involved in its genesis and progression, and the potential role of exercise in treatment.

1.2.8   Knowledge of how lifestyle factors, including nutrition and physical activity, influence lipid and lipoprotein profiles.

GENERAL POPULATION/CORE: HEALTH APPRAISAL, FITNESS, AND CLINICAL EXERCISE TESTING

1.3.1   Knowledge of and ability to discuss the physiologic basis of the major components of physical fitness: flexibility, cardiovascular fitness, muscular strength, muscular endurance, and body composition.

1.3.2   Knowledge of the value of the health/medical history.

1.3.3   Knowledge of the value of a medical clearance before exercise participation.

1.3.4   Knowledge of and the ability to perform risk stratification and its implications toward medical clearance before administration of an exercise test or participation in an exercise program.

1.3.5   Knowledge of relative and absolute contraindications to exercise testing or participation.

1.3.6   Knowledge of the limitations of informed consent and medical clearance before exercise testing.

1.3.7   Knowledge of the advantages/disadvantages and limitations of the various body-composition techniques, including but not limited to, air displacement plethysmography (BOD POD®), dual-energy x-ray absorptiometry (DEXA), hydrostatic weighing, skinfolds, and bioelectrical impedance.

1.3.8   Skill in accurately measuring heart rate and blood pressure, and obtaining rating of perceived exertion (RPE) at rest and during exercise according to established guidelines.

1.3.9   Skill in measuring skinfold sites, skeletal diameters, and girth measurements used for estimating body composition.

1.3.10   Knowledge of calibration of a cycle ergometer and a motor-driven treadmill.

1.3.11   Ability to locate the brachial artery and correctly place the cuff and stethoscope in position for blood-pressure measurement.

1.3.12   Ability to locate common sites for measurement of skinfold thicknesses and circumferences (for determination of body composition and waist-hip ratio).

1.3.13   Ability to obtain a health history and risk appraisal that includes past and current medical history, family history of cardiac disease, orthopedic limitations, prescribed medications, activity patterns, nutritional habits, stress and anxiety levels, and smoking and alcohol use.

1.3.14   Ability to obtain informed consent.

1.3.15   Ability to explain the purpose and procedures and perform the monitoring (heart rate, RPE, and blood pressure) of clients before, during, and after cardiorespiratory fitness testing.

1.3.16   Ability to instruct participants in the use of equipment and test procedures.

1.3.17   Ability to explain purpose of testing, determine an appropriate submaximal or maximal protocol, and perform an assessment of cardiovascular fitness on the treadmill or the cycle ergometer.

1.3.18   Ability to describe the purpose of testing, determine appropriate protocols, and perform assessments of muscular strength, muscular endurance, and flexibility.

1.3.19   Ability to perform various techniques of assessing body composition.

1.3.20   Ability to analyze and interpret information obtained from the cardiorespiratory fitness test and the muscular strength and endurance, flexibility, and body-composition assessments for apparently healthy individuals and those with controlled chronic disease.

1.3.21   Ability to identify appropriate criteria for terminating a fitness evaluation and demonstrate proper procedures to be followed after discontinuing such a test.

1.3.22   Ability to modify protocols and procedures for cardiorespiratory fitness tests in children, adolescents, and older adults.

1.3.23   Ability to identify individuals for whom physician supervision is recommended during maximal and submaximal exercise testing.

GENERAL POPULATION/CORE: ELECTROCARDIOGRAPHY AND DIAGNOSTIC TECHNIQUES

1.4.1   Knowledge of how each of the following arrhythmias differs from the normal condition: premature atrial contractions and premature ventricular contractions.

1.4.3   Knowledge of the basic properties of cardiac muscle and the normal pathways of conduction in the heart.

GENERAL POPULATION/CORE: PATIENT MANAGEMENT AND MEDICATIONS

1.5.1   Knowledge of common drugs from each of the following classes of medications and ability to describe the principal action and the effects on exercise testing and prescription: antianginals, antihypertensives, antiarrhythmics, anticoagulants, bronchodilators, hypoglycemics, psychotropics, and vasodilators.

1.5.2   Knowledge of the effects of the following substances on the exercise response: antihistamines, tranquilizers, alcohol, diet pills, cold tablets, caffeine, and nicotine.

GENERAL POPULATION/CORE: EXERCISE PRESCRIPTION AND PROGRAMMING

1.7.1   Knowledge of the relationship between the number of repetitions, intensity, number of sets, and rest with regard to strength training.

1.7.2   Knowledge of the benefits and precautions associated with exercise training in apparently healthy and controlled disease.

1.7.3   Knowledge of the benefits and precautions associated with exercise training across the life span (from youth to the elderly).

1.7.4   Knowledge of specific group exercise leadership techniques appropriate for working with participants of all ages.

1.7.5   Knowledge of how to select and/or modify appropriate exercise programs according to the age, functional capacity, and limitations of the individual.

1.7.6   Knowledge of the differences in the development of an exercise prescription for children, adolescents, and older participants.

1.7.7   Knowledge of and ability to describe the unique adaptations to exercise training in children, adolescents, and older participants with regard to strength, functional capacity, and motor skills.

1.7.8   Knowledge of common orthopedic and cardiovascular considerations for older partici-

pants and the ability to describe modifications in exercise prescription that are indicated.

1.7.10   Knowledge of the recommended intensity, duration, frequency, and type of physical activity necessary for development of cardiorespiratory fitness in an apparently healthy population.

1.7.11   Knowledge of and the ability to describe exercises designed to enhance muscular strength and/or endurance of specific major muscle groups.

1.7.12   Knowledge of the principles of overload, specificity, and progression and how they relate to exercise programming.

1.7.13   Knowledge of the various types of interval, continuous, and circuit training programs.

1.7.14   Knowledge of approximate METs for various sport, recreational, and work tasks.

1.7.15   Knowledge of the components incorporated into an exercise session and the proper sequence (i.e., pre-exercise evaluation, warm-up, aerobic stimulus phase, cool-down, muscular strength and/or endurance, and flexibility).

1.7.16   Knowledge of special precautions and modifications of exercise programming for participation at altitude, different ambient temperatures, humidity, and environmental pollution.

1.7.17   Knowledge of the importance of recording exercise sessions and performing periodic evaluations to assess changes in fitness status.

1.7.18   Knowledge of the advantages and disadvantages of implementation of interval, continuous, and circuit training programs.

1.7.19   Knowledge of the exercise programs that are available in the community and how these programs are appropriate for various populations.

1.7.20   Knowledge of and ability to describe activities of daily living (ADLs) and its importance in the overall health of the individual.

1.7.21   Skill to teach and demonstrate the components of an exercise session (i.e., warm-up, aerobic stimulus phase, cool-down, muscular strength/endurance, flexibility).

1.7.22   Skill to teach and demonstrate appropriate modifications in specific exercises for groups such as older adults, pregnant and postnatal women, obese persons, and persons with low back pain.

1.7.23   Skill to teach and demonstrate appropriate exercises for improving range of motion of all major joints.

1.7.24   Skill in the use of various methods for establishing and monitoring levels of exercise intensity, including heart rate, RPE, and oxygen cost.

1.7.25 Ability to identify and apply methods used to monitor exercise intensity, including heart rate and RPE.

1.7.26 Ability to describe modifications in exercise prescriptions for individuals with functional disabilities and musculoskeletal injuries.

1.7.27 Ability to differentiate between the amount of physical activity required for health benefits and/or for fitness development.

1.7.28 Knowledge of and ability to determine target heart rates using two methods: percent of age-predicted maximum heart rate and heart rate reserve (Karvonen).

1.7.29 Ability to identify proper and improper technique in the use of resistive equipment, such as stability balls, weights, bands, resistance bars, and water exercise equipment.

1.7.30 Ability to identify proper and improper technique in the use of cardiovascular conditioning equipment (e.g., stair-climbers, stationary cycles, treadmills, elliptical trainers, rowing machines).

1.7.31 Ability to teach a progression of exercises for all major muscle groups to improve muscular strength and endurance.

1.7.32 Ability to communicate appropriately with exercise participants during initial screening and exercise programming.

1.7.33 Ability to design, implement, and evaluate individualized and group exercise programs based on health history and physical fitness assessments.

1.7.34 Ability to modify exercises based on age, physical condition, and cognitive status.

1.7.35 Ability to apply energy cost, $\dot{V}O_2$, METs, and target heart rates to an exercise prescription.

1.7.36 Ability to convert between the U.S. and metric systems for length/height (inches to centimeters), weight (pounds to kilograms), and speed (miles per hour to meters per minute).

1.7.37 Ability to convert between absolute ($mL \cdot kg^{-1} \cdot min^{-1}$ or $L \cdot min^{-1}$) and relative ($mL \cdot kg^{-1} \cdot min^{-1}$, and/or METs) oxygen costs.

1.7.38 Ability to determine the energy cost for given exercise intensities during horizontal and graded walking and running stepping exercise, cycle ergometry, arm ergometry, and stepping.

1.7.39 Ability to prescribe exercise intensity based on $\dot{V}O_2$ data for different modes of exercise, including graded and horizontal running and walking, cycling, and stepping exercise.

1.7.40 Ability to explain and implement exercise prescription guidelines for apparently healthy clients, increased risk clients, and clients with controlled disease.

1.7.41 Ability to adapt frequency, intensity, duration, mode, progression, level of supervision, and monitoring techniques in exercise programs for patients with controlled chronic disease (e.g., heart disease, diabetes mellitus, obesity, hypertension), musculoskeletal problems (including fatigue), pregnancy and/or postpartum, and exercise-induced asthma.

1.7.42 Ability to design resistive exercise programs to increase or maintain muscular strength and/or endurance.

1.7.43 Ability to evaluate flexibility and prescribe appropriate flexibility exercises for all major muscle groups.

1.7.44 Ability to design training programs using interval, continuous, and circuit training programs.

1.7.45 Ability to describe the advantages and disadvantages of various commercial exercise equipment in developing cardiorespiratory fitness, muscular strength, and muscular endurance.

1.7.46 Ability to modify exercise programs based on age, physical condition, and current health status.

1.7.47 Ability to assess postural alignment and recommend appropriate exercise to meet individual needs and refer as necessary.

GENERAL POPULATION/CORE: NUTRITION AND WEIGHT MANAGEMENT

1.8.1 Knowledge of the role of carbohydrates, fats, and proteins as fuels for aerobic and anaerobic metabolism.

1.8.2 Knowledge of the following terms: obesity, overweight, percent fat, BMI, lean body mass, anorexia nervosa, bulimia nervosa, metabolic syndrome, and body-fat distribution.

1.8.3 Knowledge of the relationship between body composition and health.

1.8.4 Knowledge of the effects of diet, exercise, and behavior modification as methods for modifying body composition.

1.8.5 Knowledge of the importance of an adequate daily energy intake for healthy weight management.

1.8.6 Knowledge of the difference between fat-soluble and water-soluble vitamins.

1.8.7 Knowledge of the importance of maintaining normal hydration before, during, and after exercise.

1.8.8   Knowledge of the USDA Food Pyramid and Dietary Guidelines for Americans.

1.8.9   Knowledge of the importance of calcium and iron in women's health.

1.8.10   Knowledge of the myths and consequences associated with inappropriate weight loss methods (e.g., fad diets, dietary supplements, overexercising, starvation diets).

1.8.11   Knowledge of the number of kilocalories in one gram of carbohydrate, fat, protein, and alcohol.

1.8.12   Knowledge of the number of kilocalories equivalent to losing one pound (0.45 kg) of body fat and the ability to prescribe appropriate amount of exercise to achieve weight-loss goals.

1.8.13   Knowledge of the guidelines for caloric intake for an individual desiring to lose or gain weight.

1.8.14   Knowledge of common nutritional ergogenic aids, the purported mechanism of action, and any risk and/or benefits (e.g., carbohydrates, protein/amino acids, vitamins, minerals, herbal products, creatine, steroids, caffeine).

1.8.15   Knowledge of nutritional factors related to the female athlete triad syndrome (i.e., eating disorders, menstrual cycle abnormalities, and osteoporosis).

1.8.16   Knowledge of the NIH consensus statement regarding health risks of obesity, Nutrition for Physical Fitness Position Paper of the American Dietetic Association, and the ACSM position stand on proper and improper weight loss programs.

1.8.17   Ability to describe the health implications of variation in body-fat distribution patterns and the significance of the waist-to-hip ratio.

1.8.18   Knowledge of the nutrition and exercise effects on blood glucose levels in diabetes.

GENERAL POPULATION/CORE: HUMAN BEHAVIOR AND COUNSELING

1.9.1   Knowledge of behavioral strategies to enhance exercise and health behavior change (e.g., reinforcement, goal setting, social support).

1.9.2   Knowledge of the important elements that should be included in each behavior-modification session.

1.9.3   Knowledge of specific techniques to enhance motivation (e.g., posters, recognition, bulletin boards, games, competitions).

1.9.4   Knowledge of extrinsic and intrinsic reinforcement and ability to give examples of each.

1.9.5   Knowledge of the stages of motivational readiness.

1.9.6   Knowledge of approaches that may assist less motivated clients to increase their physical activity.

1.9.7   Knowledge of signs and symptoms of mental health states (e.g., anxiety, depression, eating disorders) that may necessitate referral to a medical or mental health professional.

1.9.8   Knowledge of the potential symptoms and causal factors of test anxiety (i.e., performance, appraisal threat during exercise testing) and how it may affect physiologic responses to testing.

1.9.9   Ability to coach clients to set achievable goals and overcome obstacles through a variety of methods (e.g., in person, on phone, and on Internet).

GENERAL POPULATION/CORE: SAFETY, INJURY PREVENTION, AND EMERGENCY PROCEDURES

1.10.1   Knowledge of and skill in obtaining basic life support, first aid, cardiopulmonary resuscitation, and automated external defibrillator certifications.

1.10.2   Knowledge of appropriate emergency procedures (i.e., telephone procedures, written emergency procedures, personnel responsibilities) in a health and fitness setting.

1.10.3   Knowledge of and skill in performing basic first-aid procedures for exercise-related injuries, such as bleeding, strains/sprains, fractures, and exercise intolerance (dizziness, syncope, heat and cold injuries).

1.10.4   Knowledge of basic precautions taken in an exercise setting to ensure participant safety.

1.10.5   Knowledge of the physical and physiologic signs and symptoms of overtraining and the ability to modify a program to accommodate this condition.

1.10.6   Knowledge of the effects of temperature, humidity, altitude, and pollution on the physiologic response to exercise and the ability to modify the exercise prescription to accommodate for these environmental conditions.

1.10.7   Knowledge of the signs and symptoms of the following conditions: shin splints, sprain, strain, tennis elbow, bursitis, stress fracture, tendonitis, patellar femoral pain syndrome, low back pain, plantar fasciitis, and rotator cuff tendonitis; the ability to recommend exercises to prevent these injuries.

1.10.8   Knowledge of hypothetical concerns and potential risks that may be associated with the use of exercises such as straight-leg sit-ups, double leg raises, full squats, hurdler's stretch, yoga plow, forceful back hyperextension, and standing bent-over toe touch.

1.10.9 Knowledge of safety plans, emergency procedures, and first-aid techniques needed during fitness evaluations, exercise testing, and exercise training.

1.10.10 Knowledge of the Health Fitness Specialist's responsibilities and limitations, and the legal implications of carrying out emergency procedures.

1.10.11 Knowledge of potential musculoskeletal injuries (e.g., contusions, sprains, strains, fractures), cardiovascular/pulmonary complications (e.g., tachycardia, bradycardia, hypotension/hypertension, tachypnea), and metabolic abnormalities (e.g., fainting/syncope, hypoglycemia/hyperglycemia, hypothermia/hyperthermia).

1.10.12 Knowledge of the initial management and first-aid techniques associated with open wounds, musculoskeletal injuries, cardiovascular/pulmonary complications, and metabolic disorders.

1.10.13 Knowledge of the components of an equipment maintenance/repair program and how it may be used to evaluate the condition of exercise equipment to reduce the potential risk of injury.

1.10.14 Knowledge of the legal implications of documented safety procedures, the use of incident documents, and ongoing safety training documentation for the purposes of safety and risk management.

1.10.15 Skill to demonstrate exercises used for people with low back pain; neck, shoulder, elbow, wrist, hip, knee and/or ankle pain; and the ability to modify a program for people with these conditions.

1.10.16 Skill in demonstrating appropriate emergency procedures during exercise testing and/or training.

1.10.17 Ability to identify the components that contribute to the maintenance of a safe environment, including equipment operation and maintenance, proper sanitation, safety and maintenance of exercise areas, and overall facility maintenance.

1.10.18 Knowledge of basic ergonomics to address daily activities that may cause musculoskeletal problems in the workplace and the ability to recommend exercises to alleviate symptoms caused by repetitive movements.

GENERAL POPULATION/CORE: PROGRAM ADMINISTRATION, QUALITY ASSURANCE, AND OUTCOME ASSESSMENT

1.11.1 Knowledge of the Health Fitness Specialist's role in administration and program management within a health/fitness facility.

1.11.2 Knowledge of and the ability to use the documentation required when a client shows signs or symptoms during an exercise session and should be referred to a physician.

1.11.3 Knowledge of how to manage a fitness department (e.g., working within a budget, interviewing and training staff, scheduling, running staff meetings, staff development).

1.11.4 Knowledge of the importance of tracking and evaluating member retention.

1.11.6 Ability to administer fitness-related programs within established budgetary guidelines.

1.11.7 Ability to develop marketing materials for the purpose of promoting fitness-related programs.

1.11.8 Ability to create and maintain records pertaining to participant exercise adherence, retention, and goal setting.

1.11.9 Ability to develop and administer educational programs (e.g., lectures, workshops) and educational materials.

1.11.10 Knowledge of basic sales techniques to promote health, fitness, and wellness services.

1.11.11 Knowledge of networking techniques with other healthcare professionals for referral purposes.

1.11.12 Ability to provide and administer appropriate customer service.

1.11.13 Knowledge of the importance of tracking and evaluating health promotion program results.

CARDIOVASCULAR: PATHOPHYSIOLOGY AND RISK FACTORS

2.2.1 Knowledge of cardiovascular risk factors or conditions that may require consultation with medical personnel before testing or training, including inappropriate changes of resting or exercise heart rate and blood pressure; new onset discomfort in chest, neck, shoulder, or arm; changes in the pattern of discomfort during rest or exercise; fainting or dizzy spells; and claudication.

2.2.2 Knowledge of the pathophysiology of myocardial ischemia and infarction.

2.2.3 Knowledge of the pathophysiology of stroke, hypertension, and hyperlipidemia.

2.2.4 Knowledge of the effects of the above diseases and conditions on the cardiorespiratory responses at rest and during exercise.

PULMONARY: PATHOPHYSIOLOGY AND RISK FACTORS

3.2.1   Knowledge of pulmonary risk factors or conditions that may require consultation with medical personnel before testing or training, including asthma, exercise-induced asthma/bronchospasm, extreme breathlessness at rest or during exercise, bronchitis, and emphysema.

METABOLIC: PATHOPHYSIOLOGY AND RISK FACTORS

4.2.1   Knowledge of metabolic risk factors or conditions that may require consultation with medical personnel before testing or training, including obesity, metabolic syndrome, thyroid disease, kidney disease, diabetes or glucose intolerance, and hypoglycemia.

ORTHOPEDIC/MUSCULOSKELETAL: PATHOPHYSIOLOGY AND RISK FACTORS

5.2.1   Knowledge of musculoskeletal risk factors or conditions that may require consultation with medical personnel before testing or training, including acute or chronic back pain, osteoarthritis, rheumatoid arthritis, osteoporosis, inflammation/pain, and low back pain.

NEUROMUSCULAR: PATHOPHYSIOLOGY AND RISK FACTORS

6.2.1   Knowledge of neuromuscular risk factors or conditions that may require consultation with medical personnel before testing or training, including spinal cord injuries and multiple sclerosis.

IMMUNOLOGIC: PATHOPHYSIOLOGY AND RISK FACTORS

7.2.1   Knowledge of immunologic risk factors or conditions that may require consultation with medical personnel before testing or training, including AIDS and cancer.

ACSM CERTIFIED CLINICAL EXERCISE SPECIALIST KNOWLEDGE, SKILLS, AND ABILITIES (KSAs)

The ACSM Certified Clinical Exercise Specialist is responsible for the mastery of the ACSM Certified Personal Trainer^{SM} KSAs, the ACSM Certified Health Fitness Specialist KSAs, and the following ACSM Certified Clinical Exercise Specialist KSAs.

GENERAL POPULATION/CORE: EXERCISE PHYSIOLOGY AND RELATED EXERCISE SCIENCE

1.1.1   **Describe and illustrate the normal cardiovascular anatomy.**

1.1.2   **Describe the physiologic effects of bed rest, and discuss the appropriate physical activities that might be used to counteract these changes.**

1.1.3   Identify the cardiorespiratory responses associated with postural changes.

1.1.5   Identify the metabolic equivalent (MET) requirements of various occupational, household, sport/exercise, and leisure-time activities.

1.1.6   Demonstrate knowledge of the unique hemodynamic responses of arm versus leg exercise, combined arm and leg exercise, and of static versus dynamic exercise.

1.1.7   Define the determinants of myocardial oxygen consumption (i.e., heart rate $\times$ systolic blood pressure = double product OR rate-pressure product) and the effects of acute exercise and exercise training on those determinants.

1.1.8   Describe the methodology for measuring peak oxygen consumption ($\dot{V}O_{2peak}$).

1.1.9   Plot the normal resting and exercise values associated with increasing exercise intensity (and how they may differ for cardiac, pulmonary, and metabolic diseased populations) for the following: heart rate, stroke volume, cardiac output, double product, arteriovenous O_2 difference, O_2 consumption, systolic and diastolic blood pressure, minute ventilation, tidal volume, breathing frequency, Vd/Vt, $\dot{V}_E/\dot{V}O_2$, $\dot{V}_E/\dot{V}CO_2$, $FEV_{1.0}$, SaO_2, and blood glucose.

1.1.10   **Discuss the effects of isometric exercise in individuals with cardiovascular, pulmonary, and/or metabolic diseases.**

1.1.11   **Demonstrate knowledge of acute and chronic adaptations to exercise for those with cardiovascular, pulmonary, and metabolic diseases.**

1.1.12   **Describe the effects of variation in environmental factors (e.g., temperature, humidity, altitude) for normal individuals and those with cardiovascular, pulmonary, and metabolic diseases.**

1.1.13   Understand the hormonal (i.e., insulin, glucagon, epinephrine, norepinephrine, angiotensin, aldosterone, renin, erythropoi-etin) responses to acute and chronic exercise.

1.1.14 Identify normal and abnormal respiratory responses during rest and exercise as assessed during a pulmonary function test (i.e., FVC, MVV, $FEV_{1.0}$, flow volume loop).

GENERAL POPULATION/CORE: PATHOPHYSIOLOGY AND RISK FACTORS

1.2.1 Summarize the atherosclerotic process, including current hypotheses regarding onset and rate of progression and/or regression.

1.2.2 Compare and contrast the differences between typical, atypical, and vasospastic angina and how these may differ in specific subgroups (i.e., men, women, people with diabetes).

1.2.3 Describe the pathophysiology of the healing myocardium and the potential complications after acute myocardial infarction (MI) (remodeling, rupture).

1.2.5 **Examine the role of lifestyle on cardiovascular risk factors, such as hypertension, blood lipids, glucose tolerance, and body weight.**

1.2.6 **Describe the lipoprotein classifications, and define their relationship to atherosclerosis.**

1.2.7 **Describe the resting and exercise cardiorespiratory and metabolic responses in those with pulmonary disease.**

1.2.8 **Describe the influence of exercise on cardiovascular, pulmonary, and metabolic risk factors.**

1.2.11 **Describe the cardiorespiratory and metabolic responses in myocardial dysfunction and ischemia at rest and during exercise.**

1.2.12 Recognize and describe the pathophysiology of the differing severities (e.g., NYHA classification) of heart failure, including cardiac output, heart rate, blood pressure, cardiac dimensions, and basic echocardiography parameters (ejection fraction, wall motion, left ventricular dimension).

1.2.13 Recognize and describe the pathophysiology of diabetes mellitus (prediabetes, types 1 and 2, gestational), including blood glucose, Hb_{A1c}, insulin sensitivity, and the risk and affect on comorbid conditions.

1.2.14 Identify the contributing factors to metabolic syndrome, their pathologic sequelae, and their affect on the primary or secondary risk of cardiovascular disease.

1.2.15 Recognize the pathologic process that various risk factors contribute for the development of cardiac, pulmonary, and metabolic diseases (e.g., smoking, hypertension, abnormal blood lipid values, obesity, inactivity, sex, genetics, diabetes).

GENERAL POPULATION/CORE: HEALTH APPRAISAL, FITNESS, AND CLINICAL EXERCISE TESTING

1.3.1 **Describe common procedures and apply knowledge of results from radionuclide imaging (e.g., thallium, technetium, sestamibi, tetrafosmin, single-photon emission computed tomography [SPECT]), stress echocardiography, and pharmacologic testing (e.g., dobutamine, adenosine, persantine).**

1.3.2 **Demonstrate knowledge of exercise testing procedures for various clinical populations, including those individuals with cardiovascular, pulmonary, and metabolic diseases in terms of exercise modality, protocol, physiologic measurements, and expected outcomes.**

1.3.3 Describe anatomic landmarks as they relate to exercise testing and programming (e.g., electrode placement, blood pressure).

1.3.4 Locate and palpate anatomic landmarks of radial, brachial, carotid, femoral, popliteal, and tibialis arteries.

1.3.5 Select an appropriate test protocol according to the age, functional capacity, physical ability, and health status of the individual.

1.3.6 Identify individuals for whom physician supervision is recommended during maximal and submaximal exercise testing.

1.3.7 Conduct pre-exercise test procedures.

1.3.8 Describe basic equipment and facility requirements for exercise testing.

1.3.9 Instruct the test participant in the use of the RPE scale and other appropriate subjective rating scales, such as the dyspnea, pain, claudication, and angina scales.

1.3.11 Describe the importance of accurate and calibrated testing equipment (e.g., treadmill, ergometers, electrocardiograph [ECG], gas analysis systems, and sphygmomanometers) and demonstrate the ability to recognize and remediate equipment that is no longer properly calibrated.

1.3.12 Obtain and recognize normal and abnormal physiologic and subjective responses (e.g., symptoms, ECG, blood pressure, heart rate, RPE and other scales, oxygen saturation, and oxygen consumption) at appropriate intervals during the test.

1.3.15   Demonstrate the ability to provide testing procedures and protocol for children and the elderly with or without various clinical conditions.

1.3.16   Evaluate medical history and physical examination findings as they relate to health appraisal and exercise testing.

1.3.17   Accurately record and interpret right and left arm pre-exercise blood pressures in the supine and upright positions.

1.3.18   Describe and analyze the importance of the absolute and relative contraindications and test termination indicators of an exercise test.

1.3.19   Select and perform appropriate procedures and protocols for the exercise test, including modes of exercise, starting levels, increments of work, ramping versus incremental protocols, length of stages, and frequency of data collection.

1.3.20   Describe and conduct immediate postexercise procedures and various approaches to cool-down and recognize normal and abnormal responses.

1.3.21   Record, organize, perform, and interpret necessary calculations of test data.

1.3.22   Describe the differences in the physiologic responses to various modes of ergometry (e.g., treadmill, cycle and arm ergometers) as they relate to exercise testing and training.

1.3.23   Describe normal and abnormal chronotropic and inotropic responses to exercise testing and training.

1.3.24   Understand and apply pretest likelihood of CAD, the positive and negative predictive values of various types of stress tests (e.g., ECG only, stress echo, radionuclide), and the potential of false positive/negative and true positive/negative results.

1.3.25   Compare and contrast obstructive and restrictive lung diseases and their effect on exercise testing and training.

1.3.26   Identify orthopedic limitations (e.g., gout, foot drop, specific joint problems, amputation, prosthesis) as they relate to modifications of exercise testing and programming.

1.3.27   Identify basic neuromuscular disorders (e.g., Parkinson's disease, multiple sclerosis) as they relate to modifications of exercise testing and programming.

1.3.28   Describe the aerobic and anaerobic metabolic demands of exercise testing and training in individuals with cardiovascular, pulmonary, and/or metabolic diseases undergoing exercise testing or training.

1.3.29   Identify the variables measured during cardiopulmonary exercise testing (e.g., heart rate, blood pressure, rate of perceived exertion, ventilation, oxygen consumption, ventilatory threshold, pulmonary circulation) and their potential relationship to cardiovascular, pulmonary, and metabolic disease.

1.3.31   Understand the basic principle and methods of coronary calcium scoring using computed-tomography (CT) methods.

1.3.32   Recognize the emergence of new imaging techniques for the assessment of heart disease (e.g., CT angiography).

1.3.33   Recognize the value of heart and lung sounds in the assessment of patients with cardiovascular and/or pulmonary disease.

1.3.34   Demonstrate the ability to perform a six-minute walk test and appropriately use the results to assess prognosis, fitness, and/or improvement.

GENERAL POPULATION/CORE: ELECTROCARDIOGRAPHY AND DIAGNOSTIC TECHNIQUES

1.4.1   Summarize the purpose of coronary angiography.

1.4.2   Describe myocardial ischemia and identify ischemic indicators of various cardiovascular diagnostic tests.

1.4.3   Describe the differences between Q-wave and non-Q-wave infarction, and ST elevation (STEMI) and non-ST elevation myocardial infarction (non-STEMI).

1.4.4   Identify the ECG patterns at rest and responses to exercise in patients with pacemakers and implantable cardiac defibrillators (ICDs). In addition, recognize the ability of biventricular pacing and possibility of pacemaker malfunction (e.g., failure to sense and failure to pace).

1.4.5   Identify resting and exercise ECG changes associated with the following abnormalities: axis; bundle-branch blocks and bifascicular blocks; atrioventricular blocks; sinus bradycardia and tachycardia; sinus arrest; supraventricular premature contractions and tachycardia; ventricular premature contractions (including frequency, form, couplets, salvos, tachycardia); atrial flutter and fibrillation; ventricular fibrillation; myocardial ischemia, injury, and infarction.

1.4.6   Define the ECG criteria for initiating and/or terminating exercise testing or training.

1.4.7 Identify ECG changes that correspond to ischemia in various myocardial regions.

1.4.8 Describe potential causes and pathophysiology of various cardiac arrhythmias.

1.4.9 Identify potentially hazardous arrhythmias or conduction defects observed on the ECG at rest, during exercise, and recovery.

1.4.10 Describe the diagnostic and prognostic significance of ischemic ECG responses and arrhythmias at rest, during exercise, or recovery.

1.4.11 Identify resting and exercise ECG changes associated with cardiovascular disease, hypertensive heart disease, cardiac chamber enlargement, pericarditis, pulmonary disease, and metabolic disorders.

1.4.12 Administer and interpret basic resting spirometric tests and measures, including $FEV_{1.0}$, FVC, and MVV.

1.4.13 Locate the appropriate sites for the limb and chest leads for resting, standard, and exercise (Mason Likar) ECGs, as well as commonly used bipolar systems (e.g., CM-5).

1.4.14 Obtain and interpret a pre-exercise standard and modified (Mason-Likar) 12-lead ECG on a participant in the supine and upright position.

1.4.15 Demonstrate the ability to minimize ECG artifact.

1.4.16 Describe the diagnostic and prognostic implications of the exercise test ECG and hemodynamic responses.

1.4.17 Identify ECG changes that typically occur as a result of hyperventilation, electrolyte abnormalities, and drug therapy.

1.4.18 Identify the causes of false-positive and false-negative exercise ECG responses and methods for optimizing sensitivity and specificity.

1.4.19 Identify and describe the significance of ECG abnormalities in designing the exercise prescription and in making activity recommendations.

GENERAL POPULATION/CORE: PATIENT MANAGEMENT AND MEDICATIONS

1.5.2 Describe mechanisms and actions of medications that may affect exercise testing and prescription (i.e., b-blockers, nitrates, calcium channel blockers, digitalis, diuretics, vasodilators, antiarrhythmic agents, bronchodilators, antilipemics, psychotropics, nicotine, antihistamines, over-the-counter [OTC] cold medications, thyroid medications, alcohol, hypoglycemic agents, blood modifiers, pentoxifylline, antigout medications, and anorexiants/diet pills).

1.5.3 Recognize medications associated in the clinical setting, their indications for care, and their effects at rest and during exercise (i.e., β-blockers, nitrates, calcium channel blockers, digitalis, diuretics, vasodilators, anitarrhythmic agents, bronchodilators, antilipemics, psychotropics, nicotine, antihistamines, OTC cold medications, thyroid medications, alcohol, hypoglycemic agents, blood modifiers, pentoxifylline, antigout medications, and anorexiants/diet pills).

1.5.4 Recognize the use of herbal and nutritional supplements, OTC medications, homeopathic remedies, and other alternative therapies often used by patients with chronic diseases.

1.5.5 Practice disease/case management responsibilities, including daily follow-up concerning patient needs, signs and symptoms, physician appointments, and medication changes for patients with chronic diseases, including cardiovascular, pulmonary, and metabolic diseases; comorbid conditions; arthritis; osteoporosis; and renal dysfunction/transplant/dialysis.

1.5.6 Direct patients actively attempting to lose weight in a formal or informal setting using behavioral, diet, exercise, or surgical methods.

1.5.7 Manage patients on oxygen therapy as needed during exercise testing or training.

1.5.8 Recognize patient clinical need for referral to other (non-ES) allied health professionals (e.g., behavioralist, physical therapist, diabetes educator, nurse).

1.5.9 Recognize patients with chronic pain who may be in a chronic pain management treatment program and who may require special adaptations during exercise testing and training.

1.5.10 Recognize exercise testing and training needs of patients with joint replacement or prosthesis.

1.5.11 Address exercise testing and training needs of elderly and young patients.

1.5.12 Recognize treatment goals and guidelines for hypertension using the most recent JNC report and other relevant evidence-based guidelines.

1.5.13 Recognize treatment goals and guidelines for dyslipidemia using the most recent NCEP report and other relevant evidence-based guidelines.

1.5.14 Demonstrate the ability to perform pulse-oximetry and blood glucose evaluations and appropriately interpret the data in a given clinical situation.

1.5.15   Demonstrate the ability to assess for peripheral edema and other indicators of fluid retention and respond appropriately in a given clinical setting.

GENERAL POPULATION/CORE: MEDICAL AND SURGICAL MANAGEMENT

1.6.1   Describe percutaneous coronary interventions (PCI) and peripheral interventions as an alternative to medical management or bypass surgery.

1.6.2   Describe indications and limitations for medical management and interventional techniques in different subsets of individuals with CAD and peripheral arterial disease (PAD).

1.6.3   Identify risk, benefit, and unique management issues of patients with mechanical, prosthetic valve replacement and valve repair.

1.6.4   Describe and recognize bariatric surgery as a therapy for obesity.

1.6.5   Recognize external counterpulsation (ECP) as a method of treating severe, difficult-to-treat chest pain (i.e., angina).

GENERAL POPULATION/CORE: EXERCISE PRESCRIPTION AND PROGRAMMING

1.7.2   Compare and contrast benefits and risks of exercise for individuals with risk factors for or established cardiovascular, pulmonary, and/or metabolic diseases.

1.7.3   Design appropriate exercise prescription in environmental extremes for those with cardiovascular, pulmonary, and metabolic diseases.

1.7.4   Design, implement, and supervise individualized exercise prescriptions for people with chronic disease and disabling conditions or for people who are young or elderly.

1.7.5   Design a supervised exercise program beginning at hospital discharge and continuing for up to six months for the following conditions: MI; angina: left ventricular assist device (LVAD); congestive heart failure; PCI; coronary artery bypass graft (surgery) (CABG[S]); medical management of CAD; chronic pulmonary disease; weight management; diabetes; metabolic syndrome; and cardiac transplants.

1.7.6   Demonstrate knowledge of the concept of activities of daily living (ADLs) and its importance in the overall rehabilitation of the individual.

1.7.7   Prescribe exercise using nontraditional modalities (e.g., bench stepping, elastic bands, isodynamic exercise, water aerobics, yoga, tai chi) for individuals with cardiovascular, pulmonary, or metabolic diseases.

1.7.8   Demonstrate exercise equipment adaptations necessary for different age groups, physical abilities, and other potential contributing factors.

1.7.9   Identify patients who require a symptom-limited exercise test before exercise training.

1.7.10   Organize graded exercise tests and clinical data to counsel patients regarding issues such as ADL, return to work, and physical activity.

1.7.11   Describe relative and absolute contraindications to exercise training.

1.7.12   Identify characteristics that correlate or predict poor compliance to exercise programs and strategies to increase exercise adherence.

1.7.13   Describe the importance of warm-up and cool-down sessions with specific reference to angina and ischemic ECG changes, and for overall patient safety.

1.7.14   Identify and explain the mechanisms by which exercise may contribute to reducing disease risk or rehabilitating individuals with cardiovascular, pulmonary, and metabolic diseases.

1.7.15   Describe common gait, movement, and coordination abnormalities as they relate to exercise testing and programming.

1.7.16   Describe the principle of specificity as it relates to the mode of exercise testing and training.

1.7.17   Design strength and flexibility programs for individuals with cardiovascular, pulmonary, and/or metabolic diseases; the elderly; and children.

1.7.18   Determine appropriate testing and training modalities according to the age, functional capacity, physical ability, and health status of the individual.

1.7.19   Describe the indications and methods for ECG monitoring during exercise testing and training.

1.7.20   Discuss the appropriate use of static and dynamic resistance exercise for individuals with cardiovascular, pulmonary, and metabolic disease.

1.7.21   Demonstrate the ability to modify exercise testing and training to the limitations of PAD.

1.7.22 Design, describe, and demonstrate specific resistance exercises for major muscle groups for patients with cardiovascular, pulmonary, and metabolic diseases and conditions.

1.7.23 Identify procedures for pre-exercise assessment of blood glucose, determining safety for exercise, and avoidance of exercise-induced hypoglycemia in patients with diabetes. Manage postexercise hypoglycemia when it occurs.

GENERAL POPULATION/CORE: NUTRITION AND WEIGHT MANAGEMENT

1.8.1 Describe and discuss dietary considerations for cardiovascular and pulmonary diseases, chronic heart failure, and diabetes that are recommended to minimize disease progression and optimize disease management.

1.8.2 Compare and contrast dietary practices used for weight reduction, and address the benefits, risks, and scientific support for each practice. Examples of dietary practices are high-protein/low-carbohydrate diets, Mediterranean diet, and low-fat diets, such as the American Heart Association recommended diet.

1.8.3 Calculate the effect of caloric intake and energy expenditure on weight management.

1.8.4 Describe the hypotheses related to diet, weight gain, and weight loss.

1.8.5 Demonstrate the ability to differentiate and educate patients between nutritionally sound diets versus fad diets and scientifically supported supplements and anecdotally supported supplements.

1.8.6 Differentiate among and understand the value of the various vegetarian diets (i.e., Ovo-lacto, vegan).

GENERAL POPULATION/CORE: HUMAN BEHAVIOR AND COUNSELING

1.9.1 List and apply behavioral strategies that apply to lifestyle modifications, such as exercise, diet, stress, and medication management.

1.9.2 Describe signs and symptoms of maladjustment and/or failure to cope during an illness crisis and/or personal adjustment crisis (e.g., job loss) that might prompt a psychological consult or referral to other professional services.

1.9.3 Describe the general principles of crisis management and factors influencing coping and learning in illness states.

1.9.4 Identify the psychological stages involved with the acceptance of death and dying and demonstrate the ability to recognize when it is necessary for a psychological consult or referral to a professional resource.

1.9.5 Recognize observable signs and symptoms of anxiety or depressive symptoms and the need for a psychiatric referral.

1.9.6 Describe the psychological issues to be confronted by the patient and by family members of patients who have cardiovascular or pulmonary disease or diseases of the metabolic syndrome.

1.9.7 Identify the psychological issues associated with an acute cardiac event versus those associated with chronic cardiac conditions.

1.9.8 Recognize and implement methods of stress management for patients with chronic disease.

1.9.9 Use common assessment tools to access behavioral change, such as the Transtheoretical Model.

1.9.10 Facilitate effective and contemporary motivational and behavior modification techniques to promote behavioral change.

1.9.11 Demonstrate the ability to conduct effective and informative group and individual education sessions directed at primary or secondary prevention of chronic disease.

GENERAL POPULATION/CORE: SAFETY, INJURY PREVENTION, AND EMERGENCY PROCEDURES

1.10.1 Respond appropriately to emergency situations (e.g., cardiac arrest, hypoglycemia and hyperglycemia; bronchospasm; sudden onset hypotension; severe hypertensive response; angina; serious cardiac arrhythmias; ICD discharge; transient ischemic attack [TIA] or stroke; MI) that might arise before, during, and after administration of an exercise test and/or exercise session.

1.10.2 List medications that should be available for emergency situations in exercise testing and training sessions.

1.10.3 Describe the emergency equipment and personnel that should be present in an exercise testing laboratory and rehabilitative exercise training setting.

1.10.4 Describe the appropriate procedures for maintaining emergency equipment and supplies.

1.10.5 Describe the effects of cardiovascular and pulmonary disease and the diseases of the

metabolic syndrome on performance of and safety during exercise testing and training.

1.10.6 **Stratify individuals with cardiovascular, pulmonary, and metabolic diseases, using appropriate risk-stratification methods and understanding the prognostic indicators for high-risk individuals.**

1.10.7 Describe the process for developing and updating emergency policies and procedures (e.g., call 911, call code team, call medical director, transport and use defibrillator).

1.10.8 Be aware of the current CPR, AED, and ACLS standards to be able to assist with emergency situations.

GENERAL POPULATION/CORE: PROGRAM ADMINISTRATION, QUALITY ASSURANCE, AND OUTCOME ASSESSMENT

1.11.1 **Discuss the role of outcome measures in chronic disease management programs, such as cardiovascular and pulmonary rehabilitation programs.**

1.11.2 Identify and discuss various outcome measurements used in a cardiac or pulmonary rehabilitation program.

1.11.3 Use specific outcome collection instruments to collect outcome data in a cardiac or pulmonary rehabilitation program.

1.11.4 **Understand the most recent cardiac and pulmonary rehabilitation Centers for Medicare Services (CMS) rules for patient enrollment and reimbursement (e.g., diagnostic current procedure terminology [CPT] codes, diagnostic related groups [DRG]).**

ACSM REGISTERED CLINICAL EXERCISE PHYSIOLOGIST KNOWLEDGE, SKILLS AND ABILITIES (KSAs)

The Registered Clinical Exercise Physiologist® is responsible for the mastery of the ACSM Certified Personal Trainer^{SM} KSAs, the ACSM Certified Health Fitness Specialist KSAs, the ACSM Certified Clinical Exercise Specialist KSAs, and the following ACSM Registered Clinical Exercise Physiologist® KSAs:

GENERAL POPULATION/CORE: EXERCISE PHYSIOLOGY AND RELATED EXERCISE SCIENCE

1.1.1 Describe the acute responses to aerobic, resistance, and flexibility training on the function of the cardiovascular, respiratory, musculoskeletal, neuromuscular, metabolic, endocrine, and immune systems.

1.1.2 Describe the chronic effects of aerobic, resistance, and flexibility training on the structure and function of the cardiovascular, respiratory, musculoskeletal, neuromuscular, metabolic, endocrine, and immune systems.

1.1.3 Explain differences in typical values between sedentary and trained persons in those with chronic diseases for oxygen uptake, heart rate, mean arterial pressure, systolic and diastolic blood pressure, cardiac output, stroke volume, rate pressure product, minute ventilation, respiratory rate, and tidal volume at rest and during submaximal and maximal exercise.

1.1.4 Describe the physiologic determinants of $\dot{V}O_2$, $m\dot{V}O_2$, and mean arterial pressure and explain how these determinants may be altered with aerobic and resistance exercise training.

1.1.5 Describe appropriate modifications in the exercise prescription that are due to environmental conditions in individuals with chronic disease.

1.1.6 Explain the health benefits of a physically active lifestyle, the hazards of sedentary behavior, and summarize key recommendations of U.S. national reports of physical activity (e.g., U.S. Surgeon General, Institute of Medicine, ACSM, AHA).

1.1.7 Explain the physiologic adaptations to exercise training that may result in improvement in or maintenance of health, including cardiovascular, pulmonary, metabolic, orthopedic/musculoskeletal, neuromuscular, and immune system health.

1.1.8 Explain the mechanisms underlying the physiologic adaptations to aerobic and resistance training, including those resulting in changes in or maintenance of maximal and submaximal oxygen consumption, lactate and ventilatory (anaerobic) threshold, myocardial oxygen consumption, heart rate, blood pressure, ventilation (including ventilatory threshold), muscle structure, bioenergetics, and immune function.

1.1.9 Explain the physiologic effects of physical inactivity, including bed rest, and methods that may counteract these effects.

1.1.10 Recognize and respond to abnormal signs and symptoms during exercise.

GENERAL POPULATION/CORE: PATHOPHYSIOLOGY AND RISK FACTORS

1.2.1 Describe the epidemiology, pathophysiology, risk factors, and key clinical findings of cardiovascular, pulmonary, metabolic, ortho-pedic/musculoskeletal, neuromuscular, and NIH diseases.

GENERAL POPULATION/CORE: HEALTH APPRAISAL, FITNESS, AND CLINICAL EXERCISE TESTING

1.3.1　Conduct pretest procedures, including explaining test procedures, obtaining informed consent, obtaining a focused medical history, reviewing results of prior tests and physical exam, assessing disease-specific risk factors, and presenting concise information to other healthcare providers and third-party payers.

1.3.2　Conduct a brief physical examination including evaluation of peripheral edema, measuring blood pressure, peripheral pulses, respiratory rate, and ausculating heart and lung sounds.

1.3.3　Calibrate lab equipment used frequently in the practice of clinical exercise physiology (e.g., motorized/computerized treadmill, mechanical cycle ergometer and arm ergometer), electrocardiograph, spirometer, respiratory gas analyzer (metabolic cart).

1.3.4　Administer exercise tests consistent with U.S. nationally accepted standards for testing.

1.3.5　Evaluate contraindications to exercise testing.

1.3.6　Appropriately select and administer functional tests to measure individual outcomes and functional status, including the six-minute walk, Get Up and Go, Berg Balance Scale, and the Physical Performance Test.

1.3.8　Interpret the variables that may be assessed during clinical exercise testing, including maximal oxygen consumption, resting metabolic rate, ventilatory volumes and capacities, respiratory exchange ratio, ratings of perceived exertion and discomfort (chest pain, dyspnea, claudication), ECG, heart rate, blood pressure, rate pressure product, ventilatory (anaerobic) threshold, oxygen saturation, breathing reserve, muscular strength, muscular endurance, and other common measures employed for diagnosis and prognosis of disease.

1.3.9　Determine atrial and ventricular rate from rhythm strip and 12-lead ECG and explain the clinical significance of abnormal atrial or ventricular rate (e.g., tachycardia, bradycardia).

1.3.10　Identify ECG changes associated with drug therapy, electrolyte abnormalities, subendocardial and transmural ischemia, myocardial injury, and infarction, and explain the clinical significance of each.

1.3.11　Identify SA, AV, and bundle-branch blocks from a rhythm strip and 12-lead ECG, and explain the clinical significance of each.

1.3.12　Identify sinus, atrial, junctional, and ventricular dysrhythmias from a rhythm strip and 12-lead ECG, and explain the clinical significance of each.

1.3.14　Determine an individual's pretest and posttest probability of coronary heart disease, identify factors associated with test complications, and apply appropriate precautions to reduce risks to the individual.

1.3.16　Identify probable disease-specific endpoints for testing in an individual with cardiovascular, pulmonary, metabolic, orthopedic/musculoskeletal, neuromuscular, and NIH disease.

1.3.17　Select and employ appropriate techniques for preparation and measurement of ECG, heart rate, blood pressure, oxygen saturation, RPE, symptoms, expired gases, and other measures as needed before, during, and following exercise testing.

1.3.18　Select and administer appropriate exercise tests to evaluate functional capacity, strength, and flexibility in individuals with cardiovascular, pulmonary, metabolic, orthopedic/musculoskeletal, neuromuscular, and NIH disease.

1.3.19　Discuss strengths and limitations of various methods of measures and indices of body composition.

1.3.20　Appropriately select, apply, and interpret body-composition tests and indices.

1.3.21　Discuss pertinent test results with other healthcare professionals.

GENERAL POPULATION/CORE: EXERCISE PRESCRIPTION AND PROGRAMMING

1.7.3　Determine the appropriate level of supervision and monitoring recommended for individuals with known disease based on disease-specific risk-stratification guidelines and current health status.

1.7.4　Develop, adapt, and supervise appropriate aerobic, resistance, and flexibility training for individuals with cardiovascular, pulmonary, metabolic, orthopedic/musculoskeletal, neuromuscular, and NIH disease.

1.7.6   Instruct individuals with cardiovascular, pulmonary, metabolic, orthopedic/musculoskeletal, neuromuscular, and NIH disease in techniques for performing physical activities safely and effectively in an unsupervised exercise setting.

1.7.7   Modify the exercise prescription or discontinue exercise based on individual symptoms, current health status, musculoskeletal limitations, and environmental considerations.

1.7.8   Extract and interpret clinical information needed for safe exercise management of individuals with cardiovascular, pulmonary, metabolic, orthopedic/musculoskeletal, neuromuscular, and NIH disease.

1.7.9   Evaluate individual outcomes from serial outcome data collected before, during, and after exercise interventions.

GENERAL POPULATION/CORE: HUMAN BEHAVIOR AND COUNSELING

1.9.1   Summarize contemporary theories of health behavior change, including social cognitive theory, theory of reasoned action, theory of planned behavior, transtheoretical model, and health belief model. Apply techniques to promote healthy behaviors, including physical activity.

1.9.2   Describe characteristics associated with poor adherence to exercise programs.

1.9.3   Describe the psychological issues associated with acute and chronic illness, such as anxiety, depression, social isolation, hostility, aggression, and suicidal ideation.

1.9.4   Counsel individuals with cardiovascular, pulmonary, metabolic, orthopedic/musculoskeletal, neuromuscular, and NIH disease on topics such as disease processes, treatments, diagnostic techniques, and lifestyle management.

1.9.6   Explain factors that may increase anxiety before or during exercise testing, and describe methods to reduce anxiety.

1.9.7   Recognize signs and symptoms of failure to cope during personal crises such as job loss, bereavement, and illness.

GENERAL POPULATION/CORE: SAFETY, INJURY PREVENTION, AND EMERGENCY PROCEDURES

1.10.1   List routine emergency equipment, drugs, and supplies present in an exercise testing laboratory and therapeutic exercise session area.

1.10.2   Provide immediate responses to emergencies, including basic cardiac life support, AED, activation of emergency medical services, and joint immobilization.

1.10.3   Verify operating status of emergency equipment, including defibrillator, laryngoscope, and oxygen.

1.10.4   Explain universal precautions procedures and apply as appropriate.

1.10.5   Develop and implement a plan for responding to emergencies.

1.10.6   Demonstrate knowledge of advanced cardiac life support procedures.

GENERAL POPULATION/CORE: PROGRAM ADMINISTRATION, QUALITY ASSURANCE, AND OUTCOME ASSESSMENT

1.11.1   Describe appropriate staffing for exercise testing and programming based on factors such as individual health status, facilities, and program goals.

1.11.2   List necessary equipment and supplies for exercise testing and programs.

1.11.3   Select, evaluate, and report treatment outcomes using individual-relevant results of tests and surveys.

1.11.4   Explain legal issues pertinent to healthcare delivery by licensed and nonlicensed healthcare professionals providing rehabilitative services and exercise testing and legal risk-management techniques.

1.11.5   Identify individuals requiring referral to a physician or allied health services such as physical therapy, dietary counseling, stress management, weight management, and psychological and social services.

1.11.6   Develop a plan for individual discharge from therapeutic exercise program, including community referrals.

CARDIOVASCULAR: EXERCISE PHYSIOLOGY AND RELATED EXERCISE SCIENCE

2.1.2   Describe the potential benefits and hazards of aerobic, resistance, and flexibility training in individuals with cardiovascular diseases.

2.1.4   Explain how cardiovascular diseases may affect the physiologic responses to aerobic and resistance training.

2.1.5   Describe the immediate and long-term influence of medical therapies for cardiovascular diseases on the responses to aerobic and resistance training.

CARDIOVASCULAR: PATHOPHYSIOLOGY AND RISK FACTORS

2.2.1   Describe the epidemiology, pathophysiology, rate of progression of disease, risk factors, and key clinical findings of cardiovascular diseases.

2.2.2   Explain the ischemic cascade and its effect on myocardial function.

2.2.4   Explain methods of reducing risk in individuals with cardiovascular diseases.

CARDIOVASCULAR: HEALTH APPRAISAL, FITNESS, AND CLINICAL EXERCISE TESTING

2.3.1   Describe common techniques used to diagnose cardiovascular disease, including graded exercise testing, echocardiography, radionuclide imaging, angiography, pharmacologic testing, and biomarkers (e.g., troponin, CK), and explain the indications, limitations, risks, and normal and abnormal results for each.

2.3.2   Explain how cardiovascular disease may affect physical examination findings.

2.3.4   Recognize and respond to abnormal signs and symptoms—such as pain, peripheral edema, dyspnea, and fatigue—in individuals with cardiovascular diseases.

2.3.5   Conduct and interpret appropriate exercise testing methods for individuals with cardiovascular diseases.

CARDIOVASCULAR: MEDICAL AND SURGICAL MANAGEMENT

2.6.2   Explain the common medical and surgical treatments of cardiovascular diseases.

2.6.3   Apply key recommendations of current U.S. clinical practice guidelines for the prevention, treatment, and management of cardiovascular diseases (e.g., AHA, ACC, NHLBI).

2.6.4   List the commonly used drugs (generic and brand names) in the treatment of individuals with cardiovascular diseases, and explain the indications, mechanisms of actions, major side effects, and the effects on the exercising individual.

2.6.5   Explain how treatments for cardiovascular disease, including preventive care, may affect the rate of progression of disease.

CARDIOVASCULAR: EXERCISE PRESCRIPTION AND PROGRAMMING

2.7.2   Design, adapt, and supervise an appropriate Exercise Prescription (e.g., aerobic, resistance, and flexibility training) for individuals with cardiovascular diseases.

2.7.4   Instruct an individual with cardiovascular disease in techniques for performing physical activities safely and effectively in an unsupervised setting.

2.7.5   Counsel individuals with cardiovascular disease on the proper uses of sublingual nitroglycerin.

PULMONARY (e.g., OBSTRUCTIVE AND RESTRICTIVE LUNG DISEASES): EXERCISE PHYSIOLOGY AND RELATED EXERCISE SCIENCE

3.1.1   Describe the potential benefits and hazards of aerobic, resistance, and flexibility training in individuals with pulmonary diseases.

3.1.2   Explain how pulmonary diseases may affect the physiologic responses to aerobic, resistance, and flexibility training.

3.1.3   Explain how scheduling of exercise relative to meals can affect dyspnea.

3.1.5   Describe the immediate and long-term influence of medical therapies for pulmonary diseases on the responses to aerobic, resistance, and flexibility training.

PULMONARY: PATHOPHYSIOLOGY AND RISK FACTORS

3.2.1   Describe the epidemiology, pathophysiology, rate of progression of disease, risk factors, and key clinical findings of pulmonary diseases.

3.2.3   Explain methods of reducing risk in individuals with pulmonary diseases.

PULMONARY: HEALTH APPRAISAL, FITNESS, AND CLINICAL EXERCISE TESTING

3.3.1   Explain how pulmonary disease may affect physical examination findings.

3.3.3   Demonstrate knowledge of lung volumes and capacities (e.g., tidal volume, residual volume, inspiratory volume, expiratory volume, total lung capacity, vital capacity, functional residual capacity, peak flow rate, diffusion capacity) and how they may differ between normals and individuals with pulmonary disease.

3.3.4   Recognize and respond to abnormal signs and symptoms to exercise in individuals with pulmonary diseases.

3.3.5   Describe common techniques and tests used to diagnose pulmonary diseases, and explain the indications, limitations, risks, and normal and abnormal results for each.

3.3.6   Conduct and interpret appropriate exercise testing methods for individuals with pulmonary diseases.

PULMONARY: MEDICAL AND SURGICAL MANAGEMENT

3.6.3   Explain how treatments for pulmonary disease, including preventive care, may affect the rate of progression of disease.

3.6.5   Explain the common medical and surgical treatments of pulmonary diseases.

3.6.6   List the commonly used drugs (generic and brand names) in the treatment of individuals with pulmonary diseases, and explain the indications, mechanisms of actions, major side effects, and the effects on the exercising individual.

3.6.7   Apply key recommendations of current U.S. clinical practice guidelines (e.g., ALA, NIH, NHLBI) for the prevention, treatment, and management of pulmonary diseases.

PULMONARY: EXERCISE PRESCRIPTION AND PROGRAMMING

3.7.2   Design, adapt, and supervise an appropriate exercise prescription (e.g., aerobic, resistance, and flexibility training) for individuals with pulmonary diseases.

3.7.4   Instruct an individual with pulmonary diseases in proper breathing techniques and exercises and methods for performing physical activities safely and effectively.

3.7.5   Demonstrate knowledge of the use of supplemental oxygen during exercise and its influences on exercise tolerance.

METABOLIC (e.g., DIABETES, HYPERLIPIDEMIA, OBESITY, FRAILTY, CHRONIC RENAL FAILURE, METABOLIC SYNDROME):

EXERCISE PHYSIOLOGY AND RELATED EXERCISE SCIENCE

4.1.1   Explain how metabolic diseases may affect aerobic endurance, muscular strength and endurance, flexibility, and balance.

4.1.2   Describe the immediate and long-term influence of medical therapies for metabolic diseases on the responses to aerobic, resistance, and flexibility training.

4.1.3   Describe the potential benefits and hazards of aerobic, resistance, and flexibility training in individuals with metabolic diseases.

METABOLIC: PATHOPHYSIOLOGY AND RISK FACTORS

4.2.1   Describe the epidemiology, pathophysiology, rate of progression of disease, risk factors, and key clinical findings of metabolic diseases.

4.2.5   Describe the probable effects of dialysis treatment on exercise performance, functional capacity, and safety, and explain methods for preventing adverse effects.

4.2.6   Describe the probable effects of hypo/hyperglycemia on exercise performance, functional capacity, and safety, and explain methods for preventing adverse effects.

4.2.7   Explain methods of reducing risk in individuals with metabolic diseases.

METABOLIC: HEALTH APPRAISAL, FITNESS, AND CLINICAL EXERCISE TESTING

4.3.1   Describe common techniques and tests used to diagnose metabolic diseases, and explain the indications, limitations, risks, and normal and abnormal results for each.

4.3.3   Explain appropriate techniques for monitoring blood glucose before, during, and after an exercise session.

4.3.4   Recognize and respond to abnormal signs and symptoms in individuals with metabolic diseases.

4.3.5   Conduct and interpret appropriate exercise testing methods for individuals with metabolic diseases.

METABOLIC: MEDICAL AND SURGICAL MANAGEMENT

4.6.2   Apply key recommendations of current U.S. clinical practice guidelines (e.g., ADA, NIH, NHLBI) for the prevention, treatment, and management of metabolic diseases.

4.6.3   Explain the common medical and surgical treatments of metabolic diseases.

4.6.4   List the commonly used drugs (generic and brand names) in the treatment of individuals with metabolic diseases, and explain the indications, mechanisms of actions, major side effects, and the effects on the exercising individual.

4.6.5   Explain how treatments for metabolic diseases, including preventive care, may affect the rate of progression of disease.

METABOLIC: EXERCISE PRESCRIPTION AND PROGRAMMING

4.7.2   Design, adapt, and supervise an appropriate exercise prescription (e.g., aerobic, resistance, and flexibility training) for individuals with metabolic diseases.

4.7.4   Instruct individuals with metabolic diseases in techniques for performing physical activities safely and effectively in an unsupervised exercise setting.

4.7.5   Adapt the exercise prescription based on the functional limits and benefits of assistive devices (e.g., wheelchairs, crutches, and canes).

ORTHOPEDIC/MUSCULOSKELETAL (e.g., LOW BACK PAIN, OSTEOARTHRITIS, RHEUMATOID ARTHRITIS, OSTEOPOROSIS, AMPUTATIONS, VERTEBRAL DISORDERS): EXERCISE PHYSIOLOGY AND RELATED EXERCISE SCIENCE

5.1.1   Describe the potential benefits and hazards of aerobic, resistance, and flexibility training in individuals with orthopedic/musculoskeletal diseases.

5.1.4   Explain how orthopedic/musculoskeletal diseases may affect aerobic endurance, muscular strength and endurance, flexibility, balance, and agility.

5.1.5   Describe the immediate and long-term influence of medical therapies for orthopedic/musculoskeletal diseases on the responses to aerobic, resistance, and flexibility training.

ORTHOPEDIC/MUSCULOSKELETAL: PATHOPHYSIOLOGY AND RISK FACTORS

5.2.1   Describe the epidemiology, pathophysiology, risk factors, and key clinical findings of orthopedic/musculoskeletal diseases.

ORTHOPEDIC/MUSCULOSKELETAL: HEALTH APPRAISAL, FITNESS, AND CLINICAL EXERCISE TESTING

5.3.1   Recognize and respond to abnormal signs and symptoms to exercise in individuals with orthopedic/musculoskeletal diseases.

5.3.2   Describe common techniques and tests used to diagnose orthopedic/musculoskeletal diseases.

5.3.3   Conduct and interpret appropriate exercise testing methods for individuals with orthopedic/musculoskeletal diseases.

ORTHOPEDIC/MUSCULOSKELETAL: MEDICAL AND SURGICAL MANAGEMENT

5.6.1   List the commonly used drugs (generic and brand names) in the treatment of individuals with orthopedic/musculoskeletal diseases, and explain the indications, mechanisms of actions, major side effects, and the effects on the exercising individual.

5.6.2   Explain the common medical and surgical treatments of orthopedic/ musculoskeletal diseases.

5.6.3   Apply key recommendations of current U.S. clinical practice guidelines (e.g., NIH, National Osteoporosis Foundation, Arthritis Foundation) for the prevention, treatment, and management of orthopedic/musculoskeletal diseases.

5.6.4   Explain how treatments for orthopedic/musculoskeletal disease may affect the rate of progression of disease.

ORTHOPEDIC/MUSCULOSKELETAL: EXERCISE PRESCRIPTION AND PROGRAMMING

5.7.1   Explain exercise training concepts specific to industrial or occupational rehabilitation, which includes work hardening, work conditioning, work fitness, and job coaching.

5.7.2   Design, adapt, and supervise an appropriate exercise prescription (e.g., aerobic, resistance, and flexibility training) for individuals with orthopedic/musculoskeletal diseases.

5.7.3   Instruct an individual with orthopedic/musculoskeletal disease in techniques for performing physical activities safely and effectively in an unsupervised exercise setting.

5.7.4   Adapt the exercise prescription based on the functional limits and benefits of assistive devices (e.g., wheelchairs, crutches, and canes).

NEUROMUSCULAR (e.g., MULTIPLE SCLEROSIS, MUSCULAR DYSTROPHY AND OTHER MYOPATHIES, ALZHEIMER DISEASE, PARKINSON DISEASE, POLIO AND POSTPOLIO SYNDROME, STROKE AND BRAIN INJURY, CEREBRAL PALSY, PERIPHERAL NEUROPATHIES): EXERCISE PHYSIOLOGY AND RELATED EXERCISE SCIENCE

6.1.1   Describe the potential benefits and hazards of aerobic, resistance, and flexibility training in individuals with neuromuscular diseases.

6.1.4   Explain how neuromuscular diseases may affect aerobic endurance, muscular strength and endurance, flexibility, balance, and agility.

6.1.5   Describe the immediate and long-term influence of medical therapies for neuromuscular diseases on the responses to aerobic, resistance, and flexibility training.

NEUROMUSCULAR: PATHOPHYSIOLOGY AND RISK FACTORS

6.2.1   Describe the epidemiology, pathophysiology, risk factors, and key clinical findings of neuromuscular diseases.

NEUROMUSCULAR: HEALTH APPRAISAL, FITNESS, AND CLINICAL EXERCISE TESTING

6.3.1   Recognize and respond to abnormal signs and symptoms to exercise in individuals with neuromuscular diseases.

6.3.2   Describe common techniques and tests used to diagnose neuromuscular diseases.

6.3.3   Conduct and interpret appropriate exercise testing methods for individuals with neuromuscular diseases.

NEUROMUSCULAR: MEDICAL AND SURGICAL MANAGEMENT

6.6.1   Explain the common medical and surgical treatments of neuromuscular diseases.

6.6.2   List the commonly used drugs (generic and brand names) in the treatment of individuals with neuromuscular disease, and explain the indications, mechanisms of actions, major side effects, and the effects on the exercising individual.

6.6.3   Apply key recommendations of current U.S. clinical practice guidelines (e.g., NIH) for the prevention, treatment, and management of neuromuscular diseases.

6.6.4   Explain how treatments for neuromuscular disease may affect the rate of progression of disease.

NEUROMUSCULAR: EXERCISE PRESCRIPTION AND PROGRAMMING

6.7.1   Adapt the exercise prescription based on the functional limits and benefits of assistive devices (e.g., wheelchairs, crutches, and canes).

6.7.3   Design, adapt, and supervise an appropriate exercise prescription (e.g., aerobic, resistance, and flexibility training) for individuals with neuromuscular diseases.

6.7.4   Instruct an individual with neuromuscular diseases in techniques for performing physical activities safely and effectively in an unsupervised exercise setting.

NEOPLASTIC, IMMUNOLOGIC, AND HEMATOLOGIC (e.g., CANCER, ANEMIA, BLEEDING DISORDERS, HIV, AIDS, ORGAN TRANSPLANT, CHRONIC FATIGUE SYNDROME, FIBROMYALGIA): EXERCISE PHYSIOLOGY AND RELATED EXERCISE SCIENCE

7.1.1   Explain how NIH diseases may affect the physiologic responses to aerobic, resistance, and flexibility training.

7.1.2   Describe the immediate and long-term influence of medical therapies for NIH on the responses to aerobic, resistance, and flexibility training.

7.1.3   Describe the potential benefits and hazards of aerobic, resistance, and flexibility training in individuals with NIH diseases.

NEOPLASTIC, IMMUNOLOGIC, AND HEMATOLOGIC: PATHOPHYSIOLOGY AND RISK FACTORS

7.2.1   Describe the epidemiology, pathophysiology, risk factors, and key clinical findings of NIH diseases.

NEOPLASTIC, IMMUNOLOGIC, AND HEMATOLOGIC: HEALTH APPRAISAL, FITNESS, AND CLINICAL EXERCISE TESTING

7.3.1   Recognize and respond to abnormal signs and symptoms to exercise in individuals with NIH diseases.

7.3.2   Describe common techniques and tests used to diagnose NIH diseases.

7.3.3   Conduct and interpret appropriate exercise testing methods for individuals with NIH diseases.

NEOPLASTIC, IMMUNOLOGIC, AND HEMATOLOGIC: MEDICAL AND SURGICAL MANAGEMENT

7.6.1   List the commonly used drugs (generic and brand names) in the treatment of individuals with NIH disease, and explain the indications, mechanisms of actions, major side effects, and the effects on the exercising individual.

7.6.2   Apply key recommendations of current U.S. clinical practice guidelines (e.g., ACS, NIH) for the prevention, treatment, and management of NIH diseases.

7.6.3   Explain the common medical and surgical treatments of NIH diseases.

7.6.4   Explain how treatments for NIH disease may affect the rate of progression of disease.

NEOPLASTIC, IMMUNOLOGIC, AND HEMATOLOGIC: EXERCISE PRESCRIPTION AND PROGRAMMING

7.7.1   Design, adapt, and supervise an appropriate exercise prescription (e.g., aerobic, resistance, and flexibility training) for individuals with NIH diseases.

7.7.4   Instruct an individual with NIH diseases in techniques for performing physical activities safely and effectively in an unsupervised exercise setting.

NOTE: The KSAs listed above for the ACSM Registered Clinical Exercise Physiologist® are the same KSAs for educational programs in clinical exercise physiology seeking graduate (master's degree) academic accreditation through the CoAES. For more information, please visit www.coaes.org.

Additional KSAs required (in addition to the ACSM Certified Health Fitness Specialist KSAs) for programs seeking academic accreditation in applied exercise physiology. The KSAs that follow, IN ADDITION TO the ACSM Certified Health Fitness Specialist KSAs above, represent the KSAs for educational programs in applied exercise physiology seeking graduate (master's degree) academic accreditation through the CoAES. For more information, please visit www.coaes.org.

GENERAL POPULATION/CORE: EXERCISE PHYSIOLOGY AND RELATED EXERCISE SCIENCE

1.1.1   Ability to describe modifications in exercise prescription for individuals with functional disabilities and musculoskeletal injuries.

1.1.2   Ability to describe the relationship between biomechanical efficiency, oxygen cost of activity (economy), and performance of physical activity.

1.1.3   Knowledge of the muscular, cardiorespiratory, and metabolic responses to decreased exercise intensity.

GENERAL POPULATION/CORE: PATHOPHYSIOLOGY AND RISK FACTORS

1.2.1   Ability to define atherosclerosis, the factors causing it, and the interventions that may

potentially delay or reverse the atherosclerotic process.

1.2.2   Ability to describe the causes of myocardial ischemia and infarction.

1.2.3   Ability to describe the pathophysiology of hypertension, obesity, hyperlipidemia, diabetes, chronic obstructive pulmonary diseases, arthritis, osteoporosis, chronic diseases, and immunosuppressive disease.

1.2.4   Ability to describe the effects of the above diseases and conditions on cardiorespiratory and metabolic function at rest and during exercise.

GENERAL POPULATION/CORE: HEALTH APPRAISAL, FITNESS, AND CLINICAL EXERCISE TESTING

1.3.1   Knowledge of the selection of an appropriate behavioral goal and the suggested method to evaluate goal achievement for each stage of change.

1.3.2   Knowledge of the use and value of the results of the fitness evaluation and exercise test for various populations.

1.3.3   Ability to design and implement a fitness testing/health appraisal program that includes, but is not limited to, staffing needs, physician interaction, documentation, equipment, marketing, and program evaluation.

1.3.4   Ability to recruit, train, and evaluate appropriate staff personnel for performing exercise tests, fitness evaluations, and health appraisals.

GENERAL POPULATION/CORE: PATIENT MANAGEMENT AND MEDICATIONS

1.5.1   Ability to identify and describe the principal action, mechanisms of action, and major side effects from each of the following classes of medications: antianginals, antihypertensives, antiarrhythmics, bronchodilators, hypoglycemics, psychotropics, and vasodilators.

GENERAL POPULATION/CORE: HUMAN BEHAVIOR AND COUNSELING

1.9.1   Knowledge of and ability to apply basic cognitive-behavioral intervention, such as shaping, goal setting, motivation, cueing, problem solving, reinforcement strategies, and self-monitoring.

1.9.2   Knowledge of the selection of an appropriate behavioral goal and the suggested method to evaluate goal achievement for each stage of change.

GENERAL POPULATION/CORE: SAFETY, INJURY PREVENTION, AND EMERGENCY PROCEDURES

1.10.1   Ability to identify the process to train the exercise staff in cardiopulmonary resuscitation.

1.10.2   Ability to design and evaluate emergency procedures for a preventive exercise program and an exercise testing facility.

1.10.3   Ability to train staff in safety procedures, risk-reduction strategies, and injury-care techniques.

1.10.4   Knowledge of the legal implications of documented safety procedures, the use of incident documents, and ongoing safety training.

GENERAL POPULATION/CORE: PROGRAM ADMINISTRATION, QUALITY ASSURANCE, AND OUTCOME ASSESSMENT

1.11.1   Ability to manage personnel effectively.

1.11.2   Ability to describe a management plan for the development of staff, continuing education, marketing and promotion, documentation, billing, facility management, and financial planning.

1.11.3   Ability to describe the decision-making process related to budgets, market analysis, program evaluation, facility management, staff allocation, and community development.

1.11.4   Ability to describe the development, evaluation, and revision of policies and procedures for programming and facility management.

1.11.5   Ability to describe how the computer can assist in data analysis, spreadsheet report development, and daily tracking of customer utilization.

1.11.6   Ability to define and describe the total quality management (TQM) and continuous quality improvement (CQI) approaches to management.

1.11.7   Ability to interpret applied research in the areas of exercise testing, exercise programming, and educational programs to maintain a comprehensive and current state-of-the-art program.

1.11.8   Ability to develop a risk factor screening program, including procedures, staff training, feedback, and follow-up.

1.11.9   Knowledge of administration, management, and supervision of personnel.

1.11.10   Ability to describe effective interviewing, hiring, and employee termination procedures.

1.11.11   Ability to describe and diagram an organizational chart and show the relationships between a health/fitness director, owner, medical advisor, and staff.

1.11.12   Knowledge of and ability to describe various staff training techniques.

1.11.13   Knowledge of and ability to describe performance reviews and their role in evaluating staff.

1.11.14   Knowledge of the legal obligations and problems involved in personnel management.

1.11.15   Knowledge of compensation, including wages, bonuses, incentive programs, and benefits.

1.11.16   Knowledge of methods for implementing a sales commission system.

1.11.17   Ability to describe the significance of a benefits program for staff and demonstrate an understanding in researching and selecting benefits.

1.11.18   Ability to write and implement thorough and legal job descriptions.

1.11.19   Knowledge of personnel time-management techniques.

1.11.20   Knowledge of administration, management, and development of a budget and of the financial aspects of a fitness center.

1.11.21   Knowledge of the principles of financial management.

1.11.22   Knowledge of basic accounting principles, such as accounts payable, accounts receivable, accrual, cash flow, assets, liabilities, and return on investment.

1.11.23   Ability to identify the various forms of a business enterprise, such as sole proprietorship, partnership, corporation, and S-corporation.

1.11.24   Knowledge of the procedures involved with developing, evaluating, revising, and updating capital and operating budgets.

1.11.25   Ability to manage expenses with the objective of maintaining a positive cash flow.

1.11.26   Ability to understand and analyze financial statements, including income statements, balance sheets, cash flows, budgets, and pro forma projections.

1.11.27   Knowledge of program-related break-even and cost/benefit analysis.

1.11.28   Knowledge of the importance of short-term and long-term planning.

1.11.29   Knowledge of the principles of marketing and sales.

1.11.30   Ability to identify the steps in the development, implementation, and evaluation of a marketing plan.

1.11.31 Knowledge of the components of a needs assessment/market analysis.

1.11.32 Knowledge of various sales techniques for prospective members.

1.11.33 Knowledge of techniques for advertising, marketing, promotion, and public relations.

1.11.34 Ability to describe the principles of developing and evaluating product and services, and establishing pricing.

1.11.35 Knowledge of the principles of day-to-day operation of a fitness center.

1.11.36 Knowledge of the principles of pricing and purchasing equipment and supplies.

1.11.37 Knowledge of facility layout and design.

1.11.38 Ability to establish and evaluate an equipment preventive maintenance and repair program.

1.11.39 Ability to describe a plan for implementing a housekeeping program.

1.11.40 Ability to identify and explain the operating policies for preventive exercise programs, including data analysis and reporting, confidentiality of records, relationships with healthcare providers, accident and injury reporting, and continuing education of participants.

1.11.41 Knowledge of the legal concepts of tort, negligence, liability, indemnification, standards of care, health regulations, consent, contract, confidentiality, malpractice, and the legal concerns regarding emergency procedures and informed consent.

1.11.42 Ability to implement capital improvements with minimal disruption of client or business needs.

1.11.43 Ability to coordinate the operations of various departments, including, but not limited to, the front desk, fitness, rehabilitation, maintenance and repair, day care, housekeeping, pool, and management.

1.11.44 Knowledge of management and principles of member service and communication.

1.11.45 Skills in effective techniques for communicating with staff, management, members, healthcare providers, potential customers, and vendors.

1.11.46 Knowledge of and ability to provide strong customer service.

1.11.47 Ability to develop and implement customer surveys.

1.11.48 Knowledge of the strategies for management conflict.

1.11.49 Knowledge of the principles of health promotion and ability to administer health-promotion programs.

1.11.50 Knowledge of health-promotion programs (e.g., nutrition and weight management, smoking cessation, stress management, back care, body mechanics, and substance abuse).

1.11.51 Knowledge of the specific and appropriate content and methods for creating a health-promotion program.

1.11.52 Knowledge of and ability to access resources for various programs and delivery systems.

1.11.53 Knowledge of the concepts of cost-effectiveness and cost-benefit as they relate to the evaluation of health-promotion programming.

1.11.54 Ability to describe the means and amounts by which health-promotion programs might increase productivity, reduce employee loss time, reduce healthcare costs, and improve profitability in the workplace.

Index

Page numbers in *italics* denote figures; those followed by *t* denote tables; those followed by *b* denote boxes.

Knowledge, Skills, Abilities (KSA) Index

Clinical Exercise Specialist (CES) KSAs are listed on pages 862–865, and Health Fitness Specialist (HFS) KSAs are on pages 865–868. Each KSA is listed by its certification-specific identifying number, followed by the KSA text and the page(s) on which information about the KSA is partially or fully presented.